POCKET
Cultural Health Assessment
Fourth Edition

CAROLYN ERICKSON D'AVANZO, RN, DNSc.
NEWPORT, NEW HAMPSHIRE

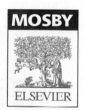

MOSBY
ELSEVIER

11830 Westline Industrial Drive
St. Louis, Missouri 63146

POCKET GUIDE TO CULTURAL
HEALTH ASSESSMENT, 4/E

ISBN-13: 978-0-323-04834-7
ISBN-10: 0-323-04834-X

Notice

Knowledge and best practice in this field are constantly changing. As new research and experience broaden our knowledge, changes in practice, treatment and drug therapy may become necessary or appropriate. Readers are advised to check the most current information provided (i) on procedures featured or (ii) by the manufacturer of each product to be administered, to verify the recommended dose or formula, the method and duration of administration, and contraindications. It is the responsibility of the practitioner, relying on their own experience and knowledge of the patient, to make diagnoses, to determine dosages and the best treatment for each individual patient, and to take all appropriate safety precautions. To the fullest extent of the law, neither the Publisher nor the Editor assumes any liability for any injury and/or damage to persons or property arising out of or related to any use of the material contained in this book.

The Publisher

Previous editions copyrighted 2003, 1998, 1994

ISBN-13: 978-0-323-04834-7
ISBN-10: 0-323-04834-X

Acquisitions Editor: Robin Carter
Senior Editorial Assistant: Mary Parker
Publishing Services Manager: John Rogers
Senior Project Manager: Kathleen L. Teal
Design Direction: Julia Dummit

Working together to grow
libraries in developing countries

www.elsevier.com | www.bookaid.org | www.sabre.org

ELSEVIER   BOOK AID International   Sabre Foundation

Printed in the United States of America

Last digit is the print number: 9   8   7   6   5   4   3

Joshua E. Abrams, MPA, MA
Consultant
International Research and
    Exchanges Board (IREX)
Fresh Meadows, New York

**Suher M. Aburawi, PhD, MPh,
    MSc, BPharm**
Associate Professor of
    Pharmacology
Department of Pharmacology and
    Clinical Pharmacy
Al-Fateh University
Tripoli, Libya

**Adebowale A. Adeyemo, MD,
    FWACP**
Senior Research Associate
Howard University
Washington, D.C.

Salim M. Adib, MD, DrPH
Professor
Faculty of Medicine
St. Joseph University
Beirut, Lebanon

Malalay Ahmadzai, MD, EMBA
Deputy Health Coordinator
Swedish Committee for
    Afghanistan (SCA)
Kabul, Afghanistan

**Mavae Nofomuli Aho-
    Redmond, BA**
Auburn, Washington

Fernando Alarçón, MD
Department of Neurology
Eugenio Espejo Hospital
Quito, Ecuador

Julia W. Albright, BS, PhD
Professor
George Washington University
    School of Medicine
Washington, D.C.

**Maydel Alfonso-Carbonell,
    Dipl.Nursing**
Gyneco-Obstetric Hospital
"Ramon González Coro"
Habana, Cuba

**Fawwaz Shakir Mahmoud
    Al-Joudi, PhD, MSc, BVMS**
Senior Lecturer,
Faculty of Allied Health Sciences
National University of Malaysia
Kuala Lumpur, Malaysia

Jason Anderson, BA, MA
Field Program Officer
USAID – Afghanistan
New York, New York

Mary Arevian, MPH, BSN
Assistant Professor
School of Nursing
American University of Beirut
Beirut, Lebanon

Edoh Azankpé, M Mgt
Elementary School Teacher
Ministry of Elementary and
    Secondary Education
Lomé, Togo

**Jorge Azofeifa, B Biol, MSc,
    DrScHum**
Profesor Escuela de Biologia
Universidad de Costa Rica
San José, Costa Rica

Akira Babazono, MD, MS, PhD
Professor
Faculty of Medical Sciences
Kyushu University
Fukuoka, Japan

Daniyar Z. Baidaralin, BA
Interior Designer
Morris Nathanson Design Inc.
Cranston,
Rhode Island

Joanne Motiño Bailey, RN, CNM, PhD
Certified Nurse Midwife
University of Michigan
Ann Arbor, Michigan

Francis Bajunirwe, MBChB, MS
Doctor
Mbarara University
Mbarara, Uganda

Virginia C.F. Ballance, BA (Hons), MA, MLS
Nursing and Health Sciences Librarian
Hilda Bowen Library
College of the Bahamas
Freeport, Bahamas

Gunay Balta, PhD
Associate Professor of Medicine
Department of Pediatrics
Hacettepe University
Ankara, Turkey

Margitta Beil-Hildebrand, PhD, MSc, NursMngt(DE), RGN
Independent Scholar
Regensburg, Germany

Ana Jovicevic Bekic, MD, MSc
Specialist in Epidemiology
Institute for Oncology and Radiology of Serbia
Belgrade, Serbia

Nissaf Bouafif Ben Alaya
Institut Pasteur de Tunis
Tunis, Tunisia

Afif Ben Salah, MD, MSc, PhD
Associate Professor and Head
Department of Epidemiology
Institut Pasteur de Tunis
Tunis, Tunisia

Abdulbari A. Bener, BSC, PhD, MFPHM, FRSS
Head
Department of Medical Statistics and Epidemiology

Hamad General Hospital
Doha, Qatar;
Advisor
World Health Organization
Geneva, Switzerland

Griffin Benjamin, MD, MPH, MBA, DM
Consultant Psychiatrist
Ministry of Health
Roseau, Dominica;
Director of Primary Health Care
Family Medical Clinic
Pottersville, Dominica

Liris Benjamin, MBBS, MPH, PhD
Lecturer and Medical Doctor
Family Medical Clinic
Pottersville, Dominica;
Ross University School of Medicine
Edison, New Jersey

Dawn Bichel, BSc
Research Services Manager
Prime Trials, Inc.
Vancouver, BC, Canada

Arûnas L. Birutis, RN
Registered Nurse
Continuum Health Partners, Inc., and Roosevelt Hospital
Neuroscience Center
New York, New York

Alexandre R. Bisdorff, MD
Neurologist
Centre Hospitalier
Emile Mayrisch
Esch-sur-Alzette, Luxembourg

Marija Bohinc, PhD, RN
Assistant Professor
College for Health Studies
University of Ljubljana
Ljubljana, Slovenia

Matthias Bopp, PhD
Institute of Social and Preventive
Medicine
University of Zurich
Zurich, Switzerland

Snezana Bosnjak, MD, PhD
Professor of Research
Institute for Oncology and
  Radiology of Serbia
Belgrade, Serbia

**Cameron Bowie, MBBS,
  MRCP, DCH, FFPHM**
Associate Professor of
Community Health College of
Medicine
University of Malawi
Blantyre, Malawi

**Richard G. Bribiescas, PhD,
  AM, BA**
Associate Professor
Department of Anthropology
Yale University
New Haven, Connecticut

**Major Franklin HG
  Bridgewater, MBBS, FRACS,
  FRCS (Eng)**
3rd Health Support Battalion,
Royal Australian Army Medical
  Corps
Australia

Emily Brounts-Hendrickx
Assistant Researcher
Maastricht University
Maastricht, The Netherlands

Catherine Bungener, PhD
Professor of Psychology
University Paris Descartes
Paris, France

**Gemma Burford, MBiochem,
  MSc**
Research Consultant
Aang Serian
Arusha, Tanzania

**Aaron G. Buseh, PhD, MPH,
  MSN**
Assistant Professor
University of Wisconsin –
  Milwaukee
Milwaukee, Wisconsin

**Hélène Carabin, DVM, MSc,
  PhD**
Associate Professor
University of Oklahoma Health
  Sciences Center
Oklahoma City, Oklahoma

Michel Carael, MD
Professor
Faculty of Social, Economical and
  Political Sciences
Free University of Brussels
Brussels, Belgium

Hugo Cardenas, PhD
Professor
Faculty of Chemistry and Biology
Universidad de Santiago de Chile
Santiago, Chile

**Francisco Javier Carod-Artal,
  MD, PhD**
Neurologist and Professor
Neurology Department
Sarah Hospital
Brasília, DF, Brazil

Conerly Casey, PhD, MSEd
Assistant Professor
American University of Kuwait
Safat, Kuwait

Santanu Chatterjee, MBBS, DTM&H
Consultant Physician
Travel and Tropical Medicine
Calcutta, India

Hsiu-Chin Chen, PhD, RN, EdD
Associate Professor
Utah Valley State College
Orem, Utah

Lee Huang Chiu, DEd, MNS, BAppSc (NrsgEd), RN, RM, OrthoCert (Hons)
Doctor and Post Graduate
Coursework Coordinator
School of Nursing and Midwifery
Victoria University
Melbourne, Victoria, Australia

Peter Ciznar, MD, PhD
Medical Doctor
1st Pediatric Department
Comenius University Medical
School
Children's Faculty Hospital
Bratislava, Slovakia

Marga Simon Coler, EdD, APRN-CS, FAAN
Professor Emeritus
University of Connecticut
Storrs, Connecticut

Maria Adriana Felix Coler, MS
Substance Abuse Counselor
Mercy/Providence Hospital
Amherst, Massachusetts

John Connell, BA, PhD
Professor
School of Geosciences
University of Sydney
Sydney, NSW, Australia

Ould El Joud Dahada, PhD, MPH
Director
Consultancy Bureau
Nouakchott, Mauritania

Georges Dahourou, Dr Pharm
Directeur
EXALAB
Burkina Faso

Akosua K. Darkwah, PhD
Department of Sociology
University of Ghana
Legon, Ghana

William D'Hoore, MD, PhD
Professor
Ecole de Santé Publique
Université Catholique de Louvain
Brussels, Belgium

John Dixon, BEcon, MEcon, PhD
Professor of Public Policy and
Management
University of Plymouth
Plymouth, United Kingdom

Josef Dolejš, PhD
National Radiation Protection
Institute
Prague, Czech Republic

Eric Dumonteil, PhD
Professor
Laboratorio de Parasitología
Centro de Investigaciones
Regionales "Dr. Hideyo
Noguchi"
Universidad Autónoma de Yucatán
Mérida, Yucatán, Mexico

Arnaud Dzeing-Ella, MD
Medical Doctor
Assistance Publique Hôpitaux
de Paris
Paris, France

Laurie Elit, MD, MSc, FRCS(c)
Associate Professor
Division of Gynecologic Oncology
Hamilton Regional Cancer Centre
Hamilton, Ontario, Canada

Angela Ellis, MA
PhD Candidate
University of Wisconsin
Madison, Wisconsin

Angel Arturo Escobedo-Carbonell, MD, MS Epid, MS Soc Comm
Medical Doctor
Academic Paediatric Hospital "Pedro Borras"
Habana, Cuba

Monique Essed-Fernandes, MA, BA
Development Policy Advisor
Paramaribo, Suriname

Ana Veríssimo Ferreira, MS
Teacher
Ministry of Education
Milharado, Portugal

Igor Y. Galaychuk, MD, DSc
Professor and Chief
Oncology Department
Ternopil State Medical University
Ternopil, Ukraine

Ximena Carrera Garese, MD
Medical Doctor
Medicaa
Montevideo, Uruguay

Adama Dodji Gbadoé, MD
Professor
University of Lomé;
Pediatrician
Ministry of High Education and Research
Lomé, Togo

Bette Gebrian, BSN, MPH, PhD
Public Health Director
Haitian Health Foundation
Jeremie, Haiti;
University of Connecticut School of Nursing
Storrs, Connecticut

Lynne S. Giddings, BA (Hons), MN, PhD, RN, RM
Associate Professor
School of Nursing and Midwifery
Auckland University of Technology
Auckland, Aotearoa, New Zealand

Eglantina Gjermeni, DSW, MSW
Doctor in Social Work
Faculty of Social Sciences
University of Tirana
Tirana Albania

Nel Glass, PhD, MHPEd, BA, Dipl Neurosci Nurs, RN
Associate Professor
School of Nursing and Health Care Practices
Southern Cross University
Lismore, NSW, Australia

Marino J. González, PhD, MSc, MD
Professor of Public Policy
Department of Economics and Administrative Sciences
Universidad Simón Bolívar
Caracas, Venezuela

Miro Gradisar, PhD
Professor
Faculty of Economics
University of Ljubljana
Ljubljana, Slovenia

Devon L. Graham, PhD
President/Scientific Director
Project Amazonas, Inc,
Florida, USA/Loreto, Peru;
Adjunct Professor
Florida International University
Miami, Florida

Bertrand Graz, MD, MPH, FMH
Doctor
DDC
Geneva, Switzerland

Elín Margrit Hallgrímsdóttir, MN, BSc, ICN, RN
Head of Continuing Education
Research Institute
University of Akureyri
Akureyri, Iceland

Marianne Hattar-Pollara, DNSc, MSN, FAAN
Associate Dean, Graduate
    Programs and Research
Chair and Professor, PhD
Program
School of Nursing
Azusa Pacific University
Azusa, California

Stephen E. Hawes, PhD
Assistant Professor, Epidemiology
School of Public Health and
    Community Medicine
University of Washington
Seattle, Washington

Edlira Haxhiymeri, PhD
Associate Professor
Faculty of Social Sciences
University of Tirana
Tirana, Albania

Anselm Hennis, MBBS, MSc, PhD, FRCP (UK)
Chronic Disease Research Centre
Tropical Medicine Research
    Institute
University of the West Indies
Bridgetown, Barbados

Eleanor Krohn Herrmann, BS, MS, MEd, EdD, FAAN
Professor Emerita
School of Nursing
University of Connecticut
Storrs, Connecticut

Geoffrey Hodgetts, MD, CCFP, FCFP
Professor of Family Medicine
Queen's University
Kingston, Ontario, Canada

David Houeto, MD, DEPA, DEA
PhD Candidate
Researcher
School of Public Health – Health
    Education Unit
Catholic University of Louvain
Brussels, Belgium

Hartwig Huemer, MD
Associate Professor
Medical University Innsbruck
Austrian Health Agency
Innsbruck, Austria

Andrew Jewell, BSc, MSc, PhD, FIBMS
Reader
Kingston University
St. George's University of London
London, United Kingdom

Lisa Johnson, MBBS, DM (Surg)
Medical Doctor
Universal Health Services
Belize City, Belize

Katja Joronen, PhD
Lecturer
Department of Nursing Science
University of Tampere
Tampere, Finland

Theano Kalavana, PhD
Department of Psychology
University of Cyprus
Nicosia, Cyprus

Irene Kalnins, RN, MSN, EdD
Associate Professor
School of Nursing
St. Louis University
St. Louis, Missouri

Chihoko Kame, MPH
Research Associate
Kyushu University
Fukuoka, Japan

Vered Kater, RN, MSN, CNS
Assistant Clinical Professor
Henriette Szold School of Nursing
Hadassah Medical Organization
Jerusalem, Israel

Marja Kaunonen, PhD, RN
Senior Assistant Professor
Department of Nursing Science
University of Tampere
Tampere, Finland

Hassina Khelladi, MS
Doctor of Physics, Teacher
University of Sciences and
    Technology "Houari
    Boumedienne"
Algiers, Algeria

Jörg Klewer, MD, PhD, FRIPH
Professor
Department of Public Health and
    Nursing Sciences
University of Applied Sciences
Zwickau, Germany

**Hester Klopper, BA CUR,
    M CUR, PhD, MBA, RN, RM**
Professor
School of Nursing Science
North-West University
Potchefstroom, South Africa

**Gennady G. Knyazev, PhD,
    Dr Sci**
Principal Research Scientist
State Research Institute of
    Physiology
Siberian Branch of the Russian
    Academy of Medical Sciences
Novosibirsk, Russia

Robert Kohn, MD, MPhil
Associate Professor of Psychiatry
    and Human Behavior
Brown University
Butler Hospital
Providence, Rhode Island

**Kenneth Y.Y. Kok, MBChB,
    FRCS, FRCSEd, FAMS, FACS**
Doctor
Ministry of Health
Bandar Seri Begawan, Brunei
    Darussalam

**K.A.L.A. Kuruppuarachchi,
    MBBS, MD, FRCPsych (UK)**
Professor of Psychiatry
Faculty of Medicine
University of Kelaniya
Ragama, Sri Lanka

Ulrike Kylberg, BNSc, MPH
Lecturer
Halmstad University
Halmstad, Sweden

Sophie Le Coeur, MD, PhD
Senior Researcher
Institut National d'Études
    Démographiques (INED)
Paris, France

Eric Ledru, MD, PhD
Agence Nationale de l'Accueil des
Etrangers et des Migrations
Marseille, France

Wai-man Lee, PhD
Assistant Professor
Department of Nursing and Health
Sciences
Hong Kong Polytechnic University
Hong Kong, China

**Miriam Rubí Gamboa Léon,
    M. EN C.**
Maestria en Ciencias
University of Tulane
Mérida, Yucatán, Mexico

Lars Lien, MD, PhD
Postdoctoral Fellow
Institute of Psychiatry
University of Oslo
Oslo, Norway

Lee Meng Lim, PhD, MN, BNsg, BA, RN-Divl, RSCN
Post Graduate Paediatric Course Coordinator
School of Nursing and Midwifery
Victoria University
Melbourne, Victoria, Australia

Moses K. Limo, PhD
Associate Professor
Egerton University
Egerton, Kenya

Julie Livingston, BA, MA, MPH, PhD
Associate Professor
Department of History
Rutgers University
New Brunswick, New Jersey

Joseph D. Lynch, MD, FACC
Medical Director
Institute for Latin American Concern (ILAC);
Associate Professor of Medicine
Creighton University
Omaha, Nebraska

Teresa L. Lynch, BSN, C, MA
Director
Institute for Latin American Concern (ILAC);
University Ministry Department
Creighton University
Omaha, Nebraska

Cheryl Cox Macpherson, BSc, PhD
Professor
School of Medicine
St. George's University
St. George's, Grenada

Jean Macq, MD, MPH, PhD
Ecole de Santé Publique
Université Libre de Bruxelles
Brussels, Belgium

Abid Mahmood, MBBS, FCPS
Classified Pathologist (Microbiologist)
Federal Government of Pakistan
Gujranwala Cantt, Pakistan

Montserrat Antonín Martín, MS, RN
Escola Universitaria d'Infermeria Gimbernat
Sant Cugat del Valles, Spain

Jérôme Maslin, MD
Director of the Laboratory
Bouffard Hospital
Ministry of Defense
French Military Hospital
Djibouti, Africa

Lawrence J. Mathers, MD
Family Physician
Rural Medical Services
Newport, Tennessee

Thubelihle Mathole, PhD, MSc, BSc (Hon)
Part Time Lecturer
University of Zimbabwe
Mt. Pleasant, Harare, Zimbabwe;
Consultant/Researcher
Avondale, Harare, Zimbabwe

Clement Ibi Mboto, PhD, MSc, FMLCN, AIBMS
Lecturer
Faculty of Science
University of Calabar
Calabar, Nigeria

Barbara Burns McGrath, RN, PhD
Research Associate Professor
School of Nursing
University of Washington
Seattle, Washington

Scott J.N. McNabb, PhD, MS
Director
Division of Integrated Surveillance
  Systems and Services (DISSS)
Centers for Disease Control and
  Prevention
Atlanta, Georgia

**Frits van Merode, MSc, MPhil,
  PhD**
Professor
Department of Health,
  Organization, Policy and
  Economics
Maastricht University
Maastricht, The Netherlands

**Charles Michelo, MD, BSc,
  MBChB, MPH**
School of Medicine
University of Zambia
Lusaka, Zambia

Amal K. Mitra, MD, MPH, DrPH
Professor
Department of Community Health
  Sciences
University of Southern Mississippi
Hattiesburg, Mississippi

Tomáš Morcinek, MD
SPS Břehová s.r.o.
Prague, Czech Republic

**Slavianka Georgieva
  Moyanova, PhD**
Associate Professor
Institute of Physiology
Bulgarian Academy of Sciences
Sofia, Bulgaria

**Tolu Mulialna, BEd, PGDDS,
  PGDEd, GCTT, MA**
School of Geography
Faculty of Islands and Oceans
The University of the South Pacific
Suva, Fiji Islands

**Jean-Claude Mwanza, MD,
  MPH, PhD**
National Academy of Sciences
National Research Council
Washington, D.C.

**Aye-Mu Myint, MB, BS,
  M Med Sc**
Research Scientist
Department of Medical Research
  (Physiology)
Myanmar

Tawfeeq Ali Naseeb, FRACGP
Assistant Professor, Family
  Medicine
College of Medicine
Arabian Gulf University
Manama, Kingdom of Bahrain

Lisa Natoli, RN, MPH
Women's and Children's Health
  Advisor
Centre for International Health
The Macfarlane Burnet Institute
  for Medical Research and
  Public Health
Melbourne, Victoria, Australia

Haq Nawaz, MD, MPH
Director/Chair
Preventive Medicine
Griffin Hospital
Derby, Connecticut

Abraham Ndiwane, EdD, RN
Assistant Professor
University of Massachusetts
Medical School
Worcester, Massachusetts

Félix Neto, PhD
Professor
Faculdade de Psicologia e de
  Ciências da Educação
Universidade do Porto
Porto, Portugal

Hoa L. Nguyen, MD, MSc
Clinical Research Coordinator
Massachusetts General Hospital
Boston, Massachusetts

**Huong T. N. Nguyen,
MA, MSW**
PhD Candidate
School of Social Service
Administration
The University of Chicago
Chicago, Illinois

**Kizito Bishikwabo Nsarhaza,
PhD**
M & E Advisor
Joint United Nations Programme
on HIV/AIDS (UNAIDS)
Geneva, Switzerland

Aceme Nyika, PhD, MPH
Nelson R. Mandela School of
Medicine
University of KwaZulu-Natal
Durban, South Africa

**Tom O'Connor, RGN, RNT, PG
Dip Ed, BSc, MSc**
Lecturer
School of Nursing, Midwifery, and
Health Systems
University College Dublin
Dublin, Ireland

**Manana Sopromadze
O'Donovan, MS**
Washington, D.C.

**Robert J. O'Donovan, Jr, BA,
MSDM**
Regional Director
South Caucasus Cooperation
Program
The Eurasia Foundation
Washington, D.C.

Nodira Ochilova, MA
Translator
Karshi, Uzbekistan

Arwa Issa Eid Oweis, DNSc, RN
Associate Professor
Faculty of Nursing
Jordan University of Science and
Technology
Irbid, Jordan

**Alvisa Palese, DNurs, MSN,
BCN, RN**
Associate Professor
Nursing Science
Udine University
Udine, Italy

Shehzad Parviz, MD (MBBS)
Medical Director
Valley Health Care, Inc.
Mill Creek, West Virginia

**Elisabeth Patiraki-Kourbani,
BSc, PhD**
Assistant Professor
Nursing Faculty
National and Kapodistrian
University of Athens
Athens, Greece

**Philayrath Phongsavan, PhD,
MPH, BA (Hons)**
Research Fellow
University of Sydney
Sydney, NSW, Australia

Bettina F. Piko, MD, PhD
Associate Professor
Department of Behavioral
Sciences
University of Szeged
Szeged, Hungary

**Maria da Conceição Paninho
Pinio, D Ed Sc**
Teacher
Ministry of Education
Setúbal, Portugal

Nurgün Platin, RN, MS, PhD
Emeritus Professor of Nursing
Ankara, Turkey

Draga Plecas, MD, PhD
Professor
Institute of Environmental Health
and Nutrition
School of Medicine
University of Belgrade
Belgrade, Yugoslavia

Ozren Polašek, MD
Research Fellow
Andrija Stampar School of Public
Health
University of Zagreb
Zagreb, Croatia

Audrey M. Pottinger, PhD
Faculty of Medical Sciences
The University of the West Indies
at Mona
Kingston, Jamaica

Anja Poulsen, MD, PhD
University of Copenhagen
Copenhagen, Denmark

Ndola Prata, MD, MSc
Assistant Adjunct Professor
School of Public Health
University of California,
Berkeley
Berkeley, California

Lien Quach, MD, MPH
Adjunct Assistant Professor
Tufts University
Medford, Massachusetts

Katharine Quanbeck, RN
Lakeville, Minnesota

**Stanley D. Quanbeck, MD,
FAAFP**
Correctional Medical Services
Lakeville, Minnesota

Marta Maturana Quijada, RN
Universidad de Santiago de Chile
Santiago, Chile

**Yahia Ahmed Raja'a, PhD,
MSc, BSc**
Associate Professor of
Community Medicine
Faculty of Medicine and Health
Sciences
Sana'a University
Sana'a, Yemen Republic

Bernd Rechel, PhD
Research Officer
World Health Organization
Aylesbury, United Kingdom

**Mary-Elizabeth Reeve, PhD,
MPH**
Director
Global Perinatal Health Education
March of Dimes Foundation
White Plains, New York

**Andrew Geoffrey Robertson,
MBBS, MPH, MHSM,
FAFPHM, FRACMA**
Chief Health Officer
Western Australian Department of
Health
East Perth, WA, Australia

**Helen D. Rodd, BDS, FDS (Paed),
PhD**
Professor
Department of Child Dental Health
University of Sheffield
Sheffield, United Kingdom

Christophe Rogier, MD, PhD
Chief
Parasite and Epidemiology
Research Department
Institute for Tropical Medicine of
the French Army (IMTSSA) – Le
Pharo
Marseille, France

**Lori Rosenstein, BA, (MA
Candidate)**
Human Resources Specialist
Travis Air Force Base
Fairfield, California

Adam Roth, MD, PhD
Afdeling for Epidemiologisk
  Forskning
Statens Serum Institut
Denmark

**Tatiana I. Ryabichenko, MD,
  PhD, DSc**
Scientific Center of Clinical &
  Experimental Medicine
Siberian Branch of the Russian
  Academy of Medical Sciences
Novosibirsk, Russia

Majid Sadeghi, MD
Associate Professor of Psychiatry
Tehran University of Medical
  Sciences
Tehran, Iran

Luisa Saiani, MNSc
Associate Professor of Nursing
  Science
Advanced Nursing Education
Faculty of Medicine
University of Verona
Verona, Italy

Hilkka Sand, PhD, RN
Principal Lecturer
Research Director
HAMK University of Applied
  Sciences
Kanta-Häme Hospital District
Hämeenlinna, Finland

**Alan Sanderson, BSc(Hons),
  CertCW, PgDip, PhD, ACMI,
  MinstLM, FHEA**
Truro College
Truro, Cornwall, United Kingdom;
University of Plymouth
Plymouth, United Kingdom

**Charles Savona-Ventura, MD,
  DScMed, FRCOG, ACertOG,
  MRCPI**
Department of Obstetrics and
  Gynaecology
Faculty of Medicine and Surgery
University of Malta
Msida, Malta

Mary G. Schaal, RN, EdD
Professor and Dean
School of Nursing
Thomas Jefferson University
Philadelphia, Pennsylvania

**Euan M. Scrimgeour, MD,
  FRACP, DTM & H**
Associate Professor in Infectious
  and Tropical Diseases
Department of Medicine
Sultan Qaboos University
Muscat, Sultanate of Oman

**Samir Shaheen, MBBS,
  Dipl Sport Med, MD**
Assistant Professor of
  Orthopaedics
Faculty of Medicine
University of Khartoum
Khartoum, Sudan

**Conrad Shamlaye, MBChB,
  MSc (Epid), MSc (Health
  Econ)**
Ministry of Health
Victoria, Mahe, Republic of
  Seychelles

**Heather Shamlaye, MBChB,
  MA**
Glasgow Caledonian University
Glasgow, Scotland, United
  Kingdom

**Nigel John Shanks, MD, PhD,
  MBA**
Chief Medical Officer
Ras Gas Co, Ltd
Doha, Qatar

Fu-Jin Shih, RN, DNSc
Professor and Acting Dean
School of Nursing
National Yang-Ming University
Taipei, Taiwan

David M. Sintasath, BS, MSc
Epidemiologist
Johns Hopkins Bloomberg School
of Public Health
Baltimore, Maryland

Kathleen Slobin, PhD
Professor
Department of Sociology-
Anthropology
North Dakota State University
Fargo, North Dakota

**Helena R. Slobodskaya, MD,
PhD, DSc**
State Research Institute of
Physiology
Siberian Branch of the Russian
Academy of Medical Sciences
Novosibirsk, Russia

**Soe-Soe, PhD, MBBS, M.Med.
Sc (Path)**
Deputy Director
Department of Medical Research
Yangon, Myanmar

Pawel Stefanoff, MD, PhD, MS
Assistant Professor
National Institute of Hygiene
Warsaw, Poland

Emil Doru Steopan, RN, MSN
University Hospital for Children
Cluj-Napoca, Romania

Sabine Stordeur, RN, MA, PhD
Clinical and Health Services
Researcher
Belgian Health Care Knowledge
Centre
Brussels, Belgium

Hamlet Suarez, MD, PhD
Laboratory of Audiology and
Vestibular Pathophysiology
School of Medicine
British Hospital
Montevideo, Uruguay

Jean Claude Tabuteau, MD
Senior Physician
Atlantic Medical Center
Delray Beach, Florida

Marika Tammaru, MD
Researcher
University of Tartu
Tartu, Estonia

Velibor B. Tasic, MD, PhD
Consultant Pediatric
Nephrologist
University Children's Hospital
Skopje, Macedonia

**Narbada Thapa, PhD,
MScEpi**
Associate Professor
Shree Birendra Hospital, Chhawni
Kathmandu, Nepal

**Suraj Bahadur Thapa, PhD,
MPhil, MD**
Doctor
Gaular Municipality, Norway

Nana Thrane, MD, PhD
Department of Pediatrics
Skejby Hospital
Aarhus, Denmark

Catherine S. Todd, MD, MPH
Assistant Professor
University of California, San Diego
San Diego, California

**Joaquín Tomás-Sábado, PhD,
NR**
Escola Universitaria Gimbernat
Sant Cugat del Valles, Spain

Chhan D. Touch, MSN, FNP
Family Nurse Practitioner
Lowell Community Health Center/
  Metta Health Center
Lowell, Massachusetts

**Mary P. Van Hook, MSW, PhD,
  ACSW, LMSW**
Professor
School of Social Work
University of Central Florida
Orlando, Florida

**Maryelena Vargas, RN, BSN,
  IBCLC, ADN**
Doctoral Candidate
Columbia University School of
  Nursing
New York, New York

Carol Vlassoff, PhD
Doctor
Pan American Health
Organization/World Health
  Organization
Quepos, Costa Rica

Jitra Waikagul, PhD
Associate Professor
Faculty of Tropical Medicine
Mahidol University
Bangkok, Thailand

Kenneth D. Ward, PhD
Associate Professor of Health
  Promotion
Director, Center for Community
  Health
University of Memphis
Memphis, Tennessee

**Frances Kam Yuet Wong, RN,
  PhD**
Professor
School of Nursing
Hong Kong Polytechnic University
Hong Kong, China

Myungsun Yi, DNS, RN
Professor
College of Nursing
Seoul National University
Seoul, Korea

Yue Zhao, PhD
Professor
School of Nursing
Tianjin Medical University
Tianjin, China

CONSULTANTS

Lesikar Ole Ngila
Director, Aang Serian, Arusha,
Tanzania

Mohamed Yunus Rafiq, BA
Co-Director, Aang Serian, Arusha,
Tanzania

**Mushfiqur R. Tarafder, MBBS,
  MPH**
University of Oklahoma Health
  Sciences Center
Oklahoma City, Oklahoma

The world is increasing in diversity while, at the same time, it is becoming more similar through the process of globalization. People and nations, increasingly, are sharing resources and exchanging ideas about political, economic, social, religious, educational, health, and other sociocultural factors. This is accomplished through mechanisms such as e-mail, the Internet, travel, cell phones, distance- and web-enhanced learning, shared production and marketing, and distribution of products. People and nations are becoming more similar in multiple ways at the macro-level of international commerce and relations. There remains great diversity, however, at the meso-level of social and ethnic/racial groups within nations, and at the micro-level of social and ethnic/racial groups within societies.

The concept of culture has been used to describe our ability to live in relative harmony in social groups through the sharing of values, beliefs, and practices. At the same time, culture can create social disharmony within and between nations and social groups due to our ethnocentric tendencies to judge others in light of our own cultural values, beliefs and practices. Intergroup and intragroup diversity is fostered through degrees of acculturation, individual life-experiences, and the situational context in which groups and individuals exist and must make decisions about life processes on a daily basis. As a result, in a world where people are becoming increasingly similar at the macro-level, great diversity exists at the meso- and micro-levels.

The revision and expansion of this pocket guide by Dr. D'Avanzo is a commendable effort to help health care providers and others understand both the diversity and similarities between and within nations. By compiling basic cultural, epidemiological, environmental, and geographic information about cultural groups throughout the world and within nations, health care providers are presented with a snapshot of existing diversity. It remains the responsibility of individual health care providers, however, to learn about the diverse cultural values, beliefs, and practices of their individual patients to fulfill their dual roles as citizens and as providers of culture competent health care.

While Dr. D'Avanzo has given us a steppingstone to culture competence, it is the individual reader who must use the information provided to put the other steppingstones in place for culture competent practice. One steppingstone is to explore the degree to which individual patients do or do not adhere to the cultural norms commonly attributed to them. This is basic to incorporating cultural beliefs and practices into health care interventions and individualizing care. Another steppingstone is to realize that the world view of a group, that is, their idea of reality and truth and how they carve up the world so that it is meaningful to them, gives rise to their health culture. Health culture is a group's beliefs about health promotion and illness prevention, disease causation and health maintenance, treatment, and care. It also forms a group's knowledge of where, when, and from whom to access care, as well as the nature of the patient-provider encounter. As a result, health care behavior cannot be readily separated from the cultural values, beliefs, and practices that shape the social structure, political and economic systems, and other sociocultural institutions of a group, including those of health care providers. A third steppingstone is to realize that health behavior is often affected by the situation at hand, such as access to care, employment responsibilities, housing conditions, transportation facilities, family structure, social support, and immigration status. As situations and the sociocultural contexts vary, so does the ability of social groups and individuals to adhere to the cultural values, beliefs, and practices that form their health-culture orientations. **Understanding the fluidity of health cultural values, beliefs, and practices should caution health care providers against stereotyping based on social or ethnic/racial group membership, analyzing behavior out of context, and acting on and interpreting situations from their own health culture point of view.**

The best way to learn about cultural groups is to use a form of participant-observation. We can learn more about social and ethnic/racial groups through: (a) reading scholarly works or viewing documentaries about groups in the region where we practice; (b) visiting ethnic neighborhoods for shopping, meals, and recreational events; (c) experiencing religious ceremonies in ethnic churches and learning about the role of religion in health and illness; and (d) sharing life-celebrations such as births, weddings, graduations, and festivals, as well as life-sorrows like death and other personal losses. We can talk with patients, their families, and their neighbors about their health culture beliefs and practices, and their explanatory models about a particular health state. We can watch as life unfolds in ethnic neighborhoods, experience its tempo, and see cultural symbols embodied in arts and crafts. By learning about others, we tend to become more cognizant of the factors that affect our patients in health and illness. We also tend to learn more about ourselves and of the health culture diversity we should address each time we assess patients.

Culture competent health care became a national imperative with the health goals set forth in *Healthy People 2010*. It is totally unacceptable that more than two centuries after the United States was founded on the principle of equality for all citizens, it is still struggling to provide its diverse national and local populations with equality in health care. We have not eliminated health disparities among population groups, or achieved cultural competence in delivery of health care. The same can be said on an international basis when one views the social, economic, and health disparities and injustices affecting population groups throughout the world. The worldwide struggle with providing equity in health care to citizens is particularly disturbing at a time when we are becoming more alike in many ways and sharing resources and ideas. Dr. D'Avanzo has provided a broad map to begin our discovery of culture competence. It is now up to each of us to fill in the highways, streets, and paths across diverse terrain to render effective and acceptable care to all of our patients.

Lydia A. DeSantis, RN, BSN, MNEd, MA, MPh, PhD, FAAN
Professor, University of Miami School of Nursing and Health Studies
Coral Gables, Florida

The present trend in transcultural theory is that individuals within any given culture vary markedly. The earth is populated with a mosaic of cultures representing every imaginable variety of learned and environmentally generated beliefs and practices. For each person, his or her own culture is deeply ingrained and comfortable, guiding both the conscious and unconscious activities and behaviors of daily life, including perspectives on health and illness. Yet, culture is also a dynamic influence, meeting changing needs of groups, as well as individuals within those groups.

In his book *Pandaemonium*, Daniel Patrick Moynihan speculated about the speed of creation of new nations on the world map: nations "created for the purpose of giving one or another ethnic group a realm of its own." True to Moynihan's vision of this, the world is indeed seeing countries broken into different entities with new names. We are all familiar with the breakdown of the Soviet Union into many smaller republics. The former Yugoslavia was broken into entities that are continuing to divide; with the latest example being the recent separation of Montenegro from Serbia. Some of these newly independent nations have little or no professional literature in the English language appropriate for use in this guide; although in many cases information could be gleaned from official sources and from experts who live in those countries.

Four major sources have been incorporated into each chapter for consistency across countries: The New York Times Almanac, The World Factbook, The World Health Organization and UNAIDS (The Joint United Nations Programme on HIV/AIDS).

The New York Times Almanac was used for data pertaining to population, language, and ethnic groups as a comparison to in-country contributor data. Ultimately, contributors selected the data they believed to be the most accurate for this guide.

The World Factbook has been used as a guide to statistics such as infant mortality, fertility rates, life expectancy, and gross domestic product (GDP) per capita income. Country statistics obtained by contributors were sometimes less or more accurate than the Factbook, and we incorporated those that were deemed most up-to-date.

The World Health Organization was used for immunization schedules. In some cases, where there was no published schedule, we had access to country statistics. In some cases there were discrepancies that could be resolved by country statistical resources.

UNAIDS, the Joint United Nations Programme on HIV/AIDS was our source for country estimates. Again, these statistics sometimes differed from in-country data and the newest, most accurate figures were used. In every case, strong efforts were made to present the reader with the most accurate data available. Because there is always lag time between finishing the manuscript and actual printing (as is true for all published books) some statistics may have changed by the time of publication.

Most of the countries of the world are incorporated into this volume; 172 countries in all. A few countries were eliminated due to their small size or the unavailability of qualified contributors who could provide a culturally accurate view of the country and its population. The Pacific Islands (also called Oceania) number in the thousands and it would be impossible to adequately represent them. In this volume, Papua New Guinea and New Zealand represent the largest Pacific Islands (since Australia is a continent unto itself). Oceania is divided into three main areas: Melanesia, Micronesia and Polynesia. We have included the Solomon Islands as an example of Melanesia; Nauru as an example of Micronesia; and Tonga as an example of Polynesia. The Caribbean Islands are represented by The Bahamas, Barbados, and Cuba.

Citations within the text have been kept to an absolute minimum for ease of reading. The reader is referred to the citations and Web addresses at the end of each chapter for source materials. Much of the cultural material is based upon contributors' personal knowledge of their culture, and may or may not be combined with information from peer-reviewed journals or documents.

The theory about the "melting pot" phenomenon that expects immigrants to become Americans, Europeans, or Scandanavians, etc. linguistically and culturally is no longer viable. Even the theory about the "salad bowl" phenomenon, in which cultures are expected to live together in peaceful coexistence, is being rejected. At this critical juncture in history the move toward cultural homogeneity is strengthening. Many of the new countries of the world came into existence because of the intense, and for some, deadly struggle for cultural homogeneity. Information relative to health and access to health care in these countries will be evolving over time, and the reader is encouraged to keep abreast of the health care literature.

One of the greatest weaknesses of a guide such as this is that of stereotyping. The reader is strongly cautioned against the false assumption that people from one country or geographic area are clones, holding the same beliefs held by their neighbors. The borders of countries are politically determined and often bear no relationship to cultural values. **The differences within one culture may be as great as variations between two different cultures.** It is helpful to make a distinction between stereotyping and generalizing. If I assume that a Latino patient will have a low tolerance for pain I am stereotyping that patient; essentially closing my mind to differences within the many Latin cultures. If I say to myself that Latino patients often express pain freely, and remind myself to closely assess the person's pain, I am generalizing and using information I have learned to provide a better assessment. The goal is to remain receptive to further questioning and evaluation of people as unique individuals. This volume grew out of day-to-day reality in the working world. When you have a patient from an unfamiliar culture, you can rarely say "Excuse me, I'll be back in a few hours after I learn about your culture." The information that you need is scattered throughout a multitude of journals and books, and most information is not readily accessible.

This guide places at your fingertips some basic information about people of the countries of our world, when and where you need it. People from countries all over the world, and health care professionals who have worked extensively abroad, provide important in-depth knowledge of respective cultures. Although some intra-ethnic differences in cultures are noted, usually only the dominant culture or aspects common to many groups are included. That limitation can be difficult to make, since most countries consist of numerous ethnic and/or racial groups. To include them all would result in a multi-volume encyclopedia that is beyond the scope of this guide. Because the United States and Canada are made up of a myriad of cultural groups from all over the world, they were not included in this guide.

The purpose of this edition is to help focus the reader's attention on the potential variations a culturally diverse client may, or may not, exhibit. It is based on generalizations that must not be mentally converted into stereotypes by the user. Pull out this guide when you are faced with someone from a culture that is unfamiliar to you. Use this guide to start quickly and efficiently increasing your awareness and understanding of **potential** similarities and differences. For unless you are conscious of the cultural patterns of behavior a patient might exhibit, you will not think to address them in your assessment. To be culturally competent with a few cultures that you routinely encounter is a **must.** To be culturally competent with the many cultures with which you may on occasion be faced is unrealistic. To not use a guide such as this for fear of stereotyping only impedes movement toward delivery of culturally relevant health care. We are willing to risk criticism for stereotyping; but in return, We ask you to thoughtfully build on the information inside these pages with an individualized cultural assessment, of which there are many in the literature.

CITED REFERENCES

Moynihan DP: Pandaemonium: ethnicity in international politics, Oxford, England, 1993, Oxford University Press.

SPECIAL RECOGNITION

The following sources were especially helpful in the preparation of this manuscript and deserve special recognition for their contributions:

Central Intelligence Agency 2006 The World Factbook.
   https://www.cia.gov/cia/publications/factbook/

UNAIDS : The Joint United Nations Programme on HIV/AIDS, 2006.
  http://www.unaids.org/en/Regions_Countries/Countries/
Wright JW editor: 2006 *The New York Times Almanac,* New York 2006, Penguin
  Group.
The World Health Organization 2006/2007.
  http://www.int/immunization_monitoring/en/globalsummary/countryprofileresult.
  cfm

◆ ACKNOWLEDGMENTS

I deeply appreciate the many contributors worldwide who contributed to this edition. Their in-depth knowledge of the countries they represent has been invaluable. Elaine Geissler's authorship of the first two editions of this book is also acknowledged and appreciated. I also warmly thank the editors and individuals at Elsevier Publishing who assisted and guided this edition, with special thanks to Robin Carter, Mary Parker, and Kathy Teal.

Carolyn Erickson D'Avanzo

• CONTENTS

◆ AFGHANISTAN (ISLAMIC REPUBLIC OF)

MAP PAGE (804)

Catherine S. Todd, and Malalay Ahmadzai

Location: Afghanistan is a landlocked country with areas isolated by rugged mountains. Covering about 647,500 km² (249,935 square miles), Afghanistan is split east to west by the Hindu Kush mountain range (the foothills of the Himalaya mountains) and wedged between Turkmenistan to the northwest, Uzbekistan and Tajikistan to the north, China to the northeast, Pakistan to the east and south, and Iran to the west. The capital is Kabul. With the exception of the southwest, which is primarily desert, most of the country is covered by high, snowcapped mountains whose valleys were characterized by lush agricultural land before recent droughts. The population is 31 million, including recently returned refugees. The gross domestic product (GDP) per capita is $800, with about 53% below the poverty line. Literacy rates are 51% for men, 21% for women.

Major Languages	Ethnic Groups	Major Religions (Islam 99%)
Dari (dialect of Farsi)	Pashtun 42%	Sunni Muslim 80%
Pashto	Tajik 27%	Shi'a Muslim 19%
Uzbek	Hazara 9%	Other (e.g., Hindu,
Other (e.g., Pashai,	Uzbek 9%	Sikh) 1%
Buruzkashi)	Other (Chahar Aimaks,	
	Turkmen, Baloch,	
	Kuchi nomads,	
	and Others) 13%	

Health Care Beliefs: Acute sick care, traditional. Acute care is the only option in many areas because of the lack of health care system infrastructure, although after implementation of the Basic Package of Health Services (BPHS) in 2003, 77% of the population has had access to health services. Health is controlled by "God's will." Depression is common, but availability of, or acknowledged need for, mental health services is lacking. The appearance of good health in men is important; therefore, they seek care less often than women do and sometimes delay care to preserve dignity. Health is considered private and rarely discussed outside the family.

Predominant Sick-Care Practices: Magical-religious. People wear charms and amulets to ward off evil spirits which manifest themselves in numerous central nervous system diseases. A medicine man *(hakim)* uses various methods for helping those with physical or psychological illnesses. Herbal medications, holy water, or visits to holy sites *(Zeyarat)* may be used to help those with ailments.

1

A

Ethnic-/Race-Specific or Endemic Diseases: About 11% of the rural population has access to safe drinking water; in urban areas, 19% has access. Approximately 86,000 children under 5 years die annually of diarrheal diseases. Measles, a vaccine-preventable disease, infects 35,000 children each year. Tuberculosis (TB) is also rampant; Afghanistan ranks 20th globally for TB prevalence, and 92 per 100,000 people die of TB annually. Other prevalent diseases include chloroquine-resistant malaria (limited to a belt in the southeast), cholera, and cutaneous leishmaniasis. As a result of land mine and other military campaign–related injuries, 3% to 4% of the population has physical disabilities. High rates of depression, suicide attempts, and suicidal ideation existed among women during the Taliban regime and persist today. There are no estimated prevalence rates for human immunodeficiency virus (HIV) and acquired immunodeficiency syndrome (AIDS) although cases have been reported.

Health-Team Relationships: The last 23 years of conflict have devastated the health care system. In 2002, only 40% of Afghans, mainly those in urban areas, had access to basic health services. Although hospitals, health posts, and clinics are listed as health care "structures," not all are staffed, supplied, or used as health care facilities. The vast majority of hospitals lack sanitation or utilities; only 74% have access to one closed source of water. In a national survey of health care facilities conducted in 2002, 16% were inactive and active facilities did not uniformly offer comprehensive services. Among facilities providing basic health services, each served an average of 25,823 people. However, this situation varied widely by geographic region, with urban areas disproportionately serviced (rural facilities had catchment populations of 145,000 or more). One third of surveyed provinces did not meet the standard of one clinic per 30,000 persons. No licensure or credentialing systems are in place for medical providers; clinical training opportunities were curtailed during the decades of war. Trained female care providers are relatively few because no female medical or nursing graduates were allowed during the Taliban period. Women entering health care are usually allowed to see only female providers, which has contributed to high maternal mortality. Since the Taliban period, emphasis has been on training female providers, particularly those dedicated to rural areas. Private doctors are concentrated in urban areas and are unaffordable for much of the population. Pharmacies, however, sell a wide variety of medications and dispense medical advice throughout the country.

Families' Role in Hospital Care: The severe shortage of health care providers (0.1 doctors per 1,000 people) means that family members must provide food, medications, comfort, and care to patients admitted to most hospitals.

Dominance Patterns: In November 2001, the Taliban was removed from power. Although women's rights were severely restricted by the Taliban, the freedoms to which women were entitled had sharply declined in the previous 23 years. In traditional Afghan society, schools are coeducational during the younger years, separate in the high school years, and again coeducational in institutes of higher learning. Because of a severe lack of female teachers, ongoing war, and the need for women and girls to help support families, many women have not been able to pursue an education during the last two decades. Eighty-five percent of the country is sustained by agriculture and in the rural areas farmed by women as well as men, even during the Taliban. Carpet weaving, needle arts, and tailoring are common skills among Afghan women. Before the Taliban regime, 40% of doctors, 70% of teachers, and 50% of civil servants were women. Family interdependence with strict obedience to elders, particularly to the father, is the norm. Dating is prohibited, arranged marriages by family members are the norm, and dowries are still common.

Eye-Contact Practices: Direct eye contact between those of the opposite sex is considered rude and immodest.

Touch Practices: Physical affection among family members is common, especially between parents and children. Affection among couples or adults is unlikely to be observed except by family members. Children are consoled by a rhythmic, coarse patting on the back or an extremity. Public displays of affection occur among same-sex friends but never among couples. Men greet each other with a fast hug in which both chests meet, somewhat off center, or they extend a hand (or both hands if they know each other well), which is held throughout the greeting. This hand gesture is not a handshake; the extended open hand is held between the other person's hands. It is also not uncommon to see friends of the same sex (men or women) holding hands as they walk. When a man greets a woman, he places one or both open hands (with the fingers together) gently on his heart as sign of respect, accompanied by a subtle nod or lowering of the eyes. Handshaking among male and female relatives is common in the eastern and southeastern parts of the country.

Perceptions of Time: Years of war have distorted time perceptions. The people of Afghanistan long for the future, but the immediacy of present needs usually eclipses futuristic thoughts or goal planning. Time is expressed as days or months before or after Ramadan, the holy month of fasting. Most people express their ages relative to the number of Ramadans that have passed in their lives.

Pain Reactions: Expressions of pain are considered signs of weakness; therefore, many are stoic and seem to have an enormous tolerance to pain. Children have not developed this ability and are uninhibited when crying because of pain. Women may describe depression (as do women in many other societies) as an all-over body pain. The desire for dignity inhibits many men from speaking of pain.

Birth Rites: Afghanistan has one of the highest infant (165 per 1000 live births) and child (<5 years) mortality rates (257 per 1000) globally; diarrheal disease is a major cause of infant deaths. One in four children dies before the fifth birthday, translating to 359,000 deaths annually. Women have no or little control over reproduction and are pressured by their families to give birth to a boy. The fertility rate is 7.4 children born per woman: life expectancy for both men and women is about 44. Divorce is very uncommon,

A

and women have little legal power to initiate divorce or support themselves afterward. Because having up to four wives is permitted, a man will marry another wife if one wife is deemed infertile. Maternal mortality is the second highest in the world, with 1,600 to 1,900 women dying per 100,000 live births, compared with 8 women per 100,000 in the United States. Peripartum hemorrhage is the most common cause of maternal death in most areas. Only 14% of births are attended by a trained provider; thus, women with any complication are likely to die. Even minor bleeding may be deadly as anemia is common resulting from closely spaced pregnancies, folate and iron insufficiencies, and malnutrition. Badahkshan, an isolated mountainous northern province, has the highest maternal mortality ratio ever measured, with 6,507 maternal deaths per 100,000 live births. Maternal deaths in this region are attributable largely to obstructed labor as a result of narrow pelvic outlets from stunted growth caused by chronic malnutrition.

Death Rites: Relatives and friends come to the home of the family to express sympathy and contribute money if needed. The body remains in the home with a *mullah* (a religious authority) or close relatives who read from the Koran throughout the night. The body is washed by relatives or *Morda Shoi* (male and female individuals who wash the body in exchange for money or goods); wrapped in new, white clothing; and placed in a simple wood coffin. The body must be buried within 24 hours (and is never cremated). Two days after the burial, a ceremony is held in the mosque or house of the deceased, followed by a meal. Headstones are usually pieces of slate. The direction of the surface or edge on the grave identifies the sex of the person in the grave.

Food Practices and Intolerances: Because food is not inspected for contaminants, water and milk products must be boiled for safety. Using the hands to eat is the norm. The diet consists primarily of nan (flat bread), rice, and meat (usually lamb). Vegetables and fruits are available seasonally, but few means of long-term food preservation are available.

Infant-Feeding Practices: Breastfeeding is not initiated until the second or third day of life, as colostrum is believed to be harmful; so the infant receives weak tea. In 1997, the United Nations Children's Fund (UNICEF) estimated that only 25% of women exclusively breastfed their infants from birth to 3 months. More recent estimates indicate that 54% of children still nurse at 20 to 23 months of age, in addition to receiving tea-soaked naan, potentially contributing to the high rates of death and malnutrition. Chronic malnutrition is common. Of children younger than 5 years, 51% are underweight and 54% have growth stunting. Children in the central and northern mountainous areas have the highest rates of malnutrition and have had to eat grasses and roots to avoid starvation during the ongoing drought. War, land mines, and lack of access to mountainous areas have presented challenges for groups attempting to deliver sustainable food products to the country.

Child-Rearing Practices: Children are an economic asset; they work to supplement the household income. Child labor (such as in carpet weaving and agricultural work) is common in rural areas, and approximately 28,000 children are working on the streets of Kabul. More children are enrolled in school (40% of girls and 66% of boys), reflecting change as

Afghanistan rebuilds. Access is still an issue for some, particularly in the southern areas, where schools have come under the attack of groups opposing development. Physical punishment as a form of discipline is customary among boys, who are valued more than girls are. There are few reported consequences for having girls, however (such as abandonment or drowning of female infants). For the most part, children are the center of the family and are attended to by both parents, although parents assume different roles.

National Childhood Immunizations: BCG at birth; OPV at 6, 10, and 14 weeks and 9 months; DPwT at 6, 10, and 14 weeks; measles at 9 and 18 months; TT, 15 to 45 years first contact, 1, +6 months, +1, +1 year. An estimated 21% of all childhood deaths are from scattered vaccine-preventable diseases. The percent of the target population vaccinated, by antigen, is: BCG (78%); DPT (66%); polio (66%); and measles (61%).

Other Characteristics: Afghans are designated the largest group of refugees globally. As of June 2005, more than 2.1 million refugees lived outside the country; 3.5 million have repatriated since 2001. One of the most heavily mined countries in the world, Afghanistan has about eight million land mines or unexploded artillery and from 2000 through 2002 had the highest number of casualties from them globally. More than half of these casualties were children under 18. Afghanistan is the world's largest opium producer, producing more than 80% of the global supply. Domestic drug use and dependence are emerging as a public health threat.

BIBLIOGRAPHY

Afghanistan National Health Resources Assessment report. Management Sciences for Health. Retrieved February 12, 2006, from http://www.msh.org/afghanistan/3.0.htm.

Bartlett LA, Mawji S, Whitehead S, et al. and the Afghan Maternal Mortality Study Team: Where giving birth is a forecast of death: maternal mortality in four districts of Afghanistan, 1999–2002. *Lancet* 365:864–70, 2005.

Bilukha OO, Brennan M: Injuries and deaths caused by unexploded ordnance in Afghanistan: review of surveillance data, 1997–2002. *BMJ* 330:127–8, 2005.

Central Intelligence Agency: 2006: *The world factbook, Afghanistan.* Retrieved September 21, 2006, from https://www.cia.gov/cia/publications/factbook/print/af.html.

Integrated Regional Information Networks (IRIN) News: Central Asia: Afghanistan: Poverty forces children to quit school to work. Retrieved February 15, 2006, from http://www.irinnews.org/report.asp?ReportID=41886&SelectRegion=Central_Asia&SelectCountry=AFGHANISTAN.

Integrated Regional Information Networks (IRIN) News: Central Asia: Afghanistan: education crisis in the South with 200 schools closed. February 8, 2006. Retrieved February 15, 2006, from http://www.irinnews.org/report.asp?ReportID=51608&SelectRegion=Asia.

Integrated Regional Information Networks (IRIN) News: Central Asia: Afghanistan: new centre for malnourished children in the north. Retrieved February 15, 2006, from http://www.irinnews.org/report.asp?ReportID=34201&SelectRegion=Central_Asia&SelectCountry=AFGHANISTAN.

ReliefWeb: UNHCR's global refugee figure lowest since 1980, internal displacement, statelessness remain high. June 17, 2005. Retrieved February 15, 2006, from http://www.reliefweb.int/rw/RWB.NSF/db900SID/EVOD-6DFDTJ?OpenDocument.

Sharp TW, Burkle FM Jr, Vaughn AF, Chotani R, Brennan RJ: Challenges and opportunities for humanitarian relief in Afghanistan. *Clin Infect Dis.* 34(suppl 5): S215–28, 2002.

UNICEF: Afghanistan—Statistics. Retrieved February 15, 2006, from http://www. unicef.org/infobycountry/afghanistan_afghanistan_statistics.html.

UNICEF: End decade databases—Breastfeeding. Retrieved February 15, 2006, from http://www.childinfo.org/eddb/brfeed/test/database.htm.

UNODC: Afghanistan opium survey 2005: executive summary. Retrieved December 3, 2006, from http://www.unodc.org/unodc/en/crop_monitoring.html#afg.

Women's E-News: Afghan women building lives amid rubble. Retrieved February 12, 2006, from http://www.womensenews.org/article.cfm?aid=2065.

World Bank: Afghanistan country update. Retrieved February 12, 2006, from http:// www.worldbank.org.af/WBSITE/EXTERNAL/COUNTRIES/SOUTHASIAEXT/AFGHA-NISTANEXTN/0,contentMDK:20143800~pagePK:141137~piPK:141127~theSite PK:305985,00.html.

World Health Organization: Tuberculosis. Retrieved September 14, 2006, from http://www.who.int/tb/publications/global_report/2006/pdf/emr.pdf.

World Health Organization: 2006: Immunization, vaccines and biologicals. Retrieved September 21, 2006, from http://www.who.int/immunization_monitoring/en/ globalsummary/countryprofileresult.cfm?C='afg'.

◆ ALBANIA (REPUBLIC OF)

MAP PAGE (798)

Eglantina Gjermeni, Edlira Haxhiymeri, and Mary P. Van Hook

Location: Albania is a mountainous country located in the southwestern part of the Balkan Peninsula. It has a total area of 28,748 km^2 (11,096 square miles): 35% forests, 15% pastures, 24% arable land, and 4% lakes. Albania borders the former Republic of Yugoslavia to the north, Greece to the south and southeast, and the Adriatic and Ionian Seas to the west. The capital is Tirana. The gross domestic product (GDP) per capita is $4,900 with about 25% below the poverty line. Literacy rates are 93% for men, 80% for women.

Major Languages	Ethnic Groups	Major Religions
Albanian (official dialect: Tosk)	Albanian 95% Greek 3% Vlach, Gypsy, Serb, Bulgarian 2%	Muslim 70% Albanian Orthodox 20% Roman Catholic 10%

The population is 5.8 million; 50% are women, and 60% are aged less than 35. Most people are employed in agriculture, followed by the public and private sectors. Religion does not have a strong influence on the life of the residents because religious practices were not allowed during the Communist regime from 1967 to 1990. Since then, the country has undergone significant social and political changes and is transitioning toward a market economy and democratic governance.

Health Care Beliefs: Acute sick care; magical-religious. Although medical treatment dominates, people believe some illnesses are caused by the supernatural power of God; therefore, they pray that God's power will heal them. Some pretend to possess special powers that can influence the course of diseases and cure people. Although this practice is illegal, these individuals purport that they can cure a malady caused by the "evil eye," an illness caused when one person looks at another with malice. Some younger people are beginning to have regular examinations for prevention purposes, although generally Albanians do not go to doctors for prevention. Health education has improved significantly in the last century. During the Communist regime, people were given lectures and courses in health care, symptoms of common diseases, and medical treatment. These efforts have improved the knowledge of the general population, so people no longer try to diagnose themselves and instead seek the advice of a doctor.

Predominant Sick-Care Practices: Biomedical; traditional. Medical care is preferred for disease treatment, even in rural and remote areas of the country. Doctors are highly respected and trusted. Although medical technology is not updated, people can go to hospitals and centers to be examined, especially in major cities. Albanians have no cultural preference for injections or oral treatment, but doctors are usually seen for crisis care only. Herbalists are popular, especially in rural areas, where people have less access to modern medicine. Most herbalists have gained their knowledge of treatments from other herbalists or family members. Some practice in arrangements with medical institutions. Herbal treatment is often successfully used for diarrhea, gastrointestinal complaints, sore throats, urinary disorders, and kidney problems. Teas of oregano, parsley, or rosemary are the most frequently used herbal treatments. Abortion once was taboo but is now legal and carried out in safe hospital-like conditions under a doctor's supervision. The abortion rate has been high (344 per 1000 births in 1999), although family planning programs have been established throughout the country.

Ethnic-/Race-Specific or Endemic Diseases: The major causes of death among adults are of cardiovascular origin, followed by cancer, accidents, violence, and respiratory system diseases. Acute respiratory tract infections, particularly pneumonia, are a leading cause of death in children. Most (83%) sick children are taken to an appropriate health care provider. Sexually transmitted diseases such as syphilis and gonorrhea are increasing in the population. Human immunodeficiency virus (HIV)/acquired immunodeficiency syndrome (AIDS) are not considered a substantial threat, but few statistical data are available. According to the Joint United Nations Programme on HIV/AIDS (UNAIDS) the prevalence rate for adults (aged 15 to 49) is less than 0.2%, with fewer than 1,000 people living with HIV. As of December 2004, 141 cases were confirmed, with 22 new that year, primarily among those aged 20 to 30 years. The percentage of women

A

with HIV is increasing (19% in 2002 to 40% in 2004), with transmission primarily through heterosexual contact. About 70% of cases are in Albanians who migrated from abroad. Prejudice has made it difficult for people to seek help, although a new medical program for health professionals is helping to reduce social stigma. Many Albanian women do not have accurate information about the transmission of HIV or where to seek testing. Whereas younger people tend to talk freely about homosexuality and preventive sexual practices, older people consider sex and homosexuality to be private issues not to be discussed openly.

Health-Team Relationships: The doctor is the primary authority in hospital settings. Nurses are subordinate and afforded more respect if they are the only health care professionals available. Doctors and nurses practice primarily in hospitals, all of which are public. Some new and well-equipped private clinics are also being set up, and the best-qualified doctors practice there after finishing their work in the public hospitals. Doctors are licensed for practice and guided by a professional code with strict guidelines for professional and patient relationships. Recently, some attempts have been made to include social workers and psychologists on hospital medical teams.

Families' Role in Hospital Care: Families and friends rally around people who are sick and play an important role in their care. Family members are expected to stay and provide food and basic hygiene, although the nurses and cleaning women offer some services.

Dominance Patterns: Until recently, a patriarchal-type family was dominant, with two to three generations living together under the same roof and males having preferential status. When Albania opened up to the international community in 1990, migration from rural to urban areas contributed to the breakdown of this structure. Gender equality is new and has not yet been embraced by a significant percentage of the population. Women do not play an important role in decision-making processes, although many are well educated and professionally trained. Women's nongovernmental organizations (NGOs) play an important role in increasing public awareness about the role of women in political and social life. Women have been identified as particularly vulnerable to abuse because of the tensions associated with this transition period. Some young women have been forced into prostitution, whereas other women experience physical violence from family members. Women's NGOs are active in helping such women. Children have also become victims of trafficking. Older adults without families can be especially vulnerable because of lack of status and support, although the number of abandoned older adults is relatively small. The pensions of older adults are important sources of financial support for many multigenerational migrant families.

Eye-Contact Practices: It is customary to sustain eye contact with other people while talking. Women (especially in rural areas) do not look at their husbands or other men and are expected to look down. In conversation with friends, not looking into their eyes signifies a lack of respect or sincerity.

Touch Practices: Touch is common, especially among individuals of the same sex. It is quite normal for men to shake hands, hug, and kiss when greeting each other. The same is true for women, who may repeat kisses on the cheeks several times, depending on how much they have missed the person. Members of the opposite sex are more restrained unless they have a close family relationship. Albanians hug and kiss children, and only in rare cases will young mothers ask people not to kiss their babies. When children are sick, touching their foreheads and holding and hugging them are ways they are comforted. Albanians believe their patterns of touch are based on their Mediterranean origins, and they are generally warm and expressive. The physical closeness that is usual for Albanians is not always welcomed by people from other cultures who are more accustomed to boundaries and privacy.

Perceptions of Time: Punctuality has not been an important value but is becoming more important and appreciated. Albanians hope for a better future, although it is difficult for them to ignore the difficulties of the present or to forget the sacrifices and hardships of the past.

Pain Reactions: Albanians typically have a high tolerance for pain and discomfort. Women are not expected to cry out in pain during labor. Loud verbal expressions in response to pain are considered shameful.

Birth Rites: Pregnancy is considered a delicate and sacred period, and the family takes great care to offer women the best quality of food they can. The fertility rate is two children born per woman, and male children are often preferred. Sexual intercourse continues during pregnancy and enjoyed as a "safe period" when no pregnancy precautions need to be taken. Tetanus toxoid injections are given to protect infants from neonatal tetanus, a major cause of infant death caused primarily by unsanitary conditions during childbirth. Professionals typically care for women during and following their deliveries, and almost all deliveries occur under the supervision of skilled personnel. Such care is more common in urban areas. Doctors assist in nearly 57% of births, nurses in 37%, and professionally trained midwives in 10%. Women are frequently treated for infections that develop at maternity hospitals, which may require that they stay in the hospital more than the usual day or two. At home, new mothers have an older woman—often their mothers or mothers-in-law, who care for them for 2 weeks. The first 40 days after birth are considered dangerous for the newborn and mother, and they are protected from the "evil eye" by not being allowed to go out or have contact with people considered by the family to be unfriendly. Mothers are warned not to become emotionally upset or to see visitors outside the door of the house because of the belief that breast milk will stop. Mothers are encouraged to breastfeed and eat food that increases milk production. Infants must be named and legally registered within the first 40 days, but if an infant dies within 40 days after birth, no ceremony accompanies the burial. Visitors, friends, and family are expected to come and visit the family and bring gifts, clothes, or money; but the mother's family of origin customarily buys most of the clothes and the crib. Parents usually decide on the name, but in rural

A

areas where traditional family structures predominate, grandparents may name the child using their or others' names. Mothers who work outside the home are allowed a 1-year leave (they are paid 80% of their salaries for 6 months and 50% for the second 6 months). Many women prefer not to stay at home for a full year because they do not want to lose their full salary. The infant mortality rate is 21.52 per 1,000 live births, and life expectancy is 75 for men, 80 for women. External migration contributes to low population increases.

Death Rites: Death is believed to be from both natural and supernatural causes. Relatives and friends expend considerable effort to be present when death nears, and the family begins expressing their grief through crying and wailing at the moment the person dies. Family members and close friends dress in black and official suits, and visits are expected from all relatives, friends, and neighbors. The body is buried within 24 hours. If the deceased is a young woman, she is dressed in a white bridal dress, and if a young man, he is dressed in a bridegroom's suit. Autopsies are not routine. The whole family is in mourning for at least 40 days, and visitors are usually given strong Turkish coffee or *raki*, a strong Albanian liquor. In turn, they are supposed to bring coffee, cigarettes, or money to help the family. The family offers meals out of respect for the dead person, and they continue to be provided during the first week after the burial, on the 40th day, and at the 6-month and 1-year anniversaries, at which time these activities are considered finished. Family members continue to visit the cemetery and bring flowers to the tomb, especially on sacred days, special anniversaries or birthdays, or to mark special family events.

Food Practices and Intolerances: Most people eat three times a day. The largest meal is generally lunch, consisting of meat and vegetables and rice, pasta, or beans. Supper in the evening is lighter, with leftovers from lunch or some light food. As the economy has undergone a transition over the past 10 years, the increasing tendency is for people to work during the day, and thus many now prefer the largest meal in the evening.

Infant-Feeding Practices: Approximately 69% of infants are exclusively breastfed at 1 month, 52% at 4 months, and 44% at 6 months. At age 6 to 9 months, 24% are receiving breast milk and solid or semisolid foods. By 12 to 23 months, only 6% are still being breastfed. Three percent of babies are born at a low birth weight. Of children younger than age 5, 14% are underweight for their age, 17% have stunted growth, and 4% are severely emaciated. Children whose mothers have a secondary education or more are least likely to be underweight and stunted compared with children of mothers with less education.

Child-Rearing Practices: The family has a very important role. Children who do not live with their families for various reasons (e.g., physical or mental handicaps, death of the parents, the inability of single parents or emigrating parents to care for them) might not be integrated into society and are at increased risk for abuse. The culture underscores the necessity for disciplining children, using corporal punishment if necessary. It is expected that when adults speak, children will remain quiet and listen. Many children have several caretakers. Maternal and paternal grandparents are usually considered the most appropriate and trustworthy caretakers, and they frequently assume this responsibility when the parents are working. Parents pay significant attention to the education of their children and often sacrifice for it. The education of girls is considered important, although worries about girls' safety have hindered the education of some. Social disruptions during the transition period from communism to independence caused some village schools to be destroyed and teachers left for more profitable occupations. Children most likely to receive an inadequate education include gypsies (Roma), children of illegal migrants to the cities, and children without families. Child labor remains high (23%) and prevents children from receiving an education. Drug abuse is a growing problem in youth because of easy access to drugs and doubts about the future. Albania has increasingly become a route for illegal drugs from Southeast Asia to Western Europe.

National Childhood Immunizations: BCG at birth; DTwP at 2, 4, 6 and 24 months; OPV at 2, 4, and 6 months and at 2 to 5 years; HepB at birth and at 2 and 6 months; MMR at 12 months and 5 years; DT at 5 years; Td 14 years; TT 15 to 45 years, first contact, +1 month. The percent of the target population vaccinated, by antigen, is: BCG, DTP1, DPT3, HepB3 (98%); MCV, Polio3 (97%); and TT2 plus (86%).

BIBLIOGRAPHY

Albanian Institute of Statistics: *Women and men in Albania, 2004*, Tirana, Albania, 2005.

Central Intelligence Agency 2006: *The World Factbook, Albania.* Retrieved September 15, 2006, from https://www.cia.gov/cia/publications/factbook/print/al.html.

Progri V, Jaupllari V: *Women and men in Albania*, Tirana, Albania, 2005, Institute of Statistics—Tirana.

United Nations Children's Fund: *Multiple indicator cluster survey*, February 2006, New York.

UNICEF, 2006: Albania, young country on the move. Retrieved February 12, 2006, from http//www.unicef.org.albania/overview.html.

US/AID, 2005: Albania, Increasing access to quality reproductive services. Retrieved February 12, 2006, from http://www.usaidalbania.org.

US/AID, 2005: Child trafficking children victims aided in Albania. Retrieved February 12, 2006, from http://www.usaidalbania.

Van Hook M, Gjermeni E, Haxhiymeri E: Sexual trafficking of women: tragic proportions and attempted solutions in Albania. *Int Social Work* 49(1):29, 2006.

Van Hook M, Haxhiymeri E, Gjermeni E: Responding to gender violence in Albania, *Int Social Work* 43(3):351–363, 2000.

World Health Organization: 2006: *Immunization, vaccines and biologicals.* Retrieved September 21, 2006 from http://www.who.int/immunization_monitoring/en/globalsummary/countryprofileresult.cfm?C'alb'

A

◆ ALGERIA (PEOPLE'S DEMOCRATIC REPUBLIC OF)

MAP PAGE (800)

Hassina Khelladi

Location: Algeria is the second-largest African country (with Sudan being the largest), with a total area of 2,381,741 km^2 (919,352 square miles). About 80% is the Sahara desert. It is bordered to the north by the Mediterranean sea, to the east by Tunisia and Libya, to the south by Niger and Mali, to the southwest by Mauritania and the Occidental Sahara, and to the west by Morocco. Algiers is the capital. The gross domestic product (GDP) per capita is $7,200, with about 25% below the poverty line. Literacy rates are 79% for men, 61% for women.

Major Languages	Ethnic Groups	Major Religions
Arabic (official)	Arab-Berber 99%	Sunni Muslim 99% (state
French	European ≤1%	religion)
Berber dialects		Christian and Jewish 1%

The population consists of Arabs and Berbers (Kabyles, Chaouias, Zénètes, Touaregs, and Mozabites). Children learn French starting in elementary school. The exact origin of the Berbers is unknown, but the Algerian population belongs to the Mediterranean race—the Ibero-Insular in the north and the Saharan (which includes Touaregs) in the south. Algeria has been dominated by many groups, resulting in a mixture of races, customs, traditions, and cultures. About 96% of the population lives in 17% of the territory, essentially in the north. Most Algerian Muslims are of the Malekite or Hanafite rite. The French population is increasing, although still not at the high levels of the 1980s. The population is about 33 million.

Health Care Beliefs: Active involvement; both health promotion and magical–religious beliefs. The emphasis is on health promotion and illness prevention; however, numerous beliefs are rooted in old-faith customs. For example, it is believed that a child who takes a long time to begin speaking must eat seven ends of sheep tongue, and the sheep must be sacrificed the day of the religious ceremony of Aid El Adha (forgiveness and fraternity day). For a quick recovery, a child with measles should wear red clothes, and sun stroke is always treated with compresses dipped into vinegar and put on the forehead. Wearing amulets inscribed with Koranic verses and putting the Fatma hand (a hand with five fingers) on a chain around the neck are believed to protect people from others with the "evil eye" (the belief that others may make them ill by looking at them). Mental illness is feared and not well understood, and psychiatric medicine is often powerless to allay the prejudices attached to this illness. An Algerian with mental illness consults a doctor only after turning to a traditional therapist *(taleb)*, and this delay in appropriate treatment may result in the need for emergency hospitalization.

A

Predominant Sick-Care Practices: Biomedical and traditional. Western medicine is generally used first, followed by traditional medicine if Western treatment fails. After becoming ill, patients first refer themselves to a doctor. If illness persists, they resort to acupuncture or mesotherapy. *Mesotherapy* consists of multiple microinjections of medications that can be given orally by means of an electronic injector at the site of the disease or pain. The absence of side effects, low cost, and encouraging results have made this treatment popular. Hydrotherapy and thalassotherapy (sea water) treatments, including the use of algae *(algotherapy)* and mud *(fangotherapy)*, are also popular for rheumatism, muscle spasms, after trauma or surgery, or for general malaise. Aqua instructors are responsible for therapy classes, swimming lessons, and exercises in the pool. Home medicine is common, and the leaves and roots of plants are made into teas. Self-medication is common. Patients pay a nominal fee for use of the public health service, but they have long waits before being seen, so patients may refer themselves to private-pay clinics. Social insurance reimburses 80% of the costs of care: the remaining 20% is paid by the mutual benefit society, a social insurance with a contribution of about $40 yearly. Patients with pain not cured by the medical system may consult healers who perform magnetism, or pious healers known as Taleb, who claim to have the power to cure with prayer and by reading Koranic verses. Both these healers are popular with individuals suffering from chronic or mental illnesses.

Ethnic-/Race-Specific or Endemic Diseases: The National Institute of Public Health of Algeria (INSP) reported the following disease cases, based on 32 million people in 2004: typhoid (1,203), dysentery (1,485), hepatitis A (681), hepatitis B (1,003), hepatitis C (421), diphtheria (8), whooping cough (68), tetanus (12), neonatal tetanus (5), acute flabby paralysis (78), measles (2,667), visceral leishmaniasis (130), skin leishmaniasis (14,822), bilharziasis (108), trachoma (860), brucellosis (3,524), rabies (24), malaria (163), tuberculosis (TB) (14,187), acquired immunodeficiency syndrome (AIDS) (28), and human immunodeficiency virus (HIV) (266). Since 1985, with the first report of HIV, the number of cases has increased from 642 to 1,721. The Joint United Nations Programme on HIV/AIDS (UNAIDS) estimates the prevalence rate for HIV in adults aged 15 to 49 to be 0.1% and that 19,000 people are living with HIV (including 4,100 women). There are no estimates for children. Total deaths attributable to AIDS are fewer than 500. The proportion of men versus women with HIV/AIDS is 3:1. Algerian women are infected most frequently through heterosexual contact with spouses, who often contract the disease while out of the country.

Health-Team Relationships: Male nurses are fairly uncommon. Nurses are trained to take care of the sick and injured, but they do not diagnose illness or prescribe treatments. Nurses are directed by doctors and provide treatments as prescribed. Patients treat health professionals with respect. If an individual's illness is considered of a sexual nature, patients are reticent to inform a health care professional. As of 2003 there were 87,791 nurses, 36,347 doctors, 8,651 dentists, and 5,705 pharmacists.

Families' Role in Hospital Care: When a family member is ill, the entire family mobilizes. At least one remains with the hospitalized person all day to keep him or her company and possibly to assist with bathing or changing linens. Food is usually prepared at home and brought in according to the patient's disease and dietary restrictions. The family is ready to give blood, organs, or money to save a relative's life, and any important decisions are decided by all family members. Their presence is an important part of the patient's therapy, and according to custom, every person who visits brings flowers, fruit, dates, or cakes.

Dominance Patterns: Algeria is a traditionally patriarchal society, although the constitution guarantees freedom to women. In theory, women are equal to men and are free citizens responsible for their own behavior. However, women continue to be cloistered by men in the name of tradition. Women are becoming aware that the patriarchal society is organized by men, often to the detriment of women, but although they resist, they also try to adapt to it and live an active lifestyle within it. Educated women believe that the misogynistic attitudes of men stem from ignorance and taboos and that the determination of men to dominate women can only be modified through knowledge and education. Despite traditional social pressures, most women want to escape the confinement and isolation of the home. Therefore, they must obtain a job or the necessary education that allows them to attain more independence and a higher rank in society. In the absence of the husband, the wife becomes the head of the family. Most Algerian women do not wear veils.

Eye-Contact Practices: Children avoid eye contact as a sign of respect for their elders, and girls and young women generally do not make direct eye contact with unfamiliar men.

Touch Practices: Touching while talking is uncommon and poorly regarded. Greetings among those with a professional relationship are limited to a handshake. An embrace signifies a very close relationship. In Islam, it is common for two people to say "Salaam" (Arabic for "peace") when they meet each other. Children asking for their parents' blessing and then kissing them on their right hand or forehead remains a popular practice among conservative families, during religious ceremonies, and as a respectful greeting.

Perceptions of Time: Algeria does not have the flexible view of time of some Mediterranean countries. In the Muslim religion, time is precious. Islam compares time with a saber—if a person does not control it, time, (i.e., the saber), will overcome the person. The older generations say that "time is money" and that "the day belongs to those who get up early." Moreover, men are judged and appreciated not by their fortunes but by their punctuality. The Algerian lifestyle is changing, so it has become more difficult to protect and preserve many of these valued customs. When talking about the future, references are made to the Koran; such discussions are always preceded by the expression "If God wills."

Pain Reactions: Koranic texts stipulate that all life events are irrevocably predestined by Allah; however, Algerians are an emotional people, sensitive to difficult and painful situations. Emotion is expressed by women through tears and lamentations and by men with heavy silence. Men do not express pain and are expected to be strong when facing painful moments.

Birth Rites: Most births occur in hospitals or in public/private clinics, but there are an estimated 50,000 home deliveries each year. The infant mortality rate is 30 deaths per 1,000 live births. Newborns are separated from their mothers except during breastfeeding. The fertility rate is 1.89 children born per woman, a reduction attributed to marrying at older ages and the educational improvement of girls. After 40 days of rest, the mother has a special bath with plants and roots at the *hammam* ("ritual bath"). Women eat meals such as lentils, sardines, and fenugreek to regain strength and increase milk production. After birth, the Algerian state allows 3 days' leave for fathers and 3 months' paid leave for working mothers. After 3 months, the law allows for flexible working hours so that breastfeeding can continue. Maternity fees (e.g., costs of hospitalization, 3 months' salary) are covered by social insurance. The seventh day after birth the Sabaa ceremony is celebrated in the presence of all family members. A special cake called *tammina* is made, which consists of honey, semolina, and spices. Early in the morning, the infant is given a bath with water that has been boiled with special plants, roots, and eggs. Afterward, the eggs are given to those present. This custom signifies hopes for the newborn's future fertility and a prosperous life. Henna is put on the infant's hands, a practice that makes the nails softer and less likely to cause injury. Kohl is put around the eyes to prevent diseases such as conjunctivitis, and the figure of a hand—the Fatma hand—is kept on a gold chain around the infant's neck to ward off illness from the evil eye. A copy of the Koran is also placed below the infant's pillow to prevent nightmares. Girls may have their ears pierced soon after birth. Algerians prefer to circumcise their male children on the 27th day of Ramadan (a holiday during which no food or drink is consumed between sunrise and sunset by anyone except the sick, children, and travelers). Contraception remains an exclusively feminine task. Modern methods include oral contraception, coils, and spermicidal creams. Traditional methods include breastfeeding and monthly timing of ovulatory periods. According to one study, about 50% use modern methods, whereas 14% use traditional methods. Life expectancy is 74 for men, 76 for women.

Death Rites: Shortly before death, a dying person must pronounce, "There is no God but Allah, and Mohammed is God's messenger." In villages the ritual may involve all the villagers, with activities suspended as a sign of respect. In cities, only the relatives and friends are involved. The body is cleaned and wrapped tightly in white cotton cloth that may have been soaked in holy water (*zemzem*). Many Muslims prefer to buy this cloth in Mecca during a pilgrimage. During transportation of the deceased to the mosque or cemetery, the body is placed in a coffin covered by a prayer carpet and is followed by the men to the cemetery. The wrapped body is carefully put into the grave without the coffin, and each man present covers the grave with soil. A meal takes place, consisting of couscous served with mutton. Food is also given to poor and needy people, an act of generosity recommended by the holy texts. Another memorial meal is held 40 days afterward. Embalming and cremation are prohibited, but an autopsy is performed when required for forensic purposes. Organ-donation transplants are acceptable.

Food Practices and Intolerances: Algerian cuisine is derived from many historic influences. Quite frugal meals of grains, such as couscous, and fresh or dried vegetables have been consumed for generations. Ottoman Empire, French, and Mediterranean influences added to the development of a varied cuisine. Favorite foods such as *méchoui* ("lamb roasted on a spit"), *bouzellouf* ("lamb's head"), and *osbane* ("lamb's intestines") are prepared during the religious ceremony of Aid El Adha. In general, Algerian cooking consists of highly seasoned dishes served with spicy sauces. Bread, butter, and apricot marmalade are common for breakfast. Vegetables, meat or fish, salad, and fruit are included in both lunch and dinner. Islam forbids consumption of any form of alcoholic drink, and only animals slaughtered according to Muslim regulations can be consumed.

Infant-Feeding Practices: A study carried out by the National Institute of Public Health with the collaboration of the United Nations Children's Fund (UNICEF) and other organizations has provided detailed information about mother and child health in Algeria. This study demonstrated that about 74% of women breastfeed during the first year of life, and 40% do so during the second year. Breastfeeding is recommended by the holy texts of the Koran for a child's first 2 years of life. Weaning usually occurs at about 2 years of age.

Child-Rearing Practices: A childless couple is doomed to failure because the Algerian man remarries to procreate. Children are treated affectionately. Grandmothers play an active role in care giving, especially when mothers are employed. Disciplining of children is carried out by the mother, and the father intervenes only at the mother's request. The father is authoritarian, and although his role becomes more prominent later in the child's life, children almost always retain a very close relationship with their mothers. Young children are enrolled in nursery school. The educational system has the mission of ensuring the development of children's personalities and their preparation for a meaningful life. All Algerians have the right to education, and school is compulsory for children aged 6 to 16 years. The educational system has three teaching levels—fundamental, secondary, and university—and is free at all levels. Classes are taught in Arabic, with the exception of university classes, in which students can choose French.

National Childhood Immunizations: BCG at birth; DTwP 3, 4, 5, and 18 months; OPV at birth and at 3, 4, 5, and 18 months and at 11 to 13 and 16 to 18 years of age; measles at 9 months and 6 years; Td at 11 to 13, 16 to 18 years; and DT at 6 years. All children born after 2001 receive hepatitis B (at birth and at 1 and 5 months). The incidence of measles has increased from 61 in 1995 to 160 more recently.Poliomyelitis has been eradicated. Vaccines are free at all public health sites. The percent of the target population vaccinated, by antigen, is: BCG (98%); DPT1 (94%); DPT3 (88%); HepB (83%); MCV (83%); MCV2 (94%); Polio3 (88%); and measles (79%).

BIBLIOGRAPHY

Bencharif A, Baba B. A propos de 1000 cas enfacts présenant des angines, rhino-paringites et bronchities à Répétition, Congrès International de Mésothérapie, São Paolo, Brasil, 1998.

Central Intelligence Agency: 2006: The World Factbook, Algeria. Retrieved September 21, 2006 from https://www.cia.gov/cia/publications/factbook/print/ag.html.

Hachid M: Les premiers Berbères entre Méditérrané, Tassili et Nil, Ina-Yas/Edisud, Aix-en-Provence, 2000, 317 pp.

Hachid M, Le Tassili des Ajjer: Aux sources de l'Afrique 50 siècles avant les Pyramides, Ed.Paris-Méditerranée, Paris, Edif2000, Alger.

http://www.ambafrance-dz.org/article.php3?id_article=256 (retrieved May 4, 2006).

Ministère de la Santé et de la Population, Institut National de Santé Publique: Enquête National sur les Objectifs de la Fin Décennie Santé Mère et Enfant EDG Algérie 2000 MICS2, Rapport de Synthèse, Alger 2001, République Algérienne Démocratique et Populaire, Retrieved July 15, 2006, from http://www.ands.dz/insp/edg.html.

Office National des Statistiques: Activité, emploi et chomage. Retrieved April 15, 2006, from http://www.ons.dz/them_sta.htm.

Office National des Statistiques: Démographie Algérienne, Retrieved May 6, 2006, from http://www.ons.dz/them_sta.htm.

Situation Epidémiologique de l'Année 2004 sur la Base des Cas Déclarés à 1'I.N.S.P, Relevé Epidémiologique Annuel, Algérie, Vol XV, Annuel 2004. Retrieved July 15, 2006, from http://www.ands.dz/insp/insp-publicat.htm.

UNAIDS, 2006 Algeria: Retrieved September 21, 2006, from http://www.unaids.org/en/Regions_Countries/Countries/algeria.asp.

World Health Organization: 2006: Immunization, vaccines and biologicals. Retrieved September 21, 2006 from http://www.who.int/immunization_monitoring/en/globalsummary/countryprofileresult.cfm?C='dza'.

◆ ANGOLA (REPUBLIC OF)

MAP PAGE (801)

Ndola Prata

Location: Angola is a former Portuguese colony on the southwest coast of Africa. The narrow coastal plain rises abruptly to a vast interior plateau. Only 30% of the total area of 1,246,700 km² (481,352 square miles) is arable. It is sparsely populated, with only nine people per square kilometer. The capital is Luanda. The province of Cabinda is an enclave separated from the rest of the country by the Democratic Republic of Congo. For the past 40 years, the country has been at war. Angola held its first multiparty general elections in 1992, but election results sparked a new bout of violence, as the opposition party contested the victory. This lasted until the signing of the Lusaka Peace Protocol November 1994. Subsequent attempts to put the peace process back on track were ineffective, and in December 1998, the war resumed and is still raging. The population is 15.4 million: 33% live in urban areas, and 44% are 0 to 14 years of age. The gross domestic product (GDP) per capita is $3,200, and 70% of the population lives below the poverty line.

Major Languages	Ethnic Groups	Major Religions
Portuguese (national)	Ovimbundu 37%	Indigenous
Bantu and other local	Kimbundu 25%	beliefs 47%
languages	Bakongo 13%	Roman Catholic
	Mestico 2%	38%
	European 1%, Other 22%	Protestant 15%

The country has many local languages: Kimbundu, Kikongo, Umbundu, Tchokwe, Ngangela, and Kuanhama. The most widely used is Portuguese. Literacy rates are 82% for men, 54% for women.

Health Care Beliefs: Acute sick care, magical-religious. Disease is generally perceived as induced by outside forces, requiring spiritual as well as medical attention, even by those who regularly use conventional health care services. When the initial signs of disease are noticed in newborns or young children, mothers and grandmothers immediately seek spiritual protection, fearing a series of problems that may end in death or disability. This usually requires a visit to a spiritual healer, who administers a small red bag of dried plants, roots, small parts of animal bones or teeth, and animal skin to be worn on a string wrapped around the waist. All these elements are thought to protect against curses. In addition, when a child is sick, parents are expected to practice sexual abstinence.

Predominant Sick-Care Practices: Biomedical; traditional. Conventional care is offered through the national health system, which includes public health and private for-profit facilities and private nonprofit organizations. Traditional medicine is offered by traditional doctors called *curandeiros*. Some focus on rituals and ceremonies calling the spirits of the dead to determine who is responsible for causing the disease. Then punishments may be prescribed or payments made to the offended person. Others treat the disease with herbs, local plants, and oils. Some healers practice in both spheres, and people of all classes frequent both types. Although herbal healers cover a vast range of diseases, spiritual healers are popular for mental health, infertility, and skin and chronic diseases. The decision to seek care is based on ethnic group norms, family values, traditions, access and affordability of care, and beliefs in the service available. Treatments for diseases such as malaria, acute respiratory tract infections, diarrhea, and measles are known to be better and faster when they involve conventional health care. For other diseases that are more difficult to self-diagnose, traditional healers are used first, and conventional medicine is used as a last resort. Public health services are free but often lack medicines, supplies, and treatments, and the person may have a long wait before being seen by a health professional. Traditional healers are not free, but prices are set based on ability to pay, and payments can also be made in kind or in installments.

Ethnic-/Race-Specific or Endemic Diseases: The most prevalent diseases are the infectious communicable diseases. These include vaccine-preventable diseases such as measles, polio, and tetanus and also diarrhea, acute respiratory tract infections, and malaria. Tuberculosis has a high annual incidence rate, and malnutrition is a major problem, especially for children younger than 5. Results from the 2001 Multiple Indicator Cluster Survey (MICS) show that approximately 45% of children under the age of 5 years have stunted growth, and 31% are underweight. Other endemic diseases that affect morbidity, but are not major killers, are trypanosomiasis, schistosomiasis, leishmaniasis, lymphatic filariasis, onchocerciasis, and other tropical diseases.The Joint United Nations Programme on HIV/AIDS (UNAIDS) has estimated the prevalence rate for human immunodeficiency virus (HIV) in adults aged 15 to 49 as 3.7%, and 320,000 are living with HIV, including 170,000 women. Around 30,000 deaths from acquired immunodeficiency syndrome (AIDS) have occurred, and there are 160,000 orphans aged 0 to 17 attributable to AIDS. In addition, 35,000 children aged 0 to 14 are living with HIV. More than 35% of all reported cases are in young people aged 15 to 29. In 1987 a National Program to Fight AIDS was created under the Ministry of Health to coordinate national prevention efforts and donor support activities. Although Angola seems to have much lower HIV prevalence rates than its neighboring countries, there is underreporting because of the limited capacities for diagnosis and the isolation of populations because of the civil war. Most men are circumcised, which might also contribute to the reduced male-to-female transmission.

Health-Team Relationships: The delivery of health care services is driven by doctors, but it is estimated that there is only one doctor for every 20,000 people. Most of the health centers are run entirely by nurses, and even in major urban areas, health centers do not have permanent doctors. Therefore, nurses are responsible for the delivery of primary health care services. The relationships between doctors and nurses are usually good. In general, public servants are not well paid, and nurses working in the public sector are in this category. Nonetheless, the work they do is so important and appreciated by their community that even though they are paid low salaries, they are committed and dedicated to their patients. Attitudes toward health professionals are generally respectful because the community considers health care workers to be authorities.

Families' Role in Hospital Care: When a person is hospitalized, at least one member of the family stays with that person 24 hours a day. Family members may help with changing linens, bathing, and other activities.

A

Some hospitals (including pediatric hospitals) do not allow family members to stay overnight, but even then family members stay within the vicinity, often in a "camping ground" in the hospital yard. This support is very important for those who are sick: although they cannot see their family for most of the day, they are reassured that somebody is always nearby. Families prepare meals for the sick person according to family norms. It is common practice to feed sick people meals that are also high in sodium and cholesterol. This practice may not be detrimental for patients who are weak from prolonged and debilitating infectious disease or after surgery and massive blood loss. It may be detrimental if a specific diet needs to be followed (e.g., for those with high blood pressure or diabetes). Lack of knowledge on the part of the family, coupled with lack of communication with health providers and hospitals' insufficient response to patient needs, can slow the recovery time.

Dominance Patterns: Angola is a male-dominated society. Most often, when a couple marries and forms a new family, the man comes from the wealthier family and thereby has decision-making and economic power over his wife. Such a man usually defers to the judgment of his own mother or another maternal figure to the extent that his decisions in family matters tend to reflect her will. These family concerns can include factors such as type of food consumed, place of residence, health-seeking behavior, family size, and child-rearing practices. In the less common scenario, in which the wife comes from a wealthier family, the situation is reversed. Because the couple tends to be financially dependent on the wife's family, the wife dominates the relationship, and her family has more of a voice in decision making. Angolan women face vastly different opportunities that depend largely on class and education. Most assume domestic responsibilities and child-rearing duties. Many serve in positions such as ministers, vice ministers, chief executive officers, and army and police officers. Tensions and contradictions accompany the changing roles of women. In general, women are respected, and their contributions to society are accepted. As a general rule, respect comes with age.

Eye-Contact Practices: Rural people do not tend to make eye contact, but it is more acceptable in urban settings. Most ethnic groups consider eye contact with the speaker a sign of defiance if an older adult or someone with higher status in the family or social hierarchy is speaking. Common practice dictates that children do not make eye contact with adults regardless of the setting.

Touch Practices: Angolans place a high premium on communicating warmth, friendliness, and welcoming greetings. Social touching is used to communicate platonic affection within and between genders. Demonstrative behavior usually involves hugging, embracing, and social kissing on the cheek, not only when greeting friends and acquaintances, but also when making first introductions. Moreover, all social groups engage in tactile behavior to express camaraderie and affection. Parents and the entire society instill such demonstrative behavior early on by teaching children to exchange social kisses during introductions and salutations with other children and adults.

Perceptions of Time: In general, the perception of time varies between urban and rural people. Unlike many countries, in general, rural people are more punctual, whereas those from urban areas have a less strict perception of time. With respect to health care (in the public sector only), it is unheard of for patients to be late for appointments because waiting to be seen is the norm.

Pain Reactions: Reactions to pain differs; for example, it is quite normal to emit loud sounds or even scream during childbirth. Screaming during other health procedures not involving anesthetics (suturing, tooth removal, cleaning of wounds, and injections) does not necessarily reflect the amount of pain being experienced but helps relieve stress and fear. In all other circumstances, pain is usually experienced in silence. The amount of a patient's pain is usually recognized through the person's facial expressions, lack of responsiveness to basic questions, and the use of pain-relieving body positions. When asked if they are in pain, it is not uncommon for patients to respond, "Just a little," and pain should be further investigated.

Birth Rites: Part of the strategy to decrease maternal mortality is to shift births from home to health centers because only 45% of home births are attended by trained personnel. This effort has not been successful, however, because of inadequate access to good-quality maternity services, an inability to carry out certain customs during and after delivery, and the lack of support from family and friends. The infant mortality rate is 185 deaths per 1,000 live births, and the fertility rate is 6.4 children born per woman. During delivery it is customary to sit on or put pressure on the woman's abdomen when it's believed she is not pushing strongly enough. In other cases a birth attendant will sweep a broom down the abdomen of the woman. When there is a delay in the expulsion of the placenta, husbands are asked to blow into an empty bottle just outside the delivery room until it is expelled. After delivery, mothers are given coconut milk and dried salted fish, which are believed to help increase milk production. Postpartum baths are very hot, and the water is boiled with special plants and roots. The arrival of a son is highly celebrated. After marriage, daughters usually live with or work close to her husband's family. Sons are expected to stay and provide for their parents in their old age by giving them shelter when they can no longer take care of themselves. Nonetheless, daughters are also celebrated. A good mix of boys and girls is considered a blessed outcome. The national family planning program began in the mid-80s to improve the well-being of mothers through child spacing. However, the program has been plagued by shortages of properly trained health workers, limited choices of contraceptive methods, and frequent interruptions in their supply. Social marketing of condoms since 2001 has increased use, especially among adolescents and young adults. The sexual behavior of young people will play a major role in the future spread of HIV, yet Angola has one of the lowest contraceptive rates in sub-Saharan Africa. The maternal mortality rate is one of the highest in the world, (1,500 per 100,000 live births). Contributing to high maternal mortality rates are the so-called indirect causes of maternal deaths: 25% from malaria; and 25% to post-abortion complications. Abortion is illegal but permitted for medical or social reasons. The personnel who do most of the illegal abortions are not properly trained,

A

and abortions are often complicated by infections and bleeding. Life expectancy is 37 for men and 40 for women.

Death Rites: Death at a young age is perceived to be caused by a curse, whereas older people die upon a call from a higher power. In both cases, the deceased are washed and nicely dressed before burial. Family members usually kiss the deceased, and only adult men and women can participate. Children and close family members are allowed in the room only for the farewell kiss. The ceremonies are attended by extended family and friends for a minimum of 7 days, when mourners dress in black, and all entertainment is prohibited. The mourning house stays open day and night, and groups of people take turns singing and dancing the death rites dance. After burial, people are given food and large amounts of alcoholic beverages. After the seventh day of the celebration of mourning, the family starts to disperse, and life is expected to resume as before.

Food Practices and Intolerances: The most important meal of the day is lunch. In the northern part of the country, the most important source of carbohydrates is the cassava root, whereas in the central and the southern regions corn is the staple. Depending on availability, people eat local vegetables and meat or fish (dried or fresh) with their cassava or corn. Both are usually eaten with a sauce that has a peanut or palm oil base. In rural areas, it is acceptable and usual practice to eat with the hands, whereas the urban population tends to use utensils.

Infant-Feeding Practices: Results from MICS-II show that 98% of children are breastfed for about 25 months. Exclusive breastfeeding does not last very long: only 14% of children younger than 4 months are solely breastfed. Mothers tend to start food supplementation between the ages of 2 and 3 months. Colostrum is perceived as weak milk, so some mothers (in urban areas) use formula in bottles, whereas mothers in rural areas may use fresh goat milk. Solid food is introduced at 3 or 4 months and consists of porridge made from corn or cassava flour. Even though children at that age are still being breastfed, at least one meal a day is solid food. These practices are often associated with diarrheal diseases because of contamination, inability to digest the food, or infants not having fully gained from the immunologic attributes of breast milk. A child is usually nursed at will, and it is not unusual to see breastfeeding in public places.

Child-Rearing Practices: Except for some urban, more Westernized families, discipline and other child-rearing duties are mainly a mother's task. Fathers are usually considered authoritarian figures and discipline the children when mothers ask. Otherwise, the role of the father starts later in the child's life. Even though fathers participate in parental decisions, mothers usually announce these decisions. Until the age of 1 or 2 years, children have a very close relationship with their mothers. They frequently sleep with their mothers (or another adult female) and are carried on their back wherever they go unless they are employed urban women. Frequently, women get pregnant while still breastfeeding, which alters these practices.

National Childhood Immunizations: BCG at birth; DTwP at 2, 4, and 6 months; OPV at birth and at 2, 4, and 6 months; measles at 9 months;

yellow fever at 9 months; TT at first contact, $+1$, $+6$ months, $+1$, $+1$ year; vitamin A at 6 and 9 months. The percent of the target population vaccinated, by antigen, is: BCG (61%); Polio3 (46%); DTP1 (62%); DTP3 (47); MCV (45%); and TT2 plus (75%).

Other Characteristics: Only 16% of the population has access to basic sanitation, 32% to safe water, and 24% to formal health care. Since hostilities resumed in 1998, more than three million people have been displaced, primarily in the provinces of Bie, Huila, Huambo, and Malanje.

BIBLIOGRAPHY

Agadjanian V, Prata N: Trends in Angola's fertility. Paper presented at the Workshop on Prospects for Fertility Decline in High Fertility Countries. Population Division, Department of Economic and Social Affairs. United Nations Secretariat. New York, 9–11, July 2001.

Agadjanian V, Prata N: War and reproduction: Angola's fertility in comparative perspective. *J S Afr Stud.* 27(2), 2001.

Central Intelligence Agency: *2006: The world factbook, Angola.* Retrieved September 1, 2006, from https://www.cia.gov/cia/publications/factbook/print/ao.html.

INE [Instituto Nacional de Estatistica]: MICS (Multiple Indicator Cluster Survey): Assessing the situation of Angolan children and women at the beginning of the millennium. INE/UNICEF, Angola, 2003.

Prata N, Vahidnia F, Fraser A: Gender and relationship differences in condom use among 15–24-year-olds in Angola. *Int Fam Plan Perspect.* 31(4):192–9, 2005.

UNAIDS: 2006. Angola: Retrieved September 1, 2006, from http://www.unaids.org/en/Regions_Countries/Countries/angola.asp.

World Bank: World Development Indicators Database. The World Bank, Washington DC, World Population Data Sheet 2005. Population Reference Bureau. Washington DC, 2001.

World Health Organization: 2006: Immunization, vaccines and biologicals. Retrieved September 1, 2006 from http://who.int/immunization_monitoring/en/globalsummary/countryprofileresult.cfm?C='ago'.

◆ ARGENTINA (ARGENTINE REPUBLIC)

MAP PAGE (797)

Carolyn M. D'Avanzo

Location: Argentina, the second largest country in South America, is a land of plains from the Atlantic Ocean to the Chilean border and contains the high peaks of the Andes. Its bordering countries are Bolivia, Brazil, Chile, Paraguay, and Uruguay. The north is swampy, and the central populated area has fertile land used for agriculture or grazing animals. The south boasts Patagonia, with its cool, arid steppes. The capital is Buenos Aires. The climate is primarily temperate—arid in the southeast and sub-Antarctic in the southwest. The total area is 2,766,890 km^2 (1,068,298 square miles). Argentina is considered a medium-income nation with a developing economy and has a gross domestic product (GDP) per capita of $13,000. The population is 39.9 million. Inflation has been a major problem and reached greater than 12% in 2005. About 38% of Argentinians live below the poverty line.

Major Languages	Ethnic Groups	Major Religions
Spanish (official)	White 97%	Roman Catholic
English	Mestizo, Amerindian,	92% (less than
Italian	Other nonwhite	2% practicing)
German	groups 3%	Protestant 2%
Amerindian languages		Jewish 2%
		Other 4%

Most white Argentinians are of European origin, primarily of Spanish and Italian descent. Argentina has 17 Amerindian languages, including Quechua, Mapuche, Guarani, Tobas, and Matacos. Literacy rates are high at greater than 97% for men and women.

Health Care Beliefs: Active involvement: health promotion is important. Since the 1990s, several bills have passed that mandate the creation of various health-promotion and disease-prevention programs, such as family planning, sex education, and sexual health services. Numerous difficulties have been encountered, particularly involving the provision of contraceptives, which seems to be primarily a result of the alliance of the country with the Roman Catholic Church. Therefore, poor women who depend on public health services for assistance with family planning are particularly vulnerable and unable to control their reproductive destiny.

Predominant Sick-Care Practices: Biomedical: curative and preventive. Reforms that took place in the 1990s opened up to competition—both internally and from private insurers—the union-administered social insurance system for workers. The current system is a combination of government-sponsored social health insurance and individual private insurance. The movement toward a managed-care approach is affecting the distribution of health care resources, with the poor receiving the least, although some free hospital clinics exist. Medical standards are highest in urban areas, and rural areas have less adequate services.

Ethnic-/Race-Specific or Endemic Diseases: Endemic diseases and conditions include malaria (regional), tuberculosis, Chagas disease, animal-borne helminthiases, intestinal parasites, histoplasmosis, paracoccidioidomycosis (northwest), leishmaniasis, trichinosis, typhoid fever and rotavirus, and severe diarrhea in children. People are at risk for Argentine hemorrhagic fever, dengue fever (endemic in neighboring countries), *Escherichia coli* infection, measles, yellow fever, cholera, hepatitis A and B, hantavirus, botulism, and *Helicobacter pylori* infection. Outbreaks of mumps and pertussis occurred and 14 cases of tetanus were reported in 2005. Argentina has one of the highest automobile accident rates in the world. High cigarette-smoking rates contribute to respiratory diseases.

A

The Joint United Nations Programme on HIV/AIDS (UNAIDS) estimates the prevalence rate for human immunodeficiency virus (HIV) in adults aged 15 to 49 years to be 0.6%, with 130,000 people living with HIV, including 36,000 women. About 4,300 have died of acquired immunodeficiency syndrome (AIDS). The Argentine-Maltese Aid Program for perinatal AIDS prevention, which has been implemented in nine public hospitals in Buenos Aires, has reduced mother-child transmission by almost 90%.

Health-Team Relationships: Population studies indicate that families are likely to protect patients from knowing their diagnosis, prognosis, and treatment. Health professionals generally prefer to discuss patients' health situations truthfully.

Dominance Patterns: The society is generally patriarchal, with deference given to the father; however, he considers the opinions of the rest of the family. Traditional gender roles are strong, particularly in rural areas and among less educated individuals.

Eye-Contact Practices: Direct eye contact is commonly maintained.

Touch Practices: Touching during conversations is quite usual, and males may touch each other without any sexual connotation.

Perceptions of Time: Argentinians have a relaxed attitude toward punctuality.

Birth Rites: The fertility rate is two children born per woman. The infant mortality rate is 15 deaths per 1,000 live births. Life expectancy is 72 for men, 80 for women.

Food Practices and Intolerances: Argentinians consume large amounts of beef. Mixed grilles *(parrillada)*, which contain almost every part of the animal, are popular, as are Italian foods such as gnocchi *(noquis)*. Argentinean ice cream is famous for its quality. Drinking mate (Paraguayan tea) from a shared gourd is a ritual of acceptance between individuals.

National Childhood Immunizations: BCG at birth and 6 years; DTPHiB at 2, 4, 6, and 18 months; OPV at 2, 4, 6, and 18 months and 6 years; IPV at 2, 4, 6, and 18 months (special cases); HepB at birth and at 2 and 6 months; Hep A at 1 year; MMR at 12 months and 6 years; DPT at 6 years; MR at 11 years and postpartum; Td at 16 years and then every 10 years; YF at 12 months (part of country). The percent of the target population vaccinated, by antigen, is: BCG and MCV (99%); DTP1 (90%); DTP3, HIB3, and Polio3 (92%).

Other Characteristics: Argentina is used as a trans-shipment country for cocaine headed for Europe; domestic consumption of drugs is increasing in the cities.

BIBLIOGRAPHY

Center for Disease Control and Prevention: International News 2006. Argentina: prevention cuts perinatal HIV/AIDS. Retrieved August 1, 2006, from http://www. thebody.com/cdc/news_updates_archive/nov4_02argentina_aids.html.
Center for HIV Information: UCSF (2006). Argentina. Retrieved August 1, 2006, from http://hivinsite.ucsf.edu/global?page+cr05-ar-00.

A

Central Intelligence Agency: 2006: The World Factbook, Argentina. Retrieved September 15, 2006, from http://www.cia.gov/cia/publications/factbook/geos/ar.html.

Grimberg M: Knowing about AIDS and sexual precautions among low-income women from the Southern area of Buenos Aires (notes for defining prevention policies), *Cad Saude Publica* 17(3):481, 2001.

Mercer R, Ramos S, Szulik D, Zamberlin N: The need for youth-oriented policies and programmes on responsible sexuality in Argentina, *Reprod Health Matters.* 9(17):184, 2001.

UNAIDS: 2006 Argentina Retrieved September 15, 2006 from http://www.unaids.org/en/Regions_Countries/Countries/argentina.asp.

World Health Organization: 2006: Immunization, vaccines and biologicals. Retrieved July 30, 2006, from http://www.who.int/immunization_monitoring/en/globalsummary/countryprofileresult.cfm?C='arg'.

World Health Organization: 2006: Retrieved July 30, 2006, from http://who.int/countries/arg/en.

◆ ARMENIA

MAP PAGE (799)

Mary Arevian

Location: The smallest of the former Soviet republics, Armenia achieved independence in 1991. It is a landlocked country in the southern Caucasus. Border countries are Azerbaijan-proper, Azerbaijan-Naxcivan enclave, Georgia, Iran, and Turkey. The capital is Yerevan. The terrain includes rugged mountains and excellent pastures. The total area is 29,800 km² (11,506 square miles). In 1988, a devastating earthquake destroyed Armenia's infrastructure and resulted in 500,000 adults and children who were homeless, had disabilities, or whose parents had been killed. In addition, about 250,000 Armenian refugees from Azerbaijan took refuge in Armenia as a consequence of problems in Nagorno Karabagh. The population of the country is about three million. The gross domestic product (GDP) is $4,500, with about 43% below the poverty line. Literacy rates are 99% for men, 98% for women.

Major Languages	Ethnic Groups	Major Religions
Armenian	Armenian 97.9%	Armenian Apostolic 94.7%
Yezidi	Yezidi (Kurd) 1.3%	Christian 0.4%
Russian	Russian 0.5%	Yezidi (monotheist and nature worship) 1.3%
Other	Other 0.3%	

Health Care Beliefs: Acute sick care; biomedical; traditional. A previous emphasis on the importance of health promotion and disease prevention is regaining impetus, due in part to the establishment of the infrastructure needed to provide public health services. It is common to see health-promotion programs on national television on stopping smoking, sensible drinking, obesity prevention, and promotion of breastfeeding. Disease is not viewed as a punishment from God for sinning, but as fate. Alternative treatments are not used for illness; people go to clinics or hospitals for biomedical treatment. Medication use is highly predominant, and doctors who do not prescribe drugs are not considered good doctors. People are used to taking medications without prescriptions. Armenia is rich in many kinds of herbs, so herbal treatments are also popular: various teas are used to treat respiratory, urinary, digestive, and other ailments. Herbs may also be used in locally prepared ointments and creams. Although some of these herbal treatments are helpful, others can be harmful. Little research has been done to determine which treatments should be encouraged. Alcohol consumption and smoking are viewed as part of the typical social and cultural behavior of men. Recently broadcasted televised programs have been relating health hazards to lifestyle choices, but the lack of public policy is a significant obstacle. Vigorous advertising campaigns promoting cigarettes and alcoholic drinks pose great challenges to the fairly insignificant health-promotion programs.

Predominant Sick-Care Practices: Biomedical. Most of the hospitals were built during the 1960s and 1970s, except for the few constructed by European countries in the area of the 1988 earthquake. Because of a persistent lack of funds, most of the hospitals have not been renovated. At present, funds are being provided by the Armenian Diaspora (especially from the United States and Europe) to renovate the hospitals and upgrade diagnostic and therapeutic equipment. The unequal distribution of health care facilities between urban and rural populations has created a large gap in health care between the two.

Ethnic-/Race-Specific or Endemic Diseases: According to the Ministry of Health, the major health problems, in order of importance, include coronary artery disease, cancer, gastrointestinal disorders, infectious diseases, diabetes, and perinatal complications. Armenians have higher rates of familial Mediterranean fever than do other countries. The Joint United Nations Programme on HIV/AIDS (UNAIDS) estimates the prevalence rate for human immunodeficiency virus (HIV) in adults (aged 15 to 49 years) is 0.1%, with 2,900 people living with HIV, including fewer than 1,000 women. Total deaths from acquired immunodeficiency syndrome (AIDS) are fewer than 500. Men constitute more than 78% of all cases. Young women are especially vulnerable: many have become sex workers to support their families owing to the high level of unemployment. Many factors contribute to problems in establishing effective prevention programs, including social attitudes, such as the "not in our country" attitude. In addition to the false belief that HIV and AIDS are not a potentially serious problem in Armenia, sex and sexual issues are taboo subjects, hindering frank and open discussions about HIV and other sexually transmitted diseases. Changing these deep-seated social attitudes will take much effort and time. Armenia has, however, adopted a national program for HIV/AIDS

A

prevention, with the help and collaboration of governmental, nongovern-mental, and international organizations.

Health-Team Relationships: The health care system is centralized, bureaucratic, medically oriented, and male dominated despite the numer-ous female physicians. Communication among health care personnel is gen-erally unidirectional, moving from doctors to therapists and nurses, and takes the form of instructions and orders. Health care service workers are paid by the government; however, if families do not pay bribes, their family members may not be admitted to a hospital or, even when admitted, may not receive basic services such as bathing, turning, and feeding. Because hospitals are paid by the government based on the amount of time a bed is occupied, the length of stay may be extended.

Families' Role in Hospital Care: Families are the sole supporters of their sick family members. They are responsible for provision of food, medications, syringes, needles, intravenous equipment, and all other necessities. It is common to see visitors carrying bags of food to the hos-pital for their relatives, and doctors and nurses are invited to eat from the food brought in for patients.

Dominance Patterns: Males are dominant. The family support system is important, so family members generally stay close. Older members are taken care of by their families, and it is a disgrace if a family institutionalizes an older family member. Women are the torchbearers and preservers of life values, religious beliefs, and motherhood customs. Throughout history the Armenian woman has had an important role in maintaining the family—and through fam-ily maintenance in preserving the nation. However, despite the fact that 60% of those who have received a higher education are women, women constitute only 3% of parliament. To really understand the status of women in Armenia, it is important to refer to historical events that had a significant impact on their role and status. For 600 years during the Turkish occupation, Armenian men saw women as inferior slaves and servants. When Armenia became part of the United Soviet Socialist Republic (1920–1991), if they were to survive, women had to learn to be rough and manage hard labor; and it was assumed that men and women were equal. However, during this period of history, while women did the hard work, men turned to the pleasures of smoking, drinking, and hav-ing extramarital sex. For a man to have an extramarital lover became a sign of prosperity and a symbol of manhood. For the sake of maintaining family peace, women silently adapted to the situation. It is now usual to see men enjoying themselves with other men and women while their wives are busy with household responsibilities as well as their work outside the home. The current status of the Armenian woman is a paradox. On one hand, she is highly educated and has entered esteemed professions such as medicine, law, and engineering. On the other hand, she is still a subordinate "slave" or "servant." Only a very small proportion of women are active in the political arena or other significant societal or community activities.

Eye-Contact Practices: Direct eye contact is usually unacceptable.

Touch Practices: Men usually greet each other and women by shaking hands. Friendly kissing between men and women is not acceptable.

Perceptions of Time: Punctuality was not important in the past. If an appointment did not take place at 9:00 AM, it could very easily occur at 9:00 PM; if not today, it could very easily be tomorrow. More recently, younger people in particular, seem to be more concerned about the value of time and the importance of being punctual.

Pain Reactions: Men are known for their stoicism, and they are not expected to express feelings of pain openly. It is acceptable for women to scream during painful experiences or to cry in a loud voice during sad occasions.

Birth Rites: Doctors typically deliver infants in hospitals. The infant mortality rate is 22 deaths per 1,000 live births. Abortion is the primary birth control method, with an average of 15 abortions for a 35-year-old woman. Vasectomy is not a culturally acceptable option for most Armenian men. As many as one in three women are infertile as the result of sexually transmitted diseases and unsafe abortions. Exempting abortions, the fertility rate is 1.33 children born per woman. Life expectancy is 68 for men, 76 for women.

Death Rites: Relatives, friends, and neighbors are required to attend at the time of death. Funeral services are held both at the church and at the place of burial. Fortunes may be spent on decorating the cemeteries. Cemeteries are visited after every family and religious occasion, such as Christmas and Easter.

Food Practices and Intolerances: Births, baptisms, marriages, and deaths have special significance. They usually celebrate happy and sad occasions with food and drink. Armenian people are very generous, and during any visit to their homes, food and drink is offered. They usually offer all that they have, even if it means that they may have nothing for the next day. Men usually get seated at the table, and women serve the meal.

Infant-Feeding Practices: Breastfeeding declined after the 1988 earthquake. Many mothers complained that their milk was not sufficient or that they were under too much stress. At that time, formula preparations were available because many charitable organizations were donating infant formula. At present, most women prefer to breastfeed their infants, and women who are not employed usually do so for about six months.

Child-Rearing Practices: Mothers are the primary caregivers for their children, but if they have to return to work, grandmothers and even great grandmothers supervise them. This shift in caregiving is not a problem because the family is usually traditional and extended. The age of marriage is generally young (about 20) for men and women. Many couples get married while still at the university studying. Because it is difficult to find housing, living with parents or even grandparents has become the norm rather then the exception. The literature describes the Armenian mother as being kind, virtuous, and sacrificial.

National Childhood Immunizations: BCG at birth and 7 years; DTwP at 3, 4.5, 6, and 18 months; Td at 6, 16, 26, 36, 46, and 56 years; OPV at

A

3, 4.5, 6, 18, and 20 months and at 6 years; MMR at 1 and 6 years; HepB at birth and 1.5 and 6 months. HIB vaccine is not yet integrated into routine schedules. The percent of the target population vaccinated, by antigen, is: BCG, MCV (94%); DTP1 (96%); DTP3 (90%); HepB3 (91%); and Polio3 (92%).

BIBLIOGRAPHY

Aztak daily, Thursday, March 21, 2002.

Aztak daily, Wednesday, March 27, 2002.

Bernal H, Maranjian O, Arevian M, Shensul S: Community health nursing in a former Soviet Union republic: a case study of change in Armenia. *Nurs Outlook* 43(2):78, 1995.

Central Intelligence Agency 2006: The World Factbook, Armenia, Retrieved September 15, 2006, from https://wwwcia.gov/cia/publications/factbook/print/am.htm.

Hertzberg DL: The interdisciplinary team: the experience in the Armenia pediatric rehabilitation program. Project HOPE Pediatric Rehabilitation Education Program. *Holistic Nurs Pract.* 7(4):42, 1993.

Jinbashian S: The woman of Armenia. *Hai Sird.* 154:32–38, 2002.

Kalayjian AS: Mental health outreach program following the earthquake in Armenia, *Issues Ment Health Nurs.* 15(6):533, 1994.

Ugularian A: HIV/AIDS in the Transcaucasus. *Hai Sird.* 155:10–12, 2001.

UNAIDS: 2006 Armenia. Retrieved September 15, 2006, from http://www.unaids.org/en/Regions_Countries/Countries/armenia.asp.

World Health Organization 2006: Immunization, vaccines and biologicals. Retrieved September 15, 2006, from http://www.int/immunization_monitoring/en/globalsummary/countryprofileresult.cfm?C='arm'.

◆ AUSTRALIA (COMMONWEALTH OF)

MAP PAGE (794)

Nel Glass

Location: Australia consists of two land masses: mainland Australia and the smaller Tasmania. It has a total area of 7,682,300 km^2 (2,965,368 square miles) and is situated in the Southern Hemisphere. Australia is surrounded by the Pacific Ocean on its east, the Southern Ocean on its south, the Indian Ocean on its west, and the Timor and Arafura Seas on the north. The closest neighboring country is Papua-New Guinea. The capital is Canberra. The population is about 20.3 million. The gross domestic product (GDP) per capita is $31,900. Literacy rates are 99%.

Major Languages	Ethnic Groups	Major Religions
English	White 95%	Anglican 26%
Aborigine	Asian 4%	Roman Catholic 26%
	Aborigine, Other 1%	Other Christian 24%
		Other 24%

Australia is a multicultural country with many immigrants; consequently, several other languages as well as English are spoken. In aboriginal cultures, children and adults can choose to learn some of the major indigenous languages, such as Ngaanyatjarra and Kariol. There has been an increasing trend toward cultural and racial diversity, but world instability and terrorism legislation may negatively affect refugee status and immigration. However, Australia is also experiencing a workplace skills shortage and actively recruiting skilled overseas workers.

Health Care Beliefs: Active involvement; health promotion. Australians are the recipients of good health care services, and underlying national health trends are consistent with health developments occurring in other developed countries. Ongoing health-promotion campaigns aim to improve physical and emotional health through the media, community health centers, hospitals, the Australian government, and schools. It is expected that individuals will take some level of responsibility for their own health care maintenance and improvement, and Australians are becoming better informed about their health status. The general population is less knowledgeable about mental illnesses, and youth suicide is still feared by some. Health-promotion campaigns have resulted in a decline in age-specific suicide rates following peaks in 1997 and 1998. The age-standardized suicide rate for men in 2003 was 17.7 per 100,000 and was lower than in any year in the previous decade. Similarly for women, there were declines in rates in many age groups, and the age-standardized suicide rate for women was 4.7 per 100,000 in 2003. Health promotion is increasingly considered to be a significant component of health care for providers and consumers.

Predominant Sick-Care Practices: Biomedical; alternative. When people are ill, most seek out traditional health care services, such as medical doctors and nurses in community health centers or hospitals. Trends toward using alternative health care are increasing, perhaps due in part to dissatisfaction with conventional medicine, regarding outcomes and encounters. It may also be associated with a desire to view health holistically. Australians are now choosing health care practitioners such as chiropractors, osteopathic doctors, masseurs, naturopathic doctors, and acupuncturists more regularly. Some choose medical doctors who combine alternative and conventional medicine in their health care approaches. For those with mental illness, most use counselors, crisis workers, and psychotherapists rather than the more traditional social workers and medical doctors. Australians increasingly are interested in understanding their physical and emotional health and being part of the decision making regarding their health care.

Ethnic-/Race-Specific or Endemic Diseases: The health status of indigenous people is much poorer than other Australians, attributed to social and economic disadvantages and racial oppression. The exact magnitude of their ill health is not known precisely, and information collected varies from state and territory. However, improvements with data collection have occurred, such that national standards for indigenous identification in hospitals have been adopted and a national advisory group for Aboriginal and Torres Strait Islander Health Information and Data has been

established. The life expectancy for indigenous Australians is also significantly lower than nonindigenous Australians. The major causes of deaths
among indigenous people are diseases of the circulatory system; trauma
such as accidents, self harm, and assault (suicide accounts for 34% of these
deaths), poisoning, cancer, respiratory diseases, and diabetes. Australia has
not reached the epidemic proportions of human immunodeficiency virus
(HIV)/acquired immunodeficiency syndrome (AIDS) that were predicted
almost two decades ago. In 2004 there were 14,840 people living with
HIV in Australia. From the start of the epidemic until the end of 2004, there
have been 24,245 diagnoses of HIV, 9,500 of AIDS, and 6,509 reported
deaths of persons living with AIDS. Compared with other countries in
2004, AIDS incidence in Australia was 1.2 per 100,000, higher than Germany (0.6) but lower than the United Kingdom (1.4), France (2.3), Spain
(4.3), and the United States (14.7). The Joint United Nations Programme
on HIV/AIDS (UNAIDS) estimates the prevalence rate for HIV in adults
(aged 15 to 49) is 0.1%, with 16,000 people living with HIV, including fewer
than 1,000 women. The estimated number of deaths from AIDS is fewer
than 500.

Health-Team Relationships: Health care providers are respected for
their knowledge and decision-making. Although in some settings health
care workers may defer more to doctors, relationships are more equitable
than previously. Because a bachelor's degree in nursing has become the
foundation education to become a registered nurse, nurses have been
recognized more for their contributions to health care. Recognition is
afforded to nurses who continue to advance their university education,
and in clinical health facilities clinical nurse specialists, clinical nurse consultants, and independent nurse practitioners are acknowledged by specific career scales.

Families' Role in Hospital Care: During the last decade, it has become
more acceptable to have significant others involved in health care decisions,
regardless of whether they are family members. It is not unusual for patients
who are terminally or acutely ill to have a family member or significant other
staying with them overnight in the hospital for support. This has been a common practice for children for more than two or three decades. It is acceptable
for family members and significant others to bring food and drinks, and
visiting hours have extended to all day in many institutions.

Dominance Patterns: Although Australia is a patriarchal society, since
the women's liberation movement of the 1960s, women have become
increasingly aware of their rights and are more assertive. A strong
women's health movement developed, and women have responded proac-
tively to improve their health status. In the past decade, the media has
paid significant attention to the nature, effects, and interventions related
to domestic violence and sexual abuse of women and children.

Eye-Contact Practices: Eye contact is considered an indicator of trust
and effective interpersonal communication. Women tend to demonstrate
and sustain eye contact more than men do. However, in many indigenous

cultures, it is considered rude for indigenous and nonindigenous people to make direct eye contact, so averting the gaze is recommended.

Touch Practices: Touching is generally perceived to indicate degrees of comfort between people, and varies according to gender. For women, touching other women during interpersonal interactions is more frequent than with men. Women touch men less often because men are likely to perceive such behaviors as having sexual connotations. Heterosexual men touch other men less frequently than they touch women, because they may be perceived as gay.

Perceptions of Time: It is considered respectful to be punctual for formal professional appointments; however, people are much more relaxed about punctuality in social engagements. In general, people do not expect others to arrive at an exact time—often within 30 minutes of the set time is considered acceptable. Australians generally focus on living in the present, but future planning for holidays and travel is common.

Pain Reactions: Pain reactions vary by gender, and it is more socially acceptable for women to speak about their feelings. Therefore, women disclose more openly the characteristics and levels of their pain than men. Australian culture is presently more accepting of men's discussing their feelings rather than expressions of pain. In an effort not to appear "weak," many men appear more stoic than women.

Birth Rites: Birth is celebrated and valued, and people focus more on the health than the sex of a newborn. The infant mortality rate is 4.63 deaths per 1,000 live births. Discussions concerning preference for the sex of the infant tend to be more implicit than explicit; nevertheless, fathers often have a desire to have a boy. Consequently, women in traditional families may keep having children until a boy is born. The fertility rate has decreased (1.76 children born per woman); however, there has been an increase in multiple births, attributable to assisted reproductive technology. In an emerging trend, more women are having children outside of traditional families. For example, lesbians are having children more than ever before, and their partner is often both a support and co-parent. Many single heterosexual women also are choosing to have children regardless of whether they have a partner. It is also evident that fewer women are choosing abortion for unplanned pregnancies, and fewer single women are choosing adoption. Whereas most births still occur in hospitals, there is a trend toward home births and births in birthing centers. Home birthing is more popular in the Far North Coast region of New South Wales, where there is a concentration of home-birth midwives and a focus on autonomy in health and healing. In home births, the mother is directly involved in major decisions regarding her antenatal and postnatal care, more so than during any other birthing practice. During hospital births, the focus is on doctor-directed care antenatally and postnatally. Although no specific diet is usually followed by pregnant women, it is common practice for women to avoid alcohol and other drugs strictly for the duration of the pregnancy. Life expectancy is 77 for men, 83 for women.

A

Death Rites: Death is usually perceived as an emotionally painful process. Women tend to speak more openly about their feelings regarding a loved one's experience of death and dying. Men tend to remain more reserved. Family and significant others are considered important parts of the dying process if the person who is dying wants them to participate. Children are often encouraged to express their feelings through art. Although more people tend to die in hospitals, more are choosing to die at home. In acute-care facility and hospital deaths, organ donation is more common, but people tend to resist autopsies because they are perceived as unnecessary. Family members and significant others are encouraged to view the body as part of their own healing process. More people are cremated because of the ever-increasing space problem created by burying people. At funerals, more family members and significant others are participating in the ceremony—for example, by speaking about the person who has died or playing their favorite music. After the service, which may or may not be held in a church, it is becoming more common for a wake to be held to celebrate the person's life.

Food Practices and Intolerances: During the last decade, Australians have focused more on healthy eating and are consuming less processed foods, saturated fats, and red meat. Although chicken, seafood, and potatoes are still very popular, most people tend to consume diets with more fiber, fresh fruits, and vegetables than in the past. Children and adolescents tend to adopt a very stable meat-eating diet; boys eat more meat than girls. During the summer months, many Australians eat meals outdoors at home and in cafes and restaurants. Dining is very social and relaxed, and cafes and restaurants usually have outdoor eating areas, which are very popular. Alcohol is readily available and consumed regularly. More cafes and restaurants have adopted either a "bring your own" alcohol policy or are licensed to serve alcohol. Beer and white wines are the most popular drinks.

Infant-Feeding Practices: Between 50% and 60% of mothers breastfeed their infants in the first 6 months, which may be linked to stronger health when they are adults. Health care organizations and associated professionals such as midwives, nurse lactation consultants, and medical doctors are strong advocates for breastfeeding. In some instances, health care professionals are even unsupportive of mothers who choose bottle feeding. Health care practitioners generally educate mothers on the benefits of breastfeeding and ultimately support their informed decisions. Breastfeeding mothers are strongly encouraged to visit family and child health centers and nursing mothers' groups for support. Although breastfeeding practices have decreased in indigenous cultures, where it was common for children to be breastfed for 2 years, it remains more prevalent in rural areas of Australia.

Child-Rearing Practices: Child-rearing practices have been changing because of several interwoven social factors. First, women are giving birth later in life. Second, married women's participation in the labor force has increased, and women are more involved in part-time than full-time work. Third, many Australians have moved away from their parents, so the notion of the extended family being available for support is diminishing. Consequently, child rearing rests with mothers rather than fathers. Because many mothers are now working several days per week, some of the child rearing is the responsibility of child-care workers. Child rearing has become less strict in that parents are more likely to reward positive behavior in children rather than punish them for negative behaviors. The old adage of "children should be seen and not heard" is not followed extensively, and parents concentrate more on improving family communication. Therefore, the ways children are responding, thinking, and feeling are critical to family stability and growth.

National Childhood Immunizations: DTaP at 15 to 17 years; DTaP-HepIPV at 2, 4, and 6 months (part of the country); DTaPHibHepIPV at 2, 4, and 6 months (part of the country); DTaPIPV at 4 years; HepA at 12 to 24 months (×2), and 18 to 30 months (part of the country); HepB at 0 to 7 days and 10 to 13 years; Hib at 2, 4, and 12 months (part of the country); Influenza >65 years; MenC conj at 12 months; MMR at 12 months and 4 years; Pneumo_conj at 2, 4, and 6 months; Varicella at 18 months, 10 to 13 years. The percent of the target population vaccinated, by antigen, is: DTP1 (97%); DTP3, Polio3 (92%); HepB3, Hib3, and MCV (94%).

BIBLIOGRAPHY

Australian Bureau of Statistics: *2003 deaths, Australia,* 2004. Retrieved November 11, 2005, from http://www.abs.gov.au/Ausstats.

Australian Bureau of Statistics: *Year book Australia population deaths,* 2004. Retrieved November 11, 2005, from http://www.abs.gov.au/ausstats.

Australian Government Department of Health and Ageing: *National immunisation program,* 2005.

Australian Institute of Health and Welfare: Australia's Health, 2004: The ninth biennial report of the Australian Institute of Health Welfare. Canberra: Australian Institute of Health and Wealth, 2004.

AVERT: *Australia HIV & AIDS statistics summary,* 2005. Retrieved November 11, 2005, from http://www.avert.org/ausstatg.htm.

Central Intelligence Agency 2006: *The World Factbook,* Australia. Retrieved September 15, 2006, from https://www.cia.gov/cia/publications/factbook/print/as.html

Davis K, Glass N: Safe sex and student nurses in rural Australia: nurses' knowledge and practices (part 1). *Cont Nurs.* 12(1), 2002.

Eastwood, H: Complementary therapies: the appeal to general practitioners, *Med J Austr.* 73:95–98, 2000.

Glass N: Interpersonal relating, Bachelor of health science in nursing, study guide, Lismore, Southern Cross University, Australia, 2004.

Glass N: Speaking feminisms and nursing. In: Greenwood J ed. *Nursing theory in Australia. development and application, Melbourne, Pearson Education,* 2000.

Gracey M: Infant feeding and weaning practices in an urbanizing traditional, Hunter-Gatherer society, *Pediatrics.* 5(2):1276–1277, 2000.

Gray E: Household work for men and women: implications for future childrearing: decisions, *J Aust Stud.* March: 85–97, 2000.

A

Siahpush M: Why do people favour alternative medicine? *Aust NZ J Pub Health.* 23 (3):266–271, 1999.

UNAIDS: 2006 Australia. Retrieved September 15, 2006, from http://www.unaids.org/en/Regions_Countries/Countries/australia.asp.

World Health Organization: 2006: Immunization, vaccines and biologicals, Retrieved September 15, 2006, from http://www.int/immunization_monitoring/en/global-summary/countryprofileresult.cfm?C='aus'.

♦ AUSTRIA (REPUBLIC OF)

MAP PAGE (798)

Hartwig Huemer

Location: Austria is a landlocked nation in central Europe. Its boundaries are Germany and the Czech Republic to the north, Hungary and the Slovak Republic to the east, Slovenia and Italy to the south, and Switzerland and Liechtenstein to the west. The total area is 83,858 km^2 (32,377 square miles) with the western part consisting mainly of snow-capped mountainous territory. The climate is temperate: cool summers and cold winters, with rain in the lowland and snow in the mountains. The population of 8.2 million is concentrated mainly in the eastern lowlands, with the capital city of Vienna accounting for 1.6 million. Austria is an aging society; 17% of the population is 65 years and older, and 68% are between 15 and 64 years of age. It has one of the highest immigration rates in Europe, which compensates for the reduced birth rate. The gross domestic product (GDP) per capita is $31,300. Although 30% of the budget is spent for the social system, 12% of the population lives below or near the official poverty level of $1,050 a month. The literacy rate is 98% for both men and women.

Major Languages	Ethnic Groups	Major Religions
German (official nationwide)	Austrian 88%	Roman Catholic 73%
Slovene (official Carynthia)	German 1%	Protestant 4.7%
Croatian, Hungarian (official in Burgenland)	Slovene	Jewish 0.1%
Czech, Slovak	Croat, Hungarian (Approx. 2 %)	None 15.2%
Bosnian	Czech, Slovak	Catholic
Serbian/Montenegro	Bosniak (1.5%)	Muslim (4.6%)
Turkish, Kurdish	Serb, Montenegrian (2%)	Eastern Orthodox (2.4%)
Other	Turk, Kurd (approx 3%)	
	Roma, Sinti (0.5%), and Others	

According to the last nationwide population count (2001), which does not register inclusion in all ethnic groups (but records religion and preferred language), about 10 % of the population was not born in Austria, and about the same percentage have foreign citizenship. Percentages of "ethnic groups" should be interpreted with care, especially among those declaring themselves as Austrians. Many well-integrated former immigrants with a good command of German as well as Austrian citizenship are included. No good data are available about the numbers of immigrants from the countries of the former eastern bloc. They are underrepresented in official statistics and form a significant part of the illegally employed workforce (1% to 2% of the overall population). The alpine Austrian "German" and Swiss "German" (the latter being used in the province of Vorarlberg) are rather different from "high German." This leads to communication problems between doctors and patients because doctors generally speak "high" German. Austrians understand the "high German" used by Germans even if they do not speak it very well, but Germans in most cases have difficulties with the Austrian or Swiss German. Most of the German-speaking Austrians originate from Slavic populations of the former Austro-Hungarian Empire (mainly Czechs, Slovaks, Hungarians, and northern Italians). The 40,000 Roma and Sinti ("gypsies") experience poorer socioeconomic conditions. Although steadily decreasing in its numbers, the Roman Catholic Church still has a powerful position, especially in educational and hospital systems run by religious orders and fraternities. Intolerance and latent anti-Semitism is associated with fundamental Catholicism but has been overstated. Ruled for 15 years by a Jewish chancellor in the 1970 to 1980s, Austria has implemented strong antiracist laws, and international surveys confirm very low rates of conflict with Jews.

Health Care Beliefs: Active involvement; health promotion important. Since the mid 1980s, health authorities have introduced a program for preventive examinations under the auspices of health insurance plans. The importance of sports and fitness for disease prevention is less emphasized.

Predominant Sick-Care Practices: Biomedical; evidence based. Austria has implemented a welfare system of guaranteed health care and social security for its citizens: 99% are covered by state required health insurance. With the exception of a flat rate charged for prescriptions, basic inpatient and outpatient treatments are free to most and covered by insurance plans. Special groups such as public servants have more extended health services. Wealthier Austrians often have additional private health insurance covering extended services, such as having the choice to be treated as "private" patients by renowned specialists, having better accommodations, or receiving expensive cures. Self-employed and retired Austrians qualify for less comprehensive plans. Austria's medical system is not "socialized" in the sense that the vast majority of physicians are not employees of the state. However, fees for basic services are regulated by negotiation between medical associations and health care providers, allowing an exceptionally high degree of coverage. With the exception of common cold medications or herbal remedies, medicines generally are not sold over the counter.

A

Ethnic-/Race-Specific or Endemic Diseases: Austria has the typical profile of an industrialized aging society, with cardiovascular diseases, cancer, respiratory problems, and liver conditions the major causes of morbidity. There are 1.3 million male and 1 million female smokers. From 1972 to 1997, rates for men decreased from 45% to 36%, whereas rates for women increased from 13% to 23%. Younger women are smoking more: about 26% of 15-year-old girls smoke cigarettes. Most adults consume alcohol (mostly wine and beer) regularly, and the incidences of cirrhosis of the liver and cardiovascular disease are some of the highest in Europe. About 8% of men and 2% of women are chronic alcoholics; these rates are also associated with a suicide rate that is 10 times higher than the general population. After Hungary and Finland, Austria has one of the highest suicide rates in the world. Death rates caused by traffic accidents are among the highest in Europe. The Alpine region is an area of iodine deficiency, but endemic goiter has been widely prevented by iodized salt. Lyme borreliosis and tick-borne encephalitis (TBE) are prevalent, the latter primarily in the eastern lowlands and river valleys. Hepatitis viruses A, B, and C are largely imported by immigrants from high-risk areas. The incidence of tuberculosis (TB) is around 12 per 100,000, with older individuals being most affected. In immigrants, TB is found in younger groups with multidrug-resistant strains from the former Soviet Union increasingly noted. Numerous sports-related injuries occur in the alpine area involving skiing and mountaineering activities, leading to excellent emergency surgery as well as advanced ambulance and air transport systems. The rate of methicillin-resistant *Staphylococcus aureus* (MRSA) in hospitals is relatively low at 10%. The rate for antibiotics use is one of the lowest in Europe, with a lower incidence of antibiotic resistance than that in neighboring countries. HIV-infected people account for less than 0.2% of the population; two thirds are males. The Joint United Nations Programme on human immunodeficiency virus (HIV)/acquired immunodeficiency syndrome (AIDS). (UNAIDS) estimates that 12,000 people are living with HIV, including 2,300 women. Since the beginning of the HIV/AIDS pandemic in 1983, only 2,427 AIDS cases have been recorded, leading to 1,400 deaths. Virtually no mother-child transmissions of HIV have been reported in recent years.

Health-Team Relationships: Most physicians are in private practice but rely on contracts with insurance agencies, which regulate fees for services. Nursing education is moving gradually from hospital-based training to university-based education. In most wards the "chief nurse" has a powerful position. Community-run hospitals tend to be more liberal than those run by religious orders or fraternities. Lengthy discussions between levels of hierarchy tend to be avoided, sometimes restricting the flow of information. Initiative is not always rewarded, and nurses are often expected to follow orders for everything except basic nursing care. There is a tendency to decrease in-hospital and increase community nursing care, primarily to reduce costs. Because of the aging population, there is a lack of nursing personnel, and additional staff is imported from Eastern Europe and overseas. Cleaning personnel often originate from southeast Europe, and communication problems often make it difficult to explain sophisticated hospital requirements and to correct different levels of perceptions of cleanliness. Confidentiality is mandatory in health care environments, and patients tend not to challenge decisions of medical authorities. Lawsuits against medical doctors are somewhat rare.

Dominance Patterns: Under the influence of Catholicism, Austria developed a very conservative patriarchal family structure with a gender-specific division of labor. Austria converted to a more egalitarian society in the 1970s. Marriage as a partnership is now more common, and the law has established equal rights and duties for married men and women that extend to child care. Discrimination against women is illegal, and the concept of equal rights extends to unpaid work by women in households as well as to single parents. Women still bear the major responsibility of child rearing and housework, however, and the income differential between sexes is significant. The employment rate of women is 63% (50% full time). Well-educated women are more likely to be employed.

Eye-Contact Practices: As in many Western countries, sustained eye contact may be regarded as being attentive, aggressive, or indication of sexual interest, depending on the situation. This does not apply to members of the immigrant population, who act according to the patterns of their countries of origin. For example, direct eye contact with a Bosnian or Turkish cleaning woman would likely make her feel uncomfortable.

Touch Practices: Touch is less common than in Mediterranean or Francophone cultures, especially between men, and the older generation. A friendly handshake is most common and is frequently used in social and business interactions. Verbal expressions have replaced the "kissing of the hand" formerly used in aristocratic circles and regarded as suitable at the Viennese Opera Ball perhaps, but not generally in other situations. In reality, the lips do not actually touch the hand of the lady. There is a clerical version of this old habit with kissing the ring of the bishop, still used by devout Roman Catholics.

Perceptions of Time: The past is valued. Traditional approaches to healing are still considered important, although Austrians emphasize biomedical approaches. Older people dominate political and economic decisions, and unemployment rates among the young are unacceptably high. It is feared that the next generation will have to bear the problems of the state-run pension systems as well as the abuse of interim pensions as a political measure to support tight labor markets. As a result of the pension system, Austria has one of the lowest rates of European countries of individuals aged 60 years and older being employed. Punctuality in business and social situations is valued.

Pain Reactions: Because the dominant Catholic belief includes acceptance of a certain degree of suffering, high vaccination coverage rates are not obtained, and the use of medications for pain is often suboptimal. Austrians have an attitude that could best be described as "forced endurance"; this is particularly true for men in that they tend not to express pain freely.

A

Birth Rites: Owing to its low birth rate, Austria can afford to have one of the most extensive maternity support systems. It is illegal for pregnant women to work 8 weeks before or after giving birth, and women receive full net pay. Natural childbirth and the father's presence in the delivery room are becoming more popular. As a consequence of an advanced pregnancy surveillance system and financial support, most births take place in hospitals, primarily attended by midwives and nurses. Parents of newborns can take 2 years of maternity or paternity leave, or it can be split between the parents. State support is received for 2 years, and mothers and fathers must be rehired at equal pay and status. More than a third of first- born children are born to single mothers, which may reflect more tolerant attitudes, or it may be a consequence of the welfare system providing higher benefits to single mothers compared with married mothers. The infant mortality rate is 4.6 deaths per 1,000 live births, and the fertility rate is 1.36 children born per woman. Life expectancy is 76 for men, 82 for women.

Death Rites: In Austrian Catholic society, death opens the door to heaven and relieves one from pain on earth. Most Austrians die in hospitals. Specialized long-term care facilities are available but tend to be prohibitively expensive. The dead are usually kept for several days, allowing the public to bid farewell, except for Muslims, who prefer immediate burial. Earth burials are most common, but cremation is becoming more popular. Sorrow is generally not expressed in public.

Food Practices and Intolerances: Breakfast usually consists of coffee or tea and bakery products. The main meal is at midday; a light meal is eaten in the early evening. The traditional Austrian diet is high in fat, carbohydrates, and sugar, which contributes to the high incidence of cardiovascular disease, diabetes, and colon cancer. Viennese cooking stands for "Austrian" cooking, which includes recipes from all over the former empire. The western parts of the country have resorted to serving mostly international food as a result of tourism. Austrians are the inventors of the "coffee house" and distributed the tradition of coffee throughout Europe after adopting it from their defeated Turkish enemies in the seventeenth century. In business, many coffee breaks are common. Eastern Austria is a traditional wine area, where mostly white wine has been cultivated since Roman times in the Danube valley, in contrast to the beer-drinking habits of the "barbarians" north of the Roman borders. Alpine populations are specialized in the creation of many kinds of distilled beverages. Through tourism, they have successfully exported their tradition of hot and spicy mulled wine. Austrians are tolerant toward legal drugs such as alcohol and tobacco but strongly object to other drug use.

Infant-Feeding Practices: Mostly industrial foodstuffs are used, but breastfeeding is encouraged. Meals for schoolchildren are usually supported by communities, and additional milk or cocoa is served in many primary schools as a calcium supplement. Fluoridation, and iodination of salt have successfully reduced the incidence of dental caries and thyroid disease.

Child-Rearing Practices: Parents of children under the age of 4 years receive stipends from the government. Maintenance allowances are provided until 8 years of age and extended if the child is living at home, in school, or unemployed. Payments are continued until the age of 27 if the person is enrolled in vocational training or the university. Despite this support, having children is expensive and a major cause of poverty. The educational system is free of fees for public schools, but many additional expenses are not covered. The lives of children are supposed to be disciplined. Physical punishment is not allowed in schools but is still used in personal practice. A "healthy" slap on the face is widely accepted as a disciplinary measure. Most cases of child abuse go unprosecuted as a result of ignorance, shame, or family pressure. Women often cannot afford to be fully employed because of the lack of available child care. In rural areas with more traditional family structures, it is common for grandparents to take part in childcare.

National Childhood Immunizations: DPT, HiB, HepB, IPV, and PNC at 3, 5, and 7 months and 2 years; two doses of MMR are scheduled within the second year. An MMR booster is given before reaching fertility age for girls only. HepB is boosted at 7 to 13 years, IPV at 7 to 9 years, and DT at 7 and 13 to 16 years. Varicella vaccine has been recommended for children older than 9 months; but is not free of charge. Middle European tick-borne encephalitis vaccine is suggested for outdoor activities in high-risk areas. The percentage of the target population vaccinated, by antigen, is: BCG (91%); DTP3, HepB, Polio3 (86%), and MCV (75%).

Other Characteristics: In opposition to the rest of Europe, Austrians ignore Santa Claus, strictly believing in the "Christkind," a small child who flies by dressed only in a white skirt in December. Reduced from a European center of power to a small republic, Austrians watch the decline with a mixture of subtle irony, humor, an unbroken sense of the good life, and the secret feeling of being still superior. Shocked by annexation by Nazi Germany in 1938, and subsequent occupation of the most populated parts by Russia from 1945 to 1955, Austrians are rather skeptical, suspicious, and xenophobic. Prejudices remain toward enemies of the former empire: Turks, Serbs, Russians, and Germans. Thus, hard-core Austrians still can become upset about the outrageous theft of the melody of their former emperor's hymn, which with a new text is now the German national anthem, and the annexation of their imperial colors. Many object to the ongoing German "colonization" of the country since Austria joined the European Union in 1999.

BIBLIOGRAPHY

AIDS/HIV statistics. Retrieved February 12, 2006, from http://www.aids.at/index. php?id=15.

Anti-Semitism worldwide. Retrieved February 15, 2006, from http://www.tau.ac.il/ Anti-Semitism/asw2004/graph-7.jpg.

Bakker A: Cardiovascular nursing in Austria, *Prog Cardiovasc Nurs*, 19(2):70–72, 2004.

A

Bienstein C: Nursing and public health within the scope of European Union integration, *Osterr Krankenpflegez.* 53(8–9):32–4, 2000.

Central Intelligence Agency: *2006: The world factbook,* Austria. Retrieved September 15, 2006, from https://www.cia.gov/cia/publications/factbook/print/au.html.

Gross D: Evidence-based nursing—a comprehensive term, *Pflege,* 17(3):196–207, 2004.

Jenull-Schiefer B, Janig H: Activities offered in nursing homes—a study of usage and satisfaction, *Z Gerontol Geriatr.* 37(5):393–401, 2004.

Ministry of Health, Infectious Diseases: Retrieved February 8, 2006, from http://www.bmgf.gv.at/cms/site/inhalte.htm?channel=CH0003&thema=CH0019.

Ministry of Health, National Vaccine Scheme. Retrieved February 10, 2006, from http://www.bmgf.gv.at/cms/site/attachments/1/4/0/CH0016/CMS1038913010412/impfplan_2006.pdf.

Nitschke I, Muller F, Ilgner A, Reiber T: Undergraduate teaching in gerodontology in Austria, Switzerland and Germany. *Gerodontology.* 21(3):123–9, 2004.

Schmidt I: Health promotion in family nursing, *Pflege Aktuell.* 59:82–5, 2005.

Soritsch A: Living with disabilities in Austria—with a special focus on the capital. *Coll Antropol.* 28(suppl 2):31–42, 2004.

Statistics Austria, "Volkszählung," 2001. Retrieved July 15, 2006, from http://www.statistik.at/gz/vz.html.

UNAIDS: 2006: Austria. Retrieved September 1, 2006, from http://www.unaids.org/en/Regions_Countries/Countries/austria.asp.

Walter I: Effects of "unification" on Austrian nursing, *Pflege.* 16(1):6–16, 2003.

◆ AZERBAIJAN (REPUBLIC OF)

MAP PAGE (799)

Lisa Natoli

Location: Azerbaijan (formerly the Azerbaijan Soviet Socialist Republic) is in Transcaucasia. It is bordered to the west by Armenia, to the south by Iran, to the north by Georgia and Daghestan, and to the east by the Caspian sea. The Republic spans 86,600 km^2 (33,436 square miles), a total area that includes the autonomous republic of Nakhchivan and the predominantly Armenian populated area of Nagorno-Karabakh. The total population is 8.3 million. The gross domestic product (GDP) per capita is $4,800, with about 49% below the poverty line.

Major Languages	Ethnic Groups	Major Religions
Azeri (official)	Azeri 90.6%	Muslim 93.4% (Both
Russian	Dagestani 2.2%	Shi'a and Sunni)
Armenian	Russian 1.8%	Russian Orthodox
Other	Other 3.9%	2.5%
		Armenian Orthodox
		2.3%
		Other 1.8%

Despite Azerbaijan's small size, cultural practices vary according to geographic location and religious trends. The Azeri language belongs to the Turkic group of languages. In 1992 its written form reverted again to Latin script for the second time in history. Some older people may prefer and better understand the Cyrillic script, an important consideration when developing health-education materials (although all official documents are required by law to be written in Latin). Russian is still widely spoken, although it is more common in and around the capital Baku compared with the regions. Literacy rates are 99% for men, 98% for women.

Health Care Beliefs: Acute sick care; traditional. Azerbaijan is far from a health-promoting society. A man living in Baku (known for its mix of nationalities, religions, and idiosyncrasies between ethnic groups) once shared the following scenario with this author to illustrate the perception of how these different groups might handle a potential health problem.

Abraham (a Jewish person) visits a hospital: "Please doctor, help! I'm afraid my heart's going to give me a pain in a few days."

Ivan (a Russian or Christian person) visits a hospital: "Please doctor, help! I have an awful heartache."

Mamed (an Azeri or a Muslim) is brought to a hospital on a stretcher, and his relatives say to the hospital personnel, "We're afraid he has already died!"

The health-promotion activities that do exist are driven largely by international agencies; local nongovernmental organizations (NGOs) are also becoming more involved in health promotion, although they depend heavily on foreign financial support to do so. At a health-systems level, the concept that health promotion should be a task of district health authorities is yet to be accepted, and heavy reliance on treatment, rather than prevention, prevails. Mental illness, although poorly understood, is not feared. It is believed that the "source of mental illness is God's will." Management continues to be based on the Soviet model, isolating the mentally ill in specialist hospitals.

Predominant Sick-Care Practices: Biomedical; traditional; magical-religious. Azeris are very focused on seeking intervention (whether medical or traditional) for even the slightest complaint. Treatment is often quite invasive (i.e., multiple, self-administered, injectable drugs), lacking in a research base, tinged with mythology, and sometimes outright dangerous. Traditional practices such as "cupping" (placing vacuumed cups on the skin) may be used in the home to treat less serious illnesses such as common colds and the flu. Health care–seeking behavior varies enormously between urban and rural areas. In Baku, people generally visit a doctor and then seek out traditional healers if they do not improve. In the rural regions, this situation is likely to be the reverse: some would argue that this relates to the lack of services in rural areas, the more widespread context of poverty, and the high costs of health care. As a whole, Azeris are secular people, but they will often ask God for help when they are sick or in difficult circumstances. However, if quality health services are made available free of charge, these will generally be accessed in preference to seeking advice

A

from family and friends or calling on God for help. Amulets may be worn by some who believe it will help keep illness away, and they may also be seen pinned to the caps of newborn infants.

Ethnic-/Race-Specific or Endemic Diseases: Many vulnerable groups have special needs, such as more than half a million internally displaced people. Poor and vulnerable groups are disproportionately impacted, and in addition to suffering complaints typical in the general population, they are at higher risk of illness because of poor hygiene and living conditions. Chronic, noncommunicable diseases such as heart disease and cancer are the most common causes of mortality, and tobacco and alcohol are know to contribute significantly to this burden of disease. Domestic violence has become more of an issue in recent years and may be linked to the consequences of unemployment and posttraumatic stress. Like other countries in the region, there was a resurgence of diphtheria and tuberculosis (TB) in the 1990s. TB continues to be a problem, especially for those subject to poor or cramped living conditions and malnutrition, such as prisoners and internally displaced people who are living in camps. Malaria was also a problem in the mid- to late 1990s, with some serious outbreaks, and transmission continues in some regions. Sexually transmitted diseases are common and underreported, as are reproductive health–related problems in women. Abortion is viewed as an acceptable form of contraception and is often performed using dangerous and unhygienic methods. As is true for other countries of the former Soviet Union, there is potential for human immunodeficiency virus (HIV) infection to become an explosive epidemic. Risk factors include a lack of awareness (particularly among adolescents), commercial sex work, population movements driven by the economic situation, increasing injecting drug use, and the inadequate supply of disposable injecting equipment. Whereas the Joint United Nations Programme on HIV/AIDS (UNAIDS) estimated the prevalence rate for HIV in adults (aged 15 to 49) is less than 0.1%, the range of risk factors coupled with poor surveillance means that this is likely to be a conservative estimate. Officially, 5,400 people are living with HIV, including fewer than 1,000 women. Fewer than 100 deaths are estimated. Men account for 80% of the cases.

Health-Team Relationships: The health team is hierarchical and doctor driven, and nurses are the subordinate group. This situation is reflected in the attitudes of patients toward the different groups of health professionals.

Families' Role in Hospital Care: Families have an important role in the support and care of hospitalized relatives. Close relatives may visit two to three times a day. It is not uncommon for the extended family and community to contribute financially to the costs of hospitalization.

Dominance Patterns: Azerbaijan is a male-dominated culture. This dominance is exemplified by practices such as the woman sitting in the back of the car or, in the case of younger women, being chaperoned by a male sibling during socializing. Men are the decision makers of the household, and generally this structure is accepted and unchallenged. These dominance patterns are less obvious in and around the capital of Baku, where women are more liberated.

Eye-Contact Practices: Eye-contact practices do not seem to have cultural significance and are individual.

Touch Practices: Azeris are warm people. In public, it is more acceptable for touching between the same sex than between males and females, although holding hands between men and women is common in Baku. It is not uncommon to see female friends walking together arm in arm or males greeting each other with a kiss (on the cheek) and an embrace. This is not to say that homosexuality is culturally accepted. In fact, it is poorly understood and remains hidden and shameful, bringing great dishonor to the family.

Perceptions of Time: Although it varies among individuals, punctuality is generally not considered important, but people are more likely to be on time for business appointments. For a wedding party, only a few guests will arrive at the precise time detailed on the invitation. Traditions are respected and maintained, more so in the rural regions. Older people complain that the younger generation is losing their traditions. However, many traditional practices, such as arranged marriages (often to cousins), still occur, even though the young people involved may not approve. They often have little choice because of family and cultural pressures.

Pain Reactions: Pain tolerance is an individual issue, although women joke that men are the weaker sex and less tolerant of pain.

Birth Rites: A male child is more celebrated than a daughter as he is seen as a source of security for aging parents and will likely continue the family name through marriage and the birth of his own sons. The fertility rate is 2.46 children born per woman. It is typical in some regions that after a home birth the mother will not take a bath for several days, believing that they are more vulnerable to certain infections at this time (although showering is acceptable). For 40 days after the delivery, mothers are protected from heavy work. They are cautious about cold water and cold in general and avoid certain foods believed to affect breastfeeding. In extremely religious, superstitious, or traditional families, women remain indoors with the baby for the first 40 days. It is believed that the infant's "aura" is weak and vulnerable to being affected by visitors and that outsiders may bring infection into the house. Only immediate family and close relatives are encouraged to visit. The infant mortality rate is 79 deaths per 1,000 live births. Life expectancy is 60 for men, 68 for women.

Death Rites: On the one hand, death is a very painful experience for those who are grieving, but it is also accepted as a part of everyday life. Family members are present, but children are usually prevented from witnessing the dying process. Tents are erected in the yard or street outside the family home of the deceased for 7 days. During this time, men come and pay their respects, and women grieve in a separate room or tent. Muslim corpses are buried with their heads facing Mecca, and, if possible, on the same day of the death before sunset. It is most common for men to visit the burial site and for women to stay and mourn outside the home of the deceased. This is meant to protect women from the pain of grief. On the third, seventh, and fortieth day after death (and on Thursdays during this period) and at each anniversary, relatives share food and tea

A

with halva (a practice called *ehsan*) with visitors who come to pay their respects. Men in mourning do not shave for 40 days after the death of a loved one. Organ donation and autopsies are strictly forbidden, although autopsies may occasionally be performed in criminal cases.

Food Practices and Intolerances: People generally eat with a spoon or fork but rarely with a knife, and it is acceptable to eat with the hands in some rural areas. Typical Azeri fare usually consists of a lot of meat—mainly lamb, beef, or mutton but not pork (although it is available in Western dining establishments). Bread is very important, and tandir bread and wafer-thin lavash are served with almost every dish. In Zoroastrian tradition, the respect for bread is real and heartfelt. Tradition says that to share bread with others opens your soul to one another, creating a bond not easily broken. A typical meal might begin with yogurt *(qatic);* a plate of seasonal garnishes such as tomatoes, cucumbers, radishes, or spring onions; cheese *(pendir);* and perhaps some sausage. The starter is often followed by soup—some variation of meat, vegetables, and potatoes (or *doghrama* in summer, which is made with yogurt, spring onions, and cucumbers and served cold). *Dolma,* leaves stuffed with lamb and herbs, are common, and *plov* (a meat/fish/chicken and rice pilaf) may also be served. *Shaslyk,* or kebabs (lamb, chicken, or *lule*—a minced kebab), follow and may include sturgeon (typically served with a delicious tart pomegranate sauce). Fruit juice, sweet carbonated drinks, beer, and vodka (essential for the endless toasts) are the typical drinks. Tea (chai) usually brings an end to the meal but is also the predominant social drink and is consumed in vast quantities throughout the day. Tea is the Azeri symbol of hospitality; it is drunk from pinch-waist glasses and sweetened with jam or sugar. It is customary to drink tea with a sugar cube in the mouth to regulate sweetness (if it is very strong tea, the sugar is kept in the mouth longer). On the street, newspaper cones of black seeds *(tum),* boiled chickpeas, sunflower seeds, or nuts are often sold. Also popular are *pirozshki*—Russian-style cold donuts filled with spiced potato—and *Azeri kutab*—thin pancakes with spinach or meat—as are the Georgian *khajapyuri,* which are cheese pastries. Seasonal fresh fruit and dried fruits and nuts are common and cheap. Street vendors also sell cakes and pastries, fruit buns, spiced cookies, nut rolls, baklava, and halva.

Infant-Feeding Practices: Numerous misconceptions about appropriate infant-feeding practices remain from the Soviet period, but they are probably more common among the less educated rural women. This is slowly improving, supported by adoption of the Baby Friendly Hospital Initiative by most maternity hospitals in recent years. Although rates of breastfeeding initiation are high, rates of exclusive breastfeeding are very low, and early introduction of non–breast milk fluids (e.g., tea, sweetened water) and complementary foods is common. These practices are driven by important beliefs, for example, that the infant needs additional fluids until the milk supply is established or that sweetened tea will protect the baby from hepatitis. It is important that these beliefs are explored and understood to modify current practices successfully.

Child-Rearing Practices: The level of discipline used with children is an individual family matter, although it is considered to be strict. Children may sleep with their parents, but this practice is often determined by living conditions. Mothers and grandmothers are responsible for disciplining children, although grandmothers are renowned, as they are in many cultures, for spoiling their grandchildren.

National Childhood Immunizations: BCG 4 to 7 days after delivery; DTwP at 2, 3, 4, and 18 months; OPV 4 to 7 days after delivery and at 2, 3, and 4 months; MMR at 12 months and 6 years; HepB at 12 hours after delivery and at 2 and 4 months; and DT at 6 years; vitamin A at 18 months and 6 years. The percent of the target population vaccinated, by antigen, is: BCG and MCV (98%); DTP1 (95%); DTP3 (93%); HepB3 (96%); and Polio3 (97%).

Acknowledgments: Shovcat Alizadeh, Azer Hasanov, Eyyub Hajiyev, Sevinj Musayeva, and Sanubar Nazarova

BIBLIOGRAPHY

Central Intelligence Agency: 2006: The world factbook, Azerbaijan. Retrieved September 15, 2006, from https://www.cia.gov/cia/publications/factbook/print/aj.html.

Claeys P, Ismailov R, Rathe S, Jabbarova A, Claeys G, Fonck K, Temmerman M: Sexually transmitted infections and reproductive health in Azerbaijan, *Sex Transm Dis.* 28(7):372, 2001.

Elliot G: *Azerbaijan with Georgia.* West Sussex, UK, 1999, Trailblazer Publications, Surrey UK, and ARC Publications.

Government of Azerbaijan. *Financial sustainability plan for National Immunoprophylaxis Programme of Azerbaijan Republic,* 2004. Retrieved November 21, 2005, from http://www.vaccinealliance.org/resources/fsp_jan04_azerbaijan.pdf.

Holley J, Akhundov O, Nolte E: *Health care systems in transition, Azerbaijan.* WHO Regional Office for Europe on behalf of European Observatory on Health Systems and Policies, 2004. Retrieved November 21, 2005, from http://www.euro.who.int/Document/E84991.pdf.

http://www.who.int/ncd_surveillance/infobase/web/InfoBasePolicyMaker/reports/reportViewer.aspx?UN_Code=31&rptCode=MOR&dm=10. Retrieved November 21, 2005.

Michaelsen K, Weaver L, Branca F, Robertson A: *Feeding and nutrition of infants and young children, guidelines for the WHO European region with emphasis on the former Soviet countries,* WHO Regional Publications, European Series, no. 87, 2000.

UNAIDS: 2006 Azerbaijan. Retrieved September 15, 2006, from http://www.unaids.org/en/Regions_Countries/Countries/azerbaijan.asp.

UNHCR: 2003. WHO. *Azerbaijan: report: country-level mortality report.* 2002. Retrieved November 21, 2005, from http://www.unhcr.ch/cgi-bin/texis/vtx/country?iso=aze.

Vitek CR, Velibekov AS: Epidemic diphtheria in the 1990s. *J Infect Dis.* 181(suppl 1):73, 2000.

WHO/UNICEF: *Review of national immunization coverage, 1980–2003, Azerbaijan.,* 2004. Retrieved November 21, 2005, from http://www.who.int/vaccines-surveillance/WHOUNICEF_Coverage_Review/pdf/azerbaijan.pdf.

World Bank: 1998–2004. http://devdata.worldbank.org/AAG/aze_aag.pdf. Retrieved November 21, 2005.

World Health Organization: 2006: Immunization, vaccines and biologicals. Retrieved September 1, 2006 from http://www.int/immunization_monitoring/en/globalsummary/countryprofileresult.cfm?C='aze'

◆ BAHAMAS (COMMONWEALTH OF)

B

MAP PAGE (796)
Virginia C.F. Ballance

Location: The Bahamas, an independent Commonwealth country, is composed of more than 700 islands, of which only 22 are inhabited. The Bahamas is located between Florida's east coast, Cuba, and Haiti. The country is spread over an area of more than 100,000 km; however, its total land mass is only 13,940 km^2 (5,382 square miles). The population is 314,000, with more than 200,000 on the urbanized New Providence Island, where the nation's capital and largest city, Nassau, is located. Much of the rest of the population lives on Grand Bahama Island in the country's second-largest city, Freeport. The balance of the population lives on the sparsely populated outlying islands of the archipelago called the Family or Out Islands. The gross domestic product (GDP) per capita is $20,200, with 9% below the poverty line.

Major Languages	Ethnic Groups	Major Religions
English (official)	Black (African	Baptist 35%
Haitian Creole	ancestry) 85%	Anglican 20%
	White 12%	Roman Catholic 20%
	Other (Asian,	Other (Protestant, Greek
	Hispanic) 3%	Orthodox, Jewish,
		Rastafarian, Muslim) 25%

About 85% of the inhabitants are of West African ancestry, descendants of slaves or freemen brought to the Caribbean directly from Africa or from the United States at the time of the American Revolution. Since the 1950s, political problems in Haiti have led a large number of Haitians to migrate to the Bahamas. The population of Haitian nationals and Bahamians of Haitian origin is estimated to be about 50,000. The balance of the population is of European and other ancestry. Smaller numbers of immigrants from other Caribbean islands, such as Barbados, Jamaica, Cuba, and Trinidad and Tobago have also settled in the Bahamas. Literacy rates are 95% for men and 97% for women.

Health Care Beliefs: Active involvement; health promotion. Diet and lifestyle-related, noncommunicable diseases (e.g., obesity, cardiovascular diseases, type 2 diabetes, hypertension, and stroke) are the leading causes of mortality and morbidity. As a result of the country's shift from communicable to preventable noncommunicable diseases, the government has implemented health-promotion and health-education campaigns that have become a vital component of the health care system. The government has launched major initiatives to educate the public about human immunodeficiency virus (HIV)/acquired immunodeficiency syndrome (AIDS) and other sexually transmitted infections, breast-feeding, family planning, drug abuse, and family violence. Also promoted are initiatives to attain a healthy lifestyle through diet and exercise and to encourage screening for cancer (mammograms, Papanicolaou (Pap) smears, prostate, and colon-cancer examinations). Alcoholism and substance abuse (especially cocaine addiction) are the major behavioral disorders, followed by depression and psychosocial disorders. Mental illness is discussed openly, although some stigma is still attached to having been treated for a psychiatric illness. Some groups are fatalistic: ill health is something that is unavoidable. Others may believe that they have been "fixed" with a spell by someone who practices *obeah,* a form of witchcraft.

Predominant Sick-Care Practices: Biomedical; traditional; magical-religious. Bahamians enjoy universal access to health care through government hospitals and clinics or from private hospitals, clinics, and doctors. Approximately 450 doctors practice in the public and private sectors, and almost all specialties are represented. Nassau and Freeport, the two major cities, have much more adequate health services than the smaller towns and cities in the Family Islands. When ill, some are inclined to self-medicate using "bush medicine"—homemade remedies of locally grown herbs and bark from trees. These remedies may be bush tea infusions, poultices, and salves or bathing in water with herbs. Self-medication may also include purchasing over-the-counter drugs. In the Family Islands, where there are no pharmacies, patients are seen at a government clinic by a nurse.

Ethnic-/Race-Specific or Endemic Diseases: Sickle cell anemia is common in people of African origin. Although malaria and dengue hemorrhagic fever are not endemic, given the large number of immigrants and frequent travel to areas where they occur (primarily Haiti and Cuba), Bahamians are at risk for these diseases. The main health problems among adults are human immunodeficiency virus/acquired immunodeficiency syndrome (HIV/AIDS), accidental injuries, substance abuse, hypertension, diabetes, heart attacks, and cancer. High rates of hypertension and diabetes in the general population result from poor eating habits, a lack of exercise, and excessive alcohol consumption. The incidence of tobacco use is the lowest in the world. Obesity is a serious health issue, and 49% of the population is classified as obese. Women (53%) are more likely to be obese than are men (43%). Food-borne illness is prevalent, usually the result of eating contaminated food sold in open-air restaurants. The World Health Organization and Joint United Nations Programme on HIV/AIDS (UNAIDS) estimate the prevalence rate for HIV in adults aged 15 to 49 years to be 3.3%, a decrease from 4.13% in 1999. The estimated number of children aged 0 to 15 years living with HIV/AIDS is fewer than 200. HIV/AIDS is the leading cause of death among Bahamian men and women aged 20 to 59. About 6,853 people are living with HIV, including 3,800 women, and there have been fewer than 500 deaths. HIV is found primarily in heterosexuals, with a male-to-female ratio of 1.2:1. Reporting procedures are stringent, and all new cases are followed up by a team of health professionals. Women reporting to government clinics for antenatal care are screened for HIV. The reduction of mother-to-child transmission is a public health success.

Health-Team Relationships: In both government-run and private hospitals, the physician dominates the health team. In the government community health clinics and some of the private walk-in clinics, nurse practitioners provide many of the services. Overall, nurse-physician relationships are good. Nurses manage the wards in hospitals. Patients' attitudes toward physicians and nurses vary. In a small country such as the Bahamas, people tend to be very familiar with one another because of family and community ties.

Families' Role in Hospital Care: Families do not stay with patients in the hospital. It is quite common, however, for families to bring food from home or outside restaurants, fruit baskets, flowers, and bottled water and other drinks. In the public hospital, male nurses and male family members are not permitted in the labor and delivery rooms. Visiting hours are observed, although families are permitted to visit for longer hours in the intensive care units and pediatric wards.

Dominance Patterns: Although Bahamian society is essentially matriarchal and most homes are headed by single mothers, men still dominate the professional and political arenas.

Eye-Contact Practices: Direct eye contact is not an issue. Bahamians are generally friendly and outgoing people and are always willing to chat with friends and family.

Touch Practices: Bahamians have no particular taboos about touching: they shake hands, embrace, or kiss when greeting friends and family.

Perceptions of Time: In the course of normal daily life, arriving on "Bahamian time," or later than scheduled, is quite acceptable. Bahamians reminisce about days gone by and former traditions and culture. Twenty-first century Bahamas is heavily influenced by the United States through television, cable, the Internet, newspapers, and family ties. Many have family members residing in the United States, attending college or university there, or visiting regularly.

Pain Reactions: Reaction to pain is individual. Whereas some may express pain openly, others are more stoic. Most Bahamians would not be reticent about expressing their level of pain to a health professional.

Birth Rites: Bahamians have many superstitions about pregnancy and birth, ranging from predictions of the sex of the infant to invocations to protect the unborn child from harm. The infant mortality rate is 25 deaths per 1,000 live births. All children are born in hospitals or clinics and unless complications occur, mothers are discharged within a day or two. Mothers are attended by midwives in the hospital and at community clinics in the islands. All new mothers are visited at home by a community health nurse and attend postnatal clinics. There is no particular preference for the gender of the child, although children generally carry the surname of the father. The fertility rate is 2.18 children born per woman, and life expectancy is 62 for men and 69 for women.

Death Rites: Death is accepted as a natural event, whether expected or unexpected. Traditionally, a funeral is scheduled at least a week after a death to allow time for family members living overseas or on remote islands to attend. Before the funeral, a wake is held at the family's residence, where food, drink, and entertainment are offered. A funeral service, often called a "home-going" service, is held in a church to offer prayers for the soul of the deceased and to celebrate that person's life. Following the service, the body is buried. Organ donation is not widely practiced, and no stigma is attached to performing autopsies.

Food Practices and Intolerances: The Bahamian diet is high in sodium, simple sugars, and fat. As a result, more than half the population is overweight, and the "full figure," which Bahamians call a "Gussiemae figure," is the norm. The diet is dominated by rice cooked with peas, grits (ground corn), bread, fried chicken, conch (a mollusc), pork, and beef. Consumption of seafood and fish is low (eaten at Christmas or on special occasions), as is consumption of fruits and vegetables. A typical meal might consist of fried or baked chicken (or conch or pork spareribs), peas and rice, macaroni and cheese, coleslaw, baked potato, or boiled corn. Breakfast typically consists of sardines, corned beef fried with tomato, or tuna fish and grits. Another favorite meal is pea soup with ham and flour dumplings. Fast-food restaurants and local establishments are heavily patronized.

Infant-Feeding Practices: Breastfeeding is not the norm. Although approximately 60% of mothers attempt breastfeeding, more than 90% introduce bottle feeding by the end of the first week of the infant's life and often before leaving the hospital or clinic.

Child-Rearing Practices: Generally, Bahamian children are raised under the edict of "spare the rod, spoil the child." In single-parent families, the mother, grandmother, or legal guardian is responsible for discipline. Children tend to be quiet and polite around adults, particularly those in authority, such as schoolteachers, clergy, or police officers.

National Childhood Immunizations: DT at 4–5, and 10–12 years; DTaPHepIPV at 2, 4 and 6 months (part of country); DTaPHibbHepIPV at 2, 4, and 6 months (part of country); DTaPHibIPV at 2, 4 and 6 months; DTwPHib at 15 months; DTwPHibHep at 2, 4 and 6 months; HepB at 5 years, +1, +6 months; Influenza at 6 and 7 months; IPV at 2, 4 and 6 months (part of country); MMR at 12 months and 4–5 years; OPV at 2,

B

4 and 6 months; Pneumo_conj at 2, 4, 6 and 15 months (part of country); Pneumo_ps at 2 years (part of country); TD at 22, 32, 42, 52, 62, 72 years. The percent of the target population vaccinated, by antigen, is: DTP1 (99%); DTP3, HepB3, Hib3, Polio3 (93%); and MCV (85%).

BIBLIOGRAPHY

Bahamas handbook and businessman's annual. Nassau, 2005, Etienne Dupuch Jr Publications.

Central Intelligence Agency: *2006: The World factbook, Bahamas,* Retrieved September 1, 2006, from https://www.cia.gov/cia/publications/factbook/print/bf.html

Craton M, Saunders G: *Islanders in the stream: a history of the Bahamian people,* Athens, Ga, 1992–1998, University of Georgia Press.

Gomez P: *19 Years of national struggle against the HIV/AIDS epidemic, 1983–2002: the Bahamas: a Caribbean success story.* Retrieved March 1, 2006, from http://www.catin.org/country/bahamas/TheBahamas_ASuccess.doc.

Pan American Health Organization: *Bahamas: Health situation analysis and trends summary:* Retrieved March 1, 2006, from http://www.paho.org/English/DD/AIS/cp_044.htm.

World Health Organization: *Bahamas: epidemiological fact sheets on HIV/AIDS and sexually transmitted infections:* Retrieved March 1, 2006, from http://www.who.int/GlobalAtlas/predefinedReports/EFS2004/EFS_PDFs/EFS2004_BS.pdf

World Health Organization: *2006: Immunization, vaccines and biologicals.* Retrieved September 15, 2006, from http://www.int/immunization_monitoring/en/globalsummary/countryprofileresult.cfm?C='bhs'.

♦ BAHRAIN (KINGDOM OF)

MAP PAGE (802)

Tawfeeq Ali Naseeb

Location: The Kingdom of Bahrain consists of an archipelago of about 36 small islands situated halfway down the Arabian Gulf, about 24 km from the eastern coast of Saudi Arabia. The total area is 720.1 km^2 (278 square miles). The population is approximately 707,160, including about 235,108 non-nationals mainly from the Indian subcontinent, Iran, the Far East, and Western countries. The capital is Manama. The gross domestic product (GDP) per capita is $23,000. English is widely used in business and banking, and Farsi (Persian) is used by families with origins in Iran. A considerable discrepancy in illiteracy rates still exists: 8% of men versus 17% of women according to the latest census.

Major Languages	Ethnic Groups	Major Religions
Arabic (official)	Bahraini 63%	Islam (Sunni, Shia)
English	Asian 19%	81%
Farsi	Other Arab groups 10%	Christian 9%
Urdu	Iranian 8%	Other 10%

B

Health Care Beliefs: Active involvement; traditional. Some Muslim nationals believe in the concept of envy as a cause of illness. For example, if someone casts an "evil eye" toward another because of jealousy, the recipient may develop an illness, a serious disease, or some misfortune as a result. If the affected person strongly believes that the cause of the disease or misfortune is the result of another's envy rather than of physiologic factors, the person is likely to go to a healer, or *shaikh,* who will use the words of the holy Koran for treatment.

Predominant Sick-Care Practices: Biomedical; magical-religious. Bahrain has two systems for health care delivery: public and a growing private sector. The government manages and finances 100% of the national health care system provided by public hospitals and health centers through the Ministries of Health and Defense. Health care services are available for everyone, even in rural areas. The government provides free primary, secondary, and tertiary health care for all nationals. Non-nationals are also eligible for care at significantly subsidized rates. The private sector is administered through private hospitals, clinics, and polyclinics and generates its own income through services provided. Alternative medicine is also increasing in popularity. Traditional medicine is rarely practiced for severe illnesses, but when a minor disease develops, some people prefer traditional healing. The number of doctors per 10,000 population increased from 15.3 in 2000 to 22.4 in 2004. Nurses have increased from 37.7 to 49.5. The number of primary health care units and centers also increased from 0.3 per 100,000 population to 0.33. The civil community has a role in health education and in the provision of care. Reproductive health education and counseling are available from various public associations.

Ethnic-/Race-Specific or Endemic Diseases: The health problems of Bahrain are typically those found in countries transitioning from developing to developed nations. Noncommunicable diseases such as cardiovascular and metabolic diseases, cancer, congenital anomalies, and accidents have taken on major roles. Circulatory-system diseases are the major cause of death (22%), followed by neoplasms (12%), conditions originating in the perinatal period (9%), respiratory system (6%), and endocrine diseases (4%). Changes in dietary habits and lifestyle have had a significant impact on the health status of the community. The rate of smoking is about 18% for men and 4% for women. Whereas infectious disease and lack of proper nutrition were previously major problems, no cases of diphtheria, pertussis, neonatal tetanus, or poliomyelitis have been reported since 1990. Although gonococcal infections dropped markedly (66 per 100,000 in 1990 to 33 per 100,000 in 2004), the incidence of syphilis has risen (191 cases, or 27

B

per 100,000 in 2004; from 37 cases, or 7 per 100,000 in 1990). Pulmonary tuberculosis incidence also rose (126 cases, or 18 per 100,000 in 2004 compared with 91 cases, or 18 per 100,000 in 1990). Human immunodeficiency virus/acquired immunodeficiency syndrome (HIV/AIDS) cases are 5, or 0.7 per 100,000. The Joint United Nations Programme on HIV/AIDS (UNAIDS) reports that injecting drug use accounted for 67% of all AIDS cases until 2000. Bahrain has an effective reporting system for HIV/AIDS. Premarital testing was introduced in 1999.

Health-Team Relationships: Nurses and doctors work together compatibly in heath services. The doctor is responsible for diagnosis and surgery, and the nurse provides support for most other needs. Doctors usually have at least a bachelor's degree in medicine and higher degrees. Nurses can either have an associate's, a bachelor's, or a master's degree. A few have a Ph.D. in nursing or a related specialty.

Families' Role in Hospital Care: Most hospitals have private rooms where one or two family members can stay with patients and take care of them. In pediatric wards, many hospitals allow mothers to stay with their children, especially when the children are quite young. Food from outside the hospital is not permitted for patients on special diets (e.g., those with diabetes, cancer, or heart disease) but is allowed for other patients. Many families bring traditional "comfort" foods for family members.

Dominance Patterns: The participation of women in social and economic life is increasing dramatically. Employed Bahraini women now account for 24% of the workforce (versus 17% in 1991). Two women have been appointed as ministers for the first time, and women have the right to vote. Women play an active role in the lifestyle of the family, especially feeding and taking care of children. Housemaids, particularly from India, Sri Lanka, Indonesia, and the Philippines also assist in child care and house management in most middle and upper class families. Premarital counseling began as optional in 1993; in 2004 it became obligatory by law.

Touch Practices: Physical touching conveys a type of congenial, in-depth feeling among friends. Touching members of the same sex is acceptable, but touching between men and women is not.

Perceptions of Time: Because of high levels of education and awareness, time perception is similar to Western standards. Being punctual is more important than in many other Arab countries.

Pain Reactions: When men or women have pain, some may seek help first from other family members or friends. Further decisions about seeking treatment are then made based on the severity and cause of the pain.

Birth Rites: Bahrainis have no taboos associated with pregnancy. After birth, special foods (*hesso* and *gellab*) are usually given to postpartum mothers with the belief that they will help them regain good health and strength. Hesso consists of eggs, watercress seeds, and fat; gellab consists of wheat flour, watercress seeds, fat, and spices. Many women no longer believe in the efficacy of these traditional foods. Bahrainis have no preference for the gender of newborns. When women marry, their children acquire the family name of the husband. As a result of improvements in socioeconomic conditions and health services, infant mortality decreased from 20 in 1990 to 17 deaths per 1,000 live births in 2006. Fertility rates are consistent at 2.6 children per woman compared with 3 in 1990. Birth weight is an indicator of the health and nutritional status of mothers as well as a prediction of infant health and development. The percentage of newborns weighing at least 2.5 kg has remained relatively constant for the past 5 years. Life expectancy increased between 1965 and 2004 and is presently 72 for men, 77 for women.

Death Rites: When a family member dies, the family usually receives condolences and consolation from others for 3 days, either in the home of a family member or in a hall linked to the mosque. Women have a separate place to receive condolences from other women. Organ donation has become extremely acceptable because Islamic leaders have increased public awareness about this topic.

Food Practices and Intolerances: Food habits have become more diversified. Breakfast usually consists of foods such as eggs, cheese, legumes, bread, jam and fermented fish *(mehiawa)*. At lunch, rice with lamb, beef, chicken, or fish, is common. On the weekend (Thursday and Friday), many families prefer to have lunch somewhere other than the home. Supper is usually diversified, and it is common for families to purchase food from outside vendors such as local and Western fast-food establishments. Food habits have changed dramatically over the past 40 years as a result of increasing oil revenues. The consumption of traditional foods such as fish, rice, dates, and vegetables has gradually decreased, and Bahrainis are consuming more beef, chicken, eggs, milk, fat, sugar, and canned and fast foods.

Infant-Feeding Practices: Prolonged breastfeeding lasting 2 years, which is promoted by Islamic culture, is no longer widely practiced. Most women breastfeed their infants for 3 to 9 months and begin to introduce solid foods at 3 to 4 months. Most women practice mixed feeding (breastfeeding and bottle feeding) because of employment or outside commitments. The percentage of children under the age of 5 years with weight-for-age values corresponding to acceptable standard reference values has significantly increased since the early 1990s, from 77% to about 92 + 0.5% for the past 5 years.

Child-Rearing Practices: Child-rearing practices are permissive but remain within the cultural context and customs of Bahrain. For example, most families do not allow their children, especially their girls, to be outside the home unattended in the evening. Physical punishment of children has decreased but is still practiced in less affluent and educated families.

National Childhood Immunizations: BCG at birth for non-Bahrainis, DT at 2, 4, 6, and 18 months and 5 to 6 years (part of country); DTaP at 5 years; IPV at 2, 4, 6 and 18 months and 5 years (part of country); OPV at 2, 4, 6, and 18 months and 5 years; HepA at 1 and 2 years; HepB at 13 years (contact, staff, school and college students); HIB at 2, 4, 6, and 18 months (part of country special cases); MMR at 1, 5 and 11 years; MenACWY 2 years; Pneumo_ps at >2 years; :Pneumo_conj at 2, 4 and 6 months (part of country); Td at 12 years, also for Haj pilgrims and after injury; TT for pregnant women. The percent of the target population vaccinated, by antigen, is: DTP1, MCV (99%); and DTP3, HepB3, Hib3, and Polio3 (98%). Immunization is provided free of charge by the public health centers. The majority of women are vaccinated for TT at an early age.

BIBLIOGRAPHY

Central Intelligence Agency: *2006: The world factbook, Bahrain,* Retrieved September 15, 2006, from https://www.cia.gov/cia/publications/factbook/print/ba.html.

Central Statistics Organization Results of 2001 census, Bahrain, 2002.

Ministry of Health Health statistics, 2004, Bahrain, 2005.

Musaiger AO: *The state of food and nutrition in Bahrain,* Riyadh, Saudi Arabia, 1993, United Nations Children's Fund—Gulf Area Office.

Musaiger AO: The state of nutrition in Bahrain, *Nutrition Health.* 14:63–74, 2000.

UNAIDS: 2006 Bahrain. Retrieved September 15, 2006, from http://www.unaids.org/en/Regions_Countries/Countries/bahrain.asp

World Health Organization 2006: Immunization, vaccines and biologicals, Retrieved September 15, 2006, from http://www.int/immunization_monitoring/en/global-summary/countryprofileresult.cfm?C='bhr'.

◆ BANGLADESH (PEOPLE'S REPUBLIC OF)

MAP PAGE (804)

Amal K. Mitra

Location: Bangladesh was liberated from Pakistan in 1971 after a 9-month war. It is bordered by India on the north, east, and west and by the Bay of Bengal and Myanmar on the south. The total area is 144,000 km^2 (55,598 square miles). The population is 1.4 million. The capital is Dhaka. It is a country of seven major rivers: Padma, Meghna, Jamuna, Brahmaputra, Madhumati, Surma, and Kushiara. Bangladesh is low lying (less than 183 m [600 ft]) and subject to tropical monsoons, frequent floods, and famine. The gross domestic product (GDP) per capita is $2,126, with 40% below the poverty line, making Bangladesh one of the poorest countries in the world. Literacy rates are 54% for men and 32% for women.

Major Languages	Ethnic Groups	Major Religions
Bangla (Bengali; official)	Bengali 98%	Muslim 83%
English (widely spoken by literate)	Bilhari and tribal 2%	Hindu 16%
		Christian and Others 1%

Health Care Beliefs: Passive role; acute sick care. Allopathic medicine is practiced throughout the country, but poor villagers still use more informal or traditional systems of medicine. Illness is considered to be caused by a curse. Rural Bangladeshis seek an explanation at several levels for unexpected life events: factors such as fate, inherited qualities, the environment, and individual behavior. For example, people usually consider miscarriages or stillbirths to be a result of "bad eye" *(ku najar)* of evil spirits *(jeen, bhut)*. This is the same phenomenon as the "evil eye" spoken of in other cultures in which a person with bad intent looks at a potential victim and causes illness; however, modern medicine is growing in popularity among literate and urban people, especially for acute illnesses.

Predominant Sick-Care Practices: Biomedical; magical-religious. Muslims and Hindus in poor communities and villages believe in wearing amulets *(tabij)* as a complementary or alternative method to cure disease or to protect themselves from illnesses. Most people believe in the efficacy of allopathic medicine, although they also use complementary and alternative treatments, such as homeopathy, ayurvedic medicine, and spiritual treatments. Those who are illiterate continue to believe that evil spirits and God's will can cause illness, and they prefer injections and intravenous fluid infusions as cures. Total withdrawal of foods or use of easily digested cereals *(sagu)* or barley water is common during fever. Faith healers, such as magic healers *(ojha)* and mystical mendicants *(fakirs)*, exorcise evil air and offer consecrated water *(pani para)* for the relief of symptoms. Poor people may prefer fakirs, herbalists *(kobiraj)*, and ojhas because these healers spend time with patients and do not always charge a fee. In villages, where most people live, untrained rural practitioners outnumber qualified allopathic doctors. Government health facilities offer modern treatments in every town and city, however. There is no health insurance, and those visiting government health centers and hospitals pay a nominal fee per visit. Those who can afford to do so pay a high cost for health care services in private clinics. People can also obtain medicines at pharmacies without a prescription.

Ethnic-/Race-Specific or Endemic Diseases: Food- and water-borne diseases such as diarrhea, dysentery, parasitic diseases, typhoid fever, and hepatitis are common among all age groups. Acute respiratory tract infections and diarrhea are the major causes of death in children under the age of 5 years. Among the insect-borne diseases, malaria is highly prevalent, especially in Chittagong Hill Tracts, Sylhet, and Mymensingh. Chloroquine-resistant malaria is a growing problem, and a recent upsurge of dengue fever caused many deaths. Arsenic poisoning has become a disaster. Arsenic concentrations in tube-well water have been found to be higher than the maximum permissible limit of 0.05 mg/L, affecting almost half of the population. Malnutrition is a major cause of death and debility in children. Low-birth-weight and malnourished children are susceptible to infections; roughly two thirds of deaths of under-5 children are attributed to malnutrition, and 75% of children have mild to moderate malnutrition. Deficiency disorders, including vitamin A, iodine, and iron deficiencies, are serious public health problems. About 30,000 children under the age of 6 years become blind each year because of vitamin A

B

deficiencies, and poor nutritional status and severe infections are important predictors. In 1973 the government instituted a plan for distributing large doses of vitamin A capsules to all children between 1 and 6 years old at 6-month intervals. More than 60% of the population has biochemical iodine deficiencies, prompting health authorities to encourage the use of iodized salt. The current goiter rate is 47%; people in the northern districts and flood-prone areas of the country are the most affected. The World Health Organization and the Joint United Nations Programme on human immunodeficiency virus/acquired immunodeficiency syndrome (HIV/AIDS) (UNAIDS) estimate the prevalence rate for HIV in adults (aged 15 to 49) to be 0.1%, with fewer than 500 deaths from AIDS. National surveillance from 1989 through 1996 reported 1.13 people with HIV per 1,000, which makes Bangladesh one of the countries with the lowest prevalence. UNAIDS estimates that 15,000 adults and children are living with HIV/AIDS. In the last round of surveillance, among the 10,445 persons tested, 35 (0.3%) were HIV infected. Among injecting drug users participating in a needle/syringe exchange program in one city, 4% were HIV infected; in one neighborhood in that city, 9% were infected.

Dominance Patterns: In this patriarchal society, women's activities may be severely restricted, and they are often physically secluded. Both years of schooling received and socioeconomic status are poorer among women than among men.

Birth Rites: The infant mortality rate is high at 61 deaths per 1,000 live births. The fertility rate is 3.11 children born per woman. About 90% of deliveries are home deliveries, which are culturally acceptable. Only about 12% are attended by skilled birth attendants. Traditional birth attendants and relatives, who attend most deliveries, sometimes use a clean inner strip of a bamboo stalk to cut the umbilical cord. A problem, especially in rural areas, is the traditional practice of using homemade *ghee* (clarified butter) to "heal" the umbilical stump. Rural traditional custom requires the mother to reach a water source unaided to wash herself and her clothing immediately after birth. After delivery, numerous rituals are performed. Plum branches are placed on the door of the home to protect against evil spirits, and the Muslim holy Imam chants the birth announcement. The mother chants prayers and stays indoors, and only the husband may visit. Traditionally, this rest period of 7, 21, or even 40 days for the mother after birth is practiced, depending on the economic status and traditional values of the family. An indicator of poor women's health is their high maternal mortality rate, which is greater than 300 per 100,000 live births. About 25% of maternal deaths are associated with anemia and hemorrhage. The use of contraceptives has increased in recent years, providing women with greater control over reproduction. Life expectancy is 62 years for both men and women.

Death Rites: A holy Imam does not have to be present at death; however, a Muslim may recite the declaration of the faith: "There is no God but God, and Muhammad is his messenger." Family members wash the body according to Islamic tradition. Autopsy is uncommon because the deceased must be buried intact. The body is wrapped in special pieces of cloth and buried in the ground without a coffin. Muslim tradition forbids organ donations or transplants. Hindus cremate the bodies of everyone except for children aged 10 years or younger, whom they bury.

Food Practices: Rice is the staple food. Most people eat two large meals of rice, vegetable curry, and lentil (*daal*) soup. Hilsa fish is very popular. The other commonly available sweet-water fishes include ruhi, katla, mrigel, kai, magur, shing, bata, baila, kachki, kajuli, khailsha, tengra, puti, and mola. Muslims eat beef but do not eat pork or turtle meat. Hindus do not eat beef, and certain castes of Hindus eat pork. Dried fish, called *sutki*, is popular among some communities, especially those from Chittagong, Cox's Bazar, Bandarban, Noakhali, Comilla, and Sylhet districts. Illiterate people have taboos against using certain food items, such as eggs and meats, during illness.

Infant-Feeding Practices: Breastfeeding is almost universal and usually continues to some degree until the child is 1 year old. For the first 3 days, the infant also is spoon-fed sugar water. Families who are economically deprived breastfeed infants until introducing supplementary foods, and then male infants may receive higher-quality supplementary nutrition. Sixty percent of mothers bottle-feed using commercial milk and starchy food by the time the infant is 3 months, and 80% do so by 5 months. This additional food is usually provided in a diluted form. Family food, such as rice and vegetables, are introduced when the infant is aged between 6 months and 1 year.

Child-Rearing Practices: Because of economic and cultural influences, boys receive preferential treatment in terms of family food allocation and health care practices, resulting in an increased mortality rate for girls after the neonatal period. Recent studies show that twice as many girls as boys die as a result of delayed initiation of care and prolonged illnesses before initiating hospital admission.

National Childhood Immunizations: BCG at birth; DTwP at 6, 10, and 14 weeks; OPV at 6, 10, 14 and 38 weeks; measles at 9 months; TT at 15 to 49 years, + 1 month + 6 months + 1 year + 1 year; Vitamin A at 38 weeks postpartum women and children 1–5. The percent of the target population vaccinated, by antigen, is: BCG (99%); DTP1 (96%); DTP3, Polio3 (88%); HepB3 (62%); MCV (81%); and TT2 plus (89%). Bangladesh adopted the Universal Program on Immunization recommended by WHO and the United Nations Children's Fund (UNICEF). Women of child-bearing age and pregnant women should be given two doses of TT during the second or third trimester of pregnancy to protect infants from tetanus, with the last dose 1 month before delivery. According to WHO, Bangladesh has had no cases of polio since 2001.

BIBLIOGRAPHY

Ahmed SM et al: Gender, socioeconomic development and health-seeking behaviour in Bangladesh, *Soc Sci Med.* 51(3):361–71, 2000.

Central Intelligence Agency: *2006: The world factbook, Bangladesh.* Retrieved September 15, 2006, from https://www.cia.gov/cia/publications/factbook/print/bg.html.

ICDDRB. HIV surveillance in Bangladesh: the present scenario. *Health Science Bull.* 3(1):1–6, 2005.

Mitra AK. et al: Predictors of serum retinol in children with shigellosis, *Am J Clin Nutr.* 68(5):1088–94, 1998.

Mitra AK, Rahman MM, Fuchs GJ: Risk factors and gender differentials for death among children hospitalized with diarrhea in Bangladesh. *J Health Popul Nutr.* 18(3):151–6, 2000.

Smith AH, Lingas EO, Rahman M: Contamination of drinking water by arsenic in Bangladesh: a public health emergency. *Bull WHO.* 78:1093–103, 2000.

UNAIDS: 2006: Bangladesh. Retrieved September 15, 2006 from http://www.unaids.org/en/Regions_Countries/Countries/bangladesh.asp.

World Health Organization: 2005: Bangladesh, Retrieved November 15, 2005, at http://www.who.int/countries/bgd/en/.

World Health Organization: 2006: Immunization, vaccines and biologicals. Retrieved September 15, 2006 from http://www.int/immunization_monitoring/en/global-summary/countryprofileresult.cfm?C='bgd'.

◆ BARBADOS

MAP PAGE (796)

Anselm Hennis

Location: Barbados is the easternmost island in the Caribbean archipelago, with a total area of approximately 430 km² (166 square miles). It lies 13 degrees north of the equator; 154 km east of Saint Vincent, its nearest neighbor; and 721 km north-northeast of Guyana. The population is 279,912, and the capital is Bridgetown. With its population density of 625 persons per km², it is the world's 10th most populous nation. Barbados ranked 31st in the 2005 United Nations Human Development Index (United Nations Development Programme, 2005), the highest rank achieved by a developing country. The gross domestic product (GDP) per capita is $17,000. The adult literacy rate exceeds 99%, and more than 80% of households have telephones.

Major Languages	Ethnic Groups	Major Religions
English	Black African 90%	Protestant 67%
	White 4%	Roman Catholic 4%
	Asian & Mixed 6%	None or Other 29%

Health Care Beliefs: Active involvement; health promotion important. The population is well educated, highly sophisticated, and informed about health and illness. They have easy access to information sources such as CNN and easy travel access to North America. Generally, the people fear mental illness and hesitate to include such individuals in the wider society. Anxiety neuroses are not uncommon, accounting for the majority of psychiatric disorders causing people to seek health care. Depression among the elderly population is reported infrequently.

Predominant Sick-Care Practices: Biomedical; traditional. The island's easily accessible health care system includes a tertiary care hospital and an island-wide ring of nine primary care polyclinics, all managed by the government and providing free care to the public. In addition, drugs listed on the national formulary are free for individuals in the public sector, whereas formulary drugs are also free privately to all nationals for chronic diseases, including diabetes, hypertension, asthma, cancer, and epilepsy. About 400 doctors live on the island, and people seek medical care from this group.

Ethnic-/Race-Specific or Endemic Diseases: Sickle cell disease occurs almost exclusively in individuals of African origin, but the overall number of cases is low. The principal illnesses are the chronic noncommunicable diseases, including cardiovascular diseases and diabetes. Most illnesses are related to nutrition and lifestyle. Approximately 50% of Barbadians aged 40 years and older suffer from hypertension, and 20% have diabetes. High rates of obesity contribute to these health problems: 10% of adult men and 30% of adult women are classified as obese, and 30% of men and 60% of women are overweight. The complications of these chronic conditions exact a significant toll on society. Data from a national stroke registry indicate that a new stroke is recorded every day in Barbados. Ongoing efforts facilitated by the Ministry of Health, the Pan American Health Organization, the Barbados Association of Medical Practitioners, the University of the West Indies, the Barbados Cancer Society, the Heart and Stroke Foundation of Barbados, the Diabetes Association, and the Diabetes Foundation of Barbados are promoting changes in risk behaviors. High rates of eye disease have also been documented; Barbadians are known to have the highest reported rates of primary open-angle glaucoma (leading to vision loss) in a national population. The Joint United Nations Programme on human immunodeficiency virus/acquired immunodeficiency syndrome (HIV/AIDS) (UNAIDS) has estimated the prevalence rate of HIV in adults (aged 15 to 49) to be 1.6%, with 2,700 people living with HIV, including fewer than 1,000 women and fewer than 100 children aged 0 to 14 years. Deaths attributed to AIDS are fewer than 500. Implementation of antiretroviral therapy in pregnancy has been demonstrated to have significantly reduced mother-to-child transmission; about 95% of infected persons receive antiretroviral therapy.

Health-Team Relationships: Health teams are more doctor-driven in hospital settings. In secondary care, polyclinic senior nurses have more significant leadership roles. Nurses are involved to a greater extent in community care and public health outreach and education.

Families' Role in Hospital Care: Families do not stay with relatives who are hospitalized, and it is considered inappropriate to bring outside food to patients.

Dominance Patterns: Although males dominate this culture, women play a principal role in the household. They are often role models and major breadwinners in many families where males "visit," the term used for single female-headed households. In a significant societal paradigm shift, women account for more than 60% of university enrollments. This translates to more women in managerial and professional positions.

Eye-Contact Practices: People do not avoid eye contact, and they are likely to assert themselves regardless of their gender or status.

Touch Practices: Excessive touching is unacceptable. Touching usually occurs only when individuals greet others and generally involves only the hands.

Perceptions of Time: Consistent with the easygoing Caribbean ethos, there is little emphasis on punctuality in contemporary life. "Arriving on Caribbean time" means arriving later than planned. People in the formal business world, however, pay more attention to timeliness. Unfortunately, the importance of past traditions is being lost rapidly. The culture is heavily influenced because of easy access to cable and satellite television and the Internet, and also because of the island's proximity to the United States.

Pain Reactions: Pain reactions vary significantly and are uniquely individual.

Birth Rites: The vast majority of births take place in a hospital. Infant mortality rates are 12 deaths per 1,000 live births. Women who have had no complications go home with their infants within a day or 2 and return for routine follow-up. Because of the progressively acculturating society, practices that were followed a generation ago have now essentially disappeared. Infant boys tend to be celebrated more than infant girls. The fertility rate is 1.65 children born per woman. Current life expectancy is 71 for men, 75 for women.

Death Rites: Perceptions of death are largely colored by religious beliefs, and in this predominantly Christian society, concepts of death and the afterlife are based on biblical perspectives. Family members will usually attend the passing of a loved one in clinical and community settings when feasible. A considerable anathema to autopsy exists, and not surprisingly the concept of organ donation has not been embraced. Therefore, the island has no established transplantation programs based on cadaveric organ donation.

Food Practices and Intolerances: The principal grain eaten is rice, often cooked with a variety of peas, and meals based on macaroni and sweet potatoes are also popular. Chicken is probably the most frequently consumed meat product. Popular local dishes include rice and peas and beef stew, with servings of vegetable salads, and the national dish is flying fish and cou cou, a dish prepared from cornmeal cooked with okra. Knives and forks are required implements for eating.

Infant-Feeding Practices: Breastfeeding is considered highly desirable and is actively promoted in the antenatal clinics.

Child-Rearing Practices: Child rearing is based on the model that children must be disciplined to respect adults, especially parents and teachers. Social class influences patterns of discipline; for example "smacking" may be more prevalent among working class groups and is accepted in the school system.

National Childhood Immunizations: BCG at 5 to 6 years; DT at 4 to 5 years; DTwP at 8 months; DTwP HiBHep at 3, 4.5, and 6 months; OPV at 3, 4.5, 6, and 18 months, 4.5 and 11 years; MMR at 1 and 3 to 5 years; and Td at 10 to 11 years. The percent of the target population vaccinated, by antigen, is: DTP1 (97%); DTP3, HepB3, Hib3 (92%); MCV (93%), and Polio3 (91%).

B

BIBLIOGRAPHY

Ministry of Health, Barbados: *Annual report of the Chief Medical Officer for the years 1997–1999.* September 2000.

Carter AO, Hambleton I, Broome H, Fraser HF, Hennis A: Prevalence and risk factors associated with obesity in the elderly in Barbados, *J Aging Health.* 18:240–8, 2006.

Corbin D, Poddar V, Hennis A, Gaskin A, Rambarat C, Wilks R, Wolfe C, Fraser H: Incidence and case fatality rates of first-ever stroke in a black Caribbean population: the Barbados Register of Strokes (BROS), *Stroke.* 35:1254–58, 2004.

Central Intelligence Agency: 2006: The world factbook, Barbados, Retrieved September 15, 2006, from https://www.cia.gov/cia/publications/factbook/print/bb.html.

Hennis A, Fraser H: Diabetes in the English-speaking Caribbean. *Rev Panam Salud Publica.* 15:90–3, 2004.

Hennis A, Fraser HS, Jonnalagadda R, Fuller J, Chaturvedi N: Explanations for the high risk of diabetes-related amputation in a Caribbean population of Black African descent, and potential for prevention, *Diabetes Care.* 27:2636–41, 2004.

Hennis A, Wu S-Y, Nemesure B, Li X, Leske MC, for the Barbados Eye Studies Group Hypertension prevalence, control and survivorship in an AfroCaribbean Population, *J Hypertens.* 20:1–7, 2002.

Hennis A, Wu S-Y, Nemesure B, Li X, Leske MC, for the Barbados Eye Studies Group: epidemiologic profile and implications of Diabetes in an African-Caribbean population, Int. *J Epidemiol.* 31:234–239, 2002.

Leske MC, Connell AMS, Schachat AP, Hyman L, the Barbados Eye Study Group: The Barbados Eye Study: prevalence of open angle glaucoma, *Arch Ophthalmol.* 112:821–9, 1994.

UNAIDS: 2006: Barbados, Retrieved September 15, 2006 from http://www.unaids.org/en/Regions_Countries/Countries/barbados.asp.

World Health Organization: 2006: Immunization, vaccines and biologicals. Retrieved September 15, 2006 from http://www.int/immunization_monitoring/en/globalsummary/countryprofileresult.cfm?C='brb'.

◆ BELARUS (REPUBLIC OF)

MAP PAGE (799)

Bernd Rechel

Location: Located in Eastern Europe, with Poland to the west, Lithuania and Latvia to the north, Russia to the east, and Ukraine to the south, Belarus is a member of the Commonwealth of Independent States (CIS). Belarus contains hilly lowlands with forests, swamps, lakes, and arable land. The total area is 207,600 km² (80,154 square miles). The population is 10.3 million; the capital is Minsk. The gross domestic product (GDP) per capita is estimated at $6,900, with about 27% below the poverty line. Literacy rates are greater than 99% for both men and women.

Major Languages	**Ethnic Groups**	**Major Religions**
Byelorussian (official)	Belarusian 81.2%	Eastern Orthodox 80%
Russian	Russian 11.4%	Other or None 20%
	Polish, Ukrainian, and	
	Other 7.4%	

Health Care Beliefs: Acute sick care; passive role. Health care is primarily crisis care. Health promotion has been neglected by the state-run sanitary-epidemiologic network, and currently people have little interest in prevention, although awareness is slowly developing. Illness and disease are still thought of fatalistically—as a normal part of life. People rarely use alternative treatments for illness and rather go to a clinic for biomedical treatment.

Predominant Sick-Care Practices: Biomedical. Ill people seek medical care in local polyclinics or hospitals. Rural areas are served by small rural health posts, and people may need to go to the nearest town for assistance, usually by infrequent bus service. In cities, polyclinics are located throughout residential neighborhoods, whereas in smaller towns they reside within the local hospital. Once treated at a clinic, a patient may be referred to a specialist for testing, provided with a prescription, or referred to a hospital if more serious treatment is needed. Hospitals are located throughout the major cities and within the principal towns of the regions or counties. Specialized hospital services, which are located mainly in Minsk, include a full range of specialist hospitals and polyclinics offering tertiary care and often specialize in certain surgical procedures or treatments. Prescriptions for medications can be filled at numerous pharmacies, and patients attempt to find the best price for unregulated pharmaceuticals because they have to pay for most medications. Services other than medications are nominally free, but under-the-table payments are widespread, restricting access to health services for the poorest of the population.

Ethnic-/Race-Specific or Endemic Diseases: Similar to developments in Russia, Belarus has faced a mortality crisis since the late 1980s, which was accelerated in the 1990s by the socioeconomic changes that followed the breakup of the Soviet Union. Life expectancy fell steeply between 1987 and 1995 and has stagnated since. Mortality is driven mainly by diseases of the circulatory system and external causes of death (such as injury, homicide, or suicide). The country also continues to suffer from the effects of nuclear fallout from the 1986 Chernobyl accident, which took place in neighboring Ukraine. After 1986, the incidence of thyroid cancer in children increased 50-fold. As is true for neighboring Russia and Ukraine, the country has witnessed an exponential increase in the cases of human immunodeficiency virus/acquired immunodeficiency syndrome (HIV/AIDS) in recent years, driven primarily by injecting drug use. Men constitute 70% of the known HIV cases. Most people with HIV (79%) are aged 15 to 29. The United Nations Joint Programme on HIV/AIDS (UNAIDS) estimated that the HIV prevalence rate at the end of 2003 was 0.2% to 0.8% of the adult (aged 15 to 49) population. It is estimated that 20,000 people are living with HIV, including 5,100 women. Deaths from AIDS are fewer than 2000.

Health-Team Relationships: Doctors are the principal authorities on health issues. Nurses play a subordinate role and have little professional autonomy.

Families' Role in Hospital Care: Inpatient drugs should nominally be provided free of charge, but families must locate and pay for many medications for their hospitalized family members. It can be difficult to find certain prescribed medications because many of the most popular drugs are not readily available. Families are also burdened by often substantial under-the-table payments.

Dominance Patterns: Belarus is a patriarchal post-Soviet society with little appreciation of democratic values. Domestic violence has not been recognized as a problem by the state or the general public, and homophobia remains widespread. The family continues to provide a mutual support system, and families are expected to look after their aging parents. Often, the parents move in with one of their children as they become less able to live on their own.

Eye-Contact Practices: Direct eye contact is acceptable.

Touch Practices: Men usually greet each other by shaking hands, and women are frequently seen walking arm in arm.

Perceptions of Time: Punctuality is not particularly important in Belarus. Although those who are involved in business with people from other countries are becoming more concerned with punctuality on a professional level, within their personal lives punctuality remains unimportant.

Pain Reactions: Although people are known for their stoicism in physically and emotionally painful situations, they openly share their experiences with family, friends, and neighbors.

Birth Rites: The infant mortality rate is 13 deaths per 1,000 live births. Birth and death rites are determined by religion rather than culture. People in Belarus are primarily Eastern Orthodox; the other primary religion is Roman Catholic. The birth and death rites practiced here are affected more by these religions than anything specific to Belarus. The fertility rate is 1.43 children born per woman. Life expectancy is 57 for men, 65 for women: child mortality rates are 11 and 9 per 1,000 for boys and girls, respectively.

Death Rites: Relatives are not required to be present at the time of death, and few specific death rites exist. Individuals who are Eastern Orthodox follow the rites of their church, which are more specific to Orthodox rituals than to the culture of Belarus. Traditional funerals involve church services, and mourners say prayers at the place of burial. Having

B

the bones of a dead person in a grave is a source of consolation and connection. Cremation is strongly discouraged, and some believe that this practice was introduced by the godless and enemies of the church. It is believed that alms in memory of the dead can bring special benefits to the deceased. Sometimes special burial funds are available to pay for burials of poor parishioners.

Food Practices and Intolerances: People primarily believe that the noon meal should be the largest meal of the day. In a society in which most families are not home for the noon meal, however, this custom can be practiced only on weekends and holidays. Belarusians, like people of many other cultures, enjoy entertaining and are extremely generous in sharing what they have with friends and family. They love to celebrate any occasion and will have a large celebratory meal—usually late in the evening—whenever possible. The staples in a Belarusian diet include potatoes, bread, and smoked sausages that come in many varieties. Tea is the most popular beverage, as is compote (a homemade fruit juice) served at room temperature. Ice is not used in cold drinks.

Infant-Feeding Practices: Breastfeeding is considered the best source of nutrition for newborns, so if possible new mothers choose to breastfeed; however, no stigma is attached to formula diets if a mother is unable to produce milk. The mother introduces mashed fruit and vegetables, creamed cereals, rice, and potatoes at about 6 months of age.

Child-Rearing Practices: Mothers are the primary caregivers for children and are allowed by law to take up to 3 years of maternity leave. However, they can return to work as soon as several weeks after the birth of their child. The mother's return to work depends almost solely on the family's financial situation, as mothers are not paid for maternity leave. In a country in which two incomes are almost essential, it is becoming much more common for mothers to take shorter leaves after the birth of a child. Parents frequently ask grandparents to look after children whose mothers have returned to work.

National Childhood Immunizations: BCG at 3 weeks and at 7 years (if tuberculin test is negative); Diptheria at 11 years; DTP at 3, 4, 5, and 18 months; HepB at birth and at 1 and 5 months; IPV at 3 and 4 months; OPV at 5, 18, and 24 months and at 7 years; MMR at 12 months and 6 years; DT at 6 years; and Td at 16, 26, 36, 46, 56, and 66 years. The percent of the target population vaccinated, by antigen, is: BCG, DTP1, DTP3, HepB3, MCV (99%); and Polio3 (98%).

BIBLIOGRAPHY

Belarus: a story of change. Press agency of the Commonwealth of Independent States Secretariat (CIS), 1999.

Central Intelligence Agency: *2006: The world factbook, Belarus.* Retrieved September 21, 2006, from https://www.cia.gov/cia/publications/factbook/print/bo.html.

Karnitski G: Health care systems in transition—Belarus (draft), Copenhagen, 1997, WHO Regional Office for Europe.

Ministry of Statistics and Analysis of the Government of Belarus: *Statistical review of Belarus,* Minsk, 2001.

UNAIDS, 2006 Belarus: Retrieved September 21, 2006, from http://www.unaids. org/en/Regions_Countries/Countries/belarus.asp.

World Health Organization: *Highlights on health in Belarus*, Copenhagen, 2000, WHO Regional Office for Europe.

World Health Organization: *WHO health for all database*, Copenhagen, 2006, WHO Regional Office for Europe.

World Health Organization: 2006: Immunization, vaccines and biologicals. Retrieved September 21, 2006, from http://www.who.int/immunization_monitoring/en/ globalsummary/countryprofileresult.cfm?C=blr'.

B

◆ BELGIUM (KINGDOM OF)

MAP PAGE (798)

Sabine Stordeur and William D'Hoore

Location: Belgium, a neighbor of France, Germany, The Netherlands, and Luxembourg, has an opening to the North Sea. Belgium has a total area of 30,000 km^2 (11,580 square miles) and is a small, highly developed, and densely populated country of over 10 million people at the crossroads of Western Europe. Although generally flat, the terrain becomes increasingly hilly and forested in the southeast (Ardennes) region. The climate is cool, temperate, and rainy. It is a federal state with three relatively autonomous regions: Flanders in the north, where the language is Dutch (Flemish); Wallonia in the south, where the language is French; and the centrally located Brussels, the capital of Belgium and Europe, an area that is officially bilingual but mostly French speaking. A small region in the east of Wallonia cites German as the official language.

Major Languages	Ethnic Groups	Major Religions
Flemish (Dutch)	Fleming 58%	Roman Catholic 75%
French	Walloon 31%	Protestant or Other 25%
German	Mixed, Other 11%	

The governing of the country is complicated by its particular structure, with three language communities and the multilingual, multicultural, and multinational status of Brussels. Flanders has about 55% of the inhabitants, Brussels 10%, and Wallonia the remaining 35%. It is a highly unionized country, and organized labor has had a powerful influence on politics. About 53% of all private-sector and public-service employees are labor union members. Belgian labor unions take positions on a wide range of political issues, including education, public finances, defense spending, environmental protection, women's rights, and abortion. They also provide a range of services, including the administration of unemployment benefits and health insurance programs. Most (73%) people work in the service sector, 25% in industry, and 2% in agriculture. Pension and other social security programs have become a major concern as the "baby boom" generation approaches retirement. The gross domestic product (GDP) per capita is $31,400, with about 4% below the poverty line. Literacy rates are over 99% for men and women.

Health Care Beliefs: Active involvement; health promotion and alternative medicine important. Medicine and medical care are based on the Western scientific model. Because science is recycled by common sense, traditional folk beliefs are replaced by pseudoscience. The "common sense model" is similar to the French model *(anthropologie de la maladie),* best described by François Laplantine, in which disease is seen as exogenous and evil. The model of health and disease is relatively rational and includes factors relating to religion and nature. Belgians believe that good food brings good health, that garlic purifies blood and spinach contains iron, which is good for growth. The use of food supplements, vitamins, and biofood is spreading among well-educated people. Healthy behaviors such as exercise, practicing safe sex, being temperate, staying lean, and refraining from smoking are promoted. Many Catholics believe that praying and going on a pilgrimage can help heal, especially severe diseases such as cancer. Other communities have their own rituals. According to the 2001 National Health Survey, 11% of the population sought help from alternative medical professionals in the year before the survey, mainly from homeopathic doctors, chiropractors, osteopathic doctors, and acupuncturists. Alternative medicine is practiced primarily but not solely by qualified doctors and physiotherapists, although most qualified doctors are skeptical about alternative medicine. Until recently, alternative medicine was a privilege enjoyed by people of high socioeconomic status because the services were not reimbursed. However, insurances now tend to cover osteopathic care.

Predominant Sick-Care Practices: Biomedical; use of alternative medical practices increasing. Health care responsibilities are shared by the national Ministry of Public Health and the Dutch-, French-, and German-speaking Community Ministries of Health. In theory, all Belgians must be covered by one of the branches of social insurance, which is based on the principle of "solidarity" (i.e., with the employed paying for the unemployed and the healthy paying for the ill). A special social security scheme exists for vulnerable groups (e.g., widows, people with disabilities, retired people, and orphans). The municipalities within each province play a part in the organization of social assistance for people with low incomes. The country now has a mean of four hospital beds per 1,000 people and an emphasis on ambulatory care. There are 3.9 physicians per 1,000 inhabitants, half of which are general practitioners. Access to health care is virtually free, and people may choose their own doctors. Most people (94%) have a family doctor, and women have more contact (seven per year) with health care practitioners than men have (4.8 per year). Frequency of contact is influenced by subjective health, not by socioeconomic status. Patients may seek help from several providers simultaneously for the same health problem. Generally, the doctors make the decision to refer their patients to hospitals, although many direct emergency admissions occur. About 6.3% of Belgians never go to the dentist.

Ethnic-/Race-Specific or Endemic Diseases: Morbidity and mortality rates are similar to those of other developed countries. The most frequent causes of death, from highest to lowest, are cardiovascular diseases (32.8% in men, 40.3% in women), cancer (31.1% in men, 22.9% in women); suicide (2.99% in men, 1.15% in women); traffic accidents (2.05% in men, 0.75% in women); falls (1.1% in men, 1.4% in women); homicide (0.19% in men, 0.15% in women) other unspecified causes (29.8% in men, 34.1% in women). For men, 37% of deaths could be prevented through primary prevention measures; for women 41%. The incidence of tuberculosis is 11 per 100,000 in Belgium (5.5 per 100,00 in native Belgians, 71.5 per 100,000 in immigrants). Broken down by area, the rates are 6.5 per 100,000 versus 9.4 in Wallonia; 13.4 per 100,000 versus 36.1 in Brussels; and 3.9 per 100,000 versus 7.6 in Flanders. In 1999 and 2000, Brussels had 23 versus 47 per 100,000 cases of meningitis, respectively (an incidence of 2.4 versus 4.8 per 100,000, respectively). The World Health Organization and UNAIDS estimate the prevalence of human immunodeficiency virus (HIV) in adults (aged 15 to 49) to be 0.3%, with 14,000 people living with HIV, including 5,400 women. Fewer than 100 deaths from acquired immunodeficiency syndrome (AIDS) have been reported.

Health-Team Relationships: Medicine, dentistry, and pharmacy, which are all classified as "healing arts," can be practiced only by those who have a doctor of medicine, surgery, or obstetrics diploma; a dentistry diploma; or a pharmacy diploma, respectively. Limited and clearly defined services can be provided by midwives and by certain people with a master's degree in sciences (e.g., clinical biology). Three types of nursing services exist: basic nursing, technical nursing, and nursing that is supervised by a doctor. Several paramedical professions (e.g., physiotherapists) are classified in a third category of health care providers. In hospitals, doctors have a dominant position because of social recognition of their clinical expertise. Signs and symbols of doctor's prominence include the length of their university studies (7 to 13 years), their salaries (which are 2 to 10 times the average nurse's salary), and their hierarchical position (as medical directors). The nursing director is generally subordinate to medical and general directors. This situation is generally accepted. More professional relationships exist among doctors (involving accountability to peers and significant commitment to patients), whereas doctors and other health care workers have more bureaucratic relationships.

Families' Role in Hospital Care: Relatives participate very little in patient care. Strict visitor schedules are followed by all hospital units to limit access of the family to the facility. The visits of close relatives are primarily courtesy visits; however, husbands and wives visit more frequently to help manage laundry, assist with personal hygiene, and provide companionship. In pediatric units, mothers frequently visit with young children, sometimes all day and night, to support them emotionally.

Dominance Patterns: Belgians love the "good life," which is reflected in their excellent food and drink, comfortable housing, reliable medical and social services, and highly developed traffic and communications infrastructure. Belgians do not want to impress other people with their achievements or convince others of their righteousness. They tend to be rather reserved and introverted during their first introductions to other people but are sincerely warm and friendly after people get to know them better. They are happy when they can enjoy a safe and comfortable life with their family and friends, and they highly value privacy. They do not like moralizing or telling other people how they should behave (an attitude for which they criticize their neighbors in Holland), and they choose "live and let live" (*chacun chez soi*) as the basis for their philosophy of life. The expression "a Belgian compromise" was created to characterize the typical solutions used by Belgians to solve their conflicts. Complex issues are settled by conceding something to all parties concerned, using an agreement so complicated that nobody completely understands all its implications. Despite the apparent inefficiency of these settlements, the compromises do seem to work in practice because they tend to stop existing conflicts and allow life to proceed with few fights or obstructions.

Eye-Contact Practices: When people talk, they look others directly in the eyes but do not sustain the gaze because a persistent look can seem inappropriate or even threatening. Conversely, an elusive look is irritating and could be perceived as a lack of attention or frankness. A handshake is accompanied by direct eye-to-eye contact.

Touch Practices: A handshake or up to three kisses on the cheek during greetings and farewells are common.

Perceptions of Time: Belgians are generally punctual, but they expect to wait about 15 minutes for medical appointments. When doctors who are not on time explain why they are late (e.g., too many patients, an emergency case), patients are generally tolerant and accept longer waiting times.

Pain Reactions: Belgians are neither extremely stoic nor excessively emphatic. They try to explain their pain, identify its origin, and ask for a remedy, although many individual differences exist. They are particularly grateful if someone helps relieve their pain. Pain is not considered a result of fate, although it is considered redemptive by some Catholics. In hospital or outpatient care settings, professional initiatives to control pain are highly individual. No "analgesic" culture yet exists, although many recent changes relative to relief of pain have occurred. Certain patients, such as children and those who are terminally ill, receive better pain management services.

Birth Rites: From the announcement of the pregnancy, the mother undergoes blood sampling for various factors (e.g., HIV, cytomegalovirus [CMV], toxoplasmosis, German measles, hepatitis B, blood type) and urine analysis (e.g., for glucose and albumin). During the 9 months of

B

pregnancy, the pregnant woman often has three ultrasounds, but she frequently has more to establish the infant's well-being. Most parents want to know the sex of the baby by about the sixth month. In the 15th week of pregnancy, various tests are done to detect possible malformations and problems (e.g., spina bifida, Down syndrome). With the onset of contractions, gynecologists perform the initial examination, and then the woman is supervised by a midwife. Mothers or the medical team frequently request epidural anesthesia, and the father often attends the delivery. Episiotomies are common, and 9.7% of deliveries are done by cesarean section. The mean hospital stay is 4 days. The first name is chosen by the parents before birth, as are the godfathers and godmothers (in Christian families). After birth, a sequence of visits begins. All bring gifts, such as baby clothes, toys, and nursery items. Infants are usually christened several months after birth. Beginning in 2002, fathers began receiving 12, rather than 3, days off after the birth of a child. Maternity leave is 14 weeks, and women are paid 90% of their salaries. Parents are equally happy with the birth of a girl or boy, and even the Belgian royal family adopted the principle of primogeniture to show equality between the sexes. Abortion is "illegal" in Belgium except under three circumstances: a threat to the mother's health, psychological or social distress, or incurable disease in the fetus. The fertility rate is 1.64 children born per woman, and the infant mortality rate is 4.7 deaths per 1,000 live births. Life expectancy is 76 for men, 82 for women.

Death Rites: Half of Belgian deaths occur in hospitals, the other 50% at home or elsewhere. A child's death is always considered unacceptable and unjust, and people feel that it simply should have been prevented. If a child dies in a hospital, parents try to incriminate medical staff members and find medical errors. Deaths of older adults are less shocking and need less explanation and justification. If death occurs after an illness, it usually occurs in the hospital. People with chronic illnesses such as cancer or AIDS often stay at home to die. People are informed of the death through notices to them personally or in the local papers. The body is often sent to a funeral home, where it is put on view for 2 to 3 days. On the day of the funeral, people wear black, and the family receives condolences. Some women wear black dresses for a year. Most deceased people are buried, but some are cremated. People are assumed to be amenable to organ donation unless they have filled out a specific document of disagreement that has been recorded in the federal database.

Food Practices and Intolerances: The main meal is the evening meal. Staples include cheese, bread, fruit, and vegetables, and beer or wine are the usual beverages. The country is famous for its mussels and fries (French-fried potatoes), waffles, and endive. Belgians have a passion for fine chocolates, and exceptional chocolatiers fill the marketplaces of every city. More beer is consumed than wine, and many are crafted by small breweries whose family recipes and techniques are generations old. Beer laces the national dish, *carbonnades flamandes,* a Flemish beef stew. Belgians love potatoes and are fond of game and meat. *Charcuterie,*

B

a basket of bread, and beer often constitute the meals, but fish and sea-food are important as well. Hearty soups play a large role in the cuisine, and the so-called *waterzooies* are the most typical soups. Medieval cookery still influences the cuisine through condiments, mustards, vinegars, and dried fruits that lend a sweet-sour and sweet-salty flavor to dishes. Almonds and spices are used in abundance, and fresh herbs lace appetizers, salads, meats, and even desserts. Belgians enjoy frogs, snails, and seafood. Seasonal foods include Christmas turkey, spring asparagus, Easter lamb, June strawberries, apples and pears, nuts, shrimp, mussels (the best of which are available from September to December), and black and white pudding for the New Year. The usual food and drinks include coffee, *rollmops* (herring rolled in vinegar), sandwiches called *pistolet fourré,* and tomato meatballs. Italian, Chinese, Vietnamese, French, and Arabian restaurants are also common. Belgians like to meet and have a beer in cafes (the popular local bars), and regular customers are known as habitués.

Infant-Feeding Practices: Breastfeeding is emphasized, although parents are not pressured about their choice. In 2000, 68% of mothers chose breastfeeding, compared with 64% in 1996. Numerous associations have been created to support mothers who breastfeed, and they can prolong their postnatal maternity leave by an additional 16 weeks.

Child-Rearing Practices: Child-rearing practices are not excessively strict or permissive. Children receive a "happy medium" between rigorous English rules and Italian permissiveness. Discipline is fundamentally the same for boys and girls; however, gender roles are acquired early. European authorities are playing a greater part in education policy. This trend is quite evident in their role in important issues, such as teaching new technologies at school, issues involving the children of immigrants, equal opportunities for boys and girls, equivalence rating of diplomas, and exchange programs.

National Childhood Immunizations: Only vaccines against poliomyelitis are compulsory. The first three doses should be administered at 2, 4, and 15 months, the last dose at 6 years. Other inoculations are recommended, particularly for children in environments such as day care: DPT at 2, 3, 4, and 15 months; DT/Td at 6 and 16 years; HiB at 2, 3, 4, and 15 months; HepB at 2, 3, 4, and 15 months; and MMR at 12 months and at 10 to 13 years. The percent of the target population vaccinated, by antigen, is: DTP1 (98%); DTP3, Polio3 (97%); HepB3 (78%); HiB3 (95%), and MCV (88%).

Other Characteristics: Belgians appreciate compliance and good manners. For example, it is generally considered impolite for men to carry on a conversation while their hands are in their pockets or while they are wearing a hat. In more formal situations (meeting one's boss or applying for a job), these would be unacceptable. Rules are based on social status, age, and hierarchy. In public, people tolerate minor expressions of love between heterosexuals (e.g., holding hands, kissing). Belgians like moderate physical exercise; football, bicycling, and tennis are all considered national sports.

BIBLIOGRAPHY

Eco-Santé OCDE: 2005: Statistiques et indicateurs pour 30 pays, Comment la Belgique se positionne, 2005. Retrieved November 23, 2005, from http://www.oecd.org/dataoecd/14/61/34983456.pdf.

Nonneman W, van Doorslaer E: The role of the sickness funds in the Belgian health care market, *Soc Sci Med.* 39(10):1483, 1994.

Office de la Naissance et de l'Enfance: *Analyse de données de la banque de données médico-sociales et d'études associées de l'ONE,* Belgique, 2002.

Szpalski M et al.: Health care utilization for low back pain in Belgium: influence of sociocultural factors and health beliefs, *Spine.* 20(4):431, 1995.

Heylingen F: Belgium, society, character and culture—an essay on the Belgain identity, 2001. Retrieved November 22, 2005, from http://pespmc1.vub.ac.be/BelgCul2.html. http://statbel.fgov.be/port/hea_fr.asp (retrieved November 19, 2005).

OECD: Available at: http://www.oecd.org/document/56/0,2340,fr_2649_37407_32566008_1_1_1_37407,00.html (retrieved November 23, 2005).

World Health Organization: Available at: http://www.who.int/countries/bel/en/ (retrieved February 27, 2006).

UNAIDS: 2006 Belgium: Retrieved September 21, 2006, from http://www.unaids.org/en/Regions_Countries/Countries/belgium.asp.

B

◆ BELIZE

MAP PAGE (795)

Lisa Johnson, and Eleanor K. Herrmann

Location: Belize is a Central American and Caribbean nation located on the east coast of the Central American mainland. The capital is Belmopan. Belize faces the Caribbean Sea to the east and is bound on the north by Mexico and on the south and west by Guatemala. The total area is 22,960 km² (8,865 square miles). The coastline, just a few feet above sea level, is flat and swampy and fringed with islets (called *cayes*) and a 185-mile coral barrier reef—the longest in the Western Hemisphere. The entire northern and southern coastal areas are lowland plains. In the south, the terrain rises gradually inland to the Maya Mountains; the highest peak is 1,259 m (3,699 ft). More than 40% of the country is protected as parks and natural reserves. The climate is subtropical, and the country lies in the path of the Atlantic hurricane belt. The population is 287,730, with a gross domestic product (GDP) per capita of $5,800, with 33% below the poverty line. Tourism is the mainstay of the economy. Literacy rates are greater than 94% for both men and women.

Major Languages	Ethnic Groups	Major Religions
English (official)	Mestizo 49%	Roman Catholic 50%
Spanish	Creole 25%	Protestant 27%

Major Languages	Ethnic Groups	Major Religions
Garifuna (Carib)	Maya 11%	Other or None 23%
Creole	Garifuna 6.1%	
	Other 8.9%	

B

Health Care Beliefs: Passive role; acute sick care. Regular physical examinations are usually not practiced, but emphasis on preventive care is increasing. Before seeking medical aid, people use home remedies or over-the-counter medications, or they consult those who offer alternative medical care, such as the *obeah man*. People believe hot coca cola or lime juice relieves diarrhea and that they should avoid consuming hot foods, cold drinks, and heavy foods at night to ward off colic and nightmares.

Predominant Sick-Care Practices: Biomedical; herbal; magical-religious. Sick care practices vary according to ethnic groups and geographic location. Women with Obeah beliefs read cards, and dream books may be consulted to interpret the significance of dreams. People believe in the power of the "evil eye" *(mal ojo)*, and among women the expression "cut your eye at someone" means to cast the evil eye. Family herbal recipes are often used before or with biomedical treatment. People seek nurses and doctors for advice and care, and each of the six districts of Belize has a government hospital. In addition, Belize has health centers and rural health posts, and most centers have a mobile clinic that periodically visits small, remote villages. A pilot project for a National Health Insurance program was launched several years ago.

Ethnic-/Race-Specific or Endemic Diseases: Malaria, especially in rural areas, and gastroenteritis caused by unsafe food handling, poor sanitation facilities, and untreated water continue to be major health threats. There are also occasional small outbreaks of dengue fever. Diabetes mellitus, hypertension, and sickle cell disease are also present in the population, the last to a much smaller degree than the previous two. Children are especially susceptible to acute respiratory tract infections and diarrheal diseases. There is limited information on human immunodeficiency virus/acquired immunodeficiency syndrome (HIV/AIDS), and it is difficult to assess its impact on population groups. The United Nations Joint Programme on HIV/AIDS (UNAIDS) and the World Health Organization estimate the prevalence rate in adults (aged 15 to 49) to be 2.5%, with 3,700 living with HIV, including 1000 women and fewer than 100 children aged 0 to 14 years. Fewer than 500 people have died of AIDS. Belize is reported to have the highest HIV prevalence rate in Central America.

Health-Team Relationships: Patients do not usually question doctors. Doctor-nurse relationships are superior-subordinate, with nurses assuming the subordinate role. There are at least two "offshore" medical schools. In 2000, the School of Nursing became a department within the University of Belize.

Families' Role in Hospital Care: Family members are now expected to provide the care that was once provided by nurses. Family members also act as advocates, and some families bring food daily. Chronically ill older adults are often cared for at home but are hospitalized for acute illnesses. At least three nursing homes are currently operating. Currently, mentally ill adults are hospitalized in Belize's only mental hospital, but psychiatric care is now being decentralized to the districts and includes acute care facilities, halfway houses, and daycare centers.

Dominance Patterns: Most households are headed by women.

Eye-Contact Practices: Many people will maintain direct eye contact, even with authority figures.

Touch Practices: Greetings are usually formal.

Perceptions of Time: People do not adhere closely to time schedules.

Pain Reactions: Expressive reactions predominate. Cancer is commonly suspected if a reason for pain is not apparent or identified. It is often believed that if the presence of pain is denied, it will go away.

Birth Rites: About 16% of children are born to mothers younger than 20 years. More than 59% of the children born are to single mothers and are referred to as "outside children." In addition to having nurse midwives, Belize has a program to train traditional birth attendants, who are recognized as primary health care workers by the Ministry of Health. The fertility rate is 3.6 children born per woman. The infant mortality rate is 25 deaths per 1,000 live births. Life expectancy is 66 for men, 70 for women.

Death Rites: People are demonstrative in their expressions of grief. Religious services are generally held for the deceased. Funeral processions include many cars and people, and burial in above-ground vaults is customary in coastal areas.

Food Practices and Intolerances: Rice, red beans, and fish are food staples and are highly seasoned with pepper. Corn is a staple among Maya Indian groups. The diet is high in carbohydrates.

Infant-Feeding Practices: Breastfeeding is encouraged, but only 24% of infants are exclusively breastfed for their first 3 months. Socioeconomic status influences the decision to breastfeed. Hospitals in Belize will bottle-feed children of HIV/AIDS mothers and mothers who have had surgery.

Child-Rearing Practices: Disposable diapers are used in most instances, except when they cannot be afforded. Toilet training begins as soon as the child can sit up. In school, sex education is presented coeducationally to 10- to 12-year-old boys and girls. About 95% of women of childbearing age (i.e., 15 to 44 years) know of at least one modern method of contraception. Grandmothers are frequently involved in child care and in many instances are the primary caregivers. Child abuse is no longer a taboo subject.

National Childhood Immunizations: BCG at birth; DTwP at 2, 4, and 6 months and at 4 years; OPV at 2, 4, and 6 months and at 4 years; DTwPHiB Hep at 2, 4, and 6 months; MMR at 1 and 2 years; IPV at 4 years; Td at over 6 years. The percent of the target population vaccinated, by antigen, is: BCG, DTP3, Polio3 (96%); DTP1 (97%); and MCV (95%). Full immunization before a child's first birthday is more likely among

B

those living in towns, Creole children, and children of mothers who have nine or more years of schooling.

Other Characteristics: Forty-one percent of the population is younger than 14 years. Skin color and physical features can influence status and opportunity.

BIBLIOGRAPHY

Central Intelligence Agency (2006). Belize. Retrieved July 12, 2006, from https://www.cia.gov/cia/publications/factbook/geos/bh.html.

UNAIDS, 2006, Belize. Retrieved September 21, 2006, from http://www.unaids.org/en/Regions_Countries/Countries/belize.asp.

World Health Organization: 2006: Immunization, vaccines and biologicals. Retrieved September 21, 2006, from http://www.who.int/immunization_monitoring/en/globalsummary/countryprofileresult.cfm?C='blz'.

◆ BENIN (REPUBLIC OF)

MAP PAGE (800)

David Houeto

Location: Benin is a small country, with a total area of 115,000 km^2 (44,390 square miles), on the western coast of Africa, with the Atlantic Ocean to the south (121 km^2 of coastline), Togo to the west, Burkina Faso and Niger to the north, and Nigeria to the east. In the south, it is humid (subtropical), in the middle it is semi-dry (semiarid), and in the north it is hot and dry (sub-Saharan). The capital is Porto-Novo. Benin has five major trading languages: Fon in the south, Yorouba in the southeast, Dendi in the central region, and Barriba and Haussa in the north, and 50 dialects. The total population is 8.4 million, with a gross domestic product (GDP) per capita of $1,100, with 33% below the poverty line. Literacy rates are 46% for men, 23% for women.

Major Languages	Ethnic Groups	Major Religions
French (official)	African 99%	Indigenous beliefs 50%
Tribal languages	European 1%	Muslim 20%
		Christian 30%

Health Care Beliefs: Passive role; traditional. Public health service and social workers participate in health promotion and disease prevention programs that are based on United Nations Children's Fund (UNICEF) suggestions: vaccination programs *(programme elargie de vaccination [PEV])*, weight control for babies, and nutritional education for mothers. During the last 10 years, health-promotion activities for the general public have increased greatly. People fear mental illness, especially where voodoo is practiced (in the south and middle of Benin). People believe in the "evil eye" (the belief that a person can make others ill by looking at them), and they protect themselves with fetish-related items called *gris-gris*.

Predominant Sick-Care Practices: Biomedical; magical-religious. People seek help from traditional healers or doctors, depending on the health problem. They frequently visit traditional healers for psychological problems and conditions such as epilepsy, fever, or cramps. Amulets are worn around the neck or limbs and are believed to ward off a variety of illnesses. Scarification, the process of cutting the skin so as to produce a pattern of scars, is sometimes believed to be a protection against evil eye. Whether to seek help from a doctor depends primarily on finances because patients have to pay for everything in advance. If it is really necessary, most attempt to visit a doctor, nurse, or midwife. Dispensaries are disseminated throughout the country and provide basic low-cost drugs because there is no health insurance. Prescription drugs, if available, are expensive and beyond the financial capability of most individuals.

Ethnic-/Race-Specific or Endemic Diseases: Sickle cell disease is race specific, affecting only black people. The most prevalent disease is malaria, followed by bacterial and protozoal diarrheal diseases, the major causes of death in children from birth to 4 years of age. Anemia is frequent, more a consequence of malaria than malnutrition. Malnutrition and certain illnesses such as measles, accompanied by nutritional taboos, put children at even greater risk. For example, in the south of Benin, children infected with measles are not allowed to have protein and red palm oil, so they often develop kwashiorkor or marasmus, and frequently they die. Disease prevalence is somewhat unclear as a result of inaccurate reporting. Hepatitis A, typhoid, and yellow fever are present in some locations, and there has been a recent outbreak of meningococcal meningitis. The United Nations Joint Programme on human immunodeficiency virus/ acquired immunodeficiency syndrome (HIV/AIDS) (UNAIDS) reports the prevalence rate of HIV in adults (aged 15 to 49) to be 1.8%, with 87,000 people living with HIV, including 45,000 women and 9,800 children aged 0 to 14 years. There have been 9,600 deaths from AIDS. About 62,000 children aged 0 to 17 have been orphaned because of AIDS. About 38% of pregnant women are receiving treatment to reduce mother-to-child transmission; overall, only 33% of HIV-infected men and women receive antiretroviral therapy. These rates may be underreported because people tend to deny the existence of HIV/AIDS. When someone dies, people say that the person died of something else, such as diarrhea or a cough. The people tend to believe HIV/AIDS is something fabricated by white people attempting to force Africans to use condoms so they will have fewer children.

Health-Team Relationships: An established hierarchy exists among doctors, nurses, and midwives. If doctors are present, they are the unquestioned leaders of the health team, and it is very difficult to criticize them. In dispensaries without doctors, a "main" nurse (who may be a man) is in charge. Health care workers tend to be very strict and dominating in their treatment of patients, and they generally do not exhibit much sympathy or pity.

Families' Role in Hospital Care: Family members usually stay with patients during hospitalization. The families provide food and clothing, change sheets, and bathe the patient. The nurses are responsible for

B

giving medications, cleansing wounds, and other ordered treatments. Compared with the role of the nurse in Western countries, the helping role of the nurse is very limited. Government support for health care is lacking.

Dominance Patterns: Men are dominant, and gender roles are strictly defined; however, men and women attempt to have independent incomes. Men are responsible for paying the fees associated with health care and education and are responsible for the family's cattle. Women are expected to raise the children, work in the fields, prepare the food, and care for the other domestic animals. Men are often unwilling to pay medical fees, so it can be difficult to convince a father to spend money on a sick child. Women have few rights regarding family planning: they cannot use birth control unless their husband agrees. The husband decides how many children his wife will have because having numerous children is considered a sign of strength or power. Having large families is also considered beneficial for women because the more children she has, the greater her social status. Things are changing, however, because children must go to school and fees are expensive.

Eye-Contact Practices: Eye contact varies in the different regions and among the various ethnicities. For example, the Bariba believe it is impolite to make direct eye contact with another person. In southern Benin, avoiding direct eye contact is a sign of respect: someone in a lower social class may avoid direct eye contact with a person of higher social status, although this is not always the case.

Touch Practices: Physical touching is acceptable and usually quite frequent. People tend to "look more with their hands than with their eyes."

Perceptions of Time: An African proverb says, "There is nothing more than time." Punctuality is not considered particularly important, so it varies significantly. Traditions also play an important role in cultural and daily life in that the future is considered far less important than the present.

Pain Reactions: Particularly in the north of Benin, most avoid expressing pain, and women are relatively quiet during labor. In certain social situations, such as being beaten at a police station, it is considered important to scream as much as possible.

Birth Rites: Infant mortality rates are high at 80 deaths per 1,000 live births. The fertility rate is 5.2 children born per woman. In certain villages, the mother takes a hot seated bath if her baby is delivered at home and continues to do so for about a month. The placenta is buried next to the family's house in a dry area. The birth of a son is often more celebrated than the birth of a daughter. Regardless, a family that already has four or five sons is usually anxious to have a daughter because daughters stay with the family and sons leave. Life expectancy is 52 for men, 54 for women.

Death Rites: The people of Benin have elaborate death ceremonies, especially for older and important people. When children or young people die, the ceremonies are small. Funerals are important ceremonies, and the deceased person is frequently celebrated on the yearly anniversary of the death. Ceremonies last at least 3 days. All family members bring money and often buy new cloth *(pagne)* for the whole family so that they can be dressed in the same material. More than 2 months' salary may

be spent on the funeral, or cattle may be sold to pay for it. Organ donations and autopsies are uncommon.

Food Practices and Intolerances: The basic foods are corn, millet, cassava, sweet potatoes, small fish, gumbo, tomatoes, onions, and meat, if
available. The food is usually eaten with the right hand, but forks are also
used. Favorite foods are corn puree *(pâte)* and meat (i.e., chicken, fish,
beef, goat, pig) in the Southern region and pounded yam and meat in
the central and northern regions. People have food taboos, such as not
eating certain foods when ill.

Infant-Feeding Practices: Infants are breastfed as long as possible.
Breastfeeding is one way a woman can delay another pregnancy. Some
people in the southern region participate in a practice called *gavage.*
When children are no longer being breastfed, their mothers may force-
feed them liquid food, which can lead to aspiration pneumonia.

Child-Rearing Practices: Children are raised in a family group in which
not only parents, but also aunts and older sisters, assume responsibilities.
In rural areas, the whole family sleeps in one room because the huts are
too small to separate children from parents; infants are always with their
mothers. Young children are not educated until they are about 3 years old
because it is more likely they will survive if they can reach this age. They
are expected to behave and follow orders given by the family. Fathers and
other men of the family are the most respected members of society.

National Childhood Immunizations: BCG at birth; DTwP at 6, 10, and
14 weeks; DTPHiBHep at 6, 10, and 14 weeks; OPV at birth and at 6,
10, and 14 weeks; measles at 9 months; and TT at first contact pregnancy
and at 1 and 6 months, at 1 year and 2 years; vitamin A at 6 months; and
YF at 9 months. The percent of the target population vaccinated, by antigen,
is: BCG, DTP1 (99%); DTP3, Polio3 (93%); HepB3 (92%); Hib3 (35%); MCV
(85%); and TT2 plus (69%). Medical staff members regularly travel to villages to provide immunizations. Social workers also monitor immunization
rates during weight-control sessions. In endemic areas, people also receive
the meningococcal meningitis vaccine.

BIBLIOGRAPHY

Central Intelligence Agency: 2006: *The world factbook, Benin.* Retrieved September
    21, 2006 from https://www.cia.gov/cia/publications/factbook/print/bn.html.
Cleland JG, Ali MM, Capo-Chichi V: Postpartum sexual abstinence in West Africa:
    implications for AIDS control and family planning programmes, *AIDS.* 13(1):125,
    1999.
INSAE: RGPH3 2002: *Caractéristiques socio-culturelles et économiques,* Tome 3,
    Oct 2003.
INSAE: *Enquête démographique et de santé 2001,* June 2002.
MSP/Benin (Ministère de la santé publique): *Annuaire statistique 2003.* Cotonou, 2004.
UNAIDS: 2006 Benin. Retrieved September 15, 2006 from http://unaids.org/en/
    Regions_Countries/Countries/benin.asp.
World Health Organization: 2006: Immunization, Vaccines and Biologicals. Retrieved
    September 21, 2006 from http://www.who.int/immunization_monitoring/en/
    globalsummary/countryprofileresult.cfm?C='ben'.

◆ BHUTAN (KINGDOM OF)

B

MAP PAGE (804)

Suraj Bahadur Thapa

Location: Bhutan is a small, mostly mountainous country on the southeast slope of the Himalayas, with China to the north and west, India to the south and east. A succession of lofty and rugged mountains reaches 7,315 m (24,000 ft), separated by deep and sometimes high fertile valleys and savannas. The climate is tropical in the southern plains and has thick forests. Most people live in the areas between the plains and the high mountains. The capital is Thimphu, and the total area is 47,000 km² (18,100 square miles). The climate in the central valleys is characterized by cool winters and hot summers, whereas the Himalaya region has severe winters and cool summers. The country's name means "land of the thunder dragon," a reference to the violent storms that originate in the Himalayas. The population is estimated at 2.2 million; however, the Bhutanese government states that the country's population is about 750,000. The discrepancy is a result of the official census, which did not count people of Nepali origin. About 40% of the population comprises children aged 0 to 14 years. Bhutan is one of the least developed economies and is based on agriculture and forestry. The gross domestic product (GDP) per capita is $1,400. Literacy rates are 60% for men, 34% for women.

Major Languages	Ethnic Groups	Major Religions
Dzongkha (official)	Bhote, Ngalop,	Lamaistic Buddhism 70%
Nepalese dialects	Sharchop 50%	Indian- and Nepalese-
Tibetan dialects	Ethnic Nepalese 35%	influenced Hinduism
	Indigenous and	25%
	migrant tribes 15%	Other 5%

Lamaistic Buddhism is the state religion, but Hindus have de facto religious freedom. Bhutan's ethnic groups include the Bhote and Ngalop, of Tibetan origin; the Sharchop, of Indo-Mongoloid origin; and ethnic Nepalese. Bhotes and Ngalops speak various Tibetan dialects; Nepalese speak various Nepalese dialects.

Health Care Beliefs: Acute sick care; passive role. Bhutan has a stable, traditional social structure. Most take a passive role regarding illness. Rather than preventing disease, people tend to seek care only when they are acutely ill. Some believe that events are determined by "the fates," or the deities, and cannot be changed. Using treatments and foods that are considered "hot" versus "cold" (according to Hindu ayurvedic classification) for illness is common in an effort to bring the body back into equilibrium. For example, herbal medicine is considered "cold," and Western medicine is considered "hot." As more Westernized medical care becomes available, beliefs about health care have begun to include both traditional and modern viewpoints. For example, a recent study attempted to evaluate traditional treatments and factors that people believed caused diarrhea. Natural causes were reported more frequently than supernatural causes, with the most important being teething (76%), followed by "cold" food (58%), stale food (53%), hot food (41%), and dirty water (38%); however, the terminology individuals used to describe dehydration indicated strong links to supernatural causes, and people had insufficient information about diarrhea management. About 83% of mothers said they continued breastfeeding when their infants had diarrhea, but 75% said that they occasionally or always withheld fluids, and 58% said that they withheld food also.

Predominant Sick-Care Practices: Biomedical; traditional; magical-religious. People believe that sickness comes to those who have been evil. Indian ayurvedic medicine and Tibetan herbal medicine are practiced, and people have faith in local healers. Bhutan's medical system improved in the 1960s with the establishment of the Department of Public Health and openings of new hospitals and dispensaries throughout the country. Western medical care has gradually been introduced since the 1980s. As of the 1990s, Bhutan had 29 general hospitals (including 5 leprosy hospitals, 3 army hospitals, and 1 mobile hospital), 46 dispensaries, and 15 malaria eradication centers. In 1997, the country had 2.03 doctors and 1.13 nurses, 0.57 pharmacists, and 0.97 dentists per 10,000 population, and 43,239 hospital beds. Training has been provided for health care assistants, nurses' aides, midwives, primary health care workers, and village volunteers. During pregnancy, 72% of women are attended by trained personnel, as are 24% of deliveries. Medical facilities are still limited, and some medications are in short supply. Individuals (primarily visitors) with serious medical problems are often sent to other countries for treatment.

Ethnic-/Race-Specific or Endemic Diseases: Endemic diseases are dengue fever, malaria in rural areas, respiratory diseases (including tuberculosis), iodine-deficiency goiter, leprosy, cholera, parasitic diseases, typhoid fever (including antibiotic-resistant strains), hepatitis A and B, and vitamin A deficiency in certain areas. People are at risk for various gastrointestinal diseases caused by parasites, altitude sickness, rabies, leprosy, and injuries from motor-vehicle accidents. Handwashing and sanitary waste disposal are not practiced in some areas, which contaminates drinking water. Young women may self-inflict burns in response to family quarrels. The United Nations Joint Programme on human immunodeficiency virus/acquired immunodeficiency syndrome (HIV/AIDS) (UNAIDS) estimates the prevalence rate for HIV in adults (aged 5 to 49) to be less than 0.01%, with fewer than 500 people living with HIV, including fewer than 100 women. No estimates have been made for children from birth to 15 years, but 45 cases in children have been reported. Fewer than 100 people have died of AIDS.

B

Dominance Patterns: Developmental programs have led to additional opportunities for women. The National Women's Association of Bhutan is working to improve the economic status of women, and opportunities have opened up in the fields of nursing, administration, and teaching. Women occupy secondary positions in business and civil service, although the Bhutanese constitution guarantees equality. Nepalese tribal and communal customs dictate women's roles, but they differ by ethnic group and are usually determined by caste. Status is measured by land ownership, occupation, and perceived religious authority. In some sense, women have a dominant social position, in that land is often passed on to daughters instead of sons. Traditional society is matriarchal and patriarchal; the head of the family is often the one held in highest esteem. Women's social status is indicated by the color of their *kira,* or ankle-length dress. Men and women wear scarves and shawls, and the specific ways of folding the scarves, as well as their designs and colors, designate status. The laws in the 1990s still allowed a man to have as many as three wives if he had the first wife's permission. The first wife also had the power to sue for divorce and alimony if her husband married additional wives without her consent.

Infant-Feeding Practices: The median duration of breastfeeding is 28 months, and infants are fed on demand. Semisolid food is introduced at about 3 months. On average, the median duration of postpartum amenorrhea is about 12 months. In general, the only reason women stop breastfeeding within 2 years is because of a new pregnancy. In a study of mothers who had given birth 30 to 36 months previously in a traditional community, infants who were weaned during a subsequent pregnancy did not gain as much weight and had more infections than infants weaned at a later date and less abruptly. People believed that the breast milk of a pregnant woman could "rot" and make a child ill. They also believed that if the mother became pregnant and the child developed diarrhea, she should immediately stop breastfeeding, a practice that deprived the child of important nutrients needed to combat diarrhea. Four of every 10 children are found to be suffering from malnutrition. The fertility rate is 5.13 infants born per woman. The infant mortality rate is high at 98 deaths per 1000 live births. Life expectancy is 55 for both men and women.

Food Practices and Intolerances: Rice and corn are staples, and yak cheese is a staple for people who live in the mountains. Meat soups, spiced chilies, beef, pork, goat, and poultry are also eaten. Beverages include beer made from cereal grains and tea with butter. People have limited access to potable water.

National Childhood Immunizations: BCG at birth; DTwPHep at 6, 10, and 14 weeks; DT at 24 months; OPV at birth and at 6, 10, and 14 weeks; measles at 9 months; vitamin A at 6, 12, 18, 24, 30, and 36 months; TT in pregnant women after first contact and at 4 weeks, 6 months, and next pregnancy. The percent of the target population vaccinated, by antigen, is:

BCG (99%); DTP1 (97%); DTP3, HepB3, Polio3 (95%), MCV (93%); and TT2 plus (86%). Because good health results from past virtue, people do not always believe immunizations can affect future health.

B

Other Characteristics: Except for members of the royal family and a few other noble families, Bhutanese do not have surnames. They may be given two names, but neither is considered to be a family name. Some people adopt their village name, wives keep their own names, and children may have names that are not connected to either parent. Approximately 100,000 Bhutanese refugees live in refugee camps in southeast Nepal. Because of ethnic persecution, these ethnic Nepalese were forced to leave after new citizenship policies were enacted by the government. Some were tortured, causing anxiety, depression, posttraumatic stress disorder, persistent somatoform pain disorder, disability and dissociative (amnesia and conversion) disorders.

BIBLIOGRAPHY

Central Intelligence Agency: *2006: The world factbook, Bhutan*. Retrieved September 21, 2006, from https://www.cia.gov/cia/publications/factbook/print/bt.html.

Encarta: http://encarta.msn.com Djibouti, Microsoft Encarta Online Encyclopedia 2005, Microsoft, (retrieved February 27, 2006).

Kingdom of Bhutan: Available at: http://www.kingdomofbhutan.com (retrieved February 27, 2006).

Thapa SB et al. Psychiatric disability among Bhutanese refugees, *Am J Psychiatry*. 60:2032–7, 2003.

Travel State of Bhutan: Available at: http://travel.state.gov/bhutan.html (retrieved February 27, 2006).

UNAIDS, 2006 Bhutan: Retrieved September 21, 2006, from http://www.unaids.org/en/Regions_Countries/Countries/bhutan.asp.

Van-Ommeren M et al: Psychiatric disorders among tortured Bhutanese refugees in Nepal. *Arch Gen Psych.* 58(5):475, 2001.

World Health Organization: 2006: Immunization, vaccines and biologicals. Retrieved September 21, 2006 from http://www.who.int/immunization_monitoring/en/globalsummary/countryprofileresult.cfm?C='ben'.

◆ BOLIVIA (REPUBLIC OF)

MAP PAGE (797)

Francisco Javier Carod-Artal

Location: Bolivia is a landlocked country in the central part of South America, bordered on the west by Peru and Chile, on the south by Argentina, and on the east by Brazil and Paraguay. The total area is 1,098,580 km² (424,162 square miles). Lake Titicaca, the highest navigable lake in the world, is on its western border with Peru. The capital is La Paz. Three distinct cultural regions divide the country. The Andean

B

mountainous area of western Bolivia (La Paz and Oruro Departments) is the most traditional, whereas the high valley area in the central portion (Cochabamba) is home to many recent immigrants because of its moderate climate. The eastern plains area (Santa Cruz de la Sierra) is modernizing rapidly, both culturally and economically. Bolivia has 8.9 million people: by some estimates, 80% to 90% of the population is Amerindian. The gross domestic product (GDP) per capita is $2,900, and about 64% live below the poverty line. Literacy rates are 93% for men, 82% for women.

Major Languages	Ethnic Groups	Major Religions
Spanish (official)	Quechua 30%	Roman Catholic 95%
Amerindian languages	Aymara 25%	Protestant
(Quechua [official]	Mestizo (White and	(Evangelical
Aymara [official]	Amerindian) 30%	Methodist) 5%
Guarani)	White 15%	

Rapid immigration from rural to urban areas has exacerbated already strained economic and residential conditions in periurban areas given that 60% of the population resides in urban areas. The Roman Catholic religion (95%) coexists with ancestral devotion to the Earth Mother (*Pachamama*) in Andean regions. In Andean rural areas, many peasants speak *quechua* or *aymara* as their only language.

Health Care Beliefs: Acute sick care; traditional. The *kallawayas*, North Andean itinerant healers, are the most famous indigenous healers, and their traditional health system has been recognized as a cultural heritage by the World Health Organization (WHO). Many of their curative tools, including charms, plants, and llama fetuses, can be found in open markets such as the La Paz witchcraft market. Herbs and other locally grown plants are widely used for their medicinal qualities. Leaves or flowers may be boiled in water to produce a *mate*, or herbal tea. The coca leaf is widely used in mate to relieve stomachaches and headache distress caused from high altitudes. Urban phytotherapy represents a medicinal alternative to treat major health problems. Ethno-botanical studies in urban Bolivia have reported that the greatest number of medicinal plants and applications are for gastrointestinal and liver disorders, rheumatism and joint dislocations, kidney and urologic problems, and gynecologic disorders. Some medicinal species have magical connotations (e.g., for cleaning and protection against witchcraft, to bring good luck, or for Andean offerings to Pachamama). Many Andean people still rely heavily on traditional practices. The cultural equivalents of certain pathologies such as headache, anxiety *(susto)*, depression, psychosomatic diseases, and witchcraft are present in Andean peoples and are treated by *wilancha*, the ritual sacrifice of a llama offered to the Pachamama.

B

Predominant Sick-Care Practices: Biomedical; magical-religious. Western and indigenous health care practices are prevalent. Modern health care is offered through the national public health system, one of several employment-linked prepaid health plans called *seguros sociales,* health nongovernmental organizations or church-affiliated services, or a small fee-for-service private sector. In the public health sector, great strides have been made in reducing infant and maternal mortality rates through immunization and a maternal reproductive health program.

Ethnic-/Race-Specific or Endemic Diseases: The most prevalent illnesses are infectious; these include vaccine-preventable diseases and acute respiratory illnesses such as pneumonia. The Bolivia Integrated Local Development Programme (PRODELI) has reduced morbidity and mortality rates from water-borne disease in children under age 5 by improving water, sanitation, and environmental factors. About 25% of children under age 3 years experience diarrhea within the first 2 weeks of life. In a 2003 survey, although 84% of mothers who were interviewed reported knowing about oral rehydration therapy (ORT) for diarrhea, only 59% of children under the age of 5 received ORT and continued feeding. Cistycercosis, an infection caused by the worm *Taenia solium,* is a highly prevalent disease and a main cause of epilepsy. Malaria, dengue, and leishmaniasis are frequently found in the Amazon basin and eastern plains areas. A significant proportion of *Leishmania* transmission is in or around houses, often close to coffee or cacao plantations. Tuberculosis (TB) is common in the Andean region, and nonadherence to TB therapy among Aymara Indians has been reported. Cost of treatment, poor access to care, ethnic discrimination, and prior maltreatment by the health system are some of the reasons for abandoning treatment. Chagas disease, a *Trypanosoma cruzi* infection resulting from the bite of an insect called vinchuca *(Triatoma infestans),* is endemic in the highland valleys. Vinchuca often live in housing roof straw in rural areas. Up to 8% of the population in endemic areas is seropositive, although most remain asymptomatic until the chronic manifestations occur up to 30 years later. Dysphagia and painful swallowing are common symptoms in chagasic mega esophagus, whereas chronic constipation is characteristic of chagasic megacolon. Chagas cardiomyopathy is characterized by congestive heart failure, arrhythmia, thromboembolism, stroke, and sudden cardiac death. Wild populations of the vector are much more widespread throughout Bolivia than previously thought. In 2005 a nationwide health campaign promoted vitamin A and other micronutrient intake in children. Goiter is an endemic metabolic disease in adults and is most prevalent near the vast salt lakes of Uyuni, where few leafy green vegetables grow and diets have insufficient iodine. Prevalence has diminished since 90% of households now consume iodized salt. The first case of acquired immunodeficiency syndrome (AIDS) was reported in 1985. The United Nations Joint Programme on human immunodeficiency virus/acquired immunodeficiency syndrome (HIV/AIDS) (UNAIDS) reports

B

the prevalence rate for HIV in adults (aged 15 to 49) to be 0.1%, with 7,000 people living with HIV, including 1,900 women. There have been fewer than 500 AIDS deaths. Where the method of transmission is known, heterosexual sex accounts for 51% of cases, men who have sex with men for 41%, and injecting drug use for 3%. Only 22% of women have a comprehensive knowledge of HIV, and only 56% know that a condom might prevent it.

Health-Team Relationships: Health care is driven by doctors. More doctors graduate each year than can be absorbed into the economy. Nursing is a low-paid, low-status profession. Graduate training in public health is offered at the University of San Andres in La Paz, at the University of San Simon in Cochabamba, and at the Real Pontificia University in Sucre. Each year, several thousand foreign students (mainly Brazilian) study medicine in Cochabamba and Santa Cruz de la Sierra. Because of the sizeable disparities in education and socioeconomic status between doctors and many of their native patients, patients commonly cite lack of trust and poor communication as barriers to quality care. Language is another barrier and is particularly a problem for native rural women and recent migrants who have settled in heavily populated periurban areas.

Families' Role in Hospital Care: In rural areas, it is not unusual for family members to stay with a hospitalized patient to prepare their food and change their linens. In more urban areas, where more resources are available, family members may supplement services offered by the hospital, although it is not required.

Dominance Patterns: Andean cultures promote male dominance and social and group integration. *Mita,* or traditional community work, is still common in rural areas. Labor organizations *(sindicatos)* have fought politically against the government in recent years. Strikes, roadblocks *(bloqueos),* and social emergency situations in 2005 resulted in serious food shortages in the cities. The literacy rate is 92% for men, 79% for women.

Eye-Contact Practices: It is common in Andean cultures to lower the eyes as a sign of respect. Because of the tremendous differences in social class and education between health care providers and patients, communication barriers can be troublesome if the providers have not been educated about how to overcome the problem.

Birth Rites: Many Andean communities are too far from a hospital for care, or they lack trust in Western medicine. Certain common beliefs surround pregnancy and childbirth. During pregnancy, women are advised to avoid sun and heat and refrain from lifting heavy objects. They do not eat spicy foods because they think these foods can cause bleeding. For Andean people, mental retardation in the infant is considered the result of a fright suffered by the mother during pregnancy. In some rural communities, childhood epilepsy is thought to be the consequence of witchcraft or abuse toward the child or mother during pregnancy. Because the first sign of pregnancy is the cessation of menstrual bleeding, women believe that blood is accumulating for the birth. Swelling of the feet and hands is regarded as a good sign; it suggests that the blood is accumulating as it should. In the rural Andes, women like a warm, intimate setting for birth. They believe that cold and wind should be avoided because they might cause fever and chills during the postpartum period. During the delivery, women drink warm teas, or mates, to stimulate the flow of blood, facilitate the birth, and aid in delivery of the placenta. After delivery, the husband or another close family member washes the placenta and buries it in a protected place, often beneath the foundation of the house. The burial of the placenta ensures that the mother and infant will live a contented life, and women, particularly those with rural origins, are reluctant to give birth in hospitals because hospitals do not respect this practice. To encourage women to deliver in hospitals, some are returning the placentas to mothers for traditional burial. Adjusted maternal (420 per 100,000 live births) and infant mortality rates (53 per 1,000 live births) are very high. As many as 30% of maternal deaths are associated with induced abortions. The fertility rate is 2.85 children born per woman. Since the National Ministry of Health has encouraged all women to give birth in hospital settings, the percentage of births that are attended by trained personnel has increased to 65%. Premarital conception rates among sexually active single women are rising. The number of women who use birth control has been estimated at 58%. Among women who know of at least one method, only 31% have used a modern method (commonly birth control pills and intrauterine devices). Some 37% reported using a traditional method (rhythm method or withdrawal before ejaculation). Fears about contraceptive use are still common, but widespread recognition of the increasing costs of raising a child is propelling many young couples to space births and to plan their family size. Life expectancy is 63 for men, 67 for women.

Death Rites: In some rural areas, newborns are not named until 7 days after birth because of fears that the infant may die. Traditionally, the body of the deceased is washed in the river. Ancient ceremonies honoring ancestors are performed every year in November at Andean cemeteries in a festival that remembers deceased family members and Catholic saints. Music, songs, and food are brought to cemeteries as symbols of respect; on some occasions, willancha and other animal sacrifices are performed. In isolated rural Indian areas, ancestors were buried beneath the houses and inside the *chullpas* (pre-Inca memorial buildings).

Food Practices: The potato is the staple of the Bolivian diet, and more than 300 varieties have been identified. Bolivians freeze-dry potatoes by soaking them in water and exposing them to the sun or the freezing nights of the June winter, making potatoes available year round. The freeze-dried potato, or *chuño*, is considered a national delicacy. Quinua *(Chenopodium quinoa)* soup is a part of the Andean dinner that provides necessary liquids.

B

Infant-Feeding Practices: Breastfeeding is prevalent. About 54% of infants younger than 6 months are breastfed exclusively, and 46% of children still receive some breast milk at 24 months. Mate is often the first food given to a newborn in Andean communities, a practice that may be related to the ancient practice of giving newborns broth made from tender corn boiled for 3 days. At high altitudes (such as in La Paz, where water boils at 88° C), the boiling temperature may not be high enough to kill water-borne bacteria, thus making the infant vulnerable to diarrhea.

Child-Rearing Practices: People who live in rural areas or who have recently migrated from a rural to an urban area swaddle their infants, and the mothers carry them on their back in brightly woven blankets. Mothers can then easily nurse their infants by simply slipping them forward under their arms.

National Childhood Immunizations: BCG at birth; DTwPHibHep at 2, 4, and 6 months; MMR at 12 to 23 months; OPV at 2, 4, and 6 months; Y Fat 1 year; vitamin A at age under 5 years; Td: CBAW (15 to 49 years) and first contact pregnancy, +1 +6 months, +1 +1 year; HepB at birth (in sentinel hospitals). The percent of the target population vaccinated, by antigen, is: BCG (93%); DPT1 (94%); DTP3, HepB3, HiB3 (81%); MCV (64%); and Polio3 (79%).

BIBLIOGRAPHY

Carod-Artal FJ, Vazquez-Cabrera CB: Ethnographic study of neurological and mental diseases among the Uru-Chipaya peoples of the Andean Altiplano, Rev Neurol. 41 (2):115–125, 2005.

Carod-Artal FJ et al. Chagasic cardiomyopathy is independently associated with ischemic stroke in Chagas disease, Stroke. 36(5):965–70, 2005.

Central Intelligence Agency: 2006: The world factbook, Bolivia. Retrieved September 21, 2006, from https://www.cia.gov/cia/publications/factbook/print/bl.html.

Frost MB et al. Maternal education and child nutritional status in Bolivia: finding the links, Soc Sci Med. 60(2):395–407, 2005.

Greene JA: An ethnography of nonadherence: culture, poverty, and tuberculosis in urban Bolivia, Cult Med Psychiatry. 28(3):401–25, 2004.

Macia MJ et al: An ethnobotanical survey of medicinal plants commercialized in the markets of La Paz and El Alto, Bolivia, J Ethnopharmacol. 97(2):337–50, 2005.

Noireau F et al: Can wild Triatoma infestans foci in Bolivia jeopardize Chagas' disease control efforts? Trends Parasitol. 21(1):7–10, 2005.

Nicoletti A et al: Epilepsy and neurocysticercosis in rural Bolivia: a population-based survey. Epilepsia. 46(7):1127–32, 2005.

UNAIDS: 2006 Bolivia. Retrieved September 21, 2006, from http://www.unaids.org/en/Regions_Countries/Countries/bolivia.asp.

UNICEF: http://www.unicef.org/infobycountry/bolivia_statistics.html, 2004 (retrieved February 23, 2006).

World Health Organization: 2006: Immunization, vaccines and biologicals. Retrieved September 21, 2006, from http://www.who.int/immunization_monitoring/en/globalsummary/countryprofileresult.cfm?C='bol'.

◆ BOSNIA-HERZEGOVINA (REPUBLIC OF BOSNIA AND HERZEGOVINA)

B

MAP PAGE (798)

Geoffrey Hodgetts

Location: Formerly part of Yugoslavia, Bosnia-Herzegovina is located on the Balkan Peninsula in southeastern Europe. It borders the Adriatic Sea (20 km), Croatia (930 km), and Serbia-Montenegro (530 km), with a total area of approximately 51,000 km^2 (19,686 square miles). The capital is Sarajevo. The terrain consists of mountains, valleys, and an area of flat, arable land in the southwest formed by the River Neretva, which flows south to the Adriatic. Two other rivers, the Vrbas and the Bosna, flow northeast into the Sava River. The Sava River, forming the border with Croatia, flows into the Danube River, which empties into the Black Sea. As a result of the Dayton Peace Accords, the country was divided into two entities, a Muslim/Croat Federation (about 51% of the country) and the Republika Srpska (49%). Bosnia-Herzegovina generally has hot summers and cold winters. The southwestern areas near the Adriatic Sea tend to have milder, wetter winters and longer summers, not unlike the climate in Italy or other northern Mediterranean countries. The gross domestic product (GDP) per capita is $6,800, with about 25% below the poverty line.

Major Languages	Ethnic Groups	Major Religions
Serbo-Croatian (also known as Serbian, Croatian, or Bosnian, depending on location in the country)	Bosniak 48.1% Serb 37% Croat 14.3% Other 0.6%	Slavic Muslim 40% Orthodox 31% Roman Catholic 15% Protestant 4% Other 10%

The population is about 4.5 million. The 1992–1995 war caused major shifts in the population; approximately 250,000 were killed, 1.5 million were internally displaced (refugees within their own country), and many thousands left the country as refugees. Approximately one quarter have returned to their original homes. The exact composition of the country by religion and ethnic groups is currently unknown. The Croatian, Bosnian, and Serbian languages are all essentially the same language with some word and phrase differences. Medical professionals often use traditional Latin terms for diagnosis, anatomic descriptions, and so on. In the former Yugoslavia, Bosnia-Herzegovina was considered a melting pot of ethnic groups. Following the war, however, the three ethnic and religious groups became more separated. The Bosnian Serbs, who are Orthodox

B

Christians, live primarily in the central northern, eastern, and southeastern parts of the country bordering on Serbia-Montenegro. The Bosnian Croats live primarily in the southwestern part bordering on Croatia and are Roman Catholic. The Bosnian Muslims, or Bosniaks (Muslims married to either Serbs or Croats), live in the central and south central part. Literacy rates are 98% for men, 91% for women.

Health Care Beliefs: Active involvement; holistic. People seek help for medical conditions primarily from doctors; however, there is a major emphasis on vitamins, traditional teas, and other home remedies, often suggested by doctors. There is much self-prescribing, and because of poor regulation of pharmacies, many prescription drugs are bought over the counter without a doctor's prescription.

Predominant Sick-Care Practices: Biomedical; traditional. The medical system is based on the eastern European polyclinic model. The major cities have very large hospitals; smaller cities and larger towns have large, outpatient, multispecialist clinics; and spread throughout the cities, towns, and rural villages are smaller clinics, or ambulantas, run by general practitioners. The primary care system is fragmented and rudimentary, and general practitioners refer most patients to specialists for the simplest conditions. This situation is changing as international aid organizations work to upgrade the skills and knowledge of local practitioners, introduce modern approaches in medical schools, and establish effective postgraduate training programs. Physician administrators, chosen for their political party affiliation, manage clinics and hospitals. Most nurses only have a high school education and lack many of the skills possessed by nurses in Western health care systems.

Ethnic-/Race-Specific or Endemic Diseases: Smoking is extremely prevalent, and the diet includes large amounts of red meat, fat, salt, and cheese. Not surprisingly, heart disease is common. Programs aimed at decreasing lifestyle risk factors for cardiovascular disease are just beginning and have been minimally effective. Post-traumatic stress disorder and depression are common because of the mental trauma experienced by so many people in the 1990s war. Poverty also affects the mental and physical health of many displaced people, who live as refugees within their own country. Tuberculosis is fairly common because of poverty and a lack of readily available treatments. Human immunodeficiency virus (HIV) and acquired immunodeficiency syndrome (AIDS) are not yet common, and blood products are not being consistently screened. The United Nations Joint Programme on HIV/AIDS (UNAIDS) estimates prevalence rates for HIV in adults (aged 15 to 49) to be less than 0.1% but rising. There are no estimates for children. Life expectancy is 74 for men, 81 for women.

Health-Team Relationships: Doctors are the dominant health care providers, and nurses serve in assistant roles. The concept of a health team has recently been successfully introduced as part of the development of a family medicine model. Specialists still make most of the important decisions about patient care, with general practitioners required to follow their recommendations with little question.

Families' Role in Hospital Care: The role taken on by the family is determined primarily by the economic situation. Hospitals have very limited resources, poorly paid staff, and a shortage of supplies and medications. Often families must make informal copayments (bribes) to hospital staff, bring food, and assist with caretaking tasks.

Dominance Patterns: As in most European societies, white men are nominally dominant. Large numbers of women are in the workforce, and they also run most aspects of home life. Women still take on the traditional role of homekeeper and childraiser, but at the same time, they often work in business or government offices or on the farm. Most roles of authority, such as heads of important governmental and nongovernmental departments and deans of colleges, tend to be male. This is less true at the primary care level, where most doctors, nurses, and leaders are women.

Eye-Contact Practices: Direct eye contact is acceptable.

Touch Practices: Regardless of gender, two people who do not know each other well greet with a handshake. A man and woman meeting for the first time usually shake hands but on subsequent meetings may greet each other with a kiss on both cheeks. *Dobar dan,* meaning "good day," is the standard verbal greeting.

Perceptions of Time: Whether because of a relaxed attitude or just because of poor organizational skills, people often forget or miss meetings. Making an appointment is not commonly done, even at the most senior levels. People tend to focus on the present and immediate future.

Pain Reactions: As in many societies, women typically express pain more freely than men.

Birth Rites: Infants are usually born in hospitals. The quality of antepartum care varies greatly across the country and is not standardized. The fertility rate is 1.22 children born per mother, and the infant mortality rate is 10 deaths per 1,000 live births. Life expectancy is 74 for men, 82 for women.

Death Rites: The treatment of the dead follows Christian and Muslim traditions. In large cities, some graves are marked by crosses and some by Islamic symbols—all in the same cemetery. Since the war, the newer cemeteries have tended to be either Christian or Muslim, but not both.

Food Practices and Intolerances: Muslims do not eat pork. Lamb is a favorite meat throughout the country, and restaurants selling only lamb dishes often line the roads between cities. Outside these restaurants, whole lambs cook outdoors over large rotisserie barbecues. The diet is high in meat overall and has strong eastern Mediterranean influences. *Civap cici* (pronounced "chevap-chee-chee"), a dish consisting of ground meat (lamb and beef) served in a bread pocket, is a favorite fast food at lunchtime, as are meat pies. They tend to be very greasy, similar to a Western hamburger. Cafes and cafe-bars are common, as are dessert and ice cream shops. Fresh vegetables and fruits are common, with yellow and red peppers a favorite, often stuffed with minced meat, as are onions and tomatoes. Fruits are readily available from the Dalmatian coast. Vegetables, fruits, meat, and fish with very reasonable prices are all readily available in large quantities in the open markets. Throughout Bosnia-Herzegovina, but especially in Herzegovina, fish is a popular dish readily available from Croatian fishermen on the Adriatic (Dalmatian) coast. Squid (*lignje*) is popular, as are trout from fish farms along the various rivers.

Child-Rearing Practices: Child rearing varies greatly. Child care ranges from loving, caring methods where children are guided (firmly if necessary); to a strict authoritarian approach in which corporal punishment is the norm. Extended family members play a large part in child care. Traditional myths or beliefs often surround the care of infants, such as not allowing infants to go outside during the first month of life.

National Childhood Immunizations: BCG at birth; HepB at birth and at 2 and 6 months; DTwP at 3, 4, and 6 months and at 2 and 5 years; DTwPHiB at 3, 4, 6, and 18 months (in part of the country); OPV at 3, 4, and 6 months and at 2, 7 and 14 years; MMR at 2 and 6 years; DT 7 years (part of country); TT at 18 years; Td at 14 years; rubella 14 years (in part of the country, girls); and HiB at 2, 4, and 18 months (in part of the country). The percent of the target population vaccinated, by antigen, is: BCG, DTP1, Polio3 (95%); DTP3, HepB3 (93%); HiB3 (50%); and MCV (90%).

Other Characteristics: In cities, adolescents and young adults who can afford to do so dress in the latest Western styles (often in black). Going out for the evening just to walk and converse is the usual social habit, particularly with high unemployment and crowded housing conditions. In the countryside, one is more likely to see a woman dressed in old but colorful clothes looking like something out of the last century; walking behind a flock of sheep and driving them along with a stick. Another common sight would be a man and his son in a horse-drawn cart full of hay, moving slowly along the narrow road as cars edge their way past. As the country rebuilds from the war and 50 years of communist rule, the contrast between those becoming wealthy and those who remain poor or are refugees is becoming more striking.

BIBLIOGRAPHY

Central Intelligence Agency: *2006: The World factbook*, Bosnia and Herzegovina. Retrieved September 21, 2006, from https://www.cia.gov/cia/publications/factbook/print/bk.html.

Office of the High Representative in Bosnia Herzegovina: Retrieved February 27, 2006, from http://www.ohr.int/.

OSCE in Bosnia and Herzegovina: Retrieved February 27, 2006 from http://www.oscebih.org/.

UNAIDS: 2006: Bosnia and Herzegovina: Retrieved September 21, 2006, from http://www.unaids.org/en/Regions_Countries/Countries/bosnia_herzegovina.asp.

UNHCR in Bosnia: Retrieved February 27, 2006, from http://www.unhcr.ba/.

World Health Organization: 2006: Immunization, vaccines and biologicals. Retrieved September 21, 2006, from http://www.who.int/immunization_monitoring/en/globalsummary/countryprofileresult.cfm?C='bih'.

B

◆ BOTSWANA (REPUBLIC OF)

MAP PAGE (801)

Julie Livingston

Location: Botswana is a semiarid, landlocked country in sub-Saharan Africa with a total area of almost 582,000 km^2 (224,652 square miles). The country has long borders with South Africa, Namibia, and Zimbabwe, and a 700-m border with the Republic of Zambia, the world's shortest international border. Most of the country's land mass is taken up by the Kalahari Desert, but the capital, Gaborone, is located in the southeast, close to the South African border. Since its independence in 1966, Botswana has become renowned for its good governance, intolerance for corruption, and respect for legal processes. It was one of the world's poorest countries before independence, but the discovery of large diamond reserves now drives the economy. The government has channeled resources into roads, schools, hospitals, clinics, health centers, and mobile clinics. Most residents identify with the village from which they came and maintain a second residence in their natal village for weekends or vacations. The population is small relative to the size of the country, is growing rapidly, and is greater than 1.7 million. The gross domestic product (GDP) per capita is $10,500, with 30% below the poverty line.

Major Languages	Ethnic Groups	Major Religions
English (official)	Batswana 95%	Christian 50%
Setswana	Bakalanga,	Indigenous beliefs
	Bakgalagadi,	50%
	Basawara,	
	Baherero 4%	
	White 1%	

Most of Botswana's people belong to the Setswana-speaking groups, or *merafe*. In the past, each *merafe* occupied a separate area, acknowledged the supremacy of the chief (*kgosi*) as the ruler in the community, and constituted a single political unit under the ruler's leadership and authority. In 1963 it was decided that to ensure national unity, people's allegiance should be to the nation rather than to individual *merafe*. The chiefs (*dikgosi*) thus lost some of their powers, and a new government was elected. *Dikgosi* were recognized by the creation of a House of Chiefs, whose major role is to advise the government on *merafe* and customary matters. The concept of *kgotla* is as old as Tswana culture and a foundation for Botswana's modern democracy. *Kgotla* is a village meeting

B

place where all matters pertaining to village policies, developments, and even disputes are discussed and agreed on. *Kgotlas* are usually situated next to the chief's home so that he or she can consult anytime as the need arises. Population migration is characterized by traditional seasonal movements between tribal villages, agricultural lands (*masimo*), and cattle posts (*meraka*). About 48.3% of the population is younger than 15 years. About 48% reside in rural areas and depend on subsistence agriculture for their livelihood. Health-services delivery has improved tremendously since independence, and Botswana has universal free education.

Health Care Beliefs: Acute sick care; traditional. Many people believe that only traditional healers are competent to treat certain diseases, one of which is mental illness. The whole family receives treatment and is encouraged to take the medicines or perform the prescribed rituals in a cohesive manner so that the sick person is cured. Older people are important for their knowledge of traditional practices relating to illness. In Tswana folk medicine, the heart is considered the central organ of the body and the primary origin of feelings, thoughts, and emotions. Episodes of illness invariably lead to questions such as, "Why has this happened to me" and "Why is this happening now?" Tswana healers may decide that a disease is caused by witchcraft, an ancestor's anger, breaking a taboo related to pollution, or God's will. Although the first three causes involve specific rituals or behavioral measures, "God's will" is often the diagnosis people resort to when treatment attempts have failed. Such a diagnosis calls for acceptance and stoic resignation. People increasingly seek cures from Christian healing prophets through rites involving prayer and water.

Predominant Sick-Care Practices: Biomedical; magical-religious. Botswana inherited a largely curative, hospital-based health care delivery system; however, most of the population had no access to any services. In 1975 a separate Ministry of Health was established. The government is committed to the idea that primary health care is the best way of improving health and promoting development. Primary health care services provide health promotion, preventive, curative, and rehabilitative services. The primary health care approach also focuses on the community, and encourages it and its individuals to take responsibility for improving their health. This encourages the community to identify health problems; set priorities for action; and plan, organize, and manage health care programs. Women, especially those in middle age, are traditionally a key resource in health care planning and implementation of programs. As mothers-in-law and grandmothers, they are the major decision makers in matters pertaining to the health of the family.

Ethnic-/Race-Specific or Endemic Diseases: The major causes of inpatient mortality and morbidity include pneumonia, pulmonary tuberculosis, cardiopulmonary diseases, malaria, intestinal infections, and obstetrical complications. Tuberculosis had ceased to be a central health concern by the mid 1990s. Despite the improvement in infant mortality rates and overall health since the late 1960s, the human immunodeficiency virus (HIV)/acquired immunodeficiency syndrome (AIDS) pandemic

B

of the late 1990s began a reversal of some gains. In 2003 the World Health Organization's (WHO) estimated prevalence rate for HIV in adults (aged 15 to 49) was 38%, one of the highest in the world. Recent United Nations Joint Programme on HIV/AIDS (UNAIDS) reports estimate the adult prevalence to be 24%, with 270,000 people living with HIV, including 140,000 women and 14,000 children aged 0 to 14. There are 120,000 orphans aged 0 to 17 as a result of AIDS, and 18,000 deaths from AIDS overall. The HIV epidemic has had large macroeconomic repercussions because of the death of many individuals in their productive years and because of the heavy investment required by the government in health care. Heterosexual intercourse has been the predominant mode of transmission. Transmission from mother to child has also contributed to the rapidly growing epidemic. Recent data indicate that 56% of infected adults are women who also have the physical and emotional burden of giving birth to infants with HIV. Women are also expected to assume much of the caregiving responsibilities for people with AIDS. Poverty, unemployment, legal and sociocultural disadvantages, dependence on partners for financial support, and lack of empowerment in negotiating sexual and reproductive matters all contribute to HIV infection rates among women. If women refuse to have unprotected sex with their partners, they may put themselves at risk for physical and sexual abuse. With 42,000 people receiving antiretroviral therapy in early 2005, and scaling up continuing, Botswana's situation is still significantly better than those of other southern African countries.

Health-Team Relationships: Nurses are the backbone of the country's health care system. They are usually the only ones in health care facilities, and they are responsible for providing preventive, curative, and rehabilitative health care services to the whole population. Their duties include supervising primary health care workers and mobilizing communities, especially women, to become responsible for self-care health tasks. Health facilities, especially ones in rural areas, have few doctors. Most doctors rely on nurses and have developed good working relationships with them. Client care is considered a team effort, with the doctor or the nurse practitioner as the team leader.

Families' Role in Hospital Care: Once admitted to a hospital, the patient becomes the responsibility of that hospital. Hospital personnel care for adults, and family members do not stay overnight with them. If a child younger than 5 years is hospitalized, a relative can stay with the child in the children's ward. Hospital food is usually good and nutritionally balanced, so relatives do not have to bring food from home.

Dominance Patterns: Literacy has been a source of empowerment for women, and at the university levels women constitute about 49% of the student body. Women make up about 35% of the formal employment sector, and most are in low-paying service jobs in education, nursing, and social and community work. Botswana has one of the highest percentages of women in government positions in Africa, but numerous women still live in poverty. Botswana has a cultural practice of unequal distribution of

B

inheritance. Sons are given the bulk of the property after their father's death, and daughters receive little or nothing. The basic assumption is that the sons will become responsible for all dependent family members, but this practice is not currently effective because the concept of the extended family is quickly disintegrating. Older adults, who are mostly women, often live in social isolation and poverty and receive little support from their children. Marriage decreases a woman's ability to acquire and control property; in most marriages, the husband is the sole administrator of their joint estate. The rising rate of divorce and single parents has created another group of women who are seriously affected by the inheritance custom: female heads of households. In 1996, 48% of rural households and 33% of urban households were headed by women. Male-headed households have three times the earning power of female-headed households because women usually have no cattle and tend to pass their poverty on from generation to generation. Young people are expected to obey anyone who is older, and although they can express themselves when they disagree, they must do so constructively and in a way that is respectful of age and experience. Older people are also expected to behave responsibly and not use their age to exploit others. Under the constitution of Botswana, every person is entitled to certain rights and liberties. In reality, certain traditional values and attitudes still dictate that women should be subordinate to their husbands and male relatives. Women are responsible for rearing children and performing household tasks. Tilling small pieces of land, sowing, weeding, and harvesting are traditionally assigned to women. The tasks of hunting, herding cattle, participation in public life, and other leadership roles are generally men's responsibilities. Although marriage under the traditional Setswana system permits a man to have more than one wife, polygamous families are actually rare. Marriage is usually consummated by the transfer of *bogadi* ("bride wealth") from the man's to the woman's family except in tribes that have abolished the practice. The marriage is considered an arrangement not only between husband and wife but also between families. After marriage, the wife moves to her husband's family home or his own home. When she lives with her parents-in-law, she becomes *ngwetsi,* or "daughter-in-law," and is expected to behave decently, bear children, and perform all the tasks that go with motherhood. Her situation in the new home depends on the relationship she has with her in-laws, which varies from family to family. The woman is expected to have a child during the first year of marriage, after which her social status goes up significantly, especially if the first child is a boy.

Eye-Contact Practices: Eye contact is a sign of honesty, but it can also be perceived as a sign of insolence and stubbornness during an emotionally charged conversation. When an adult is scolding a young person, the child is expected to be attentive and bow the head to show remorse. These behaviors are not gender specific.

Touch Practices: The almost compulsory form of touch is the handshake, which symbolizes recognition of a person's worth as a human being, even if the person is not welcome. People are considered cold and unwelcoming when they do not offer their hand while greeting others, even if the people see one another every day.

Perceptions of Time: Before the advent of the clock, time was measured by describing the position of the sun (e.g., break of dawn, midday, before or after sunset). Modern timekeeping is now the norm, and even *kgotla* meetings in rural areas are scheduled based on the clock. Punctuality has always been important, so people are usually punctual and try to complete their business on time.

Pain Reactions: From the onset of menstruation, girls are encouraged to be stoic "like proper women" in preparation for the even greater pain of childbirth. Women are expected to be quiet during childbirth and make only a few grunts. A woman who screams becomes the butt of jokes for quite a few months. This kind of pain tolerance is somewhat expected even by some nurses, who have been known to ask a screaming woman whether the elders of her household gave her proper instructions on birth. Men are also expected to be stoic and withstand pain, although, unlike women, men have no biological tests of their manhood such as childbirth.

Birth Rites: No special customs surround the birth of an infant. Circumcision of girls has never been practiced. Some ethnic groups circumcised boys during initiation in schools, but the practice halted when the schools were taken over by modern educational systems. About 98% of pregnant women go to antenatal clinics, and 92% of births are supervised by health personnel. However, only 38% of women use modern methods of family planning. Infant mortality rates are 48 per 1,000 live births, and fertility rates are 3.7 children per woman. Most Batswana believe that children's personalities and emotional dispositions are determined by the mother's physical and mental health during pregnancy. Thus, pregnant women receive as much love and care as possible. They are encouraged to eat well but not "eat for two." Trends in child mortality show that the steady expansion of health services throughout the country were associated with an impressive reduction in the mortality rate of children younger than 5 years. Life expectancy has fallen from 60+ to about 35 years because of HIV/AIDS.

Death Rites: Botswana's success in home-based care for people with AIDS and other terminal illnesses stems from the fact that most people prefer to die in the presence of supportive family members. It is believed that after death, people join the ancestors; hence it is acceptable for older people to die, but not young people, because they have not experienced life on earth. Many families are being traumatized by deaths of young people with AIDS. Autopsies are usually acceptable as the modern way of determining cause of death. Organ donation is not acceptable because of the belief that the person who had organs harvested would either be resurrected without limbs and organs or not be resurrected at all. Certain taboos and rituals surround death and family bereavement. Children are usually moved to a relative's home not only to spare them emotional turmoil but also to protect them from bad luck and contact with evil spirits.

A bereaved widow or widower undergoes cleansing rituals by a traditional doctor and is expected to abstain from sex for a year. Women are expected to wear black mourning clothes for at least 6 months but usually not more than a year. Because of increased urbanization and cross-cultural marriages, some rituals are no longer observed.

Food Practices and Intolerances: The Setswana diet has changed considerably, and people eat many foods from other cultures. However, corn, millet, and sorghum are the staples for most families. Numerous varieties of beans are eaten, usually with a relish of green leafy vegetables and meat such as beef, venison, chicken, or mutton or other meat from wild animals. Watermelons and sweet reed are particularly well liked because they are seasonal. The most popular dish is *seswaa,* meat that is cooked until it comes off the bone and then pounded. Seswaa is eaten at funerals, weddings, and other festive or solemn occasions. It is acceptable to eat with the hands as well as with knives and forks.

Infant-Feeding Practices: Breastfeeding is the norm for most women, and the median duration is 16 months for urban and 18 months for rural women. Weaning foods in the form of mashed bananas, cereals, and a special vitamin-enriched soft porridge that is supplied free at clinics are introduced at 4 months. Women who cannot breastfeed because they are infected with HIV are provided with free infant formula from the clinics for 12 months. All employed mothers whose infants are younger than 12 months are entitled to an extra hour off during the day to feed their infants.

Child-Rearing Practices: Traditionally, children were reared by the extended family and socialized by all clan members. They were taught to be well mannered, courteous, disciplined, respectful, and part of the community. This form of socialization has been taken over by the nuclear family. Although the same values are stressed, the process is not as comprehensive as it was in the past.

National Childhood Immunizations: BCG at birth; DT at 6 years; measles at 9 months; OPV at 2, 3, and 4 months; and HepB at birth and at 2 and 9 months; DtwP at 2, 3, 4, and 18 months; and TT at first contact, +1, +6 months; +1, and +1 year. No cases of polio have been reported since 1989, and HIV vaccine trials began in August 2002. The percent of the target population vaccinated, by antigen, is: BCG (99%); DTP1 (98%); DTP3, Polio3 (97%); HepB3 (85%); MCV (90%); and TT2 plus (72%).

Other Characteristics: Botswana has rapidly evolved from a poor country into a middle-income, politically stable, and multiracial country, with health indicators that are some of the best in Africa. These improvements are threatened, however, because most of the funds that could be used for development projects are being channeled toward HIV/AIDS.

BIBLIOGRAPHY

Central Intelligence Agency: *2006: The world factbook,* Botswana. Retrieved September 21, 2006, from https://www.cia.gov/cia/publications/factbook/print/bc.html.

Livingston J: *Debility and the moral imagination in Botswana*, Bloomington, 2005.

Mathebula U: *Needs and experiences of caregivers of PLWA in Francistown*, master's thesis, Gaborone, Botswana, 2000, University of Botswana.

Ministry of Health, AIDS/STD Unit: *Programme to prevent mother-to-child transmission (MTCT) of HIV in Botswana*, Gaborone, Botswana, 2000.

Ministry of Health, Family Health Division: *Botswana MTCT pilot project January 2000 review*, Gaborone, Botswana, 2000.

Tlow SD et al: *Community responses to initiatives to prevent mother-to-child transmission of HIV in Botswana*, Washington, DC, 2000, ICRW.

UNAIDS: *Report on the global HIV/AIDS epidemic*, Geneva, 2000.

UNAIDS and the World Health Organization: *HIV in pregnancy: a review*, Geneva, 1999.

UNAIDS: 2006 Botswana: Retrieved September 21, 2006, from http://www.unaids.org/en/Regions_Countries/botswana_statistics.html.

United Nations Children's Fund, Botswana statistics: Retrieved July 1, 2006, from http://www.unicef.org/infobycountry/botswana_statistics.html.

World Health Organization: Country profile, Botswana: Retrieved July 1, 2006, from http://www.who.int/countries/bwa/en/.

World Health Organization: 2006: Immunization, vaccines and biologicals. Retrieved September 21, 2006, from http://www.who.int/immunization_monitoring/en/globalsummary/countryprofileresult.cfm?C='bwa'.

World Health Organization: "3 by 5" country profile on treatment scale: Retrieved July 1, 2006. from www.who.int/3by5/support/june2005_bwa.pdf.

◆ BRAZIL (FEDERATIVE REPUBLIC OF)

MAP PAGE (797)

Marga Simon Coler and Maria Adriana Felix Coler

Location: Comprising nearly half of South America, Brazil is the fifth largest and the sixth most populous country in the world. It has 26 states distributed into five geographic regions: North (Rondônia, Acre, Amazonas, Roraima, Pará, Amapá, and Tocantins), Northeast (Alagoas, Bahia, Ceará, Maranhão, Paraíba, Pernambuco, including the Island of Fernando de Noronha, Piauí, Rio Grande do Norte, and Sergipe), Southeast (Espírito Santo, Minas Gerais, Rio de Janeiro, and São Paulo), South (Paraná, Rio Grande do Sul, and Santa Catarina), and Center-West (Goiás, Mato Grosso, and Mato Grosso do Sul) as well as the Federal District, site of Brasília, the national capital. The total area is 8,511,965 km² (3,286,475 square miles). Forests cover 60% of the country, and Brazil is the home of the Amazon River (6296 km [3,912 miles]) and the world's largest tropical rain forest.

Major Language	Ethnic Groups	Major Religions
Portuguese	White 55%	Roman Catholic (official) 95%. Other or None 0.5%

B

Major Language	Ethnic Groups	Major Religions
	Mixed White and Black 38%	(Evangelical Protestant, Afro
	Black 6%	Brazilian such as
	Other (Japanese, Arab, Amerindian) 1%	Candomblé, Umbanda and Macumba, Jewish, Islamic, and Buddhist are integral components of the culture)

The population is more than 188 million. The gross domestic product (GDP) per capita is $8,400, with 22% below the poverty line. About 84% live in urban areas. Brazil reflects African, Indian, Portuguese, and Dutch cultures in the north and northeast regions, German and Italian in the south. São Paulo has one of the largest Japanese communities in the world. A developed country, Brazil has two distinct classes (rich and poor) and a small but growing middle class. Literacy rates are 86% for men, 87% for women.

Health Care Beliefs: Active and passive involvement. There continues to be selective health promotion. The Unified Health System (SUS) places emphasis on primary health care and focuses on health promotion and illness prevention. Health agents and public health monitors are involved in community interventions. The people in the middle class are actively involved, whereas people who are poor are more passive. In 1988 the Brazilian Constitution declared that health is a constitutional right. A consequent policy was the beginning for universal and free access to active antiretroviral treatment for all human immunodeficiency virus (HIV)-infected individuals.

Predominant Sick-Care Practices: Biomedical; holistic; magical-religious (especially in interior Brazil). Pharmacies run by homeopathic doctors are common, and acupuncture is being used with increasing frequency. Pharmacists and even pharmacy owners prescribe medications and treat illnesses, especially for people in the lower socioeconomic class. Use of medicines made at home using teas made of plants, leaves, and roots is common and reflects the heritage and beliefs of Indians and ancestors. Some people seek assistance from *rezadeiras*, women who are believed to have the power to cure through prayer. The government pays about 80% of hospital costs for health problems listed in the Diagnosis-Related Group (DRG) classification system. Private health plans are common among people of the middle class. People self-medicate using over-the-counter medications, including antibiotics. Narcotics require a prescription.

Ethnic-/Race-Specific or Endemic Diseases: Endemic diseases are dengue fever, hemorrhagic dengue fever, cholera, tuberculosis, and schistosomiasis. Brazil's compulsory reportable diseases are cholera, whooping cough, dengue, diphtheria, acute cases of Chagas' disease, meningitis, yellow fever, typhoid fever, hantavirus, hepatitis B and C, visceral leishmaniasis, Hansen disease, leptospirosis, malaria (in areas where it is not endemic), *Haemophilus influenzae*, poliomyelitis, acute flaccid paralysis, pestilence, human rabies, rubeola, syndrome of congenital rubeola, congenital syphilis, human immunodeficiency virus/acquired immunodeficiency syndrome (HIV/AIDS), tetanus, tuberculosis, and chloroquine-resistant malaria. Brazilians are at risk for work-related, iatrogenic, maternal and neonatal, and asthmatic and respiratory conditions as well as malnutrition and dysentery. The United Nations Joint Programme on HIV/AIDS (UNAIDS) estimates the prevalence of HIV in adults (aged 15 to 49) to be 0.5%, with 620,000 people living with HIV, including 220,000 women. About 14,000 deaths from AIDS are recorded. Antiretroviral treatment to reduce mother-to-child transmission is being received by 58% of pregnant women with HIV. HIV carriers and AIDS patients receive the medicines necessary at each stage of the disease free of charge under the SUS.

Health-Team Relationships: The term *doctor* (or *doutor*) is used indiscriminately to express respect and affection. Nurses are addressed by their title *(enfermeira)*, followed by their first name. Within the patriarchal and capitalist health care system, nurses tend to internalize their oppressed role. Concepts of class and social status are strong.

Families' Role in Hospital Care: The family assumes some responsibility for direct care. Family members may bring food or take turns staying with the patient 24 hours a day. It is common for family members to take part in decision making about referrals and procedures such as surgeries. In some situations, such as the chronic stage of terminal diseases, one member represents the family, based on level of education, social status, and leadership skills.

Dominance Patterns: Godparents are chosen by the parents as a sign of recognition and respect for important or influential members of the community. Godparents are expected to help in the procurement of quality medical and financial care for their godchildren as needed. It is common for godparents and godchildren never to develop a relationship after the baptism. Sons and daughters address their parents in the third person (i.e., "o senhor" or "a senhora"), which is a sign of respect for older or elder members of the population. The tradition for Brazilian youth (especially young children) to ask their parents, grandparents, godparents, uncles, or aunts for a blessing, and then kissing their right hand, grows weaker as a new generation emerges, although it remains strong in small communities. When a person has more than one last name, the mother's name precedes the father's. Even if it is no longer used, a common last name, or family name, gives family members a sense of belonging.

B

Eye-Contact Practices: Direct eye contact, like other body language, is common between sexes and among social classes.

Touch Practices: Use of the body and touch to make personal and social contact is generally the "tropical" way of relating. Brazilians are perceived as warm and affectionate people. Women and men greet each other by shaking hands or kissing on both cheeks. An *abraço* ("embrace") indicates a close relationship. Greetings among those in professional relationships are limited to a handshake. Touching while talking is usual.

Perceptions of Time: Brazilians are casual about punctuality and focused on the present. The future is measured in decades or generations, and definitions of *early* and *late* are flexible. Arriving late can reflect a successful social standing. Immediate rewards are preferred to delayed gratification.

Pain Reactions: Pain is expressed vocally through moans and groans, although stoicism may be practiced. Somatization is common in people from the interior of the country.

Birth Rites: Fathers are not usually present during labor and delivery, although the presence of some family members during natural births or cesarean sections (a frequent method of delivery) is common. Circumcision of male infants is not routine. Girls may have their ears pierced soon after birth, often while they are still in the hospital. Mothers are expected to rest for 60 days, and fathers usually take a week off from work. Working parents continue to collect their salaries, and working mothers usually have flexible hours, including extra time during the day to breastfeed. Other family members may assume the role of primary caregiver while parents return to activities such as work or school. The fertility rate is 1.9 children born per woman. Tubal ligation after the birth of two children (of one boy and one girl) is a common practice for middle and upper class women. This procedure is difficult to obtain for poor mothers. The infant mortality rate is 29 deaths per 1,000 live births. The life expectancy is 68 for men, 76 for women.

Death Rites: Death rites are class dependent. People who are poor carry their dead to a cemetery, often in a cardboard casket or hammock. In small towns, the ritual may involve the entire community, and townspeople may join the procession. Small businesses are closed, and activities are suspended as a sign of sympathy and respect. Children dressed in long white robes (so that they represent angels) often lead the procession by carrying a large crown made of natural or artificial flowers. Male relatives are the pallbearers and are followed by other close relatives and friends. Brazilians sing religious or popular songs and pray during the ceremony. Individuals from the middle and upper classes are buried in wooden caskets, and hearses are often used. People who are poor can rent a plot for 2 years, after which time another body is buried on top of the one already interred. In some family graves, one body may be buried on top of another as well. Embalming and cremation are very expensive and practiced in only some regions (such as the in the south). The body is surrounded by flowers, and only the head shows during the service. The body is usually buried the day after death. In the middle and upper classes, the funeral procession is in cars rather than walking and is limited to the cemetery grounds. A cemetery worker is paid to maintain the gravesite.

Food Practices and Intolerance: Yams, bread, and couscous are common for breakfast, although cereals are becoming more popular. The main meal is eaten at noon and consists of rice, beans, mashed potatoes, pasta, and meat or fish. The consumption of vegetables and salads is increasing. The trend in middle-class families in which both parents work outside the home is to eat the noon meal at a self-service restaurant, although going home is still a popular choice because most jobs include a 2-hour lunch break. If the meal is eaten out, a coxinha, pastel, or a sandwich is not uncommon. Supper is a light meal (or soup or leftovers from lunch) and is eaten in the evening.

Infant-Feeding Practices: Breastfeeding is generally short term. Myths, especially concerns about breastfeeding ruining the shape of the woman's breast (and consequently the attitude of the father), can be the most significant factor in duration. *Mingau,* a filling formula made of a thickening agent (e.g., flour of manioc, corn, or rice) and water is used (especially by poor families) to fill the stomach of a hungry infant or toddler. Slight obesity in infants or children is considered a sign of health.

Child-Rearing Practices: Children are treated affectionately. Inhaling the scent of a child before kissing is considered a sign of intimacy and love. Warm embraces from all family members are common. Grandmothers play an active role in caregiving, especially when the mother works outside the home. Hiring a full-time housekeeper for house chores, including babysitting, is also a popular option. Children from middle and upper socioeconomic classes are enrolled in private or parochial schools. Students in lower classes receive a public education. Young children are frequently enrolled in a crèche (day care) or kindergarten. The normal school day is half a day. Children in the lowest socioeconomic bracket often work rather than go to school, and homeless children are numerous in large cities. Research on education has focused on the cognitive abilities of these homeless children and their capacity to use "street knowledge" to learn math and geography. Some of them find jobs as tour guides, demonstrating their ability to memorize historical facts (such as events, places, and famous people) even though they have poor or no reading skills.

National Childhood Immunizations: BCG birth and 6 to 10 years; DT at 2, 4, 6 and 15 months; DTwP at 15 months and at 4 to 6 years; DTwPHib at 2, 4, and 6 months; DTwPHiBHep at 2, 4, and 6 months; HepA +1 year + 6 months; HepB at birth and 1 and 6 months; HiB after 12 months; influenza after 6 + 1 month; IPV at 2, 4, 6, and 15 months; MenC_conj at 2, 4, and 6 months; MMR at 1 and 4 to 6 years; OPV at 2, 4, 6, and 15 months; Pneumo_conj before 2 and +5 years; Pneumo_ps after 2 years; Td at 7 years +2, +2 months; typhoid at >6 +3 years; varicella at 12 months or after; and YF at or after 9 months. The percent of the target

104 *Brunei (Negara Brunei Darussalam)*

population vaccinated, by antigen, is: BCG, MCV (99%); DTP1, DTP2, HiB (96%); polio (98%); and HepB3 (92%).

BIBLIOGRAPHY

Brasil, Ministério da Saúde: Datasus. Indicadores básicos de morbidade e fator de risco, 2001. File://A:\morbididade Br.htm.

Brasil, Ministério da Saúde, Fundação Nacional de Saúde, Centro Nacional de Epidemiologia: Portaria no. 1.461/GM/MS, *Informe Epidemiológico do SUS.* 9(1), 2000.

Brasil, Ministério da Saúde: Indicadores básicos de morbidade e fator de risco, 2001, File://A:\AIDS Br.htm.

Central Intelligence Agency: *2006: The world Factbook, Brazil.* Retrieved September 21, 2006, from https://www.cia.gov/cia/publications/factbook/print/br.html.

Dias J et al: Espoco geral e perspectivas da doença de Chagas no nordeste do Brasil, *Cadernos de Saúde Pública.* 16 (suppl 2), 2000.

Rachid M, Schechter M: *Manual de HIV/AIDS,* Rio de Janeiro, Brazil, 2001, Revinter, Ltda.UNICEF: http://www.unicef.org/infobycountry/brazil_statistics.html#11 updated May 1, 2006 (retrieved May 5, 2006).

UNAIDS: 2006: Brazil: Retrieved September 21, 2006, from http://www.unaids.org/en/Regions_Countries/Countries/brazil.asp.

UNICEF: http://www.unicef.org/infobycountry/brazil_statistics.html#16 updated May 1, 2006 (retrieved May 5, 2006).

World Health Organization: http://www3.who.int/idhl-rils/main.cfm?type=ByCountry&language=english WHO, 2000 (retrieved May 5, 2006).

World Health Organization: https://www.who.int/whr/2005/annex/indicators_country_a-f.pdf (retrieved April 4, 2006).

World Health Organization: http://www3.who.int/idhl-rils/frame.cfm?language=english, updated May 1, 2006 (retrieved May 5, 2006).

World Health Organization: 2006: Immunization, vaccines and biologicals. Retrieved September 21, 2006 from http://www.who.int/immunization_monitoring/en/globalsummary/countryprofileresult.cfm?'bra'.

✦ BRUNEI (NEGARA BRUNEI DARUSSALAM)

MAP PAGE (805)

Kenneth Y.Y. Kok

Location: Brunei Darussalam ("abode of peace") has a total area of 5,765 km^2 (2,230 square miles) and is situated on the northern coast of Borneo. It is a sovereign, independent, democratic, Malay Muslim monarchy according to Sunni beliefs. About 66% of the population lives in the Brunei/Muara district, where the capital, Bandar Seri Begawan, is situated.

Major Languages	Ethnic Groups	Major Religions
Malay (official)	Malay 68%	Muslim (official) 67%
English	Chinese 15%	Buddhist 13%
	Indigenous 6%	Christian 10%
	Other 11%	Indigenous, Other 10%

English is widely used in business and commerce. The population is 379,444: about 51% are younger than 25 years. The discovery of oil set Brunei on the path to economic prosperity. The gross domestic product (GDP) per capita is $23,600. Since 1984 a ministerial system of government has been in place; His Majesty the Sultan serves as the prime minister and head of state.

Health Care Beliefs: Active involvement; increasing emphasis on health promotion. With noncommunicable diseases high on the list of causes of mortality and morbidity, Brunei has identified health promotion as one of its main initiatives. Although health-promotion activities have long been in place, it is only recently that concentrated efforts have been made. Seven priority areas have been identified: nutrition, food safety, tobacco control, mental health, physical activity, healthy environment and settings, and women's health. Therefore, all prevention and promotion health services are programmed to give priority to health problems of the young. Patients with mental illness are stigmatized. With the introduction of an open-door policy in hospital psychiatric departments and improvement in the quality of care, the number of patients seeking consultation has steadily increased, with patients being more open and less worried about stigma and shame.

Predominant Sick-Care Practices: Biomedical; traditional; religious beliefs. All services provided to citizens and permanent residents are funded primarily through the general treasury. Health care is free for all citizens, permanent residents, and expatriate government employees and heavily subsidized for others. Services are accessible to the whole population. Citizens are sent overseas at the government's expense for medical care not available in Brunei. Remote areas are reached by a flying-doctor helicopter service that makes regular visits. Medicine (or *ubat kampong*) administered by traditional healers (or *bomoh*) is quite popular, but patients may not be forthcoming about consulting a bomoh.. Traditional medicine is part of the people's belief and has been practiced for centuries. Older adults, in particular, believe that disease is the work of evil entities in another realm that have disturbed them in some way. Unrealistic expectations of patients in regard to hospital care often lead to dissatisfaction, and if the patients do not have instant improvement, they resort to traditional medicine. Fear of the hospital and its unfamiliar surroundings also cause patients to seek traditional medicine; bomohs are usually well-known members of the community who reside in the same or nearby villages; bomohs use herbal concoctions, and few scientific evaluations have been done. Studies are needed not only to assess treatments' effectiveness but also to investigate drug reactions and interactions. Alternative medicine such as homeopathy and reflexology are also used.

Ethnic-/Race-Specific or Endemic Diseases: Because of the steady rise in the standard of living, mortality rates have declined. An analysis of major causes of death in the past 30 years indicates that the predominant diseases are now chronic degenerative diseases such as cancer and lifestyle diseases such as cardiovascular. The five leading causes of inpatient morbidity are acute upper respiratory infections, asthma, pregnancy with abortive outcomes, and acute lower respiratory infections. The leading causes of death are cancer, heart disease, diabetes mellitus, cerebrovascular disease, bronchitis and asthma, automobile accidents, hypertension, and pneumonia. Chickenpox continues to be the most prominent reportable disease, constituting 74% of cases in 2003. The remaining are tuberculosis, gonococcal infections, food poisoning, dengue, and others. No indigenous cases of malaria have been reported since 1969 and no poliomyelitis cases since 1978. In 1987 Brunei was entered in the World Health Organization's official register of areas where malaria has been eradicated. In 2003, a national task force on severe acute respiratory syndrome (SARS) was set up to monitor the disease, but no cases were reported. A national task force was again set up in 2005 to monitor avian flu, and to date no cases have been reported. The unabated global spread of human immunodeficiency virus (HIV)/ acquired immunodeficiency syndrome (AIDS) is a matter of grave concern. As of December 2005, the number of HIV cases reported was 640. The United Nations Joint Programme on HIV/AIDS (UNAIDS) reports the prevalence rate as less than 0.1%. Vigilance regarding AIDS is being maintained through a national control program. Most newly reported cases have occurred among immigrant workers (96%).

Health-Team Relationships: The lowest level of doctor is the medical officer; next is the senior medical officer, and heading the team is the specialist. Major decisions on patient management are solely the responsibility of the specialist. The medical staff works closely with the nursing staff and other allied health professionals. The nursing college in Brunei offers a 3-year nursing course. There is trend toward post-basic diploma courses in operating theatre, intensive care, and accident and emergency nursing. Nurses play a major role in patient management and specialized care such as infection control, diabetes management, and oncology. A patients' charter was launched in 2000, so patients are now more aware of their rights. Health care professionals are respected, trusted, and highly esteemed. In 2005, 473 medical doctors and dentists were registered to practice, with a ratio of doctors to population of 1:720. To overcome the shortage of local doctors in various disciplines, the government continues to employ expatriates on contract.

Families' Role in Hospital Care: Family ties are strong, and grown children are expected to care for aging parents. The family usually has a dominant figure, either the head of the household or the grandfather. Consultation with this person on health matters is advisable, and written consent should be obtained before any investigative or therapeutic procedure is carried out. Visiting and bringing food to hospitalized relatives are common practices. Sometimes all extended family members visit the relative at the same time, making visiting hours a noisy affair, especially on joyous occasions like childbirth. It is common for a family member to spend the night with a sick relative.

Dominance Patterns: The pattern of male dominance is slowly changing, a transition that is evident in the appointment of women to top government positions. Men are still dominant in families, however, and major family decisions are made by the head of the household, who is either the father or grandfather.

Eye-Contact Practices: Direct eye contact between opposite sexes is allowed and is expected during conversation.

Touch Practices: Public displays of affection such as kissing are unacceptable.

Perceptions of Time: Punctuality is not a major issue during festive occasions such as wedding receptions and gatherings; being 30 minutes late is acceptable. Almost all patients are on time for clinic appointments, and most arrive at least 30 minutes to an hour before the scheduled appointment.

Pain Reactions: Pain reactions seem to be related to age. Young people seek medical advice as soon as they experience pain or discomfort. Older individuals tend to keep any discomfort to themselves and do not inform their relatives, probably because they do not want to burden them or disrupt routine activities. Patients tend to be reserved in expression of pain, which is evident after surgeries when it is usually the caring relative who requests analgesics for the patient.

Birth Rites: Traditional beliefs surround pregnancy and birth. For example, it is believed that consumption of papaya and pineapples may lead to miscarriages, and consumption of squid may lead to placental deformities. The expectant mother is not allowed to wrap a towel around her neck because of the belief that this causes the umbilical cord to loop around the neck of the fetus. People believe that nailing a wall could lead to miscarriage. The pregnant woman is not allowed to sit in a doorway because this may lead to difficult labor. Nearly all births are in hospitals; childbirth at home is rare because hospitals are easily accessible. After birth, a black thread is tied at the base of both of the mother's big toes. She is advised to keep warm, is not allowed to drink cold water, and must avoid "cold" foods such as cucumber, spinach, or pineapple. She is not allowed to bathe for 3 days after birth. Some women sleep near burning charcoal to keep warm. The woman's abdomen is wrapped with herbs, and she receives traditional massages to improve her muscle tone and aid uterine involution. These activities are practiced for 40 days, during which sexual activities are prohibited. The country has experienced a significant reduction in its fertility rate. The fertility rate decreased from 3.78 children per woman in 1981 to 2.2 in 2006, with a sharp decrease in pregnancies in women under age 25 (because of later marriage and first pregnancy) and over age 40 (caused by fertility curtailment by women who have attained their desired family size). This change in the population structure will result in significant growth in the proportion of the population age 15 and older. The infant mortality rate is 12 deaths per 1,000 live births. Life expectancy is among the highest in Asia, at 75 for men, 78 for women.

B

Death Rites: Death is thought of as the path to the next world. Muslim burial is carried out within a day, and the body is wrapped in special white cloth and buried without a coffin. Cremation is not allowed. Relatives and close friends offer ritual prayers either at the home of the deceased or the mosque. Prayers are recited on three consecutive nights; 7, 14, 40, 100 days after death; and yearly thereafter. Autopsies are uncommon, and cadaveric organ donations are not allowed because the body must be buried intact. In hospitals, it is common for a dying person to request to die at home surrounded by close relatives.

Food Practices and Intolerance: Islamic law forbids the consumption of pork and alcohol, and only *halal* meat, which is slaughtered according to Muslim rites, may be consumed. Most international, Chinese, and traditional Malay foods are easily available in major hotels, in family-owned restaurants, at hawker stalls, and fast-food restaurants. After surgery, patients avoid certain foods such as prawns and shellfish because they are believed to inflame wounds and delay healing. The consumption of supplementary foods or natural tonics is common after illness, surgery, or childbirth. Among the popular tonics are fish essence with wild ginseng and cordyceps, chicken essence, and ostrich tonic with cordyceps. These tonics are believed to stimulate blood circulation, improve the complexion, reinforce the body's energy, regenerate muscle, relieve edema, and enhance the body's resistance to disease.

Infant-Feeding Practices: All mothers are encouraged to breastfeed; but because of changes in the social structure, working women are finding it increasingly difficult to continue after the first month. To re-educate women and encourage breastfeeding, the Baby-Friendly Hospital Initiative, in collaboration with the World Health Organization, has been introduced in all hospitals.

Child-Rearing Practices: Parents are quite permissive, and it is the responsibility of both to discipline the children. Corporal punishment has been abolished in schools but is still acceptable in the home. Children usually sleep with parents until about 4 or 5 years old, and they are sent to nursery schools at the age of 3. Formal religious education begins at the age of 8 or at school in grade primary 3. The *istiadat berkhatan* ("circumcision ceremony") marks a boy's coming of age and is usually performed between the ages of 10 and 12. The operation is performed at designated health clinics or hospitals. Female circumcisions are not performed.

National Childhood Immunization: BCG at birth; DT at 5 years; DTwP at 2, 3, and 4 months; DTwPHib at 2, 3, and 4 months; OPV at 2, 3, and 4 months and at 5 years; HepB at birth and at 1 and 6 months; MMR at 12 months and at 10 to 13 years; TT at 28 and 32 weeks (in pregnant women). The percent of the target population vaccinated, by antigen, is: BCG (96%); DTP1, DTP3, HepB3, Polio3 (99%); and MCV (97%).

Other Characteristics: The culture is predominantly influenced by Islam. To indicate refusal of offered food, it is polite to touch the plate lightly with the right hand. The right hand is always used to give or receive because the left is considered unclean. When sitting on the floor, a person should sit cross-legged rather than with legs stretched out in front. The polite way to summon someone is to use all four fingers of the right hand with the palm facing down and motioning the person toward you; the index finger is never used. It is customary to leave footwear at the door when entering a Muslim house.

B

BIBLIOGRAPHY

Brunei Shell Petroleum: *Annual report 2003.*

Ministry of Health, Brunei Darussalam: *The millennium report 2000,* Brunei Darussalam, 2000.

Ministry of Health, Brunei Darussalam: *National health care plan (2000-2010):* a strategic framework for action, june 2000.

Ministry of Health, Brunei Darussalam: Disease control division, Environment health services: *Cancer registry annual statistics 2002.*

Central Intelligence Agency: *2006: The world factbook, Brunei Darussalam.* Retrieved September 21, 2006, from https://www.cia.gov/cia/publications/factbook/print/bx.html http://www.moh.gov.bn. (retrieved on May 16, 2006).

UNAIDS: 2006 Brunei Darussalam: Retrieved September 21, 2006 from http://www.unaids.org/en/Regions_Countries/Countries/brunei+_darussalam.asp.

World Health Organization 2006: Immunization, Vaccines and Biologicals. Retrieved September 21, 2006, from http://www.who.int/immunization_monitoring/en/globalsummary/countryprofileresult.cfm?C='brn'.

◆ BULGARIA (REPUBLIC OF)

MAP PAGE (798)

Slavianka Moyanova

Location: Bulgaria is situated in the Balkan Peninsula in southeastern Europe and is bordered on the north by Romania, east by the Black Sea, south by Turkey and Greece, and west by Serbia and the Republic of Macedonia. The capital and largest city is Sofia. More than half of Bulgaria is hilly or mountainous. The Balkan Mountains cross the country from its northwestern corner to the Black Sea. The northern side of the Balkan Mountains slopes gradually to form the northern Bulgarian plateau, which ends at the River Danube. In the southern and southwestern parts of the country are the Rhodope and Rila mountains. The population is eight million, and the total area is 110,910 km^2 (42,822 square miles). The gross domestic product (GDP) per capita is $9,600, and 13% live below the poverty line. Literacy rates are about 99% for both men and women.

Major Languages	Ethnic Groups	Major Religions
Bulgarian	Bulgarian 84%	Christian (Bulgarian
Turkish	Turkish 9%	Orthodox) 84%
	Roma-Gypsy 5%	Muslim 12%
	Other 2%	Other 4%

B

In the Middle Ages, Bulgaria competed with the Byzantine Empire and greatly influenced the cultural life of the region. Ethnic Turks are the descendants of Osmani Turks who settled in Bulgaria during the 500 years when it was a province of the Ottoman Empire. Ethnic Bulgarians who converted to Islam are recognized as a separate group called *Pomaks*. The Bulgarian Orthodox Church is an autonomous branch of the Eastern Orthodox Church.

Health Care Beliefs: Acute sick care; some magical beliefs. Health prevention practices are ignored by a large segment of the population. Few believe that illness may be eradicated by magical intervention. Psychotherapy is not valued in the culture.

Predominant Sick-Care Practices: Biomedical; traditional and alternative. Matters of health and medicine are under the overall control of the Ministry of Health. Before the political reforms in 1989, the health care system guaranteed each resident free access to medical care. Reform in the public health system is currently under way and should result in the financial responsibility for provision of medical services being assumed by the National Insurance Fund but financed by employers and workers. Doctors and other health care practitioners in the diagnostic and consulting centers (DCCs) or medical centers contract with the fund to provide care. Patients pay a nominal fee for each visit to a general practitioner, who may refer them to a specialist if necessary. Free care is provided for all children. The hospitals also have contracts with the Fund. The numbers of private doctors working outside the government hospital system or in private health centers are increasing. In hospitals and DCCs, only standard medical treatment is offered. Bulgarians seek help from doctors only as a last resort. Although most Bulgarians trust the care they receive from doctors, they usually self-medicate and buy their drugs without a prescription. Deeply religious individuals believe that going to a priest for confession and prayer will relieve their suffering. Indigenous and alternative health care practices are used, particularly massage therapy, meditation, herbal medicine, therapeutic touch, biofeedback, and homeopathy. Such practices are often used to treat phobias, arthritis, anxiety, back problems, and headaches. Several newspapers and many books are devoted to alternative medicine. Use of medicinal herbs, especially teas, is common. Herbal treatments are based on centuries-old healing traditions, and recipes for the preparation of herb teas are passed down from mothers to family, friends, and colleagues. Although Bulgaria has many medicinal herb shops, many prefer to gather herbs themselves. Some doctors combine alternative and traditional medicine, prescribing synthetic drugs along with herbs, plant extracts, and nutrient supplements such as antioxidants.

Ethnic-/Race-Specific or Endemic Diseases: The morbidity rates of certain diseases (e.g., sexually transmitted diseases, gastrointestinal diseases, hepatitis B, tuberculosis), are much higher in the Roma (gypsy) ethnic group than in the rest of the population. Diseases related to iodine deficiencies are endemic in southeastern Bulgaria despite encouragement of the use of iodized salt. Nephritis, nephrolithiasis, and other kidney

B

diseases are endemic in northwestern Bulgaria. The most common ill-nesses are circulatory system diseases, primarily hypertension and stroke (21% of the population). The most widespread diseases among children are asthma and bronchitis, and the number affected has doubled in the past several years. Subjective opinions of health status point to deteriorat-ing health in Bulgaria. People's estimates regarding their "expected dura-tion of life in good health" have substantially decreased. By the end of 2004, Bulgaria had reported a cumulative total of 515 human immunode-ficiency virus (HIV) cases, including 145 diagnosed as acquired immuno-deficiency syndrome (AIDS). It is estimated that about 100 have died. The Joint United Nations Programme on HIV/AIDS (UNAIDS) reports that the estimated prevalence rate for HIV in adults (aged 15 to 49) is 0.1%. Among cases with a known method of transmission, more than 91% were transmitted by sexual intercourse.

Health-Team Relationships: Despite a relatively high doctor-to-patient ratio (1:283), Bulgarian doctors are overwhelmed with work, partly because of the enormous number of sick people. Since 2000, all Bulgar-ians have been allowed to choose and change their general practitioner every 6 months if desired. Everyone is at liberty to determine the qualifica-tions of doctors and dentists, which creates a market perspective and nat-ural competition among doctors. Health reforms are occurring, but Bulgaria still has many problems involving the balance between the rights and obligations of patients and doctors. Doctors and nurses work as a team, especially in preclinical centers, and the relationships are usually good because the doctors select and hire the nurses. Nurses play a sub-ordinate role. Nurses working with general practitioners do a great deal of the administrative work. In hospitals the health care teams consist of sev-eral doctors and nurses, and roles and responsibilities are strictly defined. Nurses are university educated.

Families' Role in Hospital Care: Because resources in hospitals are less than optimal, family members usually stay with patients, particularly when the illness is serious. They supplement services by bringing addi-tional food, changing linens, and buying drugs when necessary.

Dominance Patterns: In today's younger families, men and women carry equal weight in certain decision-making processes, but they do not have equal obligations at home. Women do the cooking, cleaning, washing, and most other household chores. In older families, the father is the head of the household and main decision maker. Typically, the man reads a newspaper or watches television after work and then moves to the table to wait for dinner to be served.

Eye-Contact Practices: Direct eye contact is important in social and business situations. Not maintaining a direct gaze is considered impolite or a sign of disinterest. Children are taught to make direct eye contact with teachers, friends of their parents, and during all conversations

Touch Practices: A brief, light handshake is the usual form of greeting when one is being introduced. The handshake often occurs when greeting and parting and in all social situations. If a man is seated, he stands to

B

shake hands with another person. A woman offers her hand first, but a seated woman is not obliged to stand when a man enters the room. When good male friends greet one another, a warm and long handshake may be accompanied by a light touch on the forearm or elbow or by a light embrace. Patting on the back is not totally acceptable. Close female friends who greet after not seeing each other for a long time may hug lightly, kiss one or both cheeks, or brush the cheeks as if kissing. Casual body contact among strangers (e.g., while waiting in line) is avoided.

Perceptions of Time: Punctuality is not an inherent national value. Most people are punctual in work situations, but few get to private appointments on time. Because of long lines, patients in the DCCs usually wait for long periods for previously arranged appointments with general practitioners. Patients consider long waiting times for diagnostic tests and other procedures to be a hindrance to good health care.

Pain Reactions: Bulgarians differ in their degree of response according to gender, age, and culture, although patients seek complete explanations of the meaning of their pain and its relief. Some react expressively, whereas others deny pain and display stoicism. The expressive reaction is more common. Older patients, who are more vulnerable to chronic pain, tend to feel increasingly discouraged, helpless, and hypochondriac in a system that does not adequately respond to their needs.

Birth Rites: All births occur in hospitals, and women who are at high risk for pregnancy complications are under a doctor's care. The fertility rate is 1.38 children born per woman. Women who have high-risk pregnancies may stay at home for the duration of the pregnancy. The infant mortality rate is 20 deaths per 1,000 live births. Childbirth preparation classes are not popular, and family members (including the husband) are not allowed to be present during the delivery. Women and their infants remain in the hospital for 4 to 5 days, and the infants are brought to them from the nursery four or five times daily for feedings. About 10 to 15 years ago, infants were wrapped tightly around the hips, but this practice has stopped because it was causing joint articulation problems. Life expectancy is 69 for men, 76 for women.

Death Rites: Death rites differ between urban and rural areas. The usual practice in urban areas is to hire a private funeral home to organize the burial rites. The body is dressed in nice clothing and placed inside a coffin that will be sent to a cemetery. Depending on family preference, the coffin either stays in a church or ritual home, where a priest conducts a funeral service or an official civil person reads a eulogy. Family members, friends, and colleagues of the deceased pay their last respects. One by one they walk by the coffin, putting many flowers on and around the body, after which condolences are offered to family members. At the cemetery, family and friends have one more chance to say goodbye to the deceased; then all are invited for a plate of biscuits, boiled wheat, and bread. In rural areas, family and friends say goodbye to the deceased in the person's home, where the body stays 1 or 2 days after death. The body is then transported to the cemetery in a procession, followed by a gathering.

B

Eastern Orthodox Christian practice discourages cremation, but it is practiced because of a lack of cemetery space in larger cities. Autopsies are not well accepted but are performed for forensic reasons. For other reasons, close relatives generally consult one another about the decision. Organ donation is valued, and people consider the receipt of a donated organ to be a second chance at life and a greatly valued gift. A system of registration for organ donation exists: those who object to donation of their organs record their objections so that the information can be retrieved at their death. Even when patients consent to be organ donors, doctors respect families' wishes if the families object. Parents seldom allow donations of their children's organs after death.

Food Practices and Intolerances: Large meals are eaten at midday and in the evening, and foods with ginger-flavored sauces are preferred. Popular foods include stuffed peppers, green beans, white brined cheese, meat and vegetable hash *(musaka),* hotchpotch *(guvetch),* stuffed cabbage or vine leaves, yogurt, salad with sauerkraut, mixed vegetable salad (tomatoes, roasted and peeled peppers, and cucumber) topped with grated white cheese *(Shops' salad),* and cold chopped cucumber soup *(tarator).* Because vegetables are the preferred food, most people preserve them in cans in the summer for use in winter.

Infant-Feeding Practices: All new mothers are educated about the importance of breastfeeding, not only for infant health but also for infant-mother attachment. They know that colostrum and breastfeeding help their infants resist bacteria and viruses that cause illness. Most women do their best to breastfeed as long as possible, and doctors and nurses in the hospital assist with breastfeeding techniques.

Child-Rearing Practices: Child-rearing depends on the family's culture and parental views of proper behavior. Younger families tend to be more permissive. Children usually sleep with parents until about 10 years of age. Then they move to a separate room if possible. Parents expect their children to be quiet and obedient. Because it is financially necessary for both parents to work, little time might be spent with children. Severe physical punishment or abuse is not accepted, and most parents bring their children up with loving discipline involving suggestions, explanations, and advice. According to the law, children in Bulgaria reach adulthood at age 18. Children younger than 16 may not legally consume liquor or go to disco or computer clubs without an identification card and an accompanying parent or adult. It is thought that although the teaching of moral values should come primarily from parents and school, the government has a role to play and should restrict certain activities.

National Childhood Immunizations: BCG at birth and at 7, 11, and 17 years; DT at 7 years; OPV at 2, 3, 4, 14, and 22 months and 7 years; DTwP at 2, 3, and 4 months and at 2 years; MMR at 13 months and 12 years; HepB at birth and at 1 and 6 months; Td at 12, 17, 25, 35, 45, and 55 years; and TT at 45, 55, 65, 75, and 85 years. The percent of the target population vaccinated, by antigen, is: BCG (98%); DTP1, Polio3 (97%); DTP3, HepB3, and MCV (96%).

B

Other Characteristics: The head motions for "yes" and "no" are the opposite of those used in the United States and other countries, which can cause considerable confusion between Bulgarians and foreigners.

BIBLIOGRAPHY

Central Intelligence Agency: *2006: The world factbook, Bulgaria.* Retrieved September 21, 2006, from https://www.cia.gov/cia/publications/factbook/print/bu.html.

National Statistical Institute, Bulgaria: http://www.nsi.bg National Statistical Institute, Bulgaria (retrieved on February 28, 2006).

UNAIDS: 2006: Bulgaria, Retrieved September 21, 2006 from http://www.unaids.org/en/Regions_Countries/Countries/bulgaria.asp

UNAIDS: http://www.usaid.gov/our_work/global_health/home/Countries/eande/bulgaria.pdf USAID, Country profile: Bulgaria (retrieved on February 28, 2006).

USAIDS: http://www.usaid.gov/locations/europe_eurasia/countries/bg/bulgaria.pdf USAID, Country Profile: Bulgaria (retrieved on February 28, 2006).

World Health Organization: http://www.euro.who.int/aids/ctryinfo/overview/20060118_8 Bulgaria—HIV/AIDS country profile (retrieved on February 28, 2006).

World Health Organization: 2006: Immunization, vaccines and biologicals, Retrieved September 21, 2006, from http://www.who.int/immunization_monitoring/en/globalsummary/countryprofileresult.cfm?C='bgr'.

◆ BURKINA FASO

MAP PAGE (800)

Eric Ledru, and Georges Dahourou

Location: Burkina Faso is landlocked in West Africa and consists of plains, low hills, and high savannas, with desert in the north. The total area is 274,200 km^2 (105,869 square miles). The capital is Ouagadougou. Burkina Faso is a Sahelian country with poor water resources. There is a long dry season from November to May; a hot, dry wind (Harmattan) sweeps the country and carries dust clouds from March to May. Important regional migratory flows of people occur with neighboring countries, mainly Côte d'Ivoire, Togo, and Ghana. The population is more than 13.9 million, with 7% aged between 0 and 14 years. Up to one million Burkinabe people are working outside the country. The gross domestic product (GDP) per capita is $1,300, with 45% below the poverty line. Literacy rates are 40% for men, 17% for women.

Major Languages	Ethnic Groups	Major Religions
French (official)	Mossi, Gurunsi,	Muslim 50%
Tribal languages	Senufo, Lobi,	Indigenous beliefs 40%
	Bobo, Mande,	Christian (Roman
	Funlani 40%	Catholic) 10%
	Other 60%	

Tribal languages are spoken by 90% of the population. Burkina Faso has one of the higher population densities in West Africa and is one of the poorest nations. Its economy is based primarily on agriculture, which relies on rudimentary methods. Most of the land is arid and suitable only for nomadic herders. Although 86% live in rural areas, urbanization is rapid, promoted by the high mobility of populations in search of economic opportunities. The suburbs of the main cities such as Ouagadougou and Bobo-Dioulasso are growing rapidly.

Health Care Beliefs: Acute sick care; traditional. Health promotion and disease prevention are challenges. The country is poorer and less developed than the average sub-Saharan African country and has a younger population, fewer medical facilities, low vaccination coverage, and lower quality of housing and water supply and storage. Four different modes of illness transmission can be identified in local beliefs: ingestion of improper substances, breaking of social taboos (e.g., coughing during sexual intercourse can induce chronic cough if a ritual is not respected), sorcery (sorcerers attack only friends or family members and operate at night), and improper interaction with spirits (with which diviners but also small children can communicate). For example, in the Bissa ethnic group, sexually transmitted infections (STIs) are believed to result from sexual intercourse with a twin spirit of the husband (or wife) during a dream. Animism is widespread, although there is official disapproval of such practices, and the first line of health care is often traditional indigenous healers *(tradipraticians)*. Although well accepted, access to biomedical medicine remains expensive, especially for the poorest population groups. The cost of seeking care from traditional healers is about half the cost of biomedical medicine, and in-kind payment is possible.

Predominant Sick-Care Practices: Magical-religious; traditional; biomedical where available. Burkina Faso has adopted a primary care strategy and has a five-level national health system. The Poste de Santé Primaire (PSP) is village based and staffed by paramedical staff. In parallel, most villages have tradipraticians (herbalists, bonesetters, and traditional birth attendants), but also diviners, sorcery specialists, and marabouts. Tradipraticians primarily alleviate symptoms such as abdominal and head pain but occasionally purport to cure diseases such as malaria. They use leaves, bark, and roots that are harvested according to a ritual. Some of them even refer their patients to the national health system. Others claim to cure acquired immunodeficiency syndrome (AIDS), gonorrhea, and infertility, and these only work for money. All have public offices, but the more reputable practitioners are discreet and their reputation increases based on their works. Witches and wizards are practitioners who use spells. They are renowned, and people are in awe of them. Only people with strong beliefs in animistic traditional practices consult them. The Centre de Santé et de Promotion Sociale (CSPS) provides first-level care with nurses and midwives. Family-planning methods are available and are usually provided by midwives, who have on-the-job, rather than formal, education. A doctor is available at the Centre Medical

(CM), which theoretically provides all services, including surgery. Private clinics provide the same types of services as the CM. Patients must pay for medications in both facilities, but the private practitioners often allow credits. The Centre Hospitalier Regional (CHR) provides family planning services. Burkina Faso has two national hospitals, one in Ouagadougou and the other in Bobo-Dioulasso. In addition, numerous foreign and national nongovernmental health organizations (NGOs) address particular health issues, such as water supply and the education of women. The additional disease burden caused by late-stage complications of human immunodeficiency virus (HIV), for example, wasting, opportunistic diseases, tuberculosis (TB), has been overwhelming the health care system.

Ethnic-/Race-Specific or Endemic Diseases: Endemic diseases are chloroquine-resistant malaria, meningitis, intestinal nematode infections, TB, hepatitis, cardiovascular diseases, rabies, and HIV/AIDS. About 75% of deaths in children under 5 are linked to infectious diseases (mostly diarrhea, malaria, and pneumonia). Malaria is associated with high morbidity in adults, creating disabilities that preclude working. The main zoonotic diseases (acquired by contact with livestock) are TB, brucellosis, and anthrax. Rabies is endemic and transmitted mainly through dogs. African trypanosomiasis (sleeping sickness), transmitted by the glossina fly, is a re-emerging disease, as its control has been neglected during the last decades. Water-resource development is a challenge, but hemorrhagic fever outbreaks (Rift Valley fever) and schistosomiasis (contracted by swimming in stagnant water) are linked to the proliferation of vectors (mosquitoes or molluscs, respectively) favored by irrigation systems. Furthermore, introducing rice cultivation in areas where malaria is not under control can speed its transmission. Although "old" diseases are still prolific, metabolic diseases (cerebrovascular, ischemic heart, and diabetes) associated with the occidental way of life (tobacco, nutritional imbalances, sedentary lifestyle) are emerging problems in urban areas. Strong health education remains to be done to cope with this epidemiologic transition. The estimated prevalence rate for HIV/AIDS in adults (aged 15 to 49) is 4.2%. This apparent stabilization during the last years masks a high rate of new infections associated with a high death rate (6.5 per 1,000). It is estimated that AIDS-related mortality will be equal to malaria-related mortality by 2020. AIDS cases are clustered in adults aged 25 to 45 years (i.e., the economically active individual). There are more than 250,000 orphans as a result of parents dying of AIDS. Without therapy, HIV-infected pregnant women transmit the virus to one in three children, and the estimated number of children from birth to 15 years living with HIV/AIDS is 30,000. Most HIV infections are transmitted heterosexually. Migrations and prostitution combined with infrequent use of condoms, even by those with multiple sexual partners, allow the epidemic to spread rapidly. Other STIs favor contamination by HIV, although male circumcision ensures some protection. The risk of transmission through blood transfusion, despite a strong effort to reduce it, or through ritual scarification or circumcision also exists. Chronic infection by parasitic worms may also increase susceptibility and spread of HIV. The wasting that accompanies AIDS is called *kpéréki* in the Lobi ethnic group (meaning "losing weight/dying"). The high rate of HIV-related mortality is primarily related to low access to health because of economics, but also because of social rejection of the disease. The STI/HIV/TB complex is a paradigm of the synergistic interactions among poverty, hygiene, and old and new diseases.

Health-Team Relationships: In rural areas, health workers are always respected. People are in awe of them, and they belong to the local worthies. When people distinguish among different kinds of health care workers, the doctor is always at the top of the hierarchy. In PSPs, nurses are authorized to prescribe and to perform some surgeries. In hospitals, nurses are the primary link in health care, although doctors may not always recognize their abilities.

Families' Role in Hospital Care: Some districts such as Bobo-Dioulasso have only one doctor for 20,000 inhabitants. In the hospital, family members have to carry the patient to the x-ray room when needed, provide personal care, wash bedding, and bring food to augment what is served. Most important, the family has to observe the patient and alert staff members to potential problems. If surgery is required, the family joins together to pay for the various materials (e.g., compresses, antibiotics) that are needed. Therefore, the family's contribution is vital. Traditional medicine is not practiced in hospitals.

Dominance Patterns: The rationale for determining who is worthy of receiving health care resources is based on productivity rather than gender. Women are believed to be as productive as men, so their health is valued equally. About 50% are in polygamist unions. In rural areas, it is estimated that people work about 16 hours daily between agriculture and domestic work (food processing and preparation) in the context of limited access to fuel and water. Men and older adults make the decisions, both social and economic. Public life continues to be dominated by men, and few women participate in the government. About 95% of women work in subsistence agriculture or in jobs using low levels of technology. Various NGOs have been attempting to increase women's status by teaching job skills. A commission for strengthening the roles and positions of women has existed since 1993 but has had little effect on the participation of women in the decision-making process. The 1991 constitution prohibits sexual discrimination and gives men and women equal rights in marriage, inheritance, and land access. Most women are not aware of their rights because of lack of information and education, illiteracy, and traditions. It is estimated that about 70% have been subjected to genital cutting, and the law now punishes such excision. Between men of distinct ethnic groups, the "joking relationship" persists as social cement for the society.

Eye-Contact Practices: Eye contact is related to religion. For some Muslims, the house is divided into two areas to prevent contact between males and females. When a woman talks to a man and looks at him directly, she is considered a woman of little virtue. In the presence of a hierarchical chief or someone in a clan who has higher social status, direct eye contact is avoided as a mark of respect.

Touch Practices: People walk arm in arm only in cities. Women do not shake men's hands—a constant in all ethnic groups.

Perceptions of Time: Time in West Africa involves natural references such as sunrise or sunset. It is disrespectful to shorten a discussion to go to an appointment, and the saying "time is money" has no relevance. The significance of one's current actions is determined by reference to "ancestor time." According to tradition, the present is a repetition and a recapitulation of previous acts, not a race against time.

Pain Reactions: The various ethnic groups differ in their pain reactions. The behavioral code for the Fulani ethnic group is self-discipline and stoicism for emotional or physical pain. Regardless of his ethnic group, a man does not show his feelings in public; to do so is a mark of weakness. During childbirth, it is acceptable for women of the Bobo group to express pain, whereas among the Mossi and Lobi it is not.

Birth Rites: Women generally want to have girls, and men want to have boys. Most families prefer a boy first to carry on the lineage, and large families are the norm. The fertility rate is 6.7 children born per mother. Infant mortality is 107 deaths per 1,000 live births (estimated to be 60% lower in families in which the mother has had secondary education). Maternal mortality rates (about 1,000 per 100,000 live births) are among the highest in the world. Not surprisingly, the government is placing significant emphasis on family planning activities. Life expectancy is low (46 for men, 50 for women). Young women are highly sensitive to disease because of repeated pregnancies and late weaning, which lead to micronutrient deficiencies and anemia. Use of nonsterile instruments to cut umbilical cords or application of karite nut butter results in numerous cases of neonatal tetanus. Trained birth attendants with variable knowledge, professional midwives, or traditional "old women" assist with most births. Some sick infants are treated only by the family, depending on what type of health care services are nearby, the family ethnic group, and educational level of the parents. Fulanis often keep their pregnancies secret, and the mother gives birth alone or with her mother's help. Gurmace mothers often give birth with assistance from the husband's family, and an "old woman" (or birth attendant) usually attends Rimaibe births.

Death Rites: Cremations do not take place, and burial rituals differ according to religion, social status, and ethnic group. Muslims are usually buried quickly, whereas burial of Mossi or Bobo chiefs is delayed for several days. Some ethnic groups (e.g., Dagari) bring the body back to the village. Children are buried immediately, with little ritual, whereas burials of older adults are often festive occasions.

Food Practices and Intolerances: *Tô* ("porridge of millet or maize") is the usual food of most rural Burkinabe. In Mossi country, bean and pea pastries are also eaten. Red sorghum is used mainly for beer production (*dolo*). Meat is consumed when available and may be from bush game or farm animals. Protein malnutrition is linked to the economic situation, the long dry season, inadequate cattle breeding because of sleeping sickness, inadequate use of available local foods, and poor education of mothers. The combination of numerous parasitic infections and malnutrition increases children's susceptibility to malaria and other bacterial and viral diseases. Food is believed to induce digestive diseases, even when it is quality food, if it does not conform to the perceived constitution of the person.

Infant-Feeding Practices: Breastfeeding is usual at least until 18 months. This favors vertical (mother-to-infant) transmission of AIDS, and no clear consensus exists regarding a strategy to prevent this mode of transmission. Early initiation of bottle-feeding can create nutritional problems because of lack of access to clean water. Vitamin A deficiencies are common in children and promote the development of ocular diseases.

Child-Rearing Practices: Increasing the years of school (especially for girls) is a key strategy for improving economic and health development. Vaccine coverage, for example, often parallels years of school. Girls rarely go to a formal school: adult women teach them about traditions and sex, and many taboos are involved. Boys are subjected to initiation rituals that follow strict rules and ensure perpetuation of the culture. Nearly 50% of the Burkinabe is younger than 15 years, and only about 29% of primary-school-age children receive a basic education. Lack of information about hygiene and disease influences high mortality rates: 75% of deaths of children younger than 5 are linked to preventable infectious diseases. Survey data indicate that households allocate significantly fewer resources to the care of sick children than they do to sick adults because children are not considered productive in terms of family survival.

National Childhood Immunizations: BCG at birth; DTwP at 2, 3, and 4 months; YF at 9 months; OPV at birth and at 2, 3, and 4 months; measles at 9 months; TT at first contact, +1, +6 months, +1, and +1 year. The percent of the target population vaccinated, by antigen, is: BCG, DTP1 (99%); DTP3 (96%); MCV (84%); and Polio3 (94%). Cholera cases are frequently reported and are linked to low accessibility to water, poor hygiene, and poor-quality drinking water. The "meningitis belt" (which Burkina Faso is in) is sustained by the Harmattan winds, which carry infection, and by the periodic Haj pilgrimage to crowded Muslim holy places. Immunization against meningococci is achieved through mass campaigns.

BIBLIOGRAPHY

Central Intelligence Agency: *2006: The world factbook, Burkina Faso*. Retrieved September 21, 2006 from https://www.cia.gov/cia/publications/factbook/print/uv.html.

Coulibaly ND, Yameogo KR: Prevalence and control of zoonotic diseases: collaboration between public health workers and veterinarians in Burkina Faso, *Acta Tropica*. 76:53–7, 2000.

Ledru E et al: Prevention of wasting and opportunistic infections in HIV-infected patients in West Africa: a realistic and necessary strategy before antiretroviral treatment, *Cahiers Santé*. 9:293–300, 1999.

Molyneux DH: Vector-borne infections in the tropics and health policy issues in the twenty-first century, *Trans Roy Soc Trop Med Hyg*. 95:233–8, 2001.

Morgan D, Whitworth J: The natural history of HIV-1 infection in Africa, *Nat Med*. 7:143–5, 2001.

Morten Rostrup, MSF International Council: Drugs for neglected diseases working group Retrieved March 14, 2006, from http://www.neglecteddiseases.org/> www.unaids.org.

Samuelsen H: Illness transmission and proximity: local theories of causation among the Bissa in Burkina Faso, *Med Anthropol*. 2:89–112, 2004.

World Health Organization: http://www3.who.int/whosis/country/indicators.cfm?country=bfa (retrieved March 2, 2006).

World Health Organization: 2006: Immunization, vaccines and biologicals. Retrieved September 21, 2006 from http://www.who.int/immunization_monitoring/en/globalsummary/countryprofileresult.cfm?C='bfa'.

World Health Organization: http://www3.who.int/whosis/country/indicators.cfm?country=bfa (retrieved March 2, 2006).

◆ BURUNDI (REPUBLIC OF)

MAP PAGE (801)

Jérôme Maslin

Location: Burundi is an enclaved country in the African Great Lakes region with an equatorial climate, tempered by the altitude (average of 1,700 m). The total area is 28,734 km^2, and the population is more than eight million, with about 47% aged between 0 and 14 years. The population density is 243 inhabitants per km^2, the largest in Africa after Rwanda. The capital, Bujumbura, is the most populated city. The temperatures are moderate, and the rainy season lasts 4 to 5 months. It is surrounded by Zaire to the west, Tanzania to the south and east, and Rwanda to the north. The central highlands make up most of the country. The most rainy and cold region is above an altitude of 2,000 m, and the dry season lasts from June to August. The gross domestic product (GDP) per capita is $700, with 68% below the poverty line. Literacy rates are 56% for men, 45% for women.

Major Languages	Ethnic Groups	Major Religions
French (official)	Hutu (Bantu) 85%	Roman Catholic 75%
Kirundi (official)	Tutsi (Hamitic) 14%	Protestant 15%
Swahili	Twa (Pygmy) 1%	Animist 5%
		Muslim 5%

By the nineteenth century, Burundi was ruled by the *mwami* ("king"), who was a Tutsi. After World War I, Burundi became part of the Belgian League of Nations mandate. Christianity spread, but the traditional and social culture was not altered. Christian religious practice often includes syncretism and ancestral rituals. In 1962, Burundi became independent, and the first conflicts between Hutus and Tutsis began. In 1966, the republic was established with a multiparty system. Since 1993 Burundi has been convulsed by ethnic violence in which thousands of Hutus and Tutsis died and many fled the country. In 2001 the Arusha accords, a Tutsi-Hutus power-sharing agreement, was finalized, and United Nations peacekeepers began withdrawing in 2006. One of the consequences of the civil war has been mass population movement. One in six Burundese is displaced outside the country (in neighboring countries) or inside the country (in somewhere other than their areas of residency). Most left in the first days of killing and are still in camps. The three major ethnic groups are Hutus, Tutsis, and Twas. Hutu and Tutsi are best known for their recent bloody clashes. The Twas represents only 1%, but they were the original inhabitants and were outnumbered by the Hutus. The Tutsis migrated into the country and become dominant over the Hutus. The Twas are considered pariahs and live completely outside of the dominant political, social, and economic networks of the country. All these ethnic groups share the same language and culture and worship the same God, Imaana. Kirundi is the only language spoken without regional and ethnical variants by 100% of the Burundese. French, the first official language learned in school, is used primarily by public servants and intellectuals. Swahili is spoken mainly in urban neighborhoods, markets, and commercial settings and is also widely spoken along Lake Tanganyika. English is taught in secondary school.

Health Care Beliefs: Most people acknowledge the importance of preventive and health-promotion services; however, about 90% of the population does not use modern health care services because they consider them too expensive, lacking quality drugs, and staffed by poorly prepared caregivers. Nurses tend to refer patients to traditional healers for diseases such as liver diseases, mental conditions, and those believed to be caused by sorcery. Individuals define health and illness specifically, mentioning the perceived causes of each. Being healthy is having housing, being able to conduct daily activities, and feeling well. Being ill is having too little or poor-quality food and poor hygiene. People believe that eating well and having access to good hygiene are necessary to maintaining good health. In rural areas, people would add that it is necessary to have good crop production to have good health. Crop destruction during ethnic upheaval was considered to be the worst scourge of that period.

Predominant Sick-Care Practices: A century of Christianity and many decades of colonialism have not eliminated ancestral health practices. The Burundian traditional healer is still a powerful figure in health care. The health professional wants to deal only with the specific-organic health problems of his patient. This does not satisfy the patient because, when the disease lasts, it becomes for the patient a sign of disturbance or conflict between himself, his family, his clan, or an angry ancestor. It is then necessary to seek the hidden reasons for the illness in order to manage it, and if God, "Imaana," agrees, to heal it. This perception is characteristic of African countries where the weight of tribal culture is great. People

B

alternate between imported occidental medicine with its drugs and traditional medicine with symbolic rituals and connections with the invisible world. The healer is an herbalist but also a psychologist who cures traditional "poisoning" and chases away evil aggressors. The master of divination imitates the healer in the sense that he guesses the origins of the evil or sickness and exorcises it with various plants and sacred rituals. He may produce talismans of wood or antelope horns filled with elements used as protection against evil and to ensure the good health of the user. The master of divination has no relationship with God but is connected to the spirits. The unprecedented collapse of infrastructure has broken a weak national health system lacking essential drugs, vaccines, medical instruments, and qualified personnel. Most health professionals were killed or work in urban areas for security reasons. Burundi's network of 365 health centers and about 30 referral hospitals were entirely destroyed. The health insurance system implemented by the government in 1984 is no longer effective.

Ethnic-/Race-Specific or Endemic Diseases: Burundi has a predominance of infectious and parasitic diseases. Malaria is the major public health problem: outbreaks are related to environmental factors, population movements, decreases in population immunity, and drug resistance. Respiratory tract infections are the second major problem, and third are diarrheal diseases. Diseases such as human immunodeficiency virus/acquired immunodeficiency syndrome (HIV/AIDS), epidemic meningitis, bacillary dysentery, and epidemic typhus are emerging at a time when the population has been weakened by 10 years of civil war. The Joint United Nations Programme on HIV/AIDS (UNAIDS) estimates the prevalence rate for HIV in adults (aged 15 to 49) to be 3.3%, with 150,000 living with HIV, including 79,000 women and 20,000 children aged 0 to 14. About 13,000 deaths are attributed to AIDS, and there are 120,000 orphans aged 0 to 17 as the result of parental AIDS. Since the first AIDS case in Burundi, disease progression has been rapid. AIDS is the major cause of death in adults and a major cause of infant death, and more than 70% of the beds in Bujumbura hospital are occupied by AIDS patients.

Health-Team Relationships: Relationships between doctors and nurses are hierarchical and independent of experience: the doctor dominates the interaction. In a country where the rates of those with secondary school and university educations are 6.9% and 0.7%, respectively, the doctor has considerable power. In 2000 the country had only 323 medical doctors (42 specialists) and 1,783 nurses (six specialists). Doctors have a great deal of prestige, and patient satisfaction is always limited if a patient does not see a doctor. Unlike doctors, who are difficult to approach outside the clinical setting, nurses are well integrated in their communities. Nursing education is inaccessible to the vast majority, so nurses are also well regarded. The nurses' capacity to heal, their counseling capabilities, and their presence in the community have maximized their roles as leaders. After the last elections, many nurses became deputies at the National Assembly.

Families' Role in Hospital Care: Most people reside in rural areas, and family life is given supreme importance. Inquiring about someone's health indicates a person cares for another, and Burundese show tremendous solidarity during times of illness. If someone is seriously ill and cannot walk to the health center, people will spontaneously carry the person on a traditional couch to the dispensary. This couch is used as an ambulance and hearse and is shared among families. People who are healthy and refuse to carry a sick person may have social sanctions brought against them. During hospitalizations, families and neighbors share the responsibility of patient care. Because the ill person often remains at home, the best sign of friendship and neighborly kindness is to visit and wish the person a quick recovery. Women ask whether the sick person is eating well regardless of the person's age or sex and provide the person's favorite dishes. If the patient is a man, his companions give him drinks and chat with him if he is able to converse. These moments of companionship and empathy are often significantly therapeutic. If the disease persists or the person is too weak to resume labor, neighbors work for the person, and women care for the person's children.

Dominance Patterns: Families are patriarchal. The husband is the head of the household and is responsible for providing essential needs. He usually makes important decisions in collaboration with his wife. Marriage is made legal by payment of bride wealth. The wife assumes responsibility for the family in case of the husband's absence or death. Burundese women, especially in rural areas, are still exploited. They must produce many children and provide food, fetch wood and water, and care for the health and education of the children. Some men have more than one wife, but this custom is disappearing. Women are the poorest, least educated, and least protected in the society, although new laws allow women more autonomy. Women still have very little monetary power, however, because husbands determine the distribution of income and land for labor. Farming is practiced by many people, but cattle-raising is restricted to the wealthier class. When crops are plentiful, women can sell the surplus at the local market or exchange their production skills for other utilities. Higher income–producing commercial activities such as coffee growing are restricted to the husband, who harvests crops and sells them at public markets. This imbalance in the management of family income leaves women in a vulnerable position. They must often ask the husband to pay for health care services when they or the children need it.

Eye-Contact Practices: Eye contact is highly symbolic. A slight eye signal from a friend when in public means "beware of what you say." A Kirundi proverb says, "The enemy dissimulates his hate for you, and you dissimulate that you know his hate for you through the eyes." Direct eye contact is a sign of love among the young; however, the girl refrains from making direct eye contact with the boy because it is considered more romantic. The boy says that his lover has "the eyes of a young cow," a compliment because the cow has great symbolic value. It is strictly forbidden for young women to stare at their fathers-in-law. This practice also applies to young men and their mothers-in-law. It is strictly forbidden to call in-laws by their names, regardless of their age or social status. Children cannot stare at an adult who is eating or look at the person's mouth, both of which are considered a sign of a bad education. Direct eye contact is not an issue in either traditional or modern health care settings.

Touch Practices and Relationships: To show utmost respect toward an older adult or other socially important individual, the person gives the individual the right hand and at the same time puts the left hand around the individual's right forearm. Older women put their hands on the shoulders of younger people and recite greetings and blessings. Younger women who have not met since their weddings hold each other and sing melancholy songs recalling their childhood years. Except for usual greetings, a father does not touch his daughter, and physical contact is limited between a son and his mother. Every gesture or word about sex or sexual relationships is scandalous and shameful for the whole family. There are familial and social norms that include multiple interdictions and taboos and repression of deviant behaviors. Social status is very important, and signs of status include a person's posture, body movements, and way of speaking. Upper-class people are supposed to act with dignity and not show their emotions.

Perceptions of Time: Use of the hour as a measure of time is an almost nonexistent practice outside urban areas. The time indicators used in the countryside are *mu gitondo* ("morning"), *ku murango* ("noon"), *ku muhingamo* ("afternoon"), and *ku mugoroba* ("evening"). This division divides the day among productive (agriculture and other), domestic, and social activities. Time is not flexible except during social activities such as conversations or having drinks. The most important occasions are political and administrative meetings and Sunday mass, and it is rare for people to arrive late to these events. People also use proxies, such as the length of the shadow, position of the sun, or evolution of sleep *(mumikangura)*. The other measure of time is the squawking of the chickens, first at dawn and then throughout the day until evening. Educated people have a tendency to be late unless coerced to be on time, so events can be delayed for hours. At night, time virtually stops. The family gathers in the living room, which is where passing down of legends, herders' poems, history of the clan, and moral principles takes place. Religious rituals and incantations to placate ancestral spirits can transport participants to symbolic places such as rivers or caves.

Pain Reactions: Burundian culture tends to emphasize control of emotions. Showing pain overtly is synonymous with weakness, especially for adult men, who should never cry in public. It is acceptable for women to express their emotions when they are in physical pain (e.g., after being hurt in a domestic dispute) or emotional pain (e.g., when mourning the loss of a loved one). Midwives reprimand women if they cry when giving birth.

B

Birth Rites: Giving birth confers highly desired social status, and sterile women are stigmatized. The fertility rate is 6.55 children born per woman. More than 80% of births take place at home assisted by uneducated midwives, which largely explains a maternal mortality rate of greater than 800 per 100,000 live births and an infant mortality rate of 63 deaths per 1,000 live births. The only acceptable abortions are therapeutic ones and must be approved by two doctors. Traditional members of society still believe in ancestral spirits, so pregnant women fear evil and wicked charms directed toward their infants. Eating meat or any food hit by lightning is forbidden for all women. Marriage is made legal by payment of bridal wealth. On the eighth day after birth, a ceremony is held to honor the newborn and mother; at this point, the infant is presented to the family and neighbors. It also indicates that the woman may resume sexual relations. Lastly, the celebration means that the woman should resume her domestic work. Boys are preferred because they perpetuate the patriarchal lineage. A mother who produces only daughters is harassed by her in-laws; a practice that can lead to divorce. Giving birth to twins is considered abnormal, and the ritual after the birth is quite complicated to protect the family from bad luck. Life expectancy is 45 for men, 47 for women.

Death Rites: Rites follow Christian traditions, but traditional beliefs are also important. The spirits of dead relatives, called *Abazima,* carry messages between Imaana and the human world. The Abazima may bring bad luck to those who do not respect them, so people offer gifts for protection. Thus, the cause of death is either an "accident" (an indirect expression that means "a violent death from civil war"), a "disease" (death from natural causes rather than from violence), or from "poisoning" (a reference to traditional beliefs). When a person from a rural area dies, he or she is buried immediately. The corpse is laid on a mat and taken to the cemetery. All who attended the burial perform ritual handwashing. The cemetery is a feared place because dead people's spirits are thought to be present; no one wants to be in a cemetery at night. Mourning is strictly observed for 1 week. Wearing black clothing is common in urban areas. Members of the family shave their heads and recite incantations to calm the deceased person's spirit.

Food Practices and Intolerances: Beans are the most common dish and are eaten at least once a day. Milk, butter, and meat are the most highly valued foods. Others are cassava, potatoes, banana, peas, and corn. Meat is reserved for wealthy people. People will kill a cow only on a special occasion. Few people eat meat from sheep, and it is forbidden for children to drink cow's milk after they have eaten peas. Goat meat and goat milk are also eaten. Herders are reluctant to eat their own animals, which is a sign of social status. At least 90% of people eat with their hands. The small fish of Lake Tanganyika are found all over the country. Sweet dishes are rare. Villagers usually do not eat breakfast but have a large meal at noon. Food taboos and interdictions exist,

B

although young people rarely respect them. People wash their hands and then, according to age and occasionally gender, share a meal from the same plate. The father and the mother eat from the same plate in a separate room, and children share the same meal. People make and sell a local banana-based beer called *urwarwa*, and *impeke*, a drink made of millet, is also popular.

Infant-Feeding Practices: Almost all women in rural areas breastfeed their children. If for some reason they cannot, their infant is fed with cow's milk (and in rare situations, another woman feeds the infant). Women in towns also breastfeed, often supplementing breast milk with imported powdered infant formula or cow's milk. Feeding times are not limited or planned except by working women who must follow their employers' schedules. Maternal leave is about 3 months, but breastfeeding lasts about 2 years. Meanwhile, other nutrients are progressively introduced. If a breastfeeding woman becomes pregnant, she immediately stops.

Child-Rearing Practices: Education of small children is the responsibility of the mother. No more than half of Burundians can read and write their native language. A small number can read and write French. High school enrollment is about 7% for boys and 4% for girls. During adolescence the mother prepares her daughter for a woman's life and the son becomes closer to his father. Daughters and sons do not sleep in the same bed, but children of the same sex share beds. On certain occasions such as visits adults of the same gender sleep together. Outside of urban areas, homosexuality is completely unknown.

National Childhood Immunizations: BCG at birth; DTPHiBHep at 6, 10, and 16 weeks; DTwPHiB at 6, 10, and 14 weeks; OPV at birth and at 6, 10, and 14 weeks; measles at 9 months; HepB at 6, 10, and 14 weeks; vitamin A at 9 months; and TT CBAW after first contact + 1 month. The percent of the target population vaccinated, by antigen, is: BCG (84%); DTP1 (86%); DTP3, HepB3, HiB3 (74%); MCV (75%); Polio3 (64%); and TT2 plus (45%).

BIBLIOGRAPHY

Abdul-Rasul TM: Le pluralisme thérapeutique en psychiatrie au quartier asiatique de Bujumbura au Burundi, *Bulletin des Médecins Suisses.* 82:404–6, 2001.

Central Intelligence Agency: *2006: The world factbook, Burundi.* Retrieved September 21, 2006, from https://www.cia.gov/cia/publications/factbook/print/by.html.

International Crisis Group: Le Burundi après la suspension de l'embargo: aspects internes et régionaux, Bruxelles, 1999, ICG.

Office for the Coordination of Humanitarian Affairs—Burundi: update on the humanitarian situation, August–September 2001.

Salama P, Spiegel P, Brennan R: No less vulnerable: the internally displaced in humanitarian emergencies, *Lancet.* 357:1430–1, 2001.

France-Diplomatie>Actions de la France>Aide au développement. Lutte contre le SIDA au Burundi. Retrieved September 20, 2006, from http://www.diplomatie. gouv.fr.

Ministère de la Santé Publique du Burundi/OMS: Profil épidémiologique du Burundi. Annéé 2000. Retrieved on January 17, 2002, from http://mosquito.who.int/ docs/country_updates/burundi.htm.

ONU: Le bureau pour la coordination des affaires humanitaries 2006. Retrieved September 20, 2006, from www.IRlnews.org.

UNAIDS: 2006 Burundi: Retrieved September 21, 2006 from http://www.unaids.org/en/Regions_Countries/Countries/burundi.asp.

World Health Organization 2006: Immunization, vaccines and biologicals. Retrieved September 21, 2006 from http://www.who.int/immunization_monitoring/en/globalsummary/countryprofileresult.cfm?C='bdi'.

C

◆ CAMBODIA (KINGDOM OF)

MAP PAGE (805)

Chhan D. Touch

Location: A large alluvial plain in Southeast Asia, Cambodia is ringed by mountains and bordered by Thailand on the west, Vietnam on the east, Laos on the north, and the Gulf of Thailand on the south. The capital is Phnom Penh. The total area is 181,040 km^2 (69,900 square miles), and the population is 13.9 million. The gross domestic product (GDP) per capita is $2,200, with 40% living below the poverty line. French is spoken by the educated and elite, and different dialects of Chinese are commonly spoken for business.

Major Languages	Ethnic Groups	Major Religions
Khmer/Cambodian	Khmer (Cambodian)	Buddhist (Theravada)
Chinese	90%	95%
Vietnamese	Chinese 1%	Muslim and Other 5%
French	Vietnamese 5%	
Other	Cham and Other 4%	

Health Care Beliefs: Acute sick care; magical-religious. A serious illness after travel is thought to be caused by the wrong diet or violation of certain rituals or pledges. To resolve the problem, food and apologies are offered to the spirits. *Yin* ("cold") and yang ("hot") concepts have wide influence. Yin (female, negative forces, soul, earth, moon, night, water, cold, and darkness) and yang (male, positive forces, day, fire, heat, expansion, and daylight) must be in equilibrium for optimum health. Illness may be caused by disequilibrium in the body force, known as *chi;* and restoring equilibrium cures illness. Mental illnesses are often met with denial and may manifest themselves somatically. According to common beliefs, thinking too much *(kett-cha-roeun),* particularly during periods of stress, creates mental imbalance. Self-treatment strategies include suppressing sad thoughts, being sheltered and protected by family, being encouraged to laugh, and not being left alone. It is common to take sleeping pills or drink alcohol, and suicidal ideology is not unusual. Post-traumatic stress disorder is common in older adults who lived through the Khmer Rouge period after the Vietnam War. Seeking help from a shaman, *kru khmer* ("traditional healer"), or Buddhist monk is common.

Predominant Sick-Care Practices: Biomedical; traditional. According to traditional beliefs, illness is caused by food, the environment, or the supernatural (e.g., spells, gods, demons, evil spirits, or *neak ta*) and by violation of religious codes. Herbal medicines are considered "cold," whereas Western medicine is "hot." During an illness or the postpartum period, cold and hot food consumption rules are adhered to strictly. Some illnesses are thought to be caused by "bad air" trapped in the body. Removing it (by vacuum-cup suction) allows the body to restore itself. Traditional treatments such as skin pinching, coin rubbing, circular burning, therapeutic steam baths, acupuncture, alcohol treatment (to generate heat), and acupressure are also used, and some of these practices result in bruise marks or red lines. Cambodians believe in receiving medication each time they visit a doctor, preferably in the form of injections. Injections are considered more potent than pills, and intravenous infusions of vitamin C or B complex are a favorite way to "gain energy." If suffering is thought to be caused by past sins, treatment might be avoided.

Ethnic-/Race-Specific or Endemic Diseases: Endemic diseases include chloroquine-resistant malaria, bacterial and protozoal diarrhea, dengue hemorrhagic fever, human immunodeficiency virus (HIV)/acquired immunodeficiency syndrome (AIDS), and hepatitis A. There is risk for Japanese encephalitis and schistosomiasis in some locations. The first case of confirmed Avian influenza was discovered in 2005. The Joint United Nations Programme on HIV/AIDS (UNAIDS) estimates the prevalence of HIV in adults (aged 15 to 49 years) is 1.6% to 2.6%, with 130,000 people living with HIV, including 59,000 women (one third of childbearing age), and 3,800 to 14,000 children aged 0 to 15 years. About 16,000 have died of AIDS.

Health-Team Relationships: Because doctors are considered experts and authority figures, their decisions are not questioned; to do so would be considered rude. Patients are given little information, and they do not contradict doctors openly, regardless of whether they intend to comply with the medical recommendation. An open show of impatience, non-compliance, or anger is culturally inappropriate, and remaining controlled protects patients' self-esteem and the health professionals' status. Doctors are usually men, nurses usually women. Nurses are expected to be completely submissive, are not allowed to question orders, and are expected to carry files for doctors during rounds. A female patient may refuse care from a male health care provider, but her husband can override her decision.

Families' Role in Hospital Care: Family members are expected to provide support and comfort, including personal needs and food during hospitalization. Asking family members about the best approach to use for a patient creates positive patient-provider rapport.

Dominance Patterns: The oldest member of the family is the decision maker, with male family members given priority. Husbands are expected

C

to answer all questions about their wife's health, including past medical history, although women are allowed to answer with their husband's consent. Husbands are responsible for earning money and providing what is necessary for family survival, and women are expected to manage household affairs, including raising the children. Everyone is expected to maintain family honor. Polygamy exists, although it is illegal. Confrontations between legal wives and mistresses occasionally have devastating consequences. It is socially acceptable for married men to have extramarital affairs, but women who commit adultery are disowned.

Eye-Contact Practices: Direct eye contact is disrespectful and a sign of intentional confrontation. Cambodian patients avoid direct eye contact with health care professionals who are of higher social status. This behavior should not be interpreted as an attempt to conceal information.

Touch Practices: The head, especially of a man, is considered sacred and is revered. Touching a child's head intentionally without parental consent may make parents or relatives angry and even physically violent. It is acceptable for parents to touch their children's heads, although touching is rare in many families. Handshaking has recently gained acceptance among men in the city; but it is still unacceptable in the countryside for younger men to shake older men's hands. The *wai* (placing both palms together and slightly bowing the head) is commonly used and acceptable among all ages and sexes. Physical contact during any greeting with a person of the opposite sex is strongly discouraged.

Perceptions of Time: Time is irrelevant and flexible. Planning for the future and keeping appointments are not considered important, and tardiness is expected. Setting a deadline for a task does not guarantee completion. The concept of taking medication at a specific time is not well understood or practiced, so some take their medications only if they feel ill.

Pain Reactions: Pain may be severe before relief is requested. Traditionally, pain has been thought of as a consequence of terrible deeds (*kama* or "sin") in a previous life, so some may prefer to endure pain to ensure a better reincarnation.

Birth Rites: Prenatal care is available only for influential, well-educated, or wealthy families. The fertility rate is 3.37 children born per woman. Because of concerns that prenatal vitamins increase the weight and size of the fetus, causing a difficult delivery, they may be rejected. Women also diet during pregnancy to keep infants small. Infant mortality is high at 69 deaths per 1,000 live births. Childbirth is considered to be a "cold" process because heat is lost during delivery. Women who have just given birth may refuse cold baths, cold water, and cold foods. Hot drinks, extremely spicy foods, and heavy blankets are commonly used to retain and replenish heat. Alcohol fermented with various herbs, and animals' internal organs and blood are consumed to regenerate heat. In the countryside, some women lie on mats over burning charcoal. Certain tasks such as getting up, walking, lifting, working, and self-care are restricted. Certain foods are forbidden because of the potential for *torrs*, a form of food-induced illness. Praising a newborn is prohibited and considered a bad omen. A knife or weapon is placed above the infant's head to frighten away evil spirits and keep them from snatching the infant. Life expectancy is 57 for men, 61 for women.

Death Rites: Life, birth, and *samsara* ("the circle of life") are the main themes in Cambodian Buddhist culture. Good deeds in the current life ensure a good rebirth. Patients prefer to die at home. At the last moment of life, monks are invited to chant to help the spirit leave the body properly. Candles are lit to allow the spirit to see the path, and baskets of food, money, and other goods are placed at the foot of those who are near death—an offering to take to the next life. Neighbors join in and may bring small gifts of money. After death, the family smears the person's face, palms, and soles with thick turmeric sauce. White clothes are placed on these areas to obtain physical imprints of the person, which serve as remembrances. It is thought that the spirit of the deceased will continually protect whoever carries or keeps these items. This process is most commonly followed with parents, grandparents, or well-respected individuals. The washing ceremony is carried out by the family as a way to pay their last respects and ask for forgiveness for wrongs unknowingly done to the person while they were alive. The body is kept in the house or temple for up to 7 days. Cambodians believe that the lost spirit may return and re-enter the body. After 7 days, an elaborate ceremony and procession take place, and the body is prepared for cremation. Male family members are expected to shave their heads, and men and women must wear white with a black arm band or a small piece of attached black cloth and no jewelry. Baskets of goods, food, and money are given to the priest. A coin is placed inside the mouth, and the favorite child finds this coin after cremation. The ashes are kept at the temple for 7 days. Then the ashes can be kept in an urn and placed in the temple or family *stupa* (a small house that stores the ashes of dead ancestors). Family members continue to wear white during the 3-month mourning period, and elaborate decorations, celebrations, jewelry, or joyous activities are prohibited.

Food Practices and Intolerances: Families demonstrate love through food, and families enjoy several dishes at every meal. Meat, vegetables, and rice are the major parts of Cambodian diets; many are lactose intolerant. Meat is expensive and normally is consumed only by wealthy individuals.

Infant-Feeding Practices: Breastfeeding is common practice and may continue until the child is 3. Formula is usually unavailable and expensive. Colostrum is considered dirty and is discarded. Solid foods are introduced at about 4 months; they are chewed by the mother, aunt, or grandmother before being given to the infant. In traditional families, boys may breastfeed for as many years as they desire to enhance their power and energy, whereas girls may be weaned at 2 years to prevent them from developing those male characteristics. Weaning usually results in ending milk intake completely because no fresh milk is available. During weaning, spicy, salty, or bitter substances are smeared on the nipples to discourage the child from sucking.

Child-Rearing Practices: The character and personality of an infant are thought to be determined by the time of the day, date, month, year, and season of birth. A girl is preferred as the first child because girls are more helpful to their mothers. Babies are frequently touched, cared for, and carried about by the mother or another woman. Parents are relaxed with children under 6, but then strict upbringing begins; independence is discouraged and obedience is demanded. The oldest child, whether boy or girl, is responsible for younger siblings if the parents die, are old, or are ill. Large families are preferred, especially in poor populations because more workers are available. Boys are encouraged to obtain an education, but when girls reach puberty they are discouraged from further learning. Between puberty and marriage, the traditional girl spends 1 month in seclusion and solitude, a practice known as *choul-ma-loup*. She observes many rites, eats a vegetarian diet, remains in her room in the dark, and is visited only by her mother. Her name may be changed to confuse potential evil spirits, and she is released only after she is married. The popularity of this practice is decreasing.

National Childhood Immunizations: BCG at birth; HepB at birth; DTwP at 6, 10, and 14 weeks; DTwPHep at 6, 10, and 14 weeks; OPV at birth and at 6, 10, and 14 weeks; measles at 9 months; vitamin A at 6 to 59 months for children and lactating women; and TT after first contact, + 1 month, +1, and +1 year. The percent of the target population vaccinated, by antigen, is: BCG (87%); DTP1 (85%); DTP and Polio3 (82%); MCV (79%); and TT2 plus (53%).

Other Characteristics: Women do not assume their husbands' last name after marriage. Wrist strings or lead-wrapped waist strings are worn to prevent the soul from venturing outside the body, and infants may wear them around the neck, ankles, or waist. Speaking loudly, yelling, snapping fingers under the nose, pointing, beckoning with a finger, or holding hands outstretched with the palm up offends others.

BIBLIOGRAPHY

Central Intelligence Agency: *2006: The world factbook, Cambodia.* Retrieved September 21, 2006, from https://www.cia.gov/cia/publications/factbook/print/cb.html.

D'Avanzo C: Bridging the cultural gap with Southeast Asians, *MCN, Am J Matern Child Nurs.* 17(4):204, 1992.

D'Avanzo C: The Southeast Asian client and alcohol and other drug abuse: implications for health care providers, *Subst Abuse.* 15(2):109, 1994.

D'Avanzo C: Southeast Asians: Asian Pacific Americans at risk for substance abuse, *Subst Use Misuse.* 32:829, 1997.

D'Avanzo C, Barab S: Depression and anxiety among Cambodian refugee women in France and the United States, *Issues Ment Health Nurs.* 19:1, 1990.

D'Avanzo C, Barab S: Drinking during pregnancy: practices of Cambodian refugees in France and the United States, *Health Care Women Int.* 21(4):319, 2000.

D'Avanzo C, Frye B: Research update: stress and self medication in Cambodian refugee women, *Addictions Nurs Net.* 4(2):59, 1992.

D'Avanzo C, Frye B, Froman R: Culture, stress and substance use in Cambodian refugee women, *J Stud Alcohol.* 55(4):420, 1994.

D'Avanzo C, Frye B, Froman R: Stress in the Cambodian refugee family: perceptions reported by Cambodian women, *Image*. 26(2):99, 1994.

UNAIDS: 2006 Cambodia. Retrieved September 21, 2006, from http://www.unaids.org/en/Regions_Countries/Countries/cambodia.asp.

World Health Organization: *2006: Immunization, vaccines and biologicals*. Retrieved September 21, 2006, from http://www.who.int/immunization_monitoring/en/globalsummary/countryprofileresult.cfm?C='khm'.

C

◆ CAMEROON (REPUBLIC OF)

MAP PAGE (800)

Abraham Ndiwane

Location: The Republic of Cameroon is a triangular-shaped country, with a total area of 475,000 km^2 (183,569 square miles) on the Atlantic coastline of West Africa. It is an independent and democratic country, occupying a central, strategic position on the African continent. The population is 17.3 million, and the capital is Yaounde. The gross domestic product (GDP) per capita is $2,400, with about 48% of people living below the poverty line (as high as 86% in rural areas); however, Cameroon has better living conditions than most of its neighbors.

Major Languages	Ethnic Groups	Major Religions
English (official)	Cameroon Highlander 31%	Christian 53%
French (official)	Equatorial Bantu 19%	Traditional, Animist 25%
African languages	Other African 13%	Muslim 22%
	Kirdi 11%	
	Fulani 10%	
	Northwestern Bantu 8%	
	Eastern Sudanic 7%	
	Other 1%	

Cameroonians think that the diverse cultures of its people characterize its identity, and cultural pride has tremendous significance. Cameroon is a bilingual nation and linguistically diverse, with more than 200 distinct dialects. There are 24 major native languages, predominantly Bantu dialects. Literacy rates are 85% for men, 73% for women.

Health Care Beliefs: Acute sick care; traditional. People seek out Western medical practitioners and pay for the services themselves, especially in private and nonprofit health facilities. The major emphasis of health care is on treating diseases rather than preventing them. Those who need services the most (predominantly poor, rural inhabitants) are the least able to afford them. It is recognized that health care should concentrate on primary health facilities for villages and rural inhabitants because practitioners at these facilities can respond to local demands and conditions.

Predominant Sick-Care Practices: Biomedical; ethno-medical; magical-religious. Essential health services are frequently unavailable or difficult to access, although regional disparities have improved. In public facilities, services are subsidized but are usually not well equipped. Patients may be referred to local pharmacies for prescriptions, where they pay for the medications themselves. Traditional beliefs and value systems are strong and deeply rooted. Theories about the causes of certain diseases include witchcraft or the wrath of the gods (e.g., gods of river, forest, soil, rain, and stone), so people seek out interventions from a sorcerer, herbalist, or medicine man—a person believed to possess supernatural powers to cure and protect the sick through rituals or wearing amulets. Herbalists (often called traditional doctors) have gained national attention and acknowledgment from the government for their ability to treat people whom medical practitioners consider terminal. Although the scientific community dispels such outcomes as anecdotal, traditional herbalists have contributed significantly to health care delivery, particularly in rural communities where health services are not affordable. In the northwestern region of the country, herbalists are acknowledged for their ability to cure fevers, headaches, fractures, infertility, possession by evil spirits, and human immunodeficiency virus (HIV)/acquired immunodeficiency syndrome (AIDS). People of all income levels, from all regions of the country, and of varying educational status use the services of herbalists. The coexistence of biomedical and traditional models of care requires health professionals to be nonjudgmental. Primary health care is a fairly new concept because essential health services are still lacking in most regions. A significant decline in the health infrastructure amid budget cuts has led to poor quality and management of health services and deterioration of health indicators such as infant mortality.

Ethnic-/Race-Specific of Endemic Diseases: Malaria, tuberculosis, bacterial diarrhea, hepatitis A, childhood measles, and HIV/AIDS are significant challenges. In some areas, yellow fever, schistosomiasis and meningococcal meningitis may occur. Although these diseases are preventable, they are the major killers of children and adults. Programs to reduce disease may be thwarted by traditional beliefs, attitudes, and practices. For example, an attempt to reduce neonatal tetanus in women of childbearing age was misinterpreted as a government attempt to sterilize women. This politically charged rumor frightened women and virtually halted the initiative. The Joint United Nations Programme on HIV/AIDS (UNAIDS) reports the estimated prevalence rate for HIV in adults (aged 15 to 49 years) as 5.4%, with 510,000 people living with HIV, including 290,000 women and 43,000 children aged 0 to 14. There are 240,000 orphans aged 0 to 17 as the result of parental AIDS. Deaths from AIDS are estimated to be 46,000. Cameroon has consistently increased funding for HIV/AIDS testing and treatment as a result of the government's strong political

commitment. Presently, only 22% of those infected are receiving antiretroviral therapy.

Health-Team Relationships: Medical doctors command significant
power. When patients seek health care, they usually prefer to be screened
and treated by a doctor. Most also expect a doctor to prescribe oral or
parenteral medications and may not follow medical advice when they do
not receive them. Nurses with advanced training have an expanded role
and work collaboratively with physicians to screen and treat patients,
particularly in settings with few doctors (virtually all settings). Nurses
spend more time with patients than doctors do because doctors are
expected to address more complex cases and have heavier workloads.
Patients are gradually beginning to trust nurses and think of them as
expert caregivers, particularly in health education at the primary prevention
levels.

Families' Role in Hospital Care: Illness concerns the whole family. It is
common to find the immediate and extended family at a patient's bedside
on a 24-hour basis. The numerous family members rallying at the bedside
can be detrimental to care, but family members generally cooperate with
health care providers and observe visitation hours. Family visits are important because they provide a forum for keeping the patient updated about
the community, and family members bring home-cooked meals.

Dominance Patterns: The traditional (rural) community is closely knit;
composed of siblings and extended family members living in compounds
(large pieces of land headed by a patriarch). Although it is expected that
adult siblings will leave their compounds of birth to create new ones, particularly when they are married, they are not expected to rush to do so,
especially when illness or financial constraints develop. Siblings who move
out of their native compound live close by and can reconvene in the parent
compound at a moment's notice in the event of an illness, death, or birth.
Patients who are sick gain the respect, sympathy, and attention of all
members. This is more difficult in urban communities because men and
women have professional jobs, participate in the political structure of
government, and are often dispersed throughout the country because
of job assignments.

Eye-Contact Practices: It is considered rude to stare or maintain eye
contact with an authority figure. Children will generally look down during
verbal discipline by an authority figure, even if they are told to look at
the person who is speaking. Looking down is considered showing respect
for authority. Western health care practitioners should be aware of these
cultural traits.

Perceptions of Time: Time is particularly important to those who have
jobs because some are paid only for the time they actually spend working.
Punctuality is generally not a major concern, and people may be late
for appointments and other commitments. Some keep time by approxima-
tion—for example, by looking at the direction and the intensity of the sun
or the appearance and shape of the moon. Values and beliefs are strongly
shaped and governed by past traditions handed down from one

generation to another through nightly songs and stories when family members congregate.

Pain Reactions: It is expected that men should be stoic and not cry in public when feeling physical or emotional pain; however, women are free to express their feelings. In a rural community, a person might hear a wailing woman half a mile away as she grieves the loss of a loved one, whereas the woman's husband would be disgustedly mopping tears from his face, ashamed that he is crying.

Touch Practices: Physical touching, such as hugging or a handshake, is acceptable, but touching is also associated with rituals such as prayers and traditional healing practices. It is becoming more acceptable and common for members of the opposite sex to hold hands in public, particularly in towns and cities, but this practice is rare in rural villages, where traditional customs are stronger.

Birth Rites: Parents of newlyweds are apprehensive if a couple has no children within a year or two of marriage or cohabitation. The woman is generally alleged to be the cause of infertility, but in rare situations the man takes some of the blame. Infertile couples may seek the assistance of a traditional healer or doctor. When a woman is pregnant, she is adored by her husband and relatives. She essentially gets everything she desires, and her husband makes every effort to accommodate her wishes. Similarly, the husband enjoys feelings of manhood and admiration from his peers. The infant mortality rate is high at 64 deaths per 1,000 live births. Some Cameroonians believe that labor and birth can be delayed until a mother can get to a birthing facility. For example, a woman in labor may leave her farm, walk 3 miles, and give birth almost immediately after arriving at the nearest birthing center. Women with these beliefs wear amulets or place a medicine leaf under their tongue, which is believed to offer guidance and protection until birth. Home births are rare. In such situations, the mother and infant are taken to a medical facility for follow-up evaluations. Women are reluctant to accept analgesics, which they believe interrupts nature's processes. A female relative or friend usually accompanies a woman in labor to a health facility. Husbands are not expected to be with their wives during labor or delivery because of the husband's discomfort with the process, a respect for the wife's privacy, and society's belief that the birthing process is best handled by women. These views are slowly changing through education that encourages husbands to participate in the birth of their children. Birth is a time of celebration marked by singing, dancing, and round-the-clock cooking and feasting. It is the perfect opportunity for grandparents and others to live with the family for an extended period and assist the new mother with chores. In the past, wealthy parents preferred to have sons so that they could be heirs to the family fortune, whereas poor parents celebrated female children more because the family expected bridal gifts before marriage. These commodity-orientated perceptions have changed, however, because more parents are sending their children to school; therefore, the age of marriage tends to be older. The fertility rate decreased from 5.7% in 1992 to 4.4% in 2006. The focus on education is the result of a joint effort by the government, missionary societies, and private initiatives to encourage literacy. Cameroon has one of the highest rates of school attendance in Africa, with data indicating that 93% of 6-year-old boys and 84% of 6-year-old girls are enrolled in primary school. Life expectancy is 51 for both men and women.

Death Rites: Death, like birth, is a family event that is characterized by days or weeks of mourning. If the deceased person was old or had attained status in the community, the death ritual and celebration tends to be more prolonged and elaborate than it is for an infant. When the cause of death is poorly understood, people generally blame a dissenting family member or witchcraft rather than natural causes. The body may undergo special cleansing rituals by a traditional herbalist or someone believed to have supernatural powers. The body is buried quickly and far from commonly inhabited areas so that the ghost of the deceased does not return to hurt the living. Autopsies and organ donations are generally unacceptable. In some communities, the bodies of deceased Christians are washed and dressed according to local customs. A religious service is conducted by a priest or pastor before burial. If the deceased was a non-Christian or an atheist, traditional burial rites and celebrations take place.

Food Practices and Intolerances: Most kitchen chores are the responsibility of women. For traditional Cameroonians, a good wife is a woman who is able to prepare various dishes for her husband and his friends. A good husband should be able to work hard and provide food for his wife and family. Food choices tend to vary according to regions of the country. For instance, in the northwest the diet may consist of corn *fufu* (corn flour cooked into a paste) eaten with various vegetables that are mixed with spiced smoked meat or fish. A delicacy known as *achuh* is made from *cocoyams* (tuberous plants) that are cooked and pounded into a paste in a wooden vessel. Achuh is eaten with dried meat, "bush meat," or eggplant *njaniki* in a spicy pudding that is rich in sodium and potassium. Fufu and achuh are traditionally served on leaves, woven baskets, or wood dishes and eaten with the hands. Food may be eaten this way even when it is liquid or semi-liquid. Although other foods such as rice, beans, and plantains may be eaten sporadically, such foods may not be considered "real" foods because they do not leave people satiated for long periods unless they are supplemented with fufu or achuh. In the southwestern and coastal regions, the staple diet may include *kwacoco* (grated cocoyams cooked with palm-nut soup) and *minyado'oh* (fermented cassava tubers cooked and eaten with roasted fish).

Infant-Feeding Practices: In the past, multinational companies advertised milk products and infant formulas. In an attempt to increase the quantities of expensive formulas, people ignored instructions and diluted them. This practice, combined with poor sterilization techniques, led to infant malnutrition and diarrhea. The Ministry of Health has begun to emphasize the importance of educating parents about the benefits of breast milk and the fact that it is the best source of nutrition for infants, particularly with regard to boosting the immune system. The duration of breastfeeding may span from birth to 18 months, although semisolid foods such as cornstarch pap fortified with sweeteners such as sugar or honey may be introduced at about 6 months. The consumption of poorly processed honey by children younger than 1 year of age has been associated with botulism. Fruit such as bananas, pears, and avocados are mashed into a paste or made into porridge and fed to infants as young as 4 months.

Child-Rearing Practices: Traditional communities are especially close, and most know one another well. Children rarely get away with criminal acts because the community participates in rearing the children, and corporal discipline such as spanking is the entire community's responsibility. In fact, some children are punished twice for the same crime—first by the person who observed the crime being committed and second by the parents. At an early age, children are taught obedience and respect for older adults. Children may not carry on a conversation when older adults are talking. If an older person walks into a room, all children and young adults must rise and offer their seats, even when other seats are available. Disciplinary measures are primarily the responsibility of the father, but in some situations the mother is the dominant disciplinarian. Children are given daily tasks such as fetching wood and water for cooking after returning from school and assisting parents on the farm on days when they do not attend school. These chores encourage the development of a work ethic and inculcate a sense of skill, autonomy, and civic responsibility that will be important for later years.

National Childhood Immunizations: BCG at birth; DTPHep at 6, 10, and 14 weeks; OPV at birth and at 6, 10, and 14 weeks; measles at 9 months; vitamin A at 6 and 12 months; YF at 9 months; TT after first contact $+1$, $+6$ months, $+1$, $+1$ year. The percent of the target population vaccinated, by antigen, is: BCG (77%); DTP1 (85%); DTP3 (80%); HepB3 and Polio3 (79%); MCV (68%); and TT2 plus (65%). Coverage levels have increased by 40%, which is attributed to a stabilizing economy, improved vaccination campaigns, decentralization of the health system, and an improvement in reporting systems.

Acknowledgments: This work is dedicated to Magdalene Pekianze Ndiwane, also known as "Big Mami," the matriarch of the Ndiwane family, who died in 2001 at Bangolan-Ndop, Cameroon at the age of 91.

BIBLIOGRAPHY

Central Intelligence Agency: *2006: The world factbook, Cameroon.* Retrieved September 21, 2006, from https://www.cia.gov/cia/publications/factbook/print/cm.html.

Clark JI, Englebert P. *Regional surveys of the world, Africa south of the Sahara 2001,* ed 30, London, 2001, Europa Publications.

DeLancey MW, Delancey MD: *Historical dictionary of the Republic of Cameroon,* ed 3, Lanham, Md, 2000. Scarecrow Press.

The Economist Intelligence Unit Limited: *Country profile, Cameroon,* London, 2000, Redhouse Press.

Feldman-Savelsberg P, Ndonko FT, Schmidt-Ehry B: Sterilizing vaccines or the politics of the womb: retrospective study of a rumor in Cameroon, *Med Anthrop Quart.* 14(2):159, 2000.

Panford S, Nyaney MO, Amoah SO, Aidoo NG: Using folk media in HIV/AIDS prevention in rural Ghana, *Am J Public Health.* 91(10):1559, 2001.

UNAIDS: 2006 Cameroon: Retrieved September 21, 2006, from http://www.unaids.org/en/Regions_Countries/Countries/cameroon.asp.

World Health Organization: Immunization, vaccines and biologicals. Retrieved September 21, 2006, from http://www.who.int/immunization_monitoring/en/globalsummary/countryprofileresult.cfm?C='cmr'.

World Health Report: Cameroon: Basic indicators for population health, 2004. Retrieved November 8, 2005, from www.who.int/whr/2004/annex/country/cmr/en/print.htm.

◆ CAPE VERDE (REPUBLIC OF)

MAP PAGE (800)

Félix Neto and Ana Veríssimo Ferreira

Location: Cape Verde is in the North Atlantic Ocean, 600 km west-northwest of Senegal. It has 10 major islands and 8 islets, with a total area of 4,030 km² (1556 square miles). The six inhabited islands are characterized by mountainous landscapes, whereas the other three have long beaches. The islands are divided into two groups named after the trade winds from the African continent: windward (Barlavento) and leeward (Sotavento). Cape Verde has a milder climate than neighboring countries at the same latitude. The east winds from the African continent are extremely warm during January and February, making the climate tropical and dry. Cape Verdeans are famous for their friendliness and hospitality.

Major Languages	Ethnic Groups	Major Religions
Portuguese (official)	Creole (Mulatto) 71%	Roman Catholic 80%
Crioulo (Portuguese and West African blend)	African 28%	fused with indigenous beliefs
	European 1%	Other or None 20%

Portuguese is used for formal communication; Crioulo (Creole) is used for informal communication. The population is 434,812 (231,650 in urban and 203,162 in rural areas). Santiago is the largest island and the capital, with 50% of the population. The islands were discovered and colonized by the Portuguese in the fifteenth century and became a trading center for African slaves. Most Cape Verdeans descend from both groups. Although independence was achieved in 1975, the vestiges of

Portuguese culture are considerably more evident than are the African, except on the island of São Tiago, which has more people of African ancestry. The gross domestic product (GDP) per capita is about $6,200, and about 30% live below the poverty line. Literacy rates are 86% for men, 69% for women.

Health Care Beliefs: Acute sick care; traditional. There has been an increase in health services, and both general and infant mortality rates have improved. A primary care system needs to be developed directed toward high-risk groups, with emphasis on disease prevention and health promotion. An efficient ambulance service that can transfer patients among islands is needed. Health care access is particularly limited in socially and geographically underprivileged areas. Residents in these areas do not have good sanitary conditions because of a lack of access to potable water and deficiencies in basic sanitation and sewer systems. It is common for people either to pray or wear amulets to ward off illnesses or to bring about a cure. Mental heath has not been adequately addressed, and those afflicted are often found living on the streets, assisted only by neighbors. People tend to believe that such disorders are caused by evil spirits.

Predominant Sick-Care Practices: Biomedical; magical-religious. Cape Verde ranks fourth in Africa in the categories of health services, education, and quality of life. Patients seek help from doctors as well as from indigenous healers, who use teas and treatments made from plants and oils. These two healing systems coexist despite governmental efforts to promote and improve the Public Health Service and create more private services. Patients make appointments with doctors in either hospitals or in smaller facilities called *health units*. There are two central (Praia and Mindelo) and three regional hospitals (Santo Antão, Santa Catarina, and Fogo). All the islands have health units. In the health service, people pay a hospital fee. In the private service, people pay about $35 per visit. Since 1991, about 93 new doctors and 16 specialists trained in Cuba have been admitted. This allows more doctors per island and health services, available 24 hours a day. Cape Verde has about 300 doctors and 400 nurses. The ratio of doctors to inhabitants is 1:1,500, and the ratio of nurses is 1:1,300, with more health professionals in urban areas. The average number of hospital beds is about 650. A new infrastructure has been implemented and 2 new hospitals, 4 health centers, and 13 sanitary units are under construction. It is expected that these will improve diagnosis, medical assistance, and working conditions for health professionals.

Ethnic-/Race-Specific or Endemic Diseases: Despite being near the African continent, Cape Verde has exemplary sanitary standards and good vaccination coverage on all islands. In recent years, health officials have reported 66 cases of malaria, including one death from complications of cerebral malaria in Praia, São Tiago. Imported malaria from other countries in West Africa is believed to be the primary cause of the outbreak. In response, the Ministry of Health and local public health officials are taking measures to reduce mosquito breeding sources and have increased surveillance activities, including screening local residents and travelers from West African countries. Transmission of malaria on São Tiago is seasonal, peaking from September to November. Health officials are concerned about the spread of endemic diseases such as cholera, dysentery, meningitis, human immunodeficiency virus (HIV)/acquired immunodeficiency syndrome (AIDS), and tuberculosis. Several projects are in progress to increase access to safe water and improve living conditions. Heart disease registries did not exist before 1989; however, it is clear that cardiovascular problems are increasing. Diarrheal and respiratory system diseases are the main causes of mortality in children younger than 5 years; malnutrition and perinatal infections are also major problems. With World Health Organization (WHO) assistance, the country is attempting to increase vaccination coverage and develop better screening for diseases. Increases in technical training and the introduction of new medical specialties are being used to improve health care. WHO has no national statistics for HIV/AIDS, but some sources report an estimated prevalence rate of 0.035%, with about 778 persons living with HIV/AIDS and an estimated 225 deaths. The islands have implemented projects to measure prevalence and increase awareness of the disease. There is universal free access to antiretroviral therapy.

Health-Team Relationships: Relationships among health care professionals and patients are excellent. Despite the lack of technical and human resources in hospitals and health care settings, health professionals form a team to assist as best they can given their resources. Doctors and nurses work in cooperation in hospitals and health units in the islands. Specialized services lack enough radiology, laboratory, instrumentation, and anesthesiology technicians. Pediatricians, gynecologists, public health doctors, radiologists, and cardiologists are available. Although Cape Verde has a nursing school, the quality of education is low.

Families' Role in Hospital Care: The traditional family is extended and includes children, grandparents, uncles, aunts, parentless godchildren, and homeless children. Family members are close and provide a safety net when members are sick. They visit frequently and bring food to hospitalized patients because the meals provided are inadequate. It is often common for families to provide other necessities such as sanitary products and diapers.

Dominance Patterns: Older adults have the most knowledge and experience and are still the most respected family members. Boys are trained only to do chores that are considered men's work, and girls follow the example of their mothers. From preadolescence on, the roles of male and female are markedly different. Domestic violence against women such as spousal abuse and rape is common. People rarely report such crimes to the police, and neighbors and relatives keep silent. Women's organizations are seeking legislation to address crimes of domestic violence, but women are often reluctant to seek legal action. Despite constitutional prohibitions, sex discrimination continues. Legal provisions delineate full equality, and yet women have difficulty obtaining certain types of jobs even though they are paid less than men. The constitution prohibits discrimination against women in family and custody matters, but most women are unaware of their rights largely because they are illiterate. The Organization of Cape Verdean Women alleges disparate treatment in inheritance matters despite laws calling for equal rights. Physical and sexual child abuse and mistreatment and juvenile prostitution are continuing problems, exacerbated by chronic poverty, large (unplanned) families, and traditionally high levels of emigration of adult men. Neither women nor men are circumcised.

Eye-Contact Practices: Direct eye contact is acceptable.

Touch Practices: Touch is acceptable even between members of the opposite sex. People are gradually beginning to accept equality of the sexes as traditional ways begin to be replaced by modern ones.

Perceptions of Time: Cape Verdeans are not concerned with punctuality and consider it unimportant.

Pain Reactions: People are extremely expressive when in pain or grieving.

Birth Rites: The infant mortality rate is 47 deaths per 1,000 births. The fertility rate is 3.38 children born per woman. One third of all families are headed by single mothers, and first pregnancies often occur at a very young age. Women learn the art of being mothers from their families and must follow strict rules during pregnancy or risk being punished by super-natural forces. Mothers adhere to magico-religious traditions. For example, it is believed that eating eggs during pregnancy causes an infant to be born with a big head, which makes childbirth difficult. People believe that pregnant women should not wear mourning clothes, go to funerals or cemeteries, see corpses, or be near children with disabilities because it could kill the fetus. It is also believed that metallic objects near a pregnant woman's belly may cause the child to be born with the shape of the object on the body. Otherwise, normal daily life goes on for pregnant women—carrying heavy objects on their heads, grinding corn, cooking, washing, getting water from the spring, fetching wood, and feeding animals—until very close to delivery. Abiding by three main superstitions is believed to help a woman have an easy delivery. She should walk around a church building three times, be faithful to her husband, and have all her wishes and cravings fulfilled. Midwives deliver infants, prescribe healing treatments of plants and herbs, say prayers, dress wounds, and assist with abortive measures. Pregnant women give birth with the help of the midwife or female relatives or neighbors who have already given birth. Men wait and play cards, talk, and drink. If a mother's labor is prolonged, the midwife prays to the protecting divinities and applies herbal remedies to facilitate the delivery. They also use infusions of plants (*Salvia officinalis*) and oils (ricinus and sweet almonds) for massage. Immediately after birth, infants wear amulets to keep evil spirits away; such as a string around the neck, special beads, or charms inside a small pouch, believed to break the spell of the "evil eye" (causing a person harm just by looking at the person). On some islands after cutting umbilical cords, they place them in the infants' mouth so that they can have some drops of blood (together with sulphur). Infants are then washed with urine. The goal of both of these procedures is protection from sorcery and the "evil eye." The cord and the placenta are buried to prevent bad spirits from influencing the child. Many Cape Verdeans say that they want to return to the place "where their navel was buried." The fact that many children die during the first week has influenced people to believe that potentially evil supernatural forces such as bewitching women and werewolves surround newborns in that first week, so they need the protection of family members. The *noite dos sete* ("night of the seven") ritual is performed on the seventh day after birth. The family has a party with friends to celebrate the end of the isolation period and the infant's survival. During the period of sexual abstinence after the child's birth, women are symbolically considered virgins anew. Baptism comes a few months later, and godparents play an important role because they must raise the godchild if the parents die. Life expectancy is 67 for men, 74 for women.

Death Rites: Each culture has its own traditional funeral ceremonies. The moment a person seems close to death, a *cerimónia de perdão* ("forgiveness ceremony") is held in the presence of a priest or a person representing him. In hospitals, autopsies may be performed after medico-legal forensic procedures have been followed. When a person dies at home, the body is washed with infusions of aromatic herbs, orange peels, and rosemary and dressed for the funeral. Three rites are performed to benefit the dead person. The vital elements of water, earth, and fire must be present. The body undergoes an immersion ritual associated with hiding the body in the earth when it is buried; candlelight must be part of the funeral. If the person is Roman Catholic, the funeral is performed by a priest. As the body is lowered into the grave, they play the *morna hour di bai* ("hour of departure") as every person throws a handful of earth into the grave. Family members, who are crying out and screaming, return to the deceased person's house and have a meal together. The duration of the mourning period varies: if the family members were very close to the person, they go into deep mourning. A widow is allowed to leave the house in about 3 months. Death is associated with beliefs in ghosts, wandering souls, and many other superstitions.

Food Practices and Intolerances: The food is basically Portuguese, but some dishes are unique to the islands. One of the most unusual is *pastel com diablo dentro* ("pastry with the devil inside")—a mix of fresh tuna, onions, and tomatoes wrapped in a pastry blended from boiled potatoes and corn flour, which is deep fried and served hot. Soups are also popular, one of the most common of which is *coldo de peixe* ("fish stew"). The national dish, *catchupa*, is a stew of hominy and beans with fish or meat. The people's daily foods are made more interesting by a diverse combination of popular foods—corn, beans, sweet potatoes, manioc, fish, and various meats—that are enriched by liqueurs and traditional sweets. The people have no religious bans or intolerances to particular foods.

Infant-Feeding Practices: Mothers breastfeed their infants for about 1 year. The infant may also have a *mãe de leite*, another mother who feeds the infant when the actual mother is unable to do so. At about 4 or 5 months, mush and soup are introduced. Cape Verde Children is an organization designed to improve child and family nutrition through monthly subsidies, social services, and instruction.

Child-Rearing Practices: Children generally sleep with their parents or older brothers. Child-rearing styles are quite permissive for young children; however, they are taught to obey and respect older members of the family even though the children do not follow rigid rules.

National Childhood Immunizations: BCG at birth; DTwP at 6, 10, and 14 weeks and at 15.5 months; OPV at birth and at 6, 10, and 14 weeks and at 15.5 months; HepB at birth and at 6 and 14 weeks; measles at 9 months; and TT after first contact, +1, +6, +12, +12 months. The percent of the target population vaccinated, by antigen, is: BCG (78%); DTP1 (75%); DTP3 (73%); HepB3 (69%); MCV (65%); Polio3 (72%); and TT2 plus (55%). Special days for measles vaccination have been established following an epidemic in 1997 to 1998 that caused about 50 deaths.

Other Characteristics: The most common ways to become husband and wife are *amigarem-se* or *ajuntarem-se*, meaning to live in concubinage, and *tirar de casa* ("eloping because of economic difficulties"). Regardless, the couple is considered to be a husband and wife worthy of respect. Later, they may legally marry, frequently during the time when their children or grandchildren are being baptized. A common practice and ancient tradition is the procedure of displaying the bride's virginity to wedding guests by showing them a stained towel. When a widow gets married, there is no celebration. The couple then proceeds to the cemetery where they both cry over the dead husband's grave so that his soul will not haunt them.

BIBLIOGRAPHY

Centers for Disease Control: http://www.cdc.gov/travel/other/cape-verde.htm (retrieved March 6, 2006).

Central Intelligence Agency: 2006: *The world factbook, Cape Verde.* Retrieved September 21, 2006, from https://www.cia.gov/cia/publications/factbook/print/cv.html.

GEP/Ministério da Saúde: *Estatisticas da mortalidade,* Praia, 2000.

Instituto Nacional de Estatística de Cabo Verde: http://ine.cv/estatisticas-cvINE 1990 e 2000—Censo 90 e 2000, Perspectivas demográficas de Cabo Verde—Horizonte 2020 (retrieved April 4, 2006).

Política de saúde, de infância, e de juventude do Governo da República de Cabo Verde: http://www.governo.cv/Prog-Desenv-Social-Saúde.html (retrieved April 4, 2006).

World Health Organization: 2006: Immunization, vaccines and biologicals. Retrieved September 21, 2006, from http://www.who.int/immunization_monitoring/en/globalsummary/countryprofileresult.cfm?C='cpv'.

◆ CENTRAL AFRICAN REPUBLIC

MAP PAGE (800)

Carolyn M. D'Avanzo

C

Location: A landlocked republic 805 km (500 miles) north of the African equator, with a total area of 623,000 km² (240,535 square miles), the Republic is covered with tropical forest in the south and semi-desert land in the northeast. The country shelters the geographic heart of Africa in Bakala (Ouaka). It shares boundaries in the north with Chad, east with Sudan, south with the Democratic Republic of Congo and Congo (Brazzaville), and west with Cameroon. It has an extensive water system that flows all year long, including the Oubangui River. It is one of the poorest countries in the world. The capital is Bangui. The population is 4.3 million, with 41% of the population 0 to 14 years of age. The gross domestic product (GDP) per capita is $1,100. French is the official language; and Sango, the national language, is spoken nationwide. Though not taught in school, Sango is used by the media, at home, in church, and in public institutions. Arabic is mainly used in mosques and Islamic schools. An additional 67 living languages are spoken by 83 tribes. Literacy rates are 63% for men, 40% for women.

Major Languages	Ethnic Groups	Major Religions
French (official)	Baya 34%	Protestant and Roman
Sangho	Banda 27%	Catholic 33%
Arabic	Mandjia 21%	Muslim 44%
	Sara 10%	Indigenous beliefs 23%
	Mboum, Other 8%	

Health Care Beliefs: Acute sick care; traditional. Illness beliefs are rooted in supernatural incidents and belief in evil spirits. Traditional therapies involving abstinence from certain foods and use of laxative agents to ward off evil forces and wash off the core of the illness *(fa mama ti kobela)* are common. Minor illnesses are managed by family, relatives, and neighbors through experienced-based procedures. Traditional rituals are used, occasionally with poor results. The government is targeting such practices through extensive weekly health education campaigns on media channels. Herbal remedies are the first choice for ailments ranging from colds *(koro)* to diarrhea *(sassa)* to fractures *(herbal cast)*. Despite the fact that 40% of the population lives in urban areas, traditional remedies such as suction-pad techniques using small horns to draw out illness are still used. Mental disease is believed to originate from possession by evil spirits when an individual breaks a pact with ancestral spirits or black magic takes over. The society fears those with mental health problems and marginalizes those who are possessed. Acquired immunodeficiency syndrome (AIDS) is perceived simply as a misfortune, and people deny its actual cause. Treatment involves traditional healers and prayers rather than biomedicine. Prenatal care is insufficient outside of Bangui, and very few women comply with their full schedule of appointments. Most births in rural areas occur at home, and women prefer traditional birth attendants, relatives, or friends to hospital delivery rooms and midwives.

Predominant Sick-Care Practices: Magical-religious, with biomedicine as a last resort. Traditional healers, witch doctors, and advice from older adults or neighbors are the primary recourse because sickness is considered the result of fate or a spell. They seek help from modern medical practitioners as the last resort if it is available. The government has recognized that traditional healers are a significant part of its effort to restore and promote the health of the population. Herbal remedies are the custom across the country. For example, a "sauna" of a boiling mixture of barks and leaves is used to heal illnesses ranging from malaria to measles. Scarification plays a dual role in prevention and cures. It is considered a shield against fate and sickness. The small, black, scarred areas on the arms or chest of patients, pregnant women, and children are common. Consultation with fortune tellers and wearing amulets are integrated practices observed by Christians and Muslims. Although more people believe in the healing power of prayer and God's protective interventions, many still adopt mixed practices in which they rely on their talismans but also pray. Sunday is devoted to God, so very few patients go to health care facilities on Sundays, and most businesses are closed. Self-medication practices are also widespread despite efforts by the Ministry of Health to curtail the drug dealers, or *boubanguere,* many of whom are not qualified to give health advice or prescriptions.

Ethnic-/Race-Specific or Endemic Diseases: Malaria outbreaks rage nationwide throughout the year because of the extensive river network, hot and humid climate, and insufficient number of sewers to drain the rain—perfect conditions for mosquito breeding. The malaria strain is resistant to both chloroquine and sulfadoxine-pyrimethamine. Trypanosomiasis and schistosomiasis are rampant in some regions; the most recent trypanosomiasis outbreaks were reported in the High Mbomou area. Recent outbreaks of cholera and meningitis occurred in Kouango and Paoua, respectively. Although no yellow fever cases have been reported in the past decade, it remains a risk. Onchocerciasis is the main cause of blindness. Iodine deficiency disorders, especially goiter (la perle de beauté, or "beauty pearl"), are common among the Gbaya but occur in other regions also. The dry season is associated with acute respiratory tract infections, intestinal parasitic infestations, and diarrhea, which is one of the leading causes of death among children younger than 5 years. Childhood malnutrition is high. Tuberculosis has run rampant as an opportunistic infection in patients with human immunodeficiency virus (HIV). The Joint United Nations Programme on HIV/AIDS (UNAIDS) reports the estimated prevalence rate for HIV in adults (aged 15 to 49 years) to be 10.7%, with 250,000 people living with HIV, including 130,000 women and 7,200 to 61,000 children aged 0 to 14 years. Between 140,000 and 200,000 children under age 15 have been orphaned by acquired immuno-deficiency syndrome (AIDS). Transmission is essentially heterosexual. About 24,000 to 39,000 people have died of AIDS, and only 3% of infected people receive antiretroviral therapy.

Health-Team Relationships: Doctors head the health care system at the hospital level and are respected by nurses, midwives, and other health workers. The team relationship is well framed, and doctors' decisions are final. Complaints against doctors are not expressed openly because of fear of repercussions. The authority of the doctor stretches beyond the health facility to the community and into daily life. Midwives and the chiefs of health centers are the next level of authority and deference. Patients are not expected to openly disagree or discuss their health issues with doctors or health workers.

Families' Role in Hospital Care: Family members, relatives, and friends take turns staying at the bedside. The family provides care, whereas the nurses provide the medical treatments. Each member of the family is required to visit the patient and contribute to his or her moral, physical, and financial support by visiting, bringing food, or paying for prescriptions because health insurance does not exist. Hospitals in Bangui serve at least one meal, whereas in the provinces, hospitals cannot afford to provide food.

Dominance Patterns: The system is patriarchal. After marriage, wives yield their rights to their husbands and stay in the husband's family even after the husband's death. Children are treated equally, although some ethnic groups believe it is preferable for the first-born child to be a boy. Girls are expected to help with and master the chores of a wife in prepa-ration for her future life with her husband. A wife who cannot cook well or keep her husband's house neat is considered dishonorable. Although polygamy is legal (with a husband being allowed to have as many as four wives), not all men embrace the practice (although they may have multiple extramarital partners, and any resulting offspring bear the father's name).

Touch Practices: Touch is usual and natural. People of the same sex frequently walk holding hands or shoulders because they are friends or siblings. When two girls or women are chatting, they often touch. Adults also cuddle children as a sign of affection or appreciation. In some ethnic groups in southern areas, such as the Gbaka and Yaloma, touching has rules. For example, a son- or daughter-in-law can never shake hands with or eat in front of parents-in-law.

Eye-Contact Practices: Direct eye contact is considered impolite, dis-respectful, and disobedient in some traditional ethnic groups, such as Banda, Sara, and Gbaya. People are also expected to keep their eyes down when speaking to an older person or one in authority. This practice is not as important among contemporaries.

Perceptions of Time: In rural areas, people judge time according to the solar cycle, and being on time is not extremely important. A person can show up anytime after the scheduled hour. The *l'heure Africaine,* or "the

African hour," method of time is used in urban areas and is well known by foreigners living in the country. In other words, people are expected to arrive later than scheduled for events or meetings. Recently, people have become more concerned with being on time. For example, they are more likely to be on time for work or government-related or medical appointments. Punctuality is extremely important in school. The society lives mainly in the present.

C

Pain Reactions: Adults of all ethnic groups are expected to suppress external reactions to pain. Enduring pain is an important aspect of becoming an adult. Adults in intense pain may snap their fingers or nip certain body parts (e.g., legs, arms, abdomen). Men are not expected to express pain because it is a sign of weakness and womanhood. On the contrary, women are allowed to cry out in pain during childbirth or when bitten during a conjugal conflict. Children younger than age 10 are also allowed to express their pain loudly, but those 10 or older are reprimanded for not behaving like adults.

Birth Rites: In rural areas, mothers-in-law and close female relatives or friends assist with childbirth, whereas in urban areas they remain outside the delivery room. After birth the mother is given plenty of semiliquid food—usually soups made of fish, beef bones, or green vegetables and porridge made of rice, corn, or millet—to stimulate milk production. Muslim women usually add hot pepper to the porridge in the belief that it breaks up blood clots in the uterus after delivery. The infant mortality rate is high at 86 deaths per 1,000 live births. Members of some ethnic groups also drink alcoholic beverages such as beer and palm wine to stimulate breast-milk production. To reduce postpartum morbidity and mortality, relatives and friends take care of the mother and help with the household duties for the first 3 months. It is not unusual to see the mother-in-law move into the new mother's home after birth. In almost all ethnic groups, a new mother's care is based on traditional therapies, including squatting over or in a concoction of hot leaves, herbal massage, and wearing herbal pads. The baby shower takes place within the first month after the birth, and religious groups, co-workers, friends, and relatives bring gifts. Newborns undergo ethnic-specific rituals such as scarification identifying their ethnic group, application of makeup, head shaving, and use of amulets. The first-born son is highly celebrated because he bears the father's name and is expected to be the pillar of the family after the father's death. In rural areas, newborns are kept inside for at least a month to keep them from seeing the moon at night, which is believed to take away their beauty. The fertility rate is 4.41 children born per woman. Life expectancy is 43 for men, 44 for women.

Death Rites: All ethnic groups consider the dead to be sacred. Bodies are only allowed to be buried in the ground; cremation and organ donations are unacceptable. Burial rituals and death rites differ according to religion and ethnic group. The common practice is for family members, friends, and relatives to spend several days and nights helping the mourning family. Most ethnic groups believe that after death the dead join their ancestors in the beyond, either in water or a traditional forest. Many groups (e.g., Gbaka) perform rituals to determine whether the dead person has arrived in the afterworld. A new generation of Christian theology has revolutionized traditional concepts of death and death rites. More frequently, Christian wakes are occurring across the country. Autopsies are rare and are practiced in hospitals for legal purposes at a doctor's request.

Food Practices and Intolerances: Although great differences in food practices exist among ethnic groups, some foods are considered "national" and offered to all visitors or strangers: *koko* (dark green, thinly chopped leaves that look somewhat like grass), *ngouza* (cassava or manioc leaves), and *gozo* (cassava root). The diet is well balanced, consisting of proteins (such as peanuts, beef, wild livestock, and fish), starch (such as gozo, banana plantains, corn, potatoes, yams, and millet), leafy vegetables, and in-season tropical fruits. Milk is scarce in the north and northeastern regions where the *mbororos*, or nomad beef farmers, live. The northern ethnic groups, such as the Banda, Sara, and Kaba, consume more meat from wild livestock and starches such as gozo and millet; vegetables are a luxury and rarely available. Riverside ethnic groups, such as the Ngbanziri, Gbaka, Mondjombo, Yakoma, and Sango, eat more fish, vegetables, plantains, yams, and corn. Forbidden foods are specific to each ethnic group. Some may not eat antelope, buffalo, or a certain kind of fish or vegetable that is considered a sacred ethnic totem. A two-meal eating pattern is the norm. Rural families have one meal in the morning and the second in the evening, whereas urban families have one meal at noon and the next in the evening. People use their hands to eat in rural and urban areas. In many ethnic groups, it is proper to use only the right hand when eating. Men, women, and children have their own eating groups; in rural areas, these groups eat separately at mealtimes and do not interact. In urban areas, this practice is less common. The father may eat with the boys and the mother with the girls. In some families, fathers use a spoon to eat, a practice that is increasing in urban areas. In some restaurants, people still eat with their hands, and the staff provides water and soap.

Infant-Feeding Practices: Breast milk is the first food given to infants. Breastfeeding on demand is common and practiced by all women unless medical contraindications exist. Occasionally, the infant is bottle-fed water right after birth before the breast milk comes in. Colostrum is considered "dirty" milk that is bad for the infant, so it is purged and discarded. Exclusive breastfeeding is done only for a short period; however, the country has begun a national campaign to promote breastfeeding. Supplementation with semi-liquid cornstarch or millet porridge begins when the infant is about 3 months, but some women begin using supplementary foods with infants as young as 1 month. Bottle-feeding with formula is more common in urban areas and may begin at birth in addition to breastfeeding. Weaning begins at about 9 months or when the infant begins to walk. Some children are breastfed until they are 2 years or older.

Child-Rearing Practices: Child rearing is managed by parents, relatives, neighbors, and friends. Corporal punishment such as spanking is customary and still practiced in many elementary schools. Children are taught early to respect their parents, older siblings, and adults. They are expected to refrain from raising their voice, grumbling, or raising their hands to older adults. Children perform chores according to their abilities. For instance, a 1-year-old boy who is asked to bring a cup or broom to his mother is expected to do it. A 7-year-old girl should be able to cook simple meals, prepare the gozo, and take care of her younger siblings, whereas a 7-year-old boy is expected to be able to fix a broken stool and run errands efficiently. Circumcision of boys is the norm and is performed either by trained men in the village, male nurses at home, or interns or doctors in a health facility. The procedure usually occurs when the boy is between ages 4 and 7. Circumcision of girls is common among some groups, such as the Bandas.

National Childhood Immunizations: BCG at birth; DTwP at 6, 10, and 14 weeks; OPV at birth and at 6, 10, and 14 weeks; measles at 9 months; yellow fever at 9 months; TT pregnant women, +1, +6 months, +1, +1 year. MMR and hepatitis are provided if parents can afford them. The percent of the target population vaccinated, by antigen, is: BCG (70%); DTP1 (65%); DTP3 (40%); MCV (35%); Polio3 (40%); TT2 plus (56%); and YF (58%).

BIBLIOGRAPHY

Central Intelligence Agency: 2006: The world factbook, Central African Republic. Retrieved September 21, 2006, from https://www.cia.gov/cia/publications/factbook/print/ct.html.

Sepou A, Yanza MC, Nguembi E, Tekpa G, Ngbale R: How is breast-feeding valued in the urban and semi-urban Central African milieu? *Sante.* 11(2):85–89, 2001.

Sepou A, Enza J, Nali MN: Prenatal care in a semiurban area of Central African Republic: frequency, influential factors, maternal and neonatal prognosis, *Med Trop.* 60(3):257–261, 2000.

UNAIDS: 2006 Central Africans Republic. Retrieved September 21, 2006, from http://www.unaids.org/en/Regions_Countries/Countries/central_african_republic.asp.

World Health Organization: 2006: Immunization, vaccines and biologicals. Retrieved September 21, 2006, from http://www.who.int/immunization_monitoring/en/globalsummary/countryprofileresult.cfm='caf'.

◆ CHAD (REPUBLIC OF)

MAP PAGE (800)

Carolyn M. D'Avanzo

Location: Chad is the fifth largest country on the African continent, covering nearly 1.3 million km^2 (501,800 square miles). This landlocked country is in the northern portion of central Africa and shares a border with Libya to the north, Sudan to the east, Central African Republic and Cameroon to the

C

south, and Nigeria and Niger to the west. The northernmost third of the country is part of the Sahara Desert and includes the Tibesti Mountains and the Ennedi Plateau. The central band, part of the Sahel, includes Lake Chad and the capital city of N'Djamena to the west. The southernmost tier is the primary agricultural region of the country. Chad has a population of 9.9 million people. The gross domestic product (GDP) per capita is $1,500, with 80% of the population living under the poverty line. Most people live in rural areas; only four cities have populations of 200,000 or more: N'Djaména, Moundou, Koumra, and Kélo.

Major Languages	Ethnic Groups	Major Religions
French (official)	200 distinct Muslim	Muslim 51%
Arabic (official)	and non-Muslim	Christian 35%
Sara and Sango (in	groups	Indigenous beliefs
south)		(primarily
More than 100 other		Animism) 7%
languages and		Other 7%
dialects		

There are more than 200 distinct ethnic groups, most of whom are Muslim: Arabs, Toubou, Fulbe, Kotoko, Hausa, Kanembou, Baguirmi, Boulala, and Maba in the northern and central regions of the country. Most non-Muslims reside in the southern part of the country, groups such as the Sara, Ngambaye, Mbake, Goulaye, Moudang, Moussei, and Massa. More than 100 different languages and dialects are spoken. Newspapers are generally printed in French and Arabic, and radio and television programs are broadcast in both languages. Literacy rates are 56% for men, 39% for women.

Health Care Beliefs: Acute sick care; holistic. Health is defined by many Chadians as a state that extends beyond physical well-being and includes harmony within the family and ethnic lineage. Health care practices reflect these beliefs and include use of a mixture of treatment modalities, including Western medicine and ritual and local healing practices.

Predominant Sick-Care Practices: Biomedical where available; traditional. The public health care system is decentralized to provide basic services to as much of the population, which is mostly rural, as possible. An estimated 400 health centers function in rural areas of the country and are the primary point of care for most Chadians. People who cannot be treated at the health centers are referred to one of the approximately 36 district hospitals. Oversight of the public health care system is the responsibility of the Ministry of Health in N'Djamena, which has a health delegation in each of the country's 14 prefectures, or regional capitals. A plethora of traditional healers exist and are widely used in both rural and urban areas. Medications, including antibiotics, are available in pharmacies and markets in urban centers but are less readily available in rural areas and are not affordable to all. Many families use plants and herbs to treat themselves for common ailments and do not consult a health care practitioner.

Ethnic-/Race-Specific or Endemic Diseases: Malaria, yellow fever, and schistosomiasis are endemic. The country also has frequent epidemics of cholera and meningitis. There have been outbreaks of hepatitis A and E, cholera, bacterial and protozoal diarrhea, typhoid, and schistosomiasis. Polio has occurred near the Nigerian border. The first two cases of acquired immunodeficiency syndrome (AIDS) were documented in 1986. Since that time, the number of cases has risen rapidly. The Joint United Nations Programme on HIV/AIDS (UNAIDS) reports the prevalence rate for human immunodeficiency virus (HIV) in adults (aged 15 to 49 years) as 3.5%, with 180,000 people living with HIV, including 90,000 women and 16,000 children aged 0 to 14. There are 57,000 orphans as a result of parental AIDS. Deaths from AIDS are estimated to be 11,000. Only 17% of those infected receive antiretroviral therapy.

Health-Team Relationships: Chad has a severe shortage of doctors; and most practice in urban centers. Rural health centers are largely staffed by nurses or nurses' aides. Working relationships in the health care sector vary from setting to setting; however, given the dearth of health care providers, many practitioners work without the support of a team.

Families' Roles in Hospital Care: Families play an important role in caring for the sick. They are responsible for bringing food to those who are hospitalized or receiving inpatient treatments. Most health care facilities allow and encourage visits. In some situations, family members sleep at the hospital with the family member.

Dominance Patterns: The families of all ethnic groups are dominated by men. Living arrangements are also *patrilocal,* meaning that after women are married, they generally live in their husband's home or village. Children of parents who have been divorced or separated are generally raised by paternal aunts after the children have been weaned, although some exceptions to this practice exist, particularly in urban areas.

Eye-Contact Practices: Young men and women are expected to show respect for older adults. Although eye contact is not expressly forbidden, it is uncommon among certain people (e.g., a young woman and her mother- or father-in-law). In the southern regions, no rules prohibit eye contact between the sexes.

Touch Practices: A handshake is the most common form of greeting in all parts of the country and is considered appropriate when greeting and bidding farewell to someone.

Perceptions of Time: Punctuality is becoming increasingly important, particularly in urban areas of the country.

Pain Reactions: In most ethnic groups, pain is something to be endured. With the exception of very young children, patients are often chastised for crying or complaining about physical discomfort.

Birth Rites: The infant mortality rate is very high at 91 deaths per 1,000 live births. Most women give birth in their homes; however, the percentage varies according to the setting and other factors, such as a woman's

C

level of education. Women in urban areas are much more likely than women who live in rural areas to give birth in a hospital or other health care facility. Similarly, women who have some high school education give birth in a hospital or other health care facility more frequently than women with only a primary school education or women who have never been to school. The timing and characteristics of naming ceremonies for newborn children differ among ethnic groups. The fertility rate is 6.25 children born per woman. Life expectancy is 46 for men, 49 for women.

Death Rites: Death rites vary widely among Chad's many ethnic and religious groups. Burials, rather than cremation, are the accepted practice. Among the Sara, Chad's largest ethnic group, families gather for 3 to 4 days to mourn. The mourning ceremonies include singing, dancing, and sleeping at the home of the relatives of the deceased. Deaths are often announced on Radio Chad so that distant relatives are aware of family deaths. In recent years and in response to difficult economic times, these radio announcements have included messages asking relatives to stay at home to mourn.

Food Practices and Intolerances: Staple foods include millet, sorghum, rice, and corn, which are often consumed in the form of a paste called *boule* and eaten with a meat or vegetable sauce. Meals are communal, although children generally eat separately, as do men and women in some groups. Crops are generally harvested in December and January, a time when food is most plentiful. Planting season coincides with the onset of the rainy season in early June.

Infant-Feeding Practices: Most mothers supplement breast milk with water and porridge when infants are several months old. Exclusive breast-feeding is uncommon; however, children continue to be breastfed for extended periods—often until the mother's next pregnancy.

Child-Rearing Practices: Children are raised by the extended family and often live with different members of the family, all of whom are responsible for providing for their education and upbringing. It is therefore not uncommon for children to live with aunts, uncles, grandparents, or cousins or to move from one household to another. This practice is especially common among school-age children who need to move from villages to larger cities to continue their studies.

National Childhood Immunizations: BCG at birth; DTwP at 6, 10, and 14 weeks; OPV at birth and at 6, 10 and 14 weeks; measles at 9 months; YF at 9 months; and TT at first contact, +1, +2, +6 months, +1, +1 year. The percent of the target population vaccinated, by antigen, is: BCG (40%); DTP1 (45%); DTP3 (20%); MCV (23%); Polio3 (36%); and TT2 plus (39%).

BIBLIOGRAPHY

Central Intelligence Agency: *2006: The world factbook*, Chad. Retrieved September 21, 2006, from https://www.cia.gov/cia/publications/factbook/print/cd.html

Programme National de Lutte Contre le SIDA/MST: Chand-Santé Année 1, Numéro 00, 2000.

UNAIDS: 2006 Chad. Retrieved September 21, 2006, from http://www.unaids.org/en/Regions_Countries/Countries/chad.asp.

World Health Organization: 2006: Immunization, vaccines and biologicals. Retrieved September 21, 2006, from http://www.who.int/immunization_monitoring/en/globalsummary/countryprofileresult.cfm?C='tcd'.

C

◆ CHILE (REPUBLIC OF)

MAP PAGE (797)

Marta Maturana Quijada and Hugo Cardenas

Location: Chile fills a narrow, 2,897-km (1,800-mile) strip between the Andes Mountains and the Pacific Ocean. One third is covered by towering mountain ranges, and the southernmost city in the world is located at its tip. A 1,127-km (a 700-mile) valley in Chile's center is densely populated, and the driest desert in the world, the Atacama Desert, is located in the north. The population is 16 million; the capital is Santiago. The gross domestic product (GDP) per capita is $11,300, with 18% living below the poverty line. Literacy rates are 96% for both men and women.

Major Languages	Ethnic Groups	Major Religions
Spanish (official)	European and Mestizo 95%	Roman Catholic 89%
	Indigenous 3%	Protestant 11%
	Other 2%	

The influence of Europeans and of Jews and Arabs from Palestine and other Middle Eastern countries is evident in Chile's cultural and political life. Many groups have maintained their languages, and many bilingual schools exist. Only 3% of the population is indigenous: primary is the Mapuche, who live mostly in the rural central and southern regions. Aymara and Atacameños live in the north. Rapanu live on Easter Island (Isla de Pascua in Spanish, also known as *Rapa Nui* in the native language of the *pascuenses,* the Spanish denomination of the local people). These groups speak their original languages but are taught Spanish in public schools. Although church attendance has declined in recent years, Chilean society shows many signs of strong Catholic influence. Legal divorce was approved only last year after nearly 10 years of discussion; abortion is officially prohibited. During the last two decades, Protestant denominations have become more influential.

Health Care Beliefs: Traditional; active involvement; with high levels of self-medication. Many pharmacies in small towns and suburbs do not respect the legal requirement of medical prescriptions. Prevalent dietary practices include consumption of increasingly high levels of fast-food and high-calorie diets and low consumption of healthier alternatives. Obesity is an issue even in babies and young children. In rural areas, traditional medicine is important; and in cities a growing number use some form of alternative medicine (Reiki, acupuncture, aromatherapy). Health services are predominantly geared toward illness, but disease prevention and health promotion are increasingly important. National health education and treatment programs are used to control endemic illnesses (e.g., malnutrition, diabetes, tuberculosis, human immunodeficiency virus (HIV)/acquired immunodeficiency syndrome (AIDS) and provide services for older adults. Discrimination against people with mental illness is a significant problem.

Predominant Sick-Care Practices: Biomedical; traditional; religious. Middle- and upper-class Chileans have practices similar to North America. Poor Chileans rely more on the public health system, where care is received in public *consultorios* and hospitals. In the last 15 years, many doctors immigrated from Ecuador, Venezuela, and Cuba, and they work primarily in private practice in low-income neighborhoods. Because they charge substantially less than Chilean doctors, they are quite popular. Physicians, nurses, midwives, and other health care professionals receive a university education, so most Chileans have confidence and pride in the system. Prayer is a common adjunct to Western health care, reflecting the strong influence that Christianity has on daily life. Patients also are more willing to acknowledge a combination of folk or traditional practices with Western medicine. Chile has been a pioneer in its development of a universal health system. In the past decades, an American-style mix of public and private health service delivery has emerged. The public health system has a mandate to ensure coverage of all people unable to afford the high cost of private medical insurance. There is, however, a wait of sometimes more than a year for surgical and complex medical procedures, which has led to an agreement between the public and private systems so that patients in the public system who cannot be seen within 3 months may go to private clinics and hospitals. The same law obligates the Ministry of Health to use private facilities when medical treatments are not available in public hospitals or when public hospitals are overwhelmed by the high numbers of patients after natural disasters or accidents. Very poor people and those over age 65 have access to free health services through a nationally planned and regionally administered network of rural and urban clinics *(consultorios)* and public hospitals. A new legal framework initiated in 2005, AUGE (an acronym meaning Acceso Universal para Prestaciones Integrales y Garantías Explícitas: "Universal Access to Guarantied Health Services") obligates the public health system to provide treatment or services in the private system when people entitled to receive treatment for any of 25 listed pathologies do not have access in the public hospitals. The public system is the only one that provides free coverage for chronic and expensive illnesses such as cancer and HIV/AIDS. Last year private health insurance companies were obligated by law to provide coverage of chronic diseases that previously were not covered. In addition to the public system, the National Health Fund (*Fondo Nacional de Salud,* or FONASA) is an alternative for people with middle incomes. FONASA allows access to some levels of the private system and consists of three levels, all of which have a high-deductible payment when used in the private system but very low costs when used in the public system. The private system, administered by insurance companies known as ISAPRES (*Instituciones de Salud Previsional*), is more expensive, but provides a greater variety of services that occasionally are of higher quality. However, after users reach age 65, the cost of the private system becomes too expensive for all but the very wealthy, and most people switch to FONASA.

Ethnic-/Race-Specific or Endemic Diseases: Cystic echinococcosis and trichinosis are endemic in rural areas of the southern and central valley. Typhoid and hepatitis A and E are endemic in most of the country, and Chagas disease is endemic in the north. Diarrhea (caused by *Shigella* organisms) is frequent, and in Chileans is self-contained, lasting about 24 hours after antibiotic treatment. Visitors from other countries are encouraged to drink bottled or boiled water to avoid what is locally known as *chilenitis,* serious diarrhea caused primarily by *Shigellae,* and occasionally by *Escherichia coli.* The most common causes of illness and death are circulatory problems (high blood pressure and acute myocardial infarction), malignant neoplasms (of the stomach and respiratory system), injuries, and poisoning (with prevalent alcoholism and the highest rate of liver cirrhosis in the region), and respiratory illnesses. The incidence of gallbladder stones is one of the highest in the world and frequently leads to cancer of the gallbladder. Standard medical practice is to remove the gallbladder as a preventive measure. Respiratory illnesses in children are the major cause of illness and hospitalization, accounting for 60% of doctor visits in this age group. Malnutrition is found almost exclusively among poor children, with one study reporting a 9% incidence of goiter in school-age children (despite the fact that commercially available salt is iodized). During winters influenza is a problem of epidemic proportions. Free vaccination is provided to those at risk, including infants and older adults, as well as powdered milk for infants during the first year of life and breakfast and lunch programs for children attending public schools in economically disadvantaged communities. Obesity, alcoholism, smoking, and lack of exercise are health problems that are beginning to be recognized. Digestive problems increase during summer, when fecal contamination of food in restaurants and public places is a problem. No human or animal cases of avian influenza have been reported. The Joint United Nations Programme on HIV/AIDS (UNAIDS) reports the estimated prevalence rate for human immunodeficiency virus (HIV) in adults (aged 15 to 49 years) is 0.3%, with 33,300 people infected, including 7,600 women. Fewer than 500 deaths from acquired immunodeficiency syndrome (AIDS) have been reported. About 50% of reported AIDS cases are in men who have sex with men, followed by heterosexual transmission (30%). The government provides free antiviral tri-therapy to all infected people who are not covered by the private health system (only 10% are receiving tri-therapy). A recent law obligated private health insurance companies to cover up to 90% of tri-therapy for patients. Despite public education campaigns, discrimination against children and adults living with HIV/AIDS is very strong. Organizations caring for these patients (many of them related to the Roman Catholic Church) are usually kept secret because of past opposition by neighbors, leading to violence. Asymptomatic children with HIV are not accepted in public schools because of the strong opposition of students, parents and teachers.

Health-Team Relationships: Relationships are doctor driven, and other health professionals tend to be subordinate. The "professionals of medical collaboration" *(profesionales de colaboración médica),* such as nurses, have primary roles. For example, nurses have important administrative and educational functions for which they are primarily responsible. Patients' attitudes toward doctors and nurses are typically that of total faith and subordination, especially in more disadvantaged social groups. Until very recently, treatments were rarely discussed with the patient and family. Today, informed consent for major surgeries and treatments is enforced by local ethics committees that have the legal power to stop research and treatment procedures. Hospitals located in regions with high concentrations of indigenous people (e.g., the regional hospital of Temuco, capital of the IXth region) have instituted ethnoculturally responsive programs to orient patients and families and assist them with accessing and understanding health care services. Very few health professionals are in Mapuche or Aymara. The role of nurses in prevention is very important in the public health system. University-trained midwives have an active role in women's reproductive health, contraceptive programs, and the health of babies until weaning or the end of the first year of life.

Family's Role in Hospital Care: In public hospitals, relatives cannot stay with patients or bring them food, and visits are restricted to one or two at a time from 2:00 to 5:00 PM. In private clinics, one relative can stay all day and night with a patient if desired, but at an additional cost.

Dominance Pattern: Chile has a Latin culture with strong male dominance. Men are usually paid more, and many companies prefer male employees so that they can avoid the costs associated with childbirth. Young women experience significant discrimination, therefore, when applying for jobs in public and private sectors. In 2006 the first woman was elected president of the country after about 150 years of democracy. She promised a strong anti-discrimination policy to ensure that more women are elected to important government positions. Violence against women within the family has been a hidden problem. In 2005 about 60 women died after being shot, strangled, or beaten by their partners. Many more suffer less severe injuries that do not reach the public eye. This is a very high rate for the size of the population, and the government initiated an educational campaign encouraging abused women to seek counseling by health and legal professionals. A related problem is the frequency of sexual abuse of children by relatives, including parents. Pederasty reached levels of international concern because the Chilean law did not specifically penalize sexual relations with minors until last year.

Eye-Contact Practices: Chileans are usually open in their interactions: to look each other in the eye during conversations is considered good manners. To avoid eye contact during a conversation may be considered offensive.

Touch Practices: Both women and men shake hands rather vigorously and kiss people on the cheek in greeting, sometimes even in professional settings. It is not appropriate for a health care provider to kiss patients. A handshake is always expected, and failure to extend a hand when greeting a person is interpreted as lack of acceptance.

Perceptions of Time: Punctuality has less significance than in the United States or Germany, but it is significantly more important than in Mexico or other Latin American countries. People are typically 30 minutes late for most appointments and events.

Pain Reactions: People freely express their pain.

Birth Rites: The birth of a son is not more celebrated, but most families aim to have at least one son. Almost all births occur in public hospitals and private clinics, with prenatal care and low-risk birth services provided by university-prepared midwives. The public health system provides free surgical sterilizations for multiparous women who request it. The most common contraceptives for women with low incomes are intrauterine devices, and adolescents primarily use oral contraceptives. Abortion is illegal, but the rate of 45 abortions per 1,000 women is the highest in the region. This year the Supreme Court approved the distribution of the "morning-after" pill by the public health system (it was already available in pharmacies for women who could afford it). This generated high-profile discussion by conservative Catholic groups against emergency contraceptives.

Death Rites: When possible, family members are present when a person dies. Organ donation is an increasing practice after strong educational campaigns launched by the Ministry of Health. Autopsies are mandatory after death at home, public hospitals, and clinics, except in cases when the cause of death can be certified by a physician and there is no additional reason for autopsy. Cremation is an increasing practice.

Food Practices and Intolerances: The Chilean diet is firmly based on bread and butter and pasta and rice, all of which contribute to the problem of obesity. Meat (beef, mutton) is the preferred source of protein, followed by poultry. Although there is an extensive coastline with much fishing activity, fish has never become a primary source of protein in the diet. Repeated educational campaigns to increase fish consumption during the last decades have failed.

Infant-Feeding Practices: In rural areas, breastfeeding is the standard practice for the first year of the infant's life. In urban settings and in the middle class, breastfeeding more than the first few weeks is difficult for women who must return to work. National campaigns encourage breastfeeding; however, the practice of providing formula and milk to mothers after birth persists. It is estimated that only 24% of mothers are still breastfeeding 6 months after delivery.

Child-Rearing Practices: While the mother is at work, infants mostly stay at nurseries under the care of university-trained child care workers

C

called *parvularias*. In families with low incomes, mothers care for the children until they begin their formal education, which by law is at age 5 years. Child rearing is rather permissive. Even young children are part of the social activities of the family and attend parties in the evening, but it is expected that children will be respectful and obedient. The extended family, especially grandparents, also plays an important role in raising children. Most people value education as a means of promoting upward socioeconomic mobility and status; so male and female children are encouraged and rewarded if they do well in their studies. In families of the middle and upper classes, children sleep in their own beds. Families tend to follow the norm in Latin America, so living at home until marriage is common for men and women. Old parents usually live in their own houses or with some younger member of the family until death.

National Childhood Immunizations: BCG at birth; DT at 7 years; DTwP at 18 months and 4 years; DTwPHib at 2, 4, 6 months; HepB at 2, 4, and 6 months; MMR at 12 months and 6 years; OPV at 2, 4, 6, and 18 months. Immunizations are mandatory and provided free by the public health system. Periodically, the Ministry of Health provides free vaccinations (e.g., against *Haemophilus influenzae*) for people who are at risk. The percent of the target population vaccinated, by antigen, is: BCG (95%); DTP1 and Polio3 (92%); DTP3 and Hib3 (91%); and MCV (90%).

BIBLIOGRAPHY

Central Intelligence Agency: 2006: *The world factbook, Chile.* Retrieved September 21, 2006, from https://www.cia.gov/cia/publications/factbook/print/ci.html.

Chilean Government: www.gobierno.cl/plan_auge/que_es_auge.asp (retrieved on February 20, 2006).

Chilean Ministry of Health: www.minsal.cl (retrieved on February 20, 2006).

Ministry of Health: Piloto AUGE 2004. *Working draft of the Ministry of Health.* Version 1.2.1, April 2004.

Ministry of Health: Reglamento Orgánico de los Servicios de Salud. DTO N° 42, de 1986.

UNAIDS: 2006 Chile. Retrieved September 21, 2006, from http://www.unaids.org/en/Regions_Countries/Countries/chile.asp.

World Health Organization: 2006: Immunization, vaccines and biologicals. Retrieved September 21, 2006, from http://www.who.int/immunization_monitoring/en/globalsummary/countryprofileresult.cfm?C='chl'.

◆ CHINA (PEOPLE'S REPUBLIC OF)

MAP PAGE (803)

Yue Zhao, Wai-man Lee, and Frances Kam Wong

Location: The People's Republic of China is the world's third largest country and occupies the eastern part of Asia. The total area is 9,596,960 km² (3,705,392 square miles), and the population is 1.3 billion. The northwestern part is mountainous and arid with high plateaus, whereas southeastern China has fertile agricultural land and river deltas. Tibet is part of the People's Republic of China, and the colonies of Hong Kong and Macao were returned to Chinese sovereignty in 1997 and 1999, respectively. The gross domestic product (GDP) per capita is $6,800, with 10% living below the poverty line.

C

Major Languages	Ethnic Groups	Major Religions
Putonghua (Mandarin, official)	Han Chinese 92%	Zhuang, Uygur,
Cantonese	Zhuang, Uygur, Hui, Yi,	Atheist (officially;
Local dialects (six or	Tibetan, Miao,	however, elements
more)	Manchu, Mongol,	of Confucianism,
	Buyi, Korean 8%	Taoism, Buddhism,
		Christianity, and
		Islam can be
		found)

From an anthropologic point of view, several hundred identifiable minority groups exist, of which 55 have been officially recognized. Literacy rates are 95% for men, 87% for women.

Health Care Beliefs: Holistic; increasing interest in health promotion. Illness prevention and health promotion and maintenance are important. Children are taught at a very young age that it is necessary to be healthy and avoid damaging the body, an act of piety that pays respect to parents. The Chinese attribute disease to a disruption in body energy (*qi*/chi). Health is believed to be a state of spiritual and physical harmony with nature. Regular exercise is practiced by many throughout life. For example, Tao-chi chuan (Tai-Chi), considered "soft" exercise, is recommended for older adults and frail people because it does not strain or shock the body or result in painful muscles. Some avoid major surgery because they fear that the life force may be disturbed. Chinese may resist blood tests because of the belief that removal of blood will weaken the body. Although natural therapies are preferred, Chinese often choose dietary or herbal therapies (tonics or pills) to prevent disease. Stigma is attached to mental illness, so severe mental disturbance is the only criterion for entering the health care system. Chinese patients with psychiatric problems tend to describe their symptoms as headaches or other somatic complaints, delaying psychiatric consultation. Chinese believe that illness needs to be drawn out of the body, and a common treatment is to rub a coin vigorously over the body after the coin is heated or smeared with oil. If red welts appear, it is believed that a person is ill and that the coin rubbing helped.

Predominant Sick-Care Practices: Biomedical; traditional; passive involvement. The Chinese combine traditional Chinese (TCM) and Western medicine; however, when both types are used in treatments, drug interactions may occur. TCM includes acupuncture and moxibustion therapy, external treatments, massage therapy, pharmaceutical (herbal) therapy, and breathing exercises. Western medicine was introduced in the mid-1800s, and during the past century it has become widespread. Since the end of the nineteenth century, Chinese medical experts have successfully been integrating TCM and Western medicine. The health care system is transitioning from a free system to an insurance system with an option of fee-for-service choices. According to TCM, people have five zang and six fu organs. The heart, liver, spleen, lungs, and kidneys have completely different connotations in TCM and Western medicine. From a TCM perspective, the liver's functions include conducting and dispersing (i.e., dredging, smoothing, flowing, and dispersing life activity within the body), storing blood, promoting digestive functions, and regulating normal circulation of the *qi*, blood, and water. In addition, the liver helps regulate emotions. If the liver is diseased, its ability to conduct and disperse decreases, and sadness, moodiness, excessive worrying, belching, and sentimental sighing occurs. Chinese medical practitioners use the hot-cold dichotomy to classify the energies of diets, physical constitution, disease, and symptoms. In the Chinese medical belief system, eating foods with "hot" energy(e.g., chili pepper, ginger, cinnamon bark) causes people to experience hot sensations, and foods with "cold" energy (e.g., tea, apple, bean curd) results in cold sensations. Chinese with a "hot" constitution should consume more cold-energy foods, whereas people with a "cold" physical constitution should consume hot-energy foods. The hot-cold dichotomy concept is applied to diseases as well as symptoms. If a disease or symptom gets worse after exposure to cold surroundings, then it is a "cold" disease or symptom, and the same theory applies to hot surroundings. "Hot" diseases include constipation and rheumatism. Chinese expect that when they are ill, others are obliged to care for them, which reduces active participation in improving their own health.

Ethnic-/Race-Specific or Endemic Diseases: Endemic diseases include fluorosis, endemic goiter, tuberculosis, thalassemia, and chloroquine-resistant malaria. Chinese are also at risk for viral hepatitis, Japanese encephalitis, schistosomiasis, and alpha-thalassemia. Neurasthenia (nervous exhaustion) is a common modern Chinese psychiatric disorder; its psychological symptoms include anxiety, depression, and hypochondria. Cancer, cerebrovascular accidents (CVAs), cardiac disease, and tobacco-related diseases are the leading causes of death in cities. Respiratory diseases, cancer, and CVAs are the leading causes of death in rural areas. As the Chinese society becomes more prosperous, obesity is becoming more prevalent, especially among young children. In 2005, 18% of the population was overweight and 6% were obese. In 2002, the average smoking rate was 24%, (predominantly men), about 21% regularly drank alcohol, and only 14% said they got regular physical exercise. In 2005 the Chinese Health Department reported that about 650,000 people were infected with human immunodeficiency virus (HIV) (82% aged 20 to 39). The Joint United Nations Programme on HIV/AIDS (UNAIDS) reports the prevalence rate for HIV in adults (15–49) to be

0.1%, with 180,000 infected women, and 31,000 deaths from acquired immunodeficiency syndrome (AIDS). The ratio of male to female HIV carriers is 5.2:1, and drug users account for 44% of the cases where mode of transmission is known.

Health-Team Relationships: In 2005, China had about 1.31 million nurses. There are about 1.5 licensed doctors and 1 nurse per 1,000 people. Most nurses work in acute settings; a very small number work in community and rehabilitative settings. Patients usually are not given much information about their illnesses, medicines, or diagnostic procedures. The protection of patient's rights is of great concern, which has prompted a Law for the Protection of Consumer Rights. Patients, however, prefer not to express their concerns about interventions or treatments openly or directly and tend to express their thoughts politely, with restraint, and indirectly. The doctor or nurse is expected to read the implied messages. County hospitals, township hospitals, and village clinics form the health service network in rural areas in mainland China.

Families' Role in Hospital Care: Typically, at least one family member remains with a sick child or severely ill adult during hospitalization. The family supplies food and clean clothing and assists with feeding, bathing, and keeping the patient comfortable. In cases of serious illness, doctors often have discussions with family members who may make decisions without involving the patient. Family reunions during significant festivals are important, so hospitalized patients may ask for home leave or to be discharged to celebrate a holiday, such as the Chinese New Year during the Spring Festival.

Dominance Patterns: The family is more important than the individual. Marked role differences are based on generation, age, birth order, gender, and social status. When making decisions, the young defer to the old, and both parents make decisions about children. Older adults are not segregated from others and have a high status in the family and society. Older Chinese parents take pride in being supported and cared for by their children. Devotion to parents includes caring for them physically, psychologically, and socially. This may be changing, however, with the migration of children for better work opportunities, China's "one child only" policy, and a decline in the number of multigenerational families that live together. Father-son relationships are strong; women who are married become part of their husband's family.

Eye-Contact Practices: Direct eye contact is acceptable, but staring is inappropriate.

Touch Practices: Chinese do not like to be touched by strangers. Introductions involve a nod or a slight bow. Although patients prefer health care professionals of the same gender, personal space and confidentiality during care giving are not issues.

Perceptions of Time: Chinese have a concept of time that is inexact and involves patience. The language for the past and present tenses are the same. The past is valued, so traditional approaches to healing are preferred when modern procedures or medications are ineffective. In the traditional

Chinese calendar, the year is divided into four seasons with 24 solar periods. Wind, cold, summer heat, dampness, dryness, and fire are the "six evils" that are closely related to climate and seasonal change. The evils are occasionally considered causes of illness by TCM practitioners.

Pain Reactions: Strong negative feelings such as anger and pain are often suppressed. Chinese patients may be reluctant to report pain and may not interrupt health care professionals to ask for pain relief treatments, although analgesics and TCM such as acupuncture are available for pain control. Displays of emotion are considered character weaknesses. The Chinese language gives patients numerous descriptors to use for expressing pain, and women tend to describe pain more fully than men.

Birth Rites: In 2005 the infant mortality rate was 26 deaths per 1,000 live births. The fertility rate is 1.73 children born per woman. Acupuncture is used during labor induction, labor stimulation, and cesarean section. Fathers are not present in labor or delivery rooms or in postpartum areas. Women in labor are fully clothed and delivered in the low lithotomy position. For 30 days after childbirth, mothers are particularly careful to avoid attacks by "cold" and "wind" because according to TCM, keeping warm is important. The mother may be advised not to bathe or shampoo her hair for the first few days after giving birth. When taking a shower, women use ginger to reduce the chance of being attacked by cold and wind. New mothers are confined for a month and eat certain traditional foods to promote lactation. A celebratory feast takes place 1 month after the baby's birth. Mothers who already have a child have to use intrauterine devices, in compliance with national regulations. Life expectancy is 71 for men, 74 for women.

Death Rites: The Chinese have an aversion to anything concerning death. Autopsies and disposal of the body are individual preferences; they are not prescribed by religion. Euthanasia is illegal, but organ donation is encouraged. Cremation is performed in urban areas and encouraged in rural areas. The oldest son is responsible for making all arrangements for the deceased. The body is initially buried in a coffin but after 7 years it is exhumed and cremated, and the urn is reburied in the family tomb. White, yellow, or black clothing is worn as a sign of mourning. Very traditional Chinese may hire professional criers for funerals. Relatives visit the tomb and pay their respects to deceased relatives at the Pure Brightness Festival and the Double Ninth Festival every year.

Food Practices and Intolerances: The traditional diet is becoming higher in fat and sugar content. Excessive amounts of soy sauce and dried and preserved foods contribute to high sodium intakes. Food is used as therapy to help cure certain illnesses. The Chinese focus on different sorts of foods at different times of year to reflect the seasonal changing of the yin-yang balance. People are generally advised to avoid eating hastily or eating too much. The Chinese believe that soup helps to maintain health, especially for women who have given birth or those who are older or frail. Herbs are used with food, and many kinds of food are believed to have medicinal qualities. By means of traditional cooking such as stewing, simmering, steaming and boiling, medicinal foods are mixed with other foods so that the ailment may be treated while the family members convey their love for the person through the cooking process. Hot or warm beverages are preferred. A typical meal consists of rice with meat, fish, and vegetables. The Chinese believe eating animal organs that correspond to a human body part can improve the body part's functioning (e.g., eating a pig's heart, despite its high level of cholesterol, to revitalize cardiac functioning).

Infant-Feeding Practices: Breastfeeding is encouraged. The practice usually lasts at least 1 year and may be continued for 4 to 5 years in rural areas. Manufactured infant formulas are being marketed in China and are becoming more popular, although they are regarded as inferior to breast milk. Weaning begins when the infant is 3 months old, with the introduction of rice soup cooked with fish or minced meat. Milk is used as a supplement.

Child-Rearing Practices: Parents are permissive with young children, and grandparents help rear children of working parents. Children are frequently tightly swaddled and warmly dressed. When children are old enough to understand authority, they are required to obey. They are encouraged to receive extra training after school, such as in painting, music, and sports. When the children reach school age, they are placed in daycare facilities or are cared for by older family members. Children are taught to show respect for parents and authority figures. Parents tend to shame children or make them feel guilty as a form of discipline. Children learn to control their emotions. Aggressive behaviors are undesirable and suppressed. Children are taught to be unselfish and function competitively only in a group. Fathers are less involved in child rearing, and mother-son relationships are close and enduring. Child abuse is rare. Parents take an active role in influencing their children's educational choices and living environments.

National Childhood Immunizations: BCG at birth; DT at 6 years; DTwP at 3, 4, and 5 months; JapEnc at 8, 18 to 24 months, and 6 years; measles at 8 and 18 to 24 months; MenAC after age 2 years; OPV at 2, 3, and 4 months; and Hep B at birth and at 1 and 6 months. The percent of the target population vaccinated, by antigen, is: BCG and MCV (86%); DTP1 (95%); DTP3 and Polio3 (87%); and HepB3 (84%).

BIBLIOGRAPHY

Bowman KW, Hui EC: Bioethics for clinicians:20. Chinese bioethics, *CMAJ JAMC.* 163(11).

Central Intelligence Agency: 2006: The world Factbook, Chona. Retrieved September 21, 2006 from https://www.cia.gov/cia/publications/factbook/print/ch.html.

Chinese Center for Disease Control and Prevention: Improvement of Chinese AIDS control and prevention in 2005 (January 27, 2006). Retrieved January 27, 2006, from www.chinacdc.net.cn (in Chinese).

Liu XH: Drug food of traditional Chinese medicine and rehabilitation medicine. *Mod Rehabil.* 2001 (21) (in Chinese).

Wong FKY, Lee WM, Mok E: Educating nurses to care for the dying in Hong Kong: a problem-based learning approach, *Cancer Nurs.* 24(2):112–121, 2001.

Wu YF, Ma GS, Hu YH, et al: The current prevalence status of body overweight and obesity in China: data from the China National Nutrition and Health Survey, *Chinese J Prev Med.* 39(5):316–319, 2005 (in Chinese).

Chinese Health Department The Minister of Chinese Health Department report of Chinese Health care reform. Retrieved August 3, 2005 from www.sina.com.cn (in Chinese).

UNAIDS: 2006 China. Retrieved September 21, 2006 from http://www.unaids.org/en/Regions_Countries/Countries/china.asp.

Wang SJ: People's healthy leaving behavior in China. Retrieved January 10, 2005, from www.syd.com.cn (in Chinese).

World Health Organization: 2006: Immunization, vaccines and biologicals. Retrieved September 21, 2006, from http://www.who.int/immunization_monitoring/en/globalsummary/countryprofileresult.cfm?C='chn'.

C

◆ COLOMBIA (REPUBLIC OF)

MAP PAGE (797)

Maryelena Vargas

Location: Colombia, in the northwestern part of South America, is the only country in South America that borders the Atlantic Ocean, the Pacific Ocean, and the Caribbean Sea. Venezuela and Brazil are to the east, Peru and Ecuador to the south, and Panama and the Pacific Ocean to the West. The capital is Bogota. It is composed of low coastal plains and three parallel mountain ranges that are part of the Andes and run north to south. It is tropical along the coast and eastern plains and cooler in the high-lands. Fifty nine percent of the population lives below the national poverty line; unemployment has reached about 18% in the urban areas where 77% of the population lives. During the past 2 years, Colombia's economy has been on a recovery trend as the coffee industry pursues greater market shares in developed countries. The total area is 1,138,910 km^2 (439,734 square miles). The population is 45 million, with 30% aged 0 to 14 years. Most Colombian immigrants in the United States come from urban lower- or middle-class backgrounds. Colombia's ethnic diversity is a result of the intermingling of indigenous people, Spanish colonists, and African slaves.

Major Languages	Ethnic Groups	Major Religions
Spanish (official)	Mestizo 58%	Roman Catholic 90%
	White 20%	Other 10%
	Mulatto 14%	
	Black 4%	
	Mixed Black and Amerindian 3%	
	Amerindian 1%	

Few foreigners have immigrated to Colombia compared with immigration to several other South American countries. Religious groups such as Anglican, Jehovah's witnesses, Evangelical, and Mormon have altered the country's religious preferences. The literacy rate is 93% for men, 93% for women.

Health Care Beliefs: Acute sick care predominates; also traditional. Among Amerindian people, magical-religious practices are common, and shamans usually provide traditional remedies and care for the sick. Illness may be thought of as a punishment from God for transgressions. A drink made of unprocessed sugar and water *(agua de panela)* is believed to help cure respiratory problems and influenza.

Predominant Sick-Care Practices: Biomedical; magical-religious. During the past few years, despite significant socioeconomic differences, an increasing number of urban and rural dwellers have gained access to medical services and social security coverage. Colombia has a variety of private and public insurance companies and health care providers at all levels of health care delivery. In 1993, Colombia became one of the first middle-low income countries to adopt a managed competition strategy to reform its health care system. It has a high rate of coverage from contributory and subsidized affiliation. Sociocultural and economic factors also have allowed for the continued acceptance of folk healers *(curanderos)*, who may be consulted in addition to biomedical practitioners. Most medications can be purchased in pharmacies over the counter. This leads to self-prescribing and contributes to the global problem of antibiotic resistance.

Ethnic-/Race-Specific or Endemic Diseases: The primary endemic disease is chloroquine-resistant malaria. Colombians are also at risk for yellow fever, dengue fever, cholera, mild protein deficiency malnutrition, digestive tract parasitic diseases, malnutrition disorders, and iron deficiency anemia. Because of increased migration to the unexplored tropical hinterland, diseases such as malaria, dengue, and yellow fever have become endemic. Most infant and child deaths are linked to diarrheal diseases, digestive tract infections, nutritional disorders, and complications related to vaccine-preventable viruses. Common health problems are respiratory infections, ophthalmologic and vision problems, digestive tract parasitic diseases, acute upper respiratory tract infections, peripheral vascular problems such as varicose veins, and malnutrition disorders. Preventable and curable diseases, such as gastrointestinal disorders and certain types of respiratory ailments affect the poorest people, whereas the incidence of degenerative and chronic diseases is typical in urban dwellers and higher income earners. In addition, 7% of Colombians (three million people) are over age 60, and they experience diseases that are common in industrialized nations, such as ischemic heart disease, chronic obstructive pulmonary disease, hypertension, diabetes mellitus, and cancer. Many adult deaths result from "social pathologies," such as homicide and accidents. Violent criminal attacks and homicides, referred to in Colombia as *blood deaths,* account for a large percentage of deaths as a result of poor law enforcement, high levels of social and political violence, and criminal activities related to narcotics production and distribution. The Joint United Nations Programme on HIV/AIDS (UNAIDS) estimates the prevalence rate for human immunodeficiency virus (HIV) in adults (aged 15 to 49 years) is 0.6%, with 160,000 people living with HIV, including 45,000 women. About 8,200 have died of acquired immunodeficiency syndrome (AIDS). About three fourths of all infections are transmitted via men having sex with men as well as heterosexually.

Health-Team Relationships: Patients show enormous respect toward medical doctors. This can result in shyness and an extreme reluctance to ask questions. Patients may be very modest with care providers of the opposite sex. Hospitalized patients are expected to be passive, and family members provide most self-care activities at home. The nurses' role is extremely important. They are responsible for establishing initial contact with patients when they arrive at the hospital (although in public hospital settings, they do so after a social worker has analyzed the patient's socioeconomic and cultural situation). They are also responsible for providing most of the care a hospitalized patient requires, such as prescription management and treatment surveillance. When patients arrive at the hospital, the nurse interviews the person and performs a preliminary examination to identify the patients' needs and health status. The nurse then refers them to the appropriate medical doctor. Chief nurses are highly specialized at the graduate level and educated to establish effective health team relationships. They are in charge of planning and coordinating patient care with the team. Nursing is a regulated profession; curricula at state and private universities are controlled. Because of deficiencies in the education received by nonprofessional auxiliary personnel, however, nurses are also in charge of supervising these workers. Because new regulations in the Colombian health system have resulted in a very tight schedule that allows medical doctors to devote very little time to their patients, nurses are more accessible and spend more time with patients. Consequently, patients trust and believe them.

Families' Role in Hospital Care: Female family members may try to provide so much care that it becomes a hindrance to patients' resuming basic self-care activities. Mothers or older sisters might be expected to stay overnight. Commonly, there are many visitors, bringing home cooked meals, sweets, grapes, and flowers to the patient.

Dominance Patterns: There is a high rate of migration from rural to urban areas. With the growth of urban industrial centers and accompanying socioeconomic developments, signs of change are evident in the traditional norms and patterns of family life. The decline of the patriarchal extended family structure has become more apparent in urban society. Increased geographic and social mobility has weakened kinship ties and extended greater independence to young people. Nevertheless, the patriarchal pattern still prevails. In low- and middle-class environments, women are expected to be respectful to husbands, and the father or older sibling is expected to be the spokesperson. They take part in most decision-making discussions, including those involving health issues, such as the decision of whether or not to tell patients they have a terminal illness. Domestic violence is a high-priority problem.

Eye-Contact Practices: Citizens of peasant and urban lower-class origin may try to avoid making direct eye contact with authority figures and older adults or in awkward situations.

Touch Practices: Touch is important and used when giving bad news. Hugs are used to greet others. Handshaking is common, although some women may grasp the wrists of other women instead of their hands. In general, a narrow physical space is maintained among close friends and relatives. Indicating a person's height by extending the arm with the palm down is an insulting gesture.

Perceptions of Time: Colombians have a relaxed and flexible sense of time. Short-term planning is more common than long-term. People may be a little late for appointments, and some appointments may be cancelled at the last minute.

Birth Rites: During labor, pain relief is welcome but not expected by women in lower socioeconomic groups. The father or family members are not usually present during the delivery. Although abortion is illegal, many women—especially those in urban areas—seek out illegal abortion clinics to terminate unwanted pregnancies. Such actions put their lives at risk. When the father is involved, his decision about continuing or terminating a pregnancy is what counts. Large segments of the population believe that abortion is a sin. Colombia has an impressive record for family planning and contraception, which is used by most women. Although contraceptive methods for men are becoming more available, they are less popular because of predominant machismo attitudes. Although many women use contraceptives, sterilization is preferred after two or more children. The fertility rate is 2.54 children born per woman. Male circumcision is a personal, rather than religious, decision and is usually done close to birth. The infant mortality rate is 21 deaths per 1,000 live births. The city of Bogotá created international interest in its "kangaroo care" system of treatment for premature (low birth weight) infants. Life expectancy is 68 for men, 76 for women.

Death Rites: Family members may want to view the body before it is taken to the morgue, and burials often take place within 24 to 36 hours. Cremation has become increasingly common in the last decade. Organ donations are not common but are considered acceptable.

Food Practices and Intolerances: Breakfast is an important meal and usually includes freshly squeezed fruit juice, eggs, coffee, or chocolate with milk and regional variations of cornmeal griddle cakes *(arepas)*. The diet is composed mainly of starches, rice, potatoes, beans, plantain, cassava, and pasta. The predominant meats are chicken, beef, pork, and fish. Meats that are high in cholesterol are common. Although eaten more than they were in the past, salads consisting of lettuce, tomatoes, cucumber, carrots, and onions are not considered a complete meal on their own. For most people, lunch (which often includes fruit, soup, a main course, and dessert) may be the largest meal of the day. Sandwiches are considered a substitute for meals. Most Colombians drink coffee through-out the day. Fruit juice diluted with water or milk is offered with meals. Catholics may prefer fish on Fridays during the season of Lent.

Child-Rearing Practices: Infants are mostly breastfed. Depending on their socioeconomic status, mothers prefer to care for their children until they start school at age 4 years. Children are very dependent on their parents and may live with them until they marry. Children are expected to be obedient, respectful, and quiet in the presence of adults.

National Childhood Immunizations: BCG at birth; DTwP at 18 months and 5 years; DTwPHibHep at 2, 4, and 6 months; HepB at birth; MMR at 1 and 5 years; IPV at birth and at 2, 4, and 6 months; Td first-contact pregnancy, +1, +6months and +1, +1 year; YF at 1 and 10 years. The percent of the target population vaccinated, by antigen, is: BCG, DTP3,HepB3, Hib3, and Polio3 (87%); DTP1 (95%); MCV (89%); and TT2 plus (57%). Since BCG immunization is given at birth, most Columbians who live in or immigrate to the United States test positive for the Mantoux/PPD. This does not mean that they have tuberculosis.

BIBLIOGRAPHY

Central Intelligence Agency 2006: *The world factbook, Columbia.* Retrieved September 21, 2006, from https://www.cia.gov/cia/publications/factbook/print/co.html.

Mosquera, M: Strengthening user participation through health sector reform in Colombia: a study of institutional change and social representation, *Health Policy Plan.* 16(Suppl2):52–60, 2005.

Singla M: BCG skin reaction to Mantoux negative healthy children, *BMC Infect Dis.* 5:5–19, 2005.

Pan American Health Organization: Country Health Profile. Retrieved on February 24, 2006, from http://www.paho.org/English/DD/AIS/cp_index.htm.

UNAIDS: 2006 Columbia. Retrieved September 21, 2006, from http://www.unaids.org/en/Regions_Countries/Countries/columbia.asp.

World Health Organization: 2006: Immunization, vaccines and biologicals. Retrieved September 21, 2006, from http://www.who.int/immunization_monitoring/en/globalsummary/countryprofileresult.cfm?C='col'.

http://devdata.worldbank.org/idg/IDGProfile.asp?CCODE=COL&CNAME=Colombia&SelectedCountry=COL (retrieved on February 10, 2006).

http://familydoctor.org/120.xml (retrieved on February 21, 2006).

◆ CONGO (DEMOCRATIC REPUBLIC OF THE)

MAP PAGE (801)

Jean-Claude Mwanza

Location: With a total area of 2,345,000 km^2 (905,170 square miles), the Democratic Republic of the Congo (DRC) is the third largest country in Africa; it has been independent since 1960. The capital is Kinshasha. Located in Central Africa, it is surrounded by the Central African Republic and Sudan to the north; Uganda, Rwanda, Burundi, and Tanzania to the east; Zambia and Angola to the south; and the Republic of Congo to the west, with a narrow opening of about 35 km to the Atlantic ocean. The country can be roughly divided into three regions: the central Congo basin, a large depression occupying about one third of the country and covered by one of the world biggest forests; hills and plains of savannah with woodlands; and an eastern region covered by high mountains with large lakes. The climate is tropical with a rainy and dry season. The DRC is potentially one of the world's richest countries because of abundant mineral and forest resources, fertile soil, and the enormous hydroelectric potential of the Congo River. The gross domestic product (GDP) per capita is $700, but 80% of Congolese survive with about $1/person/day. Although the most recent nationwide census did not take place in rural areas, where about 65% of the population live, the size of the population is estimated at 63 million (48% under age 15).

Major Languages	Ethnic Groups	Major Religions
French (official)	Mongo (Bantu), Luba (Bantu),	Roman Catholic
Lingala	Kongo (Bantu), Hamitic	50%
Kiswahili	(Mangbetu and Azande)	Protestant 20%
Kikongo	51%	Kimbanguist 10%
Tshiluba	Sudanic, Pygmy, Other 49%	Muslim 10%
		Syncretic sects
		and traditional
		beliefs 10%

Syncretic sects have been evident since the 1920s; most common are Kimbanguism (The Church of Christ on Earth, inspired by the "prophet" Simon Kimbangu (an originate of the Bas-Congo region); Peve ya longo, Bima, Kitawala (first in the Katanga region before spreading to South Africa), whose followers support the existence of a black God; and the Jamaa movement, originating from the Roman Catholic church. Syncretic sects have rapidly increased over the last 5 years, although many people also have traditional religious beliefs. An estimated 200 different languages are spoken, some of which are very similar. People have shown enormous interest in learning English in recent years. The literacy rate is 84% for men, 61% for women.

Health Care Beliefs: Acute sick care; passive role. Mental illness is greatly feared because of the belief that even when treated it never disappears forever. Most think that mental illness is caused by curses from a jealous person or is a punishment from God. Grave or fatal diseases may be viewed in the same way, with people believing that the ill person has done something very wrong (e.g., stolen something, murdered someone) and is receiving God's justice. Others believe in fate—that good and bad events happen to all people. Such attitudes inhibit understanding the origin of disease. Prevention and heath promotion are the tasks of the

Ministry of Health. Although the country has a Bureau National (national office) responsible for the prevention and eradication of common infectious diseases (malaria, trypanosomiasis, tuberculosis, onchocerciasis, human immunodeficiency syndrome (HIV)/acquired immunodeficiency syndrome (AIDS), schistosomiasis, diarrheal diseases, leprosy), such activities are hampered by the size of the country, poor roads, and the poor financial state of the country. Disease prevention is currently limited to free vaccinations of children (where possible). There is an effective program against tuberculosis, with a case- detection rate of 70% to 75% and an (almost free) treatment success of 75% in Kinshasa and all major cities. The DRC was one of the first countries to implement a national program against HIV. Initially, people reacted negatively by calling HIV the "syndrome inventé pour décourager les amoureux," meaning "pure fiction" designed to discourage lovers. Some years later, well-known actors and musicians were among the first to die, and then relatives, friends, and neighbors. People quickly recognized that AIDS was more than fiction and changed their sexual behavior. These factors and an effective national program resulted in a reduction in prevalence. Information on HIV/AIDS has been made available in antenatal clinics since the start of the pandemic.

Predominant Sick-Care Practices: Traditional healing; biomedical when available; and religious. Nearly two thirds of the Congolese have no access to conventional medical health care. The 400 public hospitals have no adequate equipment or medical supplies. The whole health system is down, which has led to the re-emergence of infectious and communicable diseases eradicated in the 1960s and 1970s. The extent of the territory, combined with the lack of means of communication, worsens the situation by isolating many health centers. It is now common for inpatients to obtain their own medicines and sometimes their own medical equipment (i.e., surgical tools). Pharmacies in public hospitals are empty and closed in most cases. As a result, the very expensive, dangerous, and unaffordable (for the large majority) informal sector remains the only available choice. Worse, the fee-charging system is beyond the means of most people. Under these conditions, it is not surprising that most people use traditional health care practices, especially in rural areas. In cities, people are usually treated in health centers, but Congolese of all social and intellectual levels consult traditional healers. It is common for people to consult a doctor and traditional healer simultaneously. In some cases, hospitalized individuals continue to combine modern and traditional methods without their medical doctor's knowledge. Traditional healers are so abundant that they have asked for official recognition by state authorities, an idea supported by the Ministry of Health because traditional medicine is the first source of health care for about 80% of the population. Plants and herbs are commonly used, such as *kongo bololo* (which has a bitter taste and is believed to have the same effect as quinine) for malaria, *tangawisi* ("ginger") to cure diseases and back or hemorrhoid pain and sexual impotence (for which the cola nut is used as well) and avocado leaves for anemia. Because of the collapse of the biomedical health system, it is becoming common for sick people to avoid seeking care in health facilities and instead spend time in churches (syncretic sects) waiting and hoping to be cured miraculously by God through a prophet or priest. When the expected miracle cure does not come, the priest or prophet tries to convince the sick believer that what is important is "that they be accepted by the Lord in his kingdom, in paradise, because life has no meaning on earth."

Ethnic-/Race-Specific or Endemic Diseases: Communicable diseases such as malaria, tuberculosis, onchocerciasis (river blindness), trypanosomiasis (sleeping sickness), and diarrheal diseases are the main concerns. Malaria accounts for about 50% of childhood mortality. Onchocerciasis is endemic in almost the entire country. The DRC has the highest percentage of African trypanosomiasis cases (70% of all cases) because of poor surveillance and lack of vector control. Goiter and cretinism are endemic in the Kivu and Equator regions because of iodine insufficiency in the soil and water. Konzo is a neurologic disease associated with repeated intake of cyanide-producing compounds from consumption of poorly processed bitter cassava and the low intake of sulphur amino acids from animal protein; it is found in the Yaka (Bandundu region). Glaucoma is more prevalent in the Mongo ethnic group, and albinism is more frequent among the Luba people. Some hereditary diseases are more prevalent in the Bandundu region because of frequent consanguineous marriage. There is a stable HIV prevalence of 3.2% (1.8% to 4.9%). The Joint United Nations Programme on HIV/AIDS (UNAIDS) estimates the number of people living with HIV at one million, including 520,000 women and 120,000 children aged 0 to 14. About 680,000 children aged 0 to 17 are orphans as a result of parental AIDS. There have been 90,000 deaths. Systematic rape used as a weapon by soldiers of at least six foreign countries during the war (1996–2003), has contributed to the spread of HIV in the east, with a prevalence rate of about 20%. There are concerns that this will increase prevalence in the rest of the country as a result of mass movements of the population from and to the eastern part. Heterosexual transmission accounts for 80% of cases. The independence of the health system has been affected by weak governance; misappropriation of public funds; and deliberate poor management of resources, political instability, and war (10 years) where health centers were systematically destroyed.

Health-Team Relationships: The health care system is doctor driven. Doctors and nurses (both low paid) have friendly relationships and are trusted by patients. In remote rural areas without doctors, a nurse often is the highest authority in the region. For example, after 11 years of work at a university hospital in Kinshasa, the author of this chapter, a specialist in ophthalmology, earned approximately $19 per month (paid irregularly) for clinical, academic, and research tasks. It is not unusual for nurses to earn higher salaries than doctors.

Families' Role in Hospital Care: Because of lack of transportation to medical facilities and poor pay, nurses are not available to do tasks that were once nursing duties. Hospital pharmacies are either unavailable or lack sufficient medications. Therefore, the family plays an important role

C

in taking care of sick relatives. One or several members usually spend time at the hospital, buy food from the nearest market and cook it, change and wash clothes and bedding (which belong to the family), and occasionally administer pills. When the medical team needs a particular drug, a family member is ready to go elsewhere to buy it, and another stays with the patient. It may take several hours before the needed medicine is brought in because of the long distances and poor transportation system. In private health centers, which are run primarily by Roman Catholic churches, only one family member is allowed to stay if needed, and no cooking at the hospital is allowed. The family then brings food from home. Because of the current state of health care facilities, it is rare to find an inpatient without a relative staying at the bedside. The role of the family when a person is hospitalized is vital.

Dominance Patterns: According to state law, the society is patriarchal, so children belong to the clan of the father and only the father receives allowances for children. In most of the country's ethnic groups, married woman are entirely dominated economically by their husbands. For example, he has the right to ask his wife's employer to withdraw her work responsibilities. Although men are dominant, some matrilineal ethnic groups exist, primarily the Kongo people in the western part of the country. Among the Kongo, the women's family, especially the *noko* (maternal uncle), controls the power, including decisions about a woman's marriage. Gender-based discrimination is less common in public life, and women are found at high levels in government and hospital administrations.

Eye-Contact Practices: Although eye contact is no longer an important issue, it is still thought that making direct eye contact with parents when being scolded is impolite. The child is expected to look down.

Touch Practices: Touching is not an important issue for most Congolese. However, in some religious sects (e.g., Branhamism) it is forbidden for men to hug any woman other than their wives during greetings.

Perceptions of Time: In general, very little value is attached to punctuality. It is very uncommon for events to start on time. Any invitation to attend a given ceremony is usually followed by *"à la zaïroise or à la congolaise,"* meaning that the ceremony will start in the Congolese way, or very late. In public administration the costs of such delays have caused the current chaotic state of public administration. Time is regarded as only existing in the present and is not used for future planning. Time can be thought of as a function of the profit someone expects to get from an appointment. Therefore people tend to be on time for highly important matters such as written examinations, job interviews, consultations about health problems, or payment of salary.

Pain Reactions: Although high pain tolerance is common, men are expected to express pain less as a sign of manhood. Adults are expected to be more tolerant than are children. Pain expression may depend on whether expression is considered normal for a certain circumstance. For example, women who think that dysmenorrhea is normal pain keep it private and do not express it. Pain after a spontaneous fall is expressed moderately, whereas pain from a punch or kick from a husband tends to be expressed vigorously.

Birth Rites: Birth is an occasion for rejoicing, especially after the birth of the first child. The first event after birth is the naming of the child, usually immediately after birth. The name choice is always determined within the clans from the names of grandparents, parents, and relatives. The child is either named with a given name (from the clan) followed by the father's names, or all the children of the same family have a common first name (the father's), followed by another from the clan. In addition, a third name, usually a French name, is given according to the tradition acquired from colonization. In many ethnic groups, names have significance and are chosen according to the circumstances surrounding the birth of the child (e.g. after twins or three or more siblings of the same sex in a row or first born after many years of attempts to have a child). Special names are given to twins, depending on the ethnic groups. Among Luba, the first twin is named Mbuyi and the second Kabanga; among Kongo they are named Nsimba and Nzuzi; Mbo and Mpia by those in Bandundu region; and Mbo and Mukonkole by Songe people. Many of the birth rites are no longer practiced, and birth has become an occasion to pray and thank God. The infant mortality rate is 130 deaths per 1,000 live births. The fertility rate is 6.5 children born per woman. In most parts of the country, the mortality rate of children under age 5 is more than 2/10,000/day, a catastrophic situation. Life expectancy is 50 for men, 53 for women.

Death Rites: In the second largest city, the burial ceremony takes place 1 or 2 days after death, and the corpse is taken directly from the mortuary to the cemetery. In Kinshasa, 2 or more days may pass between death and burial. One day before burial, the corpse is taken home for the last time and memorialized by family, friends, and acquaintances. Most traditional rites have disappeared; instead, people recite prayers and sing religious songs. Usually, a final religious service is held at the home, and a funeral procession consisting of hundreds of people continuously singing or crying accompany the body to the burial. Afterwards, a family representative announces the end of mourning. People are then given mild alcoholic drinks and food. During the weeks after the death, the family of the deceased receives visitors. Although cremation is acceptable, autopsies are rare, and organ donation does not exist because of cultural beliefs about the inability to perform transplantation. When circumstances surrounding the death of a young person are not clear; other youth may make the funeral a violent event, threatening the family to give an explanation and name the responsible person.

Food Practices and Intolerances: Cassava *(Manihot esculenta)* is the staple crop for most Congolese, providing at least 60% of the total energy intake. Cassava flour is not eaten alone; it is mixed with corn flour to make *ugali* (= *fufu* = *nshima*), a kind of pasta. Rice is widely consumed, especially by Tetela people. Plantains are the main staple food in the Province Orientale, and beans are widely available. Among vegetables, cassava leaves remain the most widely consumed, but sorrel, sweet potatoes, and gourd leaves are also eaten. Because of the socioeconomic collapse of the country, most people eat only one meal daily.

Infant-Feeding Practices: Approximately 35% of newborns are exclusively breastfed until age 3 months. About half of infants aged from 6 to 9 months also receive supplementary food. Breastfeeding may continue up to 2 years, particularly in rural areas. Television and radio programs encourage mothers to breastfeed as long as possible.

Child-Rearing Practices: Educated women do not carry their children on their backs, but this is a common practice in rural areas and among uneducated women in rural and urban areas. Children are expected to be respectful and polite to older adults. The parents' friends, as well as any other mother or father, are called *papa* and *maman*, and older brothers and sisters are called *yaya*. Any child who refers to an older person by the person's name is considered ill-mannered. Grandparents are usually very kind and permissive. Children are not usually present when parents entertain guests. Girls are initiated into doing "women's work" at a young age, tasks that include helping the mother in the kitchen, cooking, serving food to the father and her brothers, removing and washing dishes after meals, washing clothes, cleaning the house, taking care of younger siblings, buying food at the market, and returning home earlier in the evening than boys. The boys are expected to do the hard-labor chores at home, but they are usually away playing football or other games with friends and only return for meals and bedtime. Girls tend to be authoritarian when it comes to kitchen matters, an attitude encouraged by parents. It would not be unusual to hear a girl saying to her brothers in the kitchen, "What are you doing here? This is not your place!" or "Do you want to be a girl?" In general, parents are more demanding with girls. Girls usually live with parents until they marry; if they do otherwise, they dishonor the family. Education is encouraged because it is believed to be the only path to a better future. It is generally accepted that boys should continue their education as long as possible, whereas education for girls is discouraged. The majority of parents who are able to do so send boys overseas for a better education. Even when educated, girls are expected to get married as soon as possible.

National Childhood Immunizations: BCG at birth; DTwP at 2, 3, 4, and 16 months; OPV at birth and 2, 3, and 4 months; measles at 9 months; vitamin A at 9 months; YF at 9 months; and TT after first contact, +1 month, +1, +1, +6 months, +1, +2 years. The percent of the target population vaccinated, by antigen, is: BCG and DTP1 (73%); DTP3, Polio3, and TT2 plus (65%); MCV (56%); and YF (54%). Although recent immunization campaigns have endeavored to reach all 321 health zones in the country, coverage rates are still low.

BIBLIOGRAPHY

African Programme for Onchocerciasis Control (APOC): Status of Onchocerciasis in APOC Countries. Rapid epidemiological mapping of onchocerciasis in countries covered by APOC as of July 2004. Retrieved July 26, from http://www.apoc.bf/en/disease_distrib_MethodeSur.htm.

Central Intelligence Agency: 2006: The world factbook, Congo, Democratic Republic of the Retrieved September 21, 2006, from https://www.cia.gov/cia/publications/factbook/print/cg.html.

Lutumba P et al: Trypanosomiasis control, Democratic Republic of Congo, 1993–2003, *Emerg Infect Dis.* 11:1382–1388, 2005.

Mwanza JCK, Kabasele PM: Corneal complications of local ocular traditional treatment in the Democratic Republic of Congo, *Med Trop.* 61:500–502, 2001.

United Nations Children's Fund statistics: Africa 2000.

UNAIDS, 2006 Congo (Democratic Republic of the): Retrieved September 21, 2006 from http://www.unaids.org/en/Regions_Countries/Countries/congo.asp.

UNPOP: *The Human Development Report,* 2000.

World Health Organization: *Health action in crises, Democratic Republic of Congo,* April 2005.

World Health Organization: 2006: Immunization, vaccines and biologicals. Retrieved September 21, 2006, from http://www.who.int/immunization_monitoring/en/globalsummary/countryprofileresult.cfm?C='cog.

◆ CONGO (REPUBLIC OF THE)

MAP PAGE (801)

Sophie Le Coeur

Location: Located in West Central Africa, the Republic of the Congo (commonly called *Congo-Brazzaville*) is a former French colony that should not to be confused with its larger neighbor, the Democratic Republic of Congo (formerly Zaire, a Belgian colony). The total area is 342,000 km² (132,012 square miles). This nation, astride the equator, is surrounded by the Central African Republic and Gabon to the north; Cameroon to the west; Cabinda (Angola) to the south; and, separated by the large Congo River, the Democratic Republic of Congo to the south and east, and the Gulf of Guinea to the southwest. The land is covered by thick rain forests, and the climate is tropical, with a rainy season (March through June) and a dry season (June through October). Temperatures and humidity are constantly high. Although no updated census has been carried out since 1984, the population is estimated at 3.9 million, 46% aged between 0 and 14 years. The population density is very low, with 12 inhabitants per km². The capital city, Brazzaville, is located on the Congo River just across from Kinshasa, the capital of the Democratic Republic of Congo, and accounts for about two thirds of the country's population.

Major Languages	Ethnic Groups	Major Religions
French (official)	Kongo 48%	Christian 50%
Lingala (trade language)	Sangha 20%	Indigenous beliefs 48%
Monokutuba (trade language)	Teke 17%	Muslim 2%
Kikongo	M'Bochi 12%	
Local languages and dialects	Others 3%	

C

After a few years of economic progress from increasing oil revenues, the Congo underwent a difficult transition in the early 1990s with a slump in oil prices and the devaluation of Franc Zone currencies by 50%. The gross domestic product (GDP) per capita is $1,300 (70% of its 1984 level), which has increased poverty; the situation has been aggravated by a civil war of tribal and ethnic rivalries. About 800,000 people (27% of the population) have been displaced. In addition to 10,000 to 50,000 deaths and great devastation, the war had a severe detrimental impact on the social cohesion of the country. According to the United Nations Children's Fund (UNICEF), 11% of children under age 15 are orphans, 60,000 women and girls were victims of rape, and 5,000 children fought during the war. Public services, such as schools, administrations, and health structures, were vastly disrupted. Literacy rates are 90% for men, 78% for women.

Health Care Beliefs: Traditional and Western medicines usually complement each other. It is widely believed that although Western medicine may treat illness, the addition of traditional medicine will allow the cure by acting on the very cause of the disease, often related to family problems or witchcraft. Mental illnesses that do not disrupt the social order are well tolerated, although families would rapidly seek medical and traditional care for patients with acute delirium. Although the Republic of Congo was one of the first countries affected by the human immunodeficiency virus (HIV) epidemic, there is still enormous denial of the disease. In a study in Pointe-Noire, among more than 600 deaths related to HIV, only 15 cases of acquired immunodeficiency syndrome (AIDS) were acknowledged by the families.

Predominant Sick-Care Practices: Ethnic violence has virtually destroyed the infrastructure of the country, including its health facilities. Although some reconstruction has taken place, facilities are in very poor condition, and there is a lack of trained medical personnel and shortages of medical equipment, diagnostic supplies, and medications. Although nongovernmental organizations (NGOs) such as *Médecins Sans Frontières* (Doctors Without Borders) and the International Red Cross have provided some relief to struggling health sector efforts, most have left the country. The maternal and child surveillance system remains quite operational as indicated by the relatively high immunization coverage.

Ethnic-/Race-Specific or Endemic Diseases: Malaria, largely chloroquine-resistant malaria, is a frequent cause of morbidity and a cause of death primarily in children younger than 5 years. Other endemic infectious diseases are tuberculosis (the most common opportunistic infection in HIV-infected individuals), schistosomiasis, sleeping sickness (which has experienced a resurgence in the last decade), and Loa Loa microfilaraemia. Several outbreaks of Ebola virus at the border with Gabon have been monitored by the World Health Organization (WHO) since 2002. Malnutrition, diarrheal diseases, malaria, respiratory infections, and measles are the most common causes of death in children. Genetic hemoglobin abnormalities such as sickle cell anemia are quite common. Only 69% of the urban and 11% of the rural population have access to tap water. Tap water is not potable and is polluted from dumped raw sewage, which increases the threat of water-borne illness. The HIV epidemic is relatively stable. According to the Joint United Nations Programme on HIV/AIDS (UNAIDS), the estimated prevalence rate for HIV in adults (aged 15 to 49 years) is 5.3%, with 120,000 people living with HIV, including 61,000 women and 15,000 children aged 0 to 14. AIDS has tripled the number of deaths among adults 15 to 44 years (about 11,000 deaths overall). About 110,000 children aged 0 to 17 are orphans because of AIDS. The percentage of pregnant women receiving treatment to reduce mother-to-child transmission, reported as 99%, is clearly overestimated. The percentage of HIV-infected women and men who are reported to be receiving antiretroviral therapy (17%) is probably also overestimated but to a lesser extent.

Health-Team Relationships: Patients are taken care of mostly by nurses, except for severe cases, which are referred to a physician or in some private clinics. The relationship between patients and health care workers is quite hierarchical, with generally little room for listening to the patients, or providing them counseling. In the public sector, nurses and doctors are very low paid and cannot make a living unless they have some private practice outside the hospital. Although it is possible to find some dedicated health care workers, most of them, working in over-crowded and deteriorated facilities, with a chronic lack of supplies and medications, express their frustration through an obvious lack of commitment.

Families' Role in Hospital Care: There is always a family member at the side of the patient. They feed, change, wash them, do the nursing care, monitor drug intakes or intravenous infusions, and provide psychological support. Most of all, the role of the family is to gather the necessary financial means to buy the drugs and pay for the biological or radiologic examinations. It would be considered very inappropriate to leave a patient alone at the hospital.

Eye-Contact Practices: Between men, between women, and between men and women, eye contact is not an issue.

Touch Practices: Congolese people touch each other often. For example, it is quite usual to see two adult men or women walking in the street hand in hand. Congolese greet each other mostly by shaking hands or sometimes forehead to forehead.

Perceptions of Time: Congolese people attach little value to punctuality, and yet people tend to be more punctual for matters they consider important. Patients rarely complain about the very long waiting lines at the outpatient clinics.

Pain Reactions: There is no special issue about pain tolerance except that men are supposed to tolerate pain better than women.

Birth Rites: Most women deliver in maternity clinics, where they usually stay less than 2 days. If they deliver at home, they usually bring their newborn to the health center as soon as possible and are charged a small fee. Traditionally, the father-to-be pays for the medical follow-up, prescriptions, maternity stay, examination and surgical gloves, newborn clothes, child follow-up, and such. The more expensive these things are, the more valued women feel they are. According to the United Nations, from 2005 to 2010, about 190,000 births and 53,000 deaths per year are expected, corresponding to a 2.94 population growth rate. The fertility rate is 6.29 children born per woman. The infant mortality rate is 85 deaths per 1,000, and the under-5 mortality is 107 per 1,000 live births. The maternal mortality rate is estimated at 810 per 100,000 live births, one of the highest in the world. Life expectancy is 52 for men, 54 for women.

Death Rites: In the Congolese culture, ancestor and dead worship is essential and requires ostentatious funerals departing from the mortuary a few days after the death. Before burial, as a mourning ritual, the extended family and social acquaintances gather every evening at the home of the deceased to pay respect,where food and drinks are provided to the gathering. Funerals represent an important financial burden to families.

Food Practices or Intolerances: Manioc roots, or *cassava,* is the basic food. It is mostly prepared as a fermented "bread," called *chikuang.* Cassava flour is used for children. Manioc leaves are cooked with palm oil, which is very rich in vitamin A, and smoked dry fish, to make a dish called *saka-saka.* French bread is very popular, and fresh bread is prepared at the many bakeries in the cities. Other foods include sweet potatoes, zucchini, grains (Nté-té), plantains, and many fruits, such as pineapples, mangos, and bananas.

Infant-Feeding Practices: Most women breastfeed their infants until they are 18 months or 2 years. Although it is encouraged for 6 months, exclusive breastfeeding is uncommon, with mothers providing early supplementary foods such as corn or manioc flour when infants are as young as 2 months. Women are compliant with regard to the tradition of sexual abstinence during the duration of breastfeeding or for at least 6 months.

Child-Rearing Practices: Children are considered precious, and mothers and infants have a very close relationship. Infants are carried on their mother's backs and sleep with them. While breastfeeding, mothers take their infants with them everywhere. Because of the postpartum abstinence, birth intervals usually exceed 18 months. After the birth of a new child, the previous one is abruptly left aside and not carried on the back anymore, causing them to feel abandoned.

National Childhood Immunizations: BCG at birth; DTwP at 2, 3, 4, and 16 months; OPV at birth and 2, 3, and 4 months; measles at 9 months; YF and vitamin A at 9 months; TT at first contact, +1, +6 months, +1, +2 years. The percent of the target population vaccinated, by antigen, is: BCG (85%); DTP1, DTP3, and Polio3 (67%); MCV and TT2 plus (65%); vitamin A (49%); and YF (54%). Coverage is much lower in rural areas.

BIBLIOGRAPHY

Central Intelligence Agency: *2006: The world factbook, Congo, Republic of the.* Retrieved September 21, 2006, from https://www.cia.gov/cia/publications/factbook/print/cf.html.

Le Cœur S, Halembokaka G, Khlat M, et al: Impact of AIDS on adult mortality: a morgue-based study in Pointe-Noire, Republic of Congo, *AIDS.* 19:1683-1687, 2005.

République du Congo/Système des Nations Unies au Congo: *Rapport national sur les objectifs du millénaire pour le développement—République du Congo,* August 2004.

Talani P, Nzaba P, Bolanda D et al: An immunization coverage survey in the Kouilou area of Congo-Brazzaville, *Sante.* 14:121–124, 2004.

UNAIDS: 2006 Congo (Republic of). Retrieved September 21, 2006, from http://www.unaids.org/en/Regions_Countries/Countries/republic_of_congo.asp.

US Committee for Refugees and Immigrants: Country reports. Retrieved August 28, 2006, from http://www.refugees.org/countryreports.aspx?subm=&ssm=&cid=1578.

World Bank: Country Brief. Republic of Congo. Retrieved August 30, 2006, from http://web.worldbank.org/WBSITE/EXTERNAL/COUNTRIES/AFRICAEXT/CONGOEXTN/0,,menuPK:349223~pagePK:141132~piPK:141107~theSitePK:349199,00.html.

World Population Prospects: The 2004 revision. New York, United Nations. 2005. Retrieved August 28, 2006, from http://esa.un.org/unpp/.

World Health Organization: The world health report 2006—working together for health. Retrieved August 28, 2006, from http://www.who.int/whr/2006/en/.

World Health Organization: 2006: Immunization, vaccines and biologicals. Retrieved September 21, 2006, from http://www.who.int/immunization_monitoring/en/globalsummary/countryprofileresult.cfm?C='cog'.

C

◆ COSTA RICA (REPUBLIC OF)

MAP PAGE (795)

Jorge Azofeifa

Location: Costa Rica, the southernmost of the Central American republics, extends 51,700 km² (19,962 square miles) from northwest to southeast. It shares borders with Nicaragua in the north and Panama on the southeast. The Caribbean Sea is on the east and northeast, the Pacific Ocean on the west and southwest. The land area is crossed by three major mountain ranges (the cordilleras de Talamanca, Volcánica Central, and Guanacaste) that have created a tropical climate and vast biological diversity. The country is divided into seven provinces: Alajuela, Cartago, Guanacaste, Heredia, Limón, Puntarenas, and San José (the capital city). The population is 4.3 million. The gross domestic product (GDP) per capita is $11,100, with 18% living below the poverty line. Costa Ricans have a multiethnic population.

Major Languages	Ethnic Groups	Major Religions
Spanish (official)	Mestizo/mixed 93.66%	Roman Catholic 85%
Jamaican dialect	AfroCosta Rican 1.91%	Evangelical
	Amerindian 1.67%	Protestant 14%
	Chinese 0.21%	Other 1%

English is spoken by many because it has been taught in most private schools since the 1970s and is obligatory in all high schools. A variant of the Jamaican dialect is also spoken because the ancestors of the black community of Puerto Limon on the Caribbean coast were Jamaicans. Amerindian languages belonging to the Chibchan Stock are also spoken: Bribri, Cabecar, the Guaymi languages Ngäwbere, and Buglere. Two others, Guatuso and Boruca, are almost extinct. Literacy rates are 96% for both men and women.

Health Care Beliefs: Active involvement; health promotion important. Western medicine and disease prevention are given priority and accepted by the people, who tend to seek doctors and medical teams for care. Some use other medical practices such as homeopathy, acupuncture, and traditional indigenous medicine.

Predominant Sick-Care Practices: Biomedical and traditional. After the abolition of the army in 1948, the government invested resources into education and health. The national health system is led by the Ministry of Health and has established prevention programs through the Primary Health Care and Rural Health Programs. In addition, the Costa Rican Social Security Program (*Caja Costarricense de Seguro Social*, or CCSS) developed clinical and hospital services that provide universal coverage to the population. Both institutions have been responsible for joint improvements in environmental sanitation: water purification and piping, waste-water disposal in urban areas and latrines in rural areas; and a vaccination program. These steps have resulted in dramatic progress: since the 1970s, Costa Rica has had health statistic profiles similar to those of developed countries. Infectious diseases are no longer the major cause of morbidity and mortality, but chronic diseases have increased. The Ministry of Health and the CCSS have transformed the primary health care system by implementing the Basic Teams of Integral Health Attention (*Equipos Básicos de Atención Integral en Salud*, or EBAIS). These teams consist of a doctor, nurse, nutritionist, and health assistant. Private medical practice has gained importance in the last decades among wealthy people desiring more timely and expert care. Despite the availability of excellent health care, some Costa Ricans continue to consult healers for incurable or intractable diseases and sentimental issues.

Ethnic-/Race-Specific or Endemic Diseases: Infections of the upper respiratory tract are the main causes of illness except in older adults, whose major health problem is hypertension. Parasitic infections are a significant problem. Rates (per 100,000) for reportable diseases in 2004 were: diarrhea, 2813.6; dengue, 221.4; malaria, 30.3; hepatitis, 22.1; gonorrhea, 36.5; tuberculosis, 16.71; syphilis, 28.65; acquired immunodeficiency syndrome (AIDS), 4.61; rubella, 0.0; measles, 0.0; pertussis, 0.3. The main causes of death (rates per 10,000) were diseases of the circulatory system, 10.8; tumors, 8.4; external causes, 4.3; diseases of the respiratory system, 3.6; and diseases of the gastrointestinal system, 2.6. The Joint United Nations Programme on HIV/AIDS (UNAIDS) estimates the prevalence rate for human immunodeficiency virus (HIV) in adults (aged 15 to 49 years) to be 0.3%, with 7,400 people living with HIV, including 2,000 women. Fewer than 100 deaths from AIDS have been reported. The first AIDS cases were reported in 1983 and were only found in people with hemophilia during the next 4 years. The first cases in homosexuals were documented in 1985: about 68% of all present cases are attributed to men who have sex with men. In the 1990s, heterosexual and vertical transmission from mother to infant emerged. Life expectancy is 77 for men, 81 for women.

Health-Team Relationships: Relationships among health professionals are hierarchical, with doctors being dominant. This situation is accepted, and working relationships are generally good. All health professionals are respected and appreciated.

Families' Role in Hospital Care: Visits to the hospitals of the CCSS are allowed once a day at scheduled times. Food is provided as directed by nutritionists, depending on the special medical needs of patients. In certain cases and with permission, favorite foods may be brought from home. Family members rarely interact with doctors. In private hospitals and clinics, visits are permitted during the day, and a relative or friend of the patient is allowed to stay overnight if necessary.

Dominance Patterns: Costa Rica has had a male-dominated society, but during the last decades, more women have gained access to higher education and are now professionals. Over time, they have promoted campaigns for gender equality, which resulted in the Law of Social Equality of Women in 1990. Women continue to be excluded in most decision-making processes, however, are limited in the exercise of power, and have unequal access to resources. Women assume the main caring role when a family member is sick, although decisions regarding treatments and therapies are discussed by the entire family.

Eye-Contact Practices: Direct eye contact is customary when talking with or greeting someone of the same or opposite sex.

Touch Practices: Shaking hands is the usual way to greet people. In comfortable situations or when greeting relatives, kissing one cheek and embracing are also customary. Touching is more common among women.

Perceptions of Time: Punctuality is not an important concept for Costa Ricans. The expression *hora tica,* or "Costa Rican time," refers to the fact that delays of 30 minutes are accepted and tolerated. In certain situations, however, such as academic and official situations, being on time is more of an issue. People live in the present but do not forget traditions, and planning for the future is not unusual.

Pain Reactions: No cultural rules exist regarding pain aside from the stereotypical belief that men should tolerate pain better. Pain reactions depend primarily on the physiologic threshold of each person; therefore, pain reactions range from stoic to very expressive.

Birth Rites: Fertility rates are 2.24 children born per woman. No particular birth rites are observed by the general population. In the facilities offered by EBAIS, about 78% of women receive prenatal care, including instruction and assistance during childbirth. If a newborn is unhealthy and might die, Catholics baptize it as soon as possible. The Bribri Amerindians of the Cordillera de Talamanca follow traditional practices related to childbirth. For example, when labor begins, the woman leaves the house and gives birth alone in a hut in the woods (ideally near a creek with calm water) that was previously built for this purpose. After the birth, the mother lives in a small hut adjacent to the lodge in the village and stays there with the child for nearly a month. Mother and infant are "cleansed" through a series of rituals, after which they go back to their home. The infant mortality rate is 9.7 per 1,000 live births, the lowest in the history of the country. Life expectancy is 74 for men, 80 for women.

Death Rites: Because most of the population is Christian, no specific death rites are observed other than the wake and church ceremonies. Extended families and friends usually participate. Death is perceived as an unfortunate and sad fact of life. The Talamancan Bribri still participate in some ceremonies that involve purification of close family members and "packing" the body before the burial. Organ donation is acceptable. When the cause of death is suspicious or unexplainable, autopsies are mandated by law.

Food Practices and Intolerances: Breakfast in the rural areas usually consists of coffee or *agua dulce* (a beverage made by diluting sugar cane molasses with hot water), *gallo pinto* (fried rice with black or red beans), tortillas, and fresh cheese or eggs. In urban areas, a breakfast of coffee or tea, bread or tortillas with cheese or sour cream and eggs, and honey or marmalade is common. Cereal with milk is becoming more popular among children, adolescents, and young adults in urban areas. For lunch and dinner, rice, beans, and tortillas are common. Other components may include potatoes; cassava; plantains (cooking bananas); chickpeas, peas, kidney beans; and pasta. Meat includes beef, pork, chicken, and fish, and salads are generally made with tomatoes, cabbage, or lettuce. A wide variety of fruits are cultivated, and they are eaten as fruit or consumed as juices and drinks with meals. During the last decades, many Costa Ricans have become vegetarians, so vegetarian restaurants are not difficult to find. International cooking is popular, and Chinese and Italian fast-food restaurants are booming. Eating with the hands is permitted only when eating certain dishes, such as tortillas or pizza.

Infant-Feeding Practices: Both breast- and bottle-feeding are common. Bottle-feeding gained popularity during the 1960s through the 1980s, but campaigns initiated in the early 1980s promoted breastfeeding. Breast-feeding has become so popular that the decrease in infant death rates observed in the last years is attributed to this practice.

Child-Rearing Practices: Familial ties are very important, and children usually live with their parents until they marry. The concept of family includes parents, grandparents, aunts, uncles, and cousins. Traditionally, women remained at home and took care of the children, and this is still common in rural areas. In urban areas, many women have careers and work outside the home, and children remain with their grandmothers or sisters. Therefore, disciplining children is mainly the task of women; respect and obedience are valued qualities. If a family can afford a house with several rooms, children sleep in their own rooms because sleeping with parents is considered a bad habit.

National Childhood Immunizations: BCG at birth; DT at 10 years; DTwP at 4 and 15 months and at 4 years; DTwPHibHep at 2 and 6 months; HepB at birth; HIB at 4 and 15 months; influenza at 4 years; MMR at 15 months and 7 years; OPV at 2, 4, and 6 months and at 4 years; and Td at 10 years. The percent of the target population vaccinated, by antigen, is: BCG (88%); DTP1, Hib3, MCV (89%); DTP3, Polio3 (91%); and HepB3 (90%).

BIBLIOGRAPHY

Central Intelligence Agency: *2006: The world factbook, Costa Rica.* Retrieved September 21, 2006, from https://www.cia.gov/cia/publications/factbook/print/cs.html.

Centro Centroamericano de Población, Universidad de Costa Rica: Retrieved April 21, 2006, from http://ccp.ucr.ac.cr.

Costa Rica Instituto Nacional de Estadísticas y Censos: 2001: IX Censo Nacional de Población y V de Vivienda del 2000: resultados generales, San José, Costa Rica. Retrieved April 10, 2006, from http://www.inec.go.cr.

Mata L, Rosero L: *National health and social development in Costa Rica: a case study of intersectoral action.* Technical paper No. 13, Washington, DC, 1988, Pan American Helath Organization.

Morera B, Barrantes R, Marin-Rojas R: Gene admixture in the Costa Rican population, *Ann Hum Genet.* 67:71–80, 2003.

Organización Panamericana de la Salud: Indicadores Básicos 2005. *Situación de la Salud en Costa Rica,* 2005.

Organización Panamericana de la Salud: *Indicadores de Género y Salud.* Costa Rica, 2005.

Programa Estado de la Nación en Desarrollo Humano Sostenible: Undécimo Informe 2005, 1ª edición, Proyecto Estado de la Nación 2005, San José, Costa Rica. Retrieved May 4, 2006, from http://www.estadonacion.or.cr/Compendio/soc_salud01_04.htm.

UNAIDS: 2006 Costa Rica. Retrieved September 21, 2006, from http://www.unaids.org/en/Regions_Countries/Countries/costa_rica.asp.

World Health Organization: 2006: Immunization, vaccines and biologicals. Retrieved September 21, 2006, from http://www.who.int/immunization_monitoring/en/globalsummary/countryprofileresult.cfm?C='cri'.

♦ CÔTE D'IVOIRE (REPUBLIC OF) (IVORY COAST)

MAP PAGE (800)

Carolyn M. D'Avanzo

Location: The Côte d'Ivoire borders the Gulf of Guinea in West Africa. Its neighbors are Liberia and Guinea to the west, Mali and Burkina Faso to the north, and Ghana to the east. The total area is 322,460 km^2 (124,470 square miles). Other than low mountains in the northwest, the country is flat with undulating plains. The 515-km coastline has heavy surf and no natural harbors. Southern Côte d'Ivoire has a tropical climate. Temperatures vary from 22° C (72° F) to 32° C (90° F), and the heaviest rains fall from April to July and in October and November. During the rainy season, torrential flooding of rivers is common. In the northern savanna, temperatures are more extreme, with nighttime lows dropping in January to 12° C (54° F) and daytime highs in the summer rising above 40° C (104° F). The population is estimated to be 17.6 million. The capital is Yamoussoukro. About 40% of the population is between 0 and 14 years old, and 47% live in urban areas. The gross domestic product (GDP) per capita is $1,600, with 37% living below the poverty line.

Major Languages	**Ethnic Groups**	**Major Religions**
French (official)	Foreign Africans,	Christian 34%
60 African languages and	mostly Burkinabe	Muslim 27%
dialects, with Dioula	and Malians 27%	None 21%
most widely spoken	More than 60 ethnic	Animist 18%
	groups 25%	
	Malinke, Juula, and	
	Bambara 17%	
	Senoufou 10%	
	Baoule 15%	
	Bété 6%	

More than 60 indigenous ethnic groups exist, grouped into four major ethnic clusters: the East Atlantic (primarily Akan), West Atlantic (primarily Kru), Voltaic, and Mandé. They share common environments, economic activity, language, and overall cultural characteristics. The East Atlantic and West Atlantic cultures are found in the southern half of the country, separated by the Bandama River, and each constitute one third of the total population. The Voltaic peoples in the northeast and Mandé in the northwest together make up the remaining one third of the indigenous population. Because its present boundaries reflect colonial rule, each of Côte d'Ivoire's large cultural groups has more members outside the country than within, and many Ivoirians have strong cultural connections with people in neighboring countries. Entrenched stereotypes among ethnic and cultural groups place blame for social ills on other rival ethnic groups and immigrants more than on socioeconomic forces. The Baoulé tend to hold high political offices and are therefore perceived by critics as dominant and arrogant. Akan groups are perceived as elitist toward other groups. Groups that tended to avoid politics, such as the Bété, Lobi, and Senoufu, are stereotyped as unsophisticated. Within the large immigrant workforce, Africans from neighboring countries are often resented and suspected of taking jobs and wealth from those born in Côte d'Ivoire. The majority of foreign migratory workers are Muslim. More than 60 native dialects are spoken, corresponding roughly to the number of ethnic groups. Dioula is the most widely spoken, followed by Baoulé. A variation of Mandékan is used throughout the country as a common commercial language. Literacy rates are 58% for men, 44% for women.

Health Care Beliefs: Acute sick care; traditional. Ivoirians in rural areas have a widespread belief that illness can be drawn out by traditional methods, which include magic, religion, and herbs. Mental illness is greatly feared and poorly understood. Family elders are often sought out for advice on traditional health care.

Predominant Sick-Care Practices: Magical-religious primary; biomedical where available. During the past decades, economic progress has outpaced improvements in general health status, despite increased public health expenditures. Traditional healers continue to provide health care for about 70% of the rural population. The country has sharp urban and rural, as well as regional imbalances in the delivery of health care. Western medical care is available for middle- and upper-class urban households; however, even in the larger cities, shortages of equipment and medicines are common.

Ethnic-/Race-Specific or Endemic Diseases: Food-, insect-, and water-borne diseases are the leading causes of illnesses, including bacterial diarrhea and vomiting (from *Escherichia coli,* salmonella, cholera, hepatitis A, and parasites), fever (from malaria, typhoid fever, and toxoplasmosis), and liver damage (from yellow fever and hepatitis). Dengue, filariasis, leishmaniasis, schistosomiasis, onchocerciasis, and trypanosomiasis (sleeping sickness) are also common. The Joint United Nations Programme on HIV/AIDS (UNAIDS) estimates the prevalence rate for human immunodeficiency virus (HIV) in adults (aged 15 to 49 years) to be 7.1% with about 65,000 deaths from acquired immunodeficiency syndrome (AIDS). They estimate that 750,000 people are living with HIV, including 400,000 women and 74,000 children aged 0 to 14. There are 450,000 orphans aged 0 to 17 as a result of parental AIDS. Public health programs are in place to discourage the spread of HIV; however, many men do not consider using condoms to be "masculine" and are resistant to the practice. In addition, discussion of HIV in rural areas is typically avoided, and a person infected with or suspected of being infected with the virus is shunned.

Health-Team Relationships: Health-team relationships tend to be doctor driven, and doctors hold a superior and respected position. They generally maintain good working relationships with nurses and auxiliary workers. Because access to health care workers is so limited, rural Ivoirians highly respect all members of the health care team, including doctors, pharmacists, nurses, and health aides. Health services have severe shortages of nurses and auxiliary health care personnel, particularly in rural areas of the north.

Families' Role in Hospital Care: Family members nearly always accompany patients to the hospital and remain with them for the duration of their hospital stay. Although food is usually provided by the hospital, portions are meager and usually are supplemented by food from home.

Dominance Patterns: Nearly all aspects of Ivoirian culture are male dominated, particularly in rural areas. The status of women is significantly lower than that of men. Women tend to direct all aspects of child rearing and food preparation, but men control household finances. Educational opportunities for women are improving, and a substantial minority of students at the university level are women. The number of salaried women in the workforce is increasing. Women make up about one third of the civil service and are employed in medicine, law, business, and university teaching: positions previously only held by men.

Eye-Contact Practices: People usually make eye contact during greetings. Eye contact may be avoided when two adults of very different social status greet one another.

Touch Practices: Among family members and close friends, physical touching is acceptable and encouraged. Among acquaintances, women exchange kisses with other women on both cheeks, men exchange kisses with women on both cheeks, but men only touch the foreheads of other men. Among new acquaintances and people who do not know each other well, people shake hands.

Perceptions of Time: Strict punctuality for meetings and appointments is not emphasized, and arriving for an appointment up to 30 minutes late is not unusual.

Pain Reactions: Pain reactions range from stoical to expressive. In general, men tend to be more stoic than women.

Birth Rites: The infant mortality rate is very high at 90 deaths per 1,000 live births. In 2001 the fertility rate was 5.7 children born per woman; it is now 4.5. After a baby is born, the new parents organize a small celebration of greetings and congratulations. Particularly in rural areas, sons are preferred because they can carry on the name of the family. In addition, sons are thought of as having greater potential and the ability to make more important decisions later in life. Infectious diseases—mainly gastrointestinal and respiratory infections, malaria, measles, and tetanus—account for most illness and death in infants and young children. Unsanitary conditions and poor maternal health also contribute to deaths of infants and preschool-age children. Life expectancy is 46 for men, 52 for women.

Death Rites: Almost always, family members and close friends are present when they think a person may die. Organ donation is not performed because most people die in rural areas under the care of a traditional healer. Autopsies are rarely performed because family and friends are usually aware of the cause of death. Alternatively, the relatives of the deceased person believe that an autopsy is unnecessary because the deceased has simply been "taken by God."

C

Food Practices and Intolerances: In the northern and western regions, cereals such as rice, millet, corn, and sorghum are the main staples. In the central region of the country, yams are the staples, and in the south, cassava and plantain are the primary foods. In urban centers, particularly Abidjan, various foods are eaten by different ethnic groups, depending on place of origin, and some imported foods are available from other West African or other countries. In rural areas and many urban households, people eat with their hands. Families on the middle and upper socioeconomic levels use forks, knives, and spoons. Inequalities in seasonal, regional, and socioeconomic factors produce widespread malnutrition in the northern regions and poorer sections of cities. Deficiencies of iron and vitamin A are common among infants, children, and women of childbearing age.

Infant-Feeding Practices: Breastfeeding is universal in rural areas and almost universal in the larger cities. Most women have no choice about feeding methods because they cannot afford formula. Breastfeeding mothers avoid or consume various foods based on whether they think the foods reduce or promote breast milk production. Breastfeeding is done openly, and most breastfed infants are weaned at around 10 to 12 months. In poor rural areas, close spacing of births contributes to high rates of malnutrition in the first 2 years of life because weaning foods tend to be of poor quality.

Child-Rearing Practices: Until children marry or are about age 15, they usually sleep close to their parents. Child rearing tends to be strict. The father and the mother discipline sons, but usually only the mother disciplines daughters. Obedience to parents and respect for older adults are emphasized. The oldest family members often meet to settle disputes and prescribe or enforce rules of etiquette and marriage. They also pressure individuals to conform to socially accepted standards. Ritual circumcision of girls and boys during early adolescence is widespread in certain ethnic groups, particularly those in the north.

National Childhood Immunizations: BCG at birth; DTwPHep at 6, 10, and 14 weeks; OPV at 6, 10, and 14 weeks; measles at 9 months; YF at 9 months; vitamin A at 6 and 12 months; TT after first contact, +1 month, +1, +1, +1 year. The percent of the target population vaccinated, by antigen, is: BCG (61%); DTP1 (71%); DTP3, HepB3, and Polio3 (56%); MCV (51%); and TT2 plus (73%).

Other Characteristics: The family of the groom pays a "bride price" to the family of the bride to compensate for the loss of their daughter. This payment legitimizes any future children of the marriage, who are considered members of their father's lineage; their mother retains her place in her father's lineage. Although not recognized by Ivoirian law, dual marriages by men in rural areas (particularly in Bété societies) are relatively common. They provide a man who can afford it the potential advantages of more children, more sexual experiences, and increased prestige. After a divorce the children retain their father's lineage, although they continue to live with their mother.

BIBLIOGRAPHY

African Studies Centre: Cote d'Ivorie. Retrieved September 21, 2006, from http://www.africa.upenn.edu/Country_Specific/Cote.html

Central Intelligence Agency: 2006: The world factbook, Côte d'Ivoire. Retrieved September 21, 2006, from https://www.cia.gov/cia/publications/factbook/print/iv.html.

Ghys PD, Diallo MO, Ettiegne-Traore V, Kale K, Tawil O, Carael M, Traroe M, Mah-Bi G, DeCock KM, Wiktor SZ, Laga M, Greenberg AE:Increase in condom use and decliIne in HIV and sexually transmitted diseases among female sex workers in Abidjan, Côte d'Ivoire, 1991-1998, *AIDS.* 16:251–258, 2002.

Larsen U, Yan S: Does female ciccumcision affect infertility and fertility? A study of the Central African Republic, Côte d'Ivoire, and Tanzania, *Demography.* 373:313–321, 2000.

Levine JA, Weissel R, Chevassus S, Martinez CD, Burlingame B, Coward WA: The work burden of women, *Science.* 294:812, 2001.

UNAIDS: 2006 Côte d'Ivoire. Retrieved September 21, 2006, from http://www.unaids.org/en/Regions_Countries/Countries/cote_d_ivoire.asp.

World Health Organization: 2006: Immunization, vaccines and biologicals. Retrieved September 21, 2006, from http://www.who.int/immunization_monitoring/en/globalsummary/countryprofileresult.cfm?C=civ'.

◆ CROATIA (REPUBLIC OF)

MAP PAGE (798)

Ozren Polašek

Location: The Republic of Croatia *(Republika Hrvatska)* is located in central and southeastern Europe, bordering the Adriatic Sea, Slovenia, Hungary, Yugoslavia, and Bosnia-Herzegovina. The country has a Mediterranean coastline with more than 200 islands, mountain areas, and a fertile agricultural area. The total area is 56,542 km^2 (21,825 square miles). The lowest point is the Adriatic Sea, and the highest is Mount Dinara, 1830 m. The population is estimated at 4.5 million. The capital is Zagreb; other major cities include Split, Rijeka, Osijek, Zadar, Dubrovnik, Pula, and Sibenik. Croatia was part of the Austrian Empire until 1918. From 1918 until World War II, it was the Kingdom of Yugoslavia, and from 1945 to 1991, it was one of the republics of Socialist Federative Yugoslavia. Independence was declared in 1991; the Republic of Croatia is a parliamentary democracy. The gross domestic product (GDP) per capita is $11,600, with 11% living below the poverty line. The literacy rate is 99% for men, 98% for women.

Major Languages	Ethnic Groups	Major Religions
Croatian	Croat 89.6%	Roman Catholic 87.3%
Minor Languages	Serb 4.5%	Orthodox 4.4%
	Bosniak 0.5%	Slavic Muslim 1.3%
	Hungarian 0.4%	Other 7.0%
	Slovenian 0.3%	
	Italian 0.4%	
	Other 4.3%	

Health Care Beliefs: Active involvement; holistic; prevention important. Alternative approaches (e.g., macrobiotics, homeopathy) are becoming more popular and accepted. Prevention programs are promoted through a strong net of primary health care services under the auspices of the Andrija Stampar School of Public Health. Awareness of the risks of smoking is increasing, and screening for breast and prostate cancers is being implemented. Mental illness is not as well understood or accepted as physical illnesses. A specific and very significant problem is post-traumatic stress disorder (PTSD) in soldiers, a result of the war (1991–1995).

Predominant Sick-Care Practices: Biomedical and alternative. Most people rely on the biomedical system. The health care system provides coverage for all citizens, and the state health system is a combination of public and private practice. The health care system employs 66,286 people, of whom 45,586 (73%) are health care personnel and 10,024 are administrative. Croatia has 10,820 medical doctors (7,675 in the public health care system, and 3,145 in private practice and private institutions),and 57% are women. The country has 23 general hospitals, 2 university hospital centers, and 29 specialized hospitals; 7 rehabilitation medical institutions; 257 polyclinics; and 163 pharmacies.

Ethnic-/Race-Specific or Endemic Diseases: The major endemic disease is nephropathy, which affects people living adjacent to the Sava River in East Croatia. The same disease is well known in river areas of the neighboring countries of Bosnia and Serbia. The most common causes of mortality are cardiovascular diseases, which are responsible for 53% of all deaths, and cancer, which is responsible for 24%.The most common cancer sites in men are lung (22%), prostate (11%), colon (8%), rectum and sigmoid (7%), stomach (7%), urinary bladder (6%), kidney (4%), and pancreas 3%). In women, the most common sites are breast (23%); colon (7%); trachea, bronchi, and lung (6%); rectum and sigmoid (6%); uterine body (6%); ovary (5%); stomach (5%); cervix (4%); and pancreas (3%). In 2003, 5,678 people were treated for drug addiction, primarily to morphine. The human immunodeficiency virus (HIV)/acquired immunodeficiency syndrome (AIDS) prevalence rate is one of the lowest in Europe, with more than 90% of infections acquired outside of Croatia.

The Joint United Nations Programme on HIV/AIDS (UNAIDS) estimates the prevalence rate of HIV in adults (aged 15 to 49 years) to be below 0.1%, with fewer than 500 people living with HIV. Most cases are attributed to men who have sex with men. A total of 114 AIDS-related deaths were recorded from 1986 to 2003. Life expectancy is 71 for men, 78 for women.

Health-Team Relationships: Education of doctors and nurses is good. Health-team relationships are similar to those in other central European countries (e.g., Slovenia, Austria, the Czech Republic) in that doctors are at the top of the hierarchy. The responsibilities of doctors and nurses are clearly defined.

Families' Role in Hospital Care: Family members may visit and bring gifts and food to hospitalized patients during visiting hours. Family members are informed regularly about medical procedures performed on patients. Parents must give their informed consent for procedures performed on children, and they may stay with the child in the hospital.

Dominance Patterns: Male and female dominance depends largely on the area of the country and educational level. Male dominance was very common until about 30 years ago. This has clearly changed in Croatia, as it has in other central European countries, particularly in cities where women are just as likely to be employed as men. In agricultural areas, the traditional lifestyle has been retained, and male dominance is the norm.

Eye-Contact Practices: Direct eye contact is acceptable between sexes and among people of various social classes. Not maintaining eye contact with someone who is talking is considered impertinent.

Touch Practices: When friends or relatives meet after a long separation, it is customary for them to kiss both cheeks twice. People usually greet each other by shaking hands. An embrace represents a close relationship or affection, and couples on the street commonly hug each other or hold hands while walking, which is socially acceptable. The sight of couples kissing in public is not unusual. Greetings among those in professional relationships are limited to shaking hands.

Perceptions of Time: Being late to a business appointment is considered rude. It is expected that individuals will be punctual, but this differs regionally. As a rule, punctuality is considered more important in the northern and western parts of the country than in the southern regions.

Pain Reactions: Pain reactions are quite individual, and no rules delineate what is acceptable. People living in the southern regions near the Mediterranean tend to be more expressive, whereas people living in northern areas are more likely to hold back their feelings.

Birth Rites: It has become more common for husbands or partners to be present in the labor room during childbirth, but it is still not a widespread practice. Male circumcision is not routine except in minority religious groups. Employed mothers are granted a 12-month leave from work, and fathers usually take some time off. In rare situations, fathers take a leave of absence rather than the mothers. It is very common for grandparents to take care of small children while the parents are working. The number of single parents is increasing. Mothers are encouraged by medical personnel to breastfeed their children. Generally, sons are not celebrated more than daughters, although this varies by educational level and region of the country. In regions that are less developed and in families with less education, sons tend to be more valued. The infant mortality rate is 6.7 deaths per 1,000 live births, and the fertility rate is 1.4 children born per woman. Life expectancy is 71 for men, 79 for women.

Death Rites: Most families bury the dead according to the rites of the Roman Catholic Church, and people of other religions follow their own customs. Bodies are usually buried in caskets, but in the last few decades cremation has become more popular. Bodies are not exposed in the caskets during the funeral. It is customary to bring flowers, and a funeral procession usually goes to the cemetery. Organ donations are acceptable and are being encouraged by the press and medical institutions. Organ-donation cards are being issued, resulting in regular heart, kidney, and liver transplantations. Permission for autopsies of people who die in hospitals or under suspicious circumstances is regulated by law.

Food Practices and Intolerances: Eating with the hands is considered impolite. The diet in the northern parts of the country is mostly continental, and in the southern parts it is Mediterranean, with abundant fish and seafood. Bread is part of most meals, and potatoes and rice are also common. Croatians consume beer and wine, and many good wines are produced throughout the country. All kinds of meat are eaten and, because of increasingly pressured lifestyles, the number of fast food restaurants has grown rapidly during the last years.

Infant-Feeding Practices: In 1994 a national plan and program was implemented to promote breastfeeding, and awareness of breastfeeding among women who have just given birth is high. Bottle-feeding is also a common supplement to breastfeeding.

Child-Rearing Practices: Children are usually treated very affectionately, and grandparents play an important role in caring for them. Working families enroll their children in kindergarten programs that are usually very well organized. Grade-school education is compulsory for all children, and every child has to complete at least the 8 years required by law. The number of homeless children is very low, and they are cared for in specialized institutions. More people are becoming interested in being foster parents, but this process is strictly regulated by law.

National Childhood Immunizations: BCG at birth and at 8 and 14 years (for those who do not react to PPD); DTaP at 3, 4, and 6 months and at 1 and 3 years; IPV at 3 months; OPV at 4 and 6 months and at 1, 6, and 14 years; HepB at 12 years (3×); Per at 3 and 4 to 5 and 6 months and at 1 and 3 years; MMR at 1 and 6 years; DT at 3, 4 to 5, and 6 months and at 1 and 3 years; Td at 7, 14, and 18 years; Hib at 2, 4 to 5 and 6 months, and 1 year. The percent of the target population vaccinated, by antigen, is: BCG (98%); DTP1, DTP3, Hib3, MCV, and Polio3 (96%).

BIBLIOGRAPHY

Baklaic Z, Rodin U, Kuzman M: *Croatian Health Service yearbook 2004.*

Batuman V. Fifty years of Balkan endemic nephropathy: daunting questions, elusive answers, *Kidney Int.* 2006 Feb;69(4):644–646.

Central Bureau of Statistics: *Statistical yearbook of Republic of Croatia 2004.* Zagreb, 2005, Central Bureau of Statistics, 840 pp. Retrieved May 4, 2006, from http://www.dzs.hr/ljetopis/LjFrameH.htm ISSN 1334-0638.

Central Intelligence Agency: 2006: *The world factbook, Croatia.* Retrieved September 21, 2006, from https://www.cia.gov/cia/publications/factbook/print/hr.html.

Croatian National Institute of Public Health: Zagreb, 2005; 318 pp. ISSN 1331-2502.

Mandatory vaccination calender for 206. Retrieved August 3, 2006, from http://www.hzjz.hr/epidemiologija/cijepljenje.htm.

Strnad M: Cancer incidence in Croatia, 2003. Bulletin no. 28. Zagreb, 2005, Croatian National Institute of Public Health. Retrieved July 29, 2006, from http://www.hzjz.hr/rak/novo.htm [in Croatian].

UNAIDS: 2006 Croatia: Retrieved September 21, 2006, from http://www.unaids.org/en/Regions_Countries/Countries/croatia.asp.

World Health Organization: 2006: Immunization, vaccines and biologicals. Retrieved September 21, 2006, from http://www.who.int/immunization_monitoring/en/globalsummary/countryprofileresult.cfm?C='hrv'.

◆ CUBA (REPUBLIC OF)

MAP PAGE (796)

Angel Arturo Escobedo-Carbonell and Maydel Alfonso-Carbonell

Location: Cuba is the largest island in the Caribbean Sea—a long and narrow archipelago, sometimes compared with a large lizard. It is located 90 miles south of the southern tip of Florida, separated by the Florida straight. Cuba's territory includes the Island of Youth and several cays and coastal islets. The total area is 110,860 km^2 (42,803 square miles), and the capital is Havana City. The total population is more than 11 million. The gross domestic product (GDP) per capita is $3,500; literacy rates are 97% for both men and women.

Major Languages	Ethnic Groups	Major Religions
Spanish (official)	Mulatto or Mestizo 25%	Roman Catholic 85%
	White 65%	Other or None 15%
	Black 10%	

Many Cubans simultaneously practice a form of African worship known as Santería, a syncretism of Catholic rites with elements of African roots. More Cubans are beginning to attend Protestant services.

Health Care Beliefs: Traditional; health promotion important. Health care beliefs are superimposed over indigenous customs—Spanish and African traditions—the foundation for today's health beliefs. Beliefs are also influenced by Chinese, North American, French, Haitian, and Arabic cultures. Supernatural forces, such as the "evil eye" (being able to look at people and make them ill), are thought to cause some illnesses, so it is not unusual for people in a doctor's office (especially babies and children), to be wearing amulets on a bracelet or necklace or pinned to clothing to help protect them. The phrase "Every Cuban is a doctor" is used to convey that people always seem to have an opinion and medical advice for other people who are ill. "It's better to prevent than to cure" is a common phrase, but knowledge is not necessarily linked to behavior change. Successful disease-control programs have had a significant impact on community involvement and participation. The health and medical system guarantees unrestricted access to health care for the entire population.

Predominant Sick-Care Practices: Biomedical; complementary and magical-religious. Cubans consult doctors when they are ill or injured, although self-medication is commonly practiced. The syncretism between the Catholic and African religions affects sick-care practices and health beliefs: for example, herbalists treat common disorders and are specialists in the treatment of "evil eye." Supernatural forces must be cured by the use of ethnic treatments or magic spells as well as concurrent biomedical treatment. Ill people may seek the aid and advice of a "godfather" who is a member of the Santería. The cure often involves becoming "santo" by performing a certain ritual, wearing white clothes for a year, obeying some food restriction, or not shaking hands. The advice of family and neighbors is also considered, and they play an important role in health beliefs and health-seeking behavior. Occasionally, they evaluate the disease according to their experience and recommend medication or herbal treatments, even when the person has consulted a doctor. The easy and free access to the health care system has contributed to dramatic improvements in health status. Although the use of some complementary therapies (acupuncture, herbal remedies, fangotherapy, massage, homeopathy) has increased, Western medical treatment is usually preferred (although they may be used simultaneously). People living in rural areas have the same access to health care as urban dwellers, and coverage includes the entire spectrum of services, from vaccinations to sophisticated interventions such as organ transplants. Other social services include maternity, sickness, disability, work, injury benefits, and old age and survivors' pensions. Cuba's health statistics are similar to those of other developed countries. Women control their reproductive destiny. Abortions are legal and take place in hospitals by qualified doctors and with accompanying family planning information. It is usually considered to be a last resort.

Ethnic-/Race-Specific or Endemic Diseases: Many of the tropical diseases have been eliminated. Cuba has no poliomyelitis, malaria, diphtheria, or filariasis. Other diseases such as leprosy and tuberculosis are controlled. The major health risks are chronic diseases. Cuba has some cancer-prevention programs, such as for breast cancer. Preventive measures have been implemented to decrease risk factors related to lifestyle and behaviors, such as smoking, alcohol consumption, poor nutrition, and lack of physical exercise. Cuba has an excellent human immunodeficiency virus (HIV)/acquired immunodeficiency disease (AIDS) control program and has one of the lowest rates of infection. The Joint United Nations Programme on HIV/AIDS (UNAIDS) estimates the prevalence rate for HIV in adults (aged 15 to 49 years) to be 0.1%, with 4,800 people living with HIV, including 2,600 women and fewer than 100 children aged 0 to 15 years. Fewer than 500 deaths are attributed to AIDS. Most new infections are in young people, and prevention programs emphasize the risks of unprotected sex. Women need to feel empowered so that they can have control over their sexual relationships and negotiate the use of condoms. Antenatal care with blood screening of parents is done to avoid transmission of HIV from mother to child. Transmission is mainly through sexual intercourse, especially among homosexual men. Interventions with men have been based on promoting responsibility for their own and their partners' sexual health. Sex and homosexuality are discussed freely and openly, primarily among young people.

Health-Team Relationships: Doctors are the primary authority; nurses are subordinate and are usually female. In situations in which nurses are the only health care professionals (e.g., in schools, day-care centers, ships), they are more respected. The professional role of the nurse has expanded as nurses are educated at universities and enrolled in specialization and master's degree programs. In hospitals, the health care team includes doctors, nurses, pharmacists, dieticians, and laboratory and radiology technicians. In the community, the family doctor (a general practitioner) and nurses live in the same community, frequently in the same building, and are available at all times. They share prevention responsibilities in the community and visit the homes of ill and healthy clients. Many other professionals are located in polyclinics in the community.

Families' Role in Hospital Care: A member of the family or a close friend stays in the hospital day and night. They may provide extra food and basic hygiene if necessary. Visitors are expected, and in some families one of the healthy members notes the people who visit. Parents can stay in the hospital all day with hospitalized children. Patients assume a passive role and expect care to be provided by the family, if at all possible. The family is prepared to donate blood, and in the case of a devastating illness, doctors consult with families about diagnosis, treatment, and prognosis and tend not to give bad news to the patient. Patients' right to know their diagnosis and treatment options is gradually becoming an accepted concept.

Dominance Patterns: Cuba is traditionally a male-dominated culture with strong, interdependent family networks for love, emotional support, material assistance, and overall well-being. Mothers are considered the primary parent, offering security and constancy. Parents do not care for girls and boys differently. Women now have occupations that were traditionally held by men, such as electricians, drivers, politicians, and doctors.

Eye-Contact Practices: Direct eye contact is considered polite. Tenderness, affinity, and confidence are shown by direct eye contact between parents and children, doctors and subordinates, and among clients. Looking away may be interpreted as a sign of disrespect, dishonesty, or loss of interest.

Touch Practices: Cubans consider themselves to be especially friendly, and close contact and touching are acceptable. Men and women, and women and women, touch each other more frequently than men and men; however, younger generations are much more open to expressing physical affection such as close hugging and kisses on the cheek. Doctors may put their arms on a patient's shoulder in a show of sympathy and support. Shaking hands and hugs are common among men.

Perceptions of Time: In general, punctuality is an important value and is considered good manners. For some, being late is a sign of elegance or glamour; people who arrive late do so intentionally. For some meetings, people are asked to arrive earlier than the actual starting time to ensure punctuality.

Pain Reactions: "Men don't cry" is one of the most frequent Cuban expressions, and it is used to discourage boys from crying. Another common phrase is, "You will deliver your baby with pain." Verbal expressions of pain are acceptable.

Birth Rites: Mothers have prenatal consultations with family doctors, gynecologists, and psychologists as necessary. Topics such as family planning and correcting nutritional deficits are discussed with women who are planning to become pregnant. Parents have no preference for boys or girls. Almost 100% of births occur at hospital facilities. Natural deliveries are the norm, and cesarean sections are performed infrequently. The infant mortality rate is 6.22 deaths per 1,000 live births. Sexual intercourse continues during pregnancy. Loud noises, looking at people with deformities, and talking about deformities are avoided during pregnancy. If possible, the woman's mother and husband are present during labor and delivery. In traditional families, the new mother moves to her parents' house for 40 days after delivery. New mothers are not allowed to wash their hair until this "quarantine" is complete. Relatives and close friends go to the hospital to meet the newborn, and most husbands celebrate the infant's arrival with male friends. Older women say that malt with milk increases breast milk production. Women are allowed to take a leave of absence from their jobs from 6 weeks before and 1 year after the birth. The fertility rate is 1.66 children born per woman. Life expectancy is 75 for men, 80 for women.

Death Rites: Fear of death is common, and people do their best to be close to their family when a death is expected. When a person dies, one or two family members prepare the body for burial, including dressing and applying makeup. Relatives and friends remain with the body through the night and express sympathy with flowers. The burial takes places within 24 hours. If someone, especially a close relative, is out of the city or the country, they make considerable efforts to be present for the burial. Cremation is uncommon.

C

Food Practices and Intolerances: The largest meal is dinner because that is when all family members are present. The typical food is *congri* (rice with black beans) and roasted pork, and the typical hot beverage is coffee. Drinking juice is considered healthy. The adult diet tends to be high in fat, cholesterol, sugar, and fried foods and low in vegetables and fiber. Occasionally Cubans make comments such as, "This is grass and is for cows," a reference to their preference for meat rather than salads and vegetables. Vegetarian restaurants are poorly visited, although a change in attitudes is being promoted. Milk is available only for pregnant women, older adults, ill people, and children younger than 7 years, unless people are able to purchase it with dollars. Rice and beans are common, especially with pork, and the intake of sweets is high. Food taboos include drinking coffee with bananas and eating unripe mangoes.

Infant-Feeding Practices: During the first moments after birth, mothers make their best effort to breastfeed their infants so that infants can benefit from colostrum. A national program promotes exclusive breast-feeding for the first 6 months. Breastfeeding may cease as early as 4 months, at which time solid foods are introduced. Some mothers like to introduce foods early to see their babies getting fatter, considered to be a sign they are healthy.

Child-Rearing Practices: Crying is undesirable because a happy, contented child is thought to be a quiet child. Children have separate rooms when possible. Physical punishment is less common today, but when adults are speaking, children are expected to be quiet. Parents pay significant attention to education, and most stay in day-care centers from ages 1 to 5. Every child must attend primary school from 5 to 11 years and secondary school until age 15. Computer and television instruction supplements school programs, and there are many extracurricular activities. The school system provides health education and assumes much of the child-rearing responsibilities. Children may remain dependent on their parents long after they are the legal age of independence.

National Childhood Immunizations: BCG at birth; HepB at birth; DTwP at 18 months; DTwPHep at 2, 4, and 6 months; OPV before age 1 and 1, 2, and 9 years; MMR at 1 and 11 years; Hib 2, 4, 6, and 18 months; DT at 6 years; typhoid at 10, 13, and 16 years; TT at 13 years. The percent of the target population vaccinated, by antigen, is: BCG, Polio3, DTP1, DTP3, and HepB3 (99%); Hib3 (94%); and MCV (98%). Adults are also vaccinated according to risk (e.g., against leptospirosis).

BIBLIOGRAPHY

Central Intelligence Agency: *2006: The world factbook, Cuba.* Retrieved September 21, 2006, from https://www.cia.gov/cia/publications/factbook/print/cu.html.

Cooper RS, Ordunez P, Iraola Ferrer MD, Munoz JL, Espinosa-Brito A: Cardiovascular disease and associated risk factors in Cuba: prospects for prevention and control, *Am J Public Health.* 96(1):94–101, 2006.

De Vos P: "No one left abandoned": Cuba's national health system since the 1959 revolution, *Int J Health Serv.* 35(1):189–207, 2005.

Diogene E, Perez PJ, Figueras A, Furones JA, Debesa F, Laporte JR: The Cuban experience in focusing pharmaceuticals policy to health population needs: initial results of the National Pharmacoepidemiology Network (1996-2001), *Pharmacoepidemiol Drug Saf.* 12(5):405–407, 2003.

Dresang LT, Bredbrick L, Murray D, Shallue A, Sullivan-Vedder L. Family medicine in Cuba: community-oriented primary care and complementary and alternative medicine. *J Am Board Fam Pract.* 2005 Jul-Aug;18(4):297–303.

Gonzalez E, Armas L, Baly A, Galvez A, Alvarez M, Ferrer G, Mesa AC. [Economic and social impact of the National Tuberculosis Control Program (NTCP) on the Cuban population] *Cad Saude Publica.* 2000 Jul-Sep;16(3):687–699. Spanish.

Herrera-Valdes R, Almaguer-Lopez M: Strategies for national health care systems and centers in the emerging world: Central America and the Caribbean—the case of Cuba, *Kidney Int Suppl.* (98):S66–S68., 2005.

Hoffman SZ: HIV/AIDS in Cuba: a model for care or an ethical dilemma? *Afr Health Sci.* 4(3):208–209, 2004.

Laden MG: Latino mortality rates, *Am J Public Health.* 90(11):1798–1799, 2000.

Nayeri K, Lopez-Pardo CM: Economic crisis and access to care: Cuba's health care system since the collapse of the Soviet Union, *Int J Health Serv.* 35(4):797–816, 2005.

UNAIDS: 2006 Cuba: Retrieved September 21, 2006, from http://www.unaids.org/en/Regions_Countries/Countries/cuba.asp.

World Health Organization: 2006: Immunization, vaccines and biologicals. Retrieved September 21, 2006, from http://www.who.int/immunization_monitoring/en/globalsummary/countryprofileresult.cfm?C='cub'.

◆ CYPRUS (REPUBLIC OF)

MAP PAGE (802)

Theano Kalavana

Location: Cyprus is on the outer border of Europe in the northeastern corner of the Mediterranean near Asia Minor and Syria. It is the third largest island in the Mediterranean (after Sicily and Sardinia) and has a total area of or 9,250 km² (3,572 square miles). The capital is Nicosia. The gross domestic product (GDP) per capita is $21,500 in the Greek Cypriot area and $7,135 in north Cyprus (Turkish Cypriot area).

Major Languages	Ethnic Groups	Major Religions
Greek	Greek 78%	Greek Orthodox 78%
Turkish	Turkish 18%	Muslim 18%
English	Armenian, Other 4%	Other 4%

Most Cypriots are Greeks who speak the Greek language. English is also widely spoken because the island was a British colony for many years. The estimated Greek-Cypriot population is 784,301. It is difficult to estimate the number of Turkish-Cypriot inhabitants who now live in the northern occupied sector, which is about 38% of the total area of Cyprus. The Turkish-Cypriots are Muslims, speak the Turkish language, and comprise about 18% of the population. Minorities such as Armenians and Maronites are mainly Catholics who speak Greek as well as their own language. Literacy rates are high at 99% for men, 96% for women. Cyprus joined the European Union in 2004.

Health Care Beliefs: Acute sick care; passive role; selective traditional. The Ministry of Health has made some positive steps in the last decade regarding disease prevention and health promotion. Every year, leaflets are printed with information about different diseases and how people can protect themselves from infections. In addition, campaigns to decrease the most frequent illnesses occur at specific times each year. Most Cypriots, however, have not established consistent health habits designed to prevent illness. In the past, Cypriots believed that illness could be drawn out by placing heated cups or coins on the back of an ill person. They also rubbed the back with alcohol made from grape kernels (*zivania*) or rubbed painful areas with hot olive oil. Today, these beliefs generally exist only in small villages and among older people who may visit a doctor first and then practice their traditional beliefs as additional therapy.

Predominant Sick-Care Practices: Biomedical; magical-religious. Medical treatment is sought primarily from biomedical practitioners. Most Cypriots believe in God (*Theos*) and go to church to pray for their health and the health of their relatives and friends. They believe that God helps them recover from illnesses and maintains their health. They also make vows to churches and specific saints. For example, if a newborn baby's health is in great danger and may die, the parents offer a likeness of a baby made of wax and pray to God to save their child's life. The amulets that Cypriots wear are small and usually made of gold in the form of crosses or images of the Virgin Mary. Amulets with blue stones in the shape of an eye are worn to protect people from evil that could harm their health or bring misfortune or bad luck.

Ethnic-/Race-Specific or Endemic Diseases: Thalassemia (*mesoyiaki anaemia*) is a group of hereditary anemias occurring in people who live along the Mediterranean Sea. The disease is becoming rare because of prenatal testing. The most prevalent diseases in Cyprus are those of the respiratory system (12%); circulatory system (28%); and musculoskeletal system and connective tissue (11%). All other disease categories account for the remaining 37%. Women seek treatment more than men: 60% versus 41%, respectively. Certain viral and respiratory system diseases develop primarily among those in younger age groups, whereas other diseases—such as malignancies and diseases of the eye and adnexa, circulatory system, and respiratory system—are found among older people. Digestive system diseases and injuries, poisoning, and consequences of other external causes are equally distributed among the various age groups. The Joint United Nations Programme on HIV/AIDS (UNAIDS) reports the estimated prevalence rate for human immunodeficiency virus (HIV) in adults (aged 15 to 49 years) to be 0.2%, with fewer than 400 people living with HIV. Where the mode of transmission is known, 46.4% of the cases are transmitted heterosexually, and 45.6% are transmitted by men who have sex with men. There are no reported deaths from acquired immunodeficiency syndrome (AIDS).

Health-Team Relationships: Nurses and doctors have good working relationships, although doctors have higher social status. Nurses are respectful to doctors and do not feel that they are equals. Patients are also very respectful towards doctors. They consider them to be intellectual authorities who can relieve them of pain and make them healthy. Patients tend to complain about pain to nurses more than to doctors and believe that nurses are there to help them follow the doctors' orders.

Families' Role in Hospital Care: Families, especially the wives and mothers of patients, usually stay overnight with hospitalized patients. Fathers and husbands usually do not stay, perhaps because they consider caring for an ill person to be a woman's job. It is also occasionally easier for women to get permission for time off from work. Families tend to disobey the rules of hospitals and clinics. They may bring food to patients, ignore posted visiting hours, or use mobile phones in the hospital (which is prohibited). Most hospitals in Cyprus contain a Christian Orthodox church or a place where patients and relatives can pray and light candles.

Dominance Patterns: In the past, women had two basic obligations: to maintain the family's honor and take care of family members' physical and emotional needs (e.g., food, cleanliness, comfort). The role of men was to protect the family, provide the means for the family's survival, and represent the family in the community. If women had to work outside the home for economic reasons (especially if they worked for a person who was not a family member), it reflected poorly on the good name of the man and damaged his reputation as a provider. Although men are still dominant, they are less so than in the past. Powerful positions in society still tend to be held by men, whether they are related to jobs, organizations, or politics. However, women are much more independent, work outside the home, and are obtaining more powerful positions in many disciplines. Many men still believe that domestic activities (e.g., shopping, cooking, cleaning) and raising children are women's responsibilities. Men think of themselves as the "hard" workers—the people who work all day to provide the family income—whereas women are responsible for the "soft" duties. Both men and women are well educated, and most have graduated from universities or colleges. Both are treated equally, and discrimination on the basis of gender is not allowed. Public and private hospitals employ many female doctors in various areas of medical specialization.

Eye-Contact Practices: Direct eye contact between patients and doctors is common. Direct eye contact is also usual when people greet one another or talk. In the past, women avoided eye contact because they were expected to behave demurely outside their homes. In contemporary society, direct eye contact is quite common among members of both sexes.

C

Touch Practices: Physical touching is acceptable, and handshaking, hugging, and kissing on the cheeks is the norm among friends. Physical touch is acceptable during examinations; however, very personal examinations are sometimes difficult for women.

Perceptions of Time: Punctuality is not a significant issue. It is generally expected that guests will arrive late, and public performances may not start on time. People must have an appointment to visit a doctor, but only a few of them arrive at appointments on time; therefore, doctors have a hard time maintaining schedules. In the past, traditional Cypriots tended to focus on the present because events happened very slowly; rushing things was considered unnatural. Even though the social rules have changed, Cypriots are still focused on the present and tend to do things slowly, with the exception of young professionals, who tend to focus on the future.

Pain Reactions: Women are much more expressive than men regarding pain. Society still believes that "real men don't cry," and men are symbols of power. Men, especially older men, are stoic and try to hide their pain.

Birth Rites: During childbirth, the husband is encouraged to be with his wife. In the past, mothers delivered their infants at home with the help of midwives while the husbands were at coffee shops, talking with their male friends. When a husband was informed about a birth, he would offer a drink to everyone in the coffee shop if the baby was a boy. If the baby was a girl, the father would say nothing and just accept the "sad" event. Today, boys and girls are equally welcomed. Children are often named after their parents, with boys being named after the husband's father, girls after the woman's mother. If an infant has a serious illness, the parents offer vows to the church and to Saint Stylianos (Ayios Stylianos) or Saint Marina (Ayia Marina), the saints who are considered the guardians of babies. Mothers do not avoid bathing or certain foods and carefully follow the doctor's advice about child care. The infant mortality rate is 7 deaths per 1,000 live births; the fertility rate is 1.82 children born per woman. Life expectancy is 75 for men, 80 for women.

Death Rites: The death of a loved one is a more terrifying prospect than a person's own death or illness. Family members are very expressive and show their grief by crying or even screaming; women are more expressive than men. Grieving may go on for months or years. Close relatives usually wear black clothes for 40 days to 6 months. Parents of a dead child may wear black clothes for years; fathers may not shave and may grow long beards for months or years, whereas mothers may stop using makeup or taking care of their appearance. Cypriots believe that when people die, their souls go to God (Theos) in heaven. If the deceased person is a child, the soul becomes an angel. According to traditional Cypriot culture, death is a process by which the soul travels from this world to heaven, so a series of ceremonies led by a priest take place to aid in this process. Funeral events start from the house of the deceased, where close relatives and friends go to support the rest of the family. A service takes place in a Christian Orthodox Church and is followed by the burial. Cremation is generally unacceptable; the corpse's eyes are closed, and the body is buried in a coffin. After the funeral, all the relatives and friends eat a piece of bread, which may be accompanied by black olives, goat cheese, and coffee. Organ donations and autopsies are acceptable. Autopsies are allowed when the cause of death is suspicious.

Food Practices and Intolerances: The phrase "your eyes are bigger than your stomach" perfectly characterizes Cypriots' eating habits. They like to have massive amounts of food on their tables. Every Christmas and Easter, people go to the emergency room with digestive problems because of the enormous amount of food they have eaten. Cypriots use frying and a great deal of oil because oil makes food tasty. Meat consumption is high. Despite the fact that Cyprus is an island, fish is not eaten regularly, and many fatty dairy products such as cheese and yogurt are consumed. Salad and bread are usually served with meals, and vegetables and legumes are eaten twice a week. The basic foods are meat, potatoes, and salads. Cypriots have many favorite foods: soups such as *avgolemono* (boiled chicken pieces or chicken stock in egg and lemon broth with rice), *trahana* (dry wheat with milk stock), pasta *(pastichion)* such as *makoronia tou fournou* (baked pasta with minced-meat filling and bechamel sauce), *pourgouri* (crushed wheat rice with spaghetti), *souvlakia* kebabs (small pieces of meat on skewers cooked over charcoal and served with salad in pita bread), *sheftalia* (marinated minced meat made into sausage and cooked over charcoal), *souvla* (large pieces of meat cooked over charcoal), *kotopoulo psito* (chicken, potatoes, tomatoes, and oil baked in an oven), *koupepia* (vine leaves stuffed with minced meat, tomato, rice, and onions), *keftedes* (minced lamb that is rolled and fried), *kalamaria* (squid cut into rings or small pieces and fried), and cheeses such as *halloumi* (white cheese made from goat's milk). It is acceptable and common to eat certain foods with the hands, although knives, forks, and spoons are preferred.

Infant-Feeding Practices: Breastfeeding is common. Infant-feeding practices are similar to most other Mediterranean cultures.

Child-Rearing Practices: Child rearing tends to be very permissive and may be inconsistent. Most parents know little about disease prevention but may become overprotective in children's daily activities. Children are allowed to sleep in the same bed with their parents if they have nightmares or are not feeling well. Both parents usually work many hours. Therefore, most of children's time is spent with grandparents and nannies from Sri Lanka and the Philippines.

National Childhood Immunizations: BCG (only if contact with TB); DT at 2, 4, 6, 15- to 20 months, and 4 to 6 years; DTwP at 2, 4, 6, 15 to 20 months and 4 to 6 years (only given in private sector); OPV at 6 and 15 to 20 months; Td at 14 to 16 years; MMR at 13 months and 4 to 6 years; IPV at 2 and 4 months; measles at 15 months; HepB at 2, 4, and 8 to 12 months; Hib at 2, 4, 6, and 12 to 18 months; influenza at or after

Czech Republic

6 months; DTaPHepIPV and DTaPHib at 2 and 4 months (only given in private sector); DTPHibIPV at 2, 4, 6, and 15 to 20 months (only given in private sector); Pneumo_conj at 2, 4, 6, and 12 to 15 months; MenC_conj at 2, 4, and 6 months. The percent of the target population vaccinated, by antigen, is: BCG (99%); DTP1, Polio3 (98%); HepB3 (88%); Hib3 (58%); and MCV (86%).

BIBLIOGRAPHY

Central Intelligence Agency: *2006: The world factbook, Cyprus.* Retrieved September 21, 2006, from http://cia.gov/cia/publications/factbook/print/cy/html.

Georgiou St N: Family dynamics and school achievement in Cyrups, *J Child Psychol Psychiatry.* 36(6):977–991, 1995.

Health and Hospital Statistics: *Cyrups statistics for health and Hospitals,* 2003. Printing office of the Republic of Cyprus. Retrieved March 19, 2006, from http://www.mof.gov.cy/mof/cystat/statistics.nsf (result in progress).

Health and Hospital Statistics: *Cyrups statistics for health and hospitals* (series I, Report no 24), 2005. Printing office of the Republic of Cyprus. Retrieved December 4, 2005, from http://www.mof.gov.cy/mof/cystat/statistics.nsf.

UNAIDS: 2006 Cyprus. Retrieved September 21, 2006, from http://www.unaids.org/en/Regions_Countries/Countries/afghanistan.asp.

World Health Organization: 2006: Immunization, vaccines and biologicals. Retrieved September 21, 2006, from http://www.who.int/immunization_monitoring/en/globalsummary/countryprofileresult.cfm?C='cyp'.

◆ CZECH REPUBLIC

MAP PAGE (798)

Josef Dolejš and Tomáš Morcinek

Location: The Czech Republic is approximately in the geographic center of Europe, with a total area of 78,866 km² (30,442 square miles). It is a landlocked country 326 km from the Baltic and 322 km from the Adriatic. It shares borders with Germany (810 km), Poland (762 km), Austria (466 km), and Slovakia (265 km). The capital is Prague (Praha) with a population of 1.1 million (of a total population of 10.2 million). The Czech Republic is a parliamentary democracy. The gross domestic product (GDP) per capita is $19,500.

Major Languages	Ethnic Groups	Major Religions
Czech (official)	Czech 94.4%	Atheist 39.8%
Slovak (minority language)	Slovak 3%	Roman Catholic 39.2%
	Polish 0.6%	Protestant 4.6%
	German 0.5%	Orthodox 3%
	Roma (Gypsy) 0.3%	Other or None 13.4%
	Hungarian 0.2%	
	Other 1%	

Of the 4.6% who claim Protestant as their religion, 1.9% are members of the Czech-founded Hussite Reform Church, 1.6% the Czech Brotherhood Evangelic Church, and 0.5% the Silesian Evangelic church. Many foreign churches have been introduced and have established small parishes around the country. There is a small Jewish community of 10,000. Literacy rates are 99% for both men and women.

Health Care Beliefs: Active role; health promotion important. The major focus of health prevention in the media is on restricting saturated fats and controlling cholesterol and on increasing exercise through sports. A focus on good mental health is stressed in prevention programs. Serious mental health disturbances requiring psychiatric care can cause one's social status to be lowered because of the stigma against mental disorders. Therefore, most people are reluctant to admit that they have a problem, and they avoid diagnosis and treatment if at all possible. In general, people think the consumption of "hard" drinks and smoking are not particularly dangerous, and they are reluctant to change these risk factors. Western biomedical medicine is believed to be omnipotent. Wearing amulets to prevent illness is not a habitual practice, whereas praying for health is common for part of the population. Folk medicine using herbs is used only for minor health problems. A small portion of the population has adopted "New Age" ideas over the last 15 years and has a more negative opinion of biomedical treatment.

Predominant Sick-Care Practices: Biomedical; alternative. Western medical treatment is regularly used in hospitals and polyclinics. A limited number of physicians offer alternative treatments such as homeopathy or acupuncture. Some consult home-based herbalists if they are dissatisfied with a diagnosis and recommended treatment. Seeking out the help of indigenous healers and folk medicine practices is limited. The system of health care is based on compulsory insurance from employers; and the government is responsible for children, students, pensioners, the unemployed, and the disabled. The majority of medicines are free of charge as is medical care. Some stomatological care and extraordinary medicines are the exceptions, and require payment from the patient. Alternative medical care (homeopathy, acupuncture) is not covered by medical insurance.

Ethnic-/Race-Specific or Endemic Diseases: The leading cause of death is disease of the cardiovascular system, which caused 54% of all deaths from 1999 to 2004. Malignant neoplasms were responsible for 25%. Seventy-two new human immunodeficiency virus (HIV)/acquired immunodeficiency syndrome (AIDS) cases were recorded in 2004, the highest annual incidence rate since 1985. By January 2005, there were a total of 737 HIV-infected persons registered in the Czech Republic. Of this number, 184 persons have already developed the clinical stage of AIDS. In 2006, the Joint United Nationals Programme on HIV/AIDS (UNAIDS) reported the prevalence rate for HIV in adults (aged 15 to 49 years) as 0.1%, with 1,500 people living with HIV, including fewer than

1,000 women. It is estimated that there have been fewer than 100 deaths from AIDS. Intravenous drug-dependent individuals are considered at highest risk. Viewed from a long-term perspective, the HIV epidemic is considered stable, although the incidence of newly diagnosed infections has increased. Further long-term monitoring will show whether this rise was part of an upward trend or a single deviation.

Health-Team Relationships: Physicians are dominant and have the most responsibility. Nurses are required to follow physicians' instructions. Nurses and physicians tend to work in teams in some health care settings (for example, psychiatry), and nurses are valued members of such teams. The relationship of clients to physicians is submissive, with patients usually afraid to ask for information regarding their diseases and health care management. Patients are usually not part of decision making. This is in transition, with efforts being made to provide a better working partnership between patient and physician. Relationships between patient and nurse are more informal, more natural, and less ceremonious.

Families' Role in Hospital Care: Families are not responsible for preparing food or attending to personal hygiene for hospitalized family members. Involvement of family members is not particularly welcomed in the hospital setting, with the exception being overnight accommodations for mothers of sick children. Family members visit hospitalized people frequently when family relations are good. Families bring snacks, fruit, mineral water, and juice. Hospital rooms are generally shared by at least two, and sometimes as many as eight patients.

Dominance Patterns: Male dominance is not a significant issue, but people are afraid of ideologies such as feminism. During Communism, women had to work in factories, and their role in taking care of children was forcibly reduced. The situation is better now, and after childbirth, mothers can be at home for 7 months, during which time her employer pays 90% of her previous salary. If she has a second child, the government will pay half the minimal state salary for 4 years. This system has not resulted in increased numbers of pregnancies. Many people prefer to have more money and individual comforts rather than to have more children.

Eye-Contact Practices: Direct eye contact is usual and is expected during interpersonal communication. Differences in eye contact involve time and circumstances. For example, in relations between a man and a woman, close and frequent eye contact is usually perceived as a sign of affection.

Touch Practices: Touch is socially acceptable in nonsexual ways, depending on the age and gender of the persons involved, the character of the relations between participants, and the professional context in which it occurs. Greeting another person with a handshake is common.

Perceptions of Time: People usually attach considerable importance to punctuality. Differences in how punctuality is perceived result from place of residence. Rural people attach less importance to being on time than do those living in large cities. Time tends to be more important to professional individuals.

Pain Reactions: It is not acceptable to express verbally that one is in pain. Pain sensation is shown by facial expressions, grimace, body position, body stature, and limited activity; this will be interpreted by the health professional. People suffering pain usually use medical methods for relieving it. The health care system upholds the principle that individuals should not suffer pain and that the role of health professionals is to relieve it.

Birth Rites: As a rule, children are delivered in hospitals. The infant mortality rate is 3.7 deaths per 1,000 live births, and the fertility rate is 1.21 children born per woman. Delivery procedures are usually typical of Western practice, but some hospitals offer different alternatives. Home delivery is rare and not accepted by physicians. It is common for fathers to be present in the maternity ward, but not other family members. Mothers can usually choose whether they want the baby to stay with them (rooming-in) or to have the baby return to the nursery after feedings. Mothers bathe their babies, usually every day, in the first month of life. In the breastfeeding period, mothers avoid gas-producing foods in their diet (beans, peas, and cabbage), but consume other vegetables and fruit. In general, there are no differences in celebrating the birth of a son or a daughter, although fathers are especially happy when a son is born. For Christians, the baptism ceremony is an important event. Life expectancy is 73 for men, 80 for women.

Death Rites: Most people die in hospitals without family members present. In villages, people may die in their homes, but it is rare. Recent surveys show an increase in cremation worldwide, and the highest ratio in Europe is in the Czech Republic, where more than 72% are cremated. Traditionally, a common part of death rites is a funeral with an oration. Up to 50% of cremations in large cities do not have accompanying funeral rites, a recent phenomenon. Autopsy is obligatory by law in some cases or is requested by physicians. Patients may opt to donate their organs after death. Postmortem, agreement of the family members is also required.

Food Practices and Intolerances: The consumption of meat is very high. Although reducing the amount of fat in the diet is strongly promoted, attention is given to this concept by only a small part of society. There are some vegetarians, but they are the exception rather than the rule. The traditional Czech kitchen plays an important role in life. The national meal is pork with dumplings and boiled cabbage. Eating with the hands is only for sandwich-type foods. It is not considered polite to eat with a fork only. Meals are usually prepared at home, even celebratory ones. Visits to restaurants are infrequent, particularly in rural areas, although there is an increase in eating out in large cities.

C

Infant-Feeding Practices: Physicians recommend breastfeeding according to the World Health Organization (WHO)/United Nations Children's Fund (UNICEF) recommendations, and it is an important focus of the national health system. Mothers try to continue to breastfeed as long as possible. Bottle-feeding is also common, but it is considered to be a substitution for breast milk.

Child-Rearing Practices: It is commonly thought that strict upbringing with positive reinforcement is the best way to rear children. The time children spend watching television is less than in some countries, but the new generation spends more time with electronic entertainment than did previous generations. The school system is not ideal for talented children. In basic school, the majority of teachers are women because of low wages. Mentally disabled children are educated in special schools. Although the highest level of education in mathematics in the world exists in the Czech Republic, the last statistical survey showed intense antipathy to math. Grandparents play an important role in the life of grandchildren given that people frequently live in one city their entire lives, and family relations are very close. Having more money is not considered a reason to change one's living arrangements.

National Childhood Immunizations: BCG at 4 days and 11 years; DT at 9 weeks and at 3, 4, and 18 months; DTaP at 5 years; DTaPHip at 9 weeks and at 3, 4, and 18 months; DTwP at 5 years; DTwPHib at 9 weeks and at 3, 4, and 18 months; HepB at 9 weeks and at 3 and 9 months; MMR at 15 and 21 months. The percent of the target population vaccinated, by antigen, is: BCG and HepT3 (99%); DTP1 (98%); DTP3, Hib3, and MCV (97%); and Polio3 (96%). Vaccinations are free of charge, and there is compulsory vaccination for all children. Dentists are vaccinated without cost against hepatitis B and influenza, and those who work with animals receive rabies immunization.

BIBLIOGRAPHY

Bohumil Fizer HE: *Twenty-sixth Special Session of the General Assembly on HIV/AIDS.* New York, 27 June 2001, Statement by H. E. Mr. Bohumil Fizer, Head of the Delegation, Minister of Health of the Czech Republic.
Central Intelligence Agency: 2006: The world factbook, Czech Republic. Retrieved September 21, 2006, from https://www.cia.gov/cia/publications/factbook/print/ez.html.
Czech Statistical Office: *Statistical yearbook of the Praque, Czech Republic, 2004.*
National Institute of Public Health: http://www.szu.cz/English/english.htm.
UNAIDS: 2006 Czech Republic. Retrieved September 21, 2006, from http://www.unaids.org/en/Regions_Countries/Countries/czech_republic.asp.
World Health Organization: The international classification of diseases-10 (revision), WHO Mortality Database. Retrieved April 10, 2006, from http://www.who.int/whosis/mort/download.htm.
World Health Organization: 2006: Immunization, vaccines and biologicals. Retrieved September 21, 2006, from http://www.who.int/immunization_monitoring/en/globalsummary/countryprofileresult.cfm.?C='cze'.

◆ DENMARK (KINGDOM OF)

MAP PAGE (798)

Nana Thrane

Location: Denmark is a part of Scandinavia and the northernmost part of Europe. It is the smallest and most level of the Scandinavian countries, with its highest point only 174 m (570 ft) above sea level. Greenland and the Faroe Islands are parts of Denmark but have very different landscapes. The Kingdom of Denmark has 5.5 million inhabitants; the total area is 43,070 km² (16,629 square miles). The gross domestic product (GDP) per capita is $34,600.

Major Languages	Ethnic Groups	Major Religions
Danish	Scandinavian	Danish National Evangelical
Faeroese	Faeroese	Lutheran 95%
Greenlandic (Inuit	Inuit (Eskimo)	Roman Catholic, Muslim,
dialect)	German	Other 5%
German		

Danish is the primary language. Children are required to attend grades 1 through 9 in school, where they learn English as well as German or French. In the Faroe Islands, a local dialect and Danish are spoken. In Greenland, an Inuit (Eskimo) dialect is spoken in addition to Danish. Literacy rates are 99% for both men and women.

Health Care Beliefs: Active involvement; health promotion important. The biomedical model is dominant, and understanding of the body, health, and illness is becoming more "medicalized." Denmark has a significant emphasis on health promotion and disease prevention, an emphasis that has been intensified by the fact that life expectancy has been and is now among the lowest in Europe. The Danish government has established a Health Promotion Program (1999 to 2008) to prevent "too-early death" among middle-aged Danes and to prevent social inequalities in health care. Health promotion and prevention of illness and disease are thought to be closely related to lifestyle choices, especially smoking and drinking alcohol, eating unhealthy food, and a lack of exercise. Critical research on daily Danish life is being carried out, for example, the consequences of working long hours. Denmark has the highest percentage of working women in the world (90%). It has been documented that the mortality rates from cancer are higher than those in other Scandinavian and northern European countries. In addition to lifestyle factors, the high mortality rates are believed to be related to inefficient cancer treatments. Therefore, a large effort is being made to improve prevention, diagnosis, and treatment of cancer. Since the 1980s, the Danish welfare program, including the health care system, has been undergoing substantial reforms, including an emphasis on cost-effectiveness and better management of resources. The focus in the hospital system is on quality assurance, evidence-based medicine, and patient satisfaction. Many believe people can be cared for better at home than in institutions, and so there is strong support for community health and home care.

Predominant Sick-Care Practices: Biomedical and alternative. The Danish health care system consists of three parallel systems: the system of daily life, the alternative system, and the professional system. Many common problems of health and illness are solved by people in their daily lives. Laypeople also seek help in the alternative system, and some alternative practices, such as chiropractic treatment and acupuncture, are being integrated into the professional system. The professional system is part of the public welfare system, which plays a major role in Scandinavian countries. The public welfare system is characterized by three distinct features: universality (free access for everyone), tax financing, and a strong public sector that supports social welfare and the health of its citizens. The professional health care system is divided into a primary sector at a local community level, with the general practitioner as the lead professional, supplemented by specialist doctors (consultants), physiotherapists, chiropractors, and home-care services; and a secondary sector at regional and national levels, primarily consisting of specialized hospitals. Denmark also has a few private hospitals and hospices.

Ethnic-/Race-Specific or Endemic Diseases: Most Danes (95%) live to be older than 45 years, and 83% live to be older than 65 years old. Most deaths are related to diseases and conditions of old age. The most common causes of death are cancer (26%), cardiovascular diseases (24%), and pulmonary diseases (9%). The increase in lung cancer incidence in women is among the largest in the world, and musculoskeletal diseases and psychiatric disorders are common. The Joint United Nations Programme on HIV/AIDS (UNAIDS) estimates the prevalence rate for human immunodeficiency virus (HIV) in adults (aged 15 to 49 years) to be 0.2% and that 5,600 people are living with HIV, including 1,300 women. Fewer than 100 deaths from acquired immunodeficiency syndrome (AIDS) are reported. There are no official figures for children aged 0 to 15.

Health-Team Relationships: Collaborative relationships among health care professionals have changed during previous decades. The dominance of the medical profession by doctors has weakened, and paramedical groups such as nurses, therapists, and others have grown. Interdisciplinary teamwork is the ideal, as is patient empowerment. Patients' rights have been legalized. Health-team relationships are rather relaxed and informal; however, they are still hierarchical, and the power of the professionals dominates the layperson's perspective. In clinical practice, doctors are the final authority. In health care research, the biomedical research models and methods are still dominant.

Families' Role in Hospital Care: The role of relatives in hospital care has changed significantly during the previous decades. Close family members are thought of as health care participants when a member is hospitalized; therefore, visiting hours have become quite liberal. Parents are expected to stay with children during their hospitalization. Family members are not expected to take care of adult hospitalized relatives. The state subsidizes leaves for relatives who take care of dying persons in their own home.

Dominance Patterns: Denmark is characterized by a tradition of democracy and an ideology of equality regardless of class, gender, ethnic background, or age. It is, however, a society built on capitalism, industrialization, and social control; and social inequality and inequality in health care are increasing. Women's rights are well established, although men still dominate positions of power, and women do most of the domestic chores. The current public debate involves equality and its relationship to ethnic background and minorities: the rights of emigrants and refugees have been reduced. Denmark has a youth-oriented culture.

Eye-Contact Practices: Direct eye contact symbolizes interest and is expected during conversation. If eye contact is held longer, it can symbolize either power or intimacy.

Touch Practices: Touching involves intimacy. Touch practices vary according to social class, gender, ethnicity, and age. Some people never do more than shake hands with someone outside the family. Others consider it quite normal to exchange hugs.

Perceptions of Time: It is considered important to get to appointments on time, although short delays are acceptable if a person has an explanation. Mainstream culture focuses on the future—to get on with life, be busy, and have a lot to do.

Pain Reactions: In general, people are expected to react stoically to pain, but it is acceptable for children and adults in great pain (physical or psychological) to react more expressively.

Birth Rites: Pregnancy and birth are thought of as natural events, and the fertility rate is 1.74 children born per woman. Women can work until the end of pregnancy or can begin their leave 4 to 8 weeks before birth. Pregnant women are advised to refrain from smoking or drinking alcohol but otherwise to live their normal lives. Most children are born in the hospital, and it is common for fathers to be present during delivery. Infant mortality rates are 4.51 deaths per 1,000 live births. The mother can stay in the hospital for a few hours or days if she prefers. Within the first few days, close relatives and friends come and visit to celebrate and see the infant. Life expectancy is 75 for men, 80 for women.

Death Rites: Despite the fact that death is ever present (e.g., in the newspaper, on television, in computer games, in movies), a person's own death is still a taboo subject. Danes try not to acknowledge the fact that they are all going to die until they are personally confronted with death through a serious illness, accident, or sudden death. Most Danes (80%) die in hospitals or care homes. For the last 10 years, the hospice movement, which focuses on palliation, has expanded, giving more attention to death and dying. Usually family members are present when a family member is close to death, but some people die alone. Organ donations and autopsies are acceptable, but Denmark has a chronic shortage of organs.

Food Practices and Intolerances: It is normal to eat three meals a day and enjoy different kinds of refreshment in between, such as coffee, fruit, or sweets. Breakfast may consist of cereal, oatmeal, or bread and cheese or jam, tea, coffee, and milk. Lunch may consist of open-faced sandwiches. The main meal is dinner, served between 6:00 and 7:00 pm and is normally hot food—meat with potatoes, pasta or rice, and salad. The evening meal has an important function because family members gather together. In recent years, fast food has become more common, especially among younger people. Danes drink quite a lot of coffee, and alcohol consumption in some population groups is high. Teenagers have the highest alcohol consumption in Europe.

Infant-Feeding Practices: Breastfeeding is the ideal, and it is encouraged and common. Beginning at 4 months of age, supplemental foods are introduced.

Child-Rearing Practices: Children are regarded as autonomous human beings with a personality and a will of their own; they are respected as such and learn to participate in decision making quite early. Almost all children over 1 year of age spend the day in some kind of care center.

National Childhood Immunizations: DTaPHibIPV at 3, 5, and 12 months; DTaPIPV at 5 years; MMR at 15 months and 12 years; rubella after age 18 years. The percent of the target population vaccinated, by antigen, is: BCG, DTP3, Hib3, and Polio3 (93%) and MCV (95%).

BIBLIOGRAPHY

Gamborg H, Madsen LD: Palliative care in Denmark, *Supp Care Cancer.* 5(2):82, 1997.
Houshian S, Poulsen S, Riegels-Nielsen P: Bone and joint tuberculosis in Denmark: increase due to immigration, *Acta Ortho Scand.* 71(3):312, 2000.
Statistics Denmark: Retrieved July 5, 2006, from www.dst.dk.
National Board of Health: Retrieved July 5, 2006, from www.sst.dk.
Central Intelligence Agency: *2006: The world factbook, Denmark.* Retrieved September 21, 2006, from https://www.cia.gov/cia/publications/factbook/print/da.html.
UNAIDS: 2006 Denmark. Retrieved September 21, 2006, from http://www.unaids.org/en/Regions_Countries/Countries/denmark.asp.
World Health Organization: 2006: Immunization, vaccines and biologicals. Retrieved September 21, 2006, from http://www.who.int/immunization_monitoring/en/globalsummary/countryprofileresult.cfm?C='dnk'.

◆ DJIBOUTI (REPUBLIC OF)

MAP PAGE (800)

Christophe Rogier

Location: The French Territory of the Afars and Issas (1967–1977) became Djibouti in 1977. This small, sparsely populated, developing country of the horn of Africa is in northeast Africa bordering the Gulf of Aden at the southern entrance to the Red Sea. The area is hot, dry, and sandy and made up of coastal plains, volcanic plateaus, and mountains in the north. Most of the country is desert, except in the mountains of the north, where it may be Mediterranean. In the cool season (October to April) the temperature is an average of 77° F, and in the hot season (May to September), it is 112° F. Rain is rare and irregular (less than 20 mm annually). There are two wet seasons (May to June and September to October) and one dry season from June through September marked by the Khamsin, a desert wind. Djibouti shares borders with Ethiopia, Somalia, and Eritrea and shares a sea border with Yemen. The total area is 23,200 km² (8,960 square miles). Djibouti, where about 70% of people live, is the capital. The population is about 486,530, including about 17,331 refugees, primarily from Somalia, who have fled war, repression, and drought in border countries. About 50% to 55% of the population is under 15. Literacy rates are 60% for men, 33% for women.

D

Major Languages	Ethnic Groups	Major Religions
French (official)	Somali 60%	Muslim 94%
Arabic (official)	Afar 37%	Christian 6%
Somali and Afar	Arab, Ethiopian, French,	
(widely used)	Italian 3%	

The Somalis are the predominant group in the south and in the capital city, and Somali is the most widely spoken language. More than 50% of Somalis belong to the Issa clan. The Afar is the predominant group in the north, where the Afar language is widely spoken. From 1991 to 2001, tension between Afars and Issas generated an Afar guerrilla movement that has been severely repressed by the government. The regime is democratic and pluralist, with an integral multiparty system since 2002. About 80,000 illegal foreign residents were deported to the borders in 2003. Outside the capital city, the primary economic activity is nomadic subsistence. The country has few natural resources and little industry. The gross domestic product (GDP) per capita is about $1,323. According to the 2004 United Nations Development Programme (UNDP), 74% of the population lives in relative poverty on less than 3 US$ per day. There is very little production of fruits and vegetables in oasis or in wadi. Only 3% of the land is suitable for farming. Geothermal resources are beginning to be exploited near the Assal Lake. The presence of numerous French and U.S. troops is an important source of income. A railway and an asphalted road connect Djibouti to Addis Ababa, the capital of Ethiopia, from which coffee, cereals, and oleaginous plants are exported. Djibouti exports coffee, hides, and salt. Unemployment rates are high.

Predominant Sick-Care Practices: Acute sick care; traditional. Medical facilities are very limited, medications are often unavailable, and there are inadequate supplies of potable water. There are very few physicians, and most of them have studied in the former USSR, Maghreb, or France. In 2004, there were only 86 physicians (13 per 100,000), 424 nurses or midwives (65 per 100,000), 12 pharmacists (1.85 per 100,000), and 10 dentists (1.54 per 100,000). When ill, the only option for most individuals is reliance on traditional practices or using mineral or livestock products.

Ethnic-/Race-Specific or Endemic Diseases: Malaria, especially the falciparum and vivax forms, is hypoendemic with low and irregular transmission. Anopheles arabiensis is the main malaria vector in the city and has been found since the 1970s, possibly from Ethiopia. Its focused distribution and the specificity of its breeding sites allow a control strategy aimed at treating larval sites with larvae-eating fish, complemented with bacterial toxins. Since the mid-1990s, vector-control activity has been reduced to indoor or outdoor spraying at irregular intervals. Djiboutians frequently travel, and the Djibouti-Ethiopian railway is suspected as a route for propagating malaria parasites. Although some chloroquine treatment failures were reported in 1990, most persons with *Plasmodium falciparum* were treated with chloroquine or quinine at the beginning of 2000. Genetic studies have suggested that parasitic strains are arriving from Ethiopia or Somalia and adding to already prevalent strains. In the capital city, most malaria transmission occurs near the Ambouli wadi, where wells and tanks are breeding sites for mosquitoes. Malaria transmission also occurs sporadically near oases and vegetable gardens along wadis. Assays point to a very high prevalence of chloroquine resistance (>90%). Other parasitic diseases endemic in Djibouti are bilharzias (*Schistosoma manso*ni and *S. haematobium*) in fresh-water lakes or waterfalls (Randa, district of Tadjourah), amebiasis (increasing incidence during past years), and mycetoma *(Streptomyces somaliensis)*. Endemic viral diseases are dengue fever (epidemics in 1991–1992 and 2002). Outbreaks tend to occur in October-November and February-June, transmitted by *Aedes aegypti*, which is present in the capital city. Others include West Nile fever, Hanta virus (3%), and polioviruses; hepatitis A (>95%), B (10%), C (0.3%), and E viruses, and human herpesvirus type 6 (HHV-6; 71% in 1988). There have been no cases of yellow fever recently, although vaccination is recommended. Enteric bacterial diseases endemic in Djibouti are cholera (epidemics in 1993, 1994, 1997–1998, 2000), shigellosis and typhoid. Brucellosis is endemo-epidemic with higher incidence observed in the district of Tadjourah (Adaïlou, Randa) and the Mabla Mountains. People in some geographical areas are at risk for meningococcal meningitis, but few cases are reported. Sexually transmitted infections (*Neisseria gonrrhoae, Chlamydia trachomatis, Gardnerella vaginalis, Candida, Trichomonas vaginalis*) are common. Tuberculosis (TB) is hyperendemic with an incidence rate higher than 320 new cases per 100,000 every year and a prevalence rate of about 1,000 per 100,000. *Mycobacterium tuberculosis* is the principal agent, but numerous cases of TB from *Mycobacterium canetii* also occur. Risk of injuries from motor-vehicle accidents is high because of poor road conditions. The Joint United Nations Programme on HIV/AIDS (UNAIDS) estimates that 15,000 people are living with human immunodeficiency virus (HIV) or acquired immunodeficiency syndrome (AIDS), of whom 8,400 are women. About 1,200 children aged 0 to 14 are living with HIV, and 5,700 children aged 0 to 17 are orphans because of HIV, and about 1200 deaths have been reported. The prevalence rate in adults (aged 15 to 49 years) is estimated at 3.1%. Tests of sex workers indicate high levels of infection (>30%).

Birth Rites: Infant and under-5 mortality rates are high (102 and 126 deaths per 1,000 live births, respectively). The total fertility rate is 5.3 children born per woman. Life expectancy is 54 for men, 53 for women. According to the Ministry of Health, the proportion of births attended by skilled personnel was 61% in 2003.

Death Rites: Autopsies are uncommon because the body must be buried intact. Cremations are not permitted. For Muslim burials, the body is wrapped in special pieces of cloth and buried in the ground without a coffin as soon as possible.

Food Practices and Intolerances: The soil is poor, and droughts are common. There is virtually no arable land, so people depend almost entirely on food imports. Typical foods are fish (especially Red Sea fish in spicy sauce), fried meat or chicken with lentils or other vegetables, and flat bread. Djibouti is a Muslim country, but alcohol is freely and widely available in the capital city, and its consumption is not prohibited. Locals frequently chew *qat,* a mild stimulant that is sold in the markets under wet cloths. Less than half of the population has access to safe drinking water. Water mains in the city are normally heavily chlorinated but still sometimes cause gastrointestinal problems. Outside the cities, the water is usually contaminated and causes various water-borne illnesses, especially in children. Milk is unpasteurized and occasionally a source of illness.

Child-Rearing Practices: Female genital mutilation (FGM) is still performed on 98% of Djiboutian women. Infibulation is the most widely used method. Even though this operation is mutilating, illegal, and sometimes results in death, it is still practiced at approximately the same rate as in the past. About 43% of the population is between infancy and 14 years of age, but only 36% of primary-school-age children attend school.

National Childhood Immunizations: BCG at birth; DTaP at 6, 10, and 14 weeks and 18 months; OPV at birth and at 6, 10, and 14 weeks; measles at 9 and 24 months; and TT at first contact, +1, +6 months, +1, and +1 year; vitamin A at 9, +15, and +21 months. The percent of the target population vaccinated, by antigen, is: BCG (52%); DTP1 (73%); DTP3 (71%); MCV (65%); and Polio3 (71%).

Other Characteristics: The government's record on human rights is poor. Land mines were known to be present in the districts of Tadjourah and Obock in the north, but they are now supposed to be cleared. Afars or Danakils were traditional nomads in North of Djibouti, South-East of Eritrea, and East of Ethiopia. They live in the Awash valley, a large depression named the Afar triangle. They are named *Afars* ("dusts") because of their large number and they are called *Danakil* ("pagan") by Muslims. They were goat, sheep, and donkey farmers and were nomads who traveled in a 50-km range, searching for water and pasture. They formerly transported salt and slaves by caravan for Yemenite merchants between the Ethiopian plateau and the Red Sea. They are organized by age class and are led by hereditary chiefs who own the title of sultan and have the role of arbitrator. The Afar society has common laws that regulate compensation in cases of adultery or homicide (vendettas are common). They are "Islamised" but remain impregnated with traditional animism. There is a distinction between members of aristocratic families, named *Asahyammara* ("red men") and their subjects, named *Adohyammara* ("white men"). Issas belong to an avant-garde branch of Somalis who have pushed away the Afars in the north of the bay of Tadjourah. They are present in Somalia, Ethiopia, and Kenya, with a supreme chief, the *Ogaz*, who lives at Dire Daoua, Ethiopia. Despite this apparent unity, they are divided in clans or tribes and subclans that have much autonomy. They have led a poor nomadic existence, farming small herds of goat, sheep, and camels in search of water and pasture. They also transport various goods. Afar and Issa nomads live in huts *(Toucoul)* made of wood branches covered with straw mats or hides. Because of years of adverse climatic conditions, as well as national border limitations, their mobility and access to resources have been restricted. Remaining nomads find that the traditional pastoralist existence is a livelihood option that is increasingly compromised by recurring drought and rain failure. As a consequence, most of the nomadic Djiboutian populations are no longer pastoralists, and at present about 84% of them live in urban areas where Afar and Somali are regularly in conflict over political power.

Acknowledgments: Dr. Christian Hupin (Institute for Tropical Medicine, IMTSSA, Marseille, France) and Dr. Fatouma Mohamed Ahmed (Director of the Hospitals at the technical direction of the Ministry of Health of Djibouti, member of the National Technical Commission for Health) for providing useful data.

BIBLIOGRAPHY

Anonymous: 2004 *Report on the global AIDS epidemic.* UNAIDS

Central Intelligence Agency: *2006: The world factbook, Djibouti.* Retrieved September 21, 2006 from https://www.cia.gov/cia/publications/factbook/print/dj.html.

Collinet P, Stein L, Vinatier D, and Leroy JL: Management of female genital mutilation in Djibouti: the Peltier General Hospital experience, *Acta Obstet Gynecol Scand.* 81(11):1074, 2002.

Fabre M, Koeck JL, Le Flèche P, Simon F, Hervé V, Vergnaud G, and Pourcel C: High genetic diversity revealed by variable-number tandem repeatgenotyping and analysis of hsp65 gene polymorphism in a large collection of *"Mycobacterium canettii"* strains indicates that the *M. tuberculosis* complex is a recently emerged clone on *"M. canettii,"* J Clin Microbiol. 42(7):3248, 2004.

Maslin J, Roqier C, Berger F, Mohamed Ali Khamil, Mattera D, Grandadam M, Caron M, and Nicand E: Epidemiology and genetic characterization of HIV-1 isolates in the general population of Djibouti (Horn of Africa), *J Acquir Immunodefic Dis Syndr.* 39:129, 2005.

Rogier C, Pradines B, Boqreau H, Koeck JL, Kamil MA, and Mercereau-Puijalon O: Malaria epidemic and drug resistance, Djibouti, *Emerging Infect Dis.* 11(2):317, 2005.

Microsoft: Djibouti. Retrieved February 20, 2006, from http://encarta.msn.com. Microsoft Encarta Online Encyclopedia 2005.

UNAIDS, 2006 Djibouti: Retrieved September 21, 2006 from http://www.unaids. org/en/Regions_Countries/Countries/djibouti.asp

UNICEF: Retrieved February 20, 2006, from http://www.unicef.org/infobycountry/djibouti.html.

World Health Organization: Retrieved February 20, 2006, from http://www.who.int/countries/dji/en/index.html.

World Health Organization: 2006: Immunization, vaccines and biologicals. Retrieved September 21, 2006, from http://www.who.int/immunization_monitoring/en/globalsummary/countryprofileresult.cfm?C='dji'.

◆ DOMINICA (COMMONWEALTH OF)

D

MAP PAGE (796)

Robert Kohn, Liris Benjamin, and Griffin Benjamin

Location: Dominica is one of the largest of the Windward Islands, located between the French islands of Guadeloupe and Martinique in the Eastern Caribbean. The total area is 754 km^2 (290 square miles). It has a population of more than 69,000, with 16,000 residing in Roseau, the capital. A former British colony that gained independence in 1978, Dominica is only 29 miles (47 km) long and 16 miles (26 km) wide. Its mountainous terrain makes access to the capital difficult for most villagers. The only surviving indigenous Carib population, estimated to be 4,500 people, lives in this country. In 1903, they were assigned a 3,700-acre territory in the northeast. The gross domestic product (GDP) per capita is $5,500, and about 30% live below the poverty line. Unemployment is about 10%.

Major Languages	Ethnic Groups	Major Religions
English (official)	Black 89%	Roman Catholic 70%
Kwéyòl	Mixed 7%	Protestant 14%
	Indigenous 2%	Other or None 16%
	White 1%	

The majority speak Kwéyòl, a French Creole, in addition to English. Literacy rates are 94% for both men and women. Dominica is primarily a Christian society, and most Christian residents are Catholics. Other religions include Seventh Day Adventist, Methodist, and Pentecostal.

Health Care Beliefs: Both active and passive involvement; selective health promotion. The definition of mental illness is narrow. Other than psychosis, behavioral disturbances are not considered by the general public or professionals to be mental illness or serious problems. Most disconcerting is the lack of knowledge revealed on surveys about attitudes toward mental illness among those directly involved in care, such as nurses, teachers, and police officers. Prevention efforts are needed in the areas of water and sanitation. About 78% of households have direct access to piped and treated water, but 22% of homes do not have an approved sewage-disposal system.

Predominant Sick-Care Practices: Biomedical. A well-developed primary care system serves each of the 10 parishes. The system has a network of seven health centers and 44 clinics throughout the island. The care in the public health centers and clinics is free. Each health district has a network of type I clinics that serve approximately 600 people in an 8-km (5-mile) radius. Type II and III clinics offer comprehensive services. Hospital care, including inpatient psychiatric treatment, is provided primarily through Princess Margaret Hospital, which has 225 beds. There are four hospital beds per 1,000 people. Private health care is limited to outpatient services.

Ethnic-/Race-Specific or Endemic Diseases: Typhoid fever, dysentery, tuberculosis, and gastroenteritis in children are the most common infectious diseases. The majority of 12-year-old children have untreated dental caries. The leading causes of death among children younger than 5 are caused by congenital abnormalities, premature births, and respiratory distress syndrome. The incidence rate for tuberculosis is 3 per 100,000. Dengue fever is the only vector-borne disease of significance: in 2004 there were only four cases caused by the *Aedes aegypti* mosquito. Diabetes is found in about 3% of the population, hypertension in 18%, and obesity in 50%. A study of the prevalence of medical disorders in 123 older adults found that 20% were dependent on others relative to activities of daily living. Hypertension was noted in 40% of the population, diabetes mellitus in 15%, impaired visual acuity in 20%, and evidence of glaucoma in 10%. More than half of older adults used their medications more than prescribed. About 9% of inpatient psychiatric admissions were a result of alcoholism, 8% a result of cannabis psychosis, and 2% a result of cocaine abuse. A national mental health report found that 90% of the patients in the prison psychiatric clinic had a history of drug abuse. The principal cause of death of adults is related to circulatory system diseases (55%). Neoplasms account for 29% of the recorded deaths, external causes 9%, and communicable diseases 4%. Human T-cell lymphocytic type-I virus (HTLV-1) is endemic and significantly associated with lymphoid malignancies. There are no prevalence rates for human immunodeficiency virus (HIV)/acquired immunodeficiency syndrome (AIDS) from the Joint United Nations Programme on HIV/AIDS (UNAIDS), and country statistics are not up to date. According to country statistics, more than half of the cases of AIDS are in people ages 20 to 29, and the prevalence is twice as high in males than in females. Currently, 69 cases of AIDS have been registered, and 26 died of AIDS between 1977 and 1999.

Health-Team Relationships: District nurses are the basis of the primary health care services and are primary health personnel in type I clinics. Types II and III clinics are staffed with a health officer and a district nurse midwife. Evaluations for hypertension, diabetes, pregnancy, and immunizations account for 40% of appointments with nurses in type I clinics. Only about 20% of patients are referred to the district medical officer. Dominica has 5 physicians, 42 nurses, and 0.6 dentists per 10,000 inhabitants.

Families' Role in Hospital Care: Families are usually supportive. Although meals are available in hospitals, relatives frequently feel it is their duty to prepare meals and do laundry for hospitalized family members.

Dominance Patterns: The nuclear family is prevalent in Dominica; however, in the rural areas, the extended family is prevalent, a pattern that may be related to the high number of older adults. Dominica has numerous residents who are 100 years or older. (Ma Pampo Israel, a Dominican who died in 2003, was the world's oldest living person at age 128.) Fathers are usually the head of the household; however, single-parent families are increasing in number. About 37% of all households are headed by women.

Eye-Contact Practices: Direct eye contact is common among members of the same or opposite sex.

Touch Practices: In general, Dominicans are very courteous. It is common to shout out a greeting to a friend while driving or walking. Occasionally, people even stop their vehicles in the middle of the road to exchange greetings, which does not seem to annoy other people held up in traffic. Handshaking and hugging are common.

Perceptions of Time: People are usually on time for work, but concerts sometimes start 30 to 45 minutes after the scheduled time.

Pain Reactions: Pain perceptions and thresholds are not based on cultural issues.

Birth Rites: Babies are usually carried to church for a blessing, and the ceremony is considered a special occasion. Catholic and Methodist parents choose godparents, who are expected to play a special role in the care and nurturing of the child. On special occasions such as birthdays, godparents usually give gifts to their godchildren, and as children get older, they bond with the godparents. Pregnant women have universal access to health care, yet only 36% of women receive prenatal care by the 16th week of pregnancy. Nearly all births are attended by trained personnel. Birth control is used by 50% of women of childbearing age (i.e., aged 15 to 44) and 33% of sexually active adolescents. About 23% of sexually active adolescents report having an abortion. As many as 50% of males and 20% of females have their first sexual encounter by age 10. About 50% of 13- to 15-year-olds have had sexual intercourse. Sexual abuse has been reported by 16% of adolescent girls and 7% of adolescent boys. The fertility rate is 1.94 children born per woman. The infant mortality rate is 14 deaths per 1,000 live births. Life expectancy is 72 for men, 78 for women.

Death Rites: Dominicans rally around families and friends at the time of a death. On the night of a death, many friends from the community gather at the home of the bereaved family for a wake. At this time, condolences are offered; religious hymns are sung; food is prepared; and coffee, ginger tea, and wine are drunk. Burial is usually within 5 days after the death.

Food Practices and Intolerances: Dominicans enjoy a wide variety of local dishes. Breakfasts include *farine* ("coarse cassava flour") and pear as well as *ackra* ("small pancakes" made from special tiny fishes called *titiwi*). Citrus juices, especially grapefruit and passion fruit, which are grown locally, are very popular. Fish broth, a soup made with fish, pickled pig snout, bananas, and yams, is a favorite for lunch and parties. Another favorite is *dasheen callaloo,* a soup made from young dasheen leaves, coconut milk, potatoes, dumplings, and occasionally crabs. Codfish and roasted breadfruit with cucumber salad are extremely common. Vendors blow conch shells to announce a sale of fish such as dolphin, jacks, and balahoo on the roadside or seaside.

Infant-Feeding Practices: Nearly 10% of all newborns are born with a low birth weight. A quarter of the children are breastfed during the first 120 days.

Child-Rearing Practices: Working parents employ a babysitter and take their children to day-care centers. Grandparents and relatives also play a role in childrearing. Although the country has no compulsory education program, enrolment in primary school is about 88%; most of these students attend secondary school. Only 16% of those completing secondary school enroll in community college.

National Childhood Immunizations: BCG at 3 months; DTwP at 3, +4, and +6 months; IPV at 3, 4.5, and +6 months; MMR at 1 year and 18 months; DT at 3 years; OPV at 3 months and at 4, 5, and +6 months; Td at 11 years. The percent of the target population vaccinated, by antigen, is: BCG, DTP1, DTP3, MCV, and Polio3 (98%). Other than measles, vaccine-preventable diseases have been eradicated.

BIBLIOGRAPHY

Adedayo OA, Shehu SM: Human T-cell lymphotropic virus type 1 (HTLV-1) and lymphoid malignancies in Dominica: a seroprevalence study, *Am J Hematol.* 77:336–339, 2004.

Central Intelligence Agency: *2006: The world factbook, Dominica.* Retrieved September 21, 2006, from https://www.cia.gov/cia/publications/factbook/print/do.html.

Kohn R, Sharma D, Camilleri CP, and Levav I: Attitudes towards mental illness in the Commonwealth of Dominica, *Rev Panam Salud Publica.* 7:148–154, 2000.

Pan American Health Organization (PAHO): *Health in the Americas 2002 edition,* Scientific Pub No. 587, Washington DC, 2002, PAHO.

Tull ES, Butler C, Wickramasuriya T, Fraser H, Chambers EC, and Brock V: Should body size preference be a target of health promotion efforts to address the epidemic of obesity in Afro-Caribbean women? *Ethn Dis* 11:652–660, 2001:

UNAIDS: 2006 Dominica: Retrieved September 21, 2006, from http://www.unaids.org/en/Regions_Countries/Countries/dominica.asp.

World Health Organization: 2006: Immunization, vaccines and biologicals. Retrieved September 21, 2006, from http://www.who.int/immunization_monitoring/en/globalsummary/countryprofileresult.cfm?C='dma'.

◆ DOMINICAN REPUBLIC

MAP PAGE (796)

Teresa L. Lynch and Joseph D. Lynch

Location: The Dominican Republic occupies the eastern two thirds of the Caribbean island of Hispaniola—the second largest island in the Caribbean—with Cuba being the largest. Hispaniola consists of the Dominican

Republic and Haiti. The island lies just west of Puerto Rico and is southeast of Cuba and Florida. The total area is 48,730 km² (18,815 square miles). The population is more than 9.1 million; the capital is Santo Domingo. The gross domestic product (GDP) per capita is $7,000 with 25% below the poverty line. Most people are of mixed European (predominately Spanish) and African descent. Literacy rates are 85% for both men and women.

Major Languages	Ethnic Groups	Major Religions
Spanish	Mixed 73%	Roman Catholic 90%
English (widely spoken)	White 16%	Other, None 10%
	Black 11%	

D

   Although the economy continues to grow at a respectable rate, inflation and unemployment remain major challenges. The Dominican Republic is the home of merengue and bachata, and music is an integral part of the culture. The climate is moderate year round; hurricane season is June to October. Internal and external migration, primarily to the United States, has been significant since the 1970s.

Health Care Beliefs: Acute sick care; traditional. Preventive health care is emphasized but is ineffective because of limited resources. Superstitious rituals are not widely practiced; although in some areas, healers *(curanderos, santeras)* are still consulted occasionally, and some people believe that a person with *mal de ojo* ("the evil eye") can harm others, especially young children. It is believed that the evil eye can cause almost any symptom and is often counteracted by a procedure called *ensalmo,* which includes blessing, massaging, and bathing the child. The "hot-cold" theory of health is occasionally encountered and is based on the concept that a healthy body is the result of balance between hot and cold. Illness is the result of a hot-cold imbalance. Other health beliefs are occasionally encountered, such as *viento,* a process that is initiated by exposure to cool air. *Empacho* is based on the idea that something spoiled (e.g., food, milk, saliva) can get stuck in the body as a mass or bolus and cause abdominal discomfort, vomiting, and weight loss. Treatment may include various teas and the help of a folk healer. Herbal and folk medicines are common, particularly in rural areas. Examples include garlic *(ajo)* for hypertension, gas, headaches, and cholesterol control; coconut juice for urinary tract infections, cleansing the kidneys, and constipation; orange leaves *(ojas de naranja)* in teas for colds, toothaches, and dizziness and applied directly for headaches; and aloe *(sabila)* for colds, tuberculosis, dry skin, and diabetes. Other customs include bathing for "cleansing" purposes or drinking water from the first rain in May *(primera agua de mayo)* for youth and good health. Some spiritually based approaches (e.g., *santeria*) may be used alone or in combination with the help of a healer to address health or other needs, especially psychological or interpersonal relationship problems or lasting illnesses. Some believe that a newborn should never be taken outside of the house at dawn or be held in the arms of a person who comes in from the outside at dawn because the "mist of the night" *(el sereno)* can make them ill with colic, stomach pain, and green stools.

This is called *lo anorta* and can be cured by *un curioso* or a *curandero*. *Padrejon* for older men and *subimiento* for older women is a term some-times used to refer to an ailment causing intestinal gas, dizziness, and weakness.

Predominant Sick-Care Practices: Biomedical and magical-religious. When available, doctors' clinics and hospitals are preferred, although poverty and lack of availability often result in self-care. People tend to be quite religious, so prayer is common, particularly in rural areas. About 44 of 1,000 children die before age 5 (five times the mortality rate in the United States). Causes of death include respiratory infections, diarrhea, measles, malnutrition, and fevers such as malaria and dengue. Cardiovas-cular diseases, cancer, and accidents are the most common causes of death in adults. Antibiotics and most other medications can be purchased without a doctor's prescription. Nearly all health indexes have improved significantly in recent years because of widespread government and non-governmental organization efforts. Currently, the government is emphasiz-ing improving maternal and child health. Since 1992, state public health policy has mandated that health care is a right of all people, and priority should be given to those who are the most disadvantaged. Lack of adequate funding has left this goal unfulfilled.

Ethnic-/Race-Specific or Endemic Diseases: Malaria risk is low except in the Haitian border areas or where construction or similar projects have attracted large numbers of foreign workers. Malaria is responsive to chloro-quine. Malaria, dengue fever, rabies, and hepatitis B are considered endemic. Giardiasis and bilharziasis (schistosomiasis) are also risks. Sexu-ally transmitted diseases are a significant problem but have been decreas-ing. Haitian *bateys* (areas where Haitian workers live, often for years) are particularly underserved. One study demonstrated that two thirds of school-children had intestinal infections, primarily *Blastomyces hominis* (27%), *Ent-amoeba coli* (27%), and *Giardia lamblia* (18%) among others. The Joint United Nations Programme on HIV/AIDS (UNAIDS) reports the prevalence rate for human immunodeficiency virus (HIV) in adults (aged 15 to 49 years) to be 1.1%, with 66,000 people living with HIV, including 31,000 women, and 3,600 children aged 0 to 14. There have been 6,700 deaths from acquired immunodeficiency syndrome (AIDS). HIV is primarily (75% of cases) transmitted heterosexually. The male-female ratio is currently 8:1, but the incidence in women is increasing.

Health-Team Relationships: Patients are generally deferential toward health care professionals and are quite accepting of the limitations of care. Accessibility to doctors is limited among the poor and in rural areas. There is a marked shortage of nurses.

Families' Role in Hospital Care: Families are very supportive and tend to stay with hospitalized patients. In public hospitals, patients and family members may have to purchase medications before they can be provided. Private hospitals generally include the cost of medications in the total bill.

Dominance Patterns: The country has a male-dominated, "machismo" culture, although women's rights groups are active and advances have been made in recent years. Women generally direct activities in the home and tend to be the caretakers of the family.

Eye-Contact Practices: Eye contact is generally accepted among people of similar status and education. As in most cultures, individuals who are poor or have a lower social status are less likely to initiate or maintain eye contact.

Perceptions of Time: The Dominicans are warm and affectionate. Greetings with hugs *(abrazos)* and cheek touching among all ages and both sexes are common. Dominicans have a smaller "personal space" than people in some other countries. Punctuality is not very important, particularly in the rural areas, and can be confusing—or funny—in various situations. Among businessmen and similar individuals, however, punctuality is expected. The poor are forced to live day by day, although many traditions are greatly respected, such as the importance of families, religious rites, and carnival.

Pain Reactions: There are no credible data on pain reactions. Occasionally, pain and other complaints are loudly and dramatically expressed, but generally the people seem somewhat stoic and accept pain as part of life.

Birth Rites: Prenatal care and birthing procedures are quite advanced. Approximately 97% of pregnant women have some form of prenatal care from doctors, and 95% of all births take place in medical facilities. Even 82% of women who are illiterate give birth in medical centers. Consequently, superstitions and ill-advised practices are uncommon. The births of sons and daughters are both celebrated, particularly in rural areas. Parents are happy to have a son who will help in the fields with manual labor, but they are also happy to have a daughter who will be able to help with the chores in a home without modern conveniences. Contraception is used by 85% of women of childbearing age. The fertility rate is 2.86 children born per woman. Life expectancy is 70 for men, 73 for women.

Death Rites: Death is accepted because most Dominicans believe in an afterlife. Family-centered funerals and burials are the norm. There is generally no embalming, especially in the rural areas, and the body is buried within 24 hours. The casket is usually handmade and carried in public accompanied by family and friends to the grave. Widows and widowers often have a long mourning period—up to 1 year or longer—during which they are not allowed to participate in festivities. Nine-day novenas with daily gatherings for prayers, food, and conversation are common.

Food Practices and Intolerances: Malnutrition is found among the poor and is estimated to affect 6% of those younger than age 5 and as many as 20% of people in rural poor areas, such as the southeast near the Haitian border. The food staple is rice and beans, also referred to as *la bandera Dominicana* ("the Dominican flag"). Favorite foods include plantains, mangos, yucca, sweet potatoes, eggplant, and chicken. Soups such as *sancocho,* which may include meat or chicken, and *asopo,* which also includes rice, are also popular. In poorer areas, the diet consists primarily of starch and little meat or protein.

Infant-Feeding Practices: The government promotes breastfeeding during the first 6 months. Most women are given 12 weeks of maternity leave from their jobs. The first foods, which are often bean or plantain broth, are frequently introduced between 4 and 5 months. Although some recent changes have taken place, mothers who live in rural areas primarily breastfeed, partly for economic reasons. In the city or in wealthier areas, bottle feeding is more common, although the recent emphasis on the benefits of breastfeeding has increased its popularity. *Campesinos* (children in rural areas) may breastfeed for as long as 4 or 5 years if the mother does not become pregnant.

Child-Rearing Practices: Rural, or *campesino*, areas tend to be stricter with children, and discipline and obedience are expected. Small children often sleep with parents, especially in poor or rural areas. Dominicans tend to treat their children with much love and are demonstratively affectionate, but many children, especially the girls, have to take on many responsibilities in the household and raise the younger children. The boys often work in the fields at a young age. Mothers are usually responsible for daily discipline, but fathers often handle more serious problems.

National Childhood Immunizations: BCG at birth; DPwP at 2, 4, 6, 8 months and 4 years; DTwPHibHep at 2, 4, and 6 months; DTwPHib at 18 months; HepB at birth; HIB at 2, 4, and 6 months; OPV at 2, 4, and 6 months; MMR at 12 months; MR at 1 and 5 years; varicella at 1 year (in part of the country); Td at first contact pregnancy, +1, +6 months, +1, +1 year; and vitamin A at 6, 12, 18, 24, 30, and 36 months. The percent of the target population vaccinated, by antigen, is: BCG and MCV (99%); DTP1 (92%); DTP3 and HepB3, Hib3 (77%); and Polio3 (73%).

Acknowledgments: We would like to express our appreciation to Leopoldo Carretero, MD, Dominican Family Practice physician in charge of a rural clinic in Comedero, supported by the Institute for Latin American Concern (ILAC) Mission, in Santiago, Dominican Republic, for his assistance in understanding the cultural and medical issues of the people he serves.

BIBLIOGRAPHY

American Red Cross, Geno Teofilo: Strategy to reduce childhood fatalities succeeds in Dominican Republic. Retrieved March 29, 2006, from https://www.cia.gov/cia/publications/factbook/print/dr.html.

Central Intelligence Agency: *2006: The world factbook, Dominican Republic.* Retrieved September 21, 2006, from https://www.cia.gov/cia/publications/factbook/print/dr.html.

Pan American Health Organization: The Pan American Health Organization promoting health in the Americas. Retrieved March 29, 2006, from http://www.paho.org.

UNAIDS: 2006 Dominican Republic. Retrieved September 21, 2006, from http://www.unaids.org/en/Regions_Countries/Countries/Dominican_Republic.asp.

UNICEF: At a glance: Dominican Republic, the big picture." Retrieved March 29, 2006, from http://www.unicef.org/infobycountry/domrepublic.htlm.

World Health Organization: 2006: Immunization, vaccines and biologicals. Retrieved September 21, 2006, from http://www.who.int/immunization_monitoring/en/globalsummary/countryprofileresult.cfm?C='dom'.

◆ ECUADOR (REPUBLIC OF)

MAP PAGE (797)

Fernando Alarçon

Location: Ecuador is a member of the Andean Community of Nations. It is named after the equator, which crosses the country, so a small part is in the northern hemisphere, and the rest is in the southern hemisphere. Ecuador is bound on the north by Colombia, on the south and east by Peru, and on the west by the Pacific Ocean. The total area is 283,560 km² (109,483 square miles), and the capital is Quito. The country's mainland territory is divided into three regions: the coastal region on the Pacific Ocean, the highlands of the Andes (the sierra), and the Amazon region, with its tropical vegetation and rain forest (the Oriente). The country's island territory comprises the Galápagos Islands, which are 1,000 miles away from Ecuador's shoreline. The total population is 13.5 million. The gross domestic product (GDP) per capita is $4,300, with 41% living below the poverty line. Literacy rates are 94% for men, 91% for women.

Major Languages	Ethnic Groups	Major Religions
Spanish (primary)	Mestizo (mixed) 77%	Catholic 90%
Kichwa	Indigenous 7%	Other 10%
English	White 11%	
	Black 5%	

Health Care Beliefs: Acute sick care; traditional. To prevent children from being spooked or hexed, mothers tie an amulet with a red string around the wrist. It is believed that when children have been spooked by the "evil eye," they lose weight, are sad and listless, and have no appetite. To cure them, a raw hen's egg is passed over the body for 3 days. When children have been frightened and cannot get past their fear, a raw hen's egg that has been dipped in medicinal waters is also passed over the body. Other ways of curing spooking is suddenly spraying water or liquor in the child's face. In certain communities, people with epilepsy are considered endowed with superhuman force and godly powers. When patients have a severe illness and little chance of recovering, it is not unusual for them to resort to traditional healers *(curanderos)* or Catholic shrines.

Predominant Sick-Care Practices: Magical-religious; alternative and biomedical when available. Muyuyo flower tea or milk boiled with garlic is popular for coughs. Homemade syrups consisting of diced red onions with sugar are also quite common. Compresses of *tomate de árbol* ("tree tomato") or honey mixed with liquor are used for sore throat. Among blacks, a cure for a migraine is a band tied around the head. Children's hair is not cut until after they are at least a year old, believed to ensure intelligence. Women prevent ovarian problems by not walking barefoot. In the Amazon region, a wide variety of natural herbs and plants, which are being studied for their special properties, are used to cure diseases.

An analgesic that is stronger than morphine can be extracted from certain varieties of frogs. Other medicinal uses can be found in plants such as *sangre de drago,* effective for healing wounds, and *ayahuasca,* known since ancestral times for its strength-giving properties and now recognized for its brain dopaminergic properties. Natural medicines in the Ecuadorian sierra are widely used—natural herbs such as matico, which has anti-inflammatory and antiseptic properties, and valeriana and pasiflora, which have hypnotic powers and are taken as tranquilizers. Cobwebs and the inner shell membranes of eggs are commonly used to treat open surface wounds; they effectively heal tissue. Chieftains, priests, and shamans think they must impress others by demonstrating supernatural powers, effects that can be obtained from hallucinogenic plants such as the coca leaf. The frequent use of plants deemed to be sacred by the shamans may inadvertently lead to psychiatric and neurologic disorders. Some Amazon communities still use curare for muscle relaxation. The tip of an arrow is dipped in curare and then shot out by a blowpipe to hunt wildlife or paralyze enemies. Ecuador has several institutions that focus on health: the Ministry of Public Health, the Social Security Institute, the armed forces, the police force, the municipal authorities, and nongovernmental organizations, each of which functions independently. This has prevented the development of a national health plan providing standardized coverage. The Ministry of Health has attempted to set up a national health plan, but it works only partially. At the grassroots level, this system relies on *puestos de salud,* local health units that can be found even in the smallest villages. At the other end of the spectrum are the specialized public hospitals in the largest cities—Quito, Guayaquil, and Cuenca—to which patients with difficult cases are referred for treatment or diagnosis. The social security system has a similar system, albeit smaller. Hospitals and services provided by the Ministry of Public Health focus on the lower income sector. The country's social security hospitals are for workers affiliated with the social security system and the campesinos (agricultural workers) who are part of the Campesino Insurance Program. For a small monthly stipend, rural workers are permitted to use social security services. Nongovernmental organizations, the hospitals of the armed forces and the police force, and private practices meet the health needs of the rest of the population. Because of low salaries, most public health professionals also have their own private practice, which are primarily for the middle- and upper-class sectors of society. In the country's modern private hospitals, state-of-the-art technology is available.

Ethnic-/Race-Specific or Endemic Diseases: In the Amazon region (Oriente), the climate is tropical, and diseases such as yellow fever are typical. The inhabitants live in temporary makeshift huts made of local plants. They subsist by fishing and hunting and rely on rivers—tributaries of the Amazon River—for communication and transport. The Ecuadorian coastal region has hot and humid tropical weather. A large part of the population in the northwestern province of Esmeraldas is black. The absence of proper medical care, clean water supply systems, and sanitary education are the major causes of endemic malaria, onchocerciasis, and dengue fever (including more severe hemorrhagic dengue). Ecuador also has diseases such as leishmaniasis in certain areas of the country's northern coastline. Infections, malnutrition, and dehydration are the main causes of death among children. In the southern part of the country near the Peruvian border is the Vilcabamba valley, noteworthy for the longevity of its dwellers. It has been the focus of in-depth studies by many universities around the world. Transmission of the human immunodeficiency virus (HIV) is still fairly low. The Joint United Nations Programme on HIV/AIDS (UNAIDS) estimates the prevalence for HIV in adults (aged 15 to 49 years) is 0.3%, with 23,000 people living with HIV, including 12,000 women and 330 children aged 0 to 15. Where the mode of transmission is known, about 59% of cases are attributed to men who have sex with men and 33% have been transmitted heterosexually. About 1,600 deaths are attributed to acquired immunodeficiency syndrome (AIDS).

Health-Team Relationships: The health care system is dominated by doctors, who are unquestioned and respected authority figures. Patients do not have the confidence to express themselves, complain, or request explanations because of this power balance. Practitioners from other regions of the country are obliged by law to provide service for 1 or 2 years in rural areas. These rural doctors are viewed as outsiders, however, and are mistrusted by rural inhabitants, which undermines the relationship. In contrast, traditional healers *(curanderos)* are widely accepted because they usually build up a special, holistic relationship with patients and involve family members and friends in the healing process. This has encouraged the government to incorporate traditional healers into the public health system, although as yet these efforts have been successful only with traditional birth attendants, or midwives *(parteras)*, who receive training from the Ministry of Public Health. Patients prefer practitioners of the same sex and older practitioners.

Families' Role in Hospital Care: The family of a hospitalized patient actively helps care for a relative who has been admitted. They often help other patients who have no relatives and participate in feeding and cleaning chores. In the health services of the Ministry of Public Health, families are required to cover all the expenses for hospitalization, tests, and medications. A government commission regulates the prices of medicines. Because of high prices, attempts are being made to introduce locally produced generic medicines as an alternative to high-cost imports.

Dominance Patterns: The family structure is patriarchal, with men dominating family decision making. Women have, however, become more independent, especially those in middle-class families. They play a major role in taking care of the household, especially in situations involving health and disease. Mothers provide homemade remedies, ensure cohesion of the extended family (especially when taking care of ill and older relatives), and decide when to resort to using a doctor or health care service.

Eye-Contact Practices: In rural sectors, direct eye contact is avoided, especially with women and children because of their vulnerability to being spooked or bewitched (from *mal de ojo,* or "evil eye"). The traditional downcast gaze of rural dwellers is gradually disappearing, especially in the cities.

Touch Practices: Closeness and touching are common among family and friends, especially with children, who are believed to receive protection from the evil eye through physical contact. Kissing and embracing are also frequent in all strata of society and among all ages to express trust, friendliness, and affection, although rural Andean dwellers tend to be more reserved, less expressive, and even brusque.

Perceptions of Time: Traditionally, time has been extremely elastic and imprecise. People arrive late for appointments and social gatherings. "Yesterday" may sometimes mean "several weeks ago," and "tomorrow" may mean "tomorrow," "in a week," "next year," or "never." A person greeting a friend after a long separation is likely to say, "Call me so we can get together" or "I'll be calling you." Often no phone call follows; however, during the last few years, urban life has required all people—of all ages and social classes—to be more punctual. People in low-income groups continue to postpone seeking medical care until their disease is quite severe.

Pain Reactions: Because people delay seeking medical care in the hopes that homemade remedies or time will heal them, they generally show great resistance to pain. They also feel uncomfortable expressing their discomfort or pain to doctors or health care personnel. During childbirth, however, women are accustomed to screaming and shouting, although they usually do so at regular intervals with rhythmic breathing that helps relieve the pain; however, these reactions are common only among rural or marginal urban people.

Birth Rites: The fertility rate is 2.68 children born per woman. In the most remote villages, births are attended by traditional birth attendants, or midwives, who are usually women who live in the village and receive periodic training from the Ministry of Public Health. The infant mortality rate is 23 deaths per 1,000 live births. Life expectancy is 74 for men, 79 for women.

Death Rites: When a person is dying, family members take turns keeping them company 24 hours a day. After death, the family often cries loudly, screams, shows expressive gestures of grief, and may even show hyperkinetic behavior and have seizures, although these reactions prevail mostly among rural or lower-income urban groups. Mourning lasts overnight and often is an opportunity for friends and family to get together and tell jokes, gossip, and talk about politics while drinking coffee or a hot cinnamon beverage with liquor, rum, or whisky, a practice that is common among all social classes. All Souls' Day is a holiday for remembering the dead and visiting the tombs of dead relatives in cemeteries or church vaults.

Food Practices and Intolerances: In the sierra, the diet is composed mainly of beef, pork, or chicken. Guinea pigs, a typical delicacy, are also eaten. On the coast, the staple foods are fish, rice, plantains and bananas, tuna, and shrimp, which are also the country's major agricultural export products. The Ecuadorian sierra has an abundance of potatoes, corn, and vegetables. An ancestral food combination, which modern nutritional experts have stated to be highly nutritional because it increases protein intake, is a mixture of cereals and legumes, such as rice with lentils or beans, grilled corn kernels *(tostado)* with edible lupine seeds *(chochos)*, and specially prepared maize kernels *(mote)* with broad beans *(habas)*. These dishes have been part of the Andean diet for millennia. Some farms are highly developed and produce high-quality meat and dairy products.

Infant-Feeding Practices: Breastfeeding is the norm among all social classes and frequently lasts until the child's first birthday.

Child-Rearing Practices: Birth control methods are widely used by all women except for the poorest rural dwellers. Children are expected to be obedient and listen to their parents, older adults, and older brothers and sisters. Boys have more freedom than girls, who are usually expected to lead more sheltered lives.

National Childhood Immunizations: BCG at birth; DT at 5 to 9 years; DTwPHibHep at 2, 4, and 6 months; OPV at 2, 4, and 6 months and 1 year; HepB at birth (in some areas); MMR at 12 to 23 months; YF at 1 year (in some areas); and Td after first contact, pregnancy, and at 1 and 6 months, 1, 1 year. The percent of the target population vaccinated, by antigen, is: BCG and DTP1 (99%); DTP3, HepB3, and Hib3 (94%); MCV and Polio3 (93%); and TT2 plus (55%).

Other Characteristics: Ecuador is a developing country with a highly imbalanced distribution of wealth. The oldest Ecuadorian culture is the Valdivia culture, which developed between 3990 and 2300 BC. It is noteworthy for its two-headed sculptures, believed to represent hallucinations induced by the consumption of various plants. During the period between 500 BC and 700 AD, the people produced a wide variety of ceramics, providing evidence of the magical and religious beliefs of the time and indications of how health and disease were viewed. They believed the head was the center of all intellectual powers and magical forces; therefore, deformation of the cranium, head shrinking, and trepanation was common.

BIBLIOGRAPHY

Cruz M: Historia de las Neurociencias en América. In *Salud: Historia y Cultura de América,* Salvador DO, ed. Quito, Ecuador, 1992, Editorial Abya Ayala, pp. 152–157.

Central Intelligence Agency: *2006: The world factbook.* Retrieved September 21, 2006, from https://www.cia.gov/cia/publications/factbook/print/ec.html.

Sixth National Population Census and Fifth Housing Census: November 2001. National Statistics and Census Institute of Ecuador, Press Release of February 7, 2003. http://www.inec.gov.ec (retrieved April 4, 2006).

UNAIDS, 2006 Ecuador: Retrieved September 21, 2006, from http://www.unaids. org/en/Regions_Countries/Countries/ecuador.asp.
World Health Organization: 2006: Immunization, vaccines and biologicals. Retrieved September 21, 2006, from http://www.who.int/immunization_monitoring/en/ globalsummary/countryprofileresult.cfm?C='ecu'.

E

◆ EGYPT (ARAB REPUBLIC OF)

MAP PAGE (800)

Marianne Hattar-Pollara

Location: Civilization began in the fertile valley of the Nile River about 5000 BC and the first of the dynasties of pharaohs was established in 3200 BC. The progressively modern Egypt is located in the northeastern corner of Africa, bordering southwestern Asia. The capital is Cairo. Its boundaries include the Mediterranean Sea to the north, the Red Sea and Israel to the east, Sudan to the south, and Libya to the west. The total area is 1,001,450 km^2 (386,660 square miles); 97% is desert. The population is 78.8 million. The gross domestic product (GDP) per capita is $3,900; 20% live below the poverty line.

Major Languages	Ethnic Groups	Major Religions
Arabic	Eastern Hamitic 99%	Sunni Muslim 94%
English	Other 1%	Other 6%
French		

Ethnic minorities include the Bedouin Arab tribes of the Sinai Peninsula and the eastern and western deserts, the Berber-speaking community of the Siwa Oasis, and the Nubian people clustered along the Nile in the southernmost part. The country was host to diverse ethnic groups during the colonial period, including Greeks, Italians, Syrians, Jews and Armenians. The country still hosts some 90,000 refugees and asylum seekers, mostly Palestinians and Sudanese. Literacy rates are 68% for men, and 47% for women.

Health Care Beliefs: Active and passive involvement: traditional healing. The health teachings of the Greeks, Christians, and Islamic religion influenced health beliefs. From Hippocrates onward, the humor theory and the hot-cold theory were, and to some degree continue to be, the most commonly held views of illness attributions. The Hippocratic theory holds that the human body is filled with four basic substances, called *humors*, which are held in balance when a person is healthy. All diseases and disabilities result from an excess or deficit in one of these. The hot-cold theory attributes one's state of health to the belief that exposure, either externally or internally, to excessive amounts of hot and cold is likely to cause illness. Achieving health often occurs through re-establishing the desired balance. The hot-cold theory is still influential in the health beliefs of most Egyptians. Islam made health a central concern and categorically rejected magic and quackery. This is illustrated by the teaching of the Islamic Prophet, who declared, "Seek treatment, for there is no disease created by God for which He has not created a cure, except aging" (Omran, 1980, pp. 26–27). Islamic teachings also endorse total reliance on God's will, influencing how Egyptians practice health promotion and disease prevention. With modernization and national health initiatives to prevent the spread of endemic parasitic diseases such as schistosomiasis (bilharziasis), the concept of health promotion is becoming more accepted; however, the prevailing cultural-religious framework of predestination and believing that life calamities, including the illnesses that one experiences in one's life, are predetermined from the moment of their birth may pose a continuous challenge. A popular Egyptian proverb may explain this notion further: "That which is written on the forehead will be seen by one's eyes," meaning that one's life's events, including those of health and illness, are going to be experienced no matter what one does. Therefore, concepts of health promotion and disease prevention require understanding of the cultural religious context for devising the accurate intervention and for assessing compliance. Although Egyptians believe that God alone grants life and death, the concept of brain death as actual death is increasingly acceptable. Life-support technology is acceptable and desirable to save lives but not to postpone death. The practice of physician-assisted death or mercy killing in terminal illness is illegal and morally prohibited on religious grounds. Although traditional health beliefs are still in practice in varying degrees, Egyptians hold high regard for Western medical practices and often seek the care of physicians and nurses first. In rural communities with low socioeconomic levels, clients may rely on traditional health practices first or may seek both traditional and modern medical practices simultaneously.

Predominant Sick-Care Practices: Egyptians generally describe their health, and symptoms of their illnesses, in vague, nonspecific and global terms. The rationale used to explain causes of illness may reveal a traditionally held framework of illness causations. For example a diagnosis of brain tumor may be attributed to beating one's face and head while grieving the loss of a loved one. Perception of pain may be considered the first reliable symptom to indicate illness. Seeking modern medical or traditional treatment may depend on the severity and the nature of the pain experience. Muscular pain may be attributed to exposure to wind or drafts and may be treated by home remedies. Persistent muscular pain that is compounded by other symptoms and is not responsive to traditional remedies may force the patient to seek modern treatment. Psychological distress or mental illnesses are often expressed as physical symptoms *(somatization)*. Physical complaints to express disorders such as anxiety, depression, and other psychologically based disorders are likely to receive the intended attention and care. Direct expressions of emotional symptoms, however, are considered a source of distress for the family because of the stigma associated with mental illnesses. Magical-religious or supernatural explanations of illness still exist, such as widespread belief in the evil eye, feared because it is believed to cause serious illnesses and death. Infants are considered particularly susceptible, and symptoms such as tremors, convulsive seizures, spells of crying, refusal to nurse, and skin-color changes have all been attributed to the evil eye. Protective devices such as charms or amulets inscribed with verses of the Koran, turquoise stones, or a horseshoe on the door of a house are believed to provide protection. Curative efforts may involve using a *raki* (traditional healer), who, by resorting to supernatural forces, becomes endowed with the power to control or change the course of events. Zar ceremonial dances (originating from Ethiopia) are another form of spiritual healing, performed through dance in an attempt to heal souls from possession. The term *zar* means the possessing spirit. In Egypt, the ceremony is performed mainly in rural and low socioeconomic areas, particularly to treat mental illnesses.

Ethnic-/Race-Specific or Endemic Diseases: Parasitic diseases such as schistosomiasis (bilharzias) are endemic, with up to 70% of the rural population affected. Schistosomiasis is responsible for 70% of chronic liver disease among adults. Fascioliasis along with schistosomiasis has been reported in several areas. Both parasites lead to liver damage, inducing periportal fibrosis. Tuberculosis (TB) is considered one of the most common public health problems. More than 12,000 new cases are reported annually, with half reported to be smear-positive pulmonary TB. The Ministry of Health confirmed the country's 14th case of human infection with the H5N1 avian influenza virus in a 75-year-old woman from the Al Minya governorate. As with all other cases in Egypt, her infection has been linked to exposure to diseased birds. Of the 14 cases in Egypt, six have been fatal. The World Health Organization (WHO) estimated the prevalence rate for human immunodeficiency virus (HIV)/acquired immunodeficiency syndrome (AIDS) in adults (aged 15 to 49 years) to be 0.02%, with 5,300 people living with HIV, including fewer than 1,000 women. WHO has no estimates for children aged 0 to 15. Fewer than 500 deaths have been attributed to AIDS. Where the mode of transmission is known, about half of the cases are transmitted by heterosexual contact.

Health-Team Relationships: Egyptians expect to be treated by the most senior and experienced physicians. Egyptians tend to describe and narrate the circumstances around the illness before addressing their actual physical complaints. Developing trust through therapeutic interaction is an essential component for success of the encounter with patients and their families. This is especially important when the illness is emotional or has intimate or sexual connotations because Egyptians are unlikely to express their thoughts and feelings openly. Egyptian men, especially the more religious, may refuse care or feel uncomfortable with physical examination and care provided by female health care providers. Women also may refuse care from male doctors for intimate health problems.

The issue of opposite-gendered care can be serious enough that they terminate treatment without disclosing the reasons for doing so.

Families' Role in Hospital Care: The Egyptian family often takes an active part in the care and decision making regarding hospitalized family members. Decisions about medical treatments are rarely the product of an autonomous decision of the patient. In situations of grave diagnosis or terminal illness, the family spares the patient from being informed and from making decisions so as to preserve hope. Family and friends visit patients as often as possible to ensure that the provisions of health care are proper and adequate. It is common for a close family member to stay with and care for a patient, especially at night. In villages or in public hospitals in the city, food may be brought to patients to ensure that they are well fed. It is not uncommon for family members to be present during patient interviews and examinations, and they may answer questions addressed to the patient. The elder or most knowledgeable member of the family is often included in discussions of treatment options and may sign the informed consent.

Dominance Patterns: The family is the dominant social institution and the center of all social and religious activities. Single-family units are characteristic of families dwelling in urban cities and towns, but in rural areas the extended family with at least three generations is the norm. The family, as is the case with all Arab Middle Eastern families, is hierarchical, patrilineal, and patrilocal. Roles and role relationships are shaped by cultural norms and generally afford men the authority and decision-making power over women. More recently, gendered roles are negotiated and redefined according to family preferences and needs.

Eye-Contact Practices: People are expected to maintain eye contact, considered a sign of respect and giving undivided attention. It also serves to read others' facial expressions and emotions. Cross-gender interactions may differ, depending on the nature of the relationship, religiosity, and the context of the interaction. Eye contact is maintained in cross-gender interaction between members of the immediate and extended family; however, if the members strictly adhere to religious teachings, then interaction occurs with evasive eye contact. Eye contact in cross-gender interaction outside the family may be maintained, transient, or totally evasive according to the religious convictions of the players.

Touch Practices: Physical contact, physical space, and touch are important forms of communication. Physical space is smaller than in Western cultures. Frequent hugs and exchanges of kisses are accepted forms of greeting and expressing affection, although physical touch is limited to members of the same sex. Same-gender interactions may involve shaking hands, hugging, and exchanging kisses on the cheeks, but cross-gender interactions may not exceed shaking hands. Some religious men and women may even refrain from shaking hands, especially when they are purified and physically cleansed in preparation for daily prayers. Women who wear gloves or cover their hands with their veils generally will refuse to shake hands with men.

Perceptions of Time: Being past and present oriented, Egyptians may focus on the moment rather than plan and anticipate future events. A verse in the *Koran* says, "Do not say for a thing that 'I'll do this tomorrow' except if God wills." Planning ahead may be seen as in defiance of God's will, and talking about the future must be preceded or ended with the expression "if God wills," as dictated by the *Koran.*

Pain Reactions: Pain is usually expressed either in private or in the presence of close relatives or friends. Men are expected to endure pain in a manly way and generally tend to be more stoic than women. Pain is considered an unpleasant experience, and medicating for pain relief is acceptable. Hospitalized patients may appear demanding in their persistent requests for medications because of expectations of immediate pain relief. Egyptian patients also believe that pain and exertion may impede recovery; therefore, they tend to assume the sick role fully, refrain from self-care activities, and rely considerably on assistance from nurses and family members.

Birth Rites: Giving birth to children soon after marriage is expected. Abortion is illegal but is practiced in secrecy. In certain circumstances, abortion may be considered necessary, such as when the pregnancy exposes the mother to high health risks or when a lactating woman becomes pregnant and her milk stops. A lactating mother's pregnancy can be terminated only before 120 days' gestational age. In situations of pregnancy that results from rape, termination of the pregnancy is also permitted. The use of birth-control methods that have minimal adverse effects and do not cause sterilization is permitted, but couples refrain from using it until they have the desired number of children. Infant mortality rates are 31 deaths per 1,000 live births, and the fertility rate is 2.83 children born per woman. Boys are favored over girls, but once a girl is born, praise and thanks are given for her health and the health of the mother. Male circumcision is expected to occur within the first week of birth if medically possible but also may be performed at the 40th day or before puberty. Female circumcision, although not legalized, is still performed in rural and low socioeconomic areas in girls when they are around 8 years of age or before puberty. Newborns are swaddled and dressed in a shirt called a *jalabiya,* which is made by relatives, and the grandmother stays close to the mother during the hospital stay. A celebration sponsored by the grandparents is held on the seventh day after birth. Life expectancy is 69 for men, 74 for women.

Death Rites: It is believed that only God knows a patient's true prognosis, so people are not supposed to speak of death, and health care professionals may be asked to keep a patient from knowing the truth. Near the time of death, Muslims help the patient recite the Declaration of the Faith: "There is no God but God, and Muhammad is God's messenger." Although expressive and vocal wailing is traditional and acceptable, it recently became inappropriate because Islam prohibits it. A family member may stay in the room with the body and recite verses of the *Koran*. God is asked to forgive the deceased and allow the person to go to heaven. Organ donations and transplants are allowed, and Muslim doctors may recommend transfusions to save lives. Autopsies are uncommon except for forensic reasons because the body must be buried intact; cremation is not permitted. After the funeral, Muslim burial practices involve wrapping the body in special pieces of cloth (preferably white) and burial without a coffin in the ground soon after death.

Food Practices and Intolerances: Breakfast and lunch are the main meals. The evening meal is generally a light snack and is consumed later in the evening at approximately 10 pm. Pork and pork products and alcoholic beverages are not allowed; however, Egyptians may consume alcohol if they are not strictly adhering to Islam (*Koran*, 5:3, Qur'an, 5:90). Meat must be prepared in the Islamic tradition known as *halal*, in which the slaughtered animal is killed while the person is reciting verses from the *Koran*; all the blood is drained out of the animal. There is no prohibition against shellfish like shrimp and lobster. Pork, carrion, and blood are forbidden.

Infant-Feeding Practices: Mothers are encouraged to breastfeed their babies; breastfeeding is extremely common and continues for about 2 years in villages. In cities, weaning occurs sooner. When a child refuses to transition to normal foods, the mother may cover her nipples with a bitter substance or put hair on them. Sugar water is introduced at a young age, with the introduction of hot beverages such as anise, peppermint, caraway, and chamomile, as soon as 40 days after birth. Soft foods such as yogurt with honey; apple, pear, and orange juices; and corn flakes with milk are introduced after 4 months. After 6 months, cooked pieces of chicken and soup with vegetables are introduced.

Child-Rearing Practices: Child rearing tends to be the responsibility of the mother, but all members of the immediate and extended family may participate. Boys have easier access to the males in the family and have more liberty and freedom. Boys and girls are generally socialized early to assume their gender roles. The respect of elders, social politeness, and modesty are often reinforced both in and outside the home. Female circumcision or female genital mutilation is believed to guarantee modest conduct of girls by way of decreasing sexual desire. It is a traditional practice that is widespread in villages. The 1995 Demographic and Health Survey revealed that 97% of Egyptian women between the ages of 15 and 49 reported having had circumcision.

National Childhood Immunizations: BCG at 1 to 3 months; DTwPHep at 2, 4, and 6 months; DTwP at 18 months; OPV at birth and 2, 4, 6, 9, and 18 months; measles at 9 months; MMR at 18 months; vitamin A at 9 and 18 months; and TT for pregnant women. The percent of the target population vaccinated, by antigen, is: BCG, DTP1, DTP3, HepB3, MCV, and Polio3 (98%); and TT2plus (80%).

BIBLIOGRAPHY

Abou-Basha LM, Salem A, Osman M, El-Hefni S, Zaki A: Hepatic fibrosis due to fascioliasis and/or schistosomiasis in Abis 1 village, Egypt. *East Mediterranean Health J.* 6(5):870–878, 2000.

Al-Adawi S, Martin RG, Al-Salmi A, Ghassani H: Zar: group distress and healing. *Mental Health, Religion & Culture.* 4(1):47–61, 2001.

Central Intelligence Agency: 2006: *The world factbook, Egypt.* Retrieved September 21, 2006, from https://www.cia.gov/cia/publications/factbook/print/eg.html.

Daar AS, Al Khitamy B: Bioethics for clinicians: 21. Islamic bioethics, *Can Med Assoc J.* 163(1):60–63, 2001.

El-Gibaly O, Ibrahim B, Mensch BS, Clark WH: The decline of female circumcision in Egypt: evidence and interpretation, *Social Sci Med.* 54(2):205–220, 2002.

El-Guindy H, Schmais C: The Zar: an ancient dance of healing, *Am J Dance Ther.* 16(2):107–120, 1994.

Hedayat K, Pirzadeh R: Issues in Islamic biomedical ethics: a primer for the pediatrician, *Pediatrics* 108(4):965–971, 2001.

Kamel MI, Moustafa YA, Foda N, Khashab S, Moemen M, Abo El Naga RM: Impact of schistosomiasis on quality of life and productivity of workers, *East Mediterranean Health J.* 8(2–3):354–362, 2002.

Komaromy C: Cultural diversity in death and dying, *Nurs Manage.* 11(8):32–36, 2004.

The Nobel Qur'an. Al-Maeda Sura, verse 3, 90. King Fahd Complex for Printing the Holy Qur'an.

The Nobel Qur'an. Al-Bakara Sura, verse 185. King Fahd Complex for Printing the Holy Qur'an.

UNAIDS: 2006 Egypt. Retrieved September 21, 2006, from http://www.unaids.org/en/Regions_Countries/Countries/egypt.asp.

World Health Organization: *Core health indicators.* Retrieved June 29, 2006, from http://www3.who.int/whosis/core/core_select_process.cfm?country=egy&indicators=nha&language=en.: 2006: Immunization, vaccines and biologicals. Retrieved September 21, 2006, from http://www.who.int/immunization_monitoring/en/globalsummary/countryprofileresult.cfm?C='egy'.

Zaher H, Tag El Din M, Van Maaren P: *Tuberculosis control and intersectoral collaboration: the experience of Egypt.* Retrieved June 21, 2006, from http://www.emro.who.int/stb/egypt/Collaboration.htm National Tuberculosis Control Programme, Ministry of Health and Population, Egypt website.

Zahr LK., Hattar-Pollara M: Nursing care of Arab children: consideration of cultural factors, *J Pediatr Nurs* 13(6):349–355, 1998.

◆ EL SALVADOR

MAP PAGE (795)

Mary-Elizabeth Reeve (Consultant: PreNatal El Salvador)

Location: The smallest of the Central American countries, El Salvador is situated along the Pacific Ocean. The total area is 21,040 km² (8,124 square miles), and the capital is San Salvador. Much of the land is fertile volcanic plateau. The country is divided into 14 departments, with a population of about 6.8 million. El Salvador experiences frequent natural disasters, including hurricanes, floods, and earthquakes. El Salvador sustained tremendous damage and loss of life due to Hurricane Mitch in 1998 and two major earthquakes in 2001. The gross domestic product (GDP) per capita is $4,700.

Major Languages	Ethnic Groups	Major Religions
Spanish	Mestizo 90%	Roman Catholic 83%
Indigenous languages	Amerindian 1%	Protestant and Other 17%
	White 9%	

Indigenous languages include Kekchi (Mayan), Lenca, and Pipil (Uto-Aztecan). Most indigenous people are Nahuat-Pipil (94%), followed by Lenca (4%) and Cacaopera (2%). Indigenous groups make up about 11%, or 684,613, of the total population. A high percentage is young; approximately 47% are living in poverty, most in urban areas. During the civil war from 1980 to 1992, more than 80,000 people died or disappeared, and more than one million became refugees. Literacy rates are 83% for men, 78% for women.

Health Care Beliefs: Acute sick care; traditional; increasing focus on prevention. Local health promoters carry out preventive care in rural areas. Where access is limited, preventive care does not exist, and traditional forms of health care continue to be practiced. Traditional beliefs about causes of illness include the idea that childhood illnesses, such as diarrhea, can be caused by "evil eye" (*mal del ojo*). To protect a child against the effects of mal del ojo, the family may put a bracelet made of specific types of seeds or a small red personal item on the child. During menstruation, women traditionally refrain from bathing because it is believed that bathing will make the abdomen cold and cause pain and coagulation. Women may also refrain from eating avocado, eggs, and onions because of the strong odors associated with these foods and menstruation. These beliefs are passed from grandmothers to mothers, mothers to their children, and between female friends. Women who have had a bad experience in the hospital during birth prefer a midwife and home birth. Mental illness is not feared, nor is it particularly stigmatized, although it is a significant cause of mortality. Alcoholism is common. Some individuals have religious beliefs that do not permit blood transfusions.

Predominant Sick-Care Practices: Biomedical and magical-religious. Health care practice is predominantly biomedical, with 12 physicians for every 10,000 inhabitants. The Ministry of Public Health and Social Welfare covers 80% of the population. Approximately 17% has access to social security (ISSS) health services. The Ministry of Public Health and Social Welfare provides care through 30 hospitals, 357 health units, 171 "health houses" (*casas de salud*), and 52 rural nutrition centers. More than half of the hospitals are over 30 years old and in need of renovation, new equipment, and updated technology. There are differences between rural and urban dwellers, age groups, and ethnic and socioeconomic groups in terms of health-seeking behaviors. In rural areas, people first use herbal remedies and rely on the advice of family members, midwives, and "curers" (*sobadores*), who see patients either in their own homes or in the patient's home. Herbal medicines play an important part in the curing tradition, and the cost is lower than pharmaceuticals. If traditional practices fail, a patient goes to the local health promoter. In urban areas, people rely on family advice and the local pharmacy, where they are given advice and can purchase medicines without a prescription. For more serious illnesses, they seek care at private or public clinics and hospitals. Older people rely on self-medication with herbal remedies, only going to the pharmacy or hospital in cases of severe illness. The young seek advice from family and friends but are also likely to go to a clinic. Indigenous groups maintain their own medicinal traditions, including the use of herbal remedies. Treatment decisions are based on the patient's physical appearance and also in part on traditional beliefs relating illness to external influences, such as phases of the moon and climatic conditions. Women prefer female doctors for gynecologic examinations. Health consequences of natural disasters include diarrhea, respiratory illnesses, skin diseases, and psychological symptoms, especially among children.

Ethnic-/Race-Specific or Endemic Diseases: Indigenous populations are the most underserved, and rural inhabitants have less access to health care than urban. As of 1998, in urban areas, 92% of the population has access to potable water and 86% to sewage disposal. In rural areas, only 25% of the population has access to potable water and 50% to sewage disposal. It has been estimated that 23% of children suffer from chronic malnutrition. Common diseases include acute respiratory infections, tuberculosis (TB) and diarrhea. Several dengue epidemics have occurred in the past few years, including one with a total of 16,697 cases. Malaria is caused predominantly by *Plasmodium vivax*. TB continues to be a serious problem: the annual TB incidence in recent years has been 27 to 28 cases per 100,000. Human immunodeficiency virus (HIV)/acquired immunodeficiency syndrome (AIDS) estimates from the Joint United Nations Programme on HIV/AIDS (UNAIDS)/World Health Organization (WHO) indicate that the prevalence rate for adults (aged 15 to 49 years) is 0.9%, with 36,000 people living with HIV, including 9,900 women. About 2,500 deaths have been attributed to AIDS. Reports indicate that 65% of all infections occur as the result of heterosexual transmission.

Health-Team Relationships: Health centers and small public hospitals are staffed by a team of a physician, nurse, several community health promoters, and sometimes a trained birth attendant. In rural areas, there are few health centers, and those that exist are underfunded and poorly equipped. More often, there are small *casas de salud*, which are attended a few days a week by a student physician completing his or her year of social work and a nurse and community health promoter. Rural communities may have only a community health promoter, and isolated communities may have no health personnel. The physician retains authority over the health team because of his or her higher level of education, but also because physicians are placed as health center and hospital directors. The role of the nurse is to attend to patients when the physician is not present and to attend referrals by the physician. Health promoters attend patients and provide preventive care.

Families' Role in Hospital Care: In cases of severe illness, the family may assist health personnel with care, but this is not common. More often, the family will help by purchasing medication that the hospital does not have and by locating people willing to donate blood, when necessary. Families are able to visit their relatives and accompany them during visiting hours. If the patient requires ongoing care and there is insufficient staff to provide it, a family member may remain. In some cases, family members bring food, but generally institutions provide it. Families also assist indirectly by providing transportation; taking care of young children if the mother is hospitalized; or looking after the house, the family business, or the farm.

Dominance Patterns: Men are dominant, particularly in the private sphere. Violence by husbands or partners against women is not uncommon. In the public sphere, there is more apparent equality. Both men and women have access to professional roles and status, although in rural areas, there may be greater preference for men in professional roles. Women's roles have expanded, and women have gained more opportunity overall; however, because women remain responsible for the care of home and children, their overall workload has increased.

Eye-Contact Practices: No particular patterns exist.

Touch Practices: A handshake is the customary greeting.

Perceptions of Time: People are usually punctual, but patients in rural areas may arrive up to 2 hours late because they must travel on foot a long distance, starting out at daybreak. Ideally, a patient receives care even if he or she has arrived late for an appointment.

Pain Reactions: Men demonstrate a high tolerance for pain. Women, especially those in urban areas, may express pain more freely. Children are expected to be courageous and to demonstrate a high tolerance for pain.

Birth Rites: The fertility rate is 3.12 children born per woman. The first 40 days after birth is traditionally a time of special precautions for the mother. To avoid contagious illnesses, women cover their heads with a cloth and wear cotton earplugs and socks. Women observe specific dietary restrictions to produce a lot of milk: the diet includes chocolate, tortillas with cheese, and various soups. Women who are lactating consume large quantities of soups and juices. There are no particular rituals for the infant. From 1999 to 2003, an estimated 53% of pregnant women received some prenatal care, and trained personnel attended 70% of deliveries. The maternal mortality rate is estimated at 150 per 100,000 live births. The infant mortality rate is 24 deaths per 1,000 live births, and the mortality rate for children younger than 5 years is 37 deaths per 1,000. Life expectancy is 68 for men, 75 for women.

Death Rites: Most of the population follows Catholic practices. The family holds an all-night vigil following the death of a family member. Organ donation is not generally accepted. An autopsy may be performed on an infant who dies in the hospital.

Food Practices and Intolerances: The basic diet consists of rice, corn, beans, eggs, coffee, plantains, cheese, and cream. Chicken is eaten when it is available. Sugary drinks are popular with children. There are no special foods for pregnant women or for children.

Infant-Feeding Practices: In rural areas, infants are breastfed for 1 to 2 years. In urban areas, breastfeeding is generally discontinued after 6 months; supplementary foods, such as rice soup or a fortified flour mix, begin at about 4 months. About 25% of infants are exclusively breastfed for 4 months, more than 50% for 12 to 15 months, and 40% until they are 2 years old. Over the past two generations, as women have entered the workforce, infants are breastfed for shorter periods, and women working outside the home rely to some extent on bottle-feeding.

Child-Rearing Practices: There are very few differences across rural/ urban and socioeconomic classes. In rural areas, households are often multigenerational, and women are less independent than urban women. The men leave for work, and women stay home to look after the house and children. In many households, women are the sole providers, and extended family members may help with childcare. Children often share sleeping quarters with siblings and parents. Older children are expected to assist in cleaning, washing, and ironing and the care of younger siblings. In rural areas and poor urban neighborhoods, children often make important economic contributions to the household. Interfamily violence, both physical and psychological, is not uncommon.

National Childhood Immunizations: BCG at birth; DTwP at 15 months and 4 years; DTwPHibHep at 2, 4, and 6 months; MMR at 12 months and 4 years; OPV at 2, 4, 6, 15 to 18 months, and 4 years; Td at $+1$, $+6$ months, $+1$, $+5$, and $+10$ years. The percent of the target population vaccinated, by antigen, is: BCG (84%); DTP1, DTP3, HepB3, Hib3, and Polio3 (89%); and MCV (99%).

BIBLIOGRAPHY

Central Intelligence Agency: *2006: The world factbook, El Salvador.* Retrieved September 21, International Planned Parenthood Federation: Country profile: El Salvador. Retrieved June 7, 2006, from http://www.ippf.org/regions/countries/ slv/index.htm.

Pan American Health Organization: El Salvador. In *Health in the Americans:* vol *II.* Pan American Health Organization Scientific Publication no. 587, Washington, DC, 2002, PAHO.

PAHO, UNFPA, UNIFEM: *Gender, health and development in the Americans, basic indicators 2005.* PAHO, 2005, Washington, DC.

Pan American Health Organization Country Health Profiles: El Salvador. Retrieved January 19, 2006 from http://www.paho.English/DD/AIS/cp_222.htm.

UNAIDS: 2006 El Salvador. Retrieved September 21, 2006 from http://www.unaids.org/en/Regions_Countries/Countries/el_salvador.asp.

UNICEF: Monitoring the situation of children and women: child nutrition—breastfeeding, country data. Retrieved February 24, 2006 from http://www.childinfo.org/eddb/brfeed/index.htm.

World Health Organization: 2006: Immunization, vaccines and biologicals. Retrieved September 21, 2006, from http://www.who.int/immunization_monitoring/en/globalsummary/countryprofileresult.cfm?C='slv'.

◆ ERITREA (STATE OF)   E

MAP PAGE (800)

David M. Sintasath

Location: Eritrea is located on the horn of Africa, with a total area of 121,320 km² (46,862 square miles) on the Red Sea coast, with Ethiopia and Sudan to the west and Djibouti to the south. The central part is mountainous with fertile agricultural valleys, whereas the coastal lowlands are hot, semiarid deserts. Eritrea is the youngest country in Africa and gained independence from Ethiopia in 1993 after 30 years of struggle. The population is 4.7 million, with 44% between 0 and 14 years of age. The country is poor, with a gross domestic product (GDP) per capita of only $1,000, with 50% below the poverty line. Eritrea is governed by the National Assembly, which was established as a transitional legislature in 1993, and also by the assembly-elected president. The capital is Asmara.

Major Languages	Ethnic Groups	Major Religions
Tigrinya (official)	Tigrinya 50%	Islam 50%
Arabic (official)	Tigre 25%	Eritrean Orthodox
English	Kunama 15%	Christianity 50%
	Afar 4%	
	Saho (inhabitants of Red Sea coast) 3%	
	Other 3%	

English is used in schools after the sixth grade, and some Italian, a result of Italian colonization from 1890 to 1941. Native languages belong to three distinct groups: Semitic languages such as Tigrinya and Tigre, both closely related to Ethiopian Amhar written by the ancient Geez characters; Cuschitic languages such as Afar, Beja, and Saho, spoken by the ethnic groups of the same names; and Nilotic langages, such as Kunama and Baria. Eritrea is a multiethnic nation with nine major ethnic groups.

The Tigrinya dominate politics and culture, and the Tigre populate the northern highlands. The smaller ethnic groups include the Afar, Kunama, Bilen, Saho, Hadarb, Nara, and Rashaida. Christianity is the religion of the Tigrinya ethnic group, who mostly reside in the central highlands, whereas Islam is the primary religion of the other ethnic groups in the lowlands and coastal regions. A few rural tribes still practice traditional African religions. Lilteracy rates are 70% for men, 48% for women.

Health Care Beliefs: Acute sick care; traditional. Traditionally, a uvulectomy is performed to prevent respiratory diseases. Scarring of the skin around the eyes is thought to prevent eye infections. Men and women are both circumcised, and genital mutilations have been reported in 95% of Eritrean women. Afflictions or illnesses may be attributed to transgressions against God or sorcery motivated by envy.

Predominant Sick-Care Practices: Biomedical and ethnic-medical beliefs. People predominantly tend to seek medical care from doctors or practitioners at local health care clinics. Because medical doctors are in short supply, minor medical assistance is provided by local knowledgeable individuals whose therapeutic arsenal may include such treatments as traditional herbs.

Ethnic-/Race-Specific or Endemic Diseases: Infectious diseases dominate: malaria in the lowlands, and tuberculosis and hepatitis B are widespread. Studies of the Rashaida minority tribe have revealed a particularly low seroprevalence of rubella and varicella, a fact that could be important when isolated tribes are incorporated into the society. Malnutrition, anemia, intestinal parasites, and respiratory disorders are common. The Joint United Nations Programme on HIV/AIDS (UNAIDS) estimates the prevalence rate for human immunodeficiency virus (HIV) in adults (aged 15 to 49 years) is 2.4%, with 59,000 people living with HIV, including 31,000 women and 6,600 children aged 0 to 14. There are 36,000 children aged 0 to 17 who are orphans as a result of acquired immunodeficiency syndrome (AIDS). About 5,600 deaths from AIDS have been reported; only 5% of infected persons are receiving antiretroviral therapy. The seroprevalence of HIV type 1 in female sex workers is reported to be 24%. No HIV has been found among the secluded Rashaidas.

Health-Team Relationships: Eritrea has few medical doctors (1 per 35,000 inhabitants), but doctors dominate the health care team nonetheless. Because time spent on consultations is limited, patients' attitudes can be repressive.

Families' Role in Hospital Care: Hospitals provide food as well as staff to help with patients' general sanitary needs in major cities. In rural areas, hospital care depends on the families, who provide food and support for the patient's basic needs.

Dominance Patterns: Eritrean families are traditionally patriarchal, and the women are primarily responsible for domestic duties. During the long war, however, women fought side by side with men (they constituted a third of the country's 100,000 soldiers), and so attitudes toward women became more permissive.

Eye-Contact Practices: Eritreans avoid direct eye contact with strangers, authority figures, and older people.

Touch Practices: Strangers of both sexes shake hands, and touching practices are liberal among friends. Men may greet each other by knocking shoulders three times and women by reciprocal kisses on the cheeks.

Perceptions of Time: Perhaps because of the long war, Eritreans anticipate the future. Public communications are fairly punctual, and punctuality in general is not disregarded.

Pain Reactions: Stoic reactions to pain are common. For instance, in the Afar culture, men are judged by the bravery with which they bear the pain of circumcision.

Birth Rites: The fertility rate is 5.08 children born per woman. Midwives and traditional birth attendants from within the community assist in childbirth. If a newborn is a boy, he is celebrated on the third day after birth (on the seventh day if a girl) by friends, neighbors, and relatives, who bring gifts to the mother and child. Traditionally, *gheat,* a dough made of flour and water and served with butter, spices, and sour milk, is served during the celebration. The infant mortality rate is very high: 48 deaths per 1,000 live births. Life expectancy is 57 for men, 61 for women.

Death Rites: Twelve days of mourning are usual. Friends, relatives, and neighbors pay their condolences. Both organ donations (which are very rare) and autopsies are accepted but require the consent of close relatives.

Food Practices and Intolerances: Food is traditionally served on a large platter on the center of the table, and people eat from it with their right hands. *Ingera,* a type of pancake, is often used to scoop up the food from the platter. The diet varies depending on religious beliefs. For example, Muslims do not eat pork.

Infant-Feeding Practices: Infants are usually breastfed for 1 or 2 years.

Child-Rearing Practices: Children have a strict upbringing. Physical punishment is used, primarily by the father. Children are expected to obey their parents, respect older adults, and help at home without being asked.

National Childhood Immunizations: BCG at birth; DTwPHep at 6, 10, and 14 weeks; OPV at birth and 6, 10, and 14 weeks; measles at 9 months; and TT for pregnant women and CBAW. The percent of the target population vaccinated, by antigen, is: BCG and DTP1 (91%); DTP3, HepB3, Polio3 (83%); MCV (84%); and TT2 plus (70%).

BIBLIOGRAPHY

Central Intelligence Agency: *2006: The world factbook, Eritrea.* Retrieved September 21, 2006, from https://www.cia.gov/cia/publications/factbook/print/er.html.

ORC Macro, Eritrea 2002: Results from the Demographic and Health Survey. Stud Fam Plann, 2005 Mar, 36(1):80–84.

Sintasath DM, Ghebremeskei T, Lyunch M, Kleinau E, Bretas G, Shililu, Brantly, Graves PM, Bejer JC: Malaria prevalence and associated risk factors, *Am J Trop Med Hyg*. 72(6):682–687, 2005.

Tolfvenstam T, Enbom M, Ghebrekidan H, Ruden U, Linde A, Grandien M, Wahren B: Seroprevalence of viral childhood infections in Eritrea, *J Clin Virol*. 16(1):49–54, 2000.

UNAIDS: 2006 Eritrea. Retrieved September 21, 2006, from http://www.unaids.org/en/Regions_Countries/Countries/eritrea.asp.

USAID: Country Health Statistical Report: September 2004. Retrieved December 23, 2005, from http://pdf.dec.org/pdf_docs/PNADC019.pdf.

World Health Organization: 2006: Immunization, vaccines and biologicals. Retrieved September 21, 2006, from http://www.who.int/immunization_monitoring/en/globalsummary/countryprofileresult.cfm?C='eri'.

◆ ESTONIA (REPUBLIC OF)

MAP PAGE (799)

Marika Tammaru

Location: Bordering on the Baltic Sea to its north and west, Estonia is mainly a lowland country with numerous lakes in northeastern Europe. The capital is Tallinn. It is bordered on the north by the Gulf of Finland, on the east by the Russian Federation, on the south by Latvia, and on the west by the Baltic Sea. The total area is 45,227 km^2 (17,385 square miles). The population is 1.3 million, two thirds of whom live in urban areas. The gross domestic product (GDP) per capita is $16,700. Literacy is almost 100% for both men and women.

Major Languages	Ethnic Groups	Major Religions
Estonian (official)	Estonian 68%	Lutheran and Orthodox
Russian	Russian 26%	Christian or some other
	Ukrainian 2%	faith 30%
	Belorussian 1%	No religious affiliation
	Finn 1%	34%
	Other 2%	Atheist 6%

Health Care Beliefs: Acute sick care; traditional. Although the need for prevention is understood and that sphere is developing, resources are first allocated to crisis care and inpatient services.

Predominant Sick-Care Practices: Biomedical and alternative (herbal medicine, faith healing, acupuncture). Most people go to practitioners with biomedical backgrounds, although alternative therapies are also used. Older adults in rural areas are more likely to consult folk healers.

Ethnic-/Race-Specific or Endemic Diseases: Cardiovascular disease is the major cause of death, followed by cancer and death from external causes. People are at risk for tuberculosis. Since 2001 Estonia has experienced the most rapid increase of new cases of human immunodeficiency virus (HIV) infection in Europe. The Joint United Nations Programme on HIV/AIDS (UNAIDS) estimates the prevalence rate in adults (aged 15 to 49 years) to be 1.3%, with 10,000 people living with HIV, including 2,400 women. Deaths from acquired immunodeficiency syndrome (AIDS) are estimated to be fewer than 2,000. Estimates within Estonia are lower: country statistics report a total of 5,084 persons diagnosed with HIV and 100 with AIDS since 1988. The number of women with HIV is rising: 24% of cases in 2001 and 37% in 2005. Most cases are among injecting drug users and their sexual partners. About 62% who abuse drugs intravenously are positive for HIV.

Health-Team Relationships: Patient care is doctor directed. Nurses and doctors are predominantly women. Nurses follow doctors' orders, but there is increasing participation of nurses in decision making. Asking questions of the health care provider is becoming common, and many people try to diagnose their own illnesses. Patients address health care professionals by title and last name; they may offer gifts to health care providers to ensure quality care.

Families' Role in Hospital Care: Family members are not expected to assist with bathing, feeding, comforting, or elimination. All health care needs are provided by doctors and nursing staff.

Dominance Patterns: Traditionally, the men assume a slightly more dominant role; however, men and women share responsibilities in decision making. Women have taken on a more prominent role as their economic status has increased.

Eye-Contact Practices: Direct eye contact is preferred in conversations between health care providers and patients.

Touch Practices: Touching is infrequent even within families. A handshake is common at the beginning and end of an interaction in a professional situation.

Perceptions of Time: People in health care are focused on the present and on crisis management. Previous traditions, including how older adults heal illnesses, are important. Awareness of prevention opportunities in the community is rising, and people have become more future oriented.

Pain Reactions: Pain tolerance is valued, although pain relief is both desired and requested. Verbal expressions of discomfort signify more severe pain. Although during labor some women express pain, many still attempt to keep silent and be stoic.

Birth Rites: Almost all births occur in hospitals and are attended by doctors and a midwife. The fertility rate is 1.4 children born per woman.

The father may choose to be present during the delivery and is permitted to coach the mother's labor. Courses for natural childbirth and prenatal and postpartum care are becoming more popular. Circumcision is not practiced. The infant mortality rate is 8 deaths per 1,000 live births. Life expectancy is 67 for men, 78 for women.

Death Rites: If an illness is fatal, the patient is usually told. Burial usually occurs during the week after death. During the funeral service, an open coffin permits people to view the body. Grief may be expressed verbally, and crying in public is acceptable. Cemeteries are often visited, and graves are cared for by relatives. Cremation is increasing in popularity, especially in urban areas.

Food Practices and Intolerances: The preferred main meal is lunch. Potatoes, seasonal vegetables, bread, meat, fish, and soups are common. Large quantities of milk and other dairy products, tea, and coffee are consumed.

Infant-Feeding Practices: Breastfeeding is encouraged more than bottle-feeding. Some women may choose not to breastfeed or will do so for a short time. Foods are introduced at 4 to 5 months.

Child-Rearing Practices: Children are cooperative and are reared using disciplinary styles ranging from logical reasoning to authoritarian. The grandmother may have a valued position in child rearing, especially in single-parent families or in families in which both parents work. Some children may have chores to do at home or may be taught to rely more on their parents. Women are entitled to maternity leave at 30 weeks' gestation and may lengthen the leave until the child is 3 years old. In the first year, maternity leave wages are close to a woman's regular salary rate but are considerably lower later, so many women choose to return to work at about one year after delivery.

National Childhood Immunizations: BCG at birth; DT at 2, 4.5, and 6 months and at 2 years; DTwP at 3, 4.5, and 6 months and at 2 years; DTwPHiB at 3, 4.5, and 6 months and at 2 years; OPV at 3, 4.5, and 6 months and at 2 and 7 years; IPV at 3, 4.5, and 6 months and at 2 and 7 years; Hib at 3 and 4.5 months and at 1 year; HepB at birth and at 1 and 6 months; MMR at 12 months and 13 years; and Td at 7, 12, and 17 years. The percent of the target population vaccinated, by antigen, is: BCG and DTP1 (99%); DTP3, MCV, and Polio3 (96%); HepB3 (95%); and Hib3 (37%).

BIBLIOGRAPHY

Central Intelligence Agency: *2006: The world factbook, Estonia.* Retrieved September 21, 2006, from https://www.cia.gov/cia/publications/factbook/print/en.html.

Maansoo S, editor: *Statistical yearbook of Estonia 2005.* Tallinn, 2005, Statistical Office of Estonia.

Ministry of Social Affairs: *Health care statistics yearbook 2003,* Tallinn, 2005, Ministry of Social Affairs of Estonia.

Statistical Office of Estonia: Estonia Population Census 2000. Retrieved March 1, 2006, from http://www.stat.ee/122279.

Thomson S, editor: *Health care system in transition: Estonia,* Copenhagen, 2005, European Observatory on Health Systems and Policies.

UNAIDS: 2006 Estonia. Retrieved September 21, 2006, from http://www.unaids.org/en/Regions_Countries/Countries/estonia.asp.

World Health Organization: 2006: Immunization, vaccines and biologicals. Retrieved September 21, 2006, from http://www.who.int/immunization_monitoring/en/globalsummary/countryprofileresult.cfm?C='est'.

http://www.tervisekaitse.ee/tkuus.php?msgid=3466 HIV infections in Estonia 1988–2005, (retrieved on March 1, 2006).

E

◆ ETHIOPIA (FEDERAL DEMOCRATIC REPUBLIC OF)

MAP PAGE (800)

Vered Kater

Location: Ethiopia is located in the northeastern horn of Africa, bordered by Eritrea to the north, Djibouti and Somalia to the east, Kenya to the south, and Sudan on the west. The capital is Addis Ababa. Ethiopians and Eritreans are similar cultural groups because Eritrea was an Ethiopian province that gained independence in 1993. The total area is 1,127,127 km (435,184 square miles). Ethiopia's population is 74.7 million. The gross domestic product (GDP) per capita is $900, with 50% below the poverty line. Literacy rates are 50% for men, 35% for women.

Major Languages	Ethnic Groups	Major Religions
Amharic (the official language only spoken by 60% of the population)	Oromo 40%	Muslim (Sunni) 45-50%
	Amhara and Tigre 32%	Orthodox Christianity (Coptic) 35%-40%
Tigrinya	Tigrean 14%	Animist 12%
Oromo	Somali 6%	Other 3%-8%
40% speak in 70 different tongues	Sidamo 9%, Afar 4%,	
Guraghe, Other	Guraghe, and Other 17%	

Health Care Beliefs: Acute sick care; traditional. Health promotion and disease prevention do not exist. Many nongovernmental organizations teach prevention of human immunodeficiency virus (HIV) and acquired immunodeficiency syndrome (AIDS) and provide free condoms, but little attention is paid to this or other prevention strategies. Vaccinations are essentially the only preventive care that is sought. Many illnesses are believed to be caused by someone with "the evil eye" (i.e., the power to harm others by looking at them). Fresh air may be considered dangerous because it is believed to cause *mitch,* a general name for mental illness. Attitudes toward mental illness are unclear because Ethiopians believe all illnesses are physical. They think that bad food, wet feet, or the wrong type of thinking can cause disasters. Ethiopians have the basic assumption that every human individual has a personal spirit, referred to as *qole* or *wegabi.* It is easy to offend or insult this spirit, and the result is a variety of physical or spiritual ailments. Mystical and physical healings are often combined. Care for acute illnesses is frequently sought from the family first, followed by traditional healers, and then, as a last resort, a modern doctor.

Predominant Sick-Care Practices: Traditional, magical-religious, and Western. Healers use Western as well as magical-religious methods. Local practices include prophylactic uvulectomy to prevent throat infections, extraction of the lower incisors to prevent diarrhea, and amulets and tattooing to drive away pathogenic agents. Modern medicine combined with traditional therapy, such as white onions with alcohol and butter, are used as treatment for malaria. Ethiopia has no system of health insurance, and each item used by a doctor is paid for separately. Even when a woman is hospitalized for childbirth, the gloves used by the midwife are brought by the expectant mother.

Ethnic-/Race-Specific and Endemic Diseases: Active and endemic diseases include bacterial and protozoal diarrhea, hepatitis A, typhoid fever, hepatitis E, cutaneous leishmaniasis, schistosomiasis, rabies, and meningococcal meningitis. In 2005, 5.4 million cases of malaria were reported. The prevalence of tuberculosis is increasing (some HIV-related): 262,944 new cases in 2004. Ethiopians are at risk for measles complications, intestinal parasites, diarrhea, eye infections, and vitamin A and B deficiencies. Malnutrition is widespread, with about 8 to 10 million at risk; 45% of children under 5 are at risk for severe malnutrition. The prevalence rate for HIV/AIDS is estimated at 4.4% (12.6% urban, 2.6% rural rates). Other estimates of the rate of HIV infections range from a low of 7% to a high of 18%. Deaths from AIDS are expected to rise in the coming years: AIDS already accounts for about one third of all young adult deaths. It is estimated that 1.5 million are living with HIV, including 200,000 children aged 0 to 14. About 720,000 children aged 0 to 17 are orphans as a result of parental deaths from AIDS.

Health-Team Relationships: Ethiopians highly respect health care professionals, so much so that patients often visit several healers and follow all their advice simultaneously, even when this advice is contradictory. Patients tend to demand injections because of the widespread belief that pills will not influence their symptoms.

Families' Role in Hospital Care: Families move into the hospital and help with patients' physical care. Patients do not want to be left alone, especially if they are gravely ill. The family has to bring food and take care of the patient's hygienic needs. Care for patients with chronic conditions is provided by the extended family, and older adults usually live at the home of one of their children.

Dominance Patterns: Fathers are traditionally the authority figures, and men are responsible for handling family contacts with the world outside the home. The woman's role is defined in terms of household management and matrimonial duties.

Eye-Contact Practices: Many Ethiopians do not make direct eye contact with doctors and nurses because of the perceived higher status of health professionals.

Touch Practices: Handshaking is customary, and it is polite to shake both hands of older adults simultaneously. Greetings do not include kissing, but people touch cheek to cheek four times when meeting close friends. Family members touch in public, and holding hands with someone of the same sex is not unusual.

Perceptions of Time: Time is not as important as it is in Western cultures. A common saying is that "each hour has 500 minutes." The concept of time varies among the different ethnic groups. In general, Ethiopians are not future oriented and, therefore, not very concerned with long-range goals to prevent future illness.

Pain Reactions: Individuals have a high pain tolerance but eventually accept pain medication when and if it is offered.

Birth Rites: Sex is not discussed. Women have no preparation for childbirth, and rectovaginal and vesicourinal fistulas are common complications. Pregnancy is considered a dangerous time because of the potential for damage from the evil eye and sorcery against the fetus. It is believed that unfulfilled cravings can cause a miscarriage, malformation, or prematurity. Childbirth is attended by a traditional birth attendant or a female family member, and the woman assumes the side-lying position. Traditionally, fathers do not participate in labor or delivery. About 1,000 women die of pregnancy-related causes per 100,000 live births. The mother remains confined for 12 days, and the newborn stays within the home for at least 40 days because sun rays are believed to cause severe illnesses. More then half of the total admissions involving obstetric problems are caused by illegal—frequently septic—abortions. The infant mortality rate is very high at 94 deaths per 1,000 live births. There are 166 deaths per 1,000 for children younger than 5 years. The fertility rate is five children born per woman. Life expectancy is 48 for men, 50 for women.

Death Rites: Autopsies are uncommon because of the belief that the body must be buried intact. Cremation is not permitted. For Muslim and Fallasha burials, the body is wrapped in special pieces of cloth and buried without a coffin in the ground. Loud wailing is a normal grief reaction for men and women, and the mourning period varies from a few days to a month.

Food Practices and Intolerances: Many children younger than 5 suffer from some degree of malnutrition—about 60% are 80% or less than expected weight. Daily caloric supply is estimated to be 76% of the recommended daily intake. The food is always very spicy, causing a high incidence of stomach ulcers. *Injera,* a flat, round bread made from teff grains that is high in iron, is the main staple and is eaten three times a day with other foods that are pureed and placed on top. The dish is eaten with one hand without utensils. Many cups of black coffee and sweet tea are consumed during the day. Some people do not eat the meat of wild animals, pigs, dogs, horses, and shellfish. Ethiopians have numerous fasting days. On some of the days, people are allowed to eat before sunrise and after sunset; on other days, they are not allowed to eat animal products or are allowed no food or water for 24 hours.

Infant-Feeding Practices: Water with butter is given to the infant immediately after delivery because it is believed that it softens the voice of the baby. This practice frequently causes aspiration pneumonia. Breastfeeding continues for several years, and solid food is not introduced until the child can walk. When an infant has diarrhea, Ethiopians believe withholding food and fluids will cure the child.

Child-Rearing Practices: Children are raised in a highly protective, indulgent atmosphere until they are about 3 years. Obedience and politeness are the goals of upbringing. Children who are ill may be kept lying in one place until they are better. About 90% of boys are circumcised, and the procedure is performed between birth and 5 years. Some girls in certain groups are circumcised.

National Childhood Immunizations: BCG at birth; DPT at 6, 10, and 14 weeks; OPV at birth and 6, 10, and 14 weeks; measles at 9 months; and TT 3 doses of tetanus vaccine to all women of childbearing age (15 to 49 years). The percent of the target population vaccinated, by antigen, is: OPV (75%); measles (71%); and TT (45%).

BIBLIOGRAPHY

Centres for Disease Control and Prevention: Ethiopia. Retrieved December 20, 2005, from http://www.cdc.gov/nchstp/od/gap/countries/ethiopia.

Central Intelligence Agency: 2006: *The world factbook, Ethiopia.* Retrieved September 21, 2006, from https://www.cia.gov/cia/publications/factbook/print/et.html.

Hockenberry MJ: *Wong's essentials of pediatric nursing.* 7th ed, St. Louis, 2005, Mosby.

Kater V: A tale of teaching in two cities, *Int Nurs Rev* 47(2):121, 2000.

Spector RE: *Cultural diversity in health and illness,* ed 6, New Jersey, 2004, Pearson.

UNAIDS: 2006 Ethiopia. Retrieved September 21, 2006, from http://www.unaids.org/en/Regions_Countries/Countries/ethiopia.asp.

UNICEF: Ethiopia. Retrieved December 10, 2005, from http://www.unicef.org/ethiopia/immunization.html.

UNICEF: Ethiopia. Retrieved December 15, 2005, from http://www.unicef.org/infobycountry/ethiopia_statistics.html.

World Health Organization: Retrieved March 6, 2006, from http://www.who.int/3by5/support/EFS2004_eth.pdf.

◆ FINLAND (REPUBLIC OF)

MAP PAGE (798)

Marja Kaunonen, Katja Joronen, and Hilkka Sand

Location: Finland, one of the Nordic countries, stretches about 1,126 km (700 miles) north and south from the Arctic Circle to the Gulf of Finland, with Sweden along its western border and Russia along its eastern border. The total area is 337,030 km^2 (130,127 square miles). It is the second northernmost country in the world, but the climate is relatively mild because of the influence of the North Atlantic current, the Baltic Sea, and more than 100,000 lakes. The capital is Helsinki. The landscape of southern Finland is characterized by its lakes and forests, and northern Finland, which is called *Lapland,* by its fjelds and wilderness areas. Lapland is north of the Arctic Circle and has unique summers during which the sun does not set and winters during which the sun does not rise. Finland has one of the highest standards of living in the world. The population is more than 5.2 million. The gross domestic product (GDP) per capita is $30,900. Literacy rates are 100% for men and women.

Major Languages	Ethnic Groups	Major Religions
Finnish (official)	Finnish 93%	Evangelical Lutheran 83%
Swedish (official)	Swedish, Lapp,	Greek Orthodox 1%
Lapp	Other 7%	Other or None 16%
Russian		

About 6% speak Swedish as their first language. There are two ethnic minorities, Sami (7,000 people) and Roma (10,000), and about 108,300 immigrants and refugees as of 2004. Finns study two to three foreign languages in school, and their command of English and Swedish is good.

Health Care Beliefs: Active involvement. Health promotion is considered important. Health is considered a subjective sense of well-being and an absence of physical complaints.

Predominant Sick-Care Practices: Biomedical and alternative. Biomedical sick-care practices are predominant. Legislation provides the right to good health care and related treatments, the right to be informed, and the right to self-determination. Public health care services are financed mainly by relatively high income taxes. In addition, health care services are provided by the private sector. In the private sector, a person can make an appointment directly with a specialist at a specified time, which differs from the "first come, first serve" approach of the public sector. Private doctors are paid in cash, but the Social Insurance Institution compensates for part of the payment. Certain forms of alternative medicine, such as acupuncture, have become more common and to some extent are accepted by the medical profession.

Ethnic-/Race-Specific or Endemic Diseases: Finns are at genetic risk for numerous congenital diseases, such as nephrosis, generalized amyloidosis syndrome, and polycystic liver disease. Cardiovascular diseases, cancer, stroke, musculoskeletal disorders, alcohol abuse, and mental disorders are common illnesses. Lifestyle diseases and depression are emerging as serious public health problems. Finland was the first country to fully implement a nationwide suicide-prevention project, from 1986 to 1996. In 1996 the number of suicides in Finland had decreased by 18%, although suicide rates continue to be high at 20 per 100,000. The Joint United Nations Programme on HIV/AIDS (UNAIDS) estimates the prevalence rate of human immunodeficiency virus (HIV) in adults (aged 15 to 49 years) to be 0.1%, with 1,900 people living with HIV, including fewer than 1,000 women and fewer than 100 children aged 0 to 15 years. When the mode of transmission is known, 40% are attributed to heterosexual transmission, 38% to men who have sex with men, ant 19% to injecting drug use.

Health-Team Relationships: Health care is doctor driven. Basic nursing education is offered at polytechnic schools. Graduate and postgraduate training in nursing education and administration is offered at five Finnish universities. In recent years, the implementation of family nursing programs has attracted increasing attention. Family nursing reinforces family strategies and resources, improving the response to changes in family structures. Family nursing has been implemented in child welfare clinics and in the care of older adults. Nurses and doctors work closely in outpatient clinics and school health services. Patients want strong, interactive relationships with nurses and doctors, and patient motivation is linked to good compliance, especially among adolescents. Successful nurse and patient collaboration involves active commitment of both parties.

Families' Role in Hospital Care: Most hospitals prefer open visiting hours, and family members and volunteers help feed patients. It is not unusual for family members to participate in the care of a hospitalized child and stay overnight.

Dominance Patterns: Men and women are considered equals, and both contribute to making health care decisions for children. Most Finnish women work outside the home.

Eye-Contact Practices: Finns greet guests and friends by shaking hands; kisses on the cheek are less common. Direct eye contact is considered polite and necessary, especially when greeting a person. Regardless of age, a confidential connection between health care personnel and patients must involve eye contact.

Touch Practices: Hugs and kisses for children in the family are common, but touch practices among adult family members depend on familial culture. Regardless of age or gender, touching is considered natural by health care professionals. The frequency of touching in nursing care situations increases with very sick patients. In the nursing care of older patients, nurses use three main types of touch: that used in performance of a procedure, to help a restless patient relax for a procedure, and touch used to comfort a patient. Because of the nature of their professional role, doctors have less overall physical contact with patients.

Perceptions of Time: People are usually punctual and may be irritated by tardiness. The impact of postmodernism and individualism on Finnish culture is characterized by the preference of careers rather than families. Laypersons have an increasing interest in genealogy. Finnish culture has some significant traditions, such as the celebration of Christmas (Finland is known as the home of Santa Claus) and Midsummer.

Pain Reactions: Finns are accustomed to expressing their pain in detail but in a matter-of-fact way. Extreme pain and suffering are often experienced tacitly. The consumption of medication for pain is relatively high, but other treatments—such as massage, physical therapy, and psychotherapy—are also used. Benefits from the Social Insurance Institution and insurance companies compensate for part of treatment costs. Hospitalized patients in pain are often reluctant to reveal their discomfort. Thus nursing and medical staff members must pay attention to nonverbal messages, changes in conduct, and certain somatic complaints such as dizziness and nausea. The subjective experience of pain is composed of physical and emotional reactions such as fear, anxiety, and guilt. In hospitals, pain is measured by using self-rated assessment forms. Doctors of all specialties treat patients with pain, but all university hospitals and numerous others have pain clinics for studying and treating chronic pain.

Birth Rites: The average age of primigravidas is 28 years. Having one or two children is common (the fertility rate is 1.73 children born per woman), and births of sons and daughters are celebrated equally. Any woman living permanently in Finland who has a doctor's examination before the end of the fourth month of her pregnancy is entitled to the "one-off" maternity benefit. This bonus is granted in the form of either a maternity package (containing basic clothing, linens, and other necessities for a newborn) or cash. The cash alternative amounts to 140 Euros tax-free per child, but the value of the package is almost three times the amount of money. Midwife-assisted hospital births predominate and are associated with one of the lowest infant mortality rates in the world (4 deaths per 1,000 live births). Positive childbirth experiences as perceived by first-time mothers are strongly related to the positive characteristics and professional skills of the attending midwife and positive attitude of the spouse toward the pregnancy. Most fathers participate in the delivery and consider their presence important for their growth into fatherhood. Infant "rooming in" (i.e., infants staying in the mother's hospital room) is prevalent in Finnish hospitals. Parental involvement with sick infants is encouraged, and the hospital has open visiting hours for siblings. "Kangaroo care" is used, and breastfeeding is the method of choice. Life expectancy is 75 for men, 83 for women.

Death Rites: Most Finns die in hospital settings. The first hospice in Scandinavia, Pirkanmaan Hoitokoti in Tampere, Finland, opened in 1987. Currently, Finland has three hospices. Family members typically want to participate in and follow the care of their ill family members. Study findings indicate that when a patient's condition deteriorates, the family's need for information increases. Family members often want to be at the bedside of the dying person to pay their final respects. Organ donations and autopsies are both acceptable. Funeral rituals are important because they allow the expression of grief because mourning customs such as wearing black clothing or black veils (for widows) have begun to disappear during the last decades. Funeral directors assist the family with postmortem care. Burial is common, but cremation is becoming more frequent. The funeral takes place 1 to 3 weeks after the death, and a memorial service is usually held following the burial. The death is announced in newspapers either after the burial or before it, when the obituary serves as an invitation to the funeral. Family members often attend a church service the day after the funeral. Family members and friends are the most important source of social support.

Food Practices and Intolerances: Finnish people eat much of the same food as other Europeans. Coffee, meat and cheese sandwiches, and porridge or cereal are common for breakfast. Lunch is the main meal. A small meal of coffee and sandwiches is eaten after work.

Infant-Feeding Practices: Breastfeeding is common. Whether the mother successfully breastfeeds is related to whether she has a positive experience breastfeeding in the maternity ward and whether she has emotional and concrete support from her social support network. In addition, whether a first-time mother successfully copes with childcare is related to her success with breastfeeding.

Child-Rearing Practices: Child-rearing practices are relatively permissive. Children express their opinions freely to parents and teachers. The family may have only one children's room, which is shared by boys and girls. Finland has ratified the United Nations convention on the Rights of the Child, and corporal punishment is forbidden by law. Single-parent families are now relatively common and constitute 19% of all families with children. Many single parents have joint custody, however, and the child meets with the other parent regularly. Mothers receive 263 working days of maternity allowance, the last 158 of which can be used by either the mother or the father. In addition, fathers receive 18 days of paid paternity leave. The mother's job is secure until the child is 3 years old—or 7 if the mother works only 6 hours a day. Each child receives a paid child benefit until 17 years of age. Free dental care is provided until age 18, free health care from birth to school age. One full meal is offered to children at school. Compulsory military service begins for boys at the age of 19 and lasts 6 to 12 months. Military service is voluntary for girls.

National Childhood Immunizations: BCG at birth; DTaP at 14 to 15 years; oral polio vaccination is not in use, but polio vaccination is given at age 3, 5, 12 months, and 4 years; Hib at 4, 6, and 14- to 18 months; MMR at 14–18 months and 6 years; Td at age 11 to 13 years; DTaPIPV at 3, 5, 12 months, and 6 years. The percent of the target population vaccinated, by antigen, is: BCG (98%); DTP1 (99%); DTP3, MCV, and Polio3 (97%); and Hib3 (98%). More than 98% of children have received BCG vaccination at birth or soon thereafter, which may cause a positive reaction to the Mantoux tuberculin test.

BIBLIOGRAPHY

Central Intelligence Agency: *2006: The world factbook, Finland*. Retrieved September 21, 2006, from https://www.cia.gov/cia/publications/factbook/print/fi.html.

Hakulinen-Viitanen T, Pelkonen M, Haapakorva A: *Maternity and child health care in Finland* [English summary]. Helsinki, 2005, Reports of the Ministry of Social Affairs and Health.

Hopia H, Paavilainen E, Åstedt-Kurki P: Promoting health for families of children with chronic conditions, Journal of Advanced Nursing *(J Adv Nurs)* 48(6):575–583, 2004.

Kaunonen M: *Support for a family in grief*, Academic dissertation. Tampere, Acta Universitatis Tamperensis 731, 2000.

Tarkka M-T, Paunonen M, Laippala P: Importance of the midwife in the first-time mother's experience of childbirth. *Scand J Caring Sci,* 14(3):184, 2000.

National Public Health Institute: *http://www.ktl.fi/portal/english/* (retrieved on March 1, 2006).

Statistics Finland: Available at: *http://www.stat.fi/index_en.html* (retrieved on March 1, 2006).

UNAIDS 2006 Finland: Retrieved September 21, 2006, from http://www.unaids.org/en/Regions_Countries/Countries/finland.asp.

World Health Organization: 2006: Immunization, vaccines and biologicals. Retrieved September 21, 2006, from http://www.who.int/immunization_monitoring/en/globalsummary/countryprofileresult.cfm?C='fin'.

F

◆ FRANCE (FRENCH REPUBLIC)

MAP PAGE (798)

Catherine Bungener

Location: As Benjamin Franklin once said, "Every man has two nations, and one of them is France." France is the second largest European nation, with a total area of 551,000 km² (214,890 miles). The English Channel lies to the northwest, the Atlantic Ocean to the west, and the Mediterranean Sea to the south. France shares borders with Germany, Luxembourg, Belgium, Switzerland, Italy, and Spain. France has 96 *départements* ("administrative units") within the country, four overseas départements (Guadeloupe, Martinique, French Guinea, and Réunion) and three overseas territories (French Polynesia, New Caledonia, and Wallis and Futuna). The French Alps include the highest peak in Europe: Mont Blanc. The climate is temperate with mild winters, except in mountainous areas and the northeast. The Atlantic impacts the western part of the country, where there is high humidity, violent westerly winds, and rain. The northeast has a classic continental climate: hot summers and cold winters. The southern area has a Mediterranean climate.

Major Languages	Ethnic Groups	Major Religions
French	Celtic	Roman Catholic 75–80%
	Latin	Muslim 2%
	Teutonic, Slavic,	Protestant 1.6%
	North African,	Jewish 1%

Major Languages	Ethnic Groups	Major Religions
	Indochinese,	Muslim 6%
	and Basque	Other 1.3%
	minorities	Unaffiliated 13%

The population is 62 million: the capital, Paris, has a population of 13 million. Although 99% speak French as their first language, there are numerous rapidly disappearing dialects, such as Provencal, Alsatian, Breton, Creole, Catalan, Corsican, and Basque. The gross domestic product (GDP) is $29,000, with 6% below the poverty line. Literacy rates are 100%.

Health Care Beliefs: Active involvement; strong health promotion. People tend to eat healthier foods, such as fruits and vegetables, and try to avoid saturated fats. They are encouraged to participate in sports regularly, and smoking, drinking, and taking drugs are strongly discouraged. The government has many initiatives in place for health-promotion activities. For the most part, religion does not influence health care beliefs, except among some minority populations. Because treatments with herbs, homeopathic, or chiropractic measures are not considered scientifically based, the costs of these treatments are not paid by national health insurance.

Predominant Sick-Care Practices: Biomedical. About 10% of the GDP is devoted to health (the highest in Europe). All French people are affiliated with the Sécurité Sociale, which gives access to free medical care in all public hospitals. Everyone who is employed or has a parent or spouse who is employed is covered by this health and accident insurance, contributions to which are automatically taken out of the salary. When people are sick, they go to their physicians, either in a private practice or in the hospital. They can freely choose their physician or the hospital where they want to be treated. If they choose a private hospital, however, only a part of the bill will be reimbursed. There are three physicians and nine hospital beds per 1,000 people.

Ethnic-/Race-Specific or Endemic Diseases: Cardiovascular diseases (32%) and cancer (28%) are the two major causes of death. The Joint United Nations Programme on HIV/AIDS (UNAIDS) reports the prevalence rate for human immunodeficiency virus (HIV) in adults (aged 15 to 49 years) to be 0.4%, with 130,000 living with HIV, including 45,000 women. About 59,495 people have acquired immunodeficiency syndrome (AIDS), and 1,500 deaths have occurred. Half of reported HIV-positive persons live in the Paris area. Where mode of transmission is known, about 69% of cases are transmitted heterosexually.

Health-Team Relationships: Doctors remain at the top of the hierarchy in hospitals, followed by physiotherapists, psychologists, social workers, and then nurses. The hierarchical domination of doctors over nurses is intact in all hospitals. Doctors study for 6 years to graduate and 4 more years to become specialists. Psychologists graduate after 5 years. Nurses begin patient care at the end of 4 years of study at the baccalaureate level.

Families' Role in Hospital Care: The mother of a child or a spouse is allowed stay overnight when a patient is severely ill. Otherwise, specific visiting times are set. Food and treatments are always provided, so families do not have to assume this responsibility.

Dominance Patterns: The father remains dominant and the head of the family, although more single-parent families are evolving, and in most cases the mother becomes the head of the family. More women are working, so moral and financial responsibilities are divided between both parents. Now fathers as well as mothers are entitled to parental leave for the education of children. Since 1999 the Solidarity Social Pact (PACS) offers legal recognition to adult cohabiting couples (either heterosexual or homosexual).

Eye-Contact Practices: As a sign of respect, the French maintain direct eye contact when talking to someone. Facial expressions and gestures tend to be quite expressive.

Touch Practices: The French touch frequently, especially in the southern part of the country, where people prefer closeness during conversation. Handshaking or giving a kiss on each cheek when greeting or leaving a person is the norm. Carrying on a conversation with the hands in the pockets is impolite. When meeting people, protocols are observed and behavior is polite. Titles and status are important. First names should not be used. Engaging in general conversation to establish social contact is acceptable. When working with patients, giving logical, sequential explanations for health-related actions is important to ensure compliance. Rules and regulations are circumvented to reach a goal.

Perceptions of Time: Strictly adhering to schedules is not routine, and changing plans at the last minute is acceptable; however, the French are becoming more time oriented with regard to their schedules. Long waiting times are common in all public administration settings, including public hospitals.

Pain Reactions: Pain is usually expressed by saying, "aïe!" or "ouille!" Women express pain and emotions more freely than most men. During the last several years, pain control has become a major concern. Every university hospital has a pain treatment department, and analgesics are freely given to patients who need them. Previously, pain tended to be underestimated and not treated correctly. Much remains to be done to improve the treatment of pain, especially for patients outside the larger cities.

Birth Rites: The fertility rate is 1.9 children born per woman, and the mean age of mothers giving birth is 29.6. The infant mortality rate is 4.7 deaths per 1,000 live births. Most women give birth in a hospital, where they stay from 1 to 5 days, usually keeping their infants with them 24 hours a day. If mothers are particularly tired or ill, infants stay in the nursery for the first few nights. Although religion does not play a very significant role in birth rituals, babies with Christian parents are baptized some time during the first year. During pregnancy, regular doctor's visits are prescribed, as are a minimum of three ultrasound scans. Many parents want to learn the sex of the baby as soon as possible rather than wait until birth. An amniocentesis is performed on all mothers age 38 or older. Cesarean sections are common and suggested to the mother when the position of the infant is anticipated to make the delivery difficult. Epidural anesthesia and episiotomies are the norm. Terminations of pregnancy are authorized until the 12th week of pregnancy. Maternity leave for the first two children begins 6 weeks before the birth and ends 10 weeks after; for additional children, it is 8 weeks before and 18 weeks after. Fathers now have 10 days of leave after the birth. Life expectancy is 76 for men, 84 for women.

Death Rites: Most people die in a hospital, and close family members are generally present. After a death, French Christians usually have a ceremony in a church. On November 1, chrysanthemums are brought to all the cemeteries, and families visit their parent's graves. Organ donations and autopsies are performed if the patient or the family has given consent.

Food Practices and Intolerances: The French are very fond of fine food and wines. At breakfast, bread with butter and jam or croissants is served with juice and tea or coffee. Lunch and dinner include a first course, main course (meat or fish and vegetables, rice, or pasta), often accompanied by a green salad, cheese if it was not served as first course, and dessert. Bread is always served; the typical baguette remains the favorite, although recently new kinds of breads with grains have become quite popular. People regularly drink wine with their meals. After the dessert, small cups of black coffee are frequently served. *Foie gras* ("goose liver") and seafood, especially oysters and snails, are considered fine food. The French eat a lot of red meat. Every region has its own specialties: *choucroute* ("sauerkraut") in Alsace; crêpes in Bretagne; foie gras and cassoulet in the southwest; *bouillabaisse* ("fish soup") or courses with tomatoes, garlic, and basil in the south; cheese meals in the Alps (fondue, raclette, or tartiflette); and seafood near the sea.

Infant-Feeding Practices: After childbirth, about 60% of women breastfeed their infants; only about 30% do so after the first 2 or 3 weeks. Relatively few mothers breastfeed their children for many weeks. In the hospital, the trend is toward bottle-feeding, and breastfeeding is not particularly encouraged unless the mother insists on it.

Child-Rearing Practices: Child-rearing practices are increasingly more permissive. Children usually have their own rooms and do not typically sleep with parents unless they are sick.

National Childhood Immunizations: DTaPHib at 3 months; DTaPIPV at 2, 4, 16 to 18 months, and 11 to 13 years; DTIPV at 6 years; HepB at birth and at 2, 4, 16 to 18 months; MMR at 9 to 12 months and at 12 to 15 months; Pneumo_conj at 2, 3, 4, and 12 months. The percent of the target population vaccinated, by antigen, is: BCG (84%); DTP1, DTP3, and Polio3 (98%); HepB3 (29%); Hib3 and MCV (87%). The only two compulsory vaccinations are BCG before 6 years and DPT at 2, 3, and 4 months. Vaccination for ROR (measles, mumps, and German measles), and pertussis/whooping cough are strongly recommended. Vaccination for hepatitis B is compulsory for health workers and typhoid fever for people working in biological analysis laboratories.

Other Characteristics: More people every year practice a sport regularly, especially football, rugby, and cycling. The French are often considered by foreigners to be chauvinists. They do a lot of walking in the countryside or mountains and ski during the winter, facilitated by the 35-hour work week. They often spend their vacations in France: the beaches of the Mediterranean Sea, the Atlantic Ocean, and the Channel are very popular during summer holidays. Most people take 1-month holidays during the summer, usually mid-July to mid-August.

G

BIBLIOGRAPHY

Central Intelligence Agency: *2006: The world factbook, France.* Retrieved September 21, from 2006, https://www.cia.gov/cia/publications/factbook/print/fr.html.

National Institute of Economic and Epidemiology: INSEE survey, 1999. Retrieved March 1, 2006 from www.sante-gouv.fr/www.oms.com.

UNAIDS: 2006: France, Retrieved September 21, 2006, from http://www.unaids.org/en/Regions_Countries/Countries/france.asp.

World Health Organization: France. Retrieved March 2, 2006, from http://www.who.int/fr.

World Health Organization: 2006: Immunization, vaccines and biologicals. Retrieved September 21, 2006, from http://www.who.int/immunization_monitoring/en/globalsummary/countryprofileresult.cfm?C='fra'.

◆ GABON (GABONESE REPUBLIC)

MAP PAGE (801)

Arnaud Dzeing

Location: This Central African republic sits astride the equator along the Atlantic seaboard. Most of the total area of 267,667 km² (103,319 square miles) is covered by dense tropical forests and savannahs. Gabon is bordered by Cameroon and Equatorial Guinea to the north and Congo-Brazzaville to the east, with a long common border. The climate is tropical: always hot and humid. Gabon is one of the more prosperous Black African countries. The gross domestic product (GDP) per capita is four times that of most nations of sub-Saharan Africa: $6,800. The population is 1.4 million. Libreville is the capital and is home to about half the population.

Major Languages	Ethnic Groups	Major Religions
French	Fang 30%	Christian 60%
Fang	Eschira-Punu 28%	Muslim 1%
Omyene	Other 42%	Indigenous, other 39%

The distribution of the different tribes is: Fang 30%, Eschira-Punu 28%, Ndzabi-Aduma 13%, Mbédé-Téké 10%, Kota-Kélé 8%, Omyéné 5%, Okande-Tsogho 4%, and pygmee 1%. Foreigners represent 20% of the population. The president is elected for 7 years, and he or she names a Prime Minister, who forms and directs the government. The legislative power is held by the national assembly and senate. Literacy rates are 74% for men, 53% for women.

Health Care Beliefs: Acute sick care. The common perception is that mental illness has an occult origin. It is believed that enemies can use an evil spell to disturb the mind because of jealousy or other reasons. The first reaction to having mental illness is to go to a traditional healer who uses plants, incantations, and prayers to chase the evil spirits from the body. Diseases may be considered divine punishment.

Predominant Sick-Care Practices: Biomedical; traditional; magical-religious. People seek doctors at hospitals and local dispensaries. Medical facilities and access to medication in Gabon's major cities are limited but generally adequate for routine or basic needs. A new drug manufacturing plant in Libreville should alleviate the drug-access problem. No prescription is required to buy medicines at pharmacies. Because oral medications are the most common type, people often share medicine if they think they have the same ailments. Medical services in rural areas are generally unavailable. The most vulnerable populations—those with low incomes—go to a dispensary only after treatment with traditional medicine has failed because traditional treatments are less expensive. Whether a person is dealing with a physical or mental illness, and even if a doctor is consulted, traditional healers are also used and herbal treatments are common. Traditional healers often use an exorcism ceremony to treat patients.

Ethnic-/Race-Specific or Endemic Diseases: Endemic diseases include malaria, human immunodeficiency virus (HIV), sickle-cell disease, schistosomiasis, tuberculosis, and yellow fever. People are at risk for loiasis, leptospirosis, onchocerciasis, hemorrhagic fevers, sleeping sickness, intestinal parasites, and hepatitis B and C. Gabon had three large outbreaks of Ebola virus, the latest in 2001. Ebola is fatal in approximately 70% of cases. Schistosomiasis from *Schistosoma haematobium* occurs, with an incidence of 8% to 55% of the adult population. The Joint United Nations Programme on HIV/AIDS (UNAIDS) estimates the prevalence rate for human immunodeficiency virus (HIV) in adults (aged 15 to 49 years) to be 7.9%, with 60,000 people living with HIV, including 33,000 women and 3,900 children aged 0 to 14. There are 20,000 orphans aged 0 to 17 from acquired immunodeficiency syndrome (AIDS). About 31,000 people have AIDS, with 4,700 deaths, a rate that is lower than many neighboring countries. HIV prevalence is very high (26% to 32%) among tuberculosis patients, and recent studies have shown that 66% of childbearing and pregnant women have herpes simplex virus type 2 (HSV-2) seropositivity. Life expectancy is 54 for men, and 57 for women.

Health-Team Relationships: Relationships between patients and caregivers are as good as can be expected given the shortages of personnel and equipment. Hospitals need medical equipment, supplies, and reagents, so it is common for patients to bring these items with them. Supplies necessary for surgical operations, such as gloves, cotton, and bandages, also must be supplied by the patients or their families. There is no health insurance system, so patients must bear the cost of treatment.

Families' Role in Hospital Care: It is always recommended that the family (particularly mothers) stay with patients in the hospital. The family is responsible for the physical care of the patient and also for supplies, food, and medications that are unavailable in the care unit.

Dominance Patterns: Men are dominant in the family and make all the important decisions; however, mothers raise the children. A marriage is considered a union between two families and a time of fun. The groom gives many presents to the bride's family so that his desire to marry the woman is convincing. Two men representing their respective families fight a lyrical duel with much style and as part of the negotiation. The groom must then find his prospective bride hidden under a sheet with other women in his family; if he makes the wrong choice, he has to pay extra to the bride's family. When the fun is concluded, the newlyweds are congratulated and everyone has a meal together.

Eye-Contact Practices: There are no restrictions relating to direct eye contact between sexes or people of different ages.

Touch Practices: Touching is not only acceptable, it is used to communicate. Hand movements punctuate discussions and are usually expressive.

Perceptions of Time: Punctuality is not an issue. People tend to be more punctual for administrative appointments. Time is never an issue for private appointments, and being late is acceptable. People tend to focus on historical traditions, such as respect for ancestors and older adults.

Pain Reactions: Reactions to pain vary among ethnic and socioeconomic groups. In general, it is more acceptable for women and children to express pain.

Birth Rites: It is uncommon for the father to be present during childbirth. This task is usually assumed by a female member of the family. Celebration of the birth is the same regardless of the infant's gender, but the celebration of twins (either girls or boys) is particularly special and important. The hair of the child is not cut until a certain time passes after the birth, usually at the celebration of the first birthday.

Gabon has the lowest fertility rate in sub-Saharan Africa, with 3.69 children born per woman. A link seems to exist between bilharzial diseases and infertility and ectopic pregnancies. Recent studies show that 14% of pregnant women have either gonococcal infections, chlamydial infections, or both, which affects the spread of other sexually transmitted diseases such as HIV/AIDS. The infant mortality rate is very high at 95 deaths per 1,000 live births. Life expectancy is 53 for men, 56 for women.

Death Rites: All members of the family are expected to be present for the death of a relative, and relatives living in another country generally come back to attend the burial ceremony. To encourage the presence of all family members at the funeral, friends of the family gather donations to provide the funds needed for people to return. Organ donations and autopsies are unusual.

Food Practices and Intolerances: People use knives, forks, or spoons to eat, although some food, such as cassava, is eaten with the hands. Meals with sauce containing peanuts, served with rice and cassava, are commonly eaten.

Infant-Feeding Practices: Breastfeeding is the most common form of infant feeding because of its health advantages and the high cost of formula. In addition, when water supplies are unclean, bottle-feeding increases the risk of the infant contracting parasites and other organisms.

Child-Rearing Practices: Education is considered important. Children are taught to obey adults, and they consider all adult women and men to be mothers and fathers. It is considered improper to contest the decision of an older person.

National Childhood Immunizations: BCG at birth; DTwP at 6, 10, and 14 weeks; OPV at birth and at 6, 10, and 14 weeks; measles at 9 months; HepB at 6, 10, and 14 weeks; yellow fever at 9 months; and TT CBAW ×5, pregnant women ×2. The percent of the target population vaccinated, by antigen, is: BCG (89%); DTP1 (69%); DTP3 (38%); HepB3 (55%); Polio3 (31%); and TT3 plus (60%).

BIBLIOGRAPHY

Ouzouaki et al: Genital shedding of herpes simplex virus type 2 in childbearing-aged and pregnant women living in Gabon, *Int J STD AIDS.* 17(2):124–127, 2006.

Central Intelligence Agency: *2006: The world factbook, Gabon.* Retrieved September 21, 2006, from https://www.cia.gov/cia/publications/factbook/print/gb.html.

UNAIDS: 2006 Gabon. Retrieved September 21, 2006, from http://www.unaids.org/en/Regions_Countries/Countries/gabon.asp.

World Health Organization: 2006: Immunization, vaccines and biologicals. Retrieved September 21, 2006, from http://www.who.int/immunization_monitoring/en/globalsummary/countryprofileresult.cfm?C='gab'.

http://www.flashgabon.com/index.php (retrieved July 1, 2006).

http://www.izf.net/izf/Guide/TableauDeBord/gabon.htm (retrieved May 4, 2006).

http://travel.stat.gov/gabon.html (retrieved April 2, 2006).

◆ GAMBIA (REPUBLIC OF THE)

MAP PAGE (800)

Clement Ibi Mboto and Andrew Jewell

Location: "The Gambia," is the smallest country in western Africa; located on the Atlantic coast, surrounded on the north, south, and east by Senegal, and on the west by the Atlantic Ocean. The vegetation is savannah on the uplands, with low hills and mangrove swamps along the region of the Gambia River. The climate is characterized by a long dry season from October to early June and a short rainy season from mid-June to early October. The river Gambia bisects the country into two sections, forming the North and South Banks. The land area is 11,300 km^2 (4362 square miles). The population is more than 1.6 million. The capital is Banjul, but many people live at a subsistence level in bush villages. The gross domestic product (GDP) per capita is $1,800. The Gambian economy is very dependent on rain-fed agriculture and is badly affected by severe drought. Literacy rates are 58% for men, 37% for women.

Major Languages	Ethnic Groups	Major Religions
English (official)	Mandinka 42%	Muslim 90%
Mandinka	Fula 18%	Christian 9%
Wolof	Wolof 16%	Indigenous beliefs 1%
Fula	Jola 10%	
Other	Serahuli 9%	
	Other 4%	
	Non-African 1%	

Health Care Beliefs: Acute sick care; health promotion important. The average Gambian believes in charms, and 50% of men wear them daily. Amulets and charms are believed to ward off evil and bring good luck.

Predominant Sick-Care Practices: Biomedical; magico-religious and traditional. Medical facilities are limited and substandard. Common medications are frequently unavailable. Emergency needs for some essential drugs, such as anti-rabies and anti-snake venom may require traveling to nearby Senegal. Distributions of major health care facilities are gradually improving with the establishment of a referral hospital in each division of the country and a teaching hospital in Banjul. Some people have to travel several kilometers and then wait for many hours to see a doctor. It is not unusual to find three children (or more during the malaria season) with a variety of infectious conditions sharing a hospital bed. Skilled manpower is very limited and often not available. Most specialist medical workers in the country are non-Gambians, and more than 80% of the doctors and 30% of the paramedical staff are non-Gambians. More than 70% of medical staff in some places are voluntary workers.

Ethnic-/Race-Specific or Endemic Diseases: Malaria is endemic, with year-round occurrence, highest between June and October. The malaria death rate is estimated at 0.31% for children younger than 5 years, with a slightly lower rate for adults. Amoebic dysentery, cholera, *Escherichia coli, Shigella, Helicobacter pylori,* giardiasis, and typhoid are routinely encountered, with a higher prevalence in the northern division of the country. Evidence abounds of arboviral diseases, such as Crimean-Congo hemorrhagic, Chikungunya, Dengue, Rift Valley, and West Nile fevers. Yellow fever is endemic, but nationwide yellow fever vaccination is believed to have reduced the incidence. Close to one fifth of the population may be infected with hepatitis B; endemicity for hepatitis A and C is lower. Risk for histoplasmosis and leishmaniasis is nationwide, and occasional reports of sporadic cases of cutaneous and visceral leishmaniasis occur. There are more stray dogs than those with owners, so sporadic cases of human rabies are reported countrywide. Both *Schistosoma haematobium* and *S. mansoni* are common, but the former has a greater prevalence rate. Respiratory synctial virus (RSV) is common and is associated with significant morbidity in children with acute lower respiratory tract infection (ALRI). Recent accurate statistics on the human immunodeficiency virus (HIV) epidemic are difficult to obtain. The Joint United Nations Programme on HIV/AIDS (UNAIDS) and World Health Organization (WHO) estimated the prevalence rate for HIV/AIDS in adults (aged 15 to 49 years) to be 1.2% to 4.2% at the end of 2003. This rate has been slowly increasing since the first case was diagnosed in the country in 1986; heterosexual contact is the predominant mode of transmission. Up to 24,000 people may be currently living with HIV or acquired immunodeficiency syndrome (AIDS). Both tuberculosis and syphilis have increased with the emerging evidence of increasing HIV prevalence.

Health-Team Relationships: Health care is provided at three levels. At the primary level, remote communities or those with a population of 400 have volunteers trained as village health workers (VHWs) and traditional birth attendants (TBAs). The VHWs and TBAs are often illiterate and unpaid. They provide primary health care in their communities and refer serious cases to hospitals or clinics. TBAs conduct deliveries. Secondary-level health services are delivered at dispensaries, health centers, mobile or trekking clinics, and referral hospitals. Dispensaries are often manned by students and community health nurses whose clinic services include labor and delivery. Health centers may be manned by nurses and midwives, with doctors visiting once or twice weekly. In addition to the services provided by dispensaries, they may admit a maximum of 20 patients based on available facilities and carry out minor surgery. All dispensaries and health centers refer serious cases to the referral hospitals. Tertiary health care services are provided in four major referral hospitals, including a teaching hospital in Banjul. These have more defined facilities and staff. At whatever level, health care services are often very poor. Services rendered by health care workers, especially in rural settings, often depend on what is possible and the facilities at one's disposal because of the crisis nature of most situations. Communication between patients and most health care workers is in the local dialect. In general, there is good cooperation between members of the health care team.

Families' Role in Hospital Care: The family is almost entirely responsible for rendering supportive care for any relation. A member of the family, often a male, donates blood if transfusion is needed. A family member stays on the hospital premises. The situation is more complex when the hospital involved is far from the patient's residence; in this case, cooking utensils and sleeping materials such as mats are brought to the hospital to provide some comfort for the relation. Family members are usually responsible for providing food and purchasing all prescribed drugs unavailable at the hospital.

Dominance Patterns: Ethnicity, tribal values, and religion are major contributors to variations in dominance. Most homes are polygamous and comprise the family head, his wives, and unmarried children. Women usually have responsibility for child care, although discipline may be meted out by any senior member of the family or community. Segregation based on sex is the norm: male children tend to accompany their fathers, and girls follow their mothers. Male dominance is further strengthened by strong Islamic affiliation. Polygamy cuts across all the tribes, and women may not oppose a husband's polygamous union. The society maintains traditional practices such as early marriage (especially the Fula), wife inheritance, and female circumcision (especially the Fula). For the Fula, female circumcision is sacred and mandatory, although the practice is declining among other tribal groups. Extremists consider an uncircumcised girl unfit for marriage. Marriages are often arranged by the father or uncle. Brothers and sisters and other extended family members often remain within a strong kinship network, even after marriage. Marriages between first cousins and a son's right to inherit the wife of a late father or brother are considered protective of women. Abortion is strictly forbidden by Sharia Law and is illegal unless a mother's life is threatened. Close to a third of the men and some religious leaders remain opposed to the use of modern contraceptives.

Eye-Contact Practices: Most Gambians maintain good eye contact, especially in the company of peer groups. Eye contact can be subjected to several interpretations and taboos. Eye contact may be used, for example, when a mother or relation does not wish a child to divulge information to those present. Traditionally, when a younger person greets an elder, direct eye contact is avoided. Making direct eye contact with persons while they are eating may be considered evil, particularly when one is not eating too.

Touch Practices: Shaking hands is the most common form of touch and must be done with the right hand even if one is left-handed. Hands are shaken many times during the day, even if one continues to meet the same person. At a distance, clasped hands may be raised in place of a handshake. It is not uncommon to find a child stretching hands first to an adult. In rural settings, women generally do not shake hands, especially with men. Women may sometimes hug themselves as an expression of emotion. Other forms of physical affection for a loved one, especially the opposite sex, are never shown in public.

Perceptions of Time: The concept of time is very flexible. In towns it is not uncommon for people to be an hour or two late; in rural settings, most people are at least that late for occasions.

Pain Reactions: Gambians are generally very emotional. Physical violence is not uncommon, especially in rural settings and among youths. The first reaction to most trauma is that of surprise along with the exclamation, "Woyayo," followed sometimes by intense anger, wailing, and crying, depending on the situation. The death of a loved one is initially accompanied by expression of strong disbelief. Women are generally more open in expressing emotions, especially where death is concerned. The resolution of most trauma is influenced by the family and by cultural, ethnic, or religious perceptions.

Birth Rites: Trained midwives deliver a large percentage of the infants, particularly because of the shortage of doctors. Outside of cities, most children are born with the assistance of TBAs, and even in cities, TBAs may be preferred. Squatting or supine positions are used for childbirth. Several taboos surround pregnancy and birth: not discussing the unborn infant (to prevent danger) and keeping the mother indoors for a week after delivery, followed by a naming ceremony on the eighth day in which a senior male member of the paternal family does the naming amidst a feast, drumming, and dancing. Guests may bring small gifts for the infant and mother if they desire. Some believe that the father must provide the razor blade used to cut the umbilical cord. In many instances, a witch doctor *(maribou)* provides holy verses in small leather pouches that are fastened on a string and worn around the infant's neck for protection. The fertility rate is six children born per woman (one of the highest in western Africa), and the infant mortality rate is very high at 72 deaths per 1,000 live births. Life expectancy is 52 for men, 56 for women.

Death Rites: The Muslim religion generally forbids organ donations or transplants but allows blood transfusions. Autopsies and embalming are uncommon because the body must be buried intact and as soon as possible. Cremation is not permitted. Burial must be simple as the body is washed and wrapped in a white shroud and is rolled in a mat or placed in a coffin awaiting prayers in the mosque or within the compound. The body must be buried in the ground without a coffin. Wailing and sobbing, often by women and children, are common means of expressing sympathy for the bereaved.

Food Practices and Intolerances: Rice is the dietary staple, and bread is almost a universal breakfast. Peanuts are grown for export and frequently are used in traditional dishes. Eating pigs is forbidden. Eating is often from a communal bowl. In large compounds, men, women, and children may have separate bowls. Others are always invited to join in meals. Even if one is left-handed, only the right hand is used for eating.

Infant-Feeding Practices: The newborn is given only warm water on the first day. Breastfeeding starts the second day. Weaning foods such as *sanyo* ("local millet") tend to be low in energy and protein. Families often have goats, but their milk is not commonly used in preparing infant food. Exclusive breastfeeding is still a rare practice.

Child-Rearing Practices: Societal and tribal values, religion, cultural beliefs, and the economy may have a significant impact in "molding" the child.

National Childhood Immunizations: BCG at birth; DTwP at 18 months; DTwPHib at 2, 3, and 4 months; OPV at birth and at 1, 2, 3, 9, and 18 months; HepB at birth and at 2 and 4 months; HIB at 2, 3, and 4 months; measles at 9 months; vitamin A from 6 months to 5 years; YF at 9 months; and TT after first contact and at +1 and +6 months and +1, +1 year. The percent of the target population vaccinated, by antigen, is: BCG (89%); DTP1 (94%); DTP3, HepB3, and Hib3 (88%); MCV (84%); Polio3 (90%); YF (87%); and TT2 plus (91%).

G

BIBLIOGRAPHY

Central Intelligence Agency: *2006: The world factbook, Gambia.* Retrieved September 21, 2006, from https://www.cia.gov/cia/publications/factbook/print/ga.html.

Cham M, Sunby J, Vangen S: Maternal mortality in the rural Gambia, a qualitative study on access to emergency obstetric care, *Reprod Health.* 2:3, 2005.

Goetghebuer T et al: Outcome of meningitis caused by *Streptococcus pneumoniae* and *Haemophilus influ*enzae type B in children in The Gambia, *Trop Med Int Health.* 5(3):207, 2000.

Isatou Jallow Semega- Janneh, Erik Bøhler, Halvor Holm, Ingrid Matheson, Gerd Holmboe-Ottesen: Promoting breastfeeding in rural Gambia: combining traditional and modern knowledge, *Health Policy and Planning.* 16(2):199–205, 2001.

Lienhardt C, Fielding K, Sillah JS, et al: Investigation of the risk factors for tuberculosis: a case-control study in three countries in West Africa, *Int J Epidemiol.* 34(4):914–23. Epub 2005, May 24, 2005.

World Health Organization: 2006: Immunization, vaccines and biologicals. Retrieved September 21, 2006, from http://www.who.int/immunization_monitoring/en/globalsummary/countryprofileresult.cfm?C='gmb'.

http://www.fco.gov.uk Foreign and Commonwealth Office, UK (retrieved February 20 2006).

http://travel.state.gov US Department of State Bureau of Consular Affairs, USA (retrieved August 5 2006).

http://www.dosh.gm/ggfpp/html/project_environment.html Department of State for Health and Social Welfare, the Gambia (retrieved February 20 2006).

http://www.nigeria-aids.org/pdf/AIDS_in_Gambia.pdf (retrieved September 17, 2006).

◆ GEORGIA (GEORGIAN REPUBLIC)

MAP PAGE (799)

Robert O'Donovan Jr and Manana O'Donovan (née Sopromadze)

Location: Part of the former Soviet Union, Georgia is located northeast of Turkey on the eastern shore of the Black Sea. The total area is 67,700 km^2 (26,911 square miles), and the population is more than 4.6 million. Snow-capped mountains, dense forests, fertile valleys, and turbulent rivers that provide abundant hydroelectric power characterize Georgia's topography. The gross domestic product (GDP) per capita is $3,300, with 54% of the population living below the poverty line. The capital is Tbilisi.

Major Languages	Ethnic Groups	Major Religions
Georgian (official)	Georgian 70%	Georgian Orthodox 65%
Russian	Armenian 8%	Russian Orthodox 10%
	Russian 6%	Armenian Apostolic 8%
	Azeri 6%	Muslim 11%
	Ossetian 3%	Other 6%
	Abkhaz 2%	
	Other 5%	

Health Care Beliefs: Acute sick care; traditional. Common colds, especially among children and older adults, are generally believed to be caused by exposure to drafts. Infants and very small children are often swaddled in many layers to protect them. Upset stomachs and headaches are treated with a glass of Borjomi mineral water. Girls and women are actively discouraged from sitting directly on cement or stone because Georgians believe that their reproductive systems will be damaged by the cold radiating from those materials. Nearly all newborns wear an eye-shaped amulet on the wrist or have one hung near their crib to ward off the "evil eye" (the ability of a person to harm others by simply looking at them). Fevers are occasionally treated by wiping vodka or rubbing alcohol on a patient's body or placing a vinegar and cabbage compress on the forehead. Socks are occasionally soaked in vinegar to reduce fever.

Predominant Sick Care Practices: Biomedical, alternative, and magical-religious. Western medical treatment is regularly sought in hospitals and polyclinics. Many people first consult a home-based herbalist because the treatment costs are lower. Georgians may also consult an herbalist if they are not satisfied with their doctor's diagnosis and recommended course of treatment. Informal monetary and nonmonetary payments are the norm and constitute a significant portion of income generated by medical staff. Costs of medications may be considerable. Children younger than 5 years are taken to a doctor for regular examinations, whereas older children and adults usually visit a doctor only if ill. Abortion is relatively common, as it is throughout the former Soviet Union. One 35-year-old woman estimated that her married female friends had each undergone four or five abortions. Persons with a nagging cough often do not seek professional health care. They ask a neighbor or co-worker for their recommendations and may experiment with a wide variety of medications before they consider visiting a doctor.

Ethnic-/Race-Specific or Endemic Diseases: Noncommunicable diseases account for 87% of all deaths, with cardiovascular disease the major cause of noninfectious disability (70%). Active immunization programs have dramatically reduced the number of infectious diseases. However, malaria and fasciola hepatica are endemic, with 160 cases of malaria reported in recent years. In 2000 through 2004, Georgia had the second highest 5-year measles incidence (second only to Moldova). Recent health-risk appraisals indicate that Georgians are in the "very-high-risk" category because of lack of seatbelt use and stressful lifestyles; in the "high-risk" category because of lack of exercise; and in the "moderate-risk" category because of hypertension and smoking. Body weight is comparable to American statistics, but the total cholesterol is lower. Alcoholism and drug addiction are significant problems, but they have yet to be addressed seriously. The Joint United Nations Programme on HIV/AIDS (UNAIDS) estimates the prevalence rate for human immunodeficiency virus (HIV) in adults (aged 15 to 49 years) to be 0.02%, with 5,600 people living with HIV, including fewer than 1,000 women and fewer than 100 children aged 0 to 14. Fewer than 500 deaths from acquired immunodeficiency syndrome (AIDS) are reported. Among HIV cases with a known mode of transmission, 67% are injecting drug users and 28% are infected heterosexually.

Health-Team Relationships: Nurses are expected to take care of tasks such as giving injections or changing surgical dressings. Doctors are responsible for providing a diagnosis, recommending a course of treatment, and administering complicated treatments. During the Soviet period, nurses provided home care for women who had recently given birth or individuals who had undergone serious surgeries. These services were provided as part of the health care system, and only nominal fees were charged. It is possible to access a similar level of care in the capital city despite the fact that the health care system is in disarray, but such services are too expensive for most people. Nurses are educated in 3-year programs in technical colleges.

Families' Role in Hospital Care: Families are responsible for preparing food and attending to patient hygiene. Because the health insurance industry is still in its infancy, families are required to cover the full cost of medications, especially in rural regions. At least one family member is always in a patient's room. Families visit pregnant women by communicating through a window that is usually closed. Hospital rooms are generally shared by at least 2 and sometimes as many as 10 patients.

Dominance Patterns: The head of the family and the central decision maker in most families is the father or patriarch. In social situations, men often dominate group conversations while pairs of women quietly discuss other issues.

Eye-Contact Practices: It is customary for men and women to make eye contact except with individuals whom they are trying to avoid, such as beggars on the street.

Touch Practices: Georgians greet each other with handshakes, hugs, and kisses on the cheek. While waiting in line, Georgians do not hesitate to bump into or occasionally shove the person ahead of them.

Perceptions of Time: Punctuality is not highly valued. In many instances, people's ability to arrive on time does not affect their access to health care. Many doctors do not require an appointment; patients simply show up, get in line, and wait. Even physicians whose offices arrange appointments will require patients to wait well beyond the appointed hour. As long as patients meet with a doctor and obtain written confirmation of the appointment *(spravka)*, they are not penalized at the workplace.

Pain Reactions: Many women (one woman estimated 60%) cry out loudly during labor. This is considered normal behavior, and women who are not particularly loud concern health professionals.

Birth Rites: The fertility rate is 1.42 children born per woman. Most women deliver their infants in a hospital. The infant mortality rate is 18 deaths per 1,000 live births. The pain of delivery is not usually eased with local anesthesia. Family members are not allowed in the maternity ward, and newborns are separated from their mothers except for three or four daily feedings. Both these practices are to ensure a sterile environment for the infant and mother. Women and their infants remain in the hospital for 5 to 7 days, barring any unusual circumstances. Life expectancy is 73 for men, 80 for women.

Death Rites: Most people die at home and are embalmed and prepared for viewing in the home. If a person is ill and dies in a hospital, the embalming and preparation of the body are conducted there. In either situation, the deceased is dressed in formal clothes and lies in state in the home, usually in the living room, where family and friends of the person visit. Often a few personal effects are placed in the coffin and eventually buried along with the deceased. A previously selected item is placed in the coffin and then withdrawn just before it is finally nailed shut. This item is said to bring good luck to the family. No pictures of the person's family members are allowed to be put in the coffin because Georgians believe that the person(s) in the photograph will die shortly after the burial. On the fifth or seventh day after death, the body is removed in a procession that can be quite short (e.g., for an older person, from the home to a waiting hearse on the curb) or very long (e.g., up to 2 km for a young person or for a person whose death was particularly tragic). When the procession concludes, the coffin is taken to a cemetery. The family leaves the site shortly thereafter so that they will not have to watch the actual burial. It is expected (particularly in rural areas) for family members to cry out loudly to show how much they grieve their loss. In fact, professional "wailers" are hired sometimes to increase the show of the family's loss.

Food Practices and Intolerances: Most people eat three times a day and have the largest meal in the evening. The staples of the diet are bread and various cheeses. Vegetables and a variety of fruits are available seasonally. Many Georgian dishes feature chicken or turkey in sauces made with spices and ground walnuts. Georgians believe that eating raspberries or raspberry jam is beneficial for people with a fever.

Infant-Feeding Practices: Breastfeeding is typical, and most women recognize that it is healthy for an infant to receive its mother's milk. Breastfeeding is not done in public; however, if breastfeeding is impossible for medical reasons or a woman chooses not to, formula is available.

Child-Rearing Practices: Parents are responsible for naming their children. They often name them after their own parents and tend to choose the paternal grandparents' names.

National Childhood Immunizations: BCG at birth; DTwP at 2, 3, 4, and 18 months; OPV at 2, 3, 4, and 18 months and at 5 years; HepB at birth and at 2 and 4 months; MMR at 12 months and at 5 years; DT at 5 years; and Td at 14 years. The percent of the target population vaccinated, by antigen, is: BCG (95%); DTP1 (94%); DTP3 and Polio3 (84%); HepB3 (74%); and MCV (92%).

G

BIBLIOGRAPHY

Central Intelligence Agency: *2006: The world factbook, Georgia.* Retrieved September 21, 2006, from https://www.cia.gov/cia/publications/factbook/print/gg.html.

Sabatinelli G: The malaria situation in the WHO European region, *Med Parazitol (Mosk).* 2:4, 2000.

Schengelia R: Georgia, country of ancient medical traditions, *Vesalius Acta Internationals Historiae Medicinae.* 6(1):64, 2000.

UNAIDS: 2006 Georgia. Retrieved September 21, 2006, from http://www.unaids.org/en/Regions_Countries/Countries/georgia.asp.

World Health Organization: 2006: Immunization, vaccines and biologicals. Retrieved September 21, 2006, from http://www.who.int/immunization_monitoring/en/globalsummary/countryprofileresult.cfm?C='geo'.

◆ GERMANY (FEDERAL REPUBLIC OF)

MAP PAGE (798)

Margitta Beil-Hildebrand

Location: Germany is Europe's most populous country and consists of 16 states. This central European country is bordered by Denmark and the Baltic Sea to the north; Poland and the Czech Republic to the east; Austria and Switzerland to the south; France, Luxembourg, Belgium, and the Netherlands to the west; and the North Sea to the northwest. Germany has lowlands in the north, uplands in the central region, and the Alps in the south. The land area is 356,910 km² (137,803 square miles). The largest city is the capital, Berlin, with 3.4 million inhabitants. Other densely populated areas are the Rhine-Ruhr region, and the Rhine-Main area. After World War II, Germany was divided; East Germany was on the frontline of the Soviet-led Warsaw Pact, and West Germany was embedded in Western economic organizations. The end of the Cold War paved the way for reunification in 1990. Germany has made significant efforts to bring the Eastern portion of the country up to Western standards of wages and productivity. The climate is temperate. The population is 82.6 million. The gross domestic product (GDP) per capita is $30,400. Literacy rates are 99% for both men and women.

Major Language	Ethnic Groups	Major Religions
German	German 91.2%	Protestant 31.8%
	Turkish 2.4%	Roman Catholic 32.1%
	Other 6.4%	Muslim 3.6%
		Unaffiliated, Other 32.5%

Germany absorbed two million refugees from Eastern European Countries and the Russian Federation. The country has small groups of ethnic minorities of Italians, Serbo-Croatians, Greeks, Spanish, and about 98,000 Jews.

Health Care Beliefs: Active involvement; health promotion. Germans are actively involved in health care, and health promotion is considered important. Former East Germans demonstrate the same responsibility for health care as the former West Germans as they have adjusted to a Western model of health care based on primary as well as specialist care. Efforts are being made toward early detection of cardiovascular disease, diabetes mellitus, and breast cancer—significant sources of morbidity and death. Over-the-counter treatment with herbal remedies is still common. Considerable attention is being given to equity of access, efficiency, and quality of health care.

Predominant Sick-Care Practices: Biomedical; alternative. Younger people tend to be more conscious of the relationship between diet and exercise and health, and have considerable interest in natural foods, including vegetarianism. Excellent medical care is readily and widely available throughout the country. Other than transplantation services, there are no formal requirements to document waiting lists.

Ethnic-/Race-Specific or Endemic Diseases: Endemic diseases include cardiovascular diseases, especially ischemic diseases. Current health concerns are related mainly to diseases associated with demographic trends, including long-term chronic-degenerative diseases. Traffic accidents are a common cause of injury and death. The high speeds permitted on the Autobahn pose a significant hazard. The German Federal Institute for Communicable and Non-communicable Diseases has estimated the prevalence rate for human immunodeficiency virus (HIV) and acquired immunodeficiency syndrome (AIDS) in adults (aged 15 to 49 years) as less than 0.1 % in 2005. The Joint United Nations Programme on HIV/AIDS (UNAIDS) estimates the prevalence to be 0.1% to 0.2%. About 49,000 people are currently living with HIV/AIDS, including 15,000 women and 300 children aged 0 to 15. Cumulative deaths from AIDS since the beginning of the epidemic are estimated to be 26,000. There were 750 deaths from AIDS in 2004 (including both children and adults).

Health-Team Relationships: Introductory social conversations may not be lengthy; the more direct approach of getting to the immediate issue is common. Patients often address the health professional by title rather than name and may not ask questions because they consider it a challenge of authority. However, information is shared freely, and patient satisfaction is a popular indicator for quality in health care. The doctor is no longer the principal communicator of patient information as nursing care becomes more professional and is partially independent from medical care. Nurses and doctors are working in relationships based on interprofessional competition as well as cooperation. Obstetricians and midwives have a long-standing conflict regarding overlap of their skills and services. As is true worldwide, the combination of high demands and low rewards are associated with burnout in nurses. A recent German study indicates that job demands, demanding patients, and time pressures are the best predictors of exhaustion in nurses. Job factors such as poor rewards and low-trust work relations are most predictive of disengagement from work.

Dominance Patterns: Germany is a fairly egalitarian society, and men and women share the responsibility in decision making at home and work. Women often carry the major responsibilities for child care and household work, even when they also work outside the home. However, unlike many other Western societies, paternity leave in Germany is such that it allows an alternative to the more traditional pattern of women staying at home to care for children.

Eye-Contact Practices: During initial introduction and ongoing conversations, it is important to maintain direct eye contact. For reasons of privacy, all the doors of patient rooms are kept closed and no one on the ward corridors can witness anything that goes on in the patients' private spaces.

Touch Practices: Touch is almost as common as it is in Mediterranean countries; Germans are friendly and hospitable. A handshake is common at the beginning and end of an interaction.

Perceptions of Time: Punctuality is an important concept and tends to be significant in all situations. People are oriented to the present and near future, although older adults have a strong sense of history. Past cultural traditions are also strong in some areas of the country as revealed in local dress and religious holidays. Businesses tend to open and close promptly, and most public transportation and events are on time.

Pain Reactions: Many individuals exhibit strong, stoic behavior, but this varies considerably. If feeling pain is perceived as part of the healing process, it may be tolerated; otherwise, pain relief is desired and welcomed.

Birth Rites: Most births occur in hospitals, although birth houses and home deliveries are becoming more common. The father may choose whether or not to be present during birth. There is a legal requirement that midwives attend births, although this is not true of obstetricians. According to the World Health Organization (WHO), 698,000 deliveries were performed by 9,506 midwives in 2003. Courses for natural childbirth, prenatal care, and postnatal care are very popular. The total fertility rate is 1.4 children born per woman. The infant mortality rate is low at

4.1 deaths per 1,000 live births. The average length of stay in hospital after birth has decreased in recent years to a couple of days. Life expectancy is 76 for men, 82 for women.

Death Rites: Mourning in private is expected after a death. Burials are still common, but cremation is also popular. A delay of 3 days to a week before burial may occur because of bureaucratic paperwork processing. This delay can create problems for Muslims, who prefer to bury the bodies soon after death. Long-term care at home for older adults and terminally ill patients is becoming increasingly popular, particularly as more people want to die at home.

Food Practices and Intolerances: Meat and potatoes are prevalent, although younger people are developing an interest in lighter diets. Breakfast is traditionally rolls, jam, cheese, cold meats, boiled eggs, and coffee or tea, although people are also eating more heart-healthy dishes such as cereal, fruits and muesli. Lunch is the preferred main meal, and working people may eat this meal in restaurants or at work canteens. It often includes meat, fish, dumplings, potatoes and other vegetables, and mixed salads or soups. Dinner is often a lighter meal consisting of food such as sausage, cold meats, cheese, bread, and mixed salads. Beer is the national beverage, and each region has its own beer with a distinctive taste and body. Before Christmas, hot and spicy mulled wine *(gluehwein)* is a favorite. Meals are the time to enjoy discussing social, political, or intellectual issues.

Infant-Feeding Practices: Breastfeeding is strongly encouraged but is often difficult to continue, even though mothers can take up to 3 years of maternity leave. Employers are obligated to provide a place where employees may breastfeed in private.

Child-Rearing Practices: Mild discipline is common. As for most Western societies, reasoning is most commonly used to influence behavior.

National Childhood Immunizations: DTaPHibHepIPV at 2, 3, 4, and 11 to 14 months; DTwPIPV at 9 to 17 years; MMR at 11 to 14 and 15 to 23 months; Td at 22 to 27 years; and varicella at 11 to 14 months. The percent of the target population vaccinated, by antigen, is: DTP1 (96%); DTP3 (90%); HepB3 (84%); Hib3 (92%); MCV (93%); and Polio3 (94%).

Other Characteristics: Privacy, formality, and social distance are highly valued. With reunification, interest in social, political and economic issues for a united Germany is important. Despite the European Union's open border policy, Germany still takes a serious view of recreational drug activity: drug use remains a problem.

BIBLIOGRAPHY

Allen P et al: What are 'third way' governments learning? Health care consumers and quality in England and Germany. *Health Pol,* 76(2):202–212, 2006.

Beil-Hildebrand M: *Instilling and distilling institutional excellence: rhetoric, reality and disparity,* Bern, 2004, Hans Huber.

Demerouti E et al: A model of burnout and life satisfaction amongst Nurses, *J Adv Nurs* 32(2):454–464, 2000.

Dent M: *Remodelling hospitals and health professions in Europe: medicine, nursing and the state,* Basingstoke, 2003, Macmillan.

OECD: *Health care at a glance: OECD indicators,* Paris, 2005, OECD.

Schulte-Peevers A et al: *Germany,* Victoria, 2004, Loneky Planet.

European Observatory in Health Systems and Policies: Health Care in Transition—Germany: Retrieved November 9, 2005 from http://www.euro.who.int/Document/E85472.pdf

Federal Health Reporting Data Base: Retrieved November 30, 2005 from http://www.gbe-bund.de

Federal Institute for Communicable and Non-communicable Diseases: Retrieved December 1, 2005 from http://www.rki.de/cln_011/nn_527010/DE/Content/InfAZ/H/HIVAIDS/Epidemiologie/Daten__und__Berichte/Eckdaten200412.html__nnn=true

Federal Ministry of Health: Retrieved November 30, 2005 from http://www.bmgs.bund.de

OECD: Retrieved November 30, 2005 from http://stats.oecd.org/wbos/viewhtml.aspx?QueryName=9&QueryType=View&Lang=en

UNAIDS 2006 Germany: Retrieved September 21, 2006 from http://www.unaids.org/en/Regions_Countries/Countries/germany.asp

World Health Organization: World Health Report 2005: Retrieved November 30, 2005 from http://www.who.int/whr/2005/annex/indicators_country_g-o.pdf (Retrieved November 30, 2005).

World Health Organization 2006: Immunization, Vaccines and Biologicals. Retrieved September 21, 2006 from http://www.who.int/immunization_monitoring/en/globalsummary/countryprofileresult.cfm?C='deu'

World Health Organization: Midwives: Retrieved November 30, 2005 from http://www.who.int/globalatlas/dataQuery/default.asp

G

◆ GHANA (REPUBLIC OF)

MAP PAGE (800)

Akosua K. Darkwah

Location: The West African nation of Ghana was the first colonial African country to gain its independence in 1957. Located only a few degrees north of the Equator, Ghana is bordered by the Ivory Coast on the west, Burkina Faso on the north, Togo in the east, and the Gulf of Guinea to the south. The total area is 238,537 km^2 (92,100 square miles). The population is 22.4 million. The gross domestic product (GDP) per capita is $2,500, with 31% below the poverty line. The vast majority of the population is Black African (99.8%), and there is a diverse mix of languages, religions, and ethnic groups. Literacy rates are 83% for men, 67% for women.

Major Languages	Ethnic Groups	Major Religions
English (Official)	Akan 49%	Indigenous 8.5%
Akan	Moshi-Dagbon 17%	Muslim 15.9%
Moshi-Dagomba	Ewe 13%	Christian 68.8%
Ewe	Ga-Dangme 8%	Other religion 0.7%
Ga	Other 14%	No religion 6.1%

Health Care Beliefs: Active involvement; traditional. Illnesses are often thought to have a spiritual origin or component and therefore to need a magical or quasi-religious treatment. Traditional beliefs typically coexist with more modern medical concepts (e.g., germ theory). Typical Ghanaians have a limited understanding of mental health issues. A public-sector system of psychiatric wards in district hospitals is inadequate by Western standards. Stigma is associated with mental illness, occasionally resulting in abandonment of mentally ill people by their family.

Predominant Sick-Care Practices: Biomedical; magical-religious. Ghana has a complex health system comprising a formal modern public sector under the Ministry of Health, a nonprofit sector of local institutions and Christian missions, a small and modern private sector of providers and pharmacies, a widespread and informal private sector that includes various traditional healers, and an informal private sector of kiosks and sellers that support the practice of self-diagnosis and treatment. Herbs, amulets, dolls, and prayer are commonly used in attempts to alleviate suffering or cure diseases. As with other health problems, treatment for mental illness can involve combinations of modern medical care, traditional medicine, and self-diagnosis and self-treatment. In recent years, increases in alcoholism and substance abuse have exacerbated mental health problems.

Ethnic-/Race-Specific or Endemic Diseases: Common diseases include cholera, typhoid, pulmonary tuberculosis, anthrax, pertussis, tetanus, chickenpox, yellow fever, measles, infectious hepatitis, trachoma, malaria, and schistosomiasis. Other diseases include dracunculiasis (guinea worm), dysentery, onchocerciasis (river blindness), pneumonia, dehydration, poliomyelitis, and various sexually transmitted infections. Malaria and measles are the leading causes of premature death. Most preventable deaths (i.e., more than 75%) are caused by water-borne vectors. Results from the Ghana Demographic and Health Survey (2003) indicate the prevalence rate of human immunodeficiency virus (HIV) and acquired immunodeficiency syndrome (AIDS) in adults (aged 15 to 49 years) to be 2.2% (2.7% for women and 1.5% for men). About 340,000 adult Ghanaians (180,000 women and 160,000 men) are living with HIV/AIDS, as well as 14,000 to 25,000 children aged 0 to 15. About 210,000 children aged 0 to 17 have lost at least one parent to AIDS. Knowledge about HIV/AIDS is nearly universal, but knowledge about transmission and prevention is poor. Fewer than half of women and three fifths of men know that AIDS cannot be transmitted by supernatural means.

Health-Team Relationships: Doctors are dominant in health care, and relationships among providers tend to be quite hierarchical. Patients seeking care from modern facilities are expected to submit to the provider's plan.

Families' Role in Hospital Care: A family member or members typically accompany a patient in the hospital. Family members visit as allowed and often cook and clean for the hospitalized person. Family members are important links to the world outside the hospital. Often, drugs or medical supplies required for treatment are not available, so family members must find and purchase them before treatment can proceed.

Dominance Patterns: Religion and culture, which are widely diverse, affect family organization. Muslims accept polygamy, whereas Christians tend officially to favor a pattern of monogamy. Families are typically patriarchal, although the Akans are matrilineal. Socialization patterns are often determined by sex. Respect for elders and support for extended families remain the norm, although this support has weakened in recent years.

Eye-Contact Practices: Staring is considered rude, although direct eye contact is used in conversation. Traditionally, children are expected to respect their elders and may avoid eye contact as a sign of deference.

Touch Practices: Men and women in a relationship are expected to be reserved about their feelings for each other, and traditionally they do not touch or kiss in public. At the same time, public touching among members of the same sex (e.g., holding hands while walking or conversing) is common and not assumed to have sexual overtones.

Perceptions of Time: Time perception is typically event oriented rather than time oriented. Continuing social interactions until an event is complete is considered more important than being punctual for another event.

Pain Reactions: Commodity shortages in health facilities may result in a complete lack of analgesics or use of an available but suboptimal analgesic. Outside of health facilities, self-diagnosis and self-treatment, often combined with advice from traditional healers, family, friends, or market sellers, may result in the use of inappropriate or ineffective analgesics.

Birth Rites: The fertility rate is four children born per woman. A little more than half of the births take place at home, whereas the remainder take place in a health facility. Thirty-one percent of deliveries are attended by traditional birth attendants, some of whom have had rudimentary training in Western medicine, some not. Of the deliveries in health facilities, most are attended by nurse midwives. Doctors are present at less than 10% of all deliveries and are usually called only for emergencies. Newborns typically are kept inside for a period after birth until they prove they are healthy and have the will to live. At this point, usually 8 days after delivery, the infant is brought outdoors and formally presented to the gods, the spirits of the ancestors, and society. This ceremony often includes a naming ritual. The infant mortality rate has been declining but is still very high at 64 deaths per 1,000 live births. Infections compounded by malnutrition are estimated to account for more than 70% of deaths among children younger than 5. Life expectancy is 58 for men, 60 for women.

Death Rites: Funerals are an occasion for mourning but also an opportunity to celebrate the life of the deceased. Funeral celebrations are in four parts: a wake preceding the burial (on the decline), a burial ceremony, a funeral ceremony, and a thanksgiving-memorial service. The burial and funeral ceremonies often take place on the same day, a Saturday, followed by the thanksgiving-memorial service on Sunday. In Accra, custom-made caskets representing some significant aspect of the deceased person's life can be commissioned. The costs of funerals can be high, but even the poorest families usually collect the funds to provide a decent burial. A significant part of the cost is recouped through donations provided by friends and family. Anniversaries of deaths are also important and may be marked by remembrance events.

Food Practices and Intolerances: The norm is to eat three meals per day; the evening meal is the most important. Common foods include cassava, yams, millet, corn, plantains, and rice. Most Ghanaians appreciate spicy foods. Meat, fish, and vegetables are commonly part of meals. Although the concept of dessert is not familiar in the traditional setting, seasonal fruits are eaten fairly often. Generally, the right hand is used to eat because the left hand is used to wipe the body after elimination. Malnutrition is quite widespread, especially among young children. In some situations, females have less access to food than males. According to the Ghana Demographic and Health Survey, access to safe water has improved in recent years and is available to approximately 75% of the population, although an urban (87%) and rural (63%) differential remains.

Infant-Feeding Practices: Breastfeeding for the first 18 months is nearly universal; 86% of children younger than 18 months continue to breastfeed even after the introduction of weaning foods. Breastfeeding steeply declines at about 2 years, and at age 3, only 6% of children are still breastfeeding. Only 65% of infants under the age of 3 months are exclusively breastfed. By the time they are 6 months old, only 14% are exclusively breastfed, and by the time they are a year old, only 0.7% are exclusively breastfed. Supplements include milk, water-based liquids, juice, plain water, and complementary foods. By the fourth month of life, 32% of infants are provided with complementary foods made from grains, tubers, animal products, fruits, and vegetables.

Child-Rearing Practices: The extended family passes down traditional values to children through numerous informal mechanisms such as music, stories, and rituals. In general, society considers acts by individuals to reflect the values of the family. Consequently, child rearing tends to emphasize compliance with group norms rather than displays of independence and individuality. Despite a 1994 ban, female genital cutting continues to be practiced among some groups in the northern part of the country.

National Childhood Immunizations: BCG at birth; DPT at 6, 10, and 14 weeks; OPV at birth and 6, 10, and 14 weeks; measles at 9 months; YFV at 9 months; and TT for pregnant women and CBAW. The percentage of the target population vaccinated, by antigen, is: BCG (92%); DTP3 (80%); and Polio3 (81%).

BIBLIOGRAPHY

Central Intelligence Agency: *2006: The world factbook, Ghana.* Retrieved September 21, 2006, from https://www.cia.gov/cia/publications/factbook/print/gh.html.

Ghana Office of West African Affairs/Bureau of African Affairs: Background notes. Retrieved January 28, 2002, from www.state.gov/background_notes/ghana_0298_bgn.html.

Ghana Statistical Service (GSS), Noguchi Memorial Institute for Medical Research (NMIMR), and ORC Macro: *Ghana demographic and health survey 2003.* Calverton, Maryland, 2004, GSS, NMIMR, and ORC Macro.

Ghana Statistical Service (GSS): *Ghana population and Housing Census,* 2000. Accra, 2002, GSS.

UNAIDS: 2006 Ghana. Retrieved September 21, 2006, from http://www.unaids.org/en/Regions_Countries/Countries/ghana.asp.

◆ GREECE (HELLENIC REPUBLIC) G

MAP PAGE (798)

Elisabeth Patiraki-Kourbani

Location: Greece is on the southern border of the Balkan Peninsula in southern Europe. The capital is Athens. Greece is surrounded by the Mediterranean Sea and has an archipelago of about 2,000 islands. It shares borders with Albania, Bulgaria, and Macedonia to the north; Turkey to the northwest; the Aegean Sea to the east; the Mediterranean Sea to the south; and the Ionian Sea to the west. Its terrain is mostly mountainous, with ranges extending into the sea as peninsulas or chains of islands. The total area is 131,940 km^2 (50,942 square miles), and the population is 10.6 million. The gross domestic product (GDP) per capita is $22,200. The number of residents who speak other languages, such as Pakistani and Bulgarian, is steadily increasing. Literacy rates are 99% for men, 97% for women.

Major Languages	Ethnic Groups	Major Religions
Greek (official)	Greek 98%	Greek Orthodox 98%
English	Turkish 1%	Muslim 1.3%
French	Other 1%	Other 0.7%

Health Care Beliefs: Acute care; traditional. The focus is on acute care rather than prevention and is occasionally saturated with religious elements. The Greek Orthodox religion can be very influential; Greeks strongly believe that God gives health and allows illnesses for a reason. Therefore, it is believed that illness may be cured through atonement and forgiveness. Some believe health is promoted by eating certain foods, wearing amulets to protect against the "evil eye" (i.e., the power of a person to harm others simply by looking at them), prayer, good nutrition, and wine. The belief in the protective power of traditional blue beads is becoming less usual, but wearing a Christian cross is common. Many Greeks still use various folk healing practices and home remedies. Preparations of herbs are used as medications, elixirs, ointments, beverages, and plasters. Roots, leaves, flowers, and seeds are used according to their special qualities (e.g., as diuretics, soothers, neuroleptics, stimulants, analgesics). Common preparations include peppermint for stomach pain; chamomile as a soother; cinnamon, zeylanicum, and cloves for the common cold; poultices made with acorus, calamus, and alcohol for alleviation of arthritic pain; willow leaves for constipation; and eucalyptus for bronchitis. In a recent study that explored the use of complementary and alternative medicine (CAM) in a sample of 956 European cancer patients including 81 Greek patients, around one third of patients were using some form of CAM, with only Greeks showing very low levels of use. Herbal medicines were the most commonly used therapy, and Greeks reported the use of a paste made from olive leaves. The low frequency of CAM use observed in Greece (15%) may reflect the lack of availability of many therapies, high compliance with conventional medical treatments, or concealing use of CAM to avoid any conflict of opinion with the health care team. About 30 years ago, mental illness was associated with significant social stigma. Today people with mental illness are easily accepted in social and economic life.

Predominant Sick-Care Practices: Biomedical; alternative; and magical-religious. The biomedical view of illness is replacing more traditional, magical-religious views. However, outside the scientific community, divine punishment and moral transgressions are traditionally considered causes of illness. Although medical care follows the Western model, Christian beliefs are also strong shapers of traditional practices. Greeks tend to withhold diagnoses of serious illness from patients to prevent anxiety, and relatives are informed before patients about their diagnosis. Greeks avoid saying the word *cancer* and prefer to refer to it as "the disease" or "the bad illness." Visiting Christian sites and monasteries is common among people with chronic and serious illnesses and is combined with established medical practices. People may also use massage, wear talismans or charms to discourage evil, and use healing rituals and prayers. Use of over-the-counter drugs, especially vitamins and antibiotics, is widespread.

Ethnic-/Race-Specific or Endemic Diseases: Greeks are at risk for Mediterranean-type G6PD deficiency, β-thalassemia, and familial Mediterranean fever. Common health problems are cardiovascular diseases, trauma from automobile accidents, hypertension, diabetes mellitus, obesity, cancer, and smoking-related diseases. The increasing incidence of cancer and cardiovascular disease in the last 30 years may be attributed to the dietary shifts of a great percentage of Greeks toward Western-style eating. The Joint United Nations Programme on HIV/AIDS (UNAIDS) reports the prevalence of human immunodeficiency virus (HIV) in adults (aged 15 to 49 years) to be 0.2%, with 9,300 people (mostly aged

25 to 44) living with HIV, including 2,000 women and 73 children aged 0 to 14. Deaths from acquired immunodeficiency syndrome (AIDS) are fewer than 100. About 80% of the reported cases are in men, 19% in women. About 67% of HIV-positive children were infected through mother-to-child transmission, and 16% were hemophiliacs infected via blood products. Cases of HIV have been decreasing, and the epidemic is stable. Greece has lower AIDS incidence rates than many countries in Europe and the Mediterranean region.

Health-Team Relationships: Doctors and administrators in the professional environment are usually dominant over nurses. The concept of a health team is practically nonexistent because the authority and expertise of nurses for clinical decision making are not recognized, and nursing needs of patients receive low priority. Multi-professionalism is still an aspiration rather than a reality in many clinical settings, as is holistic care. Poor multi-professional teamwork is a significant barrier to nursing professionalism. Conflict also occurs among nurses because of the diverse educational preparation levels. The Greek physician still plays the major role in provision of information about diagnosis, treatment, and prognosis to the patient, which may put the nurse in the difficult position of having to adhere to an ethical/philosophical position other than her own when communicating with patients about such issues.

Families' Roles in Hospital Care: Because of a nursing shortage, family members are allowed to stay at the hospital to provide practical, social, and psychological support. When a person is seriously ill, a peer or family member stays with the patient constantly. Family members bring in food that satisfies nutritional needs and meets dietary restrictions. It is still common practice that doctors do not reveal the truth of the diagnosis of a chronic disease without the family's consent. Cultural aspects of values and behaviors affect the meaning of illness for both individuals and their families as well as how they cope with a chronic disease. Thus, it is important to mention the close bonds found in a Greek family, especially toward severe problems such as cancer. Withholding the truth from a patient appears common in Greece. Frequently, it seems that caregivers take all the responsibilities and even make decisions on the patient's behalf, and the suffering person remains in ignorance. However, in a recent study, 71% of relatives of advanced cancer patients reported that they would inform their family members about treatment choices.

Dominance Patterns: Although primarily patriarchal, Greek families also have patterns of strong Mediterranean matriarchy. The accepted social norm is to fall in love with a member of the opposite sex, get married, and establish a family. Only 28% of older adults live alone. Love of family and respect for elders are strong values, and extended family relationships are close and supportive. Given the great respect for older adults, most Greeks would never consider institutional care for aging relatives. Regardless, the expanding population of older adults can create many family problems. Strong familial ties are also developed with nonfamily peers from churches and neighborhoods. Family lineage is respected, and children may be named after their grandparents. Marriage rates have decreased, divorce rates have increased slightly, and more women have entered the labor market; however, family solidarity is still very much the norm. Nearly half of all private households consist of couples with dependent children, whereas only 6% of households are single-parent households, the lowest in Europe.

Eye-Contact Practices: Staring in public is acceptable, and direct eye contact denotes interest in and care for the speaker.

Touch Practices: Close physical proximity is maintained during conversations. Patients tend to prefer nurses of the same sex.

Perceptions of Time: Health care providers consider a delay of 5 to 10 minutes for an appointment to be acceptable. For social occasions, it is expected that people will be "fashionably late" (about 30 minutes).

Pain Reactions: Expression of emotions during pain is allowed and even encouraged. Most Greeks freely express their discomfort by using facial grimaces and moaning, but some are quiet and stoic. It is often assumed that someone who does not express pain is not in a great deal of pain. Passive reactions to pain may be common among men who were taught that free expressions of pain are not masculine. Many women do not express their suffering in an attempt to spare their families from worry.

Birth Rites: The infant mortality rate is 5.43 deaths per 1,000 live births. Doctors deliver the majority of infants in hospitals. Some Greeks celebrate the birth of a son more than a daughter because of the desire to pass on the family name. The fertility rate is 1.34 children born per woman. Life expectancy is 77 for men, 82 for women.

Death Rites: With its roots in the ancient Greek language, the word *end* *(telos)* has two meanings: termination and purpose. The important role of death in Greek culture has caused strict customs to be performed throughout the centuries in order for grief to be resolved. Families and friends of the dying person respond to death with mourning and wails, depending on their education, religious faith, and cultural standards. In modern Greece, beliefs relating to grief and death are based on ancient and Christian traditions. In large cities, people find it difficult to embrace traditional burial rituals. In villages, support from the local community allows greater self-expression and manifestations of grief and mourning. As a result of increased life expectancy, smaller family units, and older people living alone, death has been moved into the hospital; thus, confession and Holy Communion often take place in that setting. People who are dying may be physically isolated from the outside world, and knowledge of their terminal diagnosis may be withheld. Close relatives travel vast distances to visit a dying person or attend a funeral. When a person is dying at home, friends, relatives, and family members gather at the bedside to pray. Icons depicting the saint after whom a person was named or one associated with the local church are commonly placed near the body. A relative or older woman washes the body with water or wine, and the body is wrapped in white cloth and placed in a coffin. When a young girl dies, it is common for her to be dressed as a bride. Coffins are often left open in church, and the face of the deceased may be kissed by friends and family. Burial in the family's traditional burial ground is preferred. Most bereaved women wear black, but the length of time they wear it varies. Rural women usually wear black for the rest of their lives. Men wear an armband or black tie for 40 days and may not shave. Rituals are not concluded until the body has been exhumed 5 years later and the bones have been placed in an urn or vault. Organ donation is legal and is gradually receiving greater acceptance. Some pagan (ancient Greek) traditions such as food offerings blend with Christian traditions.

Food Practices and Intolerances: Greeks typically eat three meals a day. Most have a light breakfast of coffee or milk and cookies. The main meal is lunch (about 3:00 PM), and dinner is usually between 8:00 and 9:00 PM. Fasting during certain periods of the year is practiced for religious reasons; for example, on certain holy days, Greeks do not consume meat, fish, milk, or eggs. During religious holidays, the extended family is usually invited to the grandparents' home for a meal. Greeks still follow the typical Mediterranean diet, characterized by numerous grains, vegetables, fruit, and a low intake of saturated fats. Sugar and fat intakes have increased, especially monounsaturated olive oil. Adults traditionally consume alcohol in moderate quantities during recreational activities and meals.

Infant-Feeding Practices: Most children are delivered in maternity hospitals, where about 77% of mothers begin breastfeeding. It is estimated that 47% are still breastfeeding at the end of the first month, 23% at the third month, and 5% by the sixth month. Introduction of foods depends on the infant's growth but usually starts at the sixth month, with fruits, vegetables, meat, eggs, and fish being introduced during the next few months. Mothers consider it an obligation to breastfeed their children.

Child-Rearing Practices: Parents are frequently overprotective of daughters, and all children depend heavily on their families. After 40 days, infants are moved from their parents' bedroom into their own. Child rearing is permissive, and spanking is not allowed but may be threatened. Mothers are responsible for most of the discipline.

National Childhood Immunizations: BCG at 6 years; DTwP at 2, 4, 6, and 18 months and at 4 to 6 years; HepB at birth and at 2 to 4 and 6 to 18 months; Hib at 2, 4, 6, and 12 to 15 months; IPV at 2, 4, and 18 months and at 4 to 6 years; MMR at 15 months and at 4 to 6 years; OPV at 2, 4, 6, and 18 months and at 4 to 6 years; Td at 14 to 16 years, after 18 years, and every 10 years thereafter. The percent of the target population vaccinated, by antigen, is: BCG, DTP3, HepB3, and Hib3 (88%); DTP1 (96%); and Polio3 (87%).

BIBLIOGRAPHY

Central Intelligence Agency: *2006: The world factbook, Greece.* Retrieved September 21, 2006, from https://www.cia.gov/cia/publications/factbook/print/gr.html.

Ministry of Health and Welfare: Half yearly edition of Hellenic Centre for Infectious Diseases Control (HCIDC), *HIV/AIDS Surveillance in Greece.* 20, June 2005.

Molassiotis A, Fernadez-Ortega P, Pud D, et al: Use of complementary and alternative medicine in cancer patients: a European survey, *Ann Oncol.* 16(4):655–663, 2005.

Mystakidou K: Interdisciplinary working: a Greek perspective, *Palliat Med*, 15:6 7-8, 2001.

Mystakidou K, Parpa E, Tsilika E, Kalaidopoulou O, Vlahos L: The families evaluation on management, care and disclosure for terminal stage cancer patients, *BMC Palliat Care*. 1:3, 2002.

Mystakidou K, Tsilika K, Parpa E, Katsouda E, Vlahos L: Death and grief in the Greek culture, *Omega*. 50(1):23–34, 2004.

UNAIDS: 2006 Greece. Retrieved September 21, 2006, from http://www.unaids.org/en/Regions_Countries/Countries/greece.asp.

World Health Organization: 2006: Immunization, vaccines and biologicals. Retrieved September 21, 2006, from http://www.who.int/immunization_monitoring/en/globalsummary/countryprofileresult.cfm?C='grc'.

http://www.keel.org.gr (retrieved September 1, 2006).

G

◆ GRENADA

MAP PAGE (796)

Cheryl Cox Macpherson

Location: Grenada is one of the Windward Islands at the southern end of the Caribbean. Within a 100-mile radius are the neighboring islands of Barbados to the east, St. Vincent and the Grenadines to the north, Trinidad to the south, and the Venezuela and Guyana coastlines to the west. Grenada is 35 km long (22 miles), with a total area of 340 km^2 (131 square miles). The population is 95,000. Most Grenadians live in and around the capital of St. George's at the southern end of the island. Areas outside of St. George's are more rural and often referred to as "the country." The gross domestic product (GDP) per capita is $5,000, with 32% living below the poverty line. In 2004, Hurricane Ivan destroyed 90% of the homes, hotels, businesses, schools, and government buildings; the long-term impact of this storm on Grenada's citizens is not known. The literacy rate is 98% for both men and women.

Major Languages	**Ethnic Groups**	**Major Religions**
English (official)	Mainly Black African descent	Roman Catholic 60% Anglican 20% Other 20%

Health Care Beliefs: Traditional; some health promotion. It is widely believed that hot, cold, and wet conditions cause illnesses that can lead to death. Grenadians avoid rain and do not let children play in the rain. Some do not touch water (which is cold and wet) after ironing (which is hot) until the next day. Some children believe that intestinal worms are caused by certain foods such as "corn curls." Traditional herbal medicine ("bush medicine" or "the bush") is based on local plants that are boiled into teas. People learn about these remedies from relatives and friends. Some Grenadians avoid bush medicine, but others use it to manage temporary or chronic illness (like colds or hypertension) or to supplement conventional biomedical treatments. Some older people drink bush tea regularly for general well-being. Imported vitamins and complementary medicines seem to be widely used. Imported "noni" products are available, and the noni plant grows locally. A locally produced analgesic spray made with nutmeg oil is available. A drink made from the bark or root of a local tree *(bois bande)* is used as an aphrodisiac, and patients sometimes present with genital symptoms attributed to its use. Certain foods and bush teas are believed to cure cancer.

Predominant Sick-Care Practices: Biomedical, religious, and traditional herbal medicine. Biomedical clinics staffed primarily by community nurses are available free of charge in each parish. The main hospital was expanded and modernized in 2003, but no intensive care or dialysis is available. Recently, a small charge has been implemented. Diabetes, hypertension, and trauma are managed effectively, but procedures like magnetic resonance imaging, or MRI, and dialysis are unavailable. There is one small private hospital. People tend to seek diagnosis or treatment abroad for cancer and ailments that cannot be managed effectively in Grenada. Some pay for their travel and treatment, whereas others take loans to cover the cost. Sometimes the government negotiates payment for treatment in neighboring island nations. Many use bush medicine along with conventional medicine; some use it if they cannot afford to pay for conventional medicine. A few prefer bush medicine because of their traditional beliefs.

Ethnic-/Race-Specific or Endemic Diseases: Seroprevalence for Dengue fever type 2 is 93%. Hypertension and diabetes are prevalent and are major contributors to morbidity and mortality. Prevalence for sickle cell trait is 9%. Rheumatic fever (RF) incidence was high before 2000, when a collaborative eradication project involving WINDREF, the Grenada Heart Foundation, Grenada's Ministries of Health and Education, and Rockefeller University significantly reduced incidence. Morbidity affects many pre-existing RF patients. Seroprevalence of toxoplasmosis in pregnant women under age 40 is 50%; in cats, seroprevalence is 30%. Intestinal protozoans have a prevalence of 4% in conjunction with *Cryptosporidium,* and 30% in conjunction with *Giardia* and *Entomeba.* Prevalence of intestinal nematodes is low. Human lymphotrophic T-cell virus (HTLV-1) prevalence is 4% in the general population and 8% in pregnant women. HTLV-1 causes tropical spastic paresis and severe morbidity. It is transmitted vertically and is often fatal. Prevalence of anemia among 1-year-olds was 57% in 1999 but is low among antenatal and postnatal women. Rabies is present in wildlife, and immunizations are routine for livestock and household pets; however, there is occasional human exposure. Hearing loss is expected to increase because people are exposed to extremely loud music for prolonged periods at public and private events. Human immunodeficiency virus (HIV) and acquired immuno-deficiency syndrome (AIDS) prevalence remains low. From 1996 to 2000, there were 121 new cases of HIV, including 43 acquired immunodefi-ciency syndrome (AIDS) cases and seven pediatric cases, each infected through vertical transmission. The male-to-female ratio for infected persons is 2.6 to 1. The AIDS unit within the Ministry of Health promotes condom use. Other sexually transmitted diseases included 47 cases of gonorrhea in 2000.

Health-Team Relationships: The team involves doctors trained abroad and nurses trained locally in a 3-year undergraduate program. Most doctors are employed by the government while also in private practice. There is a government pharmacy at the main hospital and numerous private pharmacies. The National Council for the Disabled tries to assist those with mental and physical disabilities, but social services and techni-cal support for patients with any condition are extremely limited by the scarcity of resources. There are no trained physical therapists.

Families' Role in Hospital Care: Families are expected to supplement food, drink, bed linens, and toilet paper for hospitalized patients. Nursing staff generally accept the presence of family members, but this varies with individuals. Visiting hours are restricted, even for young children.

Dominance Patterns: Women are often heads of households, but men are dominant when present.

Eye-Contact Practices: Direct eye contact is acceptable.

Touch Practices: Handshakes or other forms of touch occur commonly. Kissing and hugging are less frequent.

Perceptions of Time: In businesses and workplaces, people are gener-ally on time. Entertainment and social events typically begin 1 or 2 hours later than scheduled. Grenadians are relaxed about time. One widely used phrase is "just now," which translates to non-Grenadians as "not now."

Pain Reactions: Strong narcotics are seldom prescribed, even for the terminally ill. Patients in severe pain turn to prayer and spirituality for com-fort. Some patients with terminal diseases refuse pain medications to avoid side effects or because they believe suffering is part of life and is spiritually cleansing.

Birth Rites: The fertility rate is 2.34 children born per woman. About 80% of pregnant adult women attend prenatal clinics in community health facilities and are seen primarily by a nurse. The Grenada Planned Parenthood Association provides services to more than 1,000 women annually. Teen pregnancy and unwed mothers are socially accepted, but they are not permitted to return to public school after their babies are born. Some infants are delivered by a midwife at home or in a "maternity home," where women stay overnight. The infant mortality rate is 14 deaths per 1,000 live births. Life expectancy is 63 for men, 67 for women.

Death Rites: Many terminally ill people choose to die at home with family or friends as their caregivers, although little or no medical or social sup-port is available. Patients seek comfort from family, friends, and spiritual connections. Some use the term "happy hour" to describe a social gathering held after a funeral. Family members are expected to provide food and drink, sometimes for the entire community.

Food Practices and Intolerances: Grenadians are relying more on fast and junk foods, which are inexpensive and readily available. Grenada has a local Food and Nutrition Council, and government standards govern the sale of fresh meat and fish. Common foods include *calaloo* (which resembles spinach), *provision* (root vegetables), *oil down* (a stew of local vegetables with coconut and dried fish or meat), and *buljol* (dried fish prepared like tuna salad). *Coconut water* from green coconuts is drunk and used in cooking. Various types of beans are called "peas." *Coocoo* is primarily cornmeal. *Macaroni pie* means baked macaroni and cheese. Pumpkin is made into soup or mashed. Cakes, cookies, and juices are heavily sweetened, contributing to weight gain and diabetes.

Infant-Feeding Practices: The Ministry of Health encourages breastfeeding during the first year of life, and most women breastfeed for at least that amount of time. When women say they are giving their infants "tea," they usually mean a bottle or a feeding (but occasionally mean sugar water or a dilute solution of cereal). Solid foods are usually introduced at 4 or 5 months and consist of mashed bananas, potatoes, calalloo, or pumpkin.

Child-Rearing Practices: Conventional marriages, long-term common-law marriages, and single parent homes are all socially acceptable. Extended families are the norm. Many women have several children with different fathers. Typically, children live with their mothers, and fathers often live elsewhere. Some children are raised by women who are distantly related or unrelated, and some are in foster homes or small orphanages. Women often leave their children for a day or weekend with close friends or relatives, who enjoy having them. The term *auntie* may refer to a blood relative but is often used as a sign of respect or endearment. From a young age, children are taught to say "good morning" or otherwise greet adults. It is often said that Grenadians love children. However, people tend to turn a blind eye to violence and child sexual abuse perpetrated by family members and acquaintances. Discipline is stern; a belt, cane, or young tree branch is used to "beat" children as a form of discipline both at school and at home.

National Childhood Immunizations: DT at 4 years; DTwP at 18 months; DTwPHibHep at 6 to 8, 16 to 20, and 24 to 28 weeks; OPV at 6 to 8, 16 to 20, 24 to 28 weeks, 18 months, and 4 years; and MMR at 12 and 8 months. HepB at first contact, +1, +6 months; Td first visit, +1, +6 months, +10 years. The percent of the target population vaccinated, by antigen, is: DTP1(93%); DTP3, HepB3, Hib3, MCV and Polio3 (99%).

BIBLIOGRAPHY

Central Intelligence Agency: *2006: The world factbook, Grenada.* Retrieved September 21, 2006, from https://www.cia.gov/cia/publications/factbook/print/gj.html.

Macpherson CC: Healthcare development requires stakeholder consultation: palliative care in the Caribbean, *Cambridge Quarterly of Health Care Ethics* 15(3): 248-255, 2006.

Pan American Health Organization: Grenada: core health data and selected indicators. Retrieved February 28, 2006, from http://www.paho.org/English/DD/AIS/cp_308.htm.

Windward Islands Research and Education Foundation (WINDREF) at St. George's University, St George's, Grenada. Retrieved February 28, 2006, from http://www.sgu.edu/windref/windref.nsf/index?OpenForm.

World Health Organization: 2006: Immunization, vaccines and biologicals. Retrieved September 21, 2006, from http://www.who.int/immunization_monitoring/en/globalsummary/countryprofileresult.cfm?C='grd'.

◆ GUATEMALA (REPUBLIC OF)

MAP PAGE (795)

Lawrence J. Mathers

Location: Guatemala is bordered on the north and west by Mexico, on the east by Honduras and Belize, and on the south by El Salvador. The country is primarily mountainous, with narrow coastal plains in the south and rolling limestone plateaus and rain forests in the north. The climate is tropical: hot and humid in the lowlands and cooler in the highlands. The third largest country in Central America, Guatemala encompasses an area of 108,890 km^2 (42,042 square miles). Guatemala is the most populous country in Central America: between 13 to 15 million. About 60% are European or Mestizo (mixed Amerindian and European descent, locally referred to as *Ladinos*), and 40% indigenous Amerindian. About 42% of the population is under age 15. The gross domestic product (GDP) per capita is $4,700, and 75% live below the poverty line. Literacy rates are 75% for men, 63% for women.

Major Languages	Ethnic Groups	Major Religions
Spanish (official)	European and Ladino	Catholic 50%–60%
Amerindian	(mixed European	Protestant 40%
languages: 23	and Amerindian)	Indigenous Mayan
officially	60%	and Other 1%–10%
recognized	Indigenous Amerindian	
dialects	40%	
	Other <1%	

Health Care Beliefs: Acute sick care. Most value acute sick care and have a limited appreciation of preventive services, although screening services such as Pap smears and mammograms are becoming more available, especially in urban areas. Ladinos and those living in urban areas tend to be more accepting of Western medicine. Traditional and herbal remedies enjoy widespread use because of cultural familiarity or lack of access to Western medications or treatments. *Curanderos* ("traditional healers") are still sought by many indigenous peoples and some Ladinos. Guatemalans conceptualize health in a framework that categorizes medications and illnesses as either "hot" or "cold." According to this system, "hot" medications must be used to cure "cold" illnesses. Therefore, penicillin (which is considered "cold") could be used to cure a fever (which is "hot") but not pneumonia (a "cold" illness).

Predominant Sick-Care Practices: Many Guatemalans combine biomedical and traditional remedies. Guatemala City, the capital and most populous city in Central America, with more than 2.5 million people, offers a full range of medical services. Although public hospitals are free, they often face serious shortages of basic medications and equipment. Care in private clinics and hospitals is generally adequate for most routine injuries and illnesses, but these must be paid for by the patient. Many prefer private doctors to public facilities despite the cost. Some consider injections more effective than oral medications. Medical care outside the city is limited, although small towns generally have rudimentary health clinics and health outreach workers journey into rural areas regularly to provide immunizations. Medical clinics generally have no appointment system. Many drugs such as penicillin are available without a prescription, and traditional herbs are incorporated into some health care treatments. For example, *nervo forza* is a popular liquid vitamin taken to promote emotional and physical well-being.

Ethnic-/Race-Specific or Endemic Diseases: Endemic diseases include dengue fever, rabies, typhoid, hepatitis A and B, leishmaniasis, leptospirosis, onchocercosis, vitamin A deficiency, and diarrheal diseases including cholera, dysentery, shigella, and others. Sexually transmitted diseases such as gonorrhea, Chlamydia, and syphilis are also endemic. The prevalence of tuberculosis is 106 per 100,000 people, and an estimated 8% are also infected with human immunodeficiency virus (HIV). Travelers are cautioned to avoid buying food from street vendors, salads, uncooked vegetables, and tap water. There is high risk for malaria (prevalent in rural areas at altitudes lower than 1,500 m) in the departments of Alta Verapaz, Baja Verapaz, Petén, and San Marcos, and there is moderate risk in the departments of Escuintla, Huehuetenango, Izabal, Quiché, Retalhuleu, Suchitepéquez, and Zacapa. The World Health Organization (WHO) and Joint United Nations Programme on HIV/AIDS (UNAIDS) estimates that HIV prevalence is 1%, with 38,000 to 130,000 people living with HIV, including 16,000 women. There have been about 2,700 deaths from acquired immunodeficiency syndrome (AIDS). Although sex workers and men who have sex with men are at the greatest risk, about 75% of all cases are transmitted heterosexually. Only about 25% of those needing antiretroviral therapy currently receive it.

Health Team Relationships: The health care system is hierarchical and paternalistic. Doctors generally give orders rather than offering options or advice. Doctors' instructions are not usually questioned by nurses, pharmacists, ancillary health care staff, or patients. *Curanderos* and lay midwives tend to be more informal and personable.

Families' Role in Hospital Care: Especially in public hospitals, both nuclear and extended family are expected to assist with patients' personal needs, such as food and clothing. Family members may sleep on mats around the bed and play a predominant role in medical decision-making, particularly with elderly patients. At hospital discharge, those requiring ongoing assistance are usually cared for by relatives at home. The concept of putting older people in institutions is strongly frowned on.

Dominance Patterns: Family life occupies a central role; families tend to stay close, both emotionally and physically. Traditionally, the mother is looked to for emotional support, and the father provides financially for the family while remaining emotionally distant. In recent years, it has become more common for fathers to be openly involved with their wives and children. Social functions often include the extended family and create a sense of strength and solidarity. A double standard for marital fidelity is widely acknowledged; men expect their wives to be faithful, and women tend to ignore the extramarital affairs of their husbands.

Eye-Contact Practices: In professional, urban or upper-class social settings, direct eye contact is expected. Many Guatemalans living in rural areas tend to avoid direct eye contact, especially with those above them socioeconomically. It is common for indigenous and poor patients to avoid direct eye contact with health professionals. In traditional Guatemalan culture, it is widely believed that a strong person can drain the power or soul from a weaker person by staring, resulting in a condition known as *mal de ojo*. Fever, vomiting, diarrhea, difficulty sleeping, and inconsolable crying are symptoms attributed to this condition. Women, babies, and young children are the most susceptible. A curandero is generally sought out to cure mal de ojo.

Touch Practices: Guatemalans are expressive in their touch practices. Touching is an important part of physical examinations and treatment by curanderos and Western practitioners. For example, if a person's head hurts, it is expected that the curandero or doctor will touch the head. Without appropriate touch during the evaluation, the diagnosis and treatment may not be accepted.

Perceptions of Time: Punctuality is not emphasized. The concept of time is relaxed, especially for indigenous peoples. Guatemalans tend to focus on relationships and events more than hours and minutes. In urban areas and among Ladinos, being on time is more important.

Pain reactions: Guatemalans tend to exhibit greater pain tolerance than many Westerners. Men rarely complain about or seek medical care for pain unless it is severe. Women may consult doctors for lesser aches and pains, but in childbirth they exhibit a remarkable stoicism. Administration of analgesia or anesthesia during labor is not a common practice in public hospitals.

Birth Rites: Only 41% of births are attended by skilled health personnel. The national cesarean section rate is 12%. Traditional midwives with little or no training attend many births occurring outside the hospital setting. In rural communities, the proportion of births attended by midwives is higher than in urban areas. Some midwives are illiterate, and many do not understand basic aseptic techniques and are unfamiliar with basic lifesaving skills, putting their patients at great risk of complications. Indigenous women generally view labor complications fatalistically and express reluctance to receive hospital care even when it is available and medically necessary. The fertility rate is four children born per woman. The under-5 mortality rate is 47 per 1,000. Life expectancy is 68 for men, 71 for women and lower in indigenous populations.

Death Rites: Funeral practices usually follow either Roman Catholic or Mayan traditions or a combination of both. November 1st is the Day of the Dead, when people return to their birthplace to put food, alcoholic beverages, and flowers at the graves of family members and friends.

Food Practices and Intolerances: Traditional foods include fresh maize and flour tortillas, black beans, tomatoes, onions, meat, chicken, eggs, and coffee. Guatemalans generally eat three meals a day, with the largest meal eaten just after noon. Many also enjoy light midmorning and midafternoon snacks. Cornmeal mixed with lime is grilled to make tortillas, a staple of the diet. Fruits such as mameys, pitahayas, mangoes, and jocotes are popular. Tamales (cornmeal wrapped in a banana leaf and steamed), *chuchito* (cornmeal steamed in corn husks), *kakik* (spiced turkey soup), *jocon* (chicken in green tomato sauce), guacamole (avocado puree), and *subanik* (beef, pork, and chicken vapor-cooked in a highly spiced sauce) are traditional dishes. *Bunuelos*, small doughnuts glazed with honey and sprinkled with cinnamon, are enjoyed particularly on feast days.

Infant-Feeding Practices: Breastfeeding is the predominant means of feeding newborns and infants and is widely practiced and accepted even in public areas. Most mothers use breastfeeding not only for nutrition but also to pacify a crying infant.

Child-Rearing Practices: Mothers shoulder the great majority of day-to-day child-rearing responsibilities, and fathers are looked to for discipline and financial support. Although some day-care services are available in Guatemala City, private services are prohibitively expensive and public programs are inadequately funded to meet the overwhelming need. More than 40% of randomly surveyed mothers working in the slums of Guatemala City were caring for their children while working. Elementary education is free and compulsory. Nationwide, 80% of boys and 76% of girls attend primary school. However, only 65% of primary school entrants reach grade 5 and only 23% of children go on to attend secondary school. School attendance rates are lower in rural settings. For those who can afford it, private and faith-based schools (Catholic and Protestant) are available in some areas. On their 15th birthday, girls and their families celebrate the *quinceañero*, a rite of passage marking the attainment of womanhood. The party is often attended in formal attire and accompanied by traditional food, music, and dance. Most children do not leave the family home until they marry, regardless of their age. Living together before marriage is uncommon and frowned on.

National Childhood Immunizations: BCG at birth; DTwP at 18 months and 4 years; DTwPHibHep at 2, 3, and 4 months; MMR at 12 months; OPV at 2, 3, 4, and 18 months and at 4 years; Td booster, women of childbearing age (aged 15 to 49 years) and first contact in pregnancy, repeat at 1 and 6 months and every 10 years; vitamin A at 6, 12, 18, 24, 30, and 36 months. The percent of the target population vaccinated, by antigen, is: BCG (96%); DTP1 (93%); DTP3 and Polio3 (81%); HepB3 and Hib3 (27%); and MCV (77%).

Other Characteristics: Violent crime, including murder, rape, and armed assaults have increased. Poverty, widespread availability of weapons, and overworked, underfunded and at times corrupt law enforcement and judicial systems contribute to an atmosphere of violence; increased around the Christmas and Easter holidays. The Guatemala-Mexico border is known for drug and alien smuggling, with the area of the Sierra de Lacandon and Laguna del Tigre National Parks the most dangerous. Taking photographs of children, especially in rural areas, is risky. Rumors of foreigners stealing children circulate throughout Guatemala and may lead to violence toward strangers.

BIBLIOGRAPHY

Central Intelligence Agency: *2006: The world factbook, Guatemala*. Retrieved September 21, 2006, from https://www.cia.gov/cia/publications/factbook/print/gt.html.

International Food Policy Research Institute: Guatemala: a focus on working women and childcare. Retrieved March 18, 2006 from http://www.ifpri.org/themes/mp14/profiles/guatemalacity.pdf.

Organización Panamericana de la Salud. Manual de epidemiología para periodistas. Retrieved March 28, 2006 from http://www.ops.org.gt/EPC.htm.

UNICEF. At a glance: Guatemala. Retrieved April 25, 2006 from http://www.unicef.org/infobycountry/guatemala_statistics.html.

U.S. Department of State, Bureau of Consular Affairs: Consular information sheet. Retrieved April 20, 2006 from http://travel.state.gov/travel/cis_pa_tw/cis/cis_1129.html.

World Health Organization: Guatemala summary country profile for HIV/AIDS treatment scale-up. Retrieved May 10, 2006 from http://www.who.int/3by5/support/june2005_gtm.pdf.

World Health Organization 2006: Immunization, Vaccines and Biologicals. Retrieved September 21, 2006, from http://www.who.int/immunization_monitoring/en/globalsummary/countryprofileresult.cfm?C='gtm'.

✦ GUINEA (REPUBLIC OF)

MAP PAGE (800)

Carolyn M. D'Avanzo

Location: The Republic of Guinea covers 245,857 km² (94,925 square miles) and is situated along a 320-km (198 miles) coastline with the Atlantic Ocean in West Africa. Guinea-Bissau, Senegal, Mali, Côte d'Ivoire, Liberia, and Sierra Leone are its neighboring countries. The capital is Conakry, home to about 700,000 people. Guinea has a tropical climate with two seasons: wet season from May to November and dry season from December to April. Guinea is divided into four natural areas: lower, middle, upper, and forest Guinea.

Major Languages	Ethnic Groups	Major Religions
French (official)	Peuhl 35%	Muslim 85%
Tribal languages (Peuhl, Malinke, Soussou, Kissi, Guerze, Toma)	Soussou 30% Malinke 25% Guerze, Toma 9% Other 1%	Christian 8% Indigenous beliefs 7%

The population is 9.6 million; about 44% are aged between 0 and 14 years. The gross domestic product (GDP) per capita is $2,000, and 40% are living below the poverty line. French is spoken by 15% to 20% of the literate population, and tribal languages predominate. Literacy rates are 50% for men, 22% for women.

Health Care Beliefs: Acute sick care; traditional. The national health program is based on the principles of primary health care and includes an extensive program of immunization and essential drugs. It plays a central role in disease prevention and health promotion. Mental illness is feared and is thought to be the "work" of evil spirits, such as *marabouts* and *djinna*. A *marabout* is an erudite person with knowledge of the Holy Koran who may use his knowledge in both good and bad ways to influence a person's destiny. A *djinna* is thought to be a powerful and invisible human living in the midst of other persons and may perform either good or bad acts. Given the supposed influence of these beings, it is believed that indigenous healers are more capable of treating certain diseases. Therefore, when patients seem not to be responding to treatment in a hospital, family members often remove them so that indigenous healers may treat them.

Predominant Sick-Care Practices: Magical-religious and biomedical where available. Because of poverty and strong traditional beliefs, modern medicine is often sought only after traditional care has been unsuccessful. The predominant sick-care practice is herbal medicine used by *tradipraticiens*, or indigenous healers. Their acceptance is so strong that there is a Department of Traditional Medicine within the national health program that coordinates their activities throughout the country. The use of different amulets in the shape of a neck, hand, or leg worn under a belt or other clothing is found in all ethnic groups. People also believe that the evil spirits spread diseases, but *marabouts* can counteract them by writing cabalistic formulas on wood in a liquid medium, which is collected and used as a talisman by drinking it or spreading it on the body. This is thought to prevent and heal numerous ailments. Scarification and deeper incisions are made by certain tribes to drain "bad blood" or to cut the invisible ropes put there by witches to retain the patient in the sickness. When a woman is infertile, it is believed that throwing sheep's blood at her, followed by symbolic whipping, will chase away the cause.

Ethnic-/Race-Specific or Endemic Diseases: The most deadly diseases in childhood are malaria, followed by respiratory diseases. Tuberculosis and leprosy are major public health concerns. Geography appears to be a factor in illness in that sickle-cell disease is predominant in Middle Guinea as a result of the high rate of intrafamilial marriages in this population. High levels of goiter are found in Upper Guinea because of a lack of seafood rich in iodine, in addition to poverty. Upper Guinea is also in the onchocerciasis belt, a disease that is responsible for high levels of blindness. Forest Guinea has high levels of schistosomiasis. Guinea's population includes displaced people from Liberia and Sierra Leone who have worsened the status of health in Guinea for more than a decade. Outbreaks of cholera and shigellosis raise the death rate periodically. In the past years, yellow fever outbreaks have resulted in the deaths of hundreds of people, primarily children. Lassa hemorrhagic fever is endemic with a seroprevalence of 14%. Human immunodeficiency virus (HIV) is spreading quickly. The Joint United Nations Programme on HIV/AIDS (UNAIDS) reports the estimated prevalence rate for HIV in adults (aged 15 to 49 years) to be 3.2%, with 51,000 to 360,000 adults and children living with HIV. Prevalence is estimated at 42% in sex workers, and HIV-I seroprevalence may be 40% in urban areas. Prevalence varies by region and is highest in Conakry and Forest Guinea. HIV is spread primarily through multiple-partner heterosexual intercourse. The U.S. Agency for International Development (USAID) reports that the epidemic in Guinea is fueled by unprotected sex, multiple sex partners, illiteracy, poverty, unstable borders, refugee migration and scarce medical services. The United Nations Children's Fund estimated that by 2003 about 420,000 children less than 18 had lost one or both parents to AIDS.

Health-Team Relationships: People generally show respect and confidence toward physicians in particular and to the medical corps in general. There is also great confidence in the skills of traditional healers, and so this same positive relationship is also noted toward tradipraticiens. Nurses are in a subordinate role and usually work in good relationships with physicians.

Families' Role in Hospital Care: The notion of family is very broad, and family ties are strong. Grandparents are part of the family structure, and their advice is prized. They usually have more knowledge of traditional medicine than everyone else and advise family members on the treatment of illness. This often explains why herbal medicines are used initially rather than sending the sick as soon as possible to the hospital. If a person is hospitalized, many people visit and bring food. It is the responsibility of everyone in the neighborhood to visit the person. They are expected to contribute money to help the patient pay hospitalization fees and to cover the cost of food and drugs. This is particularly important as health costs rise and people continue to live in poverty. Patients also may receive talismans, herbal medicines, and amulets in secret during their stay.

Dominance Patterns: The elderly have the most power in all ethnic groups, and males are dominant over females. This pattern remains unchanged regardless of the circumstances.

Eye-Contact Practices: Rules regarding direct eye contact have a great deal to do with status. If an elderly person is speaking, it is impolite to maintain eye contact, and looking down is considered a sign of good education.

Touch Practices: Physical touching, such as hugging and shaking hands, is acceptable among friends and relatives, where there is no risk of any sexual connotation. Tradipraticiens touch their patients in the process of healing ceremonies to chase away pain or illness. Physicians are allowed to touch patients of both sexes, but within the professional context. The patient's permission must be sought, especially if the patient is of the opposite sex.

Perceptions of Time: The fact that people are paid little for the time spent in the workplace is one of the reasons why the notion of time is not strongly considered. Punctuality is not a major issue, so when someone needs to arrive at a particular time, one must constantly insist that it is important to do so.

Pain Reactions: Reactions to pain vary, depending on the cultural context. It is generally acceptable for girls to express pain more than for boys. Different cultural groups also have rules as to what is acceptable or not. For example, when a Peulh woman is delivering a baby, because this group is more introverted, she is expected to handle the pain quietly. When a Soussou woman is delivering, her cries alert the entire neighborhood.

Birth Rites: Having a child after marriage is the greatest wish of most women. When a woman is unable to have a child this is often interpreted negatively: the woman may be thought to be unfaithful or a witch. If she continues to be infertile, the husband may take a new wife; polygamy is accepted, and the culture authorizes up to four wives. Pregnant women avoid bathing in the evening to avoid giving birth to an infant with Down syndrome or a deformed infant. In Lower and Forest Guinea, in particular, but also in other ethnic groups, when a child has conditions such as spina bifida or a frank expression of chromosomal aberration (Djinnna or Seyinye), the child is frequently sent away and given a deadly mixture by a medicine man/woman. A son is usually more celebrated than a daughter, and at the hospital there is an extra fee when the baby is a male. During the pregnancy, certain activities and foods are avoided, which is believed to save the baby from malformations or adopting animal behaviors. Future mothers eat special meals that contain medicinal herbs. Whenever someone is cooking, the pregnant woman is offered food, which is thought to prevent black marks on her baby's skin.

Death Rites: Death is a physical separation and as such is a sad event. The body is cleaned by two or three respectable and trusted individuals and is then buried. Children are often taken away to be disposed of without formal burial. Organ donation is not approved of because the body is supposed to leave the earth intact as it arrived the first day of birth.

Food Practices and Intolerances: Most people avoid eating pork and other animals in which the blood has not been completely drained. However, Forest Guineans eat all kinds of game. The basic food throughout the country is rice. It is crushed so that the outside hull and subsequent vitamins are removed before being washed and cooked, losing important vitamins. The most important source of protein is seafood, and this is affordable by almost everyone. Generally, people eat with their hands.

Infant-Feeding Practices: Breastfeeding is always practiced, except in rare cases of sickness. Certain nongovernmental organizations and the ministry of Health actively encourage it until children are at least more than 6 months old.

Child-Rearing Practices: All adults in the same family and even siblings have the right to educate their children as did their parents. Certain tribes (Tomah, Guerze) send their child to the "sacred forest." This is a secret traditional institution where children receive their final education over a period of years far removed from their parents. Males and females usually are circumcised before 13 years. Corporal punishment is acceptable and the basis of education.

National Childhood Immunizations: BCG birth; DTwP at 6, 10, and 14 weeks; OPV birth and at 6, 10, and 14 weeks; measles at 9 months; vitamin A at 6 months; YF at 9 months, TT pregnant women first contact, +1, +6 months, +1, +1 year. The percent of the target population vaccinated, by antigen, is: BCG and DTP1 (90%); DTP3 (69%); MCV (59%); Polio3 (70%); TT2 plus (76%); and YF (85%).

BIBLIOGRAPHY

Central Intelligence Agency: *2006: The world factbook, Guinea.* Retrieved September 21, 2006, from https://www.cia.gov/cia/publications/factbook/print/gv.html.
U.S. Agency for International Development 2005: Health Profile: Guinea HIV/AIDS. Retrieved June 15, 2007 from www.usa.gov.
World Health Organization: 2006: Immunization, vaccines and biologicals. Retrieved September 21, 2006 from http://www.who.int/immunization_monitoring/en/globalsummary/countryprofileresult.cfm?C='gin'
http://www.fhi.org/en/hivaids/country/guinea/guineaprograms.htm (Retrieved September 1, 2006).

◆ GUINEA-BISSAU (REPUBLIC OF)

MAP PAGE (800)

Anja Poulsen and Adam Roth

Location: The Republic of Guinea-Bissau is one of West Africa's smaller countries. It has a total area of about 93,600 km² (36,000 square miles).

Much of the coastal part of the country is mangrove, whereas the interior is either cultivated or wooded savannah. Guinea-Bissau gained independence from Portugal in 1974. In 1998 and 1999, a military revolt evolved into a complex emergency. The country is still politically and economically unstable.

Major Languages	Ethnic Groups	Major Religions
Portuguese (official)	African 99%	Indigenous (Animist)
Criolo	European, Mulatto	56%
Numerous African	1%	Muslim 35%
languages		Christian 9%

The population is 1.4 million, a third of which live in the capital of Bissau. Almost all of the population is of African descent. The main ethnic groups are Balanta (30%), Fula (20%), Mandinka (14%), Manjaco (13%), Papel (7%), and others (16%). Each group has its own language, but in the urban setting of Bissau, it is Creole—a mixture of Portuguese and indigenous languages—that is most commonly used. Beliefs in witchcraft and sorcery and other forms of spiritual entities are usually intertwined with whatever religion people practice. Guinea-Bissau is a poor country: the gross national product (GNP) per capita is $800, and it ranks 172 of 177 nations using the United Nations Development Program (UNDP) human development index. Literacy rates are 58% for men, 27% for women.

Health Care Beliefs: Acute care; traditional. Three health sectors exist: professional, folk, and popular. They are all complementary and used in combination, particularly in the urban setting of Bissau. The folk sector consists of various types of traditional healers, whereas the popular sector involves "home medicine," which includes self-diagnosing and self-medicating because drugs are sold without prescriptions in pharmacies and local markets. The popular sector also includes the use of homemade medicines consisting of fruits, spices, herbs, and roots. Wearing amulets for health protection is a widespread practice, as is explaining the causes for illness as a result of intervention by ancestors and spirits or attributing illness to witches or sorcery.

Predominant Sick-Care Practices: Biomedical where available; self-treatment and magical-religious. Although access to the professional sector (i.e., hospitals, trained doctors, Western medicine) is available, it is much more difficult to obtain in rural areas. Because of high mortality rates resulting from poor biomedical health care access, most people who are ill tend to seek advice either at a health center from an indigenous healer or at the local pharmacy. The choice depends on where in the country the person lives, the type of disease he or she has, and their financial status. In rural areas, most villages have a "witch doctor." In the capital, the health centers are popular. Indigenous healers are often preferred for treating chronic diseases and psychiatric disorders. Wealthier families go to private clinics. Health centers are placed in larger towns and villages all over the country and in suburbs of the capital. In the countryside, the medical staff includes an analyst and a nurse. In the capital, most of the centers have a medical doctor as well. There is a lack of essential drugs and equipment because of the poor medical infrastructure. Adults can be charged a small fee for consultations: treatment of children and pregnant women is free, but it is common for them to be charged. This practice is accepted because the public wages for health personnel are very low. Drugs, needles, and dressings are usually purchased at local pharmacies or paid for at the health centers. In the countryside, a few smaller hospitals exist, but in the capital, the hospital Simao Mendes receives patients from all over the country. The hospital lacks essential equipment (e.g., oxygen, needles, medicine) and electricity. It is generally accepted that patients should pay for treatments and medicine, often directly to the health staff. About 41% of the population has access to health services.

Ethnic-/Race-Specific or Endemic Diseases: Malaria is highly endemic and can be resistant to chloroquine; yellow fever is prevalent in some locations. Schistosomiasis, bacterial and protozoal diarrhea, hepatitis A and B, typhoid and meningococcal meningitis occur. About 44% do not have sustainable access to an improved water source. In 2004 through 2005, there was a severe epidemic of cholera. Other endemic diseases include human rabies and measles. Childhood mortality for all ages is among the highest in the world. The most frequent causes of death in children are malaria, diarrhea, acute respiratory tract infections, and malnutrition—deaths that could be avoided in a functioning health system. Tuberculosis (TB) is frequent in children and adults. Both TB and acquired immunodeficiency syndrome (AIDS) are stigmatized diseases, which retards communication between doctor, patient, and family. The Joint United Nations Programme on HIV/AIDS (UNAIDS) estimates the prevalence of human immunodeficiency virus (HIV) as 3.8%, with 32,000 people infected, including 17,000 women and 3,200 children aged 0 to 14. There are 11,000 orphans aged 0 to 17 from parental AIDS. About 2,700 deaths are attributed to AIDS. HIV-2 is still more common than HIV-1. There is beginning implementation of antiretroviral treatment for HIV-1-positive persons.

Health-Team Relationships: After independence from Portugal in 1974, doctors were primarily Cuban and Portuguese in hospitals in the capital. At many health centers, nurses or assistant nurses have for many years been responsible for all medical treatment. During the 1980s and 1990s, more Guinean doctors completed their education either in Guinea-Bissau or abroad. Although the health system is hierarchical, nurses and doctors normally collaborate without any major problems, and patients are expected to be submissive and respectful. The nurses and doctors do not usually show empathy toward sick patients. Patients always expect a prescription for oral medications or, even better (from the patients' perspective), medication injections. If Guineans have a nurse or a doctor in the family, they normally seek their advice first. Although the government has clear rules for payment, it is common for health personnel to charge the ill person lesser or greater amounts for the consultation than outlined.

Families' Role in Hospital Care: Families assume responsibility for care of their hospitalized family member. Not only do they assume financial responsibility (e.g., pay for medicine and syringes), but they also care for the patient in terms of their food, water, and hygiene.

Dominance Patterns: Guinea-Bissau is a patriarchal society. In practice, however, the head of a household can be a woman, who assumes responsibility if someone in the household becomes ill. The relationship between men and women also varies according to ethnic group, age, social status, and whether the people are in an urban or a rural setting. People must be respectful of anyone who is older.

Eye-Contact Practices: Direct eye contact is not an issue between sexes or among people from different age or social groups.

Touch Practices: Physical contact between men and women is very rarely seen in public settings, whereas physical contact (e.g., holding hands) among members of the same sex is common. Women in urban settings may greet each other by kissing on the cheek, whereas men shake hands. A man may hold the wrist of a woman in a firm grip. This form of touch does not have sexual connotations but can be a way of conveying that the man has a matter he would like to discuss.

Perceptions of Time: Punctuality is not usually an issue among friends and family members, although if a person is employed, punctuality is more important. Wearing a watch is a sign of status, so it is not uncommon for some young people to wear watches even when the watches do not work. The intensity and position of the sun are widely used as a way to assess the time of day, particularly among people of older generations.

Pain Reactions: Telling a person in pain to *sufri* (suffer) is common. "Controlling the head"—displaying self-control—and controlling emotional expressions are behavioral ideals. Words are considered powerful; therefore, verbal expressions of pain are not always accompanied by the body language Westerners might expect. Being able to express pain verbally and in a controlled way is considered sufficient. This does not mean that people's reactions to pain are never expressed verbally or with body language, but it means that when people are in pain, others may try to calm them in a way that may seem harsh (e.g., by telling them to suffer or stop crying). It is more accepted for women and children to cry; men are expected to suffer stoically. Women often react to and show pain by tying a piece of cloth tightly around their foreheads (*mara kabeca*).

Birth Rites: The fertility rate is 4.86 children born per woman; the infant mortality rate is high at 105 deaths per 1,000 live births. If a woman is giving birth at home, an old woman from the family and a local midwife assist her. In the capital city, half of the deliveries occur at the hospital or at health centers; only the midwife assists, and the family must wait outside. Traditionally, the mother and child were expected to stay inside the house for the first week to avoid harm from wind (or evil spirits); however, this tradition is not strictly practiced today. Some ethnic groups have a feast for the child on the seventh day after birth. The infant receives gifts and is celebrated—and is finally considered a "real" child. Muslims circumcise boys before they begin school. Several other ethnic groups perform circumcisions when boys are 7 to 14 years of age. Men of the Balanta ethnic group have to prove that they are real men before their circumcision, so often a man has several children before the procedure. Traditionally, the circumcision is performed after a period of isolation in the forest, where the rituals of the ethnic group are taught. Girls are usually not circumcised, although Muslims may perform the procedures in rural areas. Life expectancy is 45 for men, 49 for women.

Death Rites: The body is usually buried within 24 hours. If an older person dies, the death is regarded as a happy event, and the family has a feast celebrating the person's long life. The feast lasts for at least a week, and it is the responsibility of the family to provide food and beverages. Funerals are extremely important social events (and in some cases business events) where contacts are maintained or created. It is important for people to attend a funeral if they know any of the deceased person's family members. When a child or a young person dies, it is an unhappy event. Roman Catholics have a mass at a church, and other ethnic groups perform the appropriate ceremonies, in some instances a year later. The size of the funeral represents the prosperity of the family and can be very costly for members of a poor society such as Guinea-Bissau. Muslims normally do not have long funerals. Autopsies and organ donations are generally unacceptable.

Food Practices and Intolerances: Breakfast is not a main meal, and often a little leftover rice from the day before is eaten. If the family has enough money, they may make porridge or fried eggs or have bread and margarine. Rice is the main staple. In the morning, women go to the market to shop for the day's meals and usually buy either a bit of fish, chicken, or meat. Lunch, the main meal of the day, can be eaten anytime between 1:00 and 4:00 in the afternoon. A person who is eating lunch invites anyone who passes to come and eat. This is more of a polite greeting than a real invitation. Different members of the household do not always eat at the same time. They may take turns, and the whole household is divided up according to who eats from the same bowl, divisions that are made according to age, gender, or both. People usually eat with spoons or their hands. If people eat in the evening, the meal is light.

Children may be given some boiled potatoes or soup with spaghetti or porridge. Fruits such as mangoes, oranges, and bananas are eaten as snacks, as are peanuts and cashews.

Infant-Feeding Practices: Infants are breastfed for an average of 22 months. Length of breastfeeding varies considerably according to ethnicity. The Balanta breastfeed the longest, Muslims the shortest. The Balanta often regard colostrum as "bad" milk. In the capital of Bissau, bottle-feeding is a symbol of social status but is seldom used. Supplementary food is introduced at 4 to 6 months, although the age varies according to ethnic group. The most common semi-liquid food is made of rice or corn.

Child-Rearing Practices: Children spend most of their time in or around their family's home. The use of a local form of adoption *(criacon)* is common, so children do not always live with their mother or father. It is common for older siblings to take care of younger ones, and children, especially girls, perform various chores in the house. Children usually sleep in the same room and bed with family members of their own age group until they are in their teens, at which time they sleep only with children of the same age, not the same sex.

National Childhood Immunizations: BCG at birth; DTwP at 6, 10, and 14 weeks; measles at 9 months; OPV at birth and at 6, 10, and 14 weeks; TT women at 15 to 45 years first contact, +1, +6 months, +1, +1 year. The percent of the target population vaccinated, by antigen, is: DTP1 (86%); BCG, DTP3, MCV, and Polio3 (80%); and TT2 plus (54%).

BIBLIOGRAPHY

Central Intelligence Agency: *2006: The world factbook, Guinea-Bissau*. Retrieved September 21, 2006, from https://www.cia.gov/cia/publications/factbook/print/pu.html.

Forest JB: *Guinea-Bissau, power, conflict and renewal in a West African nation*, 1992, Westview Press, Boulder, CO.

Godtfredsen U: *Disease perceptions and therapy strategies*, Interim Report no. 2, Guinea-Bissau, 1995, Projecto Saude de Bandim, Bissau.

Kovsted J, Tarp F: Guinea-Bissau: war, reconstruction and reform, Working Papers no. 168, Helsinki, Finland, 1999, UNU World Institute for Development Economics Research. Retrieved January 25, 2006, from www.ui.se/fakta/afrika/guineabi.htm.

Norrgren H: *Personal communication*, January 16, 2006.

Sodemann M, Aaby P, eds: Bandim Health Project 1978-2003. *Improving child health?* The Bandim Health Project, Denmark, 2003, pp. 13–21.

UNAIDS: 2006 Guinea-Bissau. Retrieved September 21, 2006, from http://www.unaids.org/en/Regions_Countries/Countries/guineabissau2.asp.

UNDP, HDR. Human Development Reports, 2003-2005, Retrieved January 16, 2006, from http://hdr.undp.org/reports.

World Health Organization: 2006: Immunization, vaccines and biologicals. Retrieved September 21, 2006, from http://www.who.int/immunization_monitoring/en/globalsummary/countryprofileresult.cfm?C='gnb'.

◆ GUYANA (COOPERATIVE REPUBLIC OF)

MAP PAGE (797)

Carolyn M. D'Avanzo

Location: Formerly British Guiana, the country is located on the northern coast of South America. The North Atlantic Ocean is to the north, Suriname to the east, Brazil to the south and Venezuela and Brazil to the west. Guyana has rolling highlands, a low coastal plain, and savannah in the south. An extensive network of rivers runs from north to south. The climate is tropical: hot and humid, moderated by northeast trade winds. Guyana has two rainy seasons: May through mid-August, and mid-November to mid-January. The total area is 214,970 km^2 (83,000 square miles). The low coastal areas are inhabited by 90% of the population of 767,245. The capital is Georgetown. Guyana has a gross domestic product (GDP) per capita of $4,600. About 62% of the population lives in rural areas. Literacy rates are 99% for both men and women.

Major Languages	Ethnic Groups	Major Religions
English	East Indian 51%	Christian 50%
Amerindian dialects	Black African 30%	Hindu 33%
Hindi	Mixed 14%	Muslim 9%
Urdu	Amerindian 4%	Other 8%
	European and Chinese 1%	

African slaves were brought to Guyana to work the sugar plantations, followed by workers from the Indian subcontinent. These groups make up the majority of the population. Each ethnic group has retained its own culture and lifestyle and has strong African and Indian traditions. Guyana more closely resembles the islands of the West Indies rather than South America in terms of history, culture, and economic characteristics. Guyana is tolerant of religious diversity. For example, Indians may be baptized as Christians and continue to participate in Hindu rituals.

Health Care Beliefs: Acute sick care; traditional; limited prevention. Some prevention procedures are practiced, such as blood pressure checks for individuals with hypertension. However, most visits to doctors are because of sickness. People believe in the "evil eye" as a cause of illness (the power of a person to harm others merely by looking at them), especially for infants and children. A particular brownish yellow soaplike substance or oil is rubbed on the clothes of infants; the strong smell is thought to keep illness away. When adults believe they might have been affected by the evil eye, they frequently go to a priest (if they are Hindu), who tells them which prayers they should recite to thwart the evil actions.

An amulet in the shape of the number three with another inverted three on top is also held or worn to prevent evil or sickness.

Predominant Sick-Care Practices: Limited biomedical and magical-religious. The government provides a considerable amount of social assistance in the form of old-age pensions and relief for destitute or infirm children. The public health system has been successful in eradicating malaria as an endemic disease. Medical care is available for minor health conditions, but the individual must pay for doctor's visits and hospital care. Emergency care for major medical illnesses or surgery is available but limited because of a lack of appropriately trained specialists, outdated diagnostic equipment, and poor sanitation. Ambulance service is substandard and may not be available when needed for emergencies. Some prescription medicines (mostly generic) are available in the country, but many cannot be obtained.

Ethnic-/Race-Specific or Endemic Diseases: Endemic diseases include filariasis, dengue fever, cutaneous leishmaniasis, and intestinal parasites. Chloroquine-resistant malaria has been eliminated as an endemic disease but remains a risk. People are at risk for diabetes mellitus, yellow fever, and leprosy. Water pollution from sewage and agricultural and industrial chemicals poses a health risk. The Joint United Nations Programme on HIV/AIDS (UNAIDS) estimates the prevalence rate for human immunodeficiency virus (HIV) in adults (aged 15 to 49 years) to be 2.5%, with 12,000 people living with HIV, including 6,600 women and fewer than 1,000 children aged 0 to 14 years. About 1,200 deaths are attributed to acquired immunodeficiency syndrome (AIDS). While there is little specific information available, it is known that by 1997, 44% of sex workers tested in Georgetown were HIV positive. Only 50% of infected people are receiving antiretroviral therapy, and only 18% of pregnant women with HIV are receiving antiretroviral therapy to reduce mother-to-child transmission.

Health-Team Relationships: Doctors and nurses seem to respect each other. Most people, especially those outside of cities, see private doctors rather than go to hospital clinics because of the distance to health care facilities. Doctors head the health care team, and nurses primarily provide personal care and specified treatments.

Families' Role in Hospital Care: Family members visit often and may stay with friends or family near the hospital so that they can be there early in the morning to assist their relative. It is common to bring in homemade food, even though the hospital provides food. Families make an effort to consult with health personnel so that they can bring food appropriate for the patient's medical condition.

Dominance Patterns: Men are considered the head of the household, but most consult with their wives about important decisions. Most women do not work outside the home and assume the major responsibilities for the children and household.

Eye-Contact Practices: Although children have much respect for their parents, direct eye contact is usual and acceptable. Children may also maintain direct eye contact with older adults. When children meet older adults on the street, they are expected to greet the adults politely (rather than ignore them) out of respect, regardless of whether they know them.

Touch Practices: People who know each other well commonly kiss each other in greeting or hug or shake hands. It is common for men and women to shake hands, and a handshake is the usual greeting when meeting someone for the first time.

Perceptions of Time: People look to the future, but past traditions are very important.

Pain Reactions: It is acceptable for both men and women to express pain. Men are not usually as open about the pain they are experiencing and seldom cry out. Regardless, many individual variations exist. Some women are quite stoic and silent about pain, and some men are very expressive.

Birth Rites: The fertility rate is two children born per woman. Infant mortality rates are high at 32 deaths per 1,000 live births. On the first day of an infant's birth, Hindu families go to a priest and tell him the day and time of the infant's birth. Consulting a book, the priest picks a name for the infant. A bracelet of black and white beads is put on the infant's ankle as quickly as possible to protect against the evil eye. A small black dot may also be put on the forehead of the infant for extra protection. Mother and infant usually stay at home in bed for 9 days while either a sister or older family member takes care of them. Family and friends are allowed to visit. On the ninth day, the mother says prayers privately, and mother and child go outdoors for the first time for a party with friends and family. Life expectancy is 63 for men, 69 for women.

Death Rites: Family members gather to say their final goodbyes to a person who is dying. During and after the dying process, Christians and Hindus stay up most of the night singing hymns and saying prayers to sympathize with the family. As a rule, Hindus favor cremation and Christians favor burial, but some Hindus bury and some Christians cremate their loved ones. When a person dies in the hospital, the funeral home is called to take the body for immediate cremation or to the person's home. If the body is brought home, a special metal coffin with a clear plastic area over the head is obtained from the funeral home. The climate is hot, and embalming is not done. During the several days while the body is viewed at home, ice is put under and around the person regularly by the funeral home staff, and the melted water is drawn off. Hindus obtain permission to cremate their loved ones publicly in an open area, such as the beach. Wood and other materials are gathered, and family and friends observe the ceremony. Afterward, those attending stay together for a meal. Prayers are then recited for 12 days. On the 12th day, family and friends have a service and recite additional prayers in memory of the person.

Food Practices and Intolerances: Chicken-fried rice, spicy dishes, curried chicken, yellow peas, and *dholl-puri* (a special bread) are very popular among those of East Indian descent, although people of Black African descent like these foods as well. Black Africans especially like the pepper pot, a combination of beef, vegetables, and rice, or brown stew, a combination of peas and rice with meat. Cooking is done on stoves or outside over open fires. It is common for people to have concrete squares with burners on top and a place for burning wood below, which makes practical sense in this hot country, even for people who live in cities.

Infant-Feeding Practices: Breastfeeding is very common and varies greatly in terms of duration—from 1 month to years. It is also common to breastfeed part of the time and bottle-feed part of the time. As foods begin to be introduced, it is common to make porridge out of green plantains (similar to bananas). The plantains are dried and brought to the mill to be ground into flour that is mixed with cow's milk or formula and occasionally sugar to form a thin gruel. Barley seeds are processed in the same way for infant food.

Child Rearing Practices: Most children attend school. The one source for higher education is the University of Guyana in Georgetown. Children are reared according to the practices of their ethnic group; most children are taught to be respectful to adults.

National Childhood Immunizations: BCG at birth; DTwP at 18 and 45 months; DTwPHibHep at 2, 4, and 6 months; IPV at 2, 4, 6, 18, and 45 months; MMR at 12 and 45 months; OPV at 2, 4, 6, 18, and 45 months; YFV at 12 months. The percent of the target population vaccinated, by antigen, is: BCG (96%); DTP1, DTP3, HepB3, and Hib3 (93%); and MCV (92%).

Other Characteristics: Guyana is a trans-shipment point for narcotics from South America, primarily from Venezuela, to Europe and the United States. It is also a producer of cannabis.

BIBLIOGRAPHY

Central Intelligence Agency: *2006: The world factbook, Guyana.* Retrieved September 21, 2006, from https://www.cia.gov/cia/publications/factbook/print/gy.html.

Palmer CJ et al: HIV prevalence in a gold mining camp in the Amazon region, Guyana, *Emerg Infect Dis.* 8(3):330, 2002.

Rawlins SC et al: American cutaneous leishmaniasis in Guyana, South America, *Ann Trop Med Parasitol.* 95(3):245, 2001.

UNAIDS: 2006 Guyana. Retrieved September 21, 2006, from http://www.unaids.org/en/Regions_Countries/Countries/guyana.asp.

World Health Organization: 2006: Immunization, vaccines and biologicals. Retrieved September 21, 2006, from http://www.who.int/immunization_monitoring/en/globalsummary/countryprofileresult.cfm?C='guy'.

http://encarta.msn.com/ (retrieved August 20, 2006).

http://travel.state.gov/guyana.html (retrieved August 20, 2006).

◆ HAITI (REPUBLIC OF)

MAP PAGE (796)

Bette Gebrian and Jean Claude Tabuteau

Location: Located in the West Indies of the Caribbean, Haiti occupies the western one third of the island of Hispaniola, which it shares with the Dominican Republic. The total area is 27,750 km² (10,714 square miles), and the capital is Port-Au-Prince. Much of the mountainous northern soil is denuded. Haiti is known as the poorest nation in the Western Hemisphere. The total population is 8.5 million, and the gross domestic product (GDP) per capita is $1,700, with 80% below the poverty line. Literacy rates are 55% for men, 51% for women.

Major Languages	Ethnic Groups	Major Religions
French	Black 95%	Catholic 80%
Creole	Mulatto and	Protestant 16%
	European 5%	Other 4%
		Voodoo (regardless of their religion, as many as 90% of Haitians believe in voodoo.)

Health Care Beliefs: Passive, somewhat fatalistic role; primarily acute sick care. Some evaluate their illnesses according to symptoms previously experienced by close relatives. Families play an important role in health beliefs and health-seeking behaviors. Herbal infusions are used for common complaints such as upset stomach *(te zebaklou)*, heat rash (*amidon* and *clarin*), and many others; and various teas are thought to be helpful. Some prefer injected medications rather than oral because they believe that injections are more effective in curing illness. Prevention is not a strong concept but can be integrated into family health care with empiric evidence of importance (e.g., rehydration during episodes of diarrhea).

Predominant Sick-Care Practices: Biomedical and magical-religious. Western medical treatment is sought as often as traditional medicine. Belief in the *loa* ("voodoo spirits") is important, as are prayer and the healing power and protection of the Judeo-Christian God. Illnesses that are perceived to originate supernaturally or magically can be treated predominantly by traditional healers. Ethnomedical beliefs about disease are based on maintenance of a hot/cold equilibrium within the body. Herbalists treat common disorders and specialize in the treatment of the "evil eye" (*maldyok*, or the power of a person to harm others merely by looking at them).

Ethnic-/Race-Specific or Endemic Diseases: Chloroquine-sensitive falciparum malaria is endemic, as are all four types of dengue fever.

Vitamin A deficiency is the most common cause of childhood blindness, and umbilical hernias are common. Main causes of pediatric deaths are diarrheal dehydration and bacterial pneumonia. Anemia is rampant, and iodine deficiency is endemic in parts of Haiti. The rate of chronic malnutrition in children under age 5 is the highest in the Western Hemisphere at 23%. According to the Joint United Nations Programme on HIV/AIDS (UNAIDS), the estimated prevalence rate for human immunodeficiency virus (HIV) in adults (aged 15 to 49 years) is 3.8%, and 190,000 are living with HIV, including 96,000 women. Only about 20% receive antiretroviral therapy, and 16,000 deaths have been attributed to acquired immunodeficiency syndrome (AIDS). About 17,000 children aged 0 to 14 are AIDS orphans. A Centers for Disease Control and Prevention (CDC) national seroprevalence study of HIV indicated that 3% of pregnant women in Haiti were positive for HIV infection. Homosexuality is discussed in private, and many homosexuals are married and have children. In the major cities, intense emphasis is on prevention of transmission and reduction of stigma toward people living with AIDS. In some cases, AIDS is considered to be caused by supernatural forces and unrelated to individual behaviors.

Health-Team Relationships: Doctors have primary authority in hospital settings, and nurses and nurse auxiliaries are subordinate. Where nurses are the only source of health care, they function as nurse practitioners and nurse midwives. Patients believe that expert authority should dictate care. Relationships with "granny midwives," who deliver more than 75% of the women, vary. Nontraditional "doctors" have thriving businesses because they are accessible and affordable. Pharmacists are rare, and medicines are sold in boutique fashion. Disapproval with a health care professional is not outwardly expressed, although contact is severed.

Families' Role in Hospital Care: The family is required to provide physical care and food. Some may wait to be told how they can help. *Family* is a loose term that encompasses close friends. Visiting the sick is expected, and friends and families rally around people in need.

Dominance Patterns: Haiti has a matriarchal society. The family is a mutual support system and siblings remain close, even after marriage. Girls and boys receive equal medical attention. Although girls are expected to be more proficient in homemaking skills than boys, women are taking on professional and political roles.

Eye-Contact Practices: It is customary to maintain eye contact with everyone except authority figures and the poor. Children are not supposed to look their parents in the eye and are expected to look down.

Touch Practices: Shaking hands is the customary greeting. Haitians have adopted the French custom of kissing on both cheeks when greeting a friend (but not a stranger). Children kiss one cheek of an adult when they greet them in any situation. It is considered rude for a young man to touch a woman (e.g., put his hand on her arm or shoulder). When a child or adult has a fever or a cold, families warm freshly made castor oil ($15 per gallon) and rub it on one side of the body one day and on the other side the next day. This process is repeated as many times as necessary. Traditional midwives use many traditional rubs for pregnant women.

Perceptions of Time: Punctuality is not an important value. A formal social system of publishing starting times exists in which the real starting time is later than the published time. Hope for the future promotes a future-oriented view; however, society is oriented predominantly to the present.

Pain Reactions: A high tolerance for pain and discomfort exists, although some sources indicate that Haitians have a low threshold. Loud verbal expressions may be heard during labor.

Birth Rites: The fertility rate is five children born per woman. Some women believe they must continue sexual intercourse during pregnancy to keep the birth canal lubricated. Purgatives are regularly taken during pregnancy to cleanse impurities from the blood and stomach of the fetus, and women believe they must avoid exposing themselves to cold air. A newborn or child may receive laxatives to foster health and strength. Most infants are delivered at home with the mothers in a squatting or semi-seated position. Believers in voodoo deliver their infants under a sheet because bright light during delivery is feared. Traditionalists may bury the placenta beneath the doorway at the birth site or burn it at a corner of the home. Infants are not named until after a confinement month. If they die during confinement, burial is done without ceremony. Women who have given birth do not usually leave the home after dark for the first month. Some also have continued the practice of squatting over a pot of boiling herbs to "close the birth canal," and burns can result. According to the hot/cold equilibrium theory, the postpartum period is the hottest state the body can reach, so mothers do not eat "hot" foods. Some women eat foods that are thought to increase milk production. Women believe that the postpartum period should be calm because strong emotions spoil breast milk, resulting in premature weaning unless traditional infusions are taken. Postpartum confinement practices are gradually becoming less common. Some put nutmeg, castor oil, or spider webs on the umbilical cord. Belly bands are commonly used for umbilical hernias. Haiti has seen a declining infant mortality rate, but the rate remains high at 80 deaths per 1,000 births. Abortion is never openly discussed, although hundreds of herbal concoctions reportedly induce abortions. The death rate from abortions performed by untrained persons is unknown. The overall contraceptive prevalence rate of women in relationships in Haiti is 28%. Life expectancy is 53 for men, 56 for women.

Death Rites: Death is believed to be from natural (i.e., caused by God) or supernatural (caused by spirits) factors. Relatives and friends expend considerable effort to be present when a person is near death. The family does not express grief out loud until most of the deceased person's possessions have been removed from the home, at which point the wailing and crying begins. The body is washed, dressed, and placed in a coffin. A religious representative may be summoned to conduct the burial service, usually within 24 hours. Embalming is not common, and autopsies are not routinely performed because they increase speculation about a person's cause of death. Cremation is unacceptable. A popular local belief alleges that witch doctors use herbal substances to make people appear dead so that they can bring them back to life later and enslave them. Because of this popular story, people may doubt whether a person is truly dead or merely appears dead. White clothing represents death. During mourning, some may assume the symptoms of the deceased person's last illness.

Food Practices and Intolerances: Most people eat one main meal a day in the afternoon. Water is taken after the meal is completed. Some women avoid drinking cold orange juice or pineapple while menstruating. The diet is spicy, with root crops, rice, beans, and plantains as staples; being plump is considered healthy. Iced drinks are never consumed during highly emotional times because strong emotions are associated with a "hot" condition.

Infant-Feeding Practices: Colostrum is considered bad milk. It is often used as a purgative to rid the infant's body of meconium. Some mothers stop breastfeeding if the infant develops diarrhea, believing that breast milk causes diarrhea or intestinal parasites. Breastfeeding is more common in rural areas and is continued for 9 to 18 months. A national program promotes exclusive breastfeeding for the first 6 months of life. A plantain porridge supplement is introduced to infants as young as 2 months. A fat child is believed to be a healthy child. Haitian infants and children do not routinely use pacifiers.

Child-Rearing Practices: It is customary to treat children harshly and strictly and use corporal punishment such as spanking. Children who ask questions or seek information from parents are considered disrespectful. When adults are speaking, children are expected to remain quiet. Bottle-feeding is sometimes used as a pacifier to keep children quiet. Many children have multiple caretakers (relatives or friends). Grandmothers are considered appropriate caretakers, and children can be left indefinitely with grandparents or other relatives while parents seek employment or schooling. In some cases, children work after school to help support the family. Haitians are reluctant to discuss sex education or reproduction with health care professionals who are not Haitian. Male circumcision is not encouraged. Bladder and bowel control is expected to be established between 3 and 5 years of age. Enuresis is said to run in families and is not considered a situation warranting professional help. Early independence is promoted, and very young children help with daily chores.

National Childhood Immunizations: BCG at birth; DTwP at 6, 10, and 14 weeks and at +1, +1 year; measles at 9 months; OPV at birth and at 6, 10, and 14 weeks, +1, +1 year; Td at 15 to 49 years, first contact, +1 month, +1, +1, +1 year; vitamin A at 6, +4, +4 months; and TT beginning at 15 years and through the reproductive cycle. The percent of the target population vaccinated, by antigen, is: BCG (71%); DTP1 (76%); DTP3, MCV and Polio3 (43%); TT2 plus (52%); and vitamin A

(66%). Polio has not yet been eradicated, and measles outbreaks have occurred in recent years.

BIBLIOGRAPHY

Central Intelligence Agency: *2006: The world factbook, Haiti.* Retrieved September 21, 2006, from https://www.cia.gov/cia/publications/factbook/print/ha.html.

DeSantis L, Ugarriza DN: Potential for intergenerational conflict in Cuban and Haitian immigrant families, *Arch Psychiatr Nurs.* IX(6):354, 1995.

Haiti Ministry of Health and Population (MSSP): *Demographic health survey. Port-au-Prince,* MSSP, 2000.

Haiti Ministry of Health: *Indicateurs de Base 2002.* Service d'Epidemiologie (SER), Port-au-Prince, 2002, Haiti.

UNAIDS: 2006: Haiti. Retrieved September 21, 2006, from http://www.unaids.org/en/Regions_Countries/Countries/haiti.asp.

World Health Organization: 2006: Immunization, vaccines and biologicals. Retrieved September 21, 2006, from http://www.who.int/immunization_monitoring/en/globalsummary/countryprofileresult.cfm?C='hti'.

H

◆ HONDURAS (REPUBLIC OF)

MAP PAGE (795)

Joanne Motiño Bailey

Location: Honduras is part of the north-central section of Central America. Honduran coastlines include the Caribbean Sea and the Pacific Ocean. The total area is 112,090 km^2 (43,278 square miles), and the capital is Tegucigalpa. Although Honduras is primarily mountainous, it also has fertile plateaus, a river valley, and a narrow coastal plain. The population is more than 7.3 million, and 44% live in urban areas. The gross domestic product (GDP) per capita is $2,900, and 53% live below the poverty line.

Major Languages	Ethnic Groups	Major Religions
Spanish	Mestizo 90%	Catholic 97%
Amerindian languages	Native American 7%	Protestant, Other 3%
English	Black 2%	
Garifuna	White 1%	

Honduras has eight culturally differentiated ethnic groups: the Lencas, Pech, Garifunas, Chortis, Tawahkas, Tolupanes or Xicaques, Miskitos, and an English-speaking black population. Literacy rates are 76% for both men and women.

Health Care Beliefs: Acute sick care; traditional. The use of herbs in home remedies is common, especially among the poor, who constitute the majority of the population. Most villages have at least one layperson who is knowledgeable about herbs and provides basic care for common ailments. Mental illness is not a generally accepted concept by health care professionals or laypeople. Two national psychiatric hospitals are located in Tegucigalpa, and referrals are made from outlying areas. Each general public hospital (of which Honduras has 28) has two or three beds available for patients with psychiatric problems. Preventative practices are not widespread because funds for such care are not readily available. The state provides minimal preventative services, with the exception of immunization programs. Public health care clinics have routine campaigns to raise awareness about reducing breeding sites to reduce mosquito-borne infections, Chagas disease, human immunodeficiency virus (HIV)/acquired immunodeficiency syndrome (AIDS) education, water purification, and proper latrine construction.

Predominant Sick-Care Practices: A combination of biomedical products, where available, and herbal treatments is implemented. The country has significant herbal resources and a wealth of traditional knowledge about herbal medicine, and its combination of herbal and biomedical therapies is of interest to other countries. Honduras is one of the poorest countries in the Western Hemisphere, and health-promotion practices are not a high priority to the average person. Areas populated by indigenous people are among the most severely underserved. The Honduran government has been focusing on changing public health attitudes and practices through educational communication. The availability of hospitals and clinics varies throughout the country. Public hospitals are understaffed and poorly maintained, and they often lack basic supplies and equipment. Private clinics and hospitals are preferred but are available only to those who can pay for their services. Although private clinics and hospitals are better supplied, they are not well regulated, and treatment can be substandard or financially driven.

Ethnic-/Race-Specific or Endemic Diseases: Leading causes of mortality in the under-5 population are acute diarrhea with dehydration and acute respiratory infections. Malaria affects inhabitants primarily in the country's northern areas. Endemic to Honduras since 1996, in recent years 28,064 cases of dengue fever were reported, primarily in the central and northern areas. No cases of poliomyelitis have been reported since 1989. The number of cases of neonatal tetanus has been reduced by 50% since 1994. Subclinical vitamin A deficiency affects 13% of the population aged 1 to 3 years, particularly in rural areas in the western and northern regions and in several urban areas. Iron deficiency is prevalent, particularly in children 1 to 3 years. The age at which young people begin to use tobacco and alcohol has decreased and ranges from 10 to 16 years. The Joint United Nations Programme on HIV/AIDS (UNAIDS) reports the prevalence of human immunodeficiency virus (HIV) in adults (aged 15 to 49 years) to be 1.5%, with 63,000 living with HIV, including 16,000 women and 2,400 children aged 0 to 14. Overall, 3,700 deaths are attributed to AIDS. Transmission is predominantly heterosexual (85%), followed by homosexual (3%), bisexual (5%), blood transfusions (1%), and vertical transmission (6%).

Health-Team Relationships: The National Autonomous University of Honduras (UNAH) is responsible for the education of health professionals. Medical doctors have 4 to 6 years of training after high school.

Professional nurses complete high school and 4 to 5 years of university education with an emphasis on health system management. Auxiliary nurses have 1 year of nurses training following junior high school; they are the primary health care providers in most rural clinics. Since 1990, nurse specialists in perinatal health and surgical nursing have been recognized as a distinct category of health professional. On average, Honduras has three professional nurses and nine doctors per 10,000 people. Honduras has a severe imbalance in geographic distribution of resources, with urban communities having a job market saturated with health personnel and others (usually the most remote) having many vacant positions. The public sector employs 69% of all health workers.

Families' Role in Hospital Care: Female family members generally provide whatever health care is possible for as long as possible to avoid dealing with the health care system. Home remedies are common, as is assistance from lay midwives in the villages. A family member will accompany a sick relative to help care for him or her in the hospital.

Dominance Patterns: Men are expected to carry out business transactions and work outside the home, and women are expected to remain home and care for children. In rural areas, women are generally expected to remain indoors and be silent when business matters are being discussed. This gender dynamic is shifting as more young women migrate to urban areas to work in international textile factories. Women now bring in most of the family's income. Many marriages are informal because of the expense of weddings and the dearth of priests. Men often desert their wives for other women, and extramarital affairs and sexual relations with prostitutes is expected. Physical abuse by men is common; but despite such attitudes and conditions, women are becoming more active in Honduran public life, including politics and business.

Eye-Contact Practices: Among many groups, particularly the poor and less educated, making direct eye contact is considered impolite. Women who make direct eye contact with men are thought to be inviting them to introduce themselves and solicit a date.

Touch Practices: It is common to shake hands when meeting friends or acquaintances.

Perceptions of Time: Hondurans generally do not watch the clock. It is acceptable for a Honduran to arrive late to a scheduled meeting, but it is considered rude for a North American to do so.

Pain Reactions: In general, children and adults bear pain stoically. Mild analgesics are widely available, but cost may be a barrier. Opiate analgesics are highly controlled substances, and it is essentially impossible to obtain opiate-containing analgesics even with a prescription.

Food Practices and Intolerances: Hondurans eat a light breakfast after waking, a moderate midday meal, and supper. Depending on socioeconomic status, a typical meal might consist of refried red beans, rice, and a piece of salty cheese. Meat (either chicken or beef) is preferred at meals if it is economically obtainable. Corn tortillas are served on the side. Near the coasts, seafood plays an important role in daily diets.

Infant-Feeding Practices: The percent of exclusively breastfed infants (from birth to 3 months) rose from 27% in 1991 to 42% in 1996. Among infants aged 6 to 9 months, 69% were being breastfed with supplemental feeding, and among children 20 to 23 months old, 45% continued to breastfeed. Breastfeeding continues for an average of about 2 months. Unfortunately, bottle-feeding is also common; mothers often use contaminated water for formula preparation, resulting in frequent and serious episodes of diarrhea. The infant mortality rate is 35 deaths per 1,000 live births: mortality rates for children under age 5 are 42 deaths per 1,000. The fertility rate is 3.59 children born per woman.

Child-Rearing Practices: In 2006, 43% of the population was children 0 to 15 years of age. Families must pay for their children's uniforms and books even when they attend public schools, so children of poorer families often receive little or no formal education. It is common for children of 4 or 5 to carry buckets of sand or water on their heads or bundles of firewood in their arms and to use a machete to cut brushwood for cooking fires. Life expectancy is 66 for men, 71 for women.

National Childhood Immunizations: BCG at birth; DT at 2, 4, 6, and 18 months and 4.5 years; DTwP at 18 months and 4 to 5 years; DTwPHibHep at 2, 4, and 6 months; OPV at birth, 2, 4, and 6 months and at 1 to 4 years; IPV at 2, 4, 6, and 18 months and at 4 years; HepB at +1, +1, +1 year; MMR at 12 months; YF >1 year; Td CBAW (12 to 49 years) ×5; vitamin A at 6, 12, and 18 months, 2 years, 30 months, and 3 years. The percent of the target population vaccinated, by antigen, is: BCG, DTP3, HepB3, Hib3, and Polio3 (91%); and MCV (92%). In some areas of the country, only 80% have received all vaccinations.

BIBLIOGRAPHY

Central Intelligence Agency: *2006: The world factbook, Honduras*. Retrieved September 21, 2006, from https://www.cia.gov/cia/publications/factbook/print/ho.html.

Pan American Health Organization: 2006: Honduras, Retrieved January 23, 2006, from http://www.paho.org/english/sha/honrstp.htm (retrieved January 23, 2006).

UNAIDS: 2006: Honduras, Retrieved September 21, 2006, from http://www.unaids.org/en/Regions_Countries/Countries/honduras.asp.

World Health Organization: 2006: Immunization, vaccines and biologicals. Retrieved September 21, 2006, from http://www.who.int/immunization_monitoring/en/globalsummary/countryprofileresult.cfm?C='hnd'.

◆ HUNGARY (REPUBLIC OF)

MAP PAGE (798)

Bettina F. Piko

Location: Hungary is a landlocked country in Central Europe that is characterized by fertile plains and mountains, with a famous freshwater lake called Balaton that serves as a major tourist attraction. The capital is Budapest. It is bordered by the Czech Republic, Slovakia, Ukraine, Romania, Serbia, Croatia, Slovenia, and Austria. The total area is 93,030 km^2 (35,919 square miles): the population is more than 10 million. The gross domestic product (GDP) per capita is $16,300, with 9% below the poverty line. Literacy rates are greater than 99% for both men and women.

Major Languages	Ethnic Groups	Major Religions
Hungarian	Hungarian 90%	Roman Catholic 68%
	Gypsy (Roma) 4%	Calvinist 20%
	German (3%), Serb (2%),	Lutheran 5%
	Slovak (0.8%),	Atheist and Other 8%
	Romanian (0.7%)	

Health Care Beliefs: Acute sick care; traditional; alternative. People believe in the omnipotence of biomedical science and doctors. When Hungarians are disappointed by biomedical care, however, they often turn to alternative healers. Rural elderly people who are involved in agriculture have the greatest tendency to believe in herbal medicine, and they are experienced in its use. Many start the day with a small glass of apricot brandy *(pálinka),* which is believed to cleanse and purify the body. There is more concern with treatment than actively preventing disease by changing dietary habits or increasing exercise. Prevention programs are being introduced to children in school. Social reactions to mental illness are dominated by fear. Stigma is common, and it is difficult for those recovering from mental illness to be free of this stigma. A positive approach toward mental health prevention is being promoted.

Predominant Sick-Care Practices: Western health care and medical treatments are dominant. There are three levels of health care services: primary, involving family doctors or general practitioners with a primary health care team of district nurses and assistants; outpatient care, involving polyclinics with specialist outpatient services; and hospitals, staffed by clinical specialists who treat hospitalized patients. Children under 18 are treated by services managed by pediatricians. Health care is financed by the National Social Insurance Company, and contribution payments are compulsory for all employees. Medications are partially subsidized by insurance and partially by patients. Many continue to turn to alternative healing practices, although the costs are not covered by insurance. Alternative healers are required to be licensed to practice.

Ethnic-/Race-Specific or Endemic Diseases: Cancer and diseases of the circulatory system are the leading causes of death. Alcoholism-related diseases such as cirrhosis of the liver, and smoking-related diseases such as lung cancer are also common, as are mental health problems and rheumatism (associated with cold, damp weather). Hungary's suicide rate is one of the highest in the world. Gypsies *(Roma)* are a minority group whose birth and mortality rates are much higher than the majority population. Their lower levels of education and higher unemployment rates cause them to seek medical care less frequently than Hungarians in general. Human immunodeficiency virus (HIV) and acquired immunodeficiency syndrome (AIDS) are relatively rare, and statistics reveal a stable situation. The Joint United Nations Programme on HIV/AIDS (UNAIDS) reports that the prevalence rate for HIV in adults (aged 15 to 49 years) is 0.1%, with 3,200 people living with HIV, including fewer than 1,000 women. About 81% of the registered cases are men who have sex with men, and 32% of heterosexual cases are believed imported from outside the country. There have been at least 274 AIDS-related deaths. Anonymous tests are available for everyone, and schools have supported anti-AIDS program networks for primary and high school students. Homosexuality is often considered a taboo subject. Hungarians tend to be conservative, except in larger cities, where liberal views are more common.

Health-Team Relationships: Doctors are dominant in the health care system and are responsible for the overall treatment of patients. The paramedical staff consists of nurses, assistants, midwives, community nurses, social workers, and psychologists. The relationship between nurses and doctors is guided by a hierarchical approach; doctors are in charge, and nurses follow orders. The patient-doctor relationship is often similar in that patients are expected to follow orders without much input about the course of treatment.

Families' Role in Hospital Care: Because hospital care is provided by health care services and paid by social insurance, the role of family members toward their relatives is mostly to provide psychological support. When children are hospitalized, parents are allowed to stay with their children in a special room for parents; commonly the mothers stay. Caring for family members in the home is difficult because often the husband and wife work full time. If they can afford it, families may employ a private nurse to care for infirm or older family members in their homes.

Dominance Patterns: The dominance patterns of social groups vary. In well-educated families, the responsibility for decision making is often shared by husband and wife. In working-class or farming families, it is more common for the father to be the head of the family and the central decision maker. Despite changes recognizing the equality of women during the last decades, the most prominent positions in the workplace are usually held by men. Moreover, as a result of cultural conditioning, women often think they are not competent to take part in management tasks.

Eye-Contact Practices: Eye contact plays an important communicative role, and it is customary to make eye contact during conversation. If another person avoids eye contact, it may be interpreted as embarrassment or that the two have a poor relationship.

Touch Practices: Touching and hugging during greetings or conversations is accepted among very close friends or family members. Hungarians tend to prefer a large personal space, so when individuals outside of their family or circle of friends get too close, the experience may be interpreted as threatening.

Perceptions of Time: People who work according to Western manage-ment rules usually insist on punctuality. Outside the work environment, people often do not make extensive future plans or adhere to strict time tables. This discrepancy between work habits and everyday patterns sometimes causes conflicts among individuals.

Pain Reactions: Hungarian people tend to be stoic about pain and think that not revealing suffering is a sign of strength. Even during childbirth, women in labor tend to avoid crying out loudly.

Birth Rites: The fertility rate is low (1.32 children born per woman), with a steadily decreasing population. Although family and children are valued, there is a desire to provide for children in a material sense. Therefore, Hungarians usually have only one or two children, except in Orthodox reli-gious families. Most deliveries take place in hospitals with the assistance of obstetricians and midwives. Pregnant women usually choose a doctor who takes care of her throughout pregnancy and assists delivery. Some women are choosing positions such as sitting during delivery. Female obstetricians are rare, and men receiving high salaries fill the specialty. After birth, most hospital stays are short unless complications occur. After discharge, a district pediatric nurse makes a home visit within 24 hours. Infants are usually separated from their mothers in the hospital, but more hospitals are using the "rooming-in" system, where infants and mothers stay together. Fathers are increasingly interested in attending deliveries ("labor with fathers," or *apás szülés*) and cutting the umbilical cord. Delivery at home is popular but strongly discouraged by doctors, who declare it increases the probability of complications. The infant mortality rate is 8.39 deaths per 1,000 live births. Life expectancy is 68 for men, 77 for women.

Death Rites: Most people die in hospitals, often without family members. Death and dying are not discussed, and there is little emotional care for dying people. The hospice movement has been introduced, with the major goal of providing appropriate medical and psychological care for the ter-minally ill. After death and an autopsy (usually recommended for hospital patients), the person is placed in a coffin and buried. Older adults gener-ally disapprove of cremation. Burial is usually accompanied by religious services. Organ donations are acceptable, but approval is strictly regu-lated. Older village people continue to follow socially patterned rituals of death and mourning, such as covering mirrors or wearing black dresses or suits during the mourning period. It is still customary after the funeral for family members and relatives to share a meal called the "funeral feast" *(halotti tor)*. This custom is based on a belief that the dead watch this loving family gathering from paradise, and this helps them to accept the reality of death and leaving their lives behind.

Food Practices and Intolerances: Traditional foods are usually high in carbohydrates and animal fat (e.g., meat with fried potatoes or "stuffed cabbage" *(töltött káposzta)*, which contains minced meat and rice and is a national food). Eating salad during meals is rare but is gaining in popular-ity among young people. Lunch is the main meal and is typically eaten in small restaurants or workplace canteens. It begins with soups, followed by coffee. Breakfast is often light, and dinner is typically heavy. Tea or coffee breaks with cookies and pastries or tea or coffee and fruit or cereal are eaten between main meals. Vegetarian and so-called "body-control diets" emphasizing carbohydrates or proteins are preferred by some. Vegetables and fruits are available year round for those who can afford them. Most families have vegetable gardens as a hobby.

Infant-Feeding Practices: Breastfeeding is highly encouraged by pediatricians and district nurses. Although breastfeeding used to end at 6 months, many mothers now prefer to continue for a year or longer. About 2 weeks after birth, lemon and orange juice and then apple juice are introduced in small spoonfuls between breastfeeding. Mashed fruit is introduced at 6 weeks, and mashed vegetables (primarily potatoes and carrots) are added at 4 months. Between the months 7 and 12, cow's milk and chicken are added. Infants who do not breastfeed receive cow's milk or other formulas as a substitute.

Child-Rearing Practices: Mothers who prefer to stay at home with their infants are allowed a maternity allowance of 3 years. Fathers are also entitled to this subsidy. To preserve their jobs, however, many parents return to work after a year or sooner, preferring to pay for a private day nursery. Child-rearing practices are rather permissive because parents want their children to have a better life than their own, which sometimes results in too much emphasis on material goods and too little on psychological strength and emotional security.

National Childhood Immunizations: BCG at birth or within 42 days and at 2, 3, 4, and 18 months; DT at 11 years; DTwP at 4 months, 5 months, 3 years, and 6 years; DTwPIPV at 3 months; Hib at 2, 4, and 5 months; OPV at 4, 5, and 15 months and at 3 and 6 years; MMR at 15 months and 11 years; and hepatitis B at 14 years. The percent of the target population vaccinated, by antigen, is: BCG, DTP1, DTP3, Hib3, MCV, and Polio3 (99%).

BIBLIOGRAPHY

Central Intelligence Agency: *2006: The world factbook, Hungary*. Retrieved September 21, 2006, from https://www.cia.gov/cia/publications/factbook/print/hu.html.

Delvaux T, Buekens P, Godin I, and Boutsen M: Barriers to prenatal care in Europe, *Am J Prev Med.* 21(1):52, 2001.

Hungarian Statistical Office: *Statistical yearbook of Hungary 2000*, Budapest, 2001, Hungarian Statistical Office.

Kopp MS, Skrabski A, Szedmak S: Psychosocial risk factors, inequality and self-rated morbidity in a changing society, *Soc Sci Med.* 51(9):1351, 2000.

Pikhart H, Bobak M, Sieqrist J, Pajak A, Rywik S, and Kyshegyi J: Psychosocial work characteristics and self rated health in four post-Communist countries, *J Epidemiol Community Health* 55(9):624, 2001.

Piko B: Interplay between self and community: a role for health psychology in Eastern Europe's public health. *J Health Psychol.* 9(1):111–120, 2004.

UNAIDS 2006 Hungary: Retrieved September 21, 2006 from http://www.unaids.org/en/Regions_Countries/Countries/hungary.asp

World Health Organization 2006: Immunization, Vaccines and Biologicals. Retrieved September 21, 2006 from http://www.who.int/immunization monitoring/en/globalsummary/countryprofileresult.cfm?C='hun'

◆ ICELAND (REPUBLIC OF)

MAP PAGE (798)

Elín M. Hallgrímsdóttir

Location: Iceland is Europe's westernmost country. It is the second largest island: 103,000 km² (39,758 square miles) in the North Atlantic. Iceland is sparsely populated, with only three people per km², living primarily along the coast. The interior contains stunning contrasts. Iceland is largely an arctic desert, punctuated with mountains, glaciers that cover more than 11,922 km² (4,601 square miles—11.5% of the total land area), volcanoes, and waterfalls. Most of the vegetation and agricultural areas are in the lowlands close to the coastline. The gross domestic product (GDP) per capita is $35,600, and the literacy rate is 99% for both men and women.

Major Languages	Ethnic Groups	Major Religions
Icelandic (official)	Descendants of Norwegians and Celts	Evangelical Lutheran 84% Other Protestant and Roman Catholic 14% No affiliation 2%

The ethnic groups that account for about 96% of the Icelandic nation are a homogeneous mixture of Nordic and Celtic origin. Immigration is increasing; in the rural areas of western Iceland, immigrants from approximately 38 countries make up 6% of the population (55% from Poland). The total population is 299,388; the capital is Reykjavik.

Health Care Beliefs: Active involvement; health promotion important. According to the Ministry of Health and Social Security Act of 1990, all inhabitants have the right to access the best possible health service for the protection of their mental, social, and physical health. Health promotion and illness prevention are stressed, with an emphasis on accident, tobacco, and drug prevention. Primary health care centers have the responsibility for general treatment and care, examinations, home nursing, and preventive measures such as family planning, maternity care, child health care, and school health. Many people have considerable interest in alternative practices such as acupuncture and naturopathic or homeopathic medicine. However, Icelandic law only permits medical doctors to diagnose illness. The use of prayer is common among older adults, although many others probably pray but simply do not discuss it.

Predominant Sick-Care Practices: Biomedical and alternative. The health service is financed primarily by the central government and is based on taxes. About 83% of bills for care at ambulatory care centers, primary health care centers, and emergency departments are covered. Users pay a service fee (copayment) of about 17%. The country is divided into health regions, each with its own primary health care center—some of which are run jointly with local community hospitals. The biomedical model is predominant, but numerous unorthodox options in alternative medicine may be used: aromatherapy and herbs (biological-based methods), meditation (mind-body interventions), massage (manipulative and body-based methods), and therapeutic touch (energy therapies). Availability of these therapies has increased in recent years in response to greater emphasis on holistic health: the preservation of mental, social, and physical health.

Ethnic-/Race-Specific or Endemic Diseases: Heart and coronary disease, stroke, cancer, and accidents cause most deaths. Cardiovascular disease incidence has been decreasing since 1980, the result of fewer cases of hypertension and the decreased consumption of high-fat foods. Obesity is an increasing problem in children and adults and is attributed to lack of exercise and unhealthy foods such as soft drinks and deep-fried foods, which are especially popular among young people. Many argue that accidents are the country's most serious health problem and the primary cause of death of children and young people (i.e., aged 5 to 35). Accidents are expensive and devastating for the society and family because many survivors need expensive life-long care and treatment. Cancer and respiratory diseases are increasing. Smoking cigarettes was common among people born between 1950 and 1965, resulting in increased rates of chronic obstructive pulmonary disease (COPD). The Joint United Nations Programme on HIV/AIDS (UNAIDS) estimates that the prevalence rate for human immunodeficiency virus (HIV) in adults (aged 15 to 49 years) is 0.2%, with fewer than 500 living with HIV. By the end of 2005, a total of 184 cases had been reported, of which 56 patients have developed acquired immunodeficiency syndrome (AIDS), and 36 have died. Most reported cases in recent years are among heterosexuals. Blood donors and people who are being treated for drug addiction are systematically tested.

Health-Team Relationships: Working relationships are usually good, and collaboration among different groups is increasing. Medical doctors diagnose and order treatment for illness, but inpatient hospital wards are directed by nurses. Nurses constitute the majority of the health care staff, which gives them a powerful position in the health care system. Admission and discharge of patients are based on collaborative decisions between nurses and doctors. The relationships between patients and nurses or doctors are generally open and friendly. Since 1986, all nursing education in Iceland consists of 4-year bachelor of science programs. The Ministry of Health and Social Security Act of 1997 states that patients are responsible for their own health—as they are able and if their physical condition permits. They are to participate actively in the treatment to which they have consented. Patients have the right to obtain information regarding their state of health, the risks and benefits of proposed treatments, other possible remedies, the consequences of lack of treatment, and seeking another opinion regarding treatment, condition, and prognosis.

Families' Role in Hospital Care: Patients have the right to receive support from their family, relatives, and friends during their treatment and hospital stay. Furthermore, the patients and their closest relatives have the right to spiritual, social, and religious support. Parents who have custody of children must give their consent for treatment of a patient younger than 16. If a parent who has custody of a sick child refuses to consent to treatment for acute life-sustaining measures, necessary treatment is started without their consent. The good of the child always overrides objections of the parents (e.g., refusal of blood transfusions for religious reasons) if the child's condition warrants it. Sick children are informed about their health when possible (although they cannot refuse treatment), and those over 12 are always consulted. Sick children staying in a health institution are entitled to the presence of their parents or other close relatives; and sick children of school age are provided with in-hospital education suited to their age and state of health. Surroundings and care of sick children in health institutions are matched to their age, maturity level, and condition.

Dominance Patterns: According to the Act on the Equal Status and Equal Rights of Women and Men, all individuals have an equal opportunity to benefit from their own enterprise and to develop their skills regardless of gender. Employers and labor unions make systematic efforts to equalize the participation of the sexes in the labor market, and women and men who are in the service of the same employer receive equal pay and enjoy equal terms for equal value and comparable work. In reality, men often have more prestigious titles and earn more than women, even when they do the same work. Some women have sued their employers because of this situation and have received reimbursements. According to a new survey, the average wage differential between men and women is about 14% to 17%. The fact that people live geographically close to one another fosters large, extended family connections. Decision making is cooperative between parents, but mothers still have more influence and responsibility in the area of child rearing and housework. Women also help family members who are sick or have disabilities more than men do.

Eye-Contact Practices: People are generally comfortable with direct eye contact.

Touch Practices: People in Iceland do not use touch extensively. Women touch each other more than men do, but men and women are comfortable touching and kissing small children. Friends and family members shake hands or kiss each other on one cheek, but the masculine greeting is to shake hands. Hand holding (e.g., between nurses and patients) is considered a supportive gesture.

Perceptions of Time: People are rather punctual, but a 5- to 10-minute delay at an appointment is accepted. People are present and future oriented, but the ability to tell stories and describe events from the past is considered a sign of wisdom by older adults.

Pain Reactions: People do not express their pain loudly. Patients do not complain much and often do not want to bother a nurse by asking for pain medication even when they are in considerable pain.

Birth Rites: The fertility rate is two children born per woman. Almost all births occur in hospitals, and the semi-seated position is common. The baby's father or a family member is usually present during delivery, and a shower is permitted for mothers soon after the baby is born. Most mid-wives are nurses because for many years one had to be a nurse before admission into a midwifery program. Midwives attend normal deliveries, and hospital stays range between 1 and 5 days. Infants "room in" (i.e., stay with their mothers at all times) in the hospital. Mothers who want to go home within 36 hours after birth receive follow-up visits in their homes by midwives during the days after discharge. Otherwise, health visitors (nurses in the health service) make follow-up home visits once a week for 4 or 5 weeks (more often when needed). Infant mortality is among the lowest in the world: 2.4 deaths per 1,000 live births. Average life expectancy is 83 years for women, 79 for men.

Death Rites: Most people die in health institutions and are surrounded by close family members. A funeral is conducted with a pastor and a choir and is followed by a burial. Usually, the individual is buried in a wooden casket about 1 week after death, but cremation is also practiced. Autop-sies are acceptable, if needed, to confirm the cause of death, and organ donations are acceptable. A unique Icelandic practice is decorating churchyards and cemeteries with festive lights during Christmas and New Year celebrations.

Food Practices and Intolerances: Breakfast may consist of yogurt pro-ducts, cereals, bread with cheese or ham, milk, juice, and coffee or tea; and daily consumption of cod liver oil is considered very healthy. Most people have a light lunch, such as sandwiches, salad, soup, or yogurt. The main meal is eaten in the early evening, consisting mainly of meat or fish that is boiled or fried with potatoes. Having rice, spaghetti or pasta, bread, and salad instead of potatoes is becoming more popular, and young people increasingly favor fast foods such as pizza.

Infant-Feeding Practices: Breastfeeding is encouraged and very com-mon for 4 to 6 months after birth. Only in special cases does a woman not breastfeed, such as when she is giving up an infant for adoption or is not producing breast milk. Formula is used when breastfeeding alone is not enough, and pacifiers are common. The recommended practice is to start with porridge at the age of 6 months and then add vegetables and fruits. From the age of 4 weeks, A and D vitamins are given. Sleeping outside on the balcony once or twice a day is believed to be healthy for infants, even when it is very cold.

Child-Rearing Practices: Of women aged 25 to 54, 88% are in the work-force, compared with 95% of men the same age. Maternity leave is 3 months for each parent, in addition to 3 months shared by both parents. Of children from infancy to 2 years old, 38% are in nurseries, and of chil-dren 3 to 5 years old, 94% are in nurseries (with a daily attendance of 4 to 9 hours). Both parents maintain discipline, but child-rearing practices are permissive. Children are allowed to participate in decision making that involves them, and they generally have a great deal of autonomy.

Of children from birth to 17 years, 23% are living with one adult. School is compulsory between ages 6 and 16.

National Childhood Immunizations: NeifVac-C at 6 and 8 months; DTaP at 5 years; DTaPHibIPV at 3, 5, and 12 months; IPV at 14 years; Td at 14 years; and Morbilli-MMR at 18 months and 12 years. The percent of the target population vaccinated, by antigen is: DTP1, DTP3, Hib3, Polio3 (95%); and MCV (90%).

Other Characteristics: Each member of the nuclear family can have a different last name. For example, a girl uses as her last name her father's first name with "dóttir" added, a boy uses his father's first name with "son" added, the mother keeps her maiden name, and the father uses his own last name.

BIBLIOGRAPHY

Central Intelligence Agency: *2006: The world factbook, Iceland.* Retrieved September 21, 2006, from https://www.cia.gov/cia/publications/factbook/print/ic.html.

Directorate of Health Ministry of Health and Social Security: Retrieved February 20, 2006, from http://eng.heilbrigdisraduneyti.is/.

The Public Health Institute of Iceland: Retrieved on February 20, 2006, from http://lydheilsustod.is/.

Statistic Iceland: Retrieved on February 20, 2006, from http://www.statice.is/

UNAIDS: 2006 Iceland. Retrieved September 21, 2006, from http://www.unaids.org/en/Regions_Countries/Countries/iceland.asp.

World Health Organizatio: 2006: Immunization, vaccines and biologicals. Retrieved September 21, 2006, from http://www.who.int/immunization_monitoring/en/globalsummary/countryprofileresult.cfm?C='isl'.

◆ INDIA (REPUBLIC OF)

MAP PAGE (804)

Santanu Chatterjee

Location: India is the seventh largest country in the world. The capital is New Delhi. It covers the Himalayan ranges in the north, the flat alluvium plains in the central region, and the peninsula in the south. The total area is 387,273 km^2 (149,487 square miles), accounting for 2.5% of the world's surface area but sustaining 17% of the world's population. The Himalayas comprise three almost parallel ranges interspersed with plateaus and valleys. The northern plains extend across the country; this area forms the basins of three river systems: the Ganges, Indus, and Brahmaputra. The rivers are primarily snow fed, originating in the Himalayas and ending in extensive deltas to the sea. In the south, the area is mostly flat, flanked by the ghats—low-lying hills running parallel to the coasts. The climate, though broadly tropical monsoon, ranges from almost equatorial in the south to Mediterranean in the north. India has four distinct seasons: winter, hot summer, rainy monsoon, and post-monsoon.

The population is about 1 billion, 27 million people. The gross domestic product (GDP) per capita is $3,300, and 25% live below the poverty line. Literacy rates are 70% for men, 48% for women.

Major Languages	Ethnic Groups	Major Religions
Hindi (national)	Indo-Aryan 72%	Hindu 81%
English	Dravidian 25%	Muslim 13%
Other official languages	Mongol, Other 3%	Christian 2%
(13); at least 24		Sikh 2%
languages spoken by		Buddhist, Jain, and
a million or more;		Others 2%
numerous other		
languages and		
dialects		

India has 325 languages expressed in more than 2,000 dialects and 25 scripts. Each region has its own unique social, ethnic, and linguistic characteristics. The coexistence of traditional and contemporary and the extreme contrasts of affluence and poverty are striking. Cities have modern amenities and a stressful lifestyle. Life in rural areas is more relaxed and agriculture based. About three fifths of people work in agriculture. Poverty and unemployment in rural regions result in urban migration, contributing to slums and strains on urban infrastructure.

Health Care Beliefs: Acute sick care; traditional. Generally, acute sick care is practiced; although traditional medicine is important. *Yoga*, an ancient system of physical exercises and breathing techniques, is practiced. *Ayurveda*, the knowledge of life and longevity, is a medical knowledge system and a way of life that involves not only the problems of the body and mind but also of the human spirit and consciousness. These biomedical and traditional practices focus on disease prevention. Spiritual values permeate most aspects of life and death. Allopathic medicine may be used in almost all rural communities, but poor Indians use more traditional systems. Mental illnesses have a social stigma, and concepts of insanity are culturally rooted in the community. Psychoneuroses and psychoses are more common among people in urban areas. High stress levels combined with urban complexities contribute to high levels of anxiety and depression. Believing that a person in a dissociative trance-like condition is possessed by a supernatural force (e.g., spirits, demons, ghosts, gods) is particularly common in rural settings. Emotional problems are frequently expressed as somatic symptoms in the form of headaches, sleep disturbances, or ill-defined body pain. Praying and giving offerings to religious places of worship to alleviate illness and suffering are common. Given their changing sex roles, the social milieu fosters a sense of extreme insecurity and helplessness in women, even though they have the greater share of family responsibilities. Migration to the city, disruption of the village lifestyle, and subsequent urbanization contribute to increases in emotional morbidity.

Predominant Sick-Care Practices: Biomedical; traditional Indian; magical-religious. The Indian systems of medicine have been practiced for centuries. Such systems include Ayurveda, Siddha, Unani, and drug-less therapies such as yoga, naturopathy, and homeopathy. Each has its own individual philosophy, merits, and strengths and offers a safe and cost-effective alternative to modern medicine. The government has recognized this and understands that "health for all" cannot be achieved by the allopathic system alone. Efforts have been made to develop these indigenous systems of medicine under an institutional framework—the Indian Systems of Medicine and Homeopathy (ISM&H)—and to integrate them with allopathy to address the needs of the population. Medical services are provided through an integrated system involving state and central government with nongovernmental, voluntary, and private institutions. In rural areas, health services function through a network of health and family welfare systems offering prevention, promotion, curative, and rehabilitative services as part of a primary health care approach. Private health care is booming and experiencing a steady increase in consumer spending on nongovernmental medical treatment. There is more dependence on private health care providers as household incomes increase. Public health care facilities are more frequently used for cases requiring hospitalization. Recent policies have advocated "cost-effective" strategies, leading to an overall decreased investment in health, which has created less access to health care for the poor. Most regions in the country have a mixed approach of public and private sector participation.

Ethnic-/Race-Specific or Endemic Diseases: Endemic diseases include malaria (chloroquine resistant) and visceral leishmaniasis. Indians are at risk for viral hepatitis types A, B, C, and E; Japanese encephalitis; tuberculosis; dengue fever; typhoid fever; rabies; ascariasis; hookworm infection; amoebiasis; lymphatic filariasis; poliomyelitis; measles; mumps; diphtheria; trachoma; and anemia in women. Vitamin A deficiency is the most common cause of childhood blindness. Communicable diseases account for about 27% of all reported illnesses. The country is in the midst of an epidemiologic transition, contending with communicable and non-communicable diseases. This transition is attributable to the aging population, a shift from rural to urban lifestyles, changes in dietary intake, increases in sedentary living, and increases in smoking and alcohol consumption. Cardiovascular diseases are the leading cause of noncommunicable diseases. The prevalence of diabetes is increasing in rural and urban areas. The major health problem in rural India is pneumonia, and bronchitis and asthma cause premature mortality. Pulmonary tuberculosis is also a problem, especially in the states of Bihar, Madhya Pradesh, Rajasthan, and Uttar Pradesh. Cancer is a health problem in all Indian states. Automobile accidents top the cause of death list in Rajasthan and Haryana, suicide is a major issue in Andhra Pradesh, and unipolar depression is frequent among women aged 15 to 44. People older than 60 are dealing with multiple chronic and acute illnesses and hearing and vision deficits. The National Family Health Survey II revealed that 47% of

2-year-olds were underweight, and deficiencies of vitamin A and iodine were problematic. The Joint United Nations Programme on HIV/AIDS (UNAIDS) estimates the prevalence rate for human immunodeficiency virus (HIV) in adults (aged 15 to 49 years) is 0.9%, with 5.7 million people living with HIV, including 1.6 million women. Deaths attributed to acquired immunodeficiency syndrome (AIDS) are between 270,000 and 680,000 people. Transmission is predominantly heterosexual, followed by injecting drug use. Although the overall prevalence is low, the large population size causes India to be second only to Africa in terms of the number of people living with HIV. Only 7% of infected people receive antiretroviral therapy, and only 1.6% of pregnant women with HIV are receiving treatment to reduce mother to child transmission.

Health-Team Relationships: Nurses usually work under medical supervision and have little direct influence on health care decisions; however, nursing is increasingly gaining importance, and nurses are an integral part of the health care team. Patients' attitudes toward members of the health team are generally appreciative and encouraging. Language proficiencies and communication skills are key issues for acceptance and success in such interactions.

Families' Role in Hospital Care: Some women are uncomfortable when examined by male health practitioners. Health care professionals are reluctant to discuss terminal illnesses with patients; however, they communicate with the patients' relatives. Adults do not enter into the decision-making process if older parents are present.

Dominance Patterns: In India's patriarchal society, the dominant figure is the father or male surrogate. Hierarchies are built within the family according to age, sex, and familial relationships or within the community based on caste, lineage, education, wealth, occupation, and relationship with the ruling power. The social structure is hierarchical and is based on the culture of superior and subordinate relationships, with a clear distinction of rights and duties. Unquestioned obedience to older adults is expected. In extended family households, older adults are often considered indispensable because of their experience and wisdom. Close relationships among generations is still a foundation of Indian families. The concept of a husband owning his wife is pervasive and allows men to abuse women in certain situations. Women depend on men, more so in traditional families, and they remain more vulnerable than men to exploitation and subjugation. Their lower status decreases women's access to resources because of lack of autonomous decision making, control over time, and parenting responsibilities. Women, especially in urban areas, often delay marriage and having children to complete their formal education. The cumulative effects of undernutrition in childhood combined with poor dental care, consumption of food of low nutritional value, chronic parasitic infestations, domestic chores such as carrying loads of water long distances, and indoor air pollution from smoky kitchens contribute to the lower health status of the rural poor. Urban, educated, and relatively affluent women have reaped benefits from globalization such as more opportunities for work and training; particularly in global software and information technology arenas. Poor and relatively uneducated women from rural areas have been adversely affected, because globalization has promoted conservative monetary and fiscal policies that have further reduced their income and employment opportunities. Women constitute a significant part of the workforce. Today, dominance patterns are undergoing great changes because of India's greater access to the media and the increasing influence of Western ideas and attitudes. Marriage arrangements are becoming more diverse, and individual independence within marriage is being emphasized more.

Touch Practices: Men shake hands with other men but not with women. Instead, men place their palms together and bow slightly to women. Educated upper-class men and women mingle freely and have less regard for adherence to social-strata rules. Modesty in dress is typical, and bare upper arms or shoulders are considered indecent. Public displays of affection are rare, and body contact is uncommon. Embracing is acceptable among social acquaintances, especially among men or within families. People touch the feet of older adults as a sign of respect or to seek blessings. It is unacceptable to touch another person with the feet, so apologies are offered in cases of such inadvertent contact. The right hand is used for all social interactions, especially when giving or receiving money.

Perceptions of Time: Perceptions of time are relaxed, especially in rural areas. People are more oriented to the past. The concept of time is closely related to the Indian concept of an infinite universe of unending cycles that extend beyond birth, life, and death. Respect for tradition is an integral part of society.

Pain Reactions: Patients generally quietly accept pain but accept pain-relief measures.

Birth Rites: The fertility rate is 2.73 children born per woman. Voluntary sterilization of males is encouraged through monetary incentives and prizes. Prenatal sex determination by diagnostic procedures is prohibited by law and strictly enforced. Although abortion is legal, unhygienic and unsafe abortions are major causes of maternal mortality. Fewer than half of mothers giving birth receive assistance from trained health professionals. Major regional differences exist, and some mothers are assisted by untrained traditional birth attendants or relatives at home. The infant mortality rate is very high at 55 deaths per 1,000 live births. More than a million infants die within 28 days after birth, mostly among infants with low birth weight, but also because of a lack of care at birth and subsequent infections. Cravings during pregnancy are satisfied because they are thought to be those of the unborn child. Pregnancy is a time for rest and care, and expectant mothers may return to their mother's home for the delivery. Pregnancy establishes a woman as an adult and garners respect and consideration from society. Pregnant women avoid sun, heat, and certain foods that are considered "hot." Boys are especially desired. In villages, celebration of a son's birth may include the beating of drums or blowing of conch shells, and the midwife is paid a reward.

The prevalence of anemia among pregnant women is 88%, even though strong antenatal programs promoting iron and folic acid supplementation are in place. Life expectancy is 64 for men, 66 for women.

Death Rites: Because they are accepting God's will, patients may make indirect references to their own deaths. A patient's desire to be lucid as death approaches must be considered in the medical treatment plan. Reincarnation is a Hindu belief. A time and place for prayer are essential for family members and patients because prayer helps them handle anxiety and conflict. In Hindu society, a priest reads from the holy Sanskrit books. Some priests tie strings (signifying a blessing) around the neck or wrist. After death, the son pours water on the mouth of the deceased. Blood transfusions, organ transplants, and autopsies are permitted. Cremations are preferred.

Food Practices and Intolerances: Hindus do not eat beef, but it is available in Muslim restaurants. Rice and corn constitute the staple cereals. Dinner is served late. Strict vegetarianism is confined primarily to southern India. Pork is available in areas with large Christian communities (e.g., Goa) or in the Tibetan and Nepalese communities. Northern Indians consume more meat and emphasize spices and breads. Rice is preferred by southerners, and curries are liberally spiced with chilies. Fish is a favorite in the coastal areas and eastern regions. Lentils are consumed throughout the country. Curd, or yogurt, is usually a side dish. A variety of fruits are fresh and widely available. People usually eat with their right hand because the left is considered unclean. Using a personal spoon to serve more food from a buffet is considered rude.

Infant-Feeding Practices: Breastfeeding on demand is the norm and may continue for 3 years. National surveys indicate that about 50% of mothers exclusively breastfeed for up to 3 months and 26% for 4 to 6 months. One third of the children receive regular, supplementary feedings between 6 and 9 months, and introduction of other foods starts between 6 and 12 months. Inadequate feeding practices rather than lack of food are often a cause of malnutrition. It is believed that colostrum is undesirable. Decreased rates of breastfeeding are noted among working women.

Child-Rearing Practices: The Integrated Child Welfare Scheme offers a package of services to children and expectant or nursing mothers through the Anganwadi centers. It provides supplementary nutrition, immunizations, health checkups, and preschool education. The focus is to reduce social and gender inequalities. Child rearing emphasizes protective nurturing and extreme permissiveness. The child is indulged, cuddled, and remains intimately attached to the mother until age 3 or 4. Toddlers usually sleep with parents until age 4 or 5 years and are not pushed into toilet training. Discipline in late childhood includes scolding and light spanking. Children are rarely praised for doing what is expected of them because praise may cause them to be susceptible to the "evil eye." Girls are less likely to receive appropriate health care such as immunizations.

National Childhood Immunizations: BCG at birth; DT at 5 years; DTaP at 6, 10, and 14 weeks and 16 to 24 months; HepB at 6, 10, and

14 weeks; measles at 9 to 12 months; OPV at birth and at 6, 10, and 14 weeks and at 16 to 24 months and 10 and 16 years; TT two doses first pregnancy or subsequent pregnancy beyond 3 years and one dose for subsequent pregnancies within 3 years; vitamin A at 9, 18, 24, 30, and 36 months. The percent of the target population vaccinated, by antigen, is: BCG (75%); DTP1 (81%); DTP3 (59%); HepB3 (8%); MCV and Polio3 (58%); TT2 plus (78%); and vitamin A (84%).

Other Characteristics: The Sikh religion forbids cutting or shaving any body hair. Older women enjoy heightened social prestige. No expression for "thank you" exists; a social act is a fulfillment of an obligation or a duty and requires no verbal acknowledgment. The head motions for "yes" and "no" are opposite of those used in the United States. Modern children and adolescents often follow Western customs regarding premarital sex, establishing nuclear families, and choosing their own spouses.

BIBLIOGRAPHY

Balaji LN, Abdullah D: Nutrition scenario in India: implications for clinical practice, *J Ind Med Assoc.* 9:536–542, 2000.

Burton B, Duvvury N, Varia N: Domestic violence in India: a summary report of a multi-site household survey, *ICRW.* 3:1–34, 2000.

Human development in South Asia 2001: globalisation and human development, HDC Research Team published report, Mahbub ul Haq Human Development Center, Klhadija Jaq, team leader, Karachi, Pakistan, 2002, Oxford University Press.

Indrayan A, Wysocki MJ, Kumar R, Chawla A, Singh N: Estimates of the years-of-life-lost due to the top nine causes of death in rural areas of the major states in India in 1995, *Natl Med J India.* 15:5–13, 2002.

Paul VK: The newborn health agenda: need for a village-level midwife, *Natl Med J India.* 13:281–283, 2000.

Central Intelligence Agency: *2006: The world factbook, India.* Retrieved September 21, 2006, from https://www.cia.gov/cia/publications/factbook/print/in.html.

UNAIDS: 2006: India. Retrieved September 21, 2006, from http://www.unaids.org/en/Regions_Countries/Countries/india.asp.

World Health Organization: 2006: Immunization, vaccines and biologicals. Retrieved September 21, 2006, from http://www.who.int/immunization_monitoring/en/globalsummary/countryprofileresult.cfm?C='ind'.

◆ INDONESIA

MAP PAGE (805)

Julia W. Albright

Location: The Indonesian archipelago lies between Southeast Asia and Australia, stretching from the Malay Peninsula to New Guinea. It is bordered by the South China Sea on the north, the Pacific Ocean on the north and east, and the Indian Ocean on the south and west. Indonesia consists of 13,700 islands, approximately 6,000 of which are inhabited. The total area is 1,926,852 km^2 (74,097 square miles), with a coastline of 34,000 miles. The capital is Jakarta. The population is 245.5 million. Indonesia is a tropical country with temperatures of 20 to 39°C (68 to 102°F). From June to September, the East monsoon brings dry weather. The West Monsoon brings the rainy season from December to March. The gross domestic product (GDP) per capita is $3,600, with 17% living below the poverty line. Literacy rates are 93% for men, 83% for women.

Major Languages	Ethnic Groups	Major Religions
Bahasa Indonesian (official)	Javanese 45%	Muslim 88%
English (official)	Sundanese 14%	Protestant 5%
Dutch	Madurese 8%	Catholic 3%
Local languages, such as	Coastal Malays 8%	Hindu 2%
Javanese	Other 25%	Buddhist 1%
		Other 1%

Health Care Beliefs: In the major cities and heavily populated areas, modern medicine is practiced in doctor's offices and hospitals. In small communities, villages, and rural areas, vestiges of folk medicine and mysticism remain (e.g., belief in protection provided by deceased ancestors). A fairly common practice is the traditional *tingkeban* ceremony during the seventh month of pregnancy that is believed to afford protection to the mother and fetus. Herbal remedies are common among the rural population.

Predominant Sick-Care Practices: The increasing population, real and potential epidemics, and natural diseases have triggered a demand for high-quality health services. The physical health infrastructure has improved significantly. There are approximately 8,000 health centers, more than 22,000 subcenters, and 7,000 mobile health units distributed around the country and more than 30,000 medical doctors and countless nurses and midwives. The deployment of more than 50,000 community midwives to work in villages and semirural areas increased professional assistance of childbirth from 32% in 1992 to 72% in 1998. The poorest 20% of the population do not have adequate health care or medical facilities as a result of the difficult topography, inaccessibility during the wet season, and insufficient funds and resources.

Ethnic-/Race-Specific or Endemic Diseases: Some success has been achieved in the prevention and control of locally endemic diseases such as pulmonary tuberculosis, leprosy, diarrheal diseases, and childhood pneumonia. Tuberculosis cure rates have increased significantly, and the prevalence of leprosy has declined from 0.36 in 1992 to 0.09 in 2000. Major improvements in vector-borne diseases have not occurred. The prevalence of dengue, filariasis, schistosomiasis, and intestinal helminth infestation has changed little. A recent outbreak of dengue fever was severe: 14,600 cases and a case-fatality rate of 1.8%. The Ministry of Health is on high alert for the threat of avian influenza. There have been 19 confirmed cases and 14 deaths due to H5N1 subtypes. The prevalence of human immunodeficiency virus (HIV) and acquired immunodeficiency syndrome (AIDS) is relatively low, with the number of infected adults estimated at 0.1% according to the Joint United Nations Programme on HIV/AIDS (UNAIDS). About 170,000 people are living with HIV, including 29,000 women. Deaths from AIDS are about 5,500. Where the mode of transmission is known, about 48% of HIV is transmitted heterosexually and 34% via injecting drug use.

Health-Team Relationships: In the mid-1990s, the Indonesian Ministry of Health, together with faculty from Indonesia's 14 medical schools and aided by international nongovernment organizations (INGOs), began programs to improve primary health care. A large cadre of village-level primary providers, the "village midwives" was recruited and dispersed throughout much of the country. Programs were initiated to define the roles and knowledge expected of medical doctors, on the one hand, and nurses and midlevel practitioners on the other. Efforts were made to revise and modernize medical training at all levels. Significant progress has resulted, including reductions in the high cost of drugs, revising the distrust of large segments of the population toward orally administered drugs, and strengthening the capabilities for early detection of illnesses, especially among children.

Families' Role in Hospital Care: Although the structural hierarchy of families varies among Javanese, Sundanese, Balinese, and the peoples of Sumatra, there are strong ties within families. Members who are sick, disabled, or elderly generally receive strong support as a whole. Hospitalization and institutionalization are avoided if possible. Those who are committed to hospital or institution are visited frequently by other family members, who often bring food and gifts and remain overnight.

Dominance Patterns: Among the various cultural and religious groups, the role and status of men and women vary noticeably. In the large cities, the roles of men and women are similar, with women participating at various levels in commerce and government. In the villages and rural areas of Java, frequently both men and women work in the fields. Unlike Javanese or Balinese families, in regions of Sumatra such as Aceh and other coastal and interior provinces, it is common for the male of the family to "go abroad" to gain wealth and commercial success while the women are responsible for maintaining the family and cultivating the land.

Eye-Contact Practices: Direct eye contact is considered disrespectful. Shaking hands is acceptable (but in the case of a woman, only if she offers her hand). Otherwise, touching others is unacceptable, even patting the head of a child. It is proper to rise when the host or hostess enters the room. Yawning in public is considered impolite.

Pain Reactions: Pain is tolerated without expressing emotion if possible. However, it is acceptable to cry or vocalize severe pain.

Birth Rites: In larger cities, most births occur in hospitals with obstetricians in attendance. In smaller communities and semi-rural and rural regions, births are generally at home with midwives in attendance. The fertility rate is 2.4 children born per woman. Infant mortality is high at 34 deaths per 1,000 live births. Prenatal care provided by midwives closely follows traditional practices. Prenatal care begins in the second trimester, when it is believed the soul has entered the body of the fetus. During the fourth or fifth month, the *dukun* ("midwife") gives the pregnant woman a full-body massage. During the seventh month, a pregnancy ritual called *tingkeban* is performed by the midwife, replete with symbolisms of fertility and protection from harm. The dukun formally commits to caring for the pregnant woman until delivery of the infant. The ritual is generally associated with a large subset of the Muslim population of West Java and other ethnic subgroups in Sumatra. Its prevalence is declining as modern obstetric procedures become more prevalent. It is disapproved as a mystical practice by other Muslim groups and by the government of Indonesia. Life expectancy is 67 for men, 72 for women.

Death Rites: Traditional, ancient religions still exist among the various ethnic groups. In some, all spirits are evil; in others, there are both benevolent and malevolent spirits, and certain rituals are practiced to summon the former. In some, death rituals are very important and may include several stages intended to assist the passage of the dead through the underworld. Certain mortuary rituals were believed to impart benefits to the living by the dead. The ancient religions are rapidly disappearing as a result of encroachment of Islam and Christianity. In more urbanized regions, death is viewed from a medical-clinical perspective, although autopsies are performed only for forensic purposes. Bodies must be buried intact according to Muslim beliefs; cremations are prohibited.

Food Practices and Intolerances: Rice, coconut, banana, peanut, and soy are the five basics of Indonesian cuisine. Coconut and coconut products are central to food preparation. Indonesians favor strong, spicy flavors in dishes prepared with fish, poultry, vegetables, and meat. Pork, blood, and carrion are forbidden for Muslims. A major source of protein is soybeans, which are eaten boiled, fermented, or as soybean curd.

Infant-Feeding Practices: Breastfeeding is common in urban and rural areas, where there is widespread belief in its benefits. The idea that breast milk enters the baby's bloodstream is common and is said to cultivate closeness between mother and infant. Complementary foods such as rice-milk porridge and other solid foods are often provided to infants at 4 months of age. Given the dense population, it is no surprise that multinational baby food companies indulge in intense marketing of semisolid foods and breast milk substitutes for infants even as young as 1 to 3 months.

National Childhood Immunizations: BCG at 1 to 11 months; DT at 6 years; DTwP at 2, 3, and 4 months; DTwPHep at 2, 3, and 4 months; HepB at 1 to 2 months and 3 and 4 months; OPV before 1 month and at 3 and 4 months; measles at 9 months and 6 years; TT at 7 to 8 years; vitamin A at 6 to 11 and 12 to 59 months. The percent of the target population vaccinated, by antigen, is: BCG (82%); DTP1 (88%); DTP3, HepB3, Polio3, TT2 plus (70%); and MCV (72%).

Other Characteristics: The tsunami of December 26, 2005, devastated the District of Banda Aceh and proximate offshore islands. Aid and relief provided saved thousands of lives and helped prevent outbreaks of infectious diseases. One of the most difficult tasks from a medical perspective is caring for the mental health of those who suffered injury and loss.

BIBLIOGRAPHY

Central Intelligence Agency: *2006: The world factbook, Indonesia.* Retrieved September 21, 2006, from https://www.cia.gov/cia/publications/factbook/print/id.html.

Childbirth Solutions, Inc.: Coconut belly rubs: traditional midwifery care in Malaysia and Indonesia. Retrieved February 25, 2006, from http://www.childbirthsolutions.com/articles/worldbirth/malaysia-indonesia/index.php.

Health Situation Indonesia: Retrieved February 25, 2006, from http://www.whosea.org/EN/Section 313/Section 1520.htm.

Neuland L: Under the banner of Islam: mobilizing religious identities in the West Java, *Australian J Anthropol.* 11(2):199–222, 2000.

UNAIDS: 2006 Indonesia. Retrieved September 21, 2006, from http://www.unaids.org/en/Regions_Countries/Countries/indonesia.asp.

U.S. Library of Congress: Sections on Social Classes, Religions, and Health. Retrieved February 24, 2006, from http://countrystudies.us/indonesia.

World Health Organization: 2006: Immunization, vaccines and biologicals. Retrieved September 21, 2006, from http://www.who.int/immunization_monitoring/en/globalsummary/countryprofileresult.cfm?C='ind'.

World Health Organization: Indonesia, epidemiological factsheet. Retrieved February 25, 2006, from http://www.who.int/hiv/countries/en.

◆ IRAN (ISLAMIC REPUBLIC OF)

MAP PAGE (802)

Majid Sadeghi

Location: The Islamic Republic of Iran is located in the Middle East between the Caspian Sea and the Persian Gulf. The capital is Tehran. Its neighboring countries are Armenia, Azerbaijan, and Turkmenistan to the north; Afghanistan and Pakistan to the east; and Iraq and Turkey to the west. Mountains are in the north and west; large deserts are in the middle; and fertile lands are in the north, northwestern, and southwestern regions. Iran's total area is 1,648,000 km^2 (636,294 square miles). The population is 68.9 million. About 60% of the population lives in urban areas and 40% in rural areas. The gross domestic product (GDP) per capita is $8,300, with 40% living below the poverty line.

Major Languages	Ethnic Groups	Major Religions
Farsi (Persian)	Persian 51%	Shi'a Muslim 89%
Turkic (Azerbaijani)	Azerbaijani 24%	(official)
Kurdish	Gilaki and	Sunni Muslim 10%
Other (English)	Mazandarani 8%	Baha'i, Jewish, Christian,
Arabic (Arab)	Kurd 7%	Zoroastrian

Major Languages	Ethnic Groups	Major Religions
	Arab 3%	
	Lur 2%	
	Baloch 2%	
	Turkmen 2%	
	Other 1%	

The Baha'i group is not recognized as an official and accepted religion in the constitution of Iran. Literacy rates are 86% for men, 73% for women.

Health Care Beliefs: Active health promotion; traditional. Prevention and health promotion are major components of the health care system, and Iran has a widespread primary health care program. Despite a significant decrease in discrimination and stigmatization toward mental disorders, these attitudes remain major challenges. Mental health care is integrated into the health system, although traditional healers continue to have a major role in treating psychiatric patients. Emotional problems are frequently expressed in somatic forms (e.g., headaches, gastrointestinal problems, insomnia). Beliefs that illness may be caused by a person with the "evil eye" (a person who can harm others merely by looking at them) or imbalances in "hot-cold" temperatures or foods are common and coexist with more modern concepts. The integration of such beliefs must be considered by health care professionals when they are providing care.

Predominant Sick-Care Practices: Biomedical and magical-religious. Most people go to medical facilities when they become ill, but traditional healers are also consulted, especially in rural areas. Patients are usually accompanied during doctor's visits by one or more people who listen very carefully, often answering questions directed to the patient. It is common for parents to attach amulets to their infant's clothes to prevent the effects of the evil eye, and prayer is common during times of illness.

Ethnic-/Race-Specific or Endemic Diseases: Endemic diseases include chloroquine-resistant malaria (in rural areas) and cardiovascular diseases. According to the Joint United Nations Program on HIV/AIDS (UNAIDS), the estimated prevalence rate for human immunodeficiency virus (HIV) in adults (aged 15 to 44 years) is 0.2%, with 66,000 living with HIV, including 11,000 women. About 1,600 deaths from acquired immunodeficiency syndrome (AIDS) have occurred. Iranian statistics report that there are about 579 men and 52 women with AIDS. Intravenous drug use (61% of cases), sexual transmission, and blood transfusions are the major sources of transmission. UNAIDS reports that the epidemic appears to be accelerating.

Health-Team Relationships: The doctor is usually the leader of the health team and has a dominant relationship with nurses and other staff. Patient attitudes toward health professionals are respectful, submissive, and obedient. Men may refuse care by female doctors and nurses. Conversely, women may also refuse care from male doctors and nurses.

Families' Role in Hospital Care: If a woman or child is hospitalized, family members (such as a husband) are likely to remain with them. If staying overnight is impossible, relatives visit them every day. Families are usually extremely concerned and pay significant attention to the family member. Bad news may be kept from the patient.

Dominance Patterns: The family and their position in society take precedence over individuals. Iran has a patriarchal society, and the dominant figure in the family is the father or his male surrogate (e.g., grandfather, oldest son). This is the usual pattern in extended families in small cities and rural areas, whereas in larger cities and nuclear families it is becoming more common for authority to be distributed between both parents. Traditional girls may wear a veil at about age 9. Boys and girls usually play together until the end of primary school; restrictions on boy-girl relations are usually in place after this age and are established by adolescence. Discipline of boys tends to be less strict than that of girls. Although women are not equal to men in Iran, the social status of women is considerably better than it is in some neighboring and similar countries. Women are members of parliament, and some are celebrated doctors, university teachers, and researchers. Women represent 62% of university students. Many women work outside the home and do not have to be accompanied by a male relative. Iranian women wear a scarf over their hair (a practice that is more prevalent in larger cities such as Tehran), the traditional Iranian Islamic veil (chador), or both when they are outside the home.

Eye-Contact Practices: As a sign of respect or possibly shame, a person of lower social status avoids direct eye contact when confronting a person of higher status. Women are expected to be modest and do not make direct eye contact with men who are not family members.

Touch Practices: Shaking hands and embracing are acceptable parts of social encounters during greetings and farewells. Women usually avoid shaking hands with men in public.

Perceptions of Time: Iranians are not generally very punctual, and being on time is not particularly important. However, keeping promises is very important and serious, for not doing so means that a person is unreliable. Being respectful of past traditions is a major characteristic of Iranian people.

Pain Reactions: Reactions to pain are usually quite expressive and accompanied by crying and screaming. Such behaviors are particularly acceptable in women. Emotional problems and neuroses often take somatic forms.

Birth Rites: Especially in rural areas, some families prefer to have boys so that they can help the father and eventually replace him and take care of the family. A boy is considered a gift from God, but it is also believed that girls bring health and wealth to a family. Boys and girls receive equal medical treatment when they are sick. In cities, doctors and educated midwives assist in deliveries, which occur primarily in hospitals. The infant mortality rate is 40 deaths per 1,000 live births; the fertility rate is 1.8

children born per mother. In many rural areas, mothers give birth at home with the assistance of a local midwife, who is often an old and experienced family member. Some believe that bathing too early (less than 40 days after birth) may cause puerperal infections, but sponge baths and showers are allowed. Some mothers give their infants an herbal product *(shir khest)* mixed with butter to clean out the intestines in the first few days after birth. An older male family member (usually a grandparent) whispers *Azan* (an Islamic prayer) into the infant's ear, claiming that the child has been born a Muslim and believes in Allah and his prophet Muhammad. The family member then writes down the time and place of the infant's birth on the back cover of the Koran. The infant's name is usually chosen on the sixth day after birth and may be Iranian or Islamic (Arabic). If an Iranian name is chosen, an Islamic nickname is chosen as well. Circumcisions are usually performed before 6 years and usually immediately after birth, followed by a party for all family members. Life expectancy is 69 for men, 72 for women.

Death Rites: According to Islamic beliefs, the deceased continues to live in another world after death. Family members are usually present at the time of death but do not express their emotions in the presence of the deceased person. After death, mourning is loud and expressive. The body is washed and wrapped in a special cloth *(kafan)*. A clergyman *(rowhani)* prays for the deceased, and the body is buried in the ground without a coffin. On the 3rd, 7th, and 40th days, family members and friends participate in ceremonies in the home of the deceased or a mosque and express condolences to the family. A clergyman speaks to the mourners about the nature and philosophy of death in Islam and asks Allah to accept the person, forgive sins, and place the deceased in Heaven. Anniversary ceremonies of the death also occur. Autopsies are acceptable, and organ donations are performed as permitted by religious leaders and the Supreme Leader.

Food Practices and Intolerances: The midday meal is the most important. Dinner is usually served late in the evening. Basic foods are rice with meat, vegetables, stew, wheat bread, dairy products, and broth. Fresh vegetables, fruit, yogurt, or sherbet may be served as dessert. Tea and nonalcoholic beverages are widely used, and food is usually eaten with a spoon, fork, and knife. Pork and alcohol are forbidden. Total fasting is practiced in Ramadan between sunrise and sunset, so an early meal is often eaten before sunrise. The Ramadan fast is not obligatory for children, sick individuals, or pregnant women.

Infant-Feeding Practices: Most Iranians prefer to breastfeed for up to 2 years. Some mothers also bottle-feed, especially those who work outside the home. Mothers may also work part-time or breastfeed at their workplace during established "feeding hours." Nursing mothers usually avoid foods that might change the taste of the milk, but generally there are no restrictions. The two most common liquid and semi-liquid foods introduced between the third and sixth months are made from almonds and rice, boiled in hot water and strained through a clean cloth. The resulting juice is combined with sugar and given by bottle or spoon. The juice is nourishing and helps gradually wean the infant.

Child-Rearing Practices: Until preschool, the education of children is entirely the mother's domain. The upbringing of boys and girls is clearly defined by tradition, and behaviors for each sex are well differentiated. From the age of reason, a girl is supposed to act like her mother. She performs tasks such as helping with housework and preparing for her father's return from work; thus, she fully identifies with her mother. Among boys, the oldest son is the one who identifies most with the father and is the "man of the family" during the father's absence. Child rearing is rather strict, and the father is the main authority figure. Children are expected to do what their parents say, especially what the father says, regarding life choices such as selection of a job, choice of a spouse, and where to live. Children still obey their parents even after becoming adults and having their own children. In recent years, child rearing has become more flexible, especially in larger cities and in educated families. A growing number of parents complain that compared with their own parents, they have become so permissive that their children actually rule the family.

National Childhood Immunizations: BCG at birth; DTwP at 2, 4, 6, and 18 months and at 4 to 6 years; OPV at birth, at 2, 4, 6, and 18 months and at 4 to 6 years; MMR at 12 months and at 4 to 6 years; HepB at birth, 2, 4, 6, and 18 months and at 4 to 6 years; Td repeated every 10 years; influenza for high-risk groups. The percent of the target population vaccinated, by antigen, is: BCG (99%); DTP1 (97%); DTP3 and Polio3 (95%); HepB3 and MCV (94%).

Other Characteristics: Two books are found in every Iranian home: the *Koran* and the *Diwan* (poems) of Hafiz. Hafiz was a great Iranian poet who lived in the fourteenth century AD.

BIBLIOGRAPHY

Central Intelligence Agency: *2006: The world factbook, Iran.* Retrieved September 21, 2006, from https://www.cia.gov/cia/publications/factbook/print/ir.html.

Djazayery A, Pajooyan J: Food consumption patterns and nutritional problems in the Islamic Republic of Iran, *Nutr Health.* 14(1):53, 2000.

Sadeghi M, Mirsepassi G: Psychiatry in Iran: International Psychiatry, *Bul Int Affairs-Royal Coll Psychiatrists.* 10: 10–12, October 2005.

UNICEF: At a glance: Iran (Islamic Republic of) statistics, 2006. Retrieved August 15, 2006, from http://www.unicef.org/infobycountry/iran.html.

UNAIDS: 2006 Iran. Retrieved September 21, 2006, from http://www.unaids.org/en/Regions_Countries/Countries/Iran_Islamic_Republic_of.asp.

World Health Organization: 2006: Immunization, vaccines and biologicals. Retrieved September 21, 2006, from http://www.who.int/immunization_monitoring/en/globalsummary/countryprofileresult.cfm?C='irn'.

World Health Organization: 2006: The world health report, country profiles, Iran (Islamic Republic of). Retrieved August 15, 2006, from http://www.who.int/countries/irn/en/.

◆ IRAQ (REPUBLIC OF)

MAP PAGE (802)

Fawwaz Shakir Mahmoud Al-Joudi

Location: Iraq is located in Southeast Asia and occupies the valleys of the Tigris and Euphrates Rivers. The capital is Baghdad. Northern Iraq is mainly mountainous, the central portion consists of plains, and river valleys extend south and west and fade gradually into desert. The land area is 438,317 km² (169,235 square miles). The population is 26.7 million. In 2003 Iraq was occupied by the United States and its allies, and massive numbers of Iraquis have either died or fled the country. Agriculture was halted, green lands destroyed, and natural resources are in jeopardy. The devastation of decades of war has taken a toll on the health, culture, economy, and stability of the community. The gross domestic product (GDP) per capita is $3,400. Literacy rates are 56% for men, 24% for women.

Major Languages	Ethnic Groups	Major Religions
Arabic (official and major)	Arab 75%	Shi'a Muslim 48%
Kurdish (official in northern Iraq)	Kurdish 17%	Sunni Muslim (Arabs and Kurds) 49%
Kildani (old Assyrian)	Other 8%	Christian 2%
Turkish (Turkmani)	Armenian, Turks (Turkmanis), and minor groups such as Chechnians, Sharkas, and Daghastanis	Others: Sabi'a, Yazidia 1%

Health Care Beliefs: Traditional; health promotion important. People say, "Good health is a blessing from Allah, the Creator." Iraqis believe that health care can be achieved by avoiding harmful or potentially harmful practices. A general awareness of disease has developed, primarily in urban areas. Traditional beliefs and practices prevail, such as regular prayers for health. The importance of good hygiene and cleanliness is highlighted in religious instruction. However, although this type of information is becoming better understood, many are not aware of the role of contaminated water, soil, and food in the transmission of harmful, unseen factors such as microbes. Even in remote areas, people understand the role of vaccinations, although illness is also partly attributed to the influence of fate. Mental defects are feared, and those with mental illnesses are considered cursed creatures who extend their curse to their families. They are generally sent to mental institutions for treatment and isolation. **Predominant Sick-Care Practices:** Biomedical; alternative; magical-religious. The majority receive medical care at government institutions. Some, especially those in rural communities, consult traditional healers and practitioners. Traditional medicine includes herbal medicines based on ancient recipes and use of local and imported herbs. People also consult sheikhs, who are usually old men or women who claim to have special powers. Sheikhs provide those who are ill with amulets called *doa* (meaning "to invite" or "to ask") that repel evil spirits and ask God for help—for care, a cure, forgiveness, or peace. Desperate individuals often seek such healers as a last resort—when conventional medicine fails to cure a difficult or incurable disease. Traditional medical practices were supplemented by modern medical care until the 1990s, when shortages of drugs and medical supplies increased.

Ethnic-/Race-Specific or Endemic Diseases: Endemic diseases include chloroquine-sensitive malaria (primarily northern Iraq), cutaneous leishmaniasis (Baghdad area), visceral leishmaniasis (eastern regions), and hepatitis B (throughout Iraq). Iraqis are at risk for schistosomiasis (*S. haematobium,* the urinary type), amoebiasis, cyclosporiasis, tuberculosis, cryptosporidiosis, trachoma, measles, pertussis (whooping cough), gonorrhea, and syphilis. Iraq had a pertussis outbreak in 1996 and a poliomyelitis outbreak in 1999. Zoonotic diseases include brucellosis, toxoplasmosis, and hydatidosis. Iraq's major organic diseases are cardiovascular diseases and cancer, which are on the increase. War casualties are increasing, with a whole new generation of disabled citizens. Although the Joint United Nations Programme on HIV/AIDS (UNAIDS) has no accurate figures for human immunodeficiency virus (HIV), the estimated prevalence rate in adults (aged 15 to 49 years) is below 0.2%. However, an unprecedented spread of HIV infection is becoming evident in a community with previously very low levels.

Health-Team Relationships: The doctor is the primary authority, and nursing is a woman's profession associated with low status. Patients generally abide by doctors' instructions. Men may refuse care by female doctors and nurses. Medical services are primarily state sponsored and include central and peripheral hospitals and clinics distributed throughout the country. The availability of basic care may differ among centers. Midwifery is still widely practiced in rural and remote areas; they are generally professionally trained, but most lack the skills necessary for complicated deliveries.

Families' Role in Hospital Care: A patient may be accompanied by one or more people who prefer to be present during examinations. They often answer questions for the patient. Occasionally, they perform tasks such as washing and positioning patients in bed. They also bring food, unless forbidden for medical reasons; food is shared by other patients and the hospital staff. Older adults expect to be treated with respect, and the role and expectations of the family are fulfilled through the extreme concern for and attention paid to family members. Reading verses from the Koran to very ill people is common; Muslims believe that it cleanses the soul, prepares the individual for meeting God, and may bring mercy to the suffering person.

Dominance Patterns: In the Islamic perspective, women are looked on with respect. In addition to helping with farming, they are major contributors to the teaching and bringing up of children. Since the establishment of the Independent State of Iraq in 1921, women have begun to move into professional life. Hence, although Iraq is a patriarchal society, women are allowed a great deal of autonomy in the domestic arena and within the family and assume responsibility in the absence of men. Women are achieving professional status in medicine, teaching, engineering, law, and the political sectors. Before 2003, Iraqi women under age 45 could not leave the country unless accompanied by a male escort such as a husband, father, or close male relative or with written permission from a husband or father. At present there seem to be two extremes of conduct: complete liberty versus further restrictions on women's rights.

Eye-Contact Practices: Socially and religiously, members of the opposite sex generally avoid direct eye contact, even when conversing. Eye contact between members of the same sex is the norm.

Touch Practices: Shaking hands is the formal method of greeting, whereas hugging and kissing are more intimate welcomes practiced among closely related people. In these instances, people may touch each other's cheek in a show of affection and tenderness. On arrival and departure, shaking hands, hugging, and kissing are common among family members of both sexes but only between those of the same sex when greeting people outside the family. Because of religious beliefs, many women refrain from shaking hands with men who are not family members.

Perceptions of Time: Punctuality varies according to location. In rural communities, punctuality is almost irrelevant. The situation is different in urban communities, where time has become important now that business practices have set in. Planning ahead is similar; the horizons of thinking and aspirations dictate the dimensions of plans.

Pain Reactions: Iraqis generally have a high pain threshold; however, those in severe pain expect immediate relief, and they may persistently ask for pain medication. Therapy involving exertion contraindicates the Iraqi belief in energy conservation for enhancing recovery. Pain is usually expressed privately or only to close relatives and friends. However, during labor and delivery, pain may be expressed freely and vehemently. The use of analgesics and tranquilizers is usually kept to a minimum to ensure the health and safety of the newborn.

Birth Rites: During the early days of pregnancy, women are encouraged to satisfy their cravings for desired foods. If cravings are denied, Iraqis believe the infant will be born with a birth sign *(wiham)*. Access to antenatal care is increasing. Many pregnant women prefer to have ultrasounds, primarily to discover the sex of the infant. An infant boy is preferred and is the pride of his family, particularly if he is the first child. After birth, mothers are treated as rehabilitating patients for 40 days. They are encouraged to eat nutritious foods to strengthen them for breastfeeding. Family gatherings to welcome the new infant are common. To keep their bones straight and begin training them for restraint, infants are wrapped with two layers of cloth. The inner layer is wrapped around the chest, abdomen, and legs. The second layer is a large, triangular cloth that covers every part of the body except the head. Underneath this layer is absorbent material such as cloth, cotton, or commercial disposable diapers (not affordable for every mother). The infant mortality rate is 48 deaths per 1,000 live births; the fertility rate is four children born per woman. Life expectancy is 67 for men, 70 for women.

Death Rites: Autopsies are uncommon because the body must be buried intact. Organ donations and transplants from a deceased person for the purpose of saving a life are allowed but require special approval by the authorities. If an autopsy must be performed (e.g., for forensic reasons), the body must be sutured back into one piece before it is taken to the family and buried. In Muslim burials, the body is thoroughly washed with water, wrapped in special pieces of white cloth, and buried without a coffin in the ground. Cremation is not permitted.

Food Practices and Intolerances: Pork, carrion, and blood are forbidden foods. Food tends to be spicy. Rice, bread, meat, and vegetables are the staple foods. Except for children and those who are sick, people fast during Ramadan between sunrise and sunset. Surveys by the United Nations Children's Fund (UNICEF) in 1999 in cooperation with the government of Iraq and local authorities in the "autonomous" (northern Kurdish) region provide reliable estimates of infant and child mortality—closely related to food supply. In the autonomous region, better food and resource allocation during the oil-for-food program has contributed to a decrease in childhood mortality. However, childhood mortality clearly increased in Iraq under United Nations sanctions in the 1990s. Deaths of infants have risen since 2003 as a result of diminished medical services, but no death registry is available.

Infant-Feeding Practices: Traditionally, mothers breastfeed their infants to increase the mother-child bond, and they may continue until almost the second year of life. In the past, when a mother did not produce enough milk, "foster mothers" were employed. Bottle-feeding is now an alternative. Infants are introduced to other foods after a few months, and most are consuming regular meals as they finish their first year. Some working mothers may stop breastfeeding, although they are allowed a 1 year paid leave after delivery, followed by an additional 6 months at half salary. The previous Iraqi government launched a campaign to encourage mothers to breastfeed.

Child-Rearing Practices: The father has the final word in disciplinary situations, and children must have their father's permission to travel. Muslim boys are usually circumcised during childhood, at home or in a hospital, and this is celebrated as the first step toward manhood. In accordance with Iraqi law, any child whose father is an Iraqi citizen is also considered an Iraqi citizen, even though their names are written in the mother's foreign passport. Education has always been free, but in the 1970s a large number of schools were established. At the same time, higher education programs were widely expanded. Since 2003, the infrastructure of education has been largely destroyed.

National Childhood Immunizations: BCG at birth; DTwP and OPV at 2, 4, 6, and 18 months and at 4 to 6 years; MMR at 15 months and at 6 years; HepB at birth and at 2 and 6 months; DT at 6 to 12 years; measles at 9 months; rubella at 12 years; Td after age 12 years; vitamin A at 9 and 18 months and at 6 years; TT on visit, +1, +6 months, +1, +1 year. The percent of the target vaccination vaccinated, by antigen, is: BCG and DTP1 (93%); DTP3 and HepB3 (81%); MCV (90%); Polio3 (87%); and TT2 plus (70%). Vaccination programs have been largely abandoned since 2003 along with the depreciated medical services.

Other Characteristics: Health and educational standards have decreased and narcotic drugs have become a problem, although previous use was thought to be low. Basic commodities such as water and electricity are in short supply.

BIBLIOGRAPHY

Ali MM, Shah, IH: Sanctions and childhood mortality in Iraq, *Lancet.* 355 (9218):1851–1857, 2000.

Central Intelligence Agency: *2006: The world factbook, Iraq.* Retrieved September 21, 2006, from https://www.cia.gov/cia/publications/factbook/print/iz.html.

Dixon J: A global perspective on statutory Social Security programs for the sick, *J Health Soc Policy.* 13(3):17–40, 2001.

Garfield R: Studies on young children's malnutrition in Iraq: problems and insights, 1990–1999, *Nutr Rev.* 58(9):269–277, 2000.

Squassoni SA: CRS Report for Congress. *Iraq: U.N. inspections for weapons of mass destruction.* Congressional Research Service, The Library of Congress. November 13, 2005. Retrieved September 15, 2006 from http://www,fas,irg/man/crs/RL 31671.pdf.

UNAIDS: 2006 Iraq. Retrieved September 21, 2006, from http://www.unaids.org/en/Regions_Countries/Countries/iraq.asp.

World Health Organization: 2006: Immunization, vaccines and biologicals. Retrieved September 21, 2006, from qhttp://www.who.int/immunization_monitoring/en/globalsummary/countryprofileresult.cfm?C='ir'.

www.state.gov/www/global/human_rights/1998_hrp_report/iraq.html (retrieved April 10, 2006).

◆ IRELAND (REPUBLIC OF)

MAP PAGE (798)

Tom O'Connor

Location: The Republic of Ireland is located in the extreme northwest of Europe between the Irish Sea and the North Atlantic Ocean. It occupies all but the most northeastern territory of the island, which is still part of the United Kingdom. Ireland encompasses 26 of the 32 counties on the island. The total area is 70,280 km² (43,671 square miles), of which 1,390 km (864 miles) are water. Rugged hills and low mountains run along most of the island's perimeter, whereas the inland areas are flat and undulating. Ireland has 1,448 km (900 miles) of coastline. Nearly 70% of the land is permanent pastures. More than 40% of Ireland's over four million people live within 97 km (60 miles) of Dublin, the capital city.

Major Languages	Ethnic Groups	Major Religions
English	Celtic	Roman Catholic 88%
Irish Gaelic	English minority	Anglican (Church of Ireland) 3%
		Other or None 7%
		Other Christian 2%

The gross domestic product (GDP) per capita is $41,000, with 10% living below the poverty line. Most of the population (58%) resides in urban areas. In the last few years, Ireland has had an influx of Eastern European and African immigrants. The indigenous language of the Celtic people of Ireland is Irish, also known as Gaelic, but most people speak English as their first language. In the far west and areas of the southwest, some people speak Irish. Literacy rates are 99% for both men and women.

Health-Care Beliefs: Active involvement; traditional. Ireland has a rich tradition of paganism. Although largely modernized and Catholicized, many of Ireland's inhabitants still heed the superstitious words and traditions of their ancestors. Younger generations, particularly in urban settings, subscribe to biomedical ideas about health and illness.

Predominant Sick-Care Practices: Biomedical and magical-religious. Until very recently, the absence of prevention and wellness programs resulted in people relying on secondary care, thereby overwhelming the system and causing great delays. Ireland is moving toward an interdisciplinary, team-based type of primary care. In 2001, a major policy document, "Quality and Fairness: A Health System for You," set out the Irish government's agenda with regard to health. Increased focus on a people-centered approach, the development of primary health units, and emphasis on health promotion are the main tenets. This policy aims also to tackle the inequalities in the Irish health care system, which result in markedly poorer health outcomes and indictors from lower socioeconomic backgrounds as well as inequalities that result from geographic locations. Primary care teams made up of interdisciplinary provider members will each serve between 3,000 and 7,000 people. It is estimated that 600 to 1,000 teams will be necessary to meet the needs of the population. Implementation of this policy has been slow, with figures for 2005 showing that only 10 such teams are now operational. The ways in which health services are managed and organized underwent radical change in 2005. The Health Services Executive has replaced 11 regional health authorities in an effort to streamline the bureaucracy of health service management. Entitlement to public medical care is available to all citizens. The population is divided into two groups for eligibility: medical cardholders and non–medical cardholders. Medical cardholders are entitled to free medical care based on a means test, while non–medical cardholders are entitled to medical care while incurring some charges. About 30% of the population is entitled to a medical card, and a new initiative to allow certain groups on the borders of means testing to access free general practitioner services is currently being negotiated. Differential coverage for hospitals for primary care is a distinctive feature of the system. People must be residents in a mental hospital's district to obtain psychiatric care; an effort is being made to remove this prerequisite. People not eligible for medical cards often have private health insurance (PHI); in fact, approximately 1.5 million people (about 42%) have PHI. The care and the expediency with which care is received are often far superior for PHI holders than for those who have medical cards. These factors have been a driving force behind reorganizing the system. Despite implementation of the reform program, public confidence in the Irish health system remains low, as evidenced by recent opinion polls.

Ethnic-/Race-Specific or Endemic Diseases: Circulatory disease, including heart disease, strokes, and other circulatory diseases, account for 38% of the mortality rate; cancers account for 25%. Diseases of the circulatory system have been the leading cause of death at least since 1968; nevertheless, the percentage dying from these diseases has been steadily decreasing. Smoking-related diseases were estimated to be the cause of 23% of all deaths of men and 16% of all deaths of women in 1995. The World Health Organization's estimated prevalence rate for human immunodeficiency virus (HIV) and acquired immunodeficiency syndrome (AIDS) in adults (aged 15 to 49 years) is 0.10% (the Joint United Nations Programme on HIV/AIDS [UNAIDS] estimates 0.2%). The estimated number of children from birth to 15 living with HIV-AIDS is 170. As of December 2004, 3,764 cases of HIV have been reported. The highest incidence of transmission (46%) was reported as the result of heterosexual contact, followed by those who use intravenous drugs (32%). Homosexual transmissions account for 22%. Emigrants from sub-Saharan Africa accounted for almost 50% of newly diagnosed cases in 2004.

Health-Team Relationships: Doctors occupy the dominant role on health care teams and are the most respected. The autonomy of nurses is increasing as nurses' educational levels rise. Since 2002 all pre-registration nursing courses are 4-year undergraduate degree programs run in partnership between higher education institutes (Universities and Institutes of Technology) and health service providers. One year of these programs is given over to an internship in the hospital setting. A variety of postgraduate courses are available to qualified nurses in specialized areas, qualifying postgraduates to practice as clinical nursing specialists. Significant numbers of nurses are now also taking master's degrees, which allows them to practice in some instances as advanced nurse practitioners (ANPs), with increased autonomy. ANPs enjoy admission and discharge privileges and the right to prescribe certain medications. There is also an increase in the numbers of nurses who have obtained and are following doctoral studies in nursing. While the number of applicants to nursing remains high, and the number of training places have increased, there is a shortage and a reliance on nurses from other countries (notably the Philippines and India). Irish nurses are among the most respected and in demand around the world, and as a result, many have left, despite the abundance of work at home.

Families' Role in Hospital Care: A lack of available hospital space and beds makes it difficult not only for patients to obtain beds but also for families to visit for extended periods. The people most likely to visit hospitalized patients are mothers and siblings. Ireland has made a concerted effort to develop separate health care facilities for children, who have previously been housed in adult wards. When children are hospitalized, especially for cancer and other life-threatening illnesses, the family plays a key role in recovery. The Department of Health and Children is moving toward a more family-friendly environment for patients and visitors, increasing their efforts to attend to emotional and psychological needs. Irish people have traditionally had a strong sense of family and community, and illness of a family or community member is a great concern to all involved. This has diminished somewhat, especially in large urban areas.

Dominance Patterns: Before the Famine of 1845, Ireland was predominantly a matriarchal society. The mass exodus of emigrants resulting from the famine began to alter the role of women. A gradual shift toward male dominance began to occur in the 1840s and was well established by 1940. Modern Ireland is defined by the continuing economic boom known as the Celtic Tiger, which has seen Ireland become one of the richest countries in the world. This in turn has altered the patriarchal society. More women are beginning to work outside of the home, and 26% of all households are headed by women.

Eye Contact Practices: Direct eye contact is expected because it indicates respect and honesty.

Touch Practices: A firm handshake is preferred. The Irish have a strong sense of personal space. They may feel comfortable with physical contact with members of their family or very close friends, but acquaintances and casual friends are not usually embraced.

Perceptions of Time: Although traditionally oriented to the past, the Irish have two interpretations of modern time: professional time, which applies to work and education settings, and recreational time. The Irish are expected to arrive on time and to be prepared for work or school events. Punctuality in social interactions is far different, with social events generally starting 20 to 30 minutes late, or on "Irish time."

Pain Reactions: The Irish seldom exhibit or vocalize pain because of their stoic nature.

Birth Rites: The fertility rate is 1.86 children born per woman. Most are Roman Catholic and have their children baptized on the day of a child's birth or about 40 days after. The priest pours holy water over the infant, which symbolically initiates the infant into Christianity and the mother and father into parenthood. The infant mortality rate is 5 deaths per 1,000 live births. Life expectancy is 75 for men, 80 for women.

Death Rites: In an attempt to thwart evil spirits from entering the body, the Irish have long kept vigil over the dead. The associated ritual was maintained throughout the rise of Christianity and is referred to as "waking the dead." Friends and family congregate in the home of the deceased, where they celebrate the individual's life and their passage into the next life. Participants comfort one another and dance, sing, and tell stories during this celebration.

Food Practices and Intolerances: Traditional dietary habits show a high consumption of potatoes, vegetables, and diary products, reflecting local agricultural produce. Although the number of people consuming the recommended number of fruit and vegetables has increased, many still consume large amounts of high-fat and high-salt foods. There is a marked increase in the consumption of pasta and rice, reflecting the growing multicultural nature of Irish society. Tea (usually served with milk) remains the beverage of choice. There is also growing concern for rising levels of obesity.

Infant-Feeding Practices: According to a recent survey, about 40% of mothers breastfeed their infants. The percentage decreases with the birth of each additional child, and 4 of every 10 women have stopped breastfeeding by the time the infant reaches the age of 6 months. Mothers who are more highly educated are more likely to nurse their children. In addition, the more professional the husband's career, the more likely his wife is to breastfeed. Most mothers (59%) bottle-feed their infants with formula, perhaps because almost 50% of all Irish mothers work outside the home; about 50% of children are born to unmarried mothers.

Child-Rearing Practices: The mother functions as the primary parent; the father is secondary and focuses more on being a support system. Recent studies indicate that modern fathers participate in domestic and childcare duties more than previous generations, although mothers still carry the bulk of those responsibilities. In 1998, a committee on the rights of the child expressed alarm about the level of violence in many Irish households and the absence of mandatory reporting legislation. Ireland banned corporal punishment in schools in 1982; in 1997, it was made a criminal offense. In the same year, the Parliamentary Select Committee on Social Affairs recommended that the existing defense for chastisement of children by parents, teachers, and persons having lawful control of them should be abolished. However, Ireland opted to reduce and prevent physical punishment through education rather than legislation.

National Childhood Immunizations: BCG at birth; DTaPHibIPV at 2, 4, and 6 months; DTaPIPV at 4 to 5 years; MMR at 12 to 15 months and at 4 to 5 years; Td at 11 to 14 years; HepB at 0, +1, and +6 months; MenC_conj at 2, 4, and 6 months; Pneumo_conj at 2, 4, and 6 months. The percent of the target population vaccinated, by antigen, is: BCG (93%); DTP1 (96%); DTP3, Hib3, and Polio3 (90%); and MCV (84%).

BIBLIOGRAPHY

Central Intelligence Agency: *2006: The world factbook, Ireland.* Retrieved September 21, 2006, from https://www.cia.gov/cia/publications/factbook/print/ei.html.
Department of Health and Children, Dublin: 2001 Quality and fairness—a health system for you. Retrieved February 1, 2006, from http://www.dohc.ie/publications/quality_and_fairness.html.

Department of Health and Children, Dublin: 2005 Health system achievements. Retrieved February 1, 2006, from http://www.dohc.ie/publications/health_system_achievements_oct_2005.html.

Department of Health and Children, Dublin: *2005 Nursing for public health: realising the vision.* Retrieved February 1, 2006, from http://www.dohc.ie/publications/realising_vision.html.

Fealy GM: Aspects of curriculum policy in preregistration nursing education in the Republic of Ireland: issues and reflections, *J Adv Nursing.* 37(6):558–565, 2002.

Health Services Executive: 2005 National service plan. Dublin. Retrieved January 17, 2006, from http://www.hse.ie/en/Publications/HSEPublications/FiletoUpload, 2106,en.pdf.

Treacy M, Hyde A: Developments in nursing in Ireland: the emergence of a disciplinary discourse, *J Prof Nursing.* 19(2):91–98, 2003.

World Health Organization: 2004 Epidemiological fact sheets on HIV/AIDS and sexually transmitted infections, Ireland. Retrieved March 28, 2006, from http://www.who.int/GlobalAtlas/predefinedReports/EFS2004/EFS_PDFs/EFS2004_IE.pdf.

World Health Organization: 2006: Immunization, vaccines and biologicals. Retrieved September 21, 2006, from http://www.who.int/immunization_monitoring/en/globalsummary/countryprofileresult.cfm?C='irl'.

◆ ISRAEL (STATE OF)

MAP PAGE (802)

Vered Kater

Location: Israel is located at the eastern end of the Mediterranean Sea, with Lebanon to the north, Syria to the northeast, Jordan to the east, and Egypt to the southwest. The total area is 20,770 km^2 (8,019 square miles). The coastal plain is fertile, and the southern region is primarily desert. The population is 6.9 million, including about 187,000 Israeli settlers in the West Bank, about 20,000 in the Golan Heights, more than 5,000 in the Gaza Strip, and fewer than 177,000 in East Jerusalem. The gross domestic product (GDP) per capita is $24,600, with 21% below the poverty line. The capital is Jerusalem, although most countries maintain embassies in Tel Aviv. Literacy rates are 97% for men, 94% for women.

Major Languages	**Ethnic Groups**	**Major Religions**
Hebrew (official)	Jewish 76%	Judaism 76%
Arabic (official for Arab minority)	Arab and other 20%	Muslim 11%
English (widely spoken)	Other 4%	Christian 9%
Yiddish (ultraorthodox and Ashkenazim immigrants from Europe)		Other (including Druze) 4%
Ladino (ultraorthodox Judeo-Spanish, Sephardic Jews)		

Health Care Beliefs: Active involvement; prevention important. Most individuals younger than 50 are active in self-care and complementary and alternative health care activities. Naturopathy and Feldenkrais methods, acupuncture, and homeopathy are accepted forms of treatment. Vitamins and over-the-counter food supplements are frequently used. Preventive medical examinations are not routine: the medical establishment sends notices for mammograms but not for yearly examinations. Mental health care is under the Ministry of Health, and 6% of the health budget goes to this service. In 1995, Israel instituted obligatory reporting of all mental health cases. Today, 148,000 cases are registered; 5,589 beds are available in 20 hospitals, and an additional seven centers for day care have the ability to treat 1,300 clients. Religious beliefs do not affect attitudes, but families prefer not to acknowledge mental health problems because to do so might decrease their children's marriage prospects.

Predominant Sick-Care Practices: Biomedical; alternative; and religious. Israel has a widespread public health system, and all citizens have government-provided medical insurance. All citizens have to be members of one of the "sick funds," and soldiers are insured by the army. The country has a basic package of health services, but 30% of costs are paid by patients. The average Israeli is willing to pay for complementary health care. Immigrants from the former Soviet Union often prefer to go to a healer first; if the healer cannot cure them, they go to their general practitioner. The use of religious objects, pictures, prayers, and booklets is common when someone is ill, and red-string bracelets are still placed on some newborn infants to protect them. Before signing a medical consent form, most religious families ask their leader (a rabbi) for his opinion and abide by his decision, even if the medical practitioner does not agree.

Ethnic-/Race-Specific or Endemic Diseases: Glucose-6-phosphate dehydrogenase (G6PD) and lactose deficiency are common. Eastern European Jews have a high occurrence of the *BCRA* gene, which is associated with a high incidence of breast and colon cancers. Tay-Sachs disease is now rare because of prenatal testing, and infantile Niemann-Pick disease is now uncommon as well. Familial Mediterranean fever is ethnicity specific. Adult Gaucher disease, diabetes, and atherosclerosis are prevalent, and salmonellosis is much more prevalent than shigellosis. The incidence of tuberculosis is decreasing: 7.3 cases per 100,000 in 2004 compared with 7.9 cases in 2003. The World Health Organization (WHO) estimated the prevalence rate for human immunodeficiency virus (HIV)/acquired immunodeficiency syndrome (AIDS) in adults (aged 15 to 49 years) to be 0.10% in 2003. The Joint United Nations Programme on HIV/AIDS [UNAIDS] reported a prevalence of less than 0.2% in 2006. Recent estimates report that about 4,309 persons are living with HIV/AIDS. Most cases seem to be transmitted heterosexually.

Health-Team Relationships: Israel has a high level of health care with high doctor-patient (4.6 per 1000) and nurse-patient (5.9 per 1000) ratios. A nursing law setting a legal framework for the profession has not been passed, although discussions have been ongoing since the 1970s. Perceptions of overwork, low income, and lack of control contribute to dissatisfaction within nursing. Nursing education is 3 years for a registered nurse and 4 years for a nurse with a bachelor of arts degree. Both types of nurses must take state board examinations. Israel has two schools of nursing where nurses with bachelor's degrees can obtain a master's degree in nursing. Nurses who want to continue and obtain their doctoral degree in nursing can do so at universities in Tel Aviv and Jerusalem. Israel has no nurse practitioners, so nurses with a clinical nurse specialty master's degree from the United States are not allowed to open an independent practice in Israel. Immigrant nurses must be recognized by the Ministry of Health, and many have to retake state board examinations. Almost all schools of nursing have reschooling courses for immigrant nurses, typically allowing them to qualify for state board examinations in 1 or 2 years. Nurses are considered professionals but are not thought of as independent workers.

Families' Role in Hospital Care: Most patients are accompanied by family members, and one person is allowed to stay with the patient at all times. The family often wants to bring food, but this is not allowed because of dietary laws. In reality, the family often does find a way to provide additional food. Meals in the hospitals are sound and sufficient, but patients do not always like the taste. Personal care is occasionally, but not frequently, provided by the family.

Dominance Patterns: About 230 Israeli communities are known as *kibbutzim*. These communal living areas began at the turn of the century as agricultural cooperatives protected by armed settlers. Property is shared equally, and although residents do not receive a salary, they are provided housing, pocket money, and necessities such as medical care and education. Women do the same work as men. Originally, the children lived in a separate house near their parents, but today the children spend their days with other children and only eat and sleep in their parents' quarters. Another form of communal living is the *moshav*, in which each family owns their own land and house, but purchasing and selling are cooperative. Israel has a reputation of being an egalitarian society, especially because of its common military service. Men and women are compelled to join, but women serve only 21 months, whereas men serve 38 months. Israel is a religious state, so religion is part of its politics. The religious authority (rabbinate) rules on personal and family issues. Marriage must be contracted religiously, and no civil marriages are allowed. A couple can obtain a divorce only through the rabbinical offices. Polygamy is prohibited by civil law but not by religious authorities (either Jewish or Arab). Dispensations can be granted for men to take a second wife, but this is rare. Some religious groups arrange marriages, and authorities tend to ignore the practice. Israel has a low (20%) divorce rate: only 1% of families are headed by a single parent.

The ideal woman is a wife and mother and is considered the cornerstone of the family. Israelis undergo more fertility treatments than any country in the world, and the treatments are subsidized by the government. The education levels of men and women are equal, but women still work for lower wages even when in the same job. Unemployment rates are higher for women, as are poverty rates. Ultraorthodox Israeli women are in the worst position, although they claim to be happy with the status quo. Israel remains patriarchal, with men making major decisions for their families—a fact that is true for all groups, not just for the ultraorthodox. It is important for health care personnel to realize that men and women who are not related by blood are not allowed to be alone in a room together. Therefore, when a male nurse or doctor is talking to a woman, the door to the room must be left open. Women belonging to ultraortho-dox groups have defined roles and restrictions. They must obey their husbands without questioning the rationale behind their orders. According to Jewish religious law, husbands have total control over marital rela-tionships and can grant or deny a divorce. Many women are considered *agunot* (meaning "chained"); they want a divorce but their husbands refuse to consent.

Eye-Contact Practices: Israelis maintain direct eye contact when meeting and talking with others.

Touch Practices: Handshaking and hugging are common practices among friends. First names are used with superiors and strangers. Among religious Jewish males (whether in Israel or elsewhere), a man never shakes hands with or touches a woman because she may be menstruat-ing, and contact during this period is not allowed. Female nurses should recognize the importance of this tradition and never touch male patients until they have confirmed their religious beliefs. Other females are allowed to touch or comfort children and women.

Perceptions of Time: Focus on the future decreases with age, and focus on the past increases. Because of the increase in terrorist activities, many Nazi Holocaust survivors need mental health assistance. For these older adults, recurring nightmares, tension, and an inability to cope are signifi-cant problems.

Pain Reactions: Patients can be very demanding, so if a doctor does not do what they want, patients may invent additional symptoms and exagger-ate pain to receive the drugs they believe they need. Often patients' friends tell them to take a particular drug for a certain ailment. Patients frequently ask for second and third opinions and consider numerous inva-sive and expensive tests to be very important and desirable.

Birth Rites: The fertility rate is 2.41 children born per woman. Many orthodox Jews will not utter the name of an infant until the infant is born for fear of inviting the "evil eye" *(ayin hara)*. Traditionalists believe that no one should buy anything for the infant or decorate the nursery before the birth because it may attract the evil eye or bad energy. Families rarely have baby showers, although many Jews order items before the birth and have the store send them after the infant is born. In orthodox families, no man is allowed to touch any female (including a wife or daughter) during menstruation. During the delivery, the husband is encouraged to be near his wife and make eye contact. He may sit with his back to the birth. The newborn is believed to be susceptible to evil influences during the first week of life, so a talisman such as a prayer book or knife is often put next to a newborn. Jews perform circumcision on the 8th day after birth, and Muslims perform the procedure on the 40th day. Orthodox Jews may be heard reading prayers together even at the height of labor pains, a practice that adds a uniquely Jewish dimension to an intensely physical experience. Frequently used prayers repeat a sentence from the *Amida* (a daily prayer): "Adonai sifatai tiftach u'fi yagid tehilatecha," ("Gd open up my lips and my mouth will declare your praise" [the name of God is never written with the letter o] and *Aneni* ("answer me"), which is a priestly benediction from the days of the temple. The healing process after the delivery ends with immersion in the ritual bath *(mikvah)* after termination of vaginal bleeding. Only then is the woman allowed to rejoin her husband in his bed. This ritual also is repeated after each menstrual period. The infant mortality rate is seven deaths per 1,000 live births. Life expectancy is 77 for men, 82 for women.

Death Rites: It is disrespectful to leave a dying person alone, so a relative remains with him or her to ensure that the soul does not leave the body. Rituals may start before a death has occurred. Embalming and the use of cosmetics are forbidden by the orthodox. Autopsies are forbidden except for forensic reasons in the case of a suspicious death. Many rabbis, including orthodox, encourage organ donations. The family asks their permission, and few refuse. Burial is in the ground in a shroud, and only casualties of war or people who had an accidental death are buried in a coffin. Jewish law requires burial within 24 hours unless the Sabbath intervenes. The eyes of the deceased are to be closed at death, and the body is left covered and untouched until a family member or Jewish undertaker is contacted for ritual proceedings. Seven days of mourning and an official leave from work are observed after the funeral.

Food Practices and Intolerances: Observant Jews are allowed to eat animals with hooves that chew their cud, and only fish with scales are considered fit for consumption. In addition to food, utensils must also be kosher. Milk and meat are not eaten at the same meal. Many religious people bring their own utensils and food when eating in countries other than Israel. Food preferences differ vastly among the various population groups. Eastern Europeans have a tendency to sweeten their food even when eating fish dishes. Asians add many hot spices and enjoy garlic, even for breakfast.

Infant-Feeding Practices: Breastfeeding is encouraged in all hospitals, and La Lèche groups are common. About 86% of all women begin after birth. Among Jewish women of higher educational levels, breastfeeding is increasing, whereas the opposite is occurring in Arab populations. In orthodox Jewish and Arab communities, the period of breastfeeding is slightly longer than it is in other groups. The average duration is 26 weeks for Jewish women and 37 weeks for Arab women. Breastfeeding begins immediately after delivery unless the new mother specifically states that she does not want to try it. Mothers are entitled to 12 weeks of paid maternity leave.

Child-Rearing Practices: At age 13 for boys and 12 for girls, Jewish children celebrate becoming full members of the community with a ceremony of *bar mitzvah* (for boys) or *bat mitzvah* (for girls). At age 18, all must join the armed forces (although some exemptions are allowed). Joining the military is the true rite of passage into adulthood. Education is rather permissive, and children are the center of the family. Religious families tend to be more strict. Children begin religious schooling at the age of 3 or 4 years, and the routine of daily prayers and intensive bible study adds several extra hours of lessons to the day. Education is obligatory until age 16 years and free until age 18; however, many educational items are actually bought by parents who can afford them.

National Childhood Immunizations: DT at 2, 4, and 12 months; DTaPIPV at 7 years and 18, 24 to 30 months; DTaPHibIPV at 2, 4, 6, and 12 months; MMR at 12 months and 6 years; Hep B at birth and 6 months; Td 13 years. The percent of the target population vaccinated, by antigen, is: BCG (98%); DTP1, HepB3, and MCV (95%); Hib3 (96%); and Polio3 (93%).

Other Characteristics: Israelis classify themselves as "religiously observant" or "not religiously observant" Jews. Observant Jews cannot travel, write, or turn on electric appliances on the Sabbath (Saturday). Religion is not a major part of daily life for a significant proportion of the population. Israelis are becoming increasingly concerned about cocaine and heroin abuse involving drugs from Lebanon and Jordan and alcoholism resulting from the recent waves of immigration from the former Soviet Union. Terrorists are a constant threat to the region's stability and safety.

BIBLIOGRAPHY

Central Intelligence Agency: *2006: The world factbook, Israel.* Retrieved September 21, 2006, from https://www.cia.gov/cia/publications/factbook/print/is.html.

Gilad J, Borer A, Riesenberg K, Peled N, Schlaeffer F: Epidemiology and ethnic distribution of multidrug-resistant tuberculosis in southern Israel, *Chest.* 117(3):738, 2000.

Malach-Pines A: Nurse' burnout: an existential psychodynamic perspective, *J Psychosoc Nurs Ment Health Serv.* 38(2):23, 2000.

Orpaz R, Korenblit M: Family nursing in community-oriented primary health care, *Int Nurs Rev.* 41(5):155, 1994.

Riba S, Greenberger C, Reches H: State involvement in professional nursing development in Israel: promotive or restrictive. *2004 Online Journal of Issues in Nursing* Article published August 31, 2004.

World Health Organization: 2006: Immunization, vaccines and biologicals. Retrieved September 21, 2006, from rhttp://www.who.int/immunization_monitoring/en/globalsummary/countryprofileresult.cfm?C='is'.
http://www.globalhealthreporting.org/ (Retrieved 5 March 2006).
http://he.wikipedia.org/wiki August (Retrieved 5 March 2006).
www.http//worldbank.org (Retrieved 5 March 2006).
http://www.infomed.co.il/immun.htm (Retrieved 5 March 2006).
http://www.nfc.co.il (Retrieved 5 March 2006).
http://www.btl.gov.il (Retrieved 5 March 2006).

◆ ITALY (ITALIAN REPUBLIC)

MAP PAGE (798)

Alvisa Palese and Luisa Saiani

Location: The Italian peninsula extends into the Mediterranean Sea in southern Europe and includes Sicily and Sardinia. It is bordered by Austria and Switzerland on the north, Slovenia on the northeast, the Adriatic Sea on the east, the Ionian Sea on the southeast, the Mediterranean Sea on the west, and France on the northwest. The total area is 301,230 km^2 (116,305 square miles). The Po River flowing from the Alps provides alluvial plains. The population is more than 58 million. The gross domestic product (GDP) per capita is $29,200. Literacy rates are about 99% for both men and women.

Major Languages	Ethnic Groups	Major Religions
Italian	Italian 98%	Roman Catholic 98%
German	Other 2%	Muslim 2%
French		
Slovene		

German is spoken in the northeastern region of Trentino-Alto Adige, French in Valle d'Aosta and the northwestern region of Piedmont, and Slovene in Trieste-Goriza in the northeast. Most people are ethnic Italian, but there are clusters of German, French, Greek, Slovene, and Albanian Italians. Although most define themselves as Roman Catholic, only a minority are practicing.

Health Care Beliefs: Active involvement; some traditional. In general, Italians are paying more attention to their health. Primary prevention is widespread, as is secondary prevention (such as screening for cancer). The number of cigarette smokers is decreasing with the introduction of laws that forbid smoking in public buildings. The majority of Italians use the National Health Service; some use private sector services. Most

Italians approach treatment with a positive attitude and want to be informed and involved in decision making.

Predominant Sick-Care Practices: Primarily biomedical. Some people may still follow practices such as hanging garlic or onions in the home or on the body to prevent illness, but this is uncommon. Pilgrimages to Lourdes (France) or Saint Giovanni Rotondo (in southern Italy) are popular options for those who believe in the healing powers of the Madonna and the saints. In most cases, these practices are officially approved by the Roman Catholic Church. Traditional healers and practices are still used in some places, being most common in southern Italy and among the elderly and uneducated. Some alternative therapies are available B and are employed when standard treatment is unsuccessful or unsatisfactory to the patient.

Ethnic-/Race-Specific or Endemic Diseases: Cardiovascular diseases (although somewhat less prevalent than in northern Europe because of the healthier Italian diet) and cancer are by far the most prevalent chronic diseases. The third highest cause of death is from motor-vehicle and work-related accidents. Obesity and lack of physical activity are resulting in a higher incidence of diabetes. Tuberculosis is an emerging problem, particularly among new immigrants. Endemic diseases include goiter (in Calabria), Lyme borreliosis (in northeastern Italy), tick-borne encephalitis (TBE) and hepatitis delta virus (in southern Italy). Italians are at risk for malaria imported from countries in which it is highly endemic—although it was endemic in the Sibari plain until recently. No single diseases are highly specific for Italy, with the possible exception of β-thalassemia, which is Mediterranean rather than Italian and has almost disappeared because of prenatal diagnosis methods. Hepatitis B has almost disappeared because of mass vaccination campaigns. Italians are among the healthiest people in the world and live longer than most. The World Health Organization (WHO) has estimated the prevalence rate for human immunodeficiency virus (HIV) and acquired immunodeficiency syndrome (AIDS) in adults (aged 15 to 49 years) as 0.5%: about 150,000 people, 50,000 of which are women. AIDS deaths are about 3,000.

Health-Team Relationships: The National Health Service guarantees primary and chronic care to all citizens. The quality of treatment, overall, is high. Much effort is being channeled to increasing communication skills between patients and health care professionals. Patients are requiring better explanations of illness, thereby requiring health care professionals to be better communicators. As nurses achieve advanced education, there has been an accompanying increase in professional status. This has facilitated good teamwork and a staff that can act independently. Teamwork is the exception rather than the rule and depends on the hospital, particularly the departmental leaders. Pediatric hospitals are leading a movement toward child-friendly hospitals, and a network of pediatric wards is working on building team-based relationships.

Families' Role in Hospital Care: Many families are close and provide moral and practical support to their relatives during hospitalizations. Direct or indirect care (given by a person paid for by the family) is common. In some cases, a family member stays with the patient, but some hospitals cannot accommodate this. Bad news, such as the diagnosis of cancer, is always given to the family rather than to the patient. When patients have long hospital stays (such as organ transplants), or if the hospital is not in the region where they live, some hospitals offer accommodations near the hospital.

Dominance Patterns: Italian society is fairly egalitarian. In rural areas, women may take the major responsibility for keeping the house and rearing children, whereas men assume the major responsibility for economic support of the family. In cities, this traditional role division has been abandoned. Men may now ask employers for several months of paternity leave to care for children. Women generally work and children go to day care or kindergarten as soon as possible.

Eye-Contact Practices: Direct eye contact is preferred and an important part of both formal and informal interpersonal relationships. Avoiding direct eye contact may be interpreted as embarrassment, a poor social relationship, or ignorance of local customs.

Touch Practices: Touch is common among Italians, who tend to be warm and outgoing. Shaking hands and hugging and kissing between members of the same or opposite sex are common and acceptable. It is common for women to walk arm-in-arm. Practices based on touching, such as shiatsu and massage, are popular, as are various forms of direct contact, such as massage for pregnant women, especially by midwives before and during delivery. Direct skin-to-skin contact with small, premature infants is practiced, although it is not being used in the majority of hospitals yet. Northern Italians may be somewhat less receptive to touching.

Perceptions of Time: Italians' perceptions of time cannot be characterized in a particular way. Punctuality practices are very similar to those of other European countries. Italy has had a historic trend toward attention to the present—a part of the general hedonistic trend in the Western world.

Pain Reactions: Pain relief has become a major priority for doctors and nurses, even though Roman Catholicism views pain as a natural part of life. A national project to create awareness of pain strategies in hospitals, nursing homes, institutions for elderly persons, and home care is underway. However, increased attention is being given to patient groups such as older adults, women who are giving birth, and people with chronic diseases. Nurses use a scale to assess pain during hospitalization. Pain control is regulated by the medical system, and patients have few concerns about possible addiction. The law allows home-care nurses to administer morphine when prescribed by a doctor; impossible a few years ago. Avoiding unnecessary pain and trying to alleviate it are now common in all spheres of Italian medicine and for all ages of patients, including newborns.

Birth Rites: The fertility rate is 1.28 children born per woman. Infants are born in hospitals with delivery units offering several delivery positions as well as water births. Cesarean section is not uncommon. Home births are discouraged because of the potential risks involved. The infant mortality rate is 6 deaths per 1,000 live births. Increasingly, fathers are present in delivery rooms, but they are still in the minority because of policy restrictions in some maternity units. More frequently, mothers, sisters, or friends are present at childbirths. The mother stays in the hospital for 2 or 3 days. The newborn usually stays with the mother, and breastfeeding is encouraged. The father usually decorates the home outside with either a blue or pink stork. Attitudes toward abortion for any reason are fairly liberal, and contraception is allowed by law. Circumcision is uncommon. Religious ceremonies such as baptisms are arranged later, after the infant is several weeks old. Most mothers work, so time taken off is in conjunction with the maternity benefits that are allowed: 2 months before and 3 months after the delivery. Life expectancy is 78 for men, 84 for women.

Death Rites: Most people die in hospitals, but there is a trend toward dying at home. Home-care services and hospice centers with teams competent in palliative care are increasing. Birth and death are accepted as part of life, and people speak openly about these events. In rural areas, a death announcement is attached to the wall of the house with a photograph and information on burial arrangements. A death notice is also put in the local paper. There are geographic differences in response: keeping grief to oneself in the north compared with open crying and wailing in the south. Black is worn for mourning and funerals, and the flowers are white. Religious rituals such as last rites (*estrema unzione*, blessing by a priest when death is impending) are still common among Roman Catholics. When the person dies at home, the body is usually prepared by the family. Babies are placed in white coffins. The coffin is carried into church with the priest and women following and children singing hymns. The men are at the end of the procession. Cremation is requested more frequently today, and only recently has a law been passed allowing families to keep the ashes of the deceased. Funeral and burial practices generally follow the rites of the church, followed by a meal. Autopsies are accepted when legally necessary or to determine the cause of death. Organ donations are permitted and encouraged, and all citizens have the option to carry a card declaring which organs are to be donated in case of death. The Muslim population follows Islamic death rites, in which the body is wrapped in a shroud and buried immediately without a coffin.

Food Practices and Intolerances: Most Italians follow a typical Mediterranean diet, which includes fish, vegetables, fruits, and grains, and red meat is emphasized less. Heart-healthy red wine with meals is common.

However, fast foods and foods high in saturated fat are becoming more popular, especially among young people.

Infant-Feeding Practices: Breastfeeding prevalence has increased during the last decade, mainly because of changing attitudes among health care professionals and, consequently, the public. Prevalence of initial exclusive breastfeeding now ranges from 85% to 95%. By 4 months after delivery, 35% to 45% of women are still breastfeeding. The rates are highest among educated women in higher socioeconomic classes. The need to return to work is still one of the main reasons for ending breastfeeding.

Child-Rearing Practices: Child-rearing styles vary considerably. After the previous period of permissiveness, parents have again begun considering the value of establishing clear rules and boundaries. Particularly among educated people and those in more northern parts of the country, men are taking on many traditionally female roles and activities within the family, such as food preparation and child care.

National Childhood Immunizations: aP, MenC_conj at 3, 5, and 11 to 12 months; Dip, Pneumo_conj at 3, 5, 11 to 12 months, and at 5 to 6 and 11 to 15 years; DT, DTaP, and IPV at 3, 5, and 11 to 12 months and at 5 to 6 years; DTaPHep, DTaPHepIPV, DTaPHib, DTaPHibHep, DTa-PHibHepIPV, and DTaPIPV at 3, 5, and 11 to 12 months; HepB at 5 months; Hib at 3, 5, and 11 to 12 months; measles, MM, MMR, MR, mumps at 12 to 15 months and at 5 to 12 years; Td at 11 to 15 years. The percent of the target population vaccinated, by antigen, is: DTP1 (97%); DTP3 and HepB3 (96%); Hib3 (95%); MCV (87%); and Polio3 (97%).

BIBLIOGRAPHY

a cura di Daghio MM, Di Giulio P, Scurti V, Tognoni G: Partecipare, condividere, comunicare, *Assistenza Infermieristica e Ricerca.* 4, 2005.

Briziarelli: Infortuni e morte sul lavoro, *Educazione Sanitaria e promozione della salute.* 28:257–263; 2005.

Central Intelligence Agency: 2006: *The world factbook, Ecuador.* Retrieved September 21, 2006, from https://www.cia.gov/cia/publications/factbook/print/ec.html.

Ciceroni L et al: Isolation and characterization of *Borrelia burgdorferi* sensu lato strains in an area of Italy where Lyme borreliosis is endemic, J Clin Microbiol. 39(6):2254, 2001.

Civenti ti G. Riflessioni sulla qualità nel lavoro sociale, *Prospettive sociali e sanitarie.* 2:1-5, 2006.

Modolo MA: Ancora educazione sanitaria e promozione della salute, *Educazione Sanitaria e Promozione della Salute.* 28:177–181; 2005.

Romi R, Sabatinelli G, Majori G: Malaria epidemiological situation in Italy and evaluation of malaria incidence in Italian travelers, *J Travel Med.* 8(1):6, 2001.

UNAIDS: 2006 Italy. Retrieved August 8, 2006, from http://www.unaids.org/en/Regions_Countries/Countries/italy.asp.

World Health Organization: 2006: Immunization, vaccines and biologicals. Retrieved September 21, 2006, from http://www.who.int/immunization_monitoring/en/globalsummary/countryprofileresult.cfm?C='ita'.

http://www.hivinsite.ucsf.edu/global (retrieved August 8, 2006).

♦ JAMAICA

MAP PAGE (796)

Audrey M. Pottinger

Location: The island of Jamaica covers a total area of 10,991 km^2 (4,242 square miles). It is 885 km (550 miles) south of Miami, Florida, and 145 km (90 miles) from Cuba. It is the third largest island in the region. The island is divided into 14 parishes and has two major urban centers: Kingston, the capital, on the southeast coast, and Montego Bay on the northwest coast. Jamaica has been an independent state of the Commonwealth since 1962 and is governed by a parliamentary system of democracy. The population is 2.7 million, with 40% younger than 20 years. The gross domestic product (GDP) per capita is $4,400, with 19% living below the poverty line. Literacy rates are 84% for men, 92% for women.

Major Languages	Ethnic Groups	Major Religions
English	Black 91%	Church of God 21%
Creole/Patois	Mixed 7%	Seventh-Day Adventist 9%
	East Indian 1%	Baptist 9%
	White, Chinese,	Pentecostal 8%
	Other 1%	Anglican 6%
		Roman Catholic 4%
		Other, including spiritualist cults 43%

Health Care Beliefs: Acute sick care; traditional. People are considered healthy if they are physically fit and have energy and vitality, and there is a reliance on herbs and homemade tonics. Illness is divided into two categories: "natural" and "unnatural." Natural illness is perceived to be caused by interaction with the natural environment (e.g., traumatic injuries, coughs, colds); unnatural illness is caused by the supernatural. For "natural" illness, people believe remedies such as baths, acupuncture, hot bush teas, and marijuana *(ganja)* are superior to medicine. Bush teas are made from the leaves and roots of herbs that are steeped in water and sweetened. It is believed that natural illness can also be the physical manifestation of spiritual factors, transforming it into an "unnatural" illness. For example, Obeah men and women are reputed to have a well-developed system of supernatural knowledge that is used to cause good or evil at the request of individuals. To cause an "unnatural" illness, the Obeah man or woman sends a spirit, or *duppy,* to the person who is to be made ill. The ill person must consult another Obeah person to be released from this influence. Some Obeah men and women specialize in using their spiritual knowledge to do good, whereas others do harm. The prevention and treatment of illness depend on the ability of the individual to determine the cause of the illness through its signs and symptoms. The *Bible* is usually kept open to various psalms and placed at open windows and under the pillow of sick people to ward off evil spirits that maintain poor health. Some people also plant strong-scented herbs such as basil to alert them to spiritual forces that may be entering the home. Although not openly admitted, many Jamaicans believe that the causes of mental illness include spirit possession, witchcraft, breaking of religious taboos, divine retribution, and the capture of the soul by a spirit. Some, therefore, are likely to choose traditional treatment over biomedical.

Predominant Sick-Care Practices: Biomedical; alternative; and magical-religious. Biomedical services are well established, whereas magical-religious practices are informal. Many of the latter practices derived from West African tribes brought to Jamaica as slaves. Both receive endorsement from the general populace. The individual may first consult a biomedical practitioner but usually continues treatment with a traditional practitioner if he or she believes the illness may be unnatural. Three classes of information are used to decide whether the illness should be treated by a doctor or traditional practitioner. If the illness comes on suddenly and its symptoms are severe, people seek immediate help from a doctor. If the symptoms are not sudden or severe, people wait before taking action, paying attention to any "divine cues" in the form of omens or dreams sent by divine messengers. People also consider advice from members of the community. People then select between biomedical and traditional practitioners. Traditional practitioners can be herbalists/healers or Obeah men and women (considered illegal practitioners because they are in contravention of the Obeah Act of 1898, which is still enforced). Herbalists/healers can be medical doctors and other educated persons who have studied and practiced alternative medicine, including acupuncture, healing through music, and the use of herbs.

Ethnic-/Race-Specific or Endemic Diseases: The five leading causes of death are malignant neoplasms (cancer), cerebrovascular disease, heart disease, diabetes mellitus, and assault (homicide). More women die of cerebrovascular disease and diabetes than men, more men die of neoplasms and homicides, and the male-to-female mortality ratio for heart disease is similar. Dengue hemorrhagic fever and typhoid continue to be threats. The Joint United Nations Programme on HIV/AIDS (UNAIDS) estimates the prevalence rate for human immunodeficiency virus (HIV) in adults (aged 15 to 49 years) to be 1.5%, with 25,000 people living with HIV, including 6,900 women, and fewer than 500 children aged 0 to 14. The number of deaths from acquired immunodeficiency syndrome (AIDS) is about 1,300. All parishes are affected; however, the major urban parishes; Kingston, St. Andrew, and St. James, have reported the most cases. HIV/AIDS is the leading cause of death in children 1 to 4 years of age. Seroprevalence rates among high-risk groups are as high as 25% among men who have sex with men and 20% among female commercial sex workers. The mode of transmission is primarily heterosexual.

Health-Team Relationships: There is much lip service paid to multidisciplinary team work in hospitals. In practice, medical doctors are generally at the top of the hierarchy. Nurses continue to make a pivotal contribution to health care despite the chronic shortage of registered nurses. Patients hold health practitioners in high esteem.

Families' Role in Hospital Care: Where there is a severe shortage of nursing staff, relatives are allowed to assist with patients' personal needs. Families consider the role of providing food for their relatives to be very important, despite the fact that patients may be on a special diet. The physical nature of in-patient facilities does not allow for relatives to remain 24 hours a day. Pediatric hospitals that are child friendly, however, will allow parents, usually mothers, to stay overnight.

Dominance Patterns: There is overt male dominance, although in practice Jamaica has a matrifocal tendency. The ideal is to have a man as the head of the household, although 43% of all households are headed by women. Similarly, the ideal is to be married, but this status exists in the upper and middle classes, whereas sexual relationships and courtship patterns of the lower classes show a tendency for relationships to begin as visits, proceed to common-law relationships, and later in life conclude in marriage. Men assume dominant sexual roles. They sire children with many different women, who are referred to as their baby mothers, a practice that gives them social status among their peers. Power roles between men and women are reversed during times of illness, when women, particularly older mothers and grandmothers, have the power to control the actions of men. They dictate the sick roles in the household and make decisions about health behaviors.

Touch Practices: Jamaicans are very expressive, and they greet each other with hugs and handshakes. The culture is homophobic, so men do not normally embrace each other except in prescribed situations such as church ceremonies. Among men from the lower social classes, a common greeting is to touch the closed fists by placing one fist on the top of the other and then reversing the action. Women embrace when they greet each other, particularly if they are close friends.

Perceptions of Time: Punctuality is considered the ideal, but in reality people are not always on time for social activities.

Pain Reactions: Individuals are expressive in their reactions to pain, whether physical or emotional. At funerals, loud weeping and moaning are expected from relatives.

Birth Rites: The fertility rate is 2.41 children born per woman. Many pregnant women give birth at hospitals. In some rural communities, a *nana,* or traditional birth attendant, performs deliveries at home even though the community has midwives. When the mother feels she is ready, she sends her partner or oldest child to call the nana, who usually lives in the village. The nana examines the mother and begins to prepare the birth room. All cracks and crevices are sealed with old newspapers, and the windows are closed and covered with heavy cloth to ensure that the mother does not develop a "baby cold" from drafts. The bed is prepared by laying down old newspaper to protect the mattress. The nana gives the mother a soap and water enema, and if the labor is unusually long, she offers thyme tea to hasten the process. After the birth, the mother sits on a pail to collect the afterbirth and attend to personal hygiene; the mother does not have a full bath until 9 days have passed. The baby is wiped clean with a flannel cloth. Visitors are not allowed to enter the room because they may carry infectious agents or unwittingly bring spirits into the room to which the infant may be susceptible. The infant is protected with warm clothes, and special attention is paid to its "mold"—the unclosed suture line at the crown of the head. It is important to ensure that the infant does not develop a "mold cold," which manifests as frequent discharges from the eyes and nose. In many instances, a Bible opened to Psalm 23 is placed under the pillow of the infant and an open pair of scissors under the mattress of the infant's cot to ward off evil influences. The infant is given a small external guard made with *asafetida,* a pungent substance used to keep away spirits. A red string, usually in the form of a bit of clean red cloth, is tied to the wrist. Red is the color of power and is used to ward off supernatural influences. In rural communities, the parents bury the umbilical cord and plant a fruit tree on the spot. A typical Jamaican saying states that people may travel to distant places, but they always return to the place where their "navel string is buried." This implies a permanent commitment to their relationship with their ancestral home and family. The infant mortality rate is 16 per 1,000 live births.

Death Rites: The culture has strong roots to ancestor worship. During celebrations, it is customary for people to pour a little of their beverages on the floor for "those who are not here," a way for the living to pay homage to those who have passed on. Funerals are occasionally delayed to accommodate relatives overseas. The wake involves family, friends, and the general community sitting up all night for several nights with the family. The family provides coffee, salted biscuits, and alcohol in the form of white rum (whites). If the family members belong to the more established religious groups, they tend to sing more hymns and drink less alcohol. If the family is in the Revival religious community, they play drums and sing hymns and other songs. The body is prepared for "churching," the transport of the casket to the church for the ceremony. The body is removed from the home feet first so that the person's spirit, or *duppy,* knows it cannot return. The tomb is prepared with concrete bricks for its sides and a concrete slab for the top. In rural communities, there is a procession of people walking and singing hymns. In urban settings, the hearse is followed by a motorcade to the cemetery. At the home, the family cleans the house, turns mirrors around, and removes the curtains for 3 days. Autopsies are acceptable. Organ donation is not acceptable because it is thought that removing parts of the body makes the duppy restless. These restless spirits can return and harm those who did not follow the prescribed methods of laying them to rest, resulting in possession by the spirits and loss of good fortune.

Food Practices: A typical breakfast may consist of boiled yams and green bananas (considered strengthening), and wheat flour made into dumplings, with mackerel cooked in coconut oil. The meal is served with cocoa or mint teas. Jamaicans often think that they should have something hot in the morning to remove the gas from their stomach. Another common meal consists of ackee fruit cooked with salt fish and wheat flour dumplings that are fried in oil. Ackee and codfish is the national dish of Jamaica. The ackee is a delicate pink fruit with a black seed which is boiled until it becomes soft and fried with codfish and tomatoes. It is extremely important that the ackee be properly prepared because it contains a potent water-soluble hypoglycemic agent. In rural communities, people used salt to preserve their foods, so salted meats and fish became known as *saltin,* and the word is still used in reference to salted fish, pork, and beef. A favorite snack food is pastry filled with seasoned ground meat, usually beef, and eaten hot, called a *patty.* The most common form of protein is chicken. Pork prepared in the way of the Maroons (African slaves who escaped from plantations and formed communities in the hills) with special herbs and seasonings is called jerk pork and is considered a delicacy. Seventh-Day Adventists and Rastafarians do not eat pork. The goat plays a major role in many rituals and festivities. Curried goat and a soup made from the goat's tripe and testes are delicacies regularly offered at functions.

Infant-Feeding Practices: Breastfeeding has been widely promoted and is preferred over bottle-feeding. Many mothers also concurrently give their infants water and fruit juices. Mothers have been resistant to breastfeeding because bottle-feeding with formula is a status symbol and shows that the mother can afford to purchase formula. Many mothers do not mix the formulas properly, however, and the infants become malnourished. Mothers also have concerns about the physical changes in their breasts that are caused by breastfeeding. Among children who are between infancy and 59 months of age, 6% show signs of overweight, 5% have low weight for age, 4% have low height for age (stunting), and 2% have low weights for height (wasting).

Child-Rearing Practices: Parents can be very strict, and corporal punishment, although banished by the Ministry of Education, is still a method of discipline in schools and supported by the community. Children are still expected to be seen but not heard, especially when adults are having a conversation. In many instances, the father is used as a threat for children who misbehave; the caregiver says, "Wait till your father come home." Women, however, actually provide daily discipline, particularly because so many households are headed by women.

National Childhood Immunizations: BCG at birth; DT, OPV, and IPV at 6 weeks and at 3, 5, and 18 months and at 4 to 6 years; DTwP at 18 months and at 4 to 6 years; DTwPHibHep and HIB at 6 weeks and 3 and 5 months; MMR at 1 year and at 4 to 6 years; Td at first contact, +1, +6 months, +1, +1, +1 year; HepB first contact, +1, +5 months. Malaria and tuberculosis are no longer threats except through importation. The percent of the target population vaccinated, by antigen, is: BCG (95%); DTP1 (91%); DTP3 (88%); HepB3 (87%); Hib3 (89%); MCV (84%); and Polio3 (83%).

360　Japan

BIBLIOGRAPHY

Central Intelligence Agency: *2006: The world factbook, Jamaica.* Retrieved September 21, 2006, from https://www.cia.gov/cia/publications/factbook/print/jm.html.

Ministry of Health, Jamaica: Health Information Unit, *Monthly Clinic Summary Reports and Hospital Monthly Statistics Report,* November 2005.

Ministry of Health, Jamaica: *Jamaica HIV/AIDS/STI national strategic plan 2002-2006. Time to care, time to act.* Jamaica, 2001, The Ministry.

Planning Institute of Jamaica and Statistical Institute of Jamaica: *Jamaica survey of living conditions, report 2000,* Jamaica, 2001, 2004, The Institute.

Statistical Institute of Jamaica: *Statistical year book of Jamaica, 2000,* Jamaica, 2000, The Institute.

UNAIDS: 2006 Jamaica. Retrieved September 21, 2006, from http://www.unaids.org/en/Regions_Countries/Countries/jamaica.asp.

World Health Organization: 2006: Immunization, vaccines and biologicals. Retrieved September 21, 2006, from http://www.who.int/immunization_monitoring/en/globalsummary/countryprofileresult.cfm?C='jam'.

◆ JAPAN

MAP PAGE (803)

Chihoko Kame and Akira Babazono

J

Location: Japan is separated from the eastern coast of Asia by the Japan Sea. It is an arc-shaped country, consisting of four major and more than 7,000 small islands spread over 377,835 km^2 (145,882 square miles). Most people live in densely populated urban areas. The country has many volcanoes and is often shaken by earthquakes. The population of Japan is 127.4 million; the capital is Tokyo. The gross domestic product (GDP) per capita is $31,500. Literacy rates are 99% for both men and women.

Major Languages	Ethnic Groups	Major Religions
Japanese	Japanese 99%	Shinto and Buddhist 89%
	Other 1%	Christianity 2%
		Other 9%

Health Care Beliefs: Acute sick care; traditional. People are well informed about illness factors: working too hard, smoking, high-fat diets, and stress; however, health-promotion and disease-prevention concepts are only slowly being integrated into the health care system, and people are reluctant to change their habits.

Predominant Sick-Care Practices: Biomedical and alternative. Western medicine is predominant, but Eastern medical practices, such as acupuncture and herbs, are also used. Japan has universal medical care insurance; however, people are required to pay from 10% to 30% of their medical expenses. Generally, if Japanese feel ill or have a health concern, they consult a doctor in a clinic or hospital or buy over-the-counter medicine from a pharmacy.

Ethnic-/Race-Specific or Endemic Diseases: The three main causes of death are malignant neoplasms, heart disease, and cerebrovascular diseases. The main causes of death have shifted from infectious diseases to lifestyle-related chronic diseases. In addition, emerging and reemerging infectious diseases are major concerns. Epidemics of *Escherichia coli* 0157 have been problematic, particularly in 1996. The Joint United Nations Programme on HIV/AIDS (UNAIDS) estimates the prevalence rate for human immunodeficiency virus (HIV) in adults (aged 15 to 49 years) as 0.1%, with 17,000 people living with HIV, including 9,900 women. About 1,400 deaths are attributed to acquired immunodeficiency syndrome (AIDS). Most reported cases during the early phases of the epidemic were caused by blood transfusions. As of 2006, about 80% of diagnosed HIV infections had been acquired through sexual contact: 38% heterosexual and 42% homosexual or bisexual.

Health-Team Relationships: In hospitals, the health care team consists of doctors, nurses, pharmacists, dietitians, clinical laboratory technicians, and radiology technicians. Physical therapists, occupational therapists, and speech therapists may also be available. Licensed social workers are not paid for by health insurance, limiting their availability. Respect for social rank is pervasive in the system, with doctors at the top of the hierarchy. The doctor is responsible for medical treatment, and nurses serve as caregivers. Most patients follow decisions made by their doctor, and it is uncommon to request or receive a second opinion. Patterns of thought are expressed indirectly; the listener is expected to get the point of a conversation without being explicitly told what it is. A person may divert the subject away from an embarrassing topic or avoid direct confrontations, and individual verbal agreements do not imply compliance. The family is generally consulted before medical decisions are made. Informed consent is stressed because it is the doctor's duty to explain the meaning of consent. The patients' right to know their diagnosis and treatment options is gradually becoming an accepted concept.

Families' Role in Hospital Care: Previously the family was expected to take care of their hospitalized family members. At present, nurses are responsible for care of inpatients, and the role of the family is primarily one of support. It is still common for mothers to care for their hospitalized children.

Dominance Patterns: In the past, the traditional Japanese perspective was that men should work outside the home and women should take care of family affairs. Values have changed, however, because of Western influences, the changing structure of society, and the improving economic power of women who work outside the home. Since the Equal Employment Opportunity Law for Men and Women was established, working environments for women have improved; nevertheless, it remains difficult for women to get jobs after having children because of concerns that their work will be interrupted by family responsibilities or future pregnancies. Traditionally, children take care of their aging parents, but this has been changing also as the number of women who work has increased. Workers can take a leave so that they can care for their parents. Since the establishment of long-term care insurance in 2000, it has become easier to receive assistance for the care of frail, aging parents.

Eye-Contact Practices: Direct eye contact was previously considered disrespectful. In modern Japan, this mindset has diminished, and direct eye contact has become more common between the sexes and with older adults. In very traditional families, it is still considered more polite to avert the eyes when speaking with older and other respected adults.

Touch Practices: Bowing is the customary greeting among Japanese, although handshakes are also acceptable. A pat on the back is unacceptable and considered rude. Lovers may greet each other with a kiss to express tender feelings.

Perceptions of Time: Punctuality is important, and being on time for appointments is valued. Many Japanese spend much of their time working, so work becomes a source for some social activities.

Pain Reactions: Most patients believe it is important to tolerate pain, so they are embarrassed to complain of discomfort. Crying out because of pain is considered somewhat shameful and not something one would want others to hear. The concept of pain relief as an accepted form of medicine has recently become more widely accepted, however, and the use of analgesics for pain is becoming the norm.

Birth Rites: Japan has one of the lowest infant mortality rates in the industrialized world: 3 per 1,000 live births. A newborn with a birth weight of 2,500 g is considered premature. People readily comply with prenatal care and health-promotion advice. Women in labor are silent and even eat during labor; most give birth in a hospital or clinic, assisted by doctors or midwives. Recently, more husbands have attended the birth of their children. After birth, the mother enjoys long periods of rest and recuperation and may stay in the hospital or clinic for 5 to 7 days and indoors for as long as 2 months. When an infant is 1 month of age, the grandmother takes the infant to a shrine to pray for healthy growth. The features of the population pyramid of Japan are the rapid increase in the number of older adults and the decrease in children. The population is aging more quickly than populations of other Western countries, and it is estimated that one of four people will be older than 65 in 2015. The fertility rate is 1.29 children born per woman; far lower than the level needed to maintain current population numbers. Life expectancy is 78 for men, 85 for women.

Death Rites: The Japanese tend to control public expressions of grief. Relatives and close friends attend a wake and then a funeral ceremony. In the past, ceremonies were performed according to the religion of the family, with most being Buddhist. More recently, Japanese have been more flexible about funerals and usually follow the wishes of the deceased. For example, ceremonies may be performed with no vestiges of religion but many flowers. It is customary to give the family a gift of money. Usually half is returned with green tea and cakes after 49 days—one of the customs used to recognize those who attended. Cremation is widely practiced.

Food Practices and Intolerances: Most people enjoy raw fish and mushrooms. Traditional foods (such as tofu, made from soybeans) are light and not greasy. Western-style food such as bread and meat is common, but many Japanese are returning to traditional diets that are low in fat and include numerous vegetables because of the health benefits.

Infant-Feeding Practices: Approximately 40% of mothers breastfeed, and weaning generally begins about 3 months after birth. Children are then bottle-fed with formula and begin receiving semi-liquid foods.

Child-Rearing Practices: The mother-child relationship is strong. Boys were traditionally considered more important than girls and were more likely to receive a higher education. Today, this favoritism is decreasing, providing better opportunities for women. The Tango Festival, in which people pray for boys to grow up safely, is held on May 5; the Doll Festival, celebrated on March 3, also includes prayers for the safety of girls. Decreases in fertility rates and an emphasis on nuclear rather than extended families have meant that some new mothers, especially those in urban areas, cannot find an experienced mother or consultant to guide her in child-rearing practices. Without social support, some mothers feel trapped, which occasionally causes them to mistreat their children. The community is being warned to be aware of signs of abuse and help to raise the children; however, many middle-age women are working, and the society has an insufficient number of adequate daycare centers. Students spend long hours preparing for school entrance examinations; this is a period that is particularly competitive and stressful because of the influence admission has on their future prospects.

National Childhood Immunizations: BCG before 6 months; OPV between 3 and 90 months; DTaP between 3 to 90, 6 to 90, 9 to 90 and 15 to 90 months; DT between 11 to 12 years; measles 12 to 90 months; rubella between 12 and 90 months. The percent of the target population vaccinated, by antigen, is: DTP1, DTP3, and MCV (99%); and Polio 3 (97%).

Other Characteristics: Most Japanese are fond of comparatively long, hot baths followed by a shower and take them in the winter and the summer unless they are ill. People often use nonverbal expressions to display their feelings. About 43% of men and 10% of women smoke cigarettes.

BIBLIOGRAPHY

Cabinet Office, Government of Japan: Retrieved June 20, 2006, from http://www.cao.go.jp/.

Central Intelligence Agency: *2006: The world factbook, Japan*. Retrieved September 21, 2006, from https://www.cia.gov/cia/publications/factbook/print/ja.html.

Infectious Disease Surveillance Center: Retrieved February 27, 2006, from http://idsc.nig.go.jp/vaccine/dschedule.html.

World Health Organization: Retrieved June 20, 2006, from http://www.who.int/GlobalAtlas/predefincdReports/ERS2004/EFS_PDFs/EFS2004_JP.pdf.

Ministry of Health, Labour and Welfare: Retrieved February 27, 2006, from http://www.dbtk.mhlw.go.jp/toukei/cgi/sse_kensaku

UNAIDS: 2006 Japan. Retrieved September 21, 2006 from http://www.unaids.org/
en/Regions_Countries/Countries/japan.asp.
World Health Organization: 2006: Immunization, vaccines and biologicals. Retrieved
September 21, 2006, from http://www.who.int/immunization_monitoring/en/
globalsummary/countryprofileresult.cfm?C='jpn'.

◆ JORDAN (HASHEMITE KINGDOM OF)

MAP PAGE (802)

Arwa Oweis

Location: The Hashemite Kingdom of Jordan is located in the Middle
East, bordered on the west by Israel and the Dead Sea, on the north by
Syria, on the east by Iraq, and on the south by Saudi Arabia. It has a total
area of 91,880 km^2 (35,465 square miles), most of which is arid desert.
Periods of migration have been documented in several distinct periods,
particularly after the Arab-Israeli war and crisis years in 1948, 1967,
and 1973. Immigration also occurred after the invasion of Kuwait by Iraq
in 1990. The population is 5.9 million, with 70% of the population younger
than 29 years. Three fourths of the population lives in three major cities:
Amman (the capital), Zarq'a, and Irbid. The gross domestic product
(GDP) per capita is $4,700, with 30% living below the poverty line. Literacy
rates are 96% for men, 86% for women.

Major Languages	Ethnic Groups	Major Religions
Arabic (official)	Arab 98%	Sunni Muslim 94%
English	Circassian 1%	Christian 4%
	Armenian 1%	Other 2%

Non-Arab minorities (e.g., Circassians, Armenians) also speak Arabic,
and English is widely understood among middle and upper classes. Jordanians distinguish between Transjordanians (citizens of the Amirate of
Transjordan, which existed from 1921 to 1948) and Palestinians (citizens
of the British-mandated territory of Palestine, which existed from 1922 to
1948, who comprise 55% to 60% of the population). Non-Arab ethnic
groups include Circassians, Shishans, Armenians, and Kurds. In addition,
there are other small religious groups: Shia, Druze, and B'hai.

Health Care Beliefs: Fatalistic; traditional. The use of drugs such as heroin or marijuana is strictly forbidden, but people smoke cigarettes despite
strong prohibitions by Islamic scholars. Water-pipe smoking has become
a widely practiced habit. There are special coffee shops for this practice,
and almost every home has at least one pipe. Because religion permeates
all aspects of life, Arabs face adversities and terminal illnesses with faith
in God's (Allah's) mercy and compassion. This practice leads to a more
fatalistic than activist approach to illness and greater dependence
on the family during illness than is common in many Western societies.

Psychiatric disorders are the major source of stigma in Arab countries, and they are often attributed to the "evil eye" (i.e., the power of a person to harm others merely by looking at them), evil spirits, and sorcery. Psychiatric services are often delayed, whereas traditional and religious modalities that are less stigmatizing are sought. People consult traditional therapists because of consistency between their beliefs and the healers' cultural explanations of disease.

Predominant Sick-Care Practices: Biomedical and magical-religious. The number and distribution of health care facilities has increased in rural areas since the adoption of the primary care concept—recognizing that the expense and inconvenience of travel hinders rural people from seeking advanced medical care and attention. In major cities, modern medicine is the primary choice, and alternative healing is usually thought of as a last resort. Institutions with advanced medical equipment are located in major cities such as Amman, Irbid, Ramtha, Az Zarqa, and As Salt. Most tribal citizens living in rural areas and the desert consult indigenous healers and wear amulets as an adjunct to biomedical care. Traditional healers such as those who use the Koran for healing also may be consulted. For example, people with fertility problems seek the advice of a doctor as well as a religious person *(shykh)* to obtain amulets. Traditional infertility treatments include "closing the back," where a woman healer rubs the woman's pelvis with olive oil and places suction cups on her back. Also used are abdominal and external ovarian massage and herbal vaginal suppositories. Traditional health practices are the domain of women who are known in their communities to possess skills in treating certain injuries and disorders. The most prevalent practice is massaging children with warm olive oil. Within the family, women assume responsibility for nutrition and treatment of illness. Beliefs in the efficacy of traditional healing practices occasionally prevent or postpone appropriate medical attention.

Ethnic-/Race-Specific or Endemic Diseases: The leading causes of mortality are cardiovascular—such as hypertension, coronary heart disease, and stroke—and along with cancer are responsible for more than half of all deaths. The prevalence of hypertension is estimated to be 32% among those aged 25 years and older, and 89% is uncontrolled. The prevalence of diabetes mellitus is 14%, and impaired glucose tolerance has been detected in an additional 10% of the population. More than 40% of adult men and 5% to 10% of women smoke regularly, and the prevalence of smoking among schoolchildren is 20%. In semi-urban communities, obesity affects 60% of women and 33% of men aged 25 and older. Prevalence rates of hypercholesterolemia and hypertriglyceridemia are 23% and 24%, respectively. The most recent national cancer registry indicated that this disease targets both men and women in patterns parallel to other countries undergoing modernization; breast cancer, lymphoma, and leukemia are the most common. Ministry of Health statistics show high numbers of traffic accidents. Diarrheal diseases, acute respiratory infections, and hepatitis B and C are still leading conditions. The incidence of pulmonary tuberculosis declined from 7 per 100,000 in

1993 to 3 in 2001. All malaria cases currently detected are imported. Jordan is considered to be a low-prevalence country for human immunodeficiency virus (HIV)/acquired immunodeficiency syndrome (AIDS): less than 0.02%. At the end of December 2001, the total cumulative number of all reported cases was 294 (123 were among Jordanians). In 72% of cases, the infection was acquired outside Jordan; more than 50% were from sexual contact.

Health-Team Relationships: Although professional organizations are playing a more active role in regulating nursing practice, the traditional arrangement of most health care institutions still places nurses in subordinate positions to administrators as well as to physicians. Most units do not give nurses freedom in scheduling and have numerous policies and procedures that are oppressive. Hospitals have further taken away nursing autonomy with the increased hiring of unqualified personnel to implement nursing tasks. Nursing practice is characterized by work overload, interprofessional conflicts, uncertainty regarding treatment decisions, a lack of clinical judgment, nonsupportive work environments, and feelings of inadequacy. These circumstances have contributed to dissatisfaction, burnout, and turnover.

Families' Role in Hospital Care: Family and kinship are the main sources of social support where relatives live near each other. Children are socialized to be obedient and loyal to their families, and individual interests are secondary. Families assume many roles when a member is ill: patient advocates, counselors, or long-term care providers if necessary. At the time of hospital admission, close relatives accompany the patient for support and to answer questions for the patient. Relatives often prepare and bring food to patients. Nurses rely on family members to provide basic care and for assistance with bathing, eating, walking, and changing clothes. Visitors bring food, chocolate, biscuits, or fruit. Close relatives who stay most of the day show their hospitality by serving visitors coffee, candy, or fruit. Visitors tend not to comply with visiting hours, and special security personnel control the influx of visitors, who can interfere with routine or emergency care.

Dominance Patterns: Jordan has traditionally been a family-oriented society in which people take care of their own, even if that means stretching their resources to the limit. Jordan is still a male-dominated society in which greater value is placed on boys because they perpetuate the family name and maintain economic security for aging parents (although Islamic teachings promote gender equity). The father is the head of the family and its breadwinner, whereas the mother raises the children and takes care of the house. Many educated women occupy positions in health, educational, and other institutions, however, so taking care of the children becomes the responsibility of grandmothers. Men are still reluctant to participate in household or childcare tasks. Status within the household varies, depending on sex, age, and type of household. In principle, men have greater autonomy. Within the household younger males may be subject to the authority of senior males: grandfathers, fathers, and uncles.

Decisions about education, marriage, and work remain family affairs. Older women exert substantial authority and control over children and adolescents, the most powerless sector within a household.

Eye-Contact Practices: It is considered impolite and unacceptable for women to make direct eye contact with men, or for children to make direct eye contact with parents, grandparents, or other older adults. People from the Middle East who are of the same gender are likely to stand quite close to each other, but men and women maintain a greater distance.

Touch Practices: Jordanians behave conservatively in public. They communicate modestly, and displays of affection are highly private. Between spouses, affectionate responses such as kissing or hugging do not occur in public areas and are considered inappropriate social behavior. It is unacceptable for men and women to shake hands with strangers (i.e., people who are not close relatives) of the opposite sex. It is preferable for patients to be treated by health professionals of the same sex. Islam prohibits male-female touching except in an emergency or when no competent health professional of the same sex is available.

Perceptions of Time: Schedules, deadlines, and punctuality are cornerstones of Arab life. Arabs often begin their meetings with chatting and social activities. Showing hospitality by serving tea or coffee and inquiring about people's health and families precedes attending to the business at hand. Arabs are more tuned to the past and present than to the future. Although they do think ahead and have plans for the future, economic constraints are major barriers.

Pain Reactions: Jordanian patients tend to attribute wellness and illness to God's will; therefore, they tend to use prayers and other religious practices as ways of coping. They face adversities with patience and endurance because they believe their suffering will be remembered in the afterlife. Jordanians may believe they ought to please their health care providers so that they can be labeled "good" patients (i.e., those who do not complain). Men in particular avoid overt displays of emotion because they could be considered weak. This behavior is rooted in the socialization process, in which sons are taught to be strong and to protect their sisters, whereas daughters are taught to be sources of love and emotional support. It is more acceptable for women to request pain medication.

Birth Rites: Most families believe that a mother should stay home for 40 days after birth, during which time she is cared for by her mother and sisters and occasionally by her husband's family. Circumcision is the norm for boys and is often performed during the first week. Swaddling the infant with a blanket and rope is still common and believed to strengthen the infant's muscles, prevent deformities such as scoliosis, and control movements of the hands that might frighten the infant during the night. The infant sleeps in a crib close to the mother. During the postpartum period, the mother is not allowed to perform religious rituals (i.e., recite prayers, fast during Ramadan) or have sexual intercourse until all postpartum discharge is gone. She is encouraged to consume special drinks such as boiled cinnamon sticks and boiled fenugreek *(hilbah)* seeds, believed to accelerate discharge and increase milk production. In some families, it is customary to shave the infant's head, estimate the weight of the hair, calculate the price of an equivalent weight of gold or silver, and give this amount as charity. Parents frequently slaughter a goat or lamb and invite relatives and friends to eat as a show of gratitude to God and so that all can welcome the infant. The fertility rate is 3.7 children per woman; infant mortality is 17 deaths per 1,000 live births. Islam approves of family planning for child spacing only; thus, sterilization is strictly prohibited. Life expectancy is 76 for men, 81 for women.

Death Rites: For patients with brain death whose body organs or systems are being artificially maintained, it is acceptable to discontinue life support or to take organs for transplantation. Autopsies are permissible in cases of suspected foul play or for educational purposes. Most people are reluctant to have autopsies performed because it is more common to bury the dead without delay. The body is washed, wrapped in white cloth (without a coffin), taken to the mosque for prayer, and then taken to the cemetery for burial. Relatives accept condolences for 3 days. If death occurs overseas, it is preferable to bring the body home. Cremation is forbidden.

Food Practices: Islamic law forbids eating pig and drinking alcohol; this law is followed to a greater or lesser extent throughout Jordan. In the last 30 years, the consumption of sugar, fat and oil, meat, and poultry have greatly increased. Yogurt, white cheese, olives, thyme, and olive oil dip are an integral part of breakfast, and unleavened bread, or *khobz,* is eaten with almost everything. Jordan's national dish is *mansaf,* a whole stewed lamb cooked in a yogurt sauce and served on a bed of rice. *Maglouba* is a meat or chicken dish with different types of vegetables and rice. The fried vegetables—such as cauliflower, eggplant, or green fava— and the meat or chicken are placed in the bottom of the pot and covered with the rice and then flipped over onto a big tray. *Musakhan* is chicken cooked with onions, olive oil, and pine nuts and baked on a thick loaf of Arabic bread. Also popular is Middle Eastern shish kebabs, skewered pieces of marinated lamb or chicken, tomatoes, and onions cooked over a charcoal fire. The most popular dessert is *kunafa,* two layers of shredded dough stuffed with sweet white (whole-milk) cheese. Stuffed *maamoul* is also popular and is made of mixed flour and semolina (cream of wheat) stuffed with dates or nuts. People like to prepare large amounts of maamoul to celebrate the two major feasts for Muslims: the Al-Fiter Eid feast (the morning of the next-to-last day of the Ramadan fasting month) and the Al-Adha Eid feast (on the 10th day of the pilgrimage month in which people travel to Mecca). Muslims fast during the month of Ramadan, abstaining from food, drink, and sexual intercourse between sunrise and sunset. Fasting is not mandatory for patients or older adults for whom it could have negative consequences. It is commonplace to be invited into people's homes for a cup of tea or Arabian coffee.

Infant-Feeding Practices: Breastfeeding is preferred. In urban areas, people are more flexible about bottle-feeding because of the increasing number of women who work and must leave their infants with a close relative. In rural areas, mothers breastfeed their infants according to traditional beliefs and because of advice about its benefits. Infants begin eating solid foods at about 4 months.

Child-Rearing Practices: Children may sleep in their parents' room until they are 3 to 4 years; then all young children may sleep in one room. Mothers take on more responsibility for discipline, but children perceive fathers as being stricter. Older adults live with their eldest son or daughter and may assume some responsibility for disciplining children even when it interferes with the mother's role. Deviant behaviors by one family member affect the reputation and honor of the entire family.

National Childhood Immunizations: BCG at first contact; DTwP at 18 months; DTwPHib at 3 and 4 months; DTwPHibHep at 2 months; IPV at 2 months; OPV at 2, 3, 10, and 18 months and 6 years; measles at 9 months; MMR at 18 months; DT at 2, 3, 4, and 18 months; Td at 6 and 15 years; and TT after first contact, +1, +6 months, +1, + 1 year. The percent of the target population vaccinated, by antigen, is: BCG (89%); DTP1 (98%); DTP3, HepB3, Hib3, MCV, Polio3, and TT2 plus (50%). No cases of polio have been reported for the last 7 years as a result of immunization and improved surveillance.

BIBLIOGRAPHY

Al-Ma'aitah R, Cameron S, Armstrong-Stassen M, Horsburgh M: Effect of gender and education on quality of nursing work-life of Jordanian nurses, *Nursing Health Care Perspect.* 20(2):88–94, 1999.

Central Intelligence Agency: *2006: The world factbook, Jordan.* Retrieved September 21, 2006, from https://www.cia.gov/cia/publications/factbook/print/jo.html.

Jordan Population and Family Health Survey (JPFHS): *Summary and recommendation of the population and family health survey.* Amman, Jordan, 2002, Department of Statistics.

The Jordanian Department of Statistics: *Statistical year book,* Amman, 2003.

Oweis Al, Abo Shaikha L: Jordanian women's expectations of their first childbirth experience, *Int J Nursing Pract.* 10:261–271, 2004.

Oweis Al, Thiabat K: Jordanian nurses perception of physicians' verbal abuse: findings from a questionnaire survey. *Int J Nursing Stud.* 42(8):881–888, 2005.

Oweis A: Bringing the professional challenges of nursing in Jordan to light. *Int J Nursing Pract.* 11(6):244–249, 2005.

World Health Organization: 2006: Immunization, vaccines and biologicals. Retrieved September 21, http://www.who.int/immunization_monitoring/en/globalsummary/countryprofileresult.cfm?C='jor'.

http://www.ourdialogue.com/p17.htm Postmortem (retrieved February 9, 2006).

http://www.traderscity.com/abcg/culture1.htm Arabian Business and Cultural Guide (retrieved February 14, 2006).

http://www.jordanembassyus.org/new/index.shtml Embassy of the Hashemite Kingdom of Jordan (retrieved January 15, 2006).

http://www.undp-jordan.org/jordan_hdr/jhdr.html Jordan human development report 2004. Building sustainable livelihoods (retrieved February 15, 2006).

◆ KAZAKHSTAN (REPUBLIC OF)

MAP PAGE (799)

Daniyar Z. Baidaralin

Location: The Republic of Kazakhstan, part of the former Soviet Union, is in central Asia, with Russia to the north, China to the east, Uzbekistan and Kyrgyzstan to the south, and the Caspian Sea to the west. Kazakhstan is the second largest country in the Commonwealth of Independent States, with a total area of 2,717,300 km² (1,049,151 square miles). The population is more than 15 million. The capital is Astana. Vast, often deserted steppes and dramatic mountain peaks dominate the country's topography. Horses and sheep are common pastoral animals. The gross domestic product (GDP) per capita is $8,200, with 19% living below the poverty line. Literacy rates are 99% for both men and women.

Major Languages	Ethnic Groups	Major Religions
Kazakh (Qazaq, official)	Kazakh (Qazaq) 57.2%	Muslim 47%
Russian (official)	Russian 27%	Russian Orthodox 44%
	Ukrainian 3.2%	Protestant 2%
	Uzbek 2.7%	Other 7%
	Tatar 1.6%	
	German 1.6%	
	Other 7%	

Native Kazakhs are a mixture of Mongol and Turkic nomadic tribes and are a majority of the population. Kazakh is spoken by more than 40% of the population; two thirds speak Russian, the language of everyday business. Kazakh is gradually replacing Russian as the official language of business in some cities.

Health Care Beliefs: Acute sick care; traditional. Common colds are generally believed to be caused by exposure to drafts, so infants and elderly people are often swaddled in many layers. Upset stomachs and headaches may be treated with a shot of vodka, and fevers are treated by rubbing vodka on the forehead and neck. Drinking cold beverages or iced drinks is thought to cause sore throats. Girls and women are discouraged from sitting directly on cement or stone because they believe that their reproductive systems will be damaged by the cold. Nearly all newborns either wear an amulet or have one hanging near their crib. Sometimes the amulet is a sheep's vertebra wrapped in cloth and tied with a ribbon, signifying the hope that the child will have a strong neck. Abortions (two or more) are relatively common as they are throughout much of the former Soviet Union. The topic is not openly discussed, but it is well known that it is a woman's right to choose to have an abortion.

Predominant Sick-Care Practices: Biomedical when available; magical-religious. The government began a program against unofficial medicine, which has sometimes caused more harm than good, as political upheaval has created economic problems that have affected the health care system. The old Soviet system emphasized specialist hospitalizations with long stays and unnecessary admissions, care that would normally be considered outpatient care. Western medical treatment continues to be regularly sought. Informal, surreptitious monetary and nonmonetary payments are the norm and a large portion of the income generated by medical staff. Costs of medications may be considerable. People recognize that the health care system needs to be restructured into a system of primary care that will better serve their health needs. A movement toward a model based on medical insurance is developing.

Ethnic-/Race-Specific or Endemic Diseases: The country and its water supplies are contaminated in the region around Semey (formerly Semipalatinsk) in northeast Kazakhstan, where repeated aboveground nuclear tests took place during the 1950s and 1960s. A noticeable increase in the number of cases of Hashimoto thyroiditis and thyroid cancer has been reported. The area around the Aral Sea is contaminated, and sediments heavily contaminated with fertilizers are exposed to prevailing winds, exposing people to dust laden with toxic chemicals and heavy metals, resulting in high levels of organochlorine pesticides in breast milk, posing a risk to newborns. There are occasional outbreaks of cholera in the larger cities, particularly Almaty. People often suffer from intestinal diseases caused by the use of human excrement for fertilizer. Cases of belly typhus are distributed by rodents through mites. Since the 1990s, the number of cigarette smokers has doubled, causing more respiratory diseases. The incidence of congenital abnormalities and cancer (especially stomach) is 30% to 50% higher than in Western countries. The Joint United Nations Programme on HIV/AIDS (UNAIDS) reports the estimated prevalence rate of HIV in adults (aged 15 to 49 years) to be 0.1% to 3.2%, with 12,000 people living with human immunodeficiency virus (HIV), including 6,800 women. Fewer than 1,000 deaths have been attributed to acquired immunodeficiency syndrome (AIDS). According to INTER-FAX-Kazakhstan incidence statistics, from January through November 2005, 846 new cases were registered. In 2004 during the same period, there were 633. Intravenous drug use accounted for 78%, and 14% was the result of unprotected sex. Most men and women reject condom use; therefore, other sexually transmitted diseases such as syphilis, gonorrhea, and herpes are common.

Health-Team Relationships: Nurses are educated in 3-year programs in technical colleges and are generally in a subordinate role to doctors in hospitals. They are expected to take care of tasks such as giving injections and changing surgical dressings. During the Soviet period, nurses provided home care for women who had recently given birth and for individuals after serious surgeries at very low cost. It continues to be possible to access a similar level of care in Almaty and other large cities, despite the disarray of the health care system, but such services are unaffordable for most.

Families' Role in Hospital Care: Families are responsible for preparing food and for personal care for hospitalized family members. Because the health insurance industry is still in its infancy, families are required to cover the full cost of medications, especially in rural regions. At least one family member is always in the patient's room. The exception is when women are giving birth; they are largely isolated and visited by one, usually female, relative at a time. Hospital rooms are generally shared by at least 2 and occasionally as many as 10 other patients.

Dominance Patterns: The youngest woman in Kazakh families has the lowest position and is responsible for serving tea, preparing meals, and waiting on the patriarch of the family, other family members, and guests. In most Kazakh families, the oldest person holds the position of greatest respect. Older women are treated with more respect than younger men. In the case of men and women of the same age, the man gets greater respect.

Eye-Contact Practices: It is customary for men to make eye contact with everyone except people they want to avoid, such as beggars. Girls and young women often do not make eye contact with strange men, and younger people usually do not make eye contact with older persons. Kazakh men often shake hands with other men, even if they see each other daily. They may hug and kiss each other on the cheek during greetings. Russian men tend to just shake hands. These greeting patterns apply to friends and strangers, but the greeting and physical contact are warmer with friends. Both Kazakh and Russian women tend to greet friends with a hug but do not make physical contact when greeting women they do not know well.

Perceptions of Time: Punctuality is not particularly valued. Much more emphasis is placed on maintaining relationships. If a person is late for an appointment with a health care professional, little if anything is lost.

Birth Rites: Infant mortality rates are high at 28 deaths per 1,000 live births. Kazakhstani women prefer to give birth in a hospital and remain 5 to 7 days. The pain of delivery is not usually eased with local anesthesia. No family members are allowed into the maternity ward, and newborns are separated from their mothers except during three or four daily feedings. The fertility rate is 1.89 children born per woman. Life expectancy is 62 for men, 73 for women.

Death Rites: Most people die at home regardless of their ethnic background. Kazakhs do not embalm; the body is cleaned and wrapped tightly in white cotton cloths, usually by family members. An *imam* ("Muslim clergyman") is summoned, and he conducts a series of prayers with the men, often outside the home. A group of mourners then gathers outside, and the body is carried out. The mourners, especially the women, wail loudly and cry profusely. Women who do not do so with enough sincerity may be criticized later for being unfeeling. The body is often placed in an uncovered coffin or wrapped in a rug so that it can be more easily transported. Only men follow the body to the cemetery. A 2-m-deep grave is dug, and a small burial chamber is created off the bottom. The wrapped body is carefully lowered into the small burial chamber, and the men take turns filling in the grave. A short dinner follows the men's return to the home. Another memorial meal is held 9 days, 40 days, and then 1 year after the death.

Food Practices and Intolerances: Most people eat three times a day and have the largest meal in the evening. The staple of the diet is mutton. Various vegetables and fruits are available seasonally, including tomatoes, cucumbers, onions, potatoes, watermelons, and cantaloupes.

Infant-Feeding Practices: Breastfeeding is typical. Most women recognize that it is healthy for an infant to receive its mother's milk; however, it is not done in public. If breastfeeding is impossible for medical reasons or if a woman chooses not to breastfeed, formula is available.

Child-Rearing Practices: As Muslims, ethnic Kazakhs circumcise their male children; however, Russians and other Slavic people often do not.

National Childhood Immunizations: BCG at birth and at 6 and 12 years; Dip at 12 years; DT at 6 to 7 years; DTwP at 2, 3, 4, and 18 months; HepB at birth and at 2 and 4 months; measles at 6 to 7 years; MMR at 12 years; mumps at 12 years; OPV at birth and at 2, 3, and 4 months; and Td at 17 years. The percent of the target population vaccinated, by antigen, is: BCG (69%); DTP1, MCV, and Polio3 (99%); DTP3 (98%); and HepB3 (94%).

Other Characteristics: Kazakh male patients may miss times of procedures and medicines or forget about them. Older male patients may joke or try to establish friendly connections with medical personal or other patients by asking personal questions. Kazakhs usually do not smile unless they hear a joke or are in a funny situation; it is not customary to smile automatically. Some are shy about discussing personal health conditions, especially those related to the male or female reproductive systems.

K

BIBLIOGRAPHY

Central Intelligence Agency: *2006: The world factbook, Kazakhstan.* Retrieved September 21, 2006, from https://www.cia.gov/cia/publications/factbook/print/kz.html.

UNAIDS: 2006 Kazakhstan. Retrieved September 21, 2006, from http://www.unaids.org/en/Regions_Countries/Countries/kazakhstan.asp.

World Health Organization: 2006: Immunization, vaccines and biologicals. Retrieved September 21, 2006, from http://www.who.int/immunization_monitoring/en/globalsummary/countryprofileresult.cfm?C='kaz'.

Zhumadilov Z et al: Thyroid abnormality trend over time in northeastern regions of Kazakhstan, adjacent to the Semipalatinsk nuclear test site: a case review of pathological findings for 7271 patients, *J Radiat Res.* 41(1):35, 2000.

http://www.akorda.kz, Akorda, official website of president of Kazakhstan (retrieved February 13, 2006).

http://www.kz/Firsteng3.htm, Kazakhstan (retrieved February 13, 2006).

http://www.government.kz, official website of government of Kazakhstan (retrieved February 13, 2006).

http://www.interfax.kz, INTERFAX KZ (retrieved February 13, 2006).

http://www.tribune-uz.info, Tribune-UZ (retrieved February 13, 2006).

http://news.akavita.by, AKAVITA BY (retrieved February 13, 2006).

http://www.unesco.kz, UNESCO KZ (retrieved February 13, 2006).
http://www.who.int/3by5/support/EFS2004_kaz.pdf, World Health Organization (WHO), 2003, (retrieved March 06, 2006).

◆ KENYA (REPUBLIC OF)

MAP PAGE (801)

Moses K. Limo

Location: Kenya is located on the equator on the east coast of Africa and borders part of Somalia and the Indian Ocean to the east, Uganda and Lake Victoria to the west, Ethiopia and Sudan to the north, and Tanzania to the south. Kenya is largely arid and semiarid in the north, whereas the Great Rift Valley and highlands to the east are the major farming regions. More than 71% of the arid and semiarid land is used for agriculture and pastoral activities. The capital is Nairobi. The total area is 582,650 km^2 (224,962 square miles), with 67% of the people living on less than 10% of the land. The Great Rift Valley, which extends north to south, is flanked by high mountain ranges and contains important freshwater lakes. The population is 34.7 million; 88% live in rural areas. The gross domestic product (GDP) per capita is $1,100, with 50% living below the poverty line. Literacy rates are 91% for men, 80% for women.

Major Languages	Ethnic Groups	Major Religions
English (official language)	Kikuyu 22%	Protestant 38%
Swahili (national language)	Luhya 14%	Roman Catholic 27%
Local languages	Luo 13%	Traditional 26%
	Kalenjin 12%	Muslim 7%
	Kamba 11%	Hindu, Sikh, and
	Meru 6%	Others 2%
	Kisii 6%	
	Other African 15%	
	Non-African 1%	

English is used in public and private business transactions, but Swahili is spoken by almost all tribes. In the workplace and most service occupations, communication is in Swahili, English, or ethnic languages. Kenya has about 42 other tribal languages and dialects corresponding to 42 ethnic groups; some are linguistically related. Sunday is a day of prayer, and church attendance is heavy; therefore, most businesses are closed on Sundays.

Health Care Beliefs: Traditional; health promotion is important. The Ministry of Health has given great emphasis to both curative and preventive health care by using the mass media. Disease may be considered attributable to natural phenomena or supernatural powers, so curses can induce illness, whereas blessings can enhance life. There is a general belief that mental illness is brought about by demonic possession, perhaps as a result of angry ancestral spirits that must be appeased. Most believe that witch doctors and herbalists can remove these spirits, and they pay them in cash and livestock. Because more people are attaining some basic formal education, attitudes toward mental illness are gradually changing. Groups such as the Turkana, Kisii, and Luo perform scarification using hot metal rods to draw out illness by draining "bad blood" from the sick person. Induced vomiting was used for gastrointestinal tract problems by the Kikuyu, but the practice is slowly dying. Traditional beliefs may hinder disease control. For example, in 2006 some families in Kilifi rejected mosquito nets distributed to reduce childhood malaria because people claimed they saw ghosts when they slept under the nets.

Predominant Sick-Care Practices: Traditional; magical-religious; and biomedical when available. Currently, about 70% of Kenyans in rural areas seek medical attention from traditional healers. Herbalists are considered the most helpful and use stems, barks, leaves, and roots for treatment. Snake and scorpion bites and other diseases are often treated effectively by indigenous approaches. Traditional medicine is also being promoted by the government so that it can legally augment public and private health services. Among people in rural areas, it is common to see amulets worn by some ethnic groups, particularly by children. It is believed that amulets ward off evil spirits that cause illness. In some incurable diseases, such as leprosy and tuberculosis (TB), patients have been left to die in the bush. There is a need to study indigenous practices because many have proven value. It is known, for example, that tribes such as the Marakwet and Kisii have performed brain surgery using medicinal plants as anticoagulants.

Ethnic-/Race-Specific or Endemic Diseases: Lifestyle diseases such as diabetes and hypertension that were not common in the past are increasing. Acute respiratory tract infections, intestinal parasitic infestations, and diarrheal diseases (in decreasing order of importance) are other major diseases. Water-borne diseases (viral, protozoal, and bacterial) are major problems because only 62% have clean water sources. Bacteremia is a major cause of death for children in rural hospitals, and antibiotic resistance is increasing. Typhoid, gastroenteritis (*Giardia*, cryptosporidia), amoebiasis, and dysentery are major causes of morbidity and mortality. Vector-borne diseases include malaria; yellow, Rift Valley, and Congo hemorrhagic fevers; typhus; leishmaniasis; and trypanosomiasis. Malaria is the most predominant disease, common along the coast and lake regions, where the hot, humid climate favors mosquito breeding and transmission. Schistosomiasis is also a problem in coastal areas. Cholera can occur everywhere because of lack of sanitation, especially in refugee camps. It also occurs along the Lake Victoria region, which has perennial flooding. About 56% of urban and 43% of rural people have adequate sanitation. Kenya has had outbreaks of smallpox, chickenpox, leprosy, and TB, particularly in slum areas. In urban areas, these

K

outbreaks are thought to be a result of a poor and inadequate health infrastructure, resulting from the rapid increase in population and overcrowding as people flock to cities to seek employment. In some public hospitals, more than half of the beds are occupied by human immunodeficiency virus (HIV) and acquired immunodeficiency syndrome (AIDS) patients. In 2006 the National AIDS Control Council reported a decrease in the prevalence rate of HIV in adults (aged 15 to 49 years) from 6.1% to 5.1% as a result of behavioral changes. Prevalence is 9.6% in urban areas, 4.6% in rural areas. It is higher in women (7.7%) than in men (4.4%), and 164 people are infected daily, translating to 60,000 new infections yearly. The prevalence in girls aged 15 to 24 is 4.5%; in boys aged 18 to 24, it is 0.8%. Currently, 1.27 million Kenyans are infected, half of whom are women. About 1.4 million pregnant women require testing annually to determine their status, and 64,000 need treatment to prevent mother-to-child transmission. About 1.2 million children have been orphaned by AIDS. Only 34% of people who need them are on antiretroviral drugs because of the lack of money to provide them.

Health-Team Relationships: In the main public and private hospitals, care is doctor driven. In the dispensaries that provide primary health care, nurses and paramedics are the main players. In all health care settings, the doctor-nurse relationship is fairly well defined in terms of roles and responsibilities. Patients highly regard health care workers and usually take advice promptly and without question. Since literacy levels are low, informed consent is an issue of concern. The relationship between patients and traditional healers is shrouded in secrecy. Policies and legislation are being formulated to regulate traditional medicine.

Families' Role in Hospital Care: Families are usually encouraged to visit. It is traditionally believed that family and community members are responsible for caring for their sick. Society is based on extended family and a sense of community, although this is being eroded by Western forces of individualism that have broken the family concept. Most hospitals offer food, but family members may bring food also, especially fruit and drinks. Family members do not stay overnight unless the patient is a child, although in high-cost private children's hospitals, there are more nurses and attendants to care for children. In rural settings that are served mainly by subdistrict hospitals, relatives may take food and other necessities to the patient as a matter of routine. Family care for elderly patients is lacking, and there is no policy to care for the aged.

Dominance Patterns: The culture is male dominated. During times of illness, the mother takes on the major role as caregiver. Mothers are also responsible for keeping the home clean, obtaining water and wood for fuel, preparing food, and feeding the children. Girls in the home may also help with these chores when they return from school. Although issues of discipline, security, and decision-making are generally the responsibility of the father, the mother disciplines when the father is away. Dominance patterns are changing in urban areas, where single mothers have more autonomy and own property.

Eye-Contact Practices: In the past, eye contact was generally unacceptable except between people of the same gender. For example, among the Masai, a girl cannot make eye contact with her father and mother-in-law, whereas among the Teso, the girl cannot make eye contact with her brother-in-law. Avoiding eye contact is considered a sign of respect and control over immorality among people of different relationships, age groups, and sexes.

Touch Practices: Males shake hands as sign of friendship and affection. In some ethnic groups, however, a mother-in-law cannot shake hands with a son-in-law or share a toilet seat. A father-in-law may not shake hands with his daughter-in-law. In some tribes, a person cannot touch or greet his or her great grandchildren. Adults may touch children on the forehead as a greeting and to show respect. In the Kalenjin culture, girls have been taught to kneel in front of men and are not allowed to speak with them until they have been circumcised. It is not common in rural areas for women to sit with men or for women to speak before men. These practices are less common in urban areas.

Perceptions of Time: In urban areas, punctuality is important in the work arena, and people are expected to be on time for appointments and children for school. For less important matters, being on time is of little concern. In rural areas, the traditional belief is that time is unlimited, so people only approximate the time, using the sun as a guide. Level of education, work ethics, and tradition are the major factors that influence people's attitudes toward time.

Pain Reactions: Adults generally react to pain stoically. It is rare to see adults, especially men, express pain because it is considered a sign of weakness. Practices such as circumcision are administered in a manner that will encourage them to suppress pain reactions in the future. For example, adult women with severe back pain from excessive manual labor are still expected to carry out household chores as usual. Children are allowed to express pain freely and are excused from chores and activities if they complain.

K

Birth Rites: The fertility rate is five children born per woman. Traditional birth attendants, despite not having legal status, are respected. The infant mortality rate is very high at 59 deaths per 1,000 live births. After birth, the mother is cared for by the husband and women from the neighborhood, who help with cooking and other household chores for at least a month. During the 3 months after birth, the mother's diet is supplemented with high-protein foods such as traditional soup made from bones, roots from special herbs, black beans, and milk. In most ethnic groups, the birth of a son is more celebrated because he is the recipient of the family's inheritance. It is argued that because daughters get married and leave home, they are not able to receive an inheritance and carry on the family name. If the first-born child in a family is a boy, the birth of a second son is not celebrated as much. Reproductive manipulation to choose the sex of a child is practiced by some communities using traditional herbal medicine. Virtually all the cultures, as well as the government, prohibit abortion.

Abortion is obtained illegally, however, and assisted by doctors and midwives. Life expectancy is 50 for men, 48 for women.

Death Rites: Because most Kenyans believe death is a continuation of life and that the spirit joins its ancestors in a different world, they have a sense of immortality. Modern Christian and Muslim teachings are changing traditional attitudes because they teach that doing good deeds on earth is the only way to open the entrance to heaven and that sinners go to eternal hell. In most ethnic groups, an older adult who is about to die calls all family members to bless them and reveal their inheritance. Organ donation and life-supporting systems are not practiced. Autopsy is common and acceptable in hospital settings but is requested only for legal reasons. The definition of death and respect for the death are quite similar among ethnic groups, although funeral rituals differ. Euthanasia is religiously and culturally unacceptable. Organ donation and life support to extend life are not practiced.

Food Practices and Intolerances: Food consumption varies among ethnic groups. People rely heavily on plant proteins supplemented with meat protein. People living around the lake region survive on fish and starches, especially cornmeal, or *ugali*. Those who live in the highlands depend mostly on beans and corn. Most traditional diets are balanced (e.g., *githeri* ["boiled corn and beans"], ugali, kale, and a protein source). Milk is consumed in different forms: fresh, fermented (mursik among Kalenjin), or—among Masai—mixed with blood. Traditional vegetables are now gaining wide acceptance in urban areas. Most individuals in rural communities use their hands to eat. In restaurants, spoons and other utensils are available as people become exposed to diverse cultures.

Infant-Feeding Practices: Breastfeeding is acceptable in all communities and practiced for 1 to 2 years. It is almost taboo for a mother not to breastfeed unless she has medical reasons. When a mother dies, her child usually will be breastfed by relatives (i.e., aunts). Bottle-feeding with formula is gaining in popularity among working mothers, especially in urban areas. Malnutrition is common in rural areas in particular, where 40,000 to 60,000 children are affected.

Child-Rearing Practices: Child rearing is generally strict, with instant discipline (e.g., spanking) being the most common method, although it is now against the law. Young children usually sleep with parents until age 4 or 5. It is the role of the women to discipline children and keep them quiet and obedient, especially when visitors are in the home. Female circumcision and clitoral excision are common in some groups, although the government and lobbying groups have launched major educational campaigns to discourage Kenyans from practicing female genital mutilation. The effort seems to be working through "knifeless" rites that foster self-esteem and confidence.

National Childhood Immunizations: BCG at birth; DTwPHibHep at 6, 10, and 14 weeks; OPV at birth and at 6, 10, and 14 weeks; measles at 9 months; and TT first contact pregnancy, +1 month, second, third, fourth pregnancy; vitamin A at 9, 12, 18, 24, 30, and 36 months; and

YF at 9 months. The percent of the target population vaccinated, by antigen, is: BCG and DTP1 (85%); DTP3, Hib3, and HepB (76%); MCV (69%); Polio3 (70%); TT2 plus (72%); vitamin A (50%); and YFV (52%). Herbal concoctions are still being used to boost the immune system of children in rural areas when mothers do not allow vaccination because of cultural beliefs.

BIBLIOGRAPHY

Central Intelligence Agency: *2006: The world factbook, Kenya.* Retrieved September 21, 2006, from https://www.cia.gov/cia/publications/factbook/print/ke.html.

Fonck M et al: Healthcare-seeking behavior and sexual behavior of patients with sexually transmitted diseases in Nairobi, Kenya, *Sex Transm Dis.* 28(7):367, 2001.

Government of Kenya, Central Bureau of Statistics: Ministry of Planning and National Development, Nairobi, Kenya, 2006.

Homsy J, King R, Balaba D, Kabatas K: Traditional health practitioners are the key to scaling up comprehensive care for HIV in sub-Sahara Africa, *AIDS.* 18(2):1723–1725, 2004.

Haaland A, Vlassoff C: Introducing health care workers for change: from transformation theory to health systems in developing countries, *Health Policy Plann* 16(suppl 1):1, 2001.

Macintyre K, Brown L, Sosler S: "It's not what you know, but who you knew": examining the relationship between behavioral change and AIDS mortality in Africa, *AIDS Educ Prev.* 13(2):160, 2001.

Orago A: National AIDs Control Council, Nairobi, Kenya. 2006. Retrieved October 10, 2006, from www.nacc.or.ke.

Global Health Reporting. HIV/AIDs. Retrieved October 10, 2006, from www.globalhealthreport.org/countries/kenya.

Global Alliance for Vaccines and Immunization. www.gavialliance.org (retrieved October 10, 2006).

UNAIDS 2006 Kenya. Retrieved September 21, 2006, from http://www.unaids.org/en/Regions_Countries/Countries/kenya.asp.

UNICEF. Unicef.org/infobycountry/index.html (retrieved October 10, 2006).

World Health Organization: 2006: Immunization, vaccines and biologicals. Retrieved September 21, 2006, from http://www.who.int/immunization_monitoring/en/globalsummary/countryprofileresult.cfm?C='ken'.

K

◆ KIRIBATI (REPUBLIC OF)

MAP PAGE (794)

Philayrath Phongsavan

Location: Kiribati (pronounced 'Kiribass'), formerly the Gilbert Islands, is an archipelago of approximately 33 low-lying coral atolls. Located in the central Pacific Ocean (roughly halfway between Hawaii and Australia), Kiribati atolls spread across 3.5 million km^2 (1.3 million square miles) of ocean along the Equator. The total area is 811 km^2 (313 square miles). The scattered atolls and dispersed population make telecommunications, logistics, and transport difficult and relatively expensive. Kiribati is divided into three island groups: the western Gilbert Islands (including Banaba), the Phoenix Islands, and the Line Islands. The low-lying and flat atolls are highly vulnerable to sea-level rises and climate changes. Kiribati is declared a "least developed country" by the United Nations (UN). The gross domestic product (GDP) per capita is $880. There are no literacy estimates.

Major Languages	Ethnic Groups	Major Religions
Kiribati (national language commonly used in the community)	Micronesian 99%	Roman Catholic 53%
	Other 1%	Protestant (mostly Congregational) 41%
English (official)		Other 6%

Most of the 105,432 *I-Kiribati* (pronounced "ee-Kiribass") live in the Gilbert Islands, with around 43% concentrated in the capital atoll of Tarawa. Urban overcrowding and population growth are posing serious threats to an environment already under stress from human and animal sewage disposal problems, household garbage, and pollutants. Wrecked heavy machinery, motor vehicles, household goods, office equipment, cans, bottles, and imported plastic items are left scattered on roads and beaches and littered throughout the islands. Poor sanitation, inadequate fresh water, contaminated coral reefs and lagoons, and high population density are key issues. There are widening gaps in income and resources among households and between urban and outer islands.

Health Care Beliefs: Passive role; traditional; increasing emphasis on prevention. Promoting physical, mental, and spiritual well-being is important to I-Kiribati, reflecting the strong influence of traditional culture and religion. The gradual shift from curative hospital-based treatment to public health programs that focus on prevention is partly a response to noncommunicable diseases, but it is also a strategic response to the challenges imposed by limited resources. Traditional remedies and rituals carried out by natural healers are often used as adjuncts to Western medicine. People tend to ignore early warning signs of ill health and dismiss symptoms that would result in their early diagnosis and successful treatment. For example, diabetes-related symptoms of increased urination and thirst or chest pain that might be associated with heart problems are not taken seriously until too late for early diagnosis.

Predominant Sick-Care Practices: Acute sick care. There is no private health insurance. The public health system is administered centrally, and most health services are concentrated in urban areas. All I-Kiribati are eligible to receive medical treatment and care from the government, but those who can afford to do so will usually seek specialized medical treatment abroad. The health system is stressed and under-resourced, with erratic supplies of essential drugs and basic medical equipment. Most of approximately 23 medical doctors are expatriate health practitioners. The only hospital is located in South Tarawa, and it has limited screening and diagnostic facilities. Almost all the doctors are located in Tarawa; village health workers staff the outer-island dispensaries, which provide primary health care services and are able to handle minor injuries and illnesses despite limited equipment, supplies, water, and toilet facilities. Retaining health staff in outer islands is an ongoing challenge. Access between the atolls and health clinics is limited by the high cost of transport. Logistics and communication difficulties between outer islands remain major barriers to providing timely medical care.

Ethnic-/Race-Specific or Endemic Diseases: There is risk of leprosy and dengue fever, including its hemorrhagic form. Diphtheria is also a potential risk, and the tuberculosis rate is relatively high at 60 per 100,000. Hepatitis B and C virus infections are endemic; it has been estimated that 69% to 81% of individuals infected with hepatitis B also have antibodies to the hepatitis delta virus. The prevalence of hepatic cancer among young men is estimated to be high, although no official rates are available. Kiribati has a strong hepatitis B immunization program that focuses on infants. Vitamin A deficiency results in xerophthalmia in about 15% of the population. The United Nations Children's Funds (UNICEF) and the Ministry of Health have implemented vitamin A supplementation programs to children and lactating women. Diarrheal diseases are common among infants and children. Cervical cancer is believed to be one of the most common cancers. In recent years, health services have focused efforts on preventing and controlling noncommunicable diseases such as cardiovascular and kidney disease, hypertension, diabetes, cancer, and motor-vehicle injuries. Although diarrhea, respiratory infections, and nutritional deficiency disorders continue as main causes of illness among infants and children, noncommunicable disease has become the leading contributor to adult morbidity and mortality. This "epidemiologic transition" is explained as the result of adverse lifestyle changes accompanying urbanization and globalization. Tobacco and alcohol consumption have increased significantly. In 2000, tobacco use among women ranged from 65% to 74%, one of the highest rates in the world. Decreasing levels of physical activity are leading to higher levels of body mass, fasting blood lipids, blood pressure, and diabetes. The World Health Organization (WHO) has yet to report the official estimated prevalence rates for human immunodeficiency virus (HIV) and acquired immunodeficiency syndrome (AIDS) for adults, or children infected through mother-to-child transmission. Although the first case was detected in 1991, by 2004 there were 42 recorded cases, with 19 deaths. Most people with confirmed HIV/AIDS are adult men. Transmission is predominantly heterosexual. The principal route for infection has been seafarers returning from abroad and placing their wives at high risk. Mandatory testing of all seafarers is now in place. Because of its small population, Kiribati is highly vulnerable to HIV.

Health-Team Relationships: Doctors' decisions and treatments are usually accepted with total faith, and asking questions of health care

K

workers is not the norm. Patient-centered care is becoming common, however. Nurses and traditional birth attendants (TBAs) are predominantly women.

Dominance Patterns: Boasting or considering oneself to be better than another is unacceptable. Although women are the caretakers within the household, I-Kiribati men are usually the primary decision makers about household activities. Women are under-represented in high-level positions within the community, government, and politics, but this is changing as more women have better access to education and work opportunities. Women now make up 38% of the workforce.

Eye-Contact Practices: Direct eye contact is acceptable during interactions. Walking between people's line of eye contact when they are talking is considered rude. It is preferable either to go around them or to stoop down below eye level to go past. Nonverbal gestures are used widely. For example, instead of a verbal reply, raising one's eyebrows as a way of responding to a question is a common practice.

Touch Practices: Handshaking in the professional domain is considered appropriate and polite in all occasions of greetings. The head is treated with the greatest of respect, for both adults and children. Permission should be sought first if touching the head is necessary for medical reasons.

Perceptions of Time: Life moves at a slow, deliberate pace. Time has no agenda; there is no sense of urgency. I-Kiribati have a relaxed attitude toward punctuality and promptness. Sunday is a time spent with family and friends and engaging in church and communal activities.

Birth Rites: About 47% of the population is younger than 18 years. The total fertility rate is 4.3 children born per woman; the infant mortality rate is very high at 47 deaths per 1,000 live births. Nearly one third of births are supervised by TBAs, so the Ministry of Health and UNICEF have supported training programs to improve their skills, thereby providing safe delivery practices and care of newborns and mothers in outer islands. Life expectancy is 58 for men, 67 for women.

Food Practices and Intolerances: Except for coconut and pandanus trees, there are few natural resources and no arable land on the sandy, narrow-strip atolls. Water is obtained from rainwater tanks or ground wells, and Kiribati is prone to drought. Marine life thrives around the islands, however, and an abundance of fish is consumed. Access to safe water and sanitation is reasonably adequate in urban areas. Breadfruit boiled or fried in butter is a staple. Over the past two decades, traditional foods are being replaced with imported processed foods high in fat, sugar, and salt. White rice and flour are consumed regularly, together with fatty meat and canned foods such as mutton flap. Most I-Kiribati have developed a taste for such foods, often consuming them in huge quantities. The general belief that large body weight represents a sign of prosperity adds to the increasing problems of obesity.

Infant-Feeding Practices: Around 80% of infants are breastfed in the first 4 to 6 months of life, more in rural areas. The rates of exclusive breastfeeding for the first 6 months and continued breastfeeding of up to 2 years or longer are declining in urban settings. It is estimated that only 19% of mothers are still breastfeeding children at the age of 2 years. Providing baby formula and milk to infants is becoming a common practice in urban areas, especially for women who must return to work. Despite national campaigns to encourage breastfeeding, practical reasons and the belief that baby formula is better than breast milk persist.

Child-Rearing Practices: Child nurturing builds on community, family, and cultural values. Child-rearing responsibilities are shared across extended family members, with grandparents providing valuable support. Girls are often taught by their grandmothers how to perform traditional dances and to take care of the family. It is not uncommon for children to play together in streets and on the beach without adult supervision.

National Childhood Immunizations: BCG at birth; DTwP at 6, 10, and 14 weeks; OPV at birth and at 6 and 14 weeks; measles at 12 months; HepB at birth and at 6 and 14 weeks; vitamin A at 6 to 12 months and 1 to 6 years; and TT at 5 and 12 years. The percent of the target population vaccinated, by antigen, is: BCG (94%); DTP1 (75%); DTP3 (62%); HepB3 (67%); MCV (56%); and Polio3 (61%). Kiribati was declared polio free in 2001. Immunization coverage can be uneven and vary widely because of the erratic supply of vaccines; especially in the outer islands.

Other Characteristics: I-Kiribati place great value on supporting, sharing, and distributing goods along kinship lines. Although most are materially poor, strong family support means that the island lifestyle is not one of extreme poverty, with all having adequate (although unevenly distributed) living standards. Each village is built around a traditional *maneaba* ("meeting place")—a rectangular building with no walls and covered with a thatched roof. Village feasts and cultural ceremonies take place in the maneaba. There is no formal social security system; kinship is a proxy welfare system. The I-Kiribati are friendly, hospitable, and polite, and they are naturally interested in others. Most live in large households with extended families. In outer islands, people tend to be involved in subsistence activities (copra, fishing, bêche-de-mer, and seaweed production). Tensions between Western and traditional ways are contributing to discontent among youth. Drunkenness is common and contributes to road accidents and domestic violence and places youth at greater risk of sexually transmitted infections and unwanted pregnancies. Restlessness, boredom, and hopelessness for the future are pervasive among youth. Church communities promote efforts to engage youth in the mainstream community.

K

BIBLIOGRAPHY

Basuni AA, Butterworth L, Cooksley G, Locarnini S, Carman WF: Prevalence of HBsAg mutants and impact of hepatitis B infant immunisation in four Pacific Island countries, *Vaccine.* 22(21–22):2791–2799, 2004.

Bataua B: Heavy toll for a small country: Kiribati faces HIV/AIDS threat. *Pacific Magazine.* July 29(7):14, 2004.

Central Intelligence Agency: *2006: The world factbook, Kiribati.* Retrieved September 21, 2006, from https://www.cia.gov/cia/publications/factbook/print/kr.html.

Doran C: *Economic impact assessment of non-communicable diseases on hospital resources in Tonga, Vanuatu and Kiribati.* Noumea, 2003, Pacific Action for Health Project, Secretariat of the Pacific Community.

Secretariat of the Pacific Community: *Pacific Island populations 2004.* Demography/Population Programme. June 2004. Retrieved January 10, 2006, from http://www.spc.int/demog/.

United Nations: *Common country assessment. Kiribati.* Suva, Fiji, 2002, Office of the United Nations Resident Coordinator.

World Health Organization: 2006: Immunization, Vaccines and Biologicals. Retrieved September 21, 2006, from rhttp://www.who.int/immunization_monitoring/en/globalsummary/countryprofileresult.cfm?C='ki'.

World Health Organization: *Prevalence surveys of sexually transmitted infections among seafarers and women attending antenatal clinics in Kiribati:* 2002–2003. Manila, Philippines, 2004, World Health Organization Regional Office for the Western Pacific.

World Health Organization/United Nations Children's Fund (UNICEF): *Kiribati. Review of national immunization coverage 1980–2003.* Manila, Philippines, August 2004, World Health Organization Regional Office for the Western Pacific.

http://www.spc.org.nc/AC/PublicHealth/pahp/NCD_economic_impact_report%20_Kiribati_Tonga_Vanuatu.pdf. (retrieved January 10, 2006).

◆ KOREA, NORTH (DEMOCRATIC PEOPLE'S REPUBLIC OF KOREA)

K

MAP PAGE (803)

Myungsun Yi

Location: North Korea occupies the northern part of the Korean peninsula off eastern Asia and is bordered by China, South Korea, and Russia. The total area is 120,540 km^2 (46,541 square miles). North Koreans call the country Choson, which was the last dynasty in Korea from 1392 to 1919. The capital is Pyongyang. Most of the country is covered with hills and mountains stretching from north to south, with narrow valleys and small plains between them. The gross domestic product (GDP) per capita is $1,700. The population is estimated at more than 23 million. Literacy rates are 99% for both men and women.

Major Languages	Ethnic Groups	Major Religions
Korean	Korean 99%	Atheist, unaffiliated 95%
	Other 1%	Buddhism, Confucianism, syncretic Chondogyo 5%

Few people practice any form of religion because religious practices are not encouraged by the government. Cheondogyo, which means the Religion of the Heavenly Way, is a synthesis of Confucianism, Buddhism, and zen. It is one of the traditional religions originating from the Korean culture in the early twentieth century.

Health Care Beliefs: Acute sick care; traditional. Biomedical treatments, acupuncture, herbal medicines, and acupressure are common therapies. Western and Oriental medicines may be used at the same time. The cause of an illness may be attributed to a disturbance of the body's vital energy *(ki)*. Health can be regarded as balanced and strong *ki*. Illness is considered a pattern of disharmony in which *ki* is not in balance because it is blocked or weak.

Predominant Sick-Care Practices: Biomedical and alternative. Western and oriental medicines are used simultaneously. About 70% of all medicines used are the product of oriental medicine. Because of continuous economic hardships, North Koreans depend heavily on herbal medicines. The health care situation is far below the standards of most Western countries and continues to deteriorate. Hospitals in Pyongyang and other cities lack medication, food, heat, and basic supplies and have frequent power outages. The flow of international food aid is critical for meeting basic survival needs. Malnutrition rates are among the world's highest, and mortality estimates are in the hundreds of thousands as the direct result of starvation or famine-related diseases.

Ethnic-/Race-Specific or Endemic Diseases: Localized air pollution is attributable to inadequate industrial controls. Water pollution and inadequate supplies of potable water are significant causes of disease. *Hwa-byung* is a Korean folk illness label that was categorized into a Korean culture-bound syndrome in the fourth edition of the *Diagnostic and Statistical Manual of Mental Disorders* (DSM-IV). It translates as "anger syndrome." As the result of a series of natural disasters such as famine, beginning in the 1990s, and a general economic decline, the food shortage has worsened and public health has deteriorated dramatically. Based on a recent survey, the World Food Programme reported that 40% of the children are stunted, 20% are underweight, and 8% are wasted, and the stunting rate is regarded as a severe public health problem. The incidence of communicable diseases such as typhoid fever, paratyphoid, cholera, and malaria has also increased dramatically because of a severe lack of medicine and poor epidemic measures. The incidence and prevalence rates of tuberculosis were 80 and 178, respectively, in 2004. There are no data available from the government on human immunodeficiency virus (HIV) and acquired immunodeficiency syndrome (AIDS). The Joint United Nations Programme on HIV/AIDS (UNAIDS) provides a loose estimate of less than 0.2%, with fewer than 100 infections in the country. It is difficult to estimate the future direction of cases; however, inadequate hygiene practices and inadequate blood management may pose a threat.

K

Health-Team Relationships: The medical system is in chaos, although ostensibly the country has a system in which doctors cover particular districts. In reality, access to health care is either very poor or nonexistent because few treatments are available. Doctors receive training for a period of 3 to 6 years and have the dominant role on the health care team. Nurses are educated at the technical level, ranging from 6 months to 3 years.

Dominance Patterns: In general, the ages of 30 to 31 for men and 28 to 29 for women are considered the proper ages for marriage. Women's labor is important, and women make up about 48% of the labor force. A system of public nursery schools makes it possible for women to work. At age 60 (for men) and age 55 (for women), older adults earn the status of "elder" and can retire.

Touch Practices: Hand holding and touching among friends of the same sex is acceptable.

Perceptions of Time: Punctuality is considered basic etiquette in formal and informal interpersonal meetings.

Birth Rites: Many customs relative to childbirth are similar to those in South Korea except that the economic and health circumstances differ vastly. The fertility rate is two children born per woman. The infant mortality rate is high at 39 deaths per 1,000 live births. Child mortality, which indicates the probability of dying under age 5 years, is also very high at 55 deaths per 1,000. Life expectancy is 66 years, but government statistics are not considered accurate.

Death Rites: Although similar culturally to South Korea, because of the political and economic climate, North Koreans are experiencing a trend toward more secular, rather than religious (Confucian), funerals. Funerals usually last 3 days and burial, rather than cremation, is preferred.

Food Practices and Intolerances: Economic hardship and famine have resulted in food often being in short supply. In traditional families, the father, using chopsticks and a spoon, may dine alone. After meals, which usually consist of rice, fish, soup, and vegetables, the family gathers for conversation. The diet is healthy except for a high sodium intake. The usual dessert is fruit.

National Childhood Immunizations: BCG within 1 week after birth; DTwP at 6, 10, and 14 weeks; OPV at 6, 10, and 14 weeks; HepB within 1 week after birth and at 1.5 and 3.5 months; measles at 9 months; vitamin A at 6 to 59 months, +6 months; and TT at 3 and 4 months of pregnancy. The percent of the target population vaccinated, by antigen, is: BCG (94%); Polio3 (97%); DPT1 (83%); DPT3 (79%); HepB3 and measles (92%); and MCV (96%).

Other Characteristics: Interpersonal relationships are hierarchical according to age and social status. Younger persons use honorific expressions in addressing older persons, and the full name with the title should be used. Addressing a person by first name is acceptable for parents and older family members and only for friends of the same age. Both hands are used in handing something to an older person. A woman does not change her family name when she marries.

BIBLIOGRAPHY

Central Intelligence Agency: *2006: The world factbook, Korea, North.* Retrieved September 21, 2006 from https://www.cia.gov/cia/publications/factbook/print/kn.html.

Choe MA et al: *Preparedness plan for integration of nursing service systems after unification of Korea.* Seoul, 2004, The Research Institute of Nursing Science, Seoul National University.

Joo KH: *North Korean living ways for 50 years,* Seoul, 2001, Minzokwon.

Moon OR: Operation of health care system in North Korea. Ajou Institute of Korean Unification and Health Care, 2001, Seoul.

UNAIDS: 2006 Korea (Democratic People's Republic of). Retrieved September 21, 2006, from http://www.unaids.org/en/Regions_Countries/Countries/dpr_korea.asp.

World Health Organization: 2006: Immunization, vaccines and biologicals. Retrieved September 21, 2006, from http://www.who.int/immunization_monitoring/en/globalsummary/countryprofileresult.cfm?C='prk'.

http://www.wfp.org/country_brief/indexcountry.asp?region=5&section=9&sub_section=5&country=408 (Retrieved March 23, 2006).

http://www.who.int/countries/prk/en/ (Retrieved March 23, 2006).

http://www.who.int/GlobalAtlas/predefinedReports/TB/PDF_Files/KP_2004_Brief.pdf (Retrieved March 23, 2006).

http://www3.who.int/whosis/country/indicators.cfm?country=prk&language=en#economic (Retrieved March 23, 2006).

◆ KOREA, SOUTH (REPUBLIC OF)

MAP PAGE (803)

Myungsun Yi

Location: South Korea occupies the southern part of the Korean peninsula off Manchuria and China in eastern Asia. Eastern Korea is mountainous, and the west and south have many mainland harbors and offshore islands. The total area is 98,480 km^2 (38,023 square miles). The population is 48.8 million. The capital is Seoul. The gross domestic product (GDP) per capita is $20,400, with 15% living below the poverty line. Literacy rates are 99% for men, 97% for women. Buddhism has been a major religion since the seventh century; the numbers of Protestants and Roman Catholics increased in the late twentieth century. Other religions, such as Cheondogyo, Taejonggyo, and Wonbulgyo (Won Buddhism) exist but are little practiced. Although Confucianism is not considered a religion, it rules the way of life for all Koreans because it was practiced for more than 500 years during the Yi dynasty from 1392 to 1919.

Major Languages	Ethnic Groups	Major Religions
Korean	Korean 99%	Atheist or Other 48%
	Chinese 1%	Buddhist 23%
		Protestant 18%
		Roman Catholic 11%

Health Care Beliefs: Active involvement; health promotion. The mind-body interaction is considered essential for good health. The cause of illness may be attributed to a disturbance of the body's vital energy *(ki)*.

Health can be regarded as balanced, strong *ki*. Illness is considered a pattern of disharmony in which *ki* is unbalanced because it is blocked or weak. Physical symptoms may be based on psychological factors, and improvement is frequently evaluated in terms of functional ability.

Predominant Sick-Care Practices: Biomedical (Western); holistic; traditional. Acupuncture, hand acupuncture, acupressure, herbal medicines, and cupping are traditional treatments and are used often. Eastern and Western medicine may be used simultaneously. The implementation of health insurance for the entire nation has increased the demand for health care services. Medical services are provided by general and educational hospitals and by clinics established and operated by national or local government or the private sector. Private institutions (primarily in urban areas) comprise more than 91% of all medical facilities, employ 89% of doctors, and account for 91% of total beds. Koreans have access to two systems of care: Western medicine, which is the mainstream form of care, and Oriental medicine. No referral system between the two systems has been established. Oriental (traditional Korean) medicine differs fundamentally from Western in its principles and characteristics and has a history of excellent success. The Oriental Medicine Bureau was established as one of the major bureaus of the Ministry of Health and Welfare in 1996 to fulfill public demand for Oriental medicine. A compulsory health insurance program for the entire population is in place. All insurers are members of the National Federation of Medical Insurance (NFMI). On behalf of its members, NFMI designates medical care institutions to provide service to the insured and reviews and pays all claims under the guidance and supervision of the Ministry of Health and Welfare. Major financial contributions to the system are paid by the insured and their employers and supplemented by government subsidies.

Ethnic-/Race-Specific or Endemic Diseases: *Hwa-byung* is a Korean folk illness label, and it was categorized into a Korean culture-bound syndrome in the fourth edition of the *Diagnostic and Statistical Manual of Mental Disorders* (DSM-IV). It is considered an anger syndrome. The incidence of infectious diseases has decreased, but the incidence of chronic degenerative diseases has increased. Major chronic diseases are hypertension, diabetes mellitus, cardiac and liver disease, and cancer. Cancer is the primary cause of death, followed by cerebrovascular disease, heart disease, diabetes mellitus, and chronic lower respiratory disease. These five diseases cause 57% of all deaths. Korea has a notification system for all infectious diseases and a laboratory surveillance system for influenza, Japanese encephalitis, typhoid fever, and *Vibrio* infections. The first case of acquired immunodeficiency syndrome (AIDS) was reported in 1985 and the first death from AIDS in 1987. The Republic of Korea has a low human immunodeficiency virus (HIV) prevalence rate. The Joint United Nations Programme on HIV/AIDS (UNAIDS) reports that the prevalence rate for HIV in adults (aged 15 to 49 years) is less than 0.1%, with 13,000 living with HIV, including 7,400 women. Fewer than 500 have died of AIDS. No statistics are available for children or AIDS orphans. The great majority (94%) of infections are sexually transmitted, with 21% occurring among women.

Health-Team Relationships: Since the end of the Korean War in 1953, the number of health care professionals in South Korea has increased dramatically. In the past, doctors and nurses were considered authority figures and were treated with great respect. People generally did not disagree with them. Today, however, patients are more vocal about participating in health care decisions; in hospitals, patients' rights are being more emphasized.

Families' Role in Hospital Care: When a family member becomes sick, the family prefers to give personal care, and they act as guardians for the sick family member. The family is actively involved in making major medical decisions such as do-not-resuscitate orders, and patients tend to delegate such decisions to family members. Patient education performed in hospital settings must involve family members.

Dominance Patterns: Parent-child relationships are more highly regarded than husband-wife relationships, and the oldest son inherits the patriarchal position. The father is dominant and makes decisions for all family members. As the head of the household, he is responsible for all its economic needs. The mother is the homemaker in charge of the domestic and emotional needs of the family. In addition to the traditional role of tending the home and raising children, women are responsible for managing the family's health. Men have more legal advantages than women in terms of rights to children because children traditionally belong to the husband's family. In less traditional families, decision making is more family oriented. At age 65, older adults earn the status of "elder" and can retire.

K

Eye-Contact Practices: Status determines whether direct eye contact is avoided or maintained. A person with higher status may maintain eye contact, whereas a person with lower status will avoid eye contact by looking down to show deference. Status is relative and is often determined by position, age, and gender; status increases with higher position, older age, and by being male.

Touch Practices: Hand-holding among good friends of the same sex is acceptable. Hugging is not often practiced, especially with the opposite sex. In health care situations, touching is usually minimal except with elderly patients.

Perceptions of Time: Punctuality is basic etiquette in formal and informal interpersonal interactions.

Pain Reactions: South Koreans tend to be stoic; however, expressing pain during childbirth is permissible.

Birth Rites: From conception, the mother starts prenatal training (*taegyo*). After delivery, mothers are expected to avoid exposure to cold (including air conditioning) and consume no iced drinks—only warm foods. *Sanhujori*, a period of 6 to 8 weeks after delivery, is a prevailing tradition and involves recovering strength by warming the body. It is expected that women will eat warm and soft food such as brown-seaweed soup *(miyeogguk)*; avoid salty, spicy, sweet, and sour foods; and attend to personal hygiene until their body is restored to its prepregnancy condition. Koreans used to prefer sons because, according to the Confucian value system, sons carry on the family name and must care for parents in their old age. Parents with daughters may continue to have children until they have a son, although government campaigns during the 1970s and 1980s urged couples to have only one child because of a projected critical increase in population. Birth rates dropped, and the government now employs a policy for childbirth promotion. The infant mortality rate is 6 deaths per 1,000 live births. Life expectancy is 74 for men, 81 for women.

Death Rites: Family members are summoned to observe a dying person's last breath and may respond with loud wailing and intense displays of emotion. Death rites may differ according to religious affiliation and death orientations. More simplified death rituals occur today compared with the elaborate rituals of Confucian funerals in the past. The funeral generally lasts 3 days, and burial, not cremation, is preferred. More people now die in the hospital rather than at home, so most funeral homes are located in hospitals.

Food Practices and Intolerances: The Korean diet is essentially healthy, with the exception of its high sodium content, which may contribute to the high prevalence rate of hypertension. Rice is the basic food, and many meals include *kimchi*, or pickled cabbage. Fruit snacks are frequently eaten, and dessert is usually fruit. Chopsticks and a large spoon are used to eat. Hot soup or stew is preferred at all meals, whereas cold liquids are not usually consumed.

Child-Rearing Practices: The mother tends to be careful, permissive, and affectionate, whereas the father tends to be strict. Breastfeeding is recommended for the health of mother and child, but the length of time for breastfeeding varies significantly. "Examination hell," or the pressure created by the need to excel on college entrance examinations, is blamed for the occasionally grim lives of some adolescents and their high suicide rate. College entrance examinations are thought to determine the fate of Korean students.

National Childhood Immunizations: BCG at birth; IPV at 2, 4, 6 to 18 months, and 4 to 6 years; HepB at birth, 1, 2, or 6 months; JapEnc at 12 to 24 months, 1 to 12 weeks, +1 year, and 6 and 12 years; DtaP at 2, 4, 6, 15 to 18 months, and 4 to 6 years; MMR at 12 to 15 months and 4 to 6 years; Td at 11 to 12 years; varicella 12 to 15 months. The percent of the target population vaccinated, by antigen, is: BCG (97%); DTP1 (98%); DTP3 and Polio3 (96%); and HepB3 and MCV (99%).

Other Characteristics: Koreans have three names: the family name is written first, followed by a generational name and a given name. First names (the generational name combined with the given name) are used only by parents, older relatives, friends, and intimate elders. Otherwise, the full name is used, usually in combination with the person's position or title. Korean society tends to be hierarchical, so a person's title is highly dependent on the particular situation. Age is a very important factor in interpersonal relationships; Koreans use honorifics for persons older than them. Both hands are used to hand something to an older person to show respect. When first offered, food and drinks are refused out of politeness, regardless of how much they are desired. The offer must be repeated. A woman does not change her family name when she marries.

BIBLIOGRAPHY

Ahn, S: Canonical correlation between Korean traditional postpartum care performance and postpartum health status, *J Korean Acad Nurs.* 35(1):37–46, 2005.

American Psychiatric Association: *Diagnostic and statistical manual of mental disorders,* ed 4. Washington, DC, 1994, American Psychiatric Association, pp 843–849.

Central Intelligence Agency: 2006: *The world factbook, Korea, South.* Retrieved September 21, 2006, from https://www.cia.gov/cia/publications/factbook/print/ks.html.

Chang SO: The meaning of ki related to touch in caring, *Holistic Nurs Pract.* 16(1), 2001.

Khim SY, Lee CS: Exploring the nature of "Hwa-Byung" using pragmatics, *J Korean Acad Nurs.* 33(1):104–112, 2003.

Lee SD: A study on the philosophical background and health concept in Oriental Medicine, *Korean J Health Promo.* 2(1):88–98, 2000.

Yi M, Jezewski MA: Korean nurses' adjustment to hospitals in the United States of America, *J Adv Nurs.* 32(3):721–729, 2000.

UNAIDS: 2006 Korea (Republic of). Retrieved September 21, 2006, from http://www.unaids.org/en/Regions_Countries/Countries/korea_republic.asp.

World Health Organization: 2006: Immunization, vaccines and biologicals. Retrieved September 21, 2006, from http://www.who.int/immunization_monitoring/en/globalsummary/countryprofileresult.cfm?C=kor.

http://kosis.nso.go.kr (retrieved March 03, 2006).

http://www.cdc.go.kr/webcdc/menu07/d_issue/051201.pdf (retrieved March 23, 2006).

http://www.nso.go.kr (retrieved March 03, 2006).

http://www.wpro.who.int/countries/05kor/health_situation.htm (Retrieved March 23, 2006).

◆ KUWAIT (STATE OF)

MAP PAGE (802)

Salim M. Adib

Location: Kuwait is located in the northwestern corner of the Persian Gulf. Its total area is 17,818 km² (about 7,000 square miles) and Kuwait City is the capital. The country slopes down gradually from west to east, with a few hills scattered in the eastern parts, where the country becomes primarily desert. Temperatures may be low during winter nights; the absolute low record was −4° C (30° F) in 1964. Temperatures can soar to amazing highs on summer days, often exceeding 50° C (120° F). The population is 2.7 million, including non-Kuwaiti expatriate residents

(60%), who are transient and primarily include Arabs and Southeast Asians. The gross domestic product (GDP) per capita is $19,200. Literacy rates are 85% for men, 82% for women.

Major Languages	**Ethnic Groups**	**Major Religions (Kuwaitis only)**
Arabic (official)	Kuwaiti 45%	Sunni Muslim 68%
English (widely spoken)	Other Arab 35%	Shi'a Muslim 30%
Iranian	South Asian 9%	Other 2%
Hindi	Iranian 4%	
Urdu	Other 7%	

Most Kuwaitis claim an affiliation to large Bedouin tribes, and about 30% are original urban dwellers (known as the "city dwellers" or "dira families"). About 20% of the population is of Persian origin. Tolerance of non-Kuwaiti religions is mandated by law, and there are at least eight declared Christian churches.

Health Care Beliefs: Acute sick care; traditional. In a survey of Kuwaitis, about 55% agreed that *djinns* ("evil spirits") play a role in making people sick, and an additional 29% were unsure. Of those surveyed, 65% believed some diseases can be healed only by faith-related practices. In addition to reading Koranic verses, healers ask patients to drink "blessed" water occasionally mixed with saffron, to eat blessed honey or dates, or to massage a painful area with blessed oil. Patients may be massaged by a practitioner who has spit in his hands to ensure passage of Koranic powers from his reciting mouth to his massaging hands. Patients may be told to play tapes of specific healing verses continuously until their problem vanishes. Some powerful spirits can be driven out only by some degree of physical violence, ranging from slight slapping of the hands and face to serious beating with sandals and sticks. More worrisome is that in recent years some healers have even begun giving electric shocks to patients. Use of herbal preparations is common.

Predominant Sick-Care Practices: Biomedical and magical-religious. Modern medicine has gradually supplanted traditional health practices. After the discovery of oil, resources were allocated to create a public health system that was accessible and free to all. In 1999, user fees were introduced for non-Kuwaitis. The private care system has developed in a major way since 2000 and is increasingly preferred by the more affluent segments despite out-of-pocket expenses. Although most medical care is sought within the formal care system, some traditional practices persist, often in combination with modern medicine. Traditional health practices include "Islamic" or "Koranic" healing performed by self-taught "practitioners" acting with almost no regulation. They tend to be consulted when patients or their families suspect that an evil spirit is contributing to an illness. A 2001 survey reported that about 56% continue to use the services of Koranic faith healers. Until recently, cauterization was a traditional procedure most often practiced by Bedouins. Parts of the body are marked with a hot iron or a heated wooden rod, a practice believed to draw out the offending illness. The most common areas for cauterization are the foot and belly, and the most commonly treated conditions are fevers, diarrhea, epilepsy, and headaches. Belief in the efficacy of herbal treatments has been channeled through the Islamic Center for Herbal Medicine since the mid-1980s, which ensures that herbs used by the public are not harmful.

Ethnic-/Race-Specific or Endemic Diseases: Although still maintaining many features of more traditional, less advanced societies, Kuwait has recently acquired many similarities to more advanced nations. Infectious diseases have ceased to be a public health concern since the advent of excellent immunization programs. The most prevalent diseases are diabetes (15% of the population) and asthma (13% of 9- to 12-year-old school children). Of concern is the increase in tobacco smoking, especially among young men. A survey of undergraduate men, average age 20 years, indicated that 42% were regular smokers. Other risks include obesity and anemia. Drug abuse is reportedly increasing among young adults. Cardiovascular disease is the major cause of death, followed by various cancers. Injuries from automobile accidents have been increasing. Accidental deaths are the third most common cause of death. The Joint United Nations Programme on HIV/AIDS (UNAIDS) reports a low prevalence of human immunodeficiency virus (HIV) in adults (aged 15 to 49 years): less than 0.2%, with fewer than 1,000 cases. Most common transmission appears to be heterosexual. Non-Kuwaitis are required to have a negative HIV test before obtaining permanent residency. No new cases among Kuwaiti nationals have been reported since 2002.

Health-Team Relationships: Until recently, the medical field was dominated by men. More women are now graduating from the only faculty of medicine in the country, and a more gender-collaborative medical environment is expected to emerge. Nursing is not held in high esteem by the locals; a 2003 survey of Kuwaiti high school girls indicated that only 19% might consider nursing as a future career. The only program graduating registered Kuwaiti nurses was closed in 1999 because of a lack of students.

Families' Role in Hospital Care: Family and friends are expected to be with hospitalized patients as much as possible. Families are demanding of personnel to ensure that patients receive adequate care and attention. Food services are generally highly rated in public hospitals and often include daily treats of baked goods and fresh juices. Nevertheless, gifts of sweets and chocolates (and occasionally flowers) are generally expected. News of a serious diagnosis or poor prognosis is usually delivered to families, rather than to patients, provided this lack of disclosure does not affect a patient's therapeutic course.

Dominance Patterns: By law, men and women are equal. In 2005, Kuwaiti women obtained the right to vote despite opposition from fundamentalist parties. Polygamy is a right reserved to men by Islam; however, less than 9% of married men practice it. Polygamy is slowly being replaced by serial marriages, as indicated by the increasing rate of divorce (one for every three marriages). By age 50, 95% of all Kuwaitis have been married at least once. High wedding costs and dowries have left as many as 40,000 Kuwaiti women in a socially undesirable single status. About 20% of Kuwaiti men have been opting to marry foreigners. In practice, Kuwaiti society remains highly patriarchal, and women are not expected to have prominent public or leadership roles. In many families, the surviving grandmother plays an essential role as the hostess of family events and remains the center of conflict resolution. Norms of public behavior for women differ greatly with respect to traditional dress. It is common to encounter women who are wearing very modern and trendy clothes walking next to women totally covered with a dark chador. Many women have prominent positions in academia, business, and diplomacy.

Eye-Contact Practices: Eye contact is expected during a conversation; however, when men and women converse, it is preferred that the eye contact be brief. Many women are uncomfortable with direct eye contact.

Touch Practices: Touching between the sexes is not encouraged. A man is not expected to shake hands with a woman if she does not take the initiative by stretching out her hand. If a man is uncomfortable about shaking hands with a woman, he discreetly touches his chest as a signal.

Perceptions of Time: Kuwaitis tend to glorify past traditions as reflections of a time when life was simpler and social ties were stronger and warmer. Most recognize that the "good old times" were also very harsh times—when life was often precarious and survival was often a matter of sheer luck. The rapidity with which modern prosperity and convenience has overtaken Kuwaitis may have reinforced the tendency to dwell on the past and the present with a fatalistic eye and confidence in Allah's providence. It is uncommon to hear public debate involving serious concerns about the future, but growing numbers of people are saying that maintaining the same standard of living will be more difficult and will require more effort.

Pain Reactions: It is preferable that pain be expressed only privately or with close relatives and friends.

Birth Rites: The birth of a boy is generally considered a more joyous event than the birth of a girl, especially if the infant is a first-born child. Childless women are often regarded with sorrow and pity, and they suffer from marked levels of psychological distress. Studies indicate that the preferred number of children is five: three boys and two girls. The fertility rate is decreasing, however, and was three children born per woman in 2006, perhaps related to the increasing median age of marriage. After delivery, women are considered impure for up to 40 days, when they must not pray, fast, or engage in sexual relations. According to tradition, they cannot be visited by new brides. Mothers of Bedouin and Iranian origins eat traditional foods after delivery, most of which include a mixture of spices to help the body shed excess fluids and promote lactation. Infant mortality rates have been decreasing steadily for 30 years: in 2006, the rate was 10 deaths per 1,000 live births. Life expectancy is 76 for men, 78 for women.

Death Rites: Friends and relatives are not expected to show too much grief because it is contrary to the religious belief that the person has moved on to a better place. Autopsy is uncommon because the body must be buried intact according to Muslim tradition. For Muslim burials, the body is wrapped in special pieces of cloth and buried without a coffin, usually within 1 day of death. Cremation is not permitted. Family members receive condolences for 3 days, with separate venues for men and women. Organ donations have been allowed since 1983 in accordance with current interpretations of Islamic regulations. The kidney transplant unit in Al-Sabah Hospital has already conducted hundreds of kidney and other organ transplant operations. A nongovernmental organization, the Kuwait Transplant Society, has been urging citizens since the mid-1980s to become organ donors by signing an organ donation card.

Food Practices and Intolerances: The staple food in Kuwait is rice, and fish is abundant. Kuwaiti cuisine is heavily influenced by Indian and Iranian cuisines, and they particularly enjoy lamb. All types of ethnic and international food, as well as fast-food chains, can be found all over the country. Pork, carrion, blood, and alcohol cannot be consumed by Muslims, and these items are not imported, sold, or served in public. Public observance of Ramadan fasting is mandatory for all adults. The ceremonial collective meal consisting of a mound of spiced saffron rice topped with a whole lamb and eaten from a common tray on a carpet is still common among more traditional Bedouin families, particularly during special social events such as weddings and the end of the period of condolences. Eating with the hands is common, especially during collective meals; only the right hand is used.

Infant-Feeding Practices: Breastfeeding is still the norm for most women. It can last for up to 18 months, with lactation periods decreasing with increasing numbers of children. The proportion of children exclusively breastfed in the first 6 months of life is estimated at 12%, and the rate increases up to 24% for breastfeeding along with complementary foods.

Child-Rearing Practices: Child rearing is relatively permissive, and parents tend to rely on the abundant and cheap domestic servants that are available to provide daily personal care and supervision of children. Despite this, physical abuse is common and tends to occur randomly. Many Kuwaiti parents continue to feel that physical punishment is a legitimate way to discipline children. Public denigration of children is preferred rather than praise because of fear of the evil eye. Children older than 1 year rarely sleep with their parents. Formal schooling of children begins at age 4.

National Childhood Immunizations: BCG at 4 to 5 years; OPV at birth and 2, 4, 6, and 18 months; Hep B at birth and 2 and 6 months; DTPHiB at 2, 4, 6, and 18 months; DTwP at 3.5 years; MMR at 1 and 3.5 years; rubella at 12 years for girls; DT at 10 and 18 years; and TT at fourth and seventh month of pregnancy. The percent of the target population vaccinated, by antigen, is: DTP1, DTP3, HepB3, Hib3, MCV, and Polio3 (99%).

BIBLIOGRAPHY

Alansari B: Prevalence of cigarette smoking among male Kuwait University under-graduate students, *Psychol Rep.* 96(3 Pt 2):1009–1010, 2005.

Al-Awadi E, Al-Hashel J, Al-Hajeri D: *Quranic faith-healing practices in Kuwait.* Kuwait City, 1999, Department of Community Medicine, Health Sciences Center, Kuwait University.

Al-Enezi A et al: *Postpartum beliefs and practices among Kuwaiti women.* Kuwait City, 1999, Department of Community Medicine, Health Sciences Center, Kuwait University.

Al-Kandari FH, Lew J. Kuwaiti high school students' perceptions of nursing as a profession: implications for nursing education and practice, *J Nurs Educ.* 44:533–540, 2005.

Central Intelligence Agency: *2006: The world factbook, Kuwait.* Retrieved September 21, 2006, from https://www.cia.gov/cia/publications/factbook/print/ku.html.

El-Shazly M, Makboul G, El-Sayyed A: Life expectancy and cause-of-death in the Kuwaiti population 1987–2000, *East Mediterranean Health J.* 10:45–55, 2004.

Fido A, Zahid MA: Coping with infertility among Kuwaiti women: cultural perspectives, *Int J Soc Psychiatry.* 50:294–300, 2004.

Memon A et al: Epidemiology of smoking among Kuwaiti adults: prevalence, charac-teristics and attitudes, *Bull WHO.* 78:1306–1315, 2000.

Ministry of Planning: *Annual statistical abstract,* ed. 37, Kuwait, 2000, Ministry of Planning of Kuwait.

UNAIDS: 2006 Kuwait. Retrieved September 21, 2006, from http://www.unaids.org/en/Regions_Countries/Countries/kuwait.asp.

World Health Organization: 2006: Immunization, vaccines and biologicals. Retrieved September 21, 2006, from http://www.who.int/immunization_monitoring/en/globalsummary/countryprofileresult.cfm?C='kwt'.

K

◆ KYRGYZSTAN (KYRGYZ REPUBLIC)

MAP PAGE (799)

Gunay Balta

Location: Kyrgyzstan was the first of the 12 non-Baltic Union of Soviet Socialist Republics (USSR) to declare its independence from the former Soviet Union in 1991 and has made impressive progress in building a state, a democracy, and a market-oriented economy based on private property and the rule of law. However, it remains one of the least devel-oped countries in the region. It is located in northeast Central Asia and has a total area of 198,000 km^2 (76,428 square miles). The capital is Bishkek. Most of the territory lies within the Tien Shan mountain range, which is covered with perennial snow and glaciers. Kyrgyzstan is remark-able for its natural beauty. It is a country of sunshine, snow-covered mountains, deep gorges cut by swift rivers, and 1,923 mountain lakes. Kyrgyzstan's young cosmopolitan population of 5.2 million is a unique mix of more than 80 ethnic groups. The gross domestic product (GDP) per capita is $2,100, and 48% live below the poverty line (particularly in remote areas). Literacy rates are 99% for men, 98% for women.

Major Languages	Ethnic Groups	Major Religions
Kyrgyz	Kyrgyz 67%	Muslim 75%
Russian	Russian 10%	Orthodox Christian 20%
	Uzbek 14%	Other 5%
	Ukrainian 0.7%	
	Uyghur 1%	
	Other 7.3%	

The Kyrgyz culture has been greatly influenced by its nomadic heritage, reflected in the country's customs and rituals. The masterpiece of folk creation is the Kyrgyz tent *(yurta)*, which is easy to assemble and transport from place to place and is popular with shepherds *(chabans)* who spend their summers in the high pastures. The Kyrgyz are an ancient nationality. Much of past history has been learned from the longest epic poem in the world: the story of Manas, which contains 500,000 lines of poetry transmitted orally through generations. The Manas legend gives insight into all aspects of traditional life—origins, customs, morals, general knowledge, and language. Many places and things in Kyrgyzstan bear the name of this ancient hero. Compulsory primary school lasts 9 years; additional education is available free at one of 1,922 secondary schools and 47 universities and institutes. A tuition-charging private education sector is also developing.

Health Care Beliefs: Acute sick care; traditional. Because of very low incomes and often neglect, people seek professional help only when seriously ill. For mild illnesses, they often use alternative treatments based on their beliefs and experiences; for example, they may apply melted lamb fat over the chest and stomach to treat respiratory or stomach illnesses. Disease is perceived as a part of life, not a punishment from God.

Predominant Sick-Care Practices: Biomedical and alternative. Like other former Soviet Union countries, there is a hierarchy of health services. Primary care is given by *feldsher*—midwifery posts in villages, doctors' clinics in small towns, and polyclinics in urban areas. There are village hospitals, central district hospitals, regional and national hospitals, and specialized hospitals. Because of the economic situation and poor motivation of health care personnel due to their low salaries, the system is dysfunctional. In principle, health services are free and accessible to everyone. In reality, services are no longer free because of limited state resources. Informal out-of-pocket payments constitute almost half of total health financing. Co-payments or full payments for any kind of health service and surreptitious payments to doctors, particularly specialists, are common. The high levels of patient spending are related to low levels of government spending and the overall fragility of the economy. In recent years, informal payments have, to some extent, been replaced by official co-payments through establishment of the Mandatory Health Insurance Fund (MHIF) as a single-payer system. Most drugs (97%) are imported, and foreign loans and grants—and those donated as humanitarian aid—are used to supply emergency drugs in particular. Despite improvements in drug supplies, some cannot afford required medications. Except for certain drugs, prescriptions from doctors are not mandatory; therefore, people search for the lowest price at pharmacies.

Ethnic-/Race-Specific or Endemic Diseases: A recent problem is the increase in frequency of iron-deficiency anemia and iodine-deficiency disorders. Mortality from noncommunicable diseases such as heart disease and stroke is increasing. Also increasing is the incidence of communicable diseases such as tuberculosis and syphilis. There is increasing morbidity from pertussis, brucellosis, echinococcosis, viral hepatitis, and gonorrhea. Although the number of officially registered cases of human immunodeficiency virus (HIV) and acquired immunodeficiency syndrome (AIDS) cases is still comparatively low, an exponential increase has been recorded in recent years. The Joint United Nations Programme on HIV/AIDS (UNAIDS) reports the prevalence rate for HIV in adults (aged 15 to 49 years) to be 0.1%, with 4,000 people living with HIV, including fewer than 1,000 women. When the mode of transmission is known, about 80% of cases are transmitted by injecting drug use.

Health-Team Relationships: Doctors are the principal authorities on most health issues. Nurses, who have lower levels of education, play a supporting role. In addition, feldshers and midwives provide primary care in the villages.

Families' Role in Hospital Care: Families are responsible for finding and purchasing all medications and medical supplies for hospitalized family members. They also may make full or partial payments for services and laboratory tests. Many of the most popular medications are not readily available and are difficult for families to find.

Dominance Patterns: Kyrgyzstan has a conservative, male-dominated society, and gender roles tend to be quite traditional. Although women are found in nearly all areas of the workforce, they focus primarily on the family, where their position is important and respected. The family is a mutual support system, and siblings remain close even after marriage. Families are expected to care for their aging parents; therefore, parents often move in with one of their children as they become less able to live on their own.

Eye-Contact Practices: Direct eye contact is acceptable and the norm.

Touch Practices: Men usually shake hands when greeting, but men and women rarely do. Women usually greet other women by kissing on one side of the face. While greeting, people of the same sex tend to hold each other by the shoulder. Hugging is uncommon except among close relatives. Women and couples often walk arm-in-arm in public.

Perceptions of Time: Generally, punctuality is not important in daily life, and people do not rush. Professionals, especially those working for foreign companies, must be prompt.

Pain Reactions: Kyrgyz people are calm when faced with physically or emotionally painful situations, and they usually bear misfortune with stoicism.

Birth Rites: Religion and culture influence celebrations. An interesting feast—Djengek Toi—celebrates the birth of an infant. Another ritual is the celebration day *(Tyshoo Kesuu)* for an infant who has just learned to walk, in which invited young children participate in a competition or race. Before the race, the infant's feet are tied with a black and white string, which the child who wins the race is allowed to cut. It is believed that after being released from the strings, the infant will be healthy and live confidently.

Death Rites: Kyrgyz people participate in religious and cultural rituals at the time of death, when relatives and friends gather at the home of the deceased. Even in the cities, they build a *yurta* (traditional tent) next to the house on the same day of death, in which they place the body on a special bed. Close relatives, especially women, sit inside the yurta, pray to God, and express their sorrow. Usually they sacrifice a horse, and traditional dishes are prepared from its meat and served to the visitors in memory of the dead person. The body is usually buried 3 days later. Cremation is not allowed. All belongings of the deceased are distributed to relatives in memory of the deceased.

Food Practices and Intolerances: Dinner is the largest meal and a time when family members come together. Meat (often lamb, but occasionally horse meat or beef with entrails) and pastries are the most common ingredients, and vegetables may be included. *Beshbarmak* ("five fingers") is the most popular traditional dish. The most festive soup, *shorpo*, is prepared with meat broth, vegetables, and spices. Bread, potatoes, and fruit are also important. Dessert is rare, but milk and milk products are often consumed. The favorite drinks are *kumys*—mildly alcoholic fermented mare's milk—and *maksim*—boiled and fermented wheat. Tea is the most common beverage, served at any time and place, and coffee is uncommon. People love to entertain; therefore, they like to celebrate every occasion. They congregate, usually at homes, have a large meal, and drink and dance until late at night. Most like to drink alcohol, at least with guests, and vodka is popular. Hospitality is an important part of life; people are friendly and generous and share whatever they have with others.

K

Infant-Feeding Practices: Infants are always born at hospitals and kept at least 7 days for examinations and vaccinations. During this period, infants whose mothers are unable to produce breast milk are fed with milk from other mothers. Breastfeeding is considered the best form of nutrition, so most new mothers attempt it, but formula is used if a mother is unable to produce enough milk. Mashed fruit, vegetables, creamed cereals, rice, and potatoes supplement breast milk or formula when the infant is about 6 months of age.

Child-Rearing Practices: As primary caregivers, mothers are allowed by law to take a maternity leave of up to 3 years. Maternity leaves are unpaid, so the ability of the woman to stay home depends almost entirely on her financial ability. It is becoming more common for mothers to take short leaves (several weeks) because most families depend on her income. Grandparents are most frequently called on to care for children whose mothers have returned to work.

National Childhood Immunizations: BCG at birth; DT at 6 years; DTwP at 2, 3.5, and 5 months and at 2 years; HepB at birth, 2 and 5 months; MMR at 12 months; MR at 6 years, OPV at birth, 2, 3.5, and 5 months; Td at 11, 16, 26, 36, 46, and 56 years. The percent of the target population vaccinated, by antigen, is: BCG (96%); DTP1, DTP3, and Polio3 (98%); MCV (99%); and HepB3 (97%).

Other Characteristics: One of the most important family events is a wedding. The celebration includes *kalym* payment, various clothes that are exchanged between the bride and bridegroom's parents, expensive dowries, farewell wailing, and an animal sacrifice for the couple. Kyrgyz men and women are very unlikely to marry outside their people, but women are free to choose their spouse. People get married at a young age and have relatively large families. Wedding customs include the tradition of kidnapping the bride. Usually the man plans the day of the kidnapping beforehand, and his friends and relatives help. Relatives gather at his home, set tables, and cook a festive dinner. One corner of a room is curtained off *(koshego)*. When the woman is brought to the house, her head is covered by a kerchief as a symbol of virginity, and she is placed behind the curtain. This custom is still practiced.

BIBLIOGRAPHY

Beishenova D: Personal communications, April 2002 and January 2005.
Central Intelligence Agency: *2006: The world factbook, Kyrgyzstan.* Retrieved September 21, 2006, from https://www.cia.gov/cia/publications/factbook/print/kg.html.
Meimanaliev A-S, Ibraimova A, Elebesov B, Rechel B: Health care systems in transition: Kyrgyzstan. European Observatory on Health System and Policies, WHO Regional Office for Europe, Vol 7, No 2, 2005. Retrieved January 20, 2006, from http://www.who.dk/Document/E86633.pdf.
Ozdenoglu S: Republic of Kyrgyzstan Country Report 2005. TIKA: Turkish International Cooperation Agency of Republic of Turkey. Retrieved January 28, 2006, from http://www.tika.gov.tr/Dosyalar/Kirgizistan.doc.
UNAIDS: 2006 Kyrgyzstan. Retrieved September 21, 2006, from http://www.unaids.org/en/Regions_Countries/Countries/kyrgyzstan.asp.
The United Nations Developing Programme in Kyrgyzstan. Retrieved January 20, 2006, from http://www.undp.kg.
The United Nations in Kyrgyzstan. Retrieved January 22, 2006, from http://www.un.org.kg/english/country.phtml.
World Health Organization: Country Health Indicators, Kyrgyzstan: Retrieved January 14, 2006, from www3.who.int/whosis/country/indicators.cfm?country=kgz.
World Health Organization: Global Health Atlas: Retrieved January 15, 2006, from http://www.who.int/globalatlas.
World Health Organization: 2006: Immunization, vaccines and biologicals. Retrieved September 21, 2006, from http://www.who.int/immunization_monitoring/en/globalsummary/countryprofileresult.cfm?C='kgz'.

◆ LAOS (LAO PEOPLE'S DEMOCRATIC REPUBLIC)

MAP PAGE (805)

Philayrath Phongsavan

Location: Laos is a landlocked country in Southeast Asia, surrounded by Myanmar, China, Vietnam, Cambodia, and Thailand. The total area is 236,800 km^2 (91,429 square miles), with mountainous terrain in the north, dense forest, and jungle. The capital is Vientiane. The population is 6.2 million. Laos has a communist government and is classified as a low-income country: the gross domestic product (GDP) per capita is $1,900, with 39% living below the poverty line. Literacy rates are 77% for men, 56% for women.

Major Languages	Ethnic Groups	Major Religions
Lao (official)	Lao Lum 68%	Theravada
French	Lao Theung 22%	Buddhism 60%
English	Lao Soung (including	Animism, Other 40%
Ethnic languages	Hmong and Yao) 9%	
	Ethnic Vietnamese and	
	Chinese 1%	

This chapter concentrates on Lao Lum or lowland Lao, who constitute the majority of the population, but Laos is home to more than 60 ethnic minority groups. Because of this high number and the lack of detailed ethnographic information about many groups, the population is broadly classified into four groups to reflect common historical patterns, language, and culture.

Health Care Beliefs: Acute sick care; traditional and significantly related to animistic beliefs. Because of the poor state of the health care system and lack of strong prevention programs other than immunization, crisis care is the norm. Unhealthy air currents or bad "winds" are thought to cause illness. Pinching or scratching an area affected by these winds produces marks or red lines and is believed to release the bad wind from the body, thus restoring health. Strings around the neck, ankles, or waist prevent "soul loss," which is thought to cause illness. Blood that is lost is considered irreplaceable, so having blood drawn is perceived with apprehension. Because of stigmas against mental illness, emotional disturbances may be manifested somatically by symptoms such as headache.

Predominant Sick-Care Practices: Biomedical, magical-religious, and traditional. Traditional health practices are closely linked to religious traditions. The Lao believe that 32 spirits (or *khouan*) inhabit the body and govern its functioning, health, and well-being. Losing a *khouan* by having an accident or being frightened can result in illness. In these circumstances, an elderly person, monk, or traditional healer will perform a traditional *soukhouan* of prayers and good wishes, and blessed white cotton strings are tied around the wrists to restore balance and call the *khouan* back to the body. Herbal medicine is an important traditional practice and is classified as "cool treatment," whereas Western medicine is considered "hot." Traditionally, illness is handled through self-care and self-medication. Going to the temple for prayer or to give food offerings to monks are usually the first approaches taken. Most do not place a high priority on disease prevention. Seeking medical care is often done when the person already has advanced illness. Because of inadequate and unhygienic conditions in many hospitals, these facilities may be thought of as places to die. Medical facilities and services are still very limited and poorly resourced, although most of the 16 provinces have at least one main hospital as well as health clinics in subdistricts. Seeking help from traditional healers as well as Western-trained providers is not uncommon. Thailand is easily accessible from Vientiane across the Friendship Bridge, and those who are able may seek more advanced medical care there.

Ethnic-/Race-Specific or Endemic Diseases: Endemic diseases include chloroquine-resistant malaria, melioidosis, schistosomiasis (southern Laos), and gnathostomiasis. Lao are at risk for dengue fever, iodine deficiency (mountainous regions), cholera, pulmonary paragonimiasis (lung fluke), and poliomyelitis. Laos has numerous cases of childhood malaria, a significant contributor to morbidity. Most people, especially in rural areas, do not have access to potable water, increasing the risk for water-borne illnesses. Frequent flooding in parts of Laos poses a constant threat of cholera and diarrheal disease outbreaks, especially at the beginning of the rainy season. More than 500,000 tons of unexploded ordnance is left over from the Vietnam War, causing approximately 120 casualties per year. Automobile accidents are a risk, because of hazardous driving behavior coupled with poorly maintained vehicles and roads. The Joint United Nations Programme on HIV/AIDS (UNAIDS) estimates the prevalence rate for human immunodeficiency virus (HIV) in adults (aged 15 to 49 years) to be 0.1%, with 3,700 people living with HIV, including fewer than 1,000 women. About 170 new infections have been reported. Deaths from acquired immunodeficiency syndrome (AIDS) are estimated at fewer than 200, and about 290 children have lost a parent to AIDS. About one fifth of cases are reported, most among heterosexuals. The Lao are especially vulnerable to increased risk of HIV because of cross-border migration between Laos and neighboring China and Vietnam, which have significant rates of infection.

Health-Team Relationships: In traditional families, the oldest male makes health care decisions and may answer questions directed to a female patient. Doctors are considered authority figures and experts whose advice should not be questioned. Patients are told little about their conditions, medications, or diagnostic procedures. As a result, patients may give poor medical histories. Nurses are considered subordinate to doctors, and their knowledge base is lower than their Western counterparts.

Families' Role in Hospital Care: Many family members may accompany the patient to the hospital and remain with them for the duration of the stay, providing physical care, equipment and supplies, and food.

Dominance Patterns: The basic family unit often involves three or four generations living together. Decision making is influenced by the astrological and lunar calendars. Although in some parts of Laos women defer to men's decisions in most matters of the "outside world," women frequently control home and community economies. Women are more or less equal in decision making, land ownership, inheritance, and workforce. Women must never touch a monk or his robe. When talking to a monk, a woman's head should not be higher than his, nor should she stand or sit too close. Such restrictions do not apply to men.

Eye-Contact Practices: In rural areas, looking directly and steadily into the eyes of someone who is respected, held in high esteem, or an elder is considered rude. Direct eye contact is generally accepted and not frowned upon in urban areas.

Touch Practices: A person's head is revered and not touched, except when parents touch the heads of their children. It is also impolite to touch someone's shoulder. A female's breast is accepted dispassionately as a means of feeding infants, whereas her lower torso is considered extremely private. Women cover the area between the waist and knees, even in private. Women who sit with their legs crossed are considered offensive, and pointing the sole of the foot toward anyone is extremely rude. The traditional greeting and goodbye is the *wai,* which is still widely practiced. This involves placing the palms of one's hands together as if praying and bowing the head slightly forward. Handshaking has gained wide acceptance among men, but not women. Touching or kissing between brother and sister is not allowed. Waving the hand with the palm up is unacceptable.

Perceptions of Time: Emphasis is not placed on the urgency of getting a task done. Punctuality is reserved for very important circumstances.

Pain Reactions: Pain may be severe before relief is requested. Many Buddhists believe pain and suffering (physically and emotionally) in this life may pave the way for a better reincarnation.

Birth Rites: Abandoned or relatives' children who become a family member may be inadvertently implied to be birth children. The husband may not be welcomed in the delivery room but may play a major role in traditional home births, where the preferred delivery position is squatting. Some may consider vernix to be accumulated sperm. Circumcision is generally unknown. Newborns are not given compliments so that evil spirits will not capture them; therefore, it is not unusual when a Westerner compliments a baby for the mother to say "No—ugly baby!" Traditionally, the woman and her newborn must remain inside the home for one month, but many need to return to work. Mothers may lie near or sit over a smoldering charcoal brazier for several days after delivery to help "dry up the womb" and drink boiled water and herbs for up to one month. The infant mortality rate is high at 83 deaths per 1,000 live births, and the total fertility rate is five children born per woman. Life expectancy is 54 for men, 58 for women.

Death Rites: Lao believe in reincarnation and the expectation of less suffering in the next life. Death at home is preferred, and cremation is practiced. Infants younger than 1 year are buried, not cremated. People who die in accidents are not cremated and are taken directly from the hospital or scene of the accident to a temple and buried quickly. After death, the body is cleaned and dressed in good clothes, and the face is washed with coconut water. White flowers and candles may be put in the deceased person's hands. In some areas, jewels or money (in a wealthier family) and rice (in a poorer family) are put in the mouth of the deceased in the belief that these objects will help the soul when it encounters gods or devils.

Food Practices and Intolerances: Laap (raw or cooked chicken, beef, or fish pounded together with fresh herbs and spices) and a salad called tam maak hung made of pounded shredded green papaya, chillies, lemon juice, and fish sauce are ubiquitous dishes, with laap always eaten at celebrations. Glutinous rice (sticky rice) is served at all meals, usually eaten with the fingers. Dishes are served and eaten communally. All meals are served with a meat, fish, or vegetable soup. Lao-lau, a form of locally prepared rice liquor, is particularly enjoyed by elderly men, as is Mekong whiskey. Rice-based soup occasionally served with small pieces of shellfish or meat is a popular food for the sick.

Infant-Feeding Practices: Traditional beliefs maintain that colostrum is poisonous and causes diarrhea. Newborns are not allowed to breastfeed until the mother has a full milk supply, so rice paste or boiled sugar water is substituted during this time. For several days after birth (or weeks if it is the mother's first child), the mother eats large amounts of salt. Consuming fat is practiced by ethnic Hmong. During this time, the mother does not eat red meat, fruit, or vegetables, although small amounts of chicken are allowed.

Child-Rearing Practices: A fat infant is considered healthy, and methods for calculating age may vary by as much as 2 years. At approximately age 6, a strict upbringing discouraging independence begins; although this practice does not always apply to urban youths. Children are expected to be obedient and respectful with adults and elders. The oldest child (boy or girl) is responsible for younger siblings if the parents become ill, are old, or die. It is not uncommon for children to be raised by relatives. About 42% of the population is 14 years or younger.

National Childhood Immunizations: BCG at birth; DTwPHep at 6, 10, and 14 weeks; HepB at birth; OPV at 6, 10, and 14 weeks; measles at 9 months; vitamin A at 6, 12, 18, 24, 30, and 36 months; TT for pregnant women and CBAW. The percent of the target population vaccinated, by antigen, is: BCG (65%); DTP1 (68%); DTP3 and HepB3 (49%); MCV (41%); and Polio3 (50%).

Other Characteristics: The wat (temple) is the focal point of community life. Every village or suburb in urban areas has at least one wat, where religious ceremonies and festivals take place. They are also home to Buddhist monks and novices. Many turn to the wat to conduct prayer or offer food and alms to monks and ancestors to gain merit and address illness. Given names are used almost exclusively, but most also go by their Lao nicknames. Full names are used only for formal occasions or on written documents.

BIBLIOGRAPHY

Central Intelligence Agency: 2006: The world factbook, Laos. Retrieved September 21, 2006, from https://www.cia.gov/cia/publications/factbook/print/la.html.

D'Avanzo C: Bridging the cultural gap with Southeast Asians, MCN, *Am J Matern Child Nurs.* 17:204, 1992.

United Nations Development Programme: *Human development report 2004: cultural liberty in today's diverse world.* New York, 2004, UNDP.

UNAIDS: 2006 Laos. Retrieved September 21, 2006, from http://www.unaids.org/en/Regions_Countries/Countries/laos.asp.

World Health Organization: *World health report 2006. Working together for health.* Geneva, 2006, WHO.

World Health Organization: 2006: Immunization, vaccines and biologicals. Retrieved September 21, 2006, from http://www.who.int/immunization_monitoring/en/globalsummary/countryprofileresult.cfm?C='lao'.

◆ LATVIA (REPUBLIC OF)

MAP PAGE (799)

Irene Kalnins

Location: Latvia, one of the three Baltic states, regained its independence after the dissolution of the Soviet Union and is now a member of the United Nations, North Atlantic Treaty Organization (NATO), and the European Union (EU). The capital is Riga. Estonia is to the north, the Russian Federation and Belarus to the east, and Lithuania to the south, with the western border on the Baltic Sea. The total area is 64,100 km² (24,749 square miles). The population is 2.3 million. The gross domestic product (GDP) per capita is $13,200, and literacy rates are almost 100% for both men and women.

Major Languages	Ethnic Groups	Major Religions
Latvian	Latvian 56%	Lutheran
Russian	Russian 29%	Roman Catholic
	Belarussian 4%	Russian Orthodox
	Ukrainian 3%	
	Polish 3%	
	Other (Lithuanian, Estonian, German, Roma 8%)	

Health Care Beliefs: Acute sick care; emphasis on health promotion. Pure food (additive free) and a healthy natural environment are valued for health maintenance. Many diseases—both of infants and children (asthma, allergies) and adults (cancer)—are attributed to processed food and a contaminated environment.

Predominant Sick-Care Practices: Biomedical, traditional, and magical-religious coexist. Western European medical care practices are often supplemented with herbs, and herbal pharmacology is included in medical and nursing education. Patients and families may consult a variety of psychic healers. The health care delivery system is centrally planned and operates through contracting with providers of primary, secondary, and tertiary care. The system is based on a network of primary care/ family doctors who serve as gatekeepers to specialist and inpatient care. All citizens and legal residents are entitled to a "basket of services" with small co-payments. These include emergency care, treatment of acute and chronic diseases, prevention and treatment of sexually transmitted and contagious diseases, prenatal and well-child care, immunizations, and free medications for defined groups and conditions. Because of budget constraints, patients wait for elective diagnostic and therapeutic services (i.e, nonemergency hip replacement), but patients can expedite access if they have the means to purchase additional private insurance or pay out of pocket. Palliative/hospice care is limited to a small number of adult and pediatric beds, and home care services are available only in Riga. In some areas, the Soviet practice of *patronāža*, home visits to newborns by a pediatrician or pediatric nurse, continue to be available, especially with first-time or high-risk pregnancies.

Ethnic-/Race-Specific or Endemic Diseases: Tick-borne encephalitis, diphtheria, tuberculosis, hepatitis, and human immunodeficiency virus (HIV)/acquired immunodeficiency syndrome (AIDS) are infectious disease concerns. Although cardiovascular disease and cancer are the two leading causes of death, there are also high rates of accidental injury and death, particularly motor-vehicle accidents associated with poor roads and high prevalence of driving while drinking. The water and sewage treatment systems in cities are being modernized, but summertime outbreaks of water-borne enteric disease from contaminated swimming areas are common. The Joint United Nations Programme on HIV/AIDS (UNAIDS) reports the prevalence rate for HIV in adults (aged 15 to 49 years) to be 0.8%, with 10,000 people, including 2,200 women, infected. Fewer than 500 deaths have been attributed to AIDS. In 2004 alone, the Republic reported 323 new HIV cases, 7 new AIDS cases, and 7 AIDS deaths. Since 1998, the major mode of transmission has been injecting drug use.

Health-Team Relationships: There are professional associations for nurses, physicians, and midwives that represent interests at the governmental level and also many specialty associations. Patients' rights are established by law, including the right to full informed consent. Baccalaureate education for nurses began in 1990 and is available to diploma graduates; there is also master's education in nursing. Nurses have largely replaced physicians as nursing school faculty. Physicians still dominate hospital care, but nurses assume increasing responsibility for patient teaching and nursing-care planning, limited only by chronic short staffing. In family practices, nurses work both in the office and on shared or autonomous home visits and are seen as indispensable. Both physicians and nurses make home visits, and there is a charge for the service except for newborn health supervision or *patronāža*. Physician and nurse supply is threatened by low salaries and heavy workloads, driving younger practitioners to wealthier countries or to private industry.

Families' Role in Hospital Care: Families are very much aware of the nursing shortage and provide a great deal of basic hygiene and feeding. Families bring additional food to enhance the bland fare from hospital kitchens, and they may need to bring linens and pajamas for changing. Families may also need to bring in medications that are outside the limited stocks of hospitals. Tips to nurses and aides are common, and patients and families often bring flowers, candy, cash, and other goods when visiting their doctor.

Dominance Patterns: Traditionally, men have a slightly more dominant role, and although husbands and wives both work, women have most of the responsibility for child rearing and home management. Pediatrics, obstetrics, and family medicine are specialties dominated by women, and surgeons are mostly men. Nursing is almost exclusively a female profession.

Eye-Contact Practices: Direct eye contact is necessary when discussing serious matters.

Touch Practices: Ethnic Russians are more expressive than Latvians, and hugs and cheek kisses between both men and women are common. Latvians are more reserved, but touching is common in families and among children and teenagers. Adult social touching is limited to handshakes.

Perceptions of Time: Latvians prize the virtues of thrift and planning for the future. Like many Europeans, Latvians feel the pace of life accelerating. Youth tend to leave the countryside and small towns and look for opportunities abroad or in the capital. Older adults are often nostalgic for the perceived stability and security of the Soviet era.

Pain Reactions: Stoicism in bearing pain is admired, but good medical practice includes effective pain management. Oral medications, parenteral agents, and patches are used, although there is still an excessive fear of morphine by both physicians and patients. Long-acting oral narcotic analgesics are not widely used.

Birth Rites: The fertility rate is 1.27 children born per woman. Almost all births occur in hospitals attended by obstetricians and midwives. Prenatal classes and father participation in labor and delivery are considered the norm by middle-class parents. The birthing stool is used as well as the delivery table. Infection-control practices on maternity floors are stringent, and visitors are limited. Circumcision is not common. Infant mortality rates are 9.4 deaths per 1,000 live births. Life expectancy is 66 for men, 77 for women.

Death Rites: If an illness is fatal, the family often prefers to be told first, and there may be conflict between families and younger physicians who insist on telling the patient. In cities, funeral homes prepare the body and also offer facilities for a funeral meal. In the countryside, families often wash and dress the body themselves and have viewing in a shed or other outbuilding. Nonreligious families employ musicians and dramatic readers to conduct the graveside ceremony. The dead remain members of the family; cemetery plots are artfully designed, planted, lovingly tended, and visited often, especially by the women of the family.

Food Practices and Intolerances: Traditionally, the preferred main meal has been lunch, and it still is on weekends and holidays. Potatoes and rye bread are staples, with meat (especially pork), fish, vegetables, and dairy foods. Coffee, tea, beer, milk, and kefir are consumed with meals. Families who have any land grow berries, fruits, and vegetables and put them up for the winter. Wild berries and mushrooms are popular, and many families head for the woods in season to gather them. All cities and towns have outdoor markets where growers sell their produce, and although supermarkets sell a variety of imported foods, consumers prefer domestic and home-grown produce, meat, and dairy foods.

Infant-Feeding Practices: Breastfeeding is encouraged and preferred. All types of formula and baby food are available, and cereal is generally introduced at 4 to 5 months.

Child-Rearing Practices: Children are encouraged to be cooperative and obedient to adults rather than express their own individualities. Families are often three-generational, and grandmothers in particular have a key role in caring for children while mothers work. Many children attend preschool; the age of public school entry is 7. Women are entitled to maternity leave at 32 weeks' gestation and may continue until the child is 3 years old; maternity leave stipends have risen to encourage an increase in the birth rate, but stipends progressively decrease, so most mothers return to work during the first year.

National Childhood Immunizations: BCG at birth; DTwPHibIPV and DTwPIPV at 3, 4.5 and 6 months; DT at 7 years; OPV at 18 months, 7 and 14 years; MMR at 15 months and 7 years; HepB at birth and 1 and 6–8 months; Hib at 3, 4.5, and 6 months; Td at 14 years. Tick-borne encephalitis (series of 3) is recommended, but is not part of the state-funded program. The percent of the target population vaccinated, by antigen, is: BCG, DTP1, DTP3, and Polio3 (99%); HepB3 (98%); Hib3 (94%); and MCV (95%).

BIBLIOGRAPHY

AIDS Prevention Centre: 2005 Statistics. Retrieved February 27, 2006, from http://www.aids-latvija.lv.

Central Intelligence Agency: *2006: The world factbook, Latvia.* Retrieved September 21, 2006, from https://www.cia.gov/cia/publications/factbook/print/lg.html.

Central Statistical Bureau of Latvia: 2006 Resident population by ethnicity. Retrieved February 27, 2006, from http://data.csb.lv/EN/dialog.

Kalnins I: Caring for the terminally ill: experiences of Latvian family caregivers, *Int Nurs Rev.* 53(2):129–135, 2006.

Kalnins I: Latvian community nurses practicing in a time of turmoil: a thin line of defense for children at risk, *Int Nurs Rev.* 49(2), 2002.

Kalnins I: Starting from a blank page: discovering and creating community health nursing in Post-Soviet Latvia, *Public Health Nurs.* 18(4):262–272, 2001.

Kalnins I, Barkauskas VH, Šeškevičius A: Baccalaureate nursing education development in two Baltic Countries: outcomes 10 years after initiation, *Nurs Outlook.* 49(3):142–147, 2001.

Staten Serum Institute: 2006: Childhood vaccination schedule, Latvia. Retrieved February 27, 2006, from http://www.ssi.dk/euvac/vaccination/latvia.html.

UNAIDS: 2006 Latvia. Retrieved September 21, 2006, from http://www.unaids.org/en/Regions_Countries/Countries/latvia.asp.

World Health Organization: 2006: Immunization, vaccines and biologicals. Retrieved September 21, 2006, from http://www.who.int/immunization_monitoring/en/globalsummary/countryprofileresult.cfm?C='lva'.

World Health Organization Regional Office for Europe: Highlights on health in Latvia, 2001. Retrieved February 27, 2006, from http://euro.who.int/countryinformation.

◆ LEBANON (LEBANESE REPUBLIC)

MAP PAGE (802)

Salim M. Adib

Location: Lebanon is a parliamentarian republic on the eastern shore of the Mediterranean Sea, bordered by Syria to the north and east and by Israel to the south. Lebanon has a total area of 10,452 km² (4,000 square miles). A long, narrow coastal plain runs parallel to the Mediterranean and is overshadowed by the Lebanon Mountains, which culminate at 3,088 m (with the highest point in the Middle East). Another mountain range, the Anti-Lebanon Mountains, runs parallel to the Lebanon range and creates a natural border with neighboring Syria. Between the two mountain ranges is a fertile plateau, the Bekaa Valley. The population is four million, of which about 300,000 are Palestinian refugees from the 1948 and 1967 wars. The capital is Beirut. The gross domestic product (GDP) per capita is $6,200, with up to 28% living below the poverty line. Literacy rates are 93% for men, 82% for women.

Major Languages	Ethnic Groups	Major Religions
Arabic (official)	Arab 95%	Muslim 70%
French	Armenian 4%	Christian, Other 30%
Armenian	Other 1%	
English		

Health Care Beliefs: Acute sick care; traditional. Lebanese generally understand and accept the biological mechanisms of health and disease. However, many still attribute disease at least partly to the "evil eye" of jealous acquaintances (the power of people to harm others merely by looking at them), exposure to cold air or water, or the wrong food combinations. In addition to modern drugs, the Lebanese still widely believe in the virtues of wild herbal concoctions from the mountains. Years of civil war and Israeli occupation have resulted in massive destruction to the infrastructure, including the health care system. In accordance with a liberal laissez-faire philosophy, the country has no national health policy. Health is largely a private-sector industry, and the reconstruction of health care facilities has been largely by private organizations. Obtaining health care is very expensive for most people, and the role of government is limited to operating a few small dispensaries and clinics. The government also attempts, at increasingly greater costs and with decreasing success, to provide uninsured citizens from lower socioeconomic levels subsidized access to private health care. More than 80% of the budget of the Ministry of Public Health is usually used to subsidize private hospitals for treatment of patients who can not afford health care expenses. The relative youth and lack of health awareness of the public have thus far prevented the country from facing unusual and uncontrollable public health problems.

Predominant Sick-Care Practices: Biomedical and magical-religious. Most people live in major cities and are unlikely to consult traditional healers or wear amulets as a first option for treatment. Most people seek a health care professional's help as their primary choice. People from rural areas with less access to modern care may decide to use available traditional practices. The Lebanese are superstitious and prefer to ensure additional "heavenly" support for health problems. Couples struggling with infertility consult a doctor for medical advice and a religious person *(sheikh)* for amulets. Lebanese Christians (and many non-Christians) visit shrines of the Virgin Mary and other saints and make vows to offer alms or other gifts if they are healed.

Ethnic-/Race-Specific or Endemic Diseases: Acute diarrheal diseases caused by contaminated food and water are common in the summer, particularly outside Beirut. The main causes of death are cardiovascular diseases and cancer. Leishmaniasis still persists at a low level, mostly in the rural northern region of Akkar bordering Syria. Brucellosis persists in the Bekaa, where unpasteurized milk and dairy products are consumed. Lebanon shares with other Mediterranean populations a higher prevalence of thalassemia and glucose-6-phosphate dehydrogenase (G6PD) deficiency. Lebanese have higher rates of familial Mediterranean fever than do people in other countries, and it is most often diagnosed in Armenians. Approximately 6% of about 70,000 newborns per year have minor or major congenital problems, most likely because of higher numbers of consanguineous marriages in the more traditional rural areas. The Joint United Nations Programme on HIV/AIDS (UNAIDS) estimates the prevalence rate for human immunodeficiency virus (HIV) in adults (aged 15 to 49 years) to be 0.1%; transmission is thought to be primarily heterosexual. Country statistics estimate that fewer than 5,000 have become infected since the beginning of the National AIDS Program in 1984.

Health-Team Relationships: The health care system is still largely male dominated, and patient-doctor relationships are still marked by paternalism. Doctors are dominant in doctor-nurse relationships, and interactions are limited, occurring during rounds (in the morning and evening) or when nurses call a doctor to discuss a patient.

Families' Role in Hospital Care: During hospital admission, many close relatives accompany patients to mitigate their uncertainties and worries and occasionally answer questions for them. When visiting hospitalized friends, visitors usually bring chocolate or flowers. Close relatives who stay most of the day with a patient show their hospitality to visitors by serving them coffee or candy.

Dominance Patterns: Although the father is usually the head of the family and its breadwinner, most mothers now work outside the home. Even in rural areas, the informal work of women—tending to farm animals and maintaining crops—is very valued as men try to obtain formal employment, often away from home. Caring for children whose mothers are working is the responsibility of grandmothers, but this is becoming rare as more couples move away to start nuclear families. Many urban couples rely on nurseries or on inexpensive domestic servants from Southeast Asia or East Africa to care for small children while both parents are busy earning a living. Women have equal rights, including the right to vote. Women currently have only five seats in the Parliament (of 128), but more are competing in the open election process at all levels. The civil code for marriage and inheritance varies depending on the declared religious affiliation of the individual; therefore, citizens must be affiliated with a legal religious group. Men and women intermingle in daily life and are largely free to choose their spouses. Nevertheless, up to 20% of marriages are still consanguineous, mostly among first-degree cousins in rural areas. All marriages in Lebanon must be performed by a religious minister; however, civil marriages of citizens performed outside Lebanon are duly registered in the country, allowing couples from different religious backgrounds to marry without having either spouse change his or her religion. As in all other Arab countries, Lebanon does not automatically grant nationality to non-Lebanese men who marry Lebanese women, but it does for non-Lebanese women who marry Lebanese men. All modern behaviors and dress codes are acceptable and common in and around Beirut but may be less acceptable in areas farther away. Modest dress is recommended in traditional parts of the country and is particularly important when visiting mosques and other religious places. The ethnically and religiously diverse Lebanese people are generally friendly and hospitable.

Eye-Contact Practices: People of the same gender are likely to stand quite close to each other. A wider distance is kept during male-female encounters, but this is less true in the more central areas of Lebanon.

Touch Practices: Although public displays of affection are not generally accepted, they are usually tolerated. Young couples may engage in intense displays of affection on campuses, on the beach, and in night-clubs—mostly in urban areas. Recently, some Muslims who are adopting more religiously conservative attitudes have been avoiding shaking hands with strangers of the opposite sex.

Perceptions of Time: People are expected to arrive at appointments on time, although congested urban traffic may not always allow them to do so. Like all Arabs, the Lebanese like to begin their meetings with numerous social niceties. They serve tea or coffee and inquire about the health and family of others before getting down to business. Ignoring those social rules may be perceived as rude and inconsiderate.

Pain Reactions: Pain reactions cannot be specifically characterized, although men may be less vocal than women.

Birth Rites: The fertility rate is the lowest in the Arab world, with 1.9 children born per woman. The infant mortality rate is 24 deaths per 1,000 live births. Most births occur in hospitals, and the average hospital stay is 3 to 4 days. Many families offer visitors boxes of sugar-coated almonds to mark the "sweetness" of the event. Traditionally, this was emphasized by serving a special semolina pudding heaped with dry coconut and nuts *(moghli)*. Most males are circumcised because it is part of the religious culture and for cleanliness; usually during the first week of life. During the 40-day postpartum period, Muslim mothers are not allowed to perform religious rituals (pray, fast during Ramadan), and sexual intercourse is prohibited until there is no remaining vaginal discharge. For Christians, baptism is a corollary to birth and generally takes place between 3 months and 1 year. A dinner, which may be fairly lavish and elaborate, is usually offered after the baptism. Life expectancy is 70 for men, 75 for women.

Death Rites: Donation of human organs is allowed, but bodies must be buried and cannot be cremated. Autopsy is permitted if ordered by a judge for legal reasons or recommended by doctors and allowed by the family members. Soon after the death of a Muslim, the body is washed and wrapped in a white cloth, taken by male relatives and friends to the mosque for prayer, and then buried without a coffin in the cemetery. Prayers are recited at churches by both sexes, but only men are expected to go with the coffin to the burial grounds. Cemeteries are administered by religious denominations; therefore, all deceased Lebanese must be identified as part of a denomination to be buried. Loud expressions of sorrow and grief are acceptable from male and female relatives alike. Relatives go back to the person's home and accept condolences for 3 days, when traditional sugar-free coffee, snacks, or soft drinks are served as a sign of sadness for the deceased. Christians in Lebanon invite friends and relatives to a remembrance ceremony marking the 40th day after death, after which it is acceptable to forgo the black ties and dresses of the grieving period. Some women, especially those in the mountain villages, chose to wear black dresses for the rest of their lives to mark their status as widows.

Food Practices and Intolerances: The staple food is wheat, eaten in breads and as cracked, grilled wheat *(borghoul)* in various foods. The cuisine relies heavily on vegetables, grains, and lamb. Some well-known dishes include hummus, a dip consisting of mashed chickpeas and sesame butter with lemon, garlic, and olive oil; *fatoush,* a pita bread salad seasoned with lemony summac herbs and olive oil; and *tabbouleh,* a parsley-mint salad with borghoul. For a quick breakfast, many buy oven-baked *manakish* pies covered with *zaatar* (a mix of oregano or thyme, sesame, and sumac) and olive oil. Fast sandwiches may consist of *shawarma* (gyro meat), *shish-tawouk* (chicken skewers), or deep-fried cakes of green fava or garbanzo beans known as *falafel*. Food products made of green fava may precipitate an acute anemia crisis in persons with G6PD deficiency. At a typical restaurant meal, the *mezza*, a large version of small vegetarian and meat-based dishes, is served first so that it can be slowly enjoyed with the local drink, *arak,* an alcoholic drink of distilled grapes with a hint of anise, which may remind some of the French pastis or Greek ouzo. The main course may consist of grilled skewered chicken and lamb or other more elaborate dishes. Desserts include Arabic sweets and the fresh fruits for which Lebanon is famous. Food is often scooped using pieces of pita bread. Lebanon produces several fine white, red and rosé wines from the central Bekaa valley. The *narghileh* (water pipe) may be smoked with or after meals by both sexes; it has been a tradition since the Ottoman nineteenth century. All types of specialized and ethnic restaurants are found in Beirut; there are no food or alcohol restrictions whatsoever.

Infant-Feeding Practices: Most women prefer to breastfeed their infants. Exclusive breastfeeding has been reported in 27% of children aged 0 to 4 months, and breastfeeding with some solid food added in 35% of children aged 6 to 9 months.

Child-Rearing Practices: There are no specific child-rearing practices. Such practices vary widely by socioeconomic levels, with children in rural areas having more outdoor freedom than those in urban areas, where parks and leisure spaces are almost nonexistent.

National Childhood Immunizations: DT before 8 years; DTwP at 4 to 6 years; DTwPHib at 2, 3, 4, and 15 to 18 months; Hep B at birth and 1 and 4 months; MMR at 13 months and at 4 to 5 years; OPV at 2, 3, 4, and 15 to 18 months, 4 to 5 years, and 10 to 12 years; TD at 10 to 12 and at 18 years. The percent of the target population vaccinated, by antigen, is: DTP1 (98%); DTP3, Hib3, and Polio3 (92%); HepB3 (88%); and MCV (96%).

Other Characteristics: Lebanon is one of the most pluralistic countries of the Arab world. Its population, composed of a mixture of Christians and Muslims, has historically been a cultural bridge between East and West. The Christian Maronite (Marooni) and the Muslim Druze (Durzi) communities are groups primarily specific to Lebanon. These communities compose the historical mountain core from which the modern Republic of Lebanon has emerged. Beirut and its surrounding coastal and mountain areas are sociologically cosmopolitan, where Arabic culture blends with Western influences, primarily French and American.

BIBLIOGRAPHY

Adib SM, Hamadeh GN: Attitudes regarding disclosure of serious illness in the Lebanese public, *J Med Ethics.* 25:399–403, 1999.

Beydoun MA: Marital fertility in Lebanon: a study based on the population and housing survey, *Soc Sci Med.* 53(6):759, 2001.

Central Intelligence Agency: *2006: The world factbook, Lebanon.* Retrieved September 21, 2006, from https://www.cia.gov/cia/publications/factbook/print/le.html.

Epidemiological Surveillance Program (ESP): Vaccinations in Lebanon. Retrieved February 26, 2006, from www.public-health.gov.lb/esu/welcome.shtml.

Hamadeh GN, Adib SM: Cancer truth disclosure by Lebanese doctors, *Soc Sci Med.* 47(9):1289, 1998.

Hamadeh GN, Adib SM: Changes in attitudes regarding cancer disclosure among medical students at the American University of Beirut, *J Med Ethics.* 27:354, 2001.

Kandela P: Lebanese medicine—still struggling against the odds, *Lancet.* 355 (9207):907, 2000.

Kabakian-Khasholian T et al. Women's experiences of medical care: satisfaction or passivity, *Soc Sci Med.* 51(1):103, 2000.

Ministry of Social Affairs, Higher Council for Childhood: *Situation of children in Lebanon: The third national report, 1998-2003.* Beirut, 2004, Ministry of Social Affairs.

National AIDS Program (NAP): HIV/AIDS in Lebanon. Retrieved February 18, 2006, from www.leb.emro.who.int/NationalProg-aids.htm.

UNAIDS: 2006 Lebanon: Retrieved September 21, 2006, from http://www.unaids.org/en/Regions_Countries/Countries/lebanon.asp.

World Health Organization: 2006: Immunization, vaccines and biologicals. Retrieved September 21, 2006, from http://www.who.int/immunization_monitoring/en/globalsummary/countryprofileresult.cfm?C='lbn'.

◆ LESOTHO (KINGDOM OF)

L

MAP PAGE (801)

Carolyn M. D'Avanzo

Location: Lesotho is landlocked and completely surrounded by South African territory. The country consists of high plateaus, hills, and mountains, and more than 80% of the country is 1,800 m above sea level. The climate is temperate, with cool or cold dry winters and hot, wet summers. In winter, snow often closes mountain passes, and temperatures drop below freezing at night, even in the lowlands. Most people live in rural areas, and some areas can be reached only on horseback or by airplane. About 35% of active male wage earners work in South Africa. The population is more than two million. The total area is 30,350 km² (11,718 square miles), and the capital is Maseru. Population pressures are forcing settlements in marginal areas. About 86% work in subsistence agriculture, although less than 10% of the land is arable as the result of overgrazing and soil erosion. The gross domestic product (GDP) per capita is $2,500. With a 45% unemployment rate, about 49% of the people live below the poverty line. Literacy rates are 75% for men, 95% for women. The much higher literacy rate for women is unusual, especially for African countries.

Major Languages	**Ethnic Groups**	**Major Religions**
English (official)	Sotho 99.7%	Christian 80%
Sesotho (official)	European, Asian,	Indigenous beliefs
Zulu	Other 0.3%	20%
Xhosa		

Health Care Beliefs: Acute sick care only, usually in the form of crisis care, with prevention a low priority. Although the government has attempted to promote primary health care, political unrest and social instability have damaged the health infrastructure. Diarrheal diseases in infants and children are a major cause of morbidity and mortality, and efforts have been made to teach mothers how to perform oral rehydration therapy at home, but with limited success. Rural communities often have undiagnosed human immunodeficiency virus (HIV) and acquired immunodeficiency syndrome (AIDS) and other sexually transmitted diseases. People have little knowledge of high-risk sexual behaviors. Unprotected sex, especially among men, is common. Health and safety are low priorities in this country because of the daily struggle for survival.

Predominant Sick-Care Practices: Biomedical when available; traditional. People consider biomedical treatment to be effective. Hospitals (in urban areas) and district hospitals are the highest level of care. Rural areas are serviced by health centers and clinics (usually within a 1- to 2-hour walk) and staffed primarily by nurse clinicians, nurse assistants, traditional birth attendants, and village health workers. The Queen Elizabeth II hospital in Maseru takes referrals from district hospitals, and Mohlomi hospital (also in Maseru) is a psychiatric referral hospital. The health system is structured so that people will be referred from clinics to district hospitals and, if necessary, to the hospitals in Maseru. When people are ill, they usually try to reach a hospital rather than a clinic because they believe they will receive higher quality care. This practice has overloaded the hospitals. Funding for health care comes from a variety of sources such as the Ministry of Health, and numerous grants from outside agencies such as the World Health Organization and World Bank. In general, medical facilities are minimal, and medications are often unavailable. Lesotho has limited emergency or ambulance services, but helicopters and six-seater planes assist in patient transportation. If appropriate treatment cannot be provided within Lesotho, patients can be referred for more specialized medical care in Bloemfontein, South Africa, at the Universitas Academic Hospital, which is 90 miles west of Maseru. The Lesotho government pays for the cost of treatment regardless of the person's socioeconomic status. Patients keep their own medical records in a "health book" *(Bukana)*, which is obtained at the first visit to a health facility. Magical-religious and traditional systems of care are used along with traditional healers *(Sangomas)* and herbalists. Water extracts, primarily from boiling roots of high-altitude medicinal plants, are often effective. *Bulbine narcissifolia* is used to heal wounds and as a mild purgative. Studies of medicinal plants used by healers and herbalists indicate that these plants have true healing qualities, with moderate to very high antibacterial activity against gram-positive and gram-negative bacteria.

Ethnic-/Race-Specific or Endemic Diseases: Endemic diseases include schistosomiasis, typhoid, hepatitis A, and rabies. There is risk for acute respiratory tract infections, pneumonia, tuberculosis, and diarrhea (in children). Tap water is not reliably potable and is a source of disease. Because of intertribal hostility and the widespread use of alcohol and cannabinoid drugs, violence-related injuries are common and put a strain on the health care system. Lesotho also has a large number of automobile-related deaths given the small size of the country. HIV is spreading, especially with the influx of migrant construction workers from other areas. As is true for many countries, estimates for HIV prevalence may be underreported or inaccurate. The prevalence rate for HIV in adults (aged 15 to 49 years) has been estimated as 23% by the Joint United Nations Programme for HIV/AIDS (UNAIDS) and as 30% by the Central Intelligence Agency, but it might be much higher. About 270,000 to 320,000 people are estimated as living with HIV, including at least 150,000 women and 18,000 children aged 0 to 14. From 23,000 to 29,000 deaths from AIDS have been recorded, and there are at least 97,000 orphans aged 0 to 17 as the result of parental AIDS.

Health-Team Relationships: In rural areas, the village chief is the leader and helps people make health care changes and decisions. Hospital aids perform most patient care. Because of inadequate funding for health care, there is only one doctor for more than 11,000 persons. Overwork and low wages contribute to the exodus of qualified health personnel to more affluent countries. A faculty of health sciences has been established at the National University of Lesotho for the training of nurses and paramedical personnel.

Families' Role in Hospital Care: The socioeconomic conditions make it imperative for relatives to participate in the care of their family members. Traditional birth attendants deliver many infants in rural areas, but few have knowledge of aseptic technique or how to handle emergencies. The Ministry of Health has made efforts to provide midwifery education in the form of "Safe Motherhood" modules.

Dominance Patterns: As in many developing countries, women are not men's equals and depend on their husbands for economic survival. The cultural position of women and alcoholic beverages facilitates a vicious cycle. The women usually brew and sell the alcohol and struggle with alcoholism themselves as they cope with drinking husbands. Although men can drink without censure, husbands can divorce their wives for drinking—a disastrous consequence.

Infant-Feeding Practices: Exclusive breastfeeding is not the norm, although health service providers actively promote it. Complementary feedings are introduced early, which reduces the amount of breast milk received and gives infants an irregular diet of milk and other protein-rich foods. Mothers also routinely give water to very young infants, and because potable water is not always available, this is a potential reservoir for pathogens. Fewer than 5% of the people in many areas use latrines or know how to maintain a clean water supply. Mothers have reported that about 18% of children aged 5 years or younger have episode of diarrheal illness. Unfortunately, some mothers believe food should be limited for those with diarrhea. The fertility rate is 3.3 children born per woman. The infant mortality rate is 87 deaths per 1,000 live births. Life expectancy is only 36 for men and 33 for women, primarily because of AIDS.

Child-Rearing Practices: About 37% of the population is younger than 14. Corporal punishment is common in schools, causing academic impairment, physical injuries, and psychological damage. Studies of rural children 15 and younger show stunting, a sign of chronic undernutrition, even within the first year of life, and the prevalence of iodine-deficiency goiter is high. Many health problems of children stem from a lack of resources. Although statutes state that a man must support both his legitimate and illegitimate children, weaknesses in the law make it hard to enforce. Women are also unaware of the law or are afraid of being physically abused or receiving other forms of retribution if they address the issue.

National Childhood Immunizations: BCG at birth; DTWP at 6, 10, and 14 weeks; OPV at 6, 10, and 14 weeks; measles at 9 and 18 months; DT at 18 months; and TT for first contact + 4 weeks, + 6 months, +1, +1 year; HepB at 6, 10, and 14 weeks; vitamin A at 6, 12, 18, 24, 30, and 36 months. The percent of the target population vaccinated, by antigen, is: BCG (96%); DTP1 (95%); DTP3 and HepB3 (83%); MCV (85%); and Polio3 (80%).

BIBLIOGRAPHY

Almroth S, Mohale M, Latham MC: Unnecessary water supplementation for babies: grandmothers blame clinics, *Acta Paediatr.* 89(12):1408, 2000.

Central Intelligence Agency: *2006: The world factbook, Lesotho.* Retrieved September 21, 2006, from https://www.cia.gov/cia/publications/factbook/print/lt.html.

Colvin M, Sharp B: Sexually transmitted infections and HIV in a rural community in the Lesotho highlands, *Sex Transm Infect.* 76(1):39, 2000.

Quotsokoane-Lusunzi MA, Karuso P: Secondary metabolites from Basotho medicinal plants. I. *Bulbine narcissifolia, J Natural Prod.* 64(10):1368, 2001.

Shonubi AM, Odusan O, Oloruntoba DO, Adbahowe SA, Siddique MA: Health for all in a least developed country, *J Natl Med Assoc.* 97:1020, 2005.

UNAIDS: 2006 Lesotho. Retrieved September 21, 2006, from http://www.unaids.org/en/Regions_Countries/Countries/lesotho.asp.

World Health Organization: 2006: Immunization, vaccines and biologicals. Retrieved September 21, 2006, from http://www.who.int/immunization_monitoring/en/globalsummary/countryprofileresult.cfm?C='lso'.

♦ LIBERIA (REPUBLIC OF)

MAP PAGE (800)

Abid Mahmood

Location: Liberia is located on the Atlantic coast of southwestern Africa, with Sierra Leone and Guinea to the north, Côte d'Ivoire to the east, and the Atlantic Ocean to the south and west. It is mostly flat, with rolling coastal plains rising to rolling plateau and low mountains. Much of the country is covered with dense tropical forests that experience a heavy annual rainfall. The climate is tropical—hot and humid, with dry winters that have hot days and cool or cold nights and wet, cloudy summers with frequent rain. The total area is 111,370 km² (43,000 square miles), and Monrovia is the capital. The population is more than 3.4 million. Liberia is a developing country in which 76% of the population works in agriculture. The gross domestic product (GDP) per capita was $1,100 before the civil war; it is now $152, and 80% of the population lives below the poverty line.

Major Languages	Ethnic Groups	Major Religions
English (official)	African 95%	Indigenous 40%
African languages	Americo-Liberian 2.5%	Christian 40%
	Congo people 2.5%	Muslim 20%

Most of the population is made up of indigenous African tribes (95%), including Kpelle, Bassa, Gio, Kru, Grebo, Mano, Krahn, Gola, Gbandi, Loma, Kissi, Vai, and Bella. About 2.5% are descendents of repatriated slaves known as Americo-Liberians, and 2.5% are descendents of immigrants from the Caribbean who had been slaves. African languages include more than 29 of the Niger-Congo group. Literacy rates are 56% for men, 42% for women (lower than previous levels as a result of war).

Health Care Beliefs: Acute sick care; ethno-medical beliefs predominate. Health-promotion efforts are frequently unsuccessful. For example, efforts to promote the home use of a sugar and salt solution to prevent dehydration in children with diarrhea have been minimally effective. People generally realize the importance of health and well-being and are receptive to health advice, but strong economic pressures and poor housing/unhygienic environments result in traditional ethno-medical views predominating. Notions of sorcery, witchcraft, or taboo violations are often expressed as the cause of diseases such as sexually transmitted diseases (STDs). Mental illness is attributed to supernatural forces and thought to be best treated by traditional healers.

Predominant Sick-Care Practices: Traditional medicine; biomedical treatments often preferred when they are available. Health care expenditures constitute a major part of domestic spending, particularly for those seeking Western health care. Traditional healers handle many serious diseases, such as human immunodeficiency virus (HIV) and acquired immunodeficiency syndrome (AIDS). Treatments comprise decoctions from the leaves and roots of medicinal herb plants, usually administered as teas, but they may also be given as enemas or vaginal implants over a 2- to 4-day period. Since the war, most hospitals and medical facilities are not functioning, and those that are open are poorly equipped and incapable of providing even basic services. Medications are scarce and often unavailable. Liberia's health care system totally collapsed after systematic looting and destruction of hospitals and health care clinics during the civil conflicts that have lasted more than 10 years. Of more than 200 doctors and 600 physician assistants before the war, only 25 doctors and 150 paramedics remained in place after hundreds of thousands of people fled for their lives. Only about a third of the population, even in the capital city of Monrovia, has access to some kind of health care. United Nations troops deployed in different areas, the World Health Organization, and a few nongovernmental organizations (NGOs) have renovated a few hospitals and dispensaries and have begun free medical treatment to some local residents. The facilities are still inadequate, however, and out of reach for people living in villages and far flung areas.

Ethnic-/Race-Specific or Endemic Diseases: Liberia has a high prevalence of epilepsy and parasitic infections (particularly neurocysticercosis). Endemic diseases include cholera, bacterial and protozoal diarrheas, onchocerciasis (sowda), meningitis, schistosomiasis, polio, Lassa fever, and hepatitis A and B. Liberians are also at risk for *Shigella* infection, typhoid fever, leprosy, yellow fever, and severe malnutrition. *Falciparum* malaria is hyperendemic and an important cause of febrile episodes during both the dry and the rainy seasons. In a study conducted by the author in 2004, 29% of the randomly selected febrile patients were positive for malarial parasites; most were children under age 5 years. There was a cholera epidemic in Monrovia in 2003, and there have been Ebola virus outbreaks. Dust-laden harmattan winds blow in from the Sahara Desert from December to March, causing episodes of respiratory illness. Vehicular travel is hazardous, and traffic accidents are a common cause of death and disability. The Joint United Nations Programme on HIV/AIDS (UNAIDS) reports that there is little information on the prevalence of HIV/AIDS because there is no sentinel surveillance system in place. According to recent estimates, HIV prevalence is about 6%, but this figure may be highly inaccurate. In a study conducted by the author, HIV prevalence among hospital visitors at the Tubmanburg Government Hospital was 15%. In this study, there was a high prevalence of HIV-2 and dual infection with HIV-1 and HIV-2. The estimated total number of people positive for HIV is about 100,000, and the estimated number of children and adults who have died since the beginning of the epidemic is 34,000. Liberia currently has 20,337 orphans as a result of parental AIDS.

Families' Role in Hospital Care: Tradition dictates that the family will accompany the patient to the hospital and take care of cooking and laundry. Centralized hospital services are not available as a result of the complete destruction of hospital infrastructures.

Dominance Patterns: Transactions for major health care expenditures are usually handled by men, using their personal income and whatever belongs to the couple. Women are more likely to spend their personal income on treating more minor health conditions affecting themselves and their children. Dominance differences exist among different villages and groups. For example, Kpelle wives have input into most financial decisions but defer to men on issues of health care and educational expenditures. Physical and sexual violence against women (>50%) was documented during the civil war.

Birth Rites: The traditional midwife was active in rural Liberia before the war; however, maternal mortality was high and is now worse. The infant mortality rate is very high at 157 deaths per 1,000 live births. Widespread premarital sex and lack of contraception result in illegal abortions, preg-nancy-related school dropout, and the potential for STD transmission. The total fertility rate is six children born per woman. Life expectancy is 38 for men, 41 for women.

Food Practices and Intolerances: Food shortages have been problem-atic because of continuing social upheaval. The diet generally consists of rice, fish, lots of greens, and vegetables. Liberians also consume cassava and its by-products, dumboy and fufu, but rice is king.

Infant-Feeding Practices: Most infants and children are malnourished and underweight as a result of extreme poverty. Some parents may strongly believe that Western medicine's pills or injections can cure severe malnutrition. About 20% of women breastfeed their infants for the first 6 months. Other foods like rice and cassava are introduced early or later, depending on the economic conditions and education level of the family.

Child-Rearing Practices: Female circumcision and excision are wide-spread among some groups. Seven ethnic groups (Kpelle, Bassa, Vai, Dan, Ma, Dei, and Gola) practice female circumcision. The practice is part of their cultures and traditions passed on by their ancestors. As many as a third of all children die before their fifth birthday. Women spend long hours in the fields, tend domestic livestock and vegetable gardens, gather firewood, haul water, prepare and cook food, take care of children, and manage household finances. In most cases, women use almost all their income to meet household needs. At the same time, traditional culture and land laws often prevent women and girls from gaining an education and obtaining access to communal resources and public services that would allow them to improve their families' livelihoods.

National Childhood Immunizations: BCG at birth; DTwP at 6, 10, and 14 weeks; OPV at birth and 6, 10, and 14 weeks; measles at 9 months; vitamin A at 9 months for infants; BCG, OPV0 or DTP1 for postpartum women; YFV 6 months and every 10 years; and TT every 14 years, +1, +6 months, +1, +1 year. The percent of the target population vacci-nated, by antigen, is: BCG (82%); DTP1 (92%); DTP3 (87%); MCV (94%); Polio3 (77%); TT2 plus (72%); and YF (89%). Only camps of internally displaced people have been adequately covered. Vaccination programs have begun in the rest of the country, but children in remote villages are not receiving vaccinations.

Other Characteristics: Civil war and government mismanagement have destroyed much of Liberia's economy, especially the infrastructure in and around Monrovia. Continued international sanctions on diamonds and timber exports will limit growth prospects for the foreseeable future. Many businessmen have fled, taking capital and expertise with them. Unemployment and poverty have peaked, and most of the population is devoid of basic needs. This situation is affecting the mental and physical health of the people, resulting in a crippled society.

BIBLIOGRAPHY

Centers for Disease Control and Prevention (CDC): Cholera epidemic after increased civil conflict—Monrovia, Liberia, June-September 2003, *MMWR Morb Mortal Wkly Rep.* 52(45):1093–1095, 2003.

Central Intelligence Agency: 2006: *The world factbook, Liberia.* Retrieved September 21, 2006, from https://www.cia.gov/cia/publications/factbook/print/li.html.

Cole M: Violence in Liberia, *CMAJ.* 169(8):755, 2003.

Huhn GD et al: Vaccination coverage survey versus administrative data in the assessment of mass yellow fever immunization in internally displaced persons—Liberia, 2004, *Vaccine.* 24(6):730–737, 2006.

Johnson K, Kennedy SB, Harris AO, Lincoln A, Neace W, Collins D: Strengthening the HIV/AIDS service delivery system in Liberia: an international research capacity building strategy, *J Eval Clin Pract.* 11(3):2757–2773, 2005.

Kennedy SB, Johnson K, Harris AO, Lincoln A, Neace W, Collins D: Evaluation of HIV/AIDS prevention resources in Liberia: strategy and implications, *AIDS Patient Care STDS.* 18(3):169–180, 2004.

Mahmood A, Yasir M: Combined *Schistosoma mansoni* and *Schistosoma haematobium* infection, *J Coll Physic Surg Pak.* 15(7):443–444, 2005.

Mahmood A, Haq RIU, Khan AA, Yasir M: Frequency of HIV infections amongst hospital visitors at Tubmanburg Town in Liberia, *J Coll Physic Surg Pak.* 16(4):314, 2006.

Mahmood A, Yasir M: Thrombocytopenia: a predictor of malaria among febrile patients in Liberia. *Infect Dis J Pak.* 2(02):41–44, 2005.

UNAIDS: 2006 Liberia. Retrieved September 21, 2006, from http://www.unaids.org/en/Regions_Countries/Countries/liberia.asp.

World Health Organization: 2006: Immunization, vaccines and biologicals. Retrieved September 21, 2006, from http://www.who.int/immunization_monitoring/en/globalsummary/countryprofileresult.cfm?C='lbr'.

http://www.Liberia/Liberia(01–06).htm (Retrieved April 24, 2006).

http://www.Liberia/CountryCaseStudyLiberia.htm (Retrieved April 24, 2006).

◆ LIBYA (LIBYAN ARAB JAMAHIRIYA)

MAP PAGE (800)

Suher M. Aburawi

Location: Libya is located almost at the center of northern Africa, and the capital is Tripoli. It has a total area of about 1,750,000 km² (675,500 square miles) and a northern coast of about 2000 km on the Mediterranean. Climatic conditions vary from mild Mediterranean along the coast to an extremely dry desert interior. The terrain is mainly low lying, with hilly regions in the northeast and northwest and the Tibesti Mountains in the south. The population is six million; 4% are expatriate workers, and their families are from adjacent African and Mediterranean countries. The gross domestic product (GDP) per capita is $11,400. Literacy rates are 92% for men, 72% for women.

Major Languages	Ethnic Groups	Major Religions
Arabic (official)	Berber and Arab 97%	Sunni Muslim 97%
English	Other 3%	Other 3%

Arabic is spoken by almost everyone. Old Hamitic languages are also spoken by a small percentage of the population in the northwest hilly region and among the Tuareg and Tabu tribes. English is widely used for activities relating to health care and technology (with drug prescriptions and medical records in English), and it is practically the second language in business, industry, and tourism.

Health Care Beliefs: Acute sick care; folk medicine. To Libyans, folk medicine is synonymous with herbal medicine. Herbal medicine is considered primary health care in mild cases of illness with generally known causes, especially for treatment of symptoms such as stomachaches, diarrhea, coughs, or spasms. The choice of herbs depends on previous evidence of success. Some reports indicate that diseases such as asthma, nephrolithiasis (kidney stones), some tumors, and hypertension are being effectively treated with herbs. Public awareness of psychotherapy has yet to emerge. Seeing a psychoanalyst is embarrassing and rare and is done with complete discretion (the general mind-set is that "only a crack would go to a shrink"). In rare cases when medical practitioners cannot provide a remedy, people may seek out supernatural treatments for psychological and physical ailments. Reading the Koran is generally believed to provide people with the strength to resist physical and psychological ailments and help in recovery; however, few would make that choice. Some, although very few, still use amulets for protection from malicious acts involving spirits or spells, but their use is kept secret from police for fear of prosecution. Self-prescribing treatments for illness is a common practice, to save either time or money, and individuals in pharmacies may make suggestions as well. Antibiotics are practically sold as over-the-counter drugs, although all agree that this should not be done.

Predominant Sick-Care Practices: Biomedical and magical-religious. Free health care is provided by a state-run system of hospitals (some of which are specialized) and clinics. Hospitals usually include outpatient departments. Since 1990, Libya has had a proliferation of private clinics offering their services to those who can afford them. The advantages of these clinics are better nursing and hospitality arrangements. Many doctors and surgeons also have private practices. Although state health policies emphasize the advantages of primary health care, the general public tends to consult specialists when medical services are needed. Going to a pediatric or obstetric hospital for related services is the norm, regardless of the condition. The general public complains about the quality of health care services, although they have confidence in doctors' skills. People usually complain about poor management, a lack of professional competence in nursing and paramedical staff, and a shortage of resources.

Ethnic-/Race-Specific or Endemic Diseases: An intermediate degree of risk is reported for food- and water-borne diseases such as bacterial diarrhea, hepatitis A, and typhoid fever. Vector-borne diseases may be a significant risk in some locations during the transmission season (typically April to October). Ethnic differences related to health conditions, practices, and attitudes are negligible; however, two small ethnic groups are distinct from the majority of the population—the Tuareg, who live in the southwest and frequently move between Libya, Algeria, and Niger, and the Tabu tribes in Tibesti. Differences between the Tuareg or Tabu and the rest of the population in terms of endemic diseases or susceptibility to diseases are not known. According to government sources, Libya is free or almost free of smallpox, polio, measles, and leprosy. Human immunodeficiency virus (HIV) and acquired immunodeficiency syndrome (AIDS) and hepatitis B are the major concerns of health authorities because of the trend of increasing infections. A Joint United Nations Programme on HIV/AIDS (UNAIDS)–World Health Organization (WHO) report estimates an HIV prevalence of 0.17% (10,000 cases). About 80% of these cases occurred since the turn of the century; most infections appear to be the result of injecting drug use.

Health-Team Relationships: Medical doctors, who are skeptical about the skills of nursing staff, do not delegate power or responsibility to them. The general public shares these convictions and attitudes, and so interns have the most direct contact with patients. This lack of trust in nurses' abilities should change over time, however, because university-level nursing education programs were introduced in the late 1990s. Medical technology university education also began at that time.

Families' Role in Hospital Care: Hospital food is tasteless; hence, for decades it has been the custom for families to bring food to inpatients. The lack of confidence in nursing staff has made it essential for family members to stay with the patient for as long as needed. Despite occasionally limited resources, these practices are strongly resisted by the hospital management and health care staff members, and family members are allowed to stay with a patient only when the family's presence benefits the patient.

Dominance Patterns: Traditionally, the husband/father is responsible for earning the family's income, whereas the wife is responsible for household chores. Children are the mother's responsibility, although boys become the father's responsibility when they become teenagers. The father's dominance over children is more prevalent—a fact that is a detriment in child development and may be a seed for psychological disorders. This pattern has been changing during the past 25 years because of developments in education, increasing numbers of working women, and the proliferation of nuclear families. Although still important, male dominance (i.e., of the husband, father, or boss) is becoming more moderate.

Eye-Contact Practices: Religious women are not expected to make direct eye contact with men who are not immediate family members. For most, eye contact is acceptable even between men and women, and it is permissible to make direct eye contact with seniors.

Touch Practices: Timidity, primarily for women, is a virtue and a teaching of Islam. Most of women's bodies and men's private parts are not exposed to people of the opposite sex (other than parents, children, and some siblings) unless need or necessity dictates. Similar restrictions on touching apply to the whole body. Thus, exposing or touching the body or parts of it does not hinder physical examinations or procedures of medical staff members; however, patients with diseases of the genitals prefer a doctor or a nurse of the same sex.

Perceptions of Time: The espoused theory of time is, "Time is as a sword. If you don't cut it, it cuts you." However, in practice, the theory is quite different. Although almost everyone preaches that time is precious, the time spent in social interactions is important. Those who are ill will not tolerate wasted time; they expect a prompt response to their symptoms. Although other professionals may have a fairly relaxed attitude about time, medical and health care professionals value it.

Pain Reactions: A woman's voice is considered disgraceful if it is heard by strange men; hence, women keep pain to themselves. For men, an expression of pain is a sign of weakness.

Birth Rites: The birth of an infant is usually celebrated. The fertility rate is 3.28 children born per woman. The birth of a boy—or of a girl who is born after a mother already has several boys—is more celebrated. Although Islam states that parents should be satisfied with God's gifts, whether boys or girls, parents become temporarily depressed after having a second or third female child in a row. The infant mortality rate is 24 deaths per 1,000 live births. Circumcision is a religious rite for Muslims and is performed on all males, usually during their first 5 years. Today, it is often performed at a hospital or clinic during the first week after birth because most births occur in hospitals. Female circumcision *(clitoridectomy)* is not performed. Life expectancy is 74 for men, 79 for women.

Death Rites: Muslims bury the dead as soon as possible, usually within 24 hours. Funeral rituals are short and attended by family, friends, and acquaintances. All who attend the funeral visit the family of the deceased to offer condolences, usually within the 3 days after burial.

Food Practices and Intolerances: The diet primarily contains starchy components derived from wheat (e.g., couscous, pasta, bread, rice), whereas the main protein sources are lamb, chicken, camel, and beef. Conventional Libyan dishes are fatty because of the excess of animal fat and vegetable oils (i.e., olive, sunflower, and corn oils). With improving health and fitness awareness, the consumption of fish, vegetables, and fruits is increasing, and the consumption of fats is decreasing. According to Islamic tradition, only specific meats can be eaten, and pork and carrion are forbidden. Most, if not all, fast from sunrise to sunset during Ramadan, which occurs for 1 month every lunar year.

Infant-Feeding Practices: Breastfeeding is common; about 91% of women breastfeed for 11 months, and no significant differences between urban and rural women have been noted. Most women who do not breast-feed have medical or physiologic reasons.

Child-Rearing Practices: The infant usually sleeps in a rocker in the parents' bedroom until the age of 12 to 18 months. Boys are separated from girls at about 10 years old. Libyan social rules require obedience to parents and respect for all older adults. Bad and good behaviors result in punishments or rewards. Punishments vary from mild physical repri-mands to taking away allowances. Rewards are usually candy, toys, and other items, depending on the age of the child.

National Childhood Immunizations: BCG at birth; DT at 6 years; DTwP at 6, 10, and 14 weeks and 18 months; HepB at birth, 6 weeks, and 8 months; measles at 9 months; MMR at 18 months; OPV at birth and 6, 10, and 14 weeks and at 18 months and 6 years; and TT at 12 years. The percent of the target population vaccinated, by antigen, is: BCG (99%); DTP1, DTP3, and Polio3 (98%); and MCV and HepB3 (97%). School admissions at ages 6 and 12 require a medical checkup and a review of immunization status.

BIBLIOGRAPHY

Central Intelligence Agency: *2006: The world factbook, Libya.* Retrieved September 21, 2006, from https://www.cia.gov/cia/publications/factbook/print/ly.html.

National Center for the Prevention of Epidemic and Endemic Disease. Libyan Epidemics Bulletin, 2004.

UNAIDS: 2006 Libyan Arab Jamahiriya. Retrieved September 21, 2006, from http://www.unaids.org/en/Regions_Countries/Countries/libyan_arab+_Jamahiriya.asp.

UNAIDS: Middle East and North Africa Fact Sheet, UNAIDS Epidemic Updates, UNAIDS, 2005.

World Health Organization: *Global epidemic detection and response,* Geneva, 2002. Retrieved March 15, 2006 from http://www.who.int/emc/surveill!index.htm/.

World Health Organization: 2006: Immunization, vaccines and biologicals. Retrieved September 21, 2006, from http://www.who.int/immunization_monitoring/en/globalsummary/countryprofileresult.cfm?C='lby'.

World Health Organization: *WHO report on global surveillance of epidemic-prone infectious diseases,* Geneva, 2000, WHO.

L

◆ LITHUANIA (REPUBLIC OF)

MAP PAGE (799)

Arūnas L. Birutis

Location: Lithuania is located in Eastern Europe on the eastern shore of the Baltic Sea. Latvia is to the north, Belarus to the east and south, Poland to the southwest, and the Kalingrad region of the Russian Federation to the south and southwest. The land is characterized by gentle rolling hills, forests, lakes, and rivers, and the climate is moderate. The land area is 65,200 km^2 (26,174 square miles), and the capital is Vilnius. The population is 3.6 million (of 115 different ethnic backgrounds), and the gross domestic product (GDP) per capita is $13,700. The largest and most populous of the Baltic states, Lithuania has 60 miles of sandy coastline, 24 miles of which face the open Baltic Sea.

Major Languages	Ethnic Groups	Major Religions
Lithuanian (official)	Lithuanian 83.4%	Roman Catholic 79%
Russian	Russian 6.3%	Russian Orthodox 4.1%
Polish	Polish 6.7%	Protestant (Lutheran,
	Other (Belarussian,	Evangelical Christian,
	Ukrainians,	Baptist) 1.9%
	Latvians,	Other (unspecified) 5.5%
	German,	None 9.5%
	Jewish) 3.6%	

Lithuania was annexed by the Union of Soviet Socialist Republics (USSR) in 1940. In March 1990, Lithuania became the first of the Soviet republics to declare independence, but it was not recognized until 1991. The last Russian troops withdrew in 1993. Lithuania joined both the North Atlantic Treaty Organization (NATO) and the European Union (EU) in the spring of 2004. Lithuania endured border changes, Soviet deportations, a massacre of its Jewish population, and German and Polish repatriations during and after World War II. Lithuania has one of the oldest living languages on earth, with two major dialects: *aukstaiciu* (highlander) and *zemaiciu* (lowlander). The Soviet era imposed the official use of Russian, so many speak Russian as a second language; the resident Slavic populace generally speaks Russian or Polish as a first language. Literacy is almost 100%.

Health Care Beliefs: Acute sick care; some health promotion. Limited emphasis is placed on health promotion or prevention. Resources are first allocated to inpatient care. Generally, the lifestyle does not include regular physical exercise as a common leisure-time activity. Although there is a long tradition of biomedicine, it coexists with religious and herbal healers and a strong belief in holistic medicine. When asked what they think has caused their illness, some Lithuanians may reply that their problems are simply a result of having had "a hard and difficult life." The Lithuanian patient may be extremely uneasy with patient education in great detail about the exact nature and prognosis of his or her disease: knowledge is considered the domain of the physician. There is a high incidence of hypertension, which is often viewed as a transient condition rather than a disease. Medication may be taken sporadically in the belief that the efficacy of medication is reduced if it is taken regularly. If they do not have headaches or "feel" their blood pressure, some will discontinue medication so that the doctor can see what their "true" blood pressure is and because they may also fear that they will develop low blood pressure with long-term use. Strong religious faith may support a belief in the supernatural healing powers of persons and sanctuaries, and religious items may be pinned to the patient's undergarments. These should suggest careful questioning regarding their view of the cause of the illness and what they have been doing or taking to treat the problem. In the former Soviet Union, it was considered shameful and sometimes dangerous to admit that someone in the family had mental health problems. Psychiatric institutions were unofficially under Soviet State Security (KGB) supervision, so there was always fear that one could be forcibly placed in a mental clinic. Thus, even today, fearful attitudes still extend to the subject of mental health.

Predominant Sick-Care Practices: Biomedical; traditional and holistic. Traditional home remedies include hot steam baths, salt and baking soda gargles, mineral water, leech therapy, massage, and plasters. Back pain may be treated with dry heat and headaches with strong ointment applied behind the ears, on the temples, and the back of the neck. Some traditional medical treatments include "cupping" (where cups are heated and applied to the back), said to draw evil humors out of the body. These often leave the appearance of bruises, which can be mistaken for evidence of physical abuse. *Skauda sirdi* ("heart pain") is a common complaint; in fact, most people over 40 years of age will say they have some type of chest pain or pressure they believe is heart related. A diagnosis of cancer is considered a death sentence, and there is a prohibition against telling the patient. It is challenging for the caregiver to present a realistic prognosis or enlist the family's cooperation in the treatment plan in the face of a high level of fear and denial. Holistic medicine is widely accepted, and physicians often prescribe herbal medications that are filled at pharmacies. Tincture of valerian is prescribed as a sedative, tincture of belladonna for peptic ulcer, and chamomile tea for upset stomach and externally as a disinfectant, as well as for vaginitis. Lithuanians often have a strong sense of stoicism as well as a sense that "this illness or trouble was meant for me." This attitude often leads to an acceptance of the problem that causes the person to postpone seeking treatment, sometimes too late for a cure.

Ethnic-/Race-Specific or Endemic Diseases: Heart disease, hypertension, respiratory diseases, smoking, and obesity (particularly in women) are common. Lithuanians are at risk for phenylketonuria, thyroid disorders, and nutritional deficiencies. Endemic diseases include tuberculosis, cardiac diseases, hepatitis, rabies, and influenza. The Joint United Nations Programme on HIV/AIDS (UNAIDS) reports the estimated prevalence rate of human immunodeficiency virus (HIV) in adults (aged 15 to 49 years) to be 0.2%, with 3,300 people living with HIV, including fewer than 1,000 women. The estimated number of deaths from acquired immunodeficiency syndrome (AIDS) is fewer than 100. About 89% of registered cases are in men. Where mode of transmission is known, 80% is from injecting drug use.

Health-Team Relationships: As in other post-Communist countries, the health care system was authoritarian and paternal. Physicians are still considered authority figures and, in general, patients follow medical orders carefully. The health system is organized around outpatient regional clinics and hospitals, and family health practice is slowly evolving. A Lithuanian who is sick may stay in bed and expect a clinic physician to make a house call. Hospital stays tend to be more frequent and longer than in the United States. Elderly patients may fear that they are being "used" for medical experimentation. It is uncommon to ask for a second opinion because to do so is considered highly disrespectful to the physician. Previously, patients often were not told what ailments they had or given an explanation for their treatment. The physician, not the nurse, is expected to transmit medical news to the family or patient. In the recent past, nurses had little autonomy and responsibility for treatment. A negative prognosis is almost never shared with the patient. The physician is expected to modify any form of bad news to give the patient hope for full or partial recovery. The health care provider's age is often (especially by older patients) equated with wisdom, knowledge, and experience. Salaries for physicians and nurses are so low that some sort of tip, gift, or auxiliary payment may be offered to ensure attentive care, and this practice is not considered unethical. When a nonmonetary gift is offered, it is usually accepted graciously after an explanation that gifts are not necessary or expected.

Families' Role in Hospital Care: Family members may assist with bathing, feeding, comforting, and elimination needs.

Dominance Patterns: Lithuanian women have been liberated in the sense of having equal employment opportunities for many decades (for example, most physicians are women), but salaries and authority lag behind those of men. Even though women work outside the home, they are still expected to take responsibility for all household tasks and the care of children. Men assume a slightly more dominant role; however, men and women share responsibility for decision making. Domestic violence is uncommon, even though partners may be very expressive in their disagreements.

Eye-Contact Practices: Eye-contact practices vary. Generally, Lithuanians do not like direct and sustained eye-to-eye focus with strangers, which is often viewed as a sign of impoliteness, hostility, a challenge to authority, or sexual in connotation. Direct eye contact may be used when communicating serious matters. Older adults may avoid direct eye contact when speaking to health care personnel.

Touch Practices: Touch is uncommon even within families. A handshake between men is usual at the beginning and end of interactions and for both sexes in professional situations. During health examinations, touching is expected and accepted, but before touching a patient, what will be done and why are explained. The health care provider's gender is not usually a factor, although female patients may prefer a female obstetrician/gynecologist. Modesty and privacy issues should be maintained when a patient's opposite-gender family members are present.

Perceptions of Time: Lithuanians focus on present-oriented crisis management relative to health care. Past traditions, including how older adults healed illnesses, are considered. Individuals can still meet with a practitioner if they are late for an appointment at a public institution, but this may not be true for an appointment with a practitioner in private practice. Physicians and nurses may be notoriously late and might not apologize for making patients wait for appointments or treatments.

Pain Reactions: Pain tolerance is valued, although pain relief is both desired and requested. Verbal expressions of pain indicate a higher level of pain. Administration of narcotic analgesics such as morphine may be misinterpreted as a sign of a hopeless situation and abandonment. Thus, it is recommended that caregivers explain to the relatives and to a dying patient that drugs such as morphine are not a last resort.

Birth Rites: High value is placed on family. The fertility rate is 1.2 children born per woman. Although the Catholic Church forbids birth control and abortion, the primary method of birth control during the 1970s and 1980s was abortion. Most Lithuanians find it very embarrassing and difficult to discuss details of the marital relationship with a third party, and couples tend to wait before seeking medical assistance for infertility. A pregnant woman will make every effort to eat well, get adequate rest, and comply with medical advice to ensure a healthy baby. Because of the traditional belief that the pregnant woman is "eating for two," caregivers carefully monitor weight gain. Women are expected to rest for several weeks after delivery, and the mother or mother-in-law may commit to childcare duties. Childbirth was considered a "woman's" affair, but the father's involvement is now encouraged, although men do not coach labor. Almost all births occur in hospitals in the semi-seated position, attended by a midwife and an obstetrician. The infant mortality rate is seven deaths per 1,000 live births. Circumcisions are not performed. Life expectancy is 69 for men, 79 for women.

Death Rites: If an illness is fatal, health care information is shared with family members by the doctor first, and they make decisions that may or may not include the patient. When death is impending, family members stand vigil so they are not alone. Relatives and friends are expected to visit and often bring food and gifts for clinicians. Prayer is often an important healing tool, and religious items may be brought into the room. Efforts are made not to grieve openly in front of the dying person. A pastor, priest, or rabbi may be present at the moment of death, and patient and family may want all mirrors covered during this time. The family closes the eyes and mouth of the deceased; to do otherwise is considered a bad omen. Autopsy may be accepted, but organ donation and withholding or withdrawing treatment are usually declined. The coffin may be taken to the patient's home so that the deceased can visit their home for the last time. Wailing and other displays of grief are reserved for expression in the home and are expected. It is customary to hold a wake followed by a mass and religious burial. In accordance with Jewish tradition, the dead are generally buried within 24 hours. Cremation is not practiced. The dead continue to be honored on All Souls Day (November 1), when the family attends mass and makes special offerings to the church.

Food Practices and Intolerances: The availability and consumption of vegetable oil and fresh fruits and vegetables have increased. The cuisines of various regions differ. Samogitians eat porridge, stew, and *kastinis* (similar to cottage cheese). Aukstaitijans enjoy various pancake and curd dishes. Dzukijans are very fond of buckwheat, which grows well in their sandy soil; they are also skilled in collecting and drying mushrooms. Suvalkijans enjoy smoked meat, especially pork. Bread has special significance and is put on the table at the beginning of the meal and never upside down, which is considered disrespectful. The oldest Lithuanian foodstuff is rye, and bakeries produce more than 15 kinds of rye bread. Some are baked with nuts, raisins, whole grains, caraway, and sunflower seeds; others are baked over marsh reeds. More than 70% of the bread consumed is dark rye. Pork is the most popular meat, and it is eaten fresh, salted, or smoked. Lithuanians make a great variety of sausages and seafood. *Saltitibarsciai,* "cold beet soup," is a favorite dish on hot summer days and is served with sour cream and dill, with hot potatoes on the side. Potato pancakes, covered with bacon or sour cream, are universal favorites. Lithuania is a beer-loving country. Strong alcohol consumption by women has increased, but it has decreased among men.

Infant-Feeding Practices: Breastfeeding is encouraged more than bottle-feeding. Many women state that although they want to breastfeed, they do not produce enough milk, so most transfer to bottle feeding between 3 and 30 days after birth. Infants are fed every 4 hours (not on demand). Non–breast-milk fluids (cow's milk, goat's milk, kefir) are introduced before age 5 months. Fruit, berries, and vegetable juice are introduced at 3 months; curd, egg yolk, oil, butter, and cereals at 5 to 6 months; and meat and broth at 6 months.

Child-Rearing Practices: The typical family is very close, and the mother is revered. Family structure is strong, and the divorce rate is unusually low. Several generations live under the same roof because of housing scarcity, so their dependence on one another for services such as childcare and management of the household are significant. The grandmother has a valued position in child rearing, especially in single-parent families or families in which both parents work. Women are entitled to paid maternity leave of 72 days before and 56 days after uncomplicated childbirth or 70 days after childbirth if the delivery was complicated or in cases of multiple births. By law, the child's mother or father is entitled to unpaid leave until the child is 3 years old.

National Childhood Immunizations: BCG at birth; DT at 6 years; DTwPHibIPV at 2, 4, 6, and 18 months; HepB at birth and 1 and 6 months [or 12 years (×3)] ; MMR at 15 months and at 6 to 12 years; OPV at 6 and 12 years; and Td at 15 years. The percent of the target population vaccinated, by antigen, is: BCG (99%); DTP1 (98%); DTP3 (94%); HepB3 (95%); Hib3 (61%); MCV (97%); and Polio3 (93%).

BIBLIOGRAPHY

Birutis A, and Čiočienė A: *Cultural aspects of Lithuanian nursing. LNA's workshop on cultural competency,* Vilnius, 2005, Lithuanian Nurses Association.

Central Intelligence Agency: *2006: The world factbook, Lithuania.* Retrieved February 27, 2006, from https://www.cia.gov/cia/publications/factbook/print/lh.html.

European Committee: *Lithuania,* ed 3, 2002, Artlora Publishing, Vilnius.

Gelazis R: Lithuanian Americans and culture care. In: Leininger M, McFarland M, editors: *Transcultural nursing: concepts, theories, research and practice,* ed 3. New York, 2002, McGraw-Hill.

Grabauskas V-J, Zaborskis A, Klumbienė J, Petkevičienė J, Žemaitienė N: Changes in health behavior of Lithuanian adolescents and adults over 1994–2002, *Medicina (Kaunas).* 40(9):884–890, 2004.

Michaelsen KF, Weaver L, Branca F, and Robertson A: *Feeding and nutrition of infants and young children,* Copenhagen, 2003, WHO Regional Publications.

Salimbene S: *What Language does your patient hurt? A practical guide to culturally competent patient care,* ed 2, Amherst, 2005, Diversity Resources.

Semaska A: The beauty of Lithuania, Vilnius 2005, Algimantas Publishing.

University of Washington Medical Center (UWMC): *Culture clue series,* Seattle, 2004, University of Washington Medical Center.

Lithuanian Health Information Centre: *Heath statistic,* Vilnius, 2004, LHIC Database. http://www.lsic.lt/. (retrieved February 27, 2006).

UNAIDS: 2006 Lithuania. Retrieved September 21, 2006, from http://www.unaids.org/en/Regions_Countries/Countries/lithuania.asp.

World Health Organization: 2006: Immunization, vaccines and biologicals. Retrieved September 21, 2006, from http://www.who.int/immunization_monitoring/en/globalsummary/countryprofileresult.cfm?C='ltu'.

✦ LUXEMBOURG (GRAND DUCHY OF)

MAP PAGE (798)

Alexandre R. Bisdorff

Location: Luxembourg is a small country in Western Europe with a temperate climate. The capital is Luxembourg. It borders France (to the south), Belgium (to the west), and Germany (to the east). The total area is 2586 km² (998 square miles) with a population of 474,413, resulting in a relatively high population density of more than 180 inhabitants per km². Most people work in services and industry, and 1.3% work in agriculture. Each day, 39% of the working population commutes from neighboring countries to work in Luxembourg. Luxembourg also has a very high percentage (39%) of foreigners living in the country. Luxembourg is a constitutional monarchy headed by the Grand Duke. The state is organized like a modern democracy, with a parliament voted for by general elections and based on the principle of separation of powers. The gross domestic product (GDP) per capita is $55,600. Literacy rates are 100% for both men and women.

Major Languages	Ethnic Groups	Major Religions
Luxembourgish (official)	Celtic base with French and German blend	Roman Catholic 97%
French (official)		Protestant and Jewish 3%
German (official)		

The main spoken language is Luxembourgish (Lëtzebuergesch), a language with Germanic roots going back to the fourth century, which is specific to the region of Luxembourg and neighboring areas in Belgium, France, and Germany. Lëtzebuergesch has sufficiently differentiated itself from its parent language such that it is no longer readily understood by Germans. The language used for official and legal documents is French, and German is used in daily newspapers. This unusual situation of the simultaneous use of several languages developed because the territory and population of the country is small and involved in permanent exchanges with neighboring countries. Every Luxembourger who grew up in this country speaks at least Luxembourgish, French, and German. English is taught in secondary schools.

Health Care Beliefs: Active participation; health promotion important. All schoolchildren are seen once a year by a doctor, who informs the parents of any problems. Vaccination programs are suggested by the Ministry of Health, and social security pays for most vaccines. Certain health-promotion activities are actively encouraged, such as yearly mammography for women in middle age and yearly Pap tests for women of every age. Some private initiatives offer programs for back exercises and injury prevention. In general, the trust in scientific medicine is relatively high; however, many patients use alternative practices, particularly if they have chronic or progressive diseases or ill-defined symptoms. Care for mental illness is provided by general practitioners and psychiatrists. Psychological, and to some extent, neurologic diseases are still associated with stigma. Fear associated with these diseases was much stronger during and after World War II because of the eugenics practiced by the Nazis who had occupied Luxembourg.

Predominant Sick-Care Practices: Biomedical and alternative. Luxembourg has 1,591 doctors: 411 general practitioners, 840 specialists, and 340 dentists. This corresponds to 3.5 doctors per 1,000 inhabitants. Most doctors have trained for at least a few years in neighboring countries because Luxembourg has no medical school offering a complete medical education. All doctors working in Luxembourg must show that they have achieved the European Union standards of skills. Doctors work in hospitals, and most specialists in hospitals also have a practice in the community. Patients may be referred abroad for rare or highly specialized services. It is mandatory that every doctor practicing in Luxembourg is automatically in the public social security system covering most of the population. Patients have free access to general and specialized practitioners and do not need a referral. Doctors and some other health professionals work as self-employed individuals and are paid on a fee-for-service basis. Tariffs are strictly regulated and the object of regular negotiations among doctors or other health professionals and the social security system. Generally, patients pay the doctor first and then receive a refund from social security. Unfounded health practices are a marginal phenomenon, but some doctors offer alternative medicine, which is not covered by social security.

Ethnic-/Race-Specific or Endemic Diseases: The most common illnesses are cardiovascular diseases, cancer, hypertension, and diabetes mellitus. Orthopedic problems such as chronic backaches and hip and knee arthrosis are also common as well as dementia and stroke in older adults. Major differences in causes of disease of the various nationalities living in Luxembourg are unknown. The incidence of human immuno-deficiency virus (HIV) infection has been between 9 and 10 cases per year (about 2.5 cases per 100,000) in the years from 1990 to 2000: 4 in 2001, 6 in 2002, 8 in 2003, and 12 in 2004. The Joint United Nations Programme on HIV/AIDS (UNAIDS) estimates the prevalence rate for HIV to be 0.2%, with fewer than 1,000 people living with HIV and fewer than 100 deaths from acquired immunodeficiency syndrome (AIDS). Among reported AIDS cases, 57% are attributed to men who have sex with men, 22% to heterosexual transmission, and 20% to injecting drug use. Of cases acquired heterosexually, about one third originate from other countries.

Health-Team Relationships: The health system is doctor driven. Because of the free access to any doctor, patients have free choice in outpatient and inpatient settings except in emergencies. Therefore, popular doctors have a big workload and fill hospital beds and surgical rooms. Hospitals have an interest in recruiting busy doctors of different specialties to ensure excellent services and to justify the pay for nurses and other personnel. Paramedics work as requested by doctors, but the system does not encourage analytic and decision-making skills by these providers.

Families' Role in Hospital Care: The role of the families is mainly to serve as a source of emotional support and help to make medical decisions regarding invasive tests and treatments for patients who are unable to do so. Families often bring food to their relatives, although it is unnecessary. Visitors for inpatients may arrive in the afternoon and stay overnight in special circumstances (e.g., when a patient is dying). One parent often stays overnight with children. The number of visitors may be limited when a patient is in intensive care or has an infectious disease.

Dominance Patterns: By law, men and women have equal rights and duties. Mothers tend to play a more important role in care of ill children because they stay with them at home or in the hospital. Currently, most doctors are men, but the number of women entering medicine is increasing in general medicine and a growing number of specialties.

Eye-Contact Practices: Eye contact is direct when people, including doctors and patients, talk to each other. A patient who avoids eye contact immediately causes the health professional to wonder whether the patient is extremely anxious, is shy, or has a mental disorder.

Touch Practices: Shaking hands is the normal way of greeting patients and their relatives before a medical consultation. Physical touching is quite acceptable during a physical examination. Touch practices do not vary between sexes, regardless of whether a male doctor is treating a female patient or vice versa.

Perceptions of Time: People value their cultural heritage because it is part of their identity. Most perceive that the ever-increasing European integration will result in many changes that will decrease national self-determination. On the whole, this is considered positive. Patients like to take advantage of the latest achievements of scientific medicine and find it quite normal that the social security system will pay for such services as it has during the last few decades. Many hope that scientific progress will result in better options for health care or cures for fatal diseases. On the other hand, some are concerned that future developments in molecular biology and embryology could lead to discrimination and abuse. Patients usually make appointments to see doctors, and doctors who are on a schedule may charge a small supplemental fee. Waiting times of several hours are not the norm. Luxembourg has no significantly long waiting lists for specialists or elective surgeries such as cataract procedures or joint replacements.

Pain Reactions: The spectrum of pain reactions reflects the multicultural nature of Luxembourg. Luxembourgers behave much like other Northern Europeans, tending to be stoic, but many patients with Mediterranean backgrounds are more expressive. Professionals need to consider cultural differences in the expression of suffering to make adequate assessments.

Birth Rites: Nearly all births occur in hospitals, and fathers may be present during childbirth. The fertility rate is 1.78 children born per woman. After birth, the father registers the newborn and its name with the local authorities. Whether the couple was married or not, the child's surname in the past was always the father's. A new law, however, allows a choice between either names, or the parents may opt for a double name. Relatives bring flowers to the mother in the hospital, where she usually stays for several days. Every newborn is examined by a pediatrician, and some screening tests for common genetic diseases are performed. Life expectancy is 76 for men, 82 for women.

Death Rites: Death is not a topic most people consider during their lives. Only a few people carry or write "do not resuscitate" (DNR) statements. Most people die in hospitals or nursing homes; if a person's death is expected, family members often ask to stay with him or her. Most Luxembourgers declare being Roman Catholic, although only a small minority actively practice. However, religious celebrations of baptism, marriage, and funerals are common. By law, doctors are allowed to take organs for transplantation from patients who are brain dead if no statement of refusal has been written by the person. In practice, most people have written such a statement, and close relatives are asked for their consent. It is usually unacceptable to overrule a family's wishes.

Luxembourg rarely does autopsies. Most are requested by attorneys for forensic reasons: cases of violent death, deaths with unknown causes, or deaths that occurred under suspicious circumstances.

Food Practices and Intolerances: Carefully preparing food and matching it with the correct wines is highly regarded and takes inspiration from France. The many foreign communities, especially the French, Italian, and Belgian, also have enriched the local cuisine.

Infant-Feeding Practices: Breastfeeding is encouraged for at least 6 weeks after birth because of scientific evidence of benefits. No attitudes are specific to the culture.

Child-Rearing Practices: Most children have their own rooms and do not sleep in their parents' room after infancy. Many parents allow their children to come to their bed at night but try to stop the habit gently. Child rearing is not particularly strict or authoritarian, and physical punishment is largely rejected. Ideally, children are supposed to grow up to become responsible adults, not submissive subjects. Most families are small. In many families, grandparents take over a part of the child's rearing, allowing both parents to work. Some children become spoiled under these circumstances, and lines of authority can become unclear when too many adults are involved in their upbringing.

National Childhood Immunizations: BCG at 1 to 2 months, if indicated; OPV at 2, 3, 4 to 6, 11 to 12 months and at 5 to 7 and 12 to 15 years and every 10 years; DTP at 2, 3, 4 to 6, and 11 to 12 months; pertussis at 12 to 15 years; MMR at 14 to 15 months and 5 to 7 years; HepB at 2, 3, and 4 to 6 months; HIB at 2, 3, 4 to 6, and 11 to 12 months; tetanus at 5 to 7 and 12 to 15 years and every 10 years. (Official recommendations of the Ministry of Health of Luxembourg, but the program is voluntary). The percent of the target population vaccinated, by antigen, is: BCG, DTP1, and Polio3 (99%); HepB3 and MCV (95%); and Hib3 (98%).

BIBLIOGRAPHY

Autier P, Shannoun F, Scharpantgen A, Lux C, Back C, Severi G, Steil S, Hansen-Koenig D: The Luxembourg Mammography Programme: a breast cancer screening programme operating in a liberal health care system: 1992-1997, *Int J Cancer.* 20:97(6):828-832, 2002.

Central Intelligence Agency: 2006: *The world factbook, Luxembourg.* Retrieved September 21, 2006, from https://www.cia.gov/cia/publications/factbook/print/lu.html.

Lynch J, Smith GD, Hillemeier M, Shaw M, Raghunathan T, Kaplan G: Income inequality, the psychosocial environment, and health: comparisons of wealthy nations, *Lancet.* 21:358(9277):194–200, 2001.

Service Central de la Statistique et des Etudes Economiques (STATEC): 2004. 6, Boulevard Royal L-2013 Luxembourg. Retrieved June 10, 2006, from http://www.statec.lu.

UNAIDS: 2006 Luxembourg. Retrieved September 21, 2006, from http://www.unaids.org/en/Regions_Countries/Countries/luxembourg.asp.

World Health Organization: 2006: Immunization, vaccines and biologicals. Retrieved September 21, 2006, from http://www.who.int/immunization_monitoring/en/globalsummary/countryprofileresult.cfm?C='lux'.

◆ MACEDONIA (THE FORMER YUGOSLAV REPUBLIC OF)

MAP PAGE (798)

Velibor B. Tasic

Location: Macedonia is located in the southeast part of the Balkan Peninsula; the capital is Skopje. It borders Yugoslavia on the north, Bulgaria on the east, Greece on the south, and Albania on the west. The total area is 25,333 km^2 (9,781 square miles). Macedonia has lakes, many mountains, and rivers. It is a country rich in culture, tradition, and history. The ethnic majority are Macedonians, followed by people of Albanian descent. Ethnic minorities include Romas (Gypsies), Turks, Serbs, and Vlahos. The country is mainly agricultural. The population is more than two million. The gross domestic product (GDP) per capita is $7,800, with 30% living below the poverty line. Literacy rates are 98% for men, 94% for women.

Major Languages	Ethnic Groups	Major Religions

Macedonian (official-
  Cyrillic alphabet)
Albanian
Turkish
	Macedonian 66%
	Albanian 23%
	Turkish 4%
	Serb 2%
	Roma (Gypsy) and
	  Other 7%
		Eastern Orthodox
		  Christian 67%
		Muslim 30%
		Other 3%

Health Care Beliefs: Acute sick care; traditional. Under the communist system, the state was active in health promotion and disease prevention. People no longer receive regular examinations for prevention purposes; even health care workers are poor role models. For example, most of those at professional risk for hepatitis B infection have not been vaccinated. Tuberculosis is a significant problem, although mobile stations are available for early detection. Many people are prejudiced toward people with mental illness, and even families might not want them back after hospitalization. Mentally ill patients are isolated during prolonged hospitalizations and often receive inadequate treatment. In rural communities, traditional practices are common. For example, coffee powder is put on an umbilical cord that will not stop bleeding; a practice with practical benefits because coffee is rich in vitamin K, which is important for clotting. It may also cause infection. When an infant has jaundice, a traditional treatment is to make a small incision on the forehead to release it, and they are dressed in yellow clothes so that their yellow skin is less noticeable. Infants wear amulets on their hands and fingers and special pieces of velvet on their eyes to protect them from the "evil eye" (the power of a person to harm others by looking at them). After delivery, infants are kept in the house for 6 weeks to protect them from infections. Pregnant women are discouraged from going to cemeteries because evil spirits might take the fetus; in some rural communities, only a mother-in-law can deliver a woman's baby.

Predominant Sick-Care Practices: Alternative; magical-religious; biomedical when available. Under the previous regime, the health system was structured, and the medical field was held in high esteem. During the past decade, after the separation of the former Yugoslav Republic, significant transitional changes took place. Health insurance was previously almost free but now is tied to employment. Because many people are currently unemployed, few people can go to a doctor. Until recently, medications could be bought without a prescription. Because access was easy, self-treatment was common and based on information from news, television, friends, or colleagues. This practice led to abuse of drugs, particularly antibiotics, with resultant drug resistance (e.g., the resistance of *Escherichia coli* against co-trimoxazole is 48%). If initial self-treatment was unsuccessful, people then consulted a doctor. Scheduled doctors visits are unusual, examinations are considered poor, and often little discretion between doctor and patient exists, especially in public facilities. People are not satisfied with public health services and prefer to consult doctors working in private offices or hospitals. If patients have their own health insurance, they pay a small amount to participate in the public system. In the private system, the entire fee must be paid, and prices are high compared to average salaries. Some consult with nonmedical staff members, or paramedics, who claim to cure people with herbs, bioenergy, or semimagical treatments. At times, the actions of these practitioners have serious consequences. A paramedic using herbs or special teas may forbid a person to use doctor-prescribed drugs. If a person has insulin-dependent diabetes, the cessation of insulin can lead to serious consequences such as diabetic ketoacidosis or coma and death. Circumcisions, which are ritually performed in Muslim communities are frequently done without anesthesia by nonprofessionals, most of whom are religious leaders. In addition to causing great pain, a frequent complication is meatal stenosis. A rare complication, poststreptococcal glomerulonephritis, is a consequence of an infected circumcision wound. Treatment with bioenergy is especially popular, and all cities or villages have a bioenergy practitioner. Diseases treated with bioenergy include nocturnal enuresis, lumboishialgia (back pain from spinal compression of the sciatic nerve), epilepsy, certain types of cancer, and many central nervous system diseases. Treatment with herbs or tea is popular for the flu, diarrhea, kidney stones, and menstrual problems. Macrobiotic diets are particularly popular among patients with cancer. Those with incurable diseases may undergo some very unpleasant procedures; for example, some believe that drinking blood from a turtle can help to cure patients with leukemia.

Ethnic-/Race-Specific and Endemic Diseases: After World War II, malaria and syphilis were eradicated. The southern part of the country still has cases of hereditary Mediterranean anemia (thalassemia), a specific hematologic disease affecting those of Macedonian ethnicity. Certain parts of the country still have cases of kalaazar (leishmaniasis). The worsening economy and low educational level have been instrumental in the increased incidence of tuberculosis, acute post-streptococcal glomerulonephritis, and rheumatic fever, particularly among Albanians. Iron-deficiency anemia is common among children, and occasionally children develop kwashiorkor. During the summer, diarrhea is common and lately has been known to progress to toxicosis with bad outcomes, especially in malnourished children. Macedonia has had occasional epidemics of hepatitis A. The prevalence of hepatitis B carriers in the population has been estimated to be up to 8%. Hepatitis C infection has become a serious problem, especially among patients on dialysis. The main causes of death are cardiovascular diseases (57%); malignant diseases (18%); symptoms, signs, and undefined situations (6%); respiratory diseases (4%); poisoning and trauma (4%); endocrine diseases (4%); digestive system diseases (2%); and others (5%). The Joint United Nations Programme on HIV/AIDS (UNAIDS) estimates the prevalence rate for human immunodeficiency virus (HIV) to be 0.1%. The first HIV-positive case was registered in 1987, the first acquired immunodeficiency syndrome (AIDS) case in 1989 (initially in hemophiliacs infected via imported blood products). By December 2005, the total number of officially registered HIV/AIDS cases since the beginning of the epidemic was 79 (63 sick, 16 seropositive). Fifty people have died of AIDS. In 2005, 12 new AIDS cases were registered. The statistics are far from the real situation given that 99% of all registered HIV/AIDS patients were not seen by health providers. Cases have been recorded in all areas of the country and in all ethnic groups. The most dominant age group is 30 to 39 years, and about 70% of all cases are in men. Transmission is recorded as primarily heterosexual (61%), followed by men who have sex with men (11%) and injecting drug users (9%). Speaking openly about sexual orientation is difficult because of the country's culture, religion, and traditions.

Health-Team Relationships: The new health care system is focusing on teamwork between nurses and doctors. A harmonious relationship exists for the most part, influenced by social and cultural environments. Patients generally respect medical staff. An initiative has been developed to create special programs for the health care of children, particularly children with special problems—those for whom communication among general doctors, pediatricians, and parents is crucial. The system is moving toward greater integration of patient needs with needs of health care professionals, and better overall communication among parties.

Families' Role in Hospital Care: Hospitals cannot provide the level of care for patients that is common in Western European countries. Food, drugs, accommodations, and hygiene are all inadequate, so relatives accompany and care for patients. Mothers of children younger than 3 years are allowed to stay in the hospital without charge. Parents may accompany older children if a bed is available. Food is usually brought to the hospital but does not always meet therapeutic recommendations; for example, if a family of a child who has acute glomerulonephritis brings fruit, drinks, or salted meals, the food could result in increased blood pressure and worsening of the child's health. During the transition into a new health care system, efforts toward open communication among patients, family, and staff members are being made, even among those in intensive care.

Dominance Patterns: In the urban environment, differences between sexes are not as important. However, in some rural areas, women continue to be predestined to remain in the home, where cooking, cleaning, and the education of children have been traditionally primarily women's tasks. Men's roles relate to making money for the family and doing more difficult physical labor.

Eye-Contact Practices: Making direct eye contact signifies trust, and avoidance of eye contact is interpreted as shame or lying. Direct eye contact might be avoided when the authority of one individual intimidates the other.

Touch Practices: Youths have more freedom in expressing their feelings, and differences exist between those in rural and urban surroundings and those who are modern or conservative. The relationship between male doctors and female patients is delicate. In some rural areas, women still go to a doctor accompanied by their husbands or someone else, especially when a gynecologic examination is performed. Some women, particularly women from Muslim areas, prefer to be examined by female doctors.

Perceptions of Time: Punctuality is not typical, and most people are late, even to doctors' appointments, frequently causing chaos. Macedonians tend to live in the present, facing only daily social, economic, and political problems. They often think about the past with nostalgia. This is true particularly for young people who feel hopeless about future prospects for employment, living conditions, or travel. Many young people look to their future by emigrating to Canada or Australia.

Pain Reactions: Men are expected to be strong when in pain, whereas women are expected to cry and yell. Children are trained to cope with pain in early childhood. Children's rights are not fully recognized, and poor pain control and prescription of intramuscular injections in the hospital make many children permanently frightened of hospital care. People in general still strongly believe that injections have more power than drugs taken orally. Many painful procedures, such as bronchoscopies and colonoscopies, are performed without any medication or analgesic relief. The problem of pain has rarely been seriously considered, especially in the public system. In private practice, somewhat more attention is paid to this issue.

Birth Rites: The fertility rate is 1.57 children born per woman. Macedonians are not actively involved in birth control, and the number of abortions far exceeds the number of deliveries, estimated as at least three abortions to one birth. Most women have three ultrasounds during pregnancy and deliver infants in hospitals with the assistance of professionals. Newborns are kept in the hospital for several days. In the past, newborn tetanus was common because the umbilical cord would be cut with a razor or unclean scissors. Since 2000, some obstetric hospitals have started rooming-in programs, where newborns are kept with their mothers constantly unless mother or child has serious complications. Some families are happier when a boy is born, and his birth may be celebrated by shooting a gun. In some cases, the father does not even want to take his infant home when it is a girl. Few deliveries are performed at home, but when infants have complications, people attempt to transport the mother to the hospital. Too frequently, infants come too late or die on the way to the hospital. Macedonia has the second highest infant mortality rate in Europe at 10 deaths per 1,000 live births (Albania has the highest.) A new project by the World Bank has been established to decrease perinatal mortality, and Macedonia has also initiated a program to prevent morbidity and mortality by using standard protocols. Surfactant also has become available and has been effective in reducing the mortality of premature infants with respiratory distress syndrome. Life expectancy is 72 for men, 77 for women.

Death Rites: Customs differ between Muslim and Eastern orthodox populations. For orthodox burials, candles are lit in the home, and family, relatives, and close friends spend the night with the body. A priest conducts the burial ceremony, the coffin is lowered into the ground, and people throw earth on it. After the funeral ceremony, participants are invited to have a meal at the home of the deceased. It is still believed that the spirit of the person is present during the 40 days after the death. Because of this belief, on the 40th day after a death, the family invites relatives and friends to a lunch to celebrate the presentation of the person to God. According to Muslim custom, men carry the coffin, and women follow behind, separated from the men. If a death occurs in the hospital, Muslims forbid autopsy; the orthodox do not have such rules. According to Macedonian law, an autopsy must be performed if a death occurs within 24 hours of admission or when the cause of the death is unclear. Organ donations are not performed. The only option for people with renal failure is kidney transplantation from a living relative. Liver and heart transplantations are not available.

Food Practices and Intolerances: Basic foods are bread, dairy products (e.g., yogurt, milk, cheese), and meat. Sheep and cows are raised in the mountains and villages, so meat and milk are inexpensive. Milk, rather than formula, is generally given to infants, since formula is expensive relative to the low incomes of most individuals. This practice leads to a higher incidence of rickets and sideropenic anemia. The country is mainly agricultural and produces many vegetables and fruits. The women prepare meals, and on Friday families have a traditional bean dish. On Sunday, people have a traditional family lunch of baked meat—usually chicken, pork or beef, with vegetables. The most typical Macedonian food is ajvar-mild paprika peppers which are baked, chopped into very small pieces, and fried in oil (often with tomato and other spices). Ajvar is also put into glass bottles or cans and sterilized (i.e., canned) for the winter.

Infant-Feeding Practices: Because of difficult social and economic conditions, children generally do not have very nutritious diets. The dominant foods are carbohydrates and fats. Breastfeeding is encouraged by health professionals but is not practiced or accepted by many modern mothers.

The United Nations Children's Fund (UNICEF) strongly promotes exclusive breastfeeding, emphasizing its advantages over artificial (formula) feeding. Various formulas are on the market, but they are expensive.

Child-Rearing Practices: Macedonians still have conservative views of proper family behavior. The father controls power and discipline, and the mother devotes her time to the education and care of the children. Parents expect children to be calm and obey rules. Children are not employed before they are 18 and therefore are economically dependent on their parents until that age.

National Childhood Immunizations: Hepatitis B at birth; HepB at 1 and 6 months; MMR at 13 months; TBC at 3 days and at 7 and 14 years; DTP at 4 months and at 2 and 4 years; DT at 7 and 14 years; tetanus at 18 years; polio at 4 months for three doses (with a 40-day interval between doses) and at 2, 7, and 14 years; and rubella at 14 years for girls. The percent of the target population vaccinated, by antigen, is: BCG (99%); DTP1 and MCV (96%); DTP3 (97%); HepB3 (91%); MCV2 (95%); and Polio3 (98%). Macedonia is certified as free of polio.

BIBLIOGRAPHY

Central Intelligence Agency: 2006: The world factbook, Macedonia. Retrieved September 21, 2006, from https://www.cia.gov/cia/publications/factbook/print/mk.html.

Chkaleska D et al: *Annual report for health status and health protection in Republic of Macedonia,* 2004.

European Observatory on Health Care Systems: *Health care systems in transition: Republic of Macedonia.* Copenhagen, 2000, European Observatory on Health Care Systems.

Karadzovski Z: *Annual report on HIV/AIDS in the country for 2005.* Skopje, 2005, Republic Institute for Health Protection.

Republic Institute for Health Protection. *Annual report 2000,* Skopje.

Tasic V: PhD thesis. University Sv.Kiril i Metodij, Skopje, 1997.

Tasic V, Polenakovic M: Poststreptococcal glomerulonephritis following circumcision, *Pediatr Nephrol.* 15:274–275, 2000.

UNAIDS: 2006 Macedonia. Retrieved September 21, 2006, from http://www.unaids.org/en/Regions_Countries/Countries/macedonia.asp.

http://www.who.int/immunization_monitoring/en/globalsummary/timeseries/tscoveragebycountry.cfm?country=The%20former%20Yugoslav%20Republic%20of%20Macedonia (retrieved September 20, 2006).

M

◆ MADAGASCAR (REPUBLIC OF)

MAP PAGE (801)

Katharine Quanbeck and Stanley D. Quanbeck

Location: Madagascar is situated in the Indian Ocean across the Mozambique Channel from southeast Africa. The capital is Antananarivo. Lining the vast coast are regions varying from semiarid and grassy grazing lands to spiny forests, sharp cliffs, and white intermingled with black (titanium) sandy beaches connecting with the expanses of coral reefs. The total area is 587,041 km^2 (226,597 square miles). This "great red island" gained independence from France and became the Malagasy Republic in 1960. The population is about 18.5 million. The literacy rate varies widely, from 5% in the coastal regions to 90% in the highlands. The gross domestic product (GDP) per capita is $900, with 73% living below the poverty line in rural areas and 53% in urban. Many Malagasy people practiced endogamy within their own clan who had come by dugout canoe or *dhow*; some intermarried with many nationalities. The Malagasy language varies widely.

Major Languages	Ethnic Groups	Major Religions
Malagasy	All are immigrants from	Traditional
French	the Near, Middle,	(syncretism with
English	and Far East, Pacific	other, i.e.,
	Islands, and Africa.	animism) 43%
		Roman Catholic 25%
		Protestant 25%
		Muslim 7%

Health Care Beliefs: Acute sick care; traditional. Since about 1975 mobile teams have worked with villagers encouraging vaccinations and promoting nutrition, breastfeeding, disease recognition, maternal and child care, preventive practices, sanitation and hygiene principles. In many areas, training of community health workers has been taking place since 1980. Community health workers (primarily women) do monthly growth monitoring and nutritional counseling, teach use of hand-grinding mills, teach women about solar cooking, distribute food to underweight children, and distribute food during famines. They also do door-to-door visiting in their villages to remind people about vaccination days, to check on use of oral rehydration gruels for those with diarrhea, and to remind those being treated for tuberculosis to show up for medication or intermittent sputum checks. Mass projects, such as mebendazole for intestinal parasite control or surveying sexually transmitted diseases (STDs), can best be carried out with the involvement of these workers. Even shamans and herbalists in villages work in coordination with them, and it is not unusual for villagers to choose their shamans to be the people who are trained to be their health workers.

Predominant Sick-Care Practices: Magical-religious; biomedical when available. It is not uncommon for people first to consult with a shaman or herbalist or to receive treatment from them simultaneously with treatment from a doctor, nurse, or medical assistant. Depending on the healer, who can be a man or woman, the person may use sticks or pieces of wood and coins mixed with rum. This is coupled with "calling on a healer spirit" to possess the healer. If a patient enters a hospital wearing a silver bracelet attached to the hair, it indicates that he or she has an indwelling spirit (i.e., is possessed, or *tromba*). Spirit possession syndromes are widespread, and the interplay between these and overt mental illness is being studied. If harmful, traditional practices are addressed, often through role-plays followed by questions and dialogue; otherwise, traditions are respected. Medications are easier to obtain than previously.

Ethnic-/Race-Specific or Endemic Diseases: Although Madagascar has some cases of chloroquine-resistant malaria, chloroquine is still the drug of choice. Tuberculosis and mental illness are major problems. Infection with human immunodeficiency virus (HIV) is suspected in persons found to be resistant to the tuberculosis regimen. Schistosomiasis (bilharzias) is prevalent; and pigs are permitted to run loose, creating the perfect environment for cysticercosis and cysticercosis-based epilepsy. Oral rehydration for the control of diarrhea has not yet reached all remote areas. Lack of clean water, lack of education, and taboos against defecating in the same place more than once all contribute to the problem. Drives to encourage exclusive breastfeeding for the first 6 months after birth have not prevented malnutrition and stunted growth in all regions. It is common to favor the boy of fraternal twins; boys are offered breast milk and food supplements first. Parasites are a continual problem, although better-educated, wealthier individuals are more apt to treat themselves. STDs are pervasive in all areas but the central highlands, where sex workers receive weekly checkups and where sex before marriage is less common. In the rain forest, filariasis leads to scrotal elephantiasis (hydroceles) as large as basketballs; in other regions, it leads to disfiguring elephantiasis of the leg. Filariasis can lead to chronic ill health. If all village homes had at least one bed net with insecticide in their homes, it would affect the endemic properties of filariasis, malaria, dengue fever, Chikungunya, and suffering due to fleas, bedbugs, and lice. The numbers of leprosy cases are decreasing. Goiter and cretinism are problems in regions of iodine deficiency. The Joint United Nations Programme on HIV/AIDS (UNAIDS) estimates the prevalence rate for human immunodeficiency virus (HIV) to be 0.5% (0.2% to 1.2%), with 49,000 living with HIV, including 13,000 women and 1,600 children aged 0 to 14. There are 13,000 orphans as a result of parental death from acquired immunodeficiency syndrome (AIDS). About 2,900 deaths have been reported.

Health-Team Relationships: Doctors receive higher salaries and are at the top of the echelon. In remote areas, where physicians often do not want to work, nurses and even untrained people are addressed as *radoko* ("doctor") by villagers, and care by such a person is sought, trusted, and followed. This is particularly true in regions with high nonliteracy rates, especially if a nurse has developed rapport with villagers. Nearly half of Malagasy doctors are women. Far too many doctors seem to be associated with an unspoken attitude of dominance and condescension about which nurses, sociologists, and paramedical professionals often complain.

Families' Role in Hospital Care: In rural clinics, family members assist relatives who are hospitalized by cooking for them at hospital guest-housing quarters. In more modern hospitals, food is cooked in the hospital. The word of elders is law and followed exactly regardless of whether they are right or wrong. The practice of "I respect you unquestioningly, so you care for me completely" can lead to the financial ruin of those who earn a living (yet must pay for the care and treatment of many clan members) and has led to the ruin of more than one self-supporting hospital. This occurs when traditional practices dictate that the income in the hospital must be used for the functioning of families, institutions, or groups related to the hospital in any way.

Dominance Patterns: Elders and ancestral spirits are respected and honored, as are traditional consecrated elders who perform sacrifices, and high priests who guard the clan's worship place. Clans are primarily patriarchal. In some clans, wives are the advisors of their husbands; in other clans a woman may be the leading elder, and it is not unusual for her to be the judge for her clan's people. For royalty clans, a son's ability to become king depends completely on his mother's identity. Royalty clans have also had queens. Women usually hold the family's money. Well-educated women leaders exist in every walk of life and in many regions. The emphasis is on the entire clan; often cousins are called "siblings" and nieces and nephews are called "children," therefore one person can have several "mothers."

Eye-Contact Practices: In some clans, eye contact is avoided with people in authority: such avoidance is uncommon in others. When children are being disciplined, they may have difficulty looking into the eyes of the adult who is speaking, even when requested to do so. The issue of eye contact varies among clans, even clans who are neighbors.

Touch Practices: Boys and girls and even husbands and wives may avoid physical contact in public. It is taboo for a couple for whom a marriage is being considered to be seen together in public. Traditional healers called *mpitsapa* are believed by many to have the power to heal by stroking, lightly massaging, or touching. It is said that a broken bone can be healed by a mpitsapa touching and manipulating the bone. In many clans, it is common for two female friends or two male friends to walk holding hands. Preschool-age children often sleep packed together in one bed. Handshaking is common, but some groups kiss the cheek three times. Parents are affectionate and dote on children. Children tend to be raised to depend on their parents and each other rather than to think and act independently. Extended family members assume major roles in child rearing. It is not unusual for a grandmother to demand that she be permitted to raise a grandchild.

Perceptions of Time: Punctuality holds no value for most clans. It is far more important to give adequate attention to politeness—to inquire about each family member and show respect by chatting—than it is to remember to reach an appointment on time. Some clans tend to focus on past traditions almost totally. Some never consider the future (tomorrow does not yet exist). Some live completely in the present. Educated individuals are the best at planning, ordering medications ahead of time, training others to be in charge in the future, and writing reports so that future efforts and activities acknowledge past mistakes or successes. Many believe that how an event occurs is preordained by God; and some believe in astrology, divination, and geomancy.

Pain Reactions: Pain is shown and expressed by many clans, although some train boys and girls to be tough and repress discomfort, pain, and fear. If children express pain, they are unworthy of their clan title (which always begins with "of the family of..." or "descendant of..."). These clans tend to express toughness bluntly and freely and use a method of relating called *mifampiziva*, a teasing, insulting pleasantry that never reaches violence.

Birth Rites: Taboos during pregnancy can involve eggs, chicken, or seafood. In most clans, sons are much more celebrated. If money is a problem, it is the sons who receive education. In remote villages in some regions, the mother squats and gives birth under a tree, occasionally alone. She cuts the cord with a shell or other sharp object and is then expected to go back and work the fields. In other clans, it is customary for the mother to *mifana*, that is, to sit beside a fire, bundled up in a heavy blanket with the infant. The mother is fed a milky sauce of small fish so that she can produce breast milk. If a woman is admired, she may sit beside the fire for up to 6 months, growing fatter and fatter. Most remote rural clans insist that only women can assist with childbirth. In some royalty clans, it is still forbidden for a king's wives to be treated by a male health worker. Many rural villagers do not name their infants for up to a year after birth because of the high infant mortality rate. In remote villages, it is not unusual for a woman who has been in labor for a day or two to ride in a wooden-wheeled ox cart for 2 or 3 days to reach a surgical center. It is a miracle when such a mother survives the delivery of a dead infant after so much time. The infant mortality rate is high at 75 deaths per 1,000 live births. The fertility rate is 6.6 children born per woman. Contraceptive use is 19%, and the percentage of mothers receiving prenatal care is 77%. Life expectancy is 52 for men, 57 for women.

M

Death Rites: It is not unusual for a family or clan member to thank a doctor when a family member dies, saying, "You have done all you can, and we have done our best as well, to care for our loved one." Many tend to place death in the hands of Zanahary or Andriananahary, their almighty and omnipotent creator god. Organ donation would be taboo if it were possible, and autopsies are rarely permitted. If a leg is surgically amputated, the body part must be buried in its own tomb. In clans who use large family tombs built above the ground, the clan elder reviews the names of those buried in the tomb and on which shelf they are resting. He also informs the family about the shelves where they will eventually go to "lie with their fathers." Some bury the dead in caves or holes, some under a large pile of rocks on a high place. *Alo-alo*—carved, wooden markers somewhat similar to totem poles—mark the tops of many graves, in addition to cow horns indicating the number of cows that were slaughtered for the funeral. The whole clan is expected to contribute money, food (e.g., a cow) and labor for the making of the grave. In some clans who reopen the grave periodically, the corpse is taken around the ancestral village and given new grave cloths. Before an elder dies, they designate who is to become the clan elder or leader. In many regions, the more important a person is, the more cattle are killed. For royalty, it is not uncommon to wait 6 months or a year or longer before the burial. The common lamentation at burials involves sharp, startling cries, wailing, and weeping by women, which begins anew every time new visitors arrive. In some clans, the king may be buried in the trunk of the largest tree they can find; clansmen often have to go scores of kilometers to find it and then have to spend much money hiring a truck to carry it to the village. Dancing en route to the burial site is not uncommon and is accompanied by revelry and singing.

Food Practices and Intolerances: In the central highlands and wherever it can be grown, rice is the staple food and eaten with a little topping *(laoka)* of meat, dried beans, lentils, greens or other vegetables, and tomatoes. The Malagasy believe they cannot feel full and have not eaten a meal unless they have eaten rice. Cassava, sweet potato, other locally available greens, and watercress are also commonly combined with beans or meat and served as a topping. A favorite snack is rice cakes *(mokary)*, which may be sweetened, *sambosse* (an Indian triangular-shaped snack), or meatballs. Most enjoy fruit in season. Staples such as cassava, sweet potato, taro root, and corn may be the primary foods eaten, combined with greens, soured milk *(habobo)*, lentils, or dried beans. Garbanzo beans (cooked to a milky consistency) are widely used to supplement breast milk.

Infant-Feeding Practices: In some clans, mothers spoon herbal teas into the mouths of their newborns and believe that colostrum is unhealthy. Mothers convinced of the benefits of breastfeeding tend to brag that their infants are so healthy and have only been fed breast milk. Gruels are introduced by 6 months and consist of rice or two parts carbohydrate food, one part lentil or dried bean, and one part peanut. The three-foods gruel is especially used to feed children who show stunted growth or who are malnourished. Mashed fruit is also used to supplement the gruel and breast milk after the infant is 6 months old. Infants who do not have an appetite are fed a mixture made of egg yolk beaten into orange or tomato juice. About 48% of children below the age of 3 years have stunted growth.

Child-Rearing Practices: Children are loved and carried almost constantly. Discipline usually involves guidance, talking, urging, and distracting rather than outright confrontation or castigation. Toilet training is often begun within the first few months after birth. The mother or another female is expected to take the child outside and sit on the ground, night or day, with her legs straight out in front of her, so that she can cradle the infant on the anterior aspect of her ankles until the infant eliminates. Health is affected by taboos and regulations imposed by shamans. Children who are allowed to begin school are often forced to quit, either to take care of siblings, to plant and harvest the fields, or—in the worst-case scenario—travel to the nearby city to become a prostitute because the family is starving. All but one clan circumcises infants—an event often accompanied by feasting, merriment, and dancing. For some clans, it is a duty or privilege of the maternal uncle to eat, with a banana, the foreskin of a child who has just been circumcised. In other clans, the foreskin is inserted into the muzzle of a shotgun and fired into the air as a symbol of future virility.

National Childhood Immunizations: BCG at birth; DTPHep at 6, 10, and 14 weeks; OPV at birth and at 6, 10, and 14 weeks; measles at 9 months; vitamin A at 9, 15, 21, 27, 31, and 39 months; and TT for pregnant women at first contact pregnancy; +1, +6 months; +1, +1 year. The percent of the target population vaccinated, by antigen is: BCG (72%); DPT1 (71%); DPT3 (61%); MCV (59%); and Polio3 (63%).

BIBLIOGRAPHY

Central Intelligence Agency: *2006: The world factbook, Madagascar.* Retrieved September 21, 2006, from https://www.cia.gov/cia/publications/factbook/print/ma.html.

Ralaimihoatra-Nicole G: Et si la lune ne revenait pas? Madagascar—le secret des Vazimba, Saint-Denis de la Réunion, Editions Grand Océan, St-Denis, Reunion (island), 2001.

Randriamihajanirina D: FISAKANA—Tsa Hanim-boay ... ! Antananarivo, Madagascar, 1999.

Tishkoff SA, Varkonyi R, Cahinhinan N, Abbes S, Argyropoulos G, Destro-Bisol G, et al: Haplotype diversity and linkage disequilibrium at human G6PD: recent origin of alleles that confer malarial resistance, *Science.* 293(5529):455–462, 2001.

UNAIDS: 2006 Madagascar. Retrieved September 21, 2006, from http://www.unaids.org/en/Regions_Countries/Countries/madagascar.asp.

UNAIDS/WHO Working Group on Global HIV/AIDS and STI Surveillance: UNAIDS/WHO epidemiological fact sheet: 2004 Update. Retrieved March 27, 2006, from http://www.who.int/hiv; http://www.unaids.org.

Underhill PA, Passarino G, Lin AA, Marzuki S, Oefner PJ, Cavalli-Sforza LL, et al: Maori origins, Y-chromosome haplotypes and implications for human history in the Pacific, *Hum Mutat.* 17:271–280, 2001.

World Health Organization: 2006: Immunization, vaccines and biologicals. Retrieved September 21, 2006, from http://www.who.int/immunization_monitoring/en/globalsummary/countryprofileresult.cfm?C='mdg'.

M

◆ MALAWI (REPUBLIC OF)

MAP PAGE (801)

Cameron Bowie

Location: Malawi is a small African country occupying a southern part of the East African Rift Valley. It has a total area of 119,140 km² (45,988 square miles). The capital is Lilongwe. Malawi is landlocked and borders Mozambique, Tanzania, and Zambia. Its topography is varied, ranging from the Rift Valley floor at sea level to the majestic Mulanje Mountain at

3,000 m. Malawi attained its independence from Britain in 1964. After being a one-party dictatorship, elections were held in 1994, and a new democratically elected government came to power. Malawi has a population of more than 13 million. It is the second poorest country in the world, with a gross domestic product (GDP) per capita of $600, with 55% living below the poverty line. The country is predominantly agriculturally based, and 85% of the population lives in rural areas. English is the official language in government, parliament, the judiciary system, and secondary and tertiary educational systems. Literacy rates are 76% for men, 50% for women.

Major Languages	Ethnic Groups	Major Religions
English (official)	Chewa, Nyanja,	Christian 75%
Chichewa (national)	Tumbuko,	Islam 20%
Chitumbuka	Yao, Lomwe, Sena,	Other 5%
	Tonga,	
	Ngoni, Ngonde, Asian,	
	European	

Health Care Beliefs: Acute sick care; traditional. Social psychologists who have studied Malawians argue that they are able to maintain two different belief systems about health and well-being without any sense of conflict or contradiction. Malawians understand the causes of diseases according to both Western scientific (biomedical) and traditional explanations (which involve mysticism and the role of spirits and ancestors in the cause of disease). Hence most people seek out both traditional healers and Western-trained medical doctors. An increasing number are also turning to prayer as a result of strong Pentecostal Christian emphasis. People primarily attribute mental illness to traditional factors such as being bewitched.

M

Predominant Sick-Care Practices: Biomedical and magico-religious. Primary health care is the major focus of the health services delivery system. The Malawi government's information, education, and communication activities are guided by health education strategies. It is believed that increased public awareness "facilitates involvement and participation, and promotes activities which will foster health and encourage people to want to be healthy, know how to stay healthy and do what they can individually or collectively to maintain health and seek help when needed" (Bomba, 1991). Because of material and financial resource limitations, the government has had to focus on activities that directly affect vulnerable groups, especially women and children. The country has one national mental hospital, and common causes for admission include substance abuse and schizophrenia.

Ethnic-/Race-Specific or Endemic Diseases: Lower respiratory tract disease is the second most common cause of death (11%), followed by malaria (8%). Malaria is the leading cause of outpatient visits and in-patient admissions Other illnesses, in decreasing order of importance, include diarrheal diseases, diseases occurring at childbirth, tuberculosis, malnutrition, and traffic accidents. Human immunodeficiency virus (HIV) and acquired immunodeficiency syndrome (AIDS) is the most important disease affecting Malawi, accounting for 34% of deaths. The most recent prevalence rate estimated by means of antenatal blood tests is 14.4%, but research indicates that this underestimates the true prevalence (likely to be about 20%). Since the first case in 1982, HIV-related diseases have precipitated an epidemic of unprecedented proportions. The total number of people infected was recently estimated to be 700,000 to one million people. This figure includes 60,000 to 91,000 children under the age of 15 and 500,000 women. One third of those infected live in urban and two thirds in rural areas. About 160,000 have AIDS and are in need of anteretroviral therapy. Some 800,000 children are orphans as a result of parental AIDS. The epidemic seems to be levelling off despite limited changes in the practice of safe sex.

Health-Team Relationships: Because of the low doctor-patient ratio (1 per 85,000), doctors are not the authoritative health care workers in most health settings. Clinical officers, medical assistants, nurses, and health surveillance assistants play the key roles. The mental health care system is actually run by psychiatric nurses because Malawi has no psychiatrists. In the eyes of the community, medical personnel have a high social status.

Families' Role in Hospital Care: The family plays a critical role in the health care of hospitalized patients. Usually the wife or the mother stays in the hospital with the patient. Because of this practice, most public hospitals have guardian shelters built near them. They are responsible for moment-to-moment care of patients in a health care sector that is severely understaffed.

Dominance Patterns: Men are usually dominant. Even in matrilineal societies, it is the uncle or brother on the maternal side who has the decision-making responsibilities.

Eye-Contact Practices: Modesty is the rule.

Touch Practices: Physical touch among men is restricted to handshakes or holding hands. Hugs, even among close traditional family members, are rare. Many men hold hands with each other as they walk down the road, which has no sexual connotations whatsoever. Women are more expressive and often hug each other in public. Traditional men and women do not touch in public, and the sexes are kept separate. Some urban men and women who have been exposed to Western influences may hold hands.

Perceptions of Time: Time is the servant, not the master; the focus is therefore on relationships, not on time. Malawians often spend a considerable amount of time greeting others and asking about their families rather than just getting down to business. Time in Malawi is not linear; it is cyclical and based on the seasons of the calendar year. Time is tied to events. Because of the relatively low literacy rate, many rural women think of history in relation to particular events (e.g., a child's birth being "before the great drought").

Pain Reactions: It is not shameful to express physical pain. Men are expected not to express emotional pain, but it is acceptable for women to cry.

Birth Rites: The fertility rate is six children born per woman. The birth of an infant is an important event. During the seventh month of pregnancy, women give the mother advice. The father is told to refrain from sexual intercourse from this time until 4 months after birth. Traditional birth attendants play an important role in the delivery of the child. The naming process of the infant is taken seriously. The infant is normally named after an ancestor who was highly regarded. Infant mortality rates are high at 94 deaths per 1,000 live births. Life expectancy is 42 for men, 41 for women. The mother's educational level is associated with compliance with immunizations.

Death Rites: An overnight vigil is held until the day of the burial. Men spend the time outside the house, whereas women remain inside the house and usually sing if the deceased person had any church affiliation. Burial takes place within 2 to 3 days. Death causes the community to feel fractured, and people participate in funeral rituals regardless of whether they personally knew the deceased person. Malawians believe the spirit moves on to the spirit world. The grave is dug on the day of the funeral, and the ceremony usually takes place in the afternoon after everyone has eaten at the deceased's house, which is where the funeral takes place. The funeral ceremony itself does not end until the coffin is lowered and the grave has been filled with soil. Women openly wail, and men put their hands on one side of their face. Health care facilities lack the technical resources for organ donation. Autopsies are acceptable; however, because the person's spirit is moving on to the next world, those conducting the autopsy have to assure the family that they will leave the body intact afterwards.

Food Practices and Intolerances: The basic foods are corn, rice, cassava, groundnuts, dark-green leafy vegetables, sorghum, millet, fish, and fruit (which vary by season). The stable diet is *nsima,* a solidified crushed corn. Men and young children get first choice of the available food, and the most popular foods include beef and fried chicken. Especially when eating nsima, Malawians eat with their hands. Men and women in rural areas usually eat separately.

Infant-Feeding Practices: Breastfeeding is almost universal. The period of weaning in rural Malawi is normally extended until about 9 months, when children are introduced to other foods.

Child-Rearing Practices: Young children are tied to the back of their mother or another female relative. At night they usually sleep in the mother's bed or on the floor beside her bed. Child rearing is a communal responsibility. Children who are old enough move in to live with their peers. *Chinamwali* is the period of transition from childhood to adulthood. Children have a traditional "training school," during which time girls and boys go separately to an isolated location and are taught the ways of adulthood. This training involves songs and various rituals. Politeness and obedience are encouraged in girls, whereas boys are encouraged to be bold and take leadership positions.

National Childhood Immunizations: BCG at birth or during first clinic appointment; pentavaccine (including DTP, *Haemophilus influenza* and hepatitis B vaccines) at 6, 10, and 14 weeks; OPV at birth and 6, 10, and 14 weeks; measles at 9 months; vitamin A at 6 to 12 months; and TT at 15 to 45 years, +4 weeks, +6 months, +1, +1 year. The percent of the target population vaccinated, by antigen is: BCG and DTP1 (99%); DTP3 and HepB3 (93%); MCV (82%); and Polio3 (94%).

BIBLIOGRAPHY

Bomba GW, Tembo KC: Historical development of health education in Malawi from 1891–1976. The Society of Malawi Journal, 44:43–46, 1991.

Central Intelligence Agency: *2006: The world factbook, Malawi.* Retrieved September 21, 2006, from https://www.cia.gov/cia/publications/factbook/print/mi.html.

Malawi Government and World Bank: *Malawi AIDS assessment study*, vol I, Lilongwe, Malawi, 1998, NACP.

Malawi Government and World Bank: *Malawi AIDS assessment study*, vol II. Lilongwe, Malawi, 1998, NACP.

Ministry of Health and Population: *Malawi national health plan: 1999–2004*, Lilongwe, Malawi, 1999, The Ministry.

Ministry of Health: *Human resources for health sector strategic plan, 2003 to 2013*, Lilongwe, Malawi, 2003, The Ministry.

National Statistical Office (Malawi) and ORC Macro: *Malawi demographic and health survey 2000.* Zomba, Malawi, and Calverton, Maryland, National Statistic Office, 2001.

UNAIDS: 2006 Malawi. Retrieved September 21, 2006, from http://www.unaids.org/en/Regions_Countries/Countries/malawi.asp.

World Health Organization 2006: Immunization, vaccines and biologicals. Retrieved September 21, 2006, from http://www.who.int/immunization_monitoring/en/globalsummary/countryprofileresult.cfm?C='mwi'.

◆ MALAYSIA M

MAP PAGE (805)

Lee Huang Chiu and Lee Meng Lim

Location: Malaysia is situated in South East Asia, surrounded by Thailand, Indonesia, Singapore, and Brunei Darussalam. Malaysia comprises West Malaysia, the southern part of the Malay Peninsula, and East Malaysia (which consists of the states of Sabah and Sarawak on the island of Borneo). Almost 80% of the country is covered by tropical rain forests. The capital is Kuala Lumpur. Malaysia has a mountain range stretching from north to south and is surrounded by a very long coastline. The total area is 330,252 km^2 (127,520 square miles). Malaysia has 13 states, 3 federal territories, and an elected constitutional monarch, His Majesty, The Yang di-Pertuan Agong. The gross domestic product (GDP) per capita is $12,000, with 8% living below the poverty line. Literacy rates are 92% for men, 85% for women.

Major Languages	Ethnic Groups	Major Religions
Malay (official, national)	Malay and other	Muslim (Malays)
Mandarin and Chinese	indigenous 51%	Tao Buddhist
dialects (eg. Hokkien,	Chinese 24%	(Chinese)
Cantonese)	Indian 7%	Hindu (Indians)
Tamil	Other 7%	Others:
English	Indigenous 11%	Christianity,
Indigenous		Baha'i,Sikhism

    The population is 25.5 million, about 62% of whom live in urban areas. Malaysia is a multicultural and multilingual country; although the national religion is Islam, other religions are practiced freely. In addition to the major ethnic groups, Malaysia also has the tribal groups of Iban, Bidayuh, Kadazan, Dusun, and Malanau. Peninsular Malaysia names all the tribal groups under the single term *Orange Asli or Original People.* The Malays that are part of the oldest indigenous group are called *bumiputera,* which translates as "sons or princes of the soil." Ethnic groups are free to maintain their own cultures and traditions and have blended together to create Malaysia's uniquely diverse heritage.

Health Care Beliefs: Modern, traditional, herbal; other complementary medicine. Although modern medicine is the most popular, all major ethnic groups have their own traditional medicine practices. The Malays practice *bomoh,* the Chinese *sinseh,* and the Indians *ayurveda.* Herbal medicine is becoming more popular, and some herbs are considered functional or healthy foods. Complementary medicines, such as homeopathy and acupuncture, are often used as alternatives to modern medicine.

Predominant Sick-Care Practices: Biomedical and traditional. The Vision for Health, which was formulated as part of the government's Vision 2020 plan to make Malaysia a fully developed nation by the year 2020, is geared toward achieving health for all by the year 2020. It emphasizes quality, innovation, and health promotion, and stresses the importance of individual responsibility and community participation in the enhancement of the quality of life. Basic health is accessible to communities through an extensive network of health facilities ranging from flying doctor services, mobile clinics, community health clinics, hospitals, and regional referral centers. Private clinics and hospitals are mainly concentrated in urban areas. Community clinics are available in every 5-km radius to ensure access. The primary health care team plays a central role in the prevention and early detection of diseases or health problems. Doctors lead health center staff, but the main service activities such as antenatal and postnatal care, immunizations, child health care, family planning, health and nutritional education, and treatment of minor ailments are the responsibility of community nurses. Public health inspectors oversee other environmental health factors such as water supply, waste and sewage disposal, and sanitary latrines.

Ethnic-/Race-Specific or Endemic Diseases: The epidemiology and endemicity of diseases seem to relate more to geographic location, stage of community development, and seasonal variations (e.g., rainy or dry season) than to ethnicity or tribal distribution. For example, dengue and dengue hemorrhagic fevers commonly occur in urban areas, whereas malaria is more common in rural areas, especially in the swampy coastal areas or jungle fringes. Vector-borne diseases peak in dry seasons, whereas water- and food-borne diseases increase after flooding. Cholera and typhoid outbreaks are related to water supply. Rural and poor urban areas are at high risk for water contamination. The ten leading causes of mortality in Ministry of Health hospitals are septicemia; diseases of the heart and pulmonary circulation; malignant neoplasms; cerebrovascular diseases; accidents; pneumonia; conditions originating in the perinatal period; digestive system diseases; nephritis, nephrotic syndrome, and nephrosis; and chronic lower respiratory disease. The prevalence of cardiovascular disease is associated with sedentary lifestyles, fat- and cholesterol-laden food, and cigarette smoking. Malaysia is in a period of transition. It has the diseases of developed nations, such as cardiovascular diseases, diabetes mellitus, hypertension, and obesity, and also those of developing countries, such as tuberculosis, sexually transmitted diseases, food and water-borne diseases, and chronic energy deficiency. The Joint United Nations Programme on HIV/AIDS (UNAIDS) estimates the prevalence rate for human immunodeficiency virus (HIV) in adults (aged 15 to 49 years) to be 0.5%, and 69,000 are living with HIV, including 17,000 women. About 4,000 deaths are attributed to acquired immunodeficiency syndrome (AIDS).

Families' Role in Hospital Care: Community and family support is strong when it comes to caring for the sick, those with disabilities, and older adults. Hospitalization or institutionalization is only used as a last resort. Visiting the sick in hospitals, bringing them food, and accompanying them in their rooms are the norm. Family members take turns spending the night with hospitalized relatives.

Dominance Patterns: Traditionally, the head of the family is a man, although the dominant person may vary. For example, the grandfather may have the most power, and the mother-in-law may have some input into decision-making. Gender issues do not affect dominance patterns of the family significantly. Taboos for menstruating women are quite common. However, the Malays, who previously referred to menstruation as "dirty" now refer to it as "a monthly affair." With changes in modern lifestyles, women have more freedom.

Touch Practices: Medical examinations by the opposite sex are acceptable, although some patients prefer to be examined by same-sex doctors. Eye contact and physical touching during taking a patient's history and performing a physical examination are normal. Exposure of private body parts such as women's breasts and genitalia is minimized. A chaperone is often a must if a male doctor examines a female patient.

Perceptions of Time: Generally speaking, punctuality depends on the occasion. Malaysians are usually punctual for prayers, business appointments, and job interviews. On other occasions, especially those involving larger groups—such as wedding ceremonies, public speeches, meetings, and festive parties—being 30 minutes to an hour late is common. Being on time for personal appointments or dates depends on the individual. Although time perceptions change with time, many Malaysians, except city dwellers, still move at a leisurely pace.

Pain Reactions: Pain tolerance and reactions seem to be related to ethnicity. Indians seem to have the lowest threshold of pain, followed by the Malays and Chinese. During labor, Indian women tend to cry out the most. The Chinese immediately seek medical advice for any pain or discomfort. Malays, on the other hand, usually wait for a while and then consult traditional practitioners, with modern practitioners a last resort.

Birth Rites: Primigravida women, grand-multipara women, and women with medical problems must give birth in a hospital. Home deliveries are encouraged for mothers with uncomplicated second, third, or fourth pregnancies and are usually attended by trained personnel. Pregnant women with potential complications who go to community clinics or health centers are referred to district or general hospitals for further assistance. The fertility rate is three children born per woman, and the infant mortality rate is 17 deaths per 1,000 live births. When the abdomen of a pregnant woman becomes obviously larger in the seventh month of gestation, some Malay families throw a small party *(melenggang perut)* for first-time mothers to announce the expected arrival of an additional family member. Food supplementation with vitamins or iron is avoided because the Malays believe they may cause the infant to become too large and result in a difficult delivery. During pregnancy, it is generally believed that certain foods must be avoided; for example, pineapple and papayas are "sharp" and may cause abortion. Pumpkins and leafy vegetables produce flatulence and are also avoided. A pregnant mother is not allowed to participate in certain activities, such as sewing, or killing or injuring an animal because these activities might deform the infant. Pregnant women must have their food cravings fulfilled; otherwise, their infants could develop mental problems or a "watery mouth." Eating freshwater fish is encouraged because it helps to heal wounds. Participation in household activities is encouraged to promote an easy delivery. During labor, traditional birth attendants and trained midwives *(bidan)* are called to assist in home deliveries. The traditional birth attendant performs the necessary rituals, and the midwives assist in the birth by cutting the cord, bathing the infant, and taking care of the perineum. After childbirth, the mother is encouraged to eat "heaty food" such as ginger, garlic and pepper to keep the body warm. Ignoring the medical establishment's denigration of this care, pregnant women still flock to midwives for massage, herbs, and emotional support, a testimony to its effectiveness. Women appreciate how midwives respect both their bodies and the families' spiritual connection with their newborns.

During the postpartum period, the new mother is forbidden to leave the house or participate in cooking and cleaning and coming in contact with cold water, but she is expected to move around the house as soon as she feels well; too much rest is believed to prolong the flow of the "contaminating" blood. Traditional massages are still performed to improve uterine contractions and involution. Birth attendants do the massage as midwives bathe the mother and infant daily for a week. On the 7th day after birth, a small party is organized by some Malays to name the infant and is followed by another party on the 40th day after birth to mark the end of the puerperium. On the 30th day, the Chinese usually celebrate the baby's 1-month birthday. Life expectancy is 70 for men, 75 for women.

Death Rites: Death is thought of as a journey into the next world. The family and community members gather to pay their last respects and bid farewell to the deceased. Death rites differ according to religion. Muslim burials are carried out as soon as possible, preferably on the day of death. Other religions may have funerals a few days later. Cremation is not allowed for Muslims, although people of other religions may choose cremation. In a Muslim burial, the body is wrapped in a white cloth and buried without a coffin in the ground. Malaysian Muslims forbid organ donation after death, although giving blood or other parts of the body, such as skin, bone marrow, or kidneys, while a person is alive, is acceptable. Autopsies are uncommon and performed only for forensic reasons, as the body must be buried intact.

Food Practices and Intolerances: Staple foods are rice and bread, but the average diet includes a large variety of foods. Rice and bread are eaten with meat, fish, poultry, and vegetables, with fruit as dessert. Food restrictions primarily involve those who are fasting during Ramadan. Muslims do not consume pork, carrion, blood, or alcoholic beverages. Hindus do not eat beef, and Buddhists are often vegetarians. Traditional Malaysians sit on the floor and eat with their fingers from an individual plate. The right hand is used, as it is considered taboo to use the left, which is kept for less clean functions. Today, most eat at a table and use forks and spoons. The Chinese use chopsticks.

M

Infant-Feeding Practices: Most mothers breastfeed their infants. Mixed feeding (breast and bottle feeding) usually starts when mothers resume working. Breastfeeding usually lasts for 18 months, but exclusive breastfeeding may only last for 4 months. Solid foods are given to infants as young as 4 months. Mashed banana and rice porridge are common infant foods.

Child-Rearing Practices: Traditionally, children sleep with parents for the first few years. Toilet training can occur earlier or after a child learns to talk, depending on the individual family. Disciplining children is usually the father's duty because he is considered the person of authority. Most parents expect their children to be obedient, and corporal punishment is acceptable. Male circumcision is usually performed between the ages of 6 to 15 years for Muslims, although it can be done as young as at birth or as old as 20 years old.

National Childhood Immunizations: BCG at birth and 6 years if no scar; DTwP at 18 months; DTwPHib at at 2, 3, and 5 months; OPV at 2, 3, 5, and 18 months and at 7 years; HepB at birth and at 2, 3, and 5 months; measles at 6 months (in Sabah only); Japanese B encephalitis at 9, 10, and 18 months and at 4 and 7 years (in Sarawak only); MMR at 12 months and at 7 years; rubella at 12 years; DT at 7 years; and TT at 15 years and for pregnant women at 18 weeks' gestation. The percent of the target population vaccinated, by antigen is: BCG (99%); and DTP1, DTP3, HepB3, Hib3, MCV, and Polio3 (90%). Malaysia was certified as being polio-free in 2000 and has achieved elimination of neonatal tetanus.

Other Characteristics: Malaysian Chinese have a family name or surname, and it comes first before the given names. Malaysian Chinese are usually addressed by their first name, which is the surname. However, other Malaysians do not have a family name. Their last name is the father's name, but they are always addressed by the first name, which is their name. Women do not change their names after marriage.

BIBLIOGRAPHY

Central Intelligence Agency: *2006: The world factbook, Malaysia.* Retrieved September 21, 2006, from https://www.cia.gov/cia/publications/factbook/print/my.html.

Department of Statistics: Retrieved January 19, 2006, from http://www/statistics. gov.my/index.php.

Malaysia, Culture & People: Retrieved January 19, 2006, from http://www.geographia.com/malaysia/cultures.html.

Ministry of Health Malaysia: *Immunization schedule for Malaysia.* Retrieved March 22, 2006, from http://www.mpaeds.org.my/Paediatric/Protocals/0.2.%20Immunisation.pdf.

NATO Secretary General: Visits/daily press brief. Bureau of East Asia and Pacific Affairs, September 2005. Retrieved March 21, 2006, from http://www.state. gov/r/pa/ei/bgn/2777.htm.

UNAIDS: 2006 Malaysia. Retrieved September 21, 2006, from http://www.unaids. org/en/Regions_Countries/Countries/malaysia.asp.

World Health Organization (WHO) Regional Office for the Western Pacific: Malaysia environmental health country profile, 2005. Retrieved January 24, 2006, from http://www.wpro.who.int/countries/05maa/.

M

◆ MALDIVES (REPUBLIC OF)

MAP PAGE (804)

Andrew Robertson

Location: Formerly the Maldive Islands, the country is made up of atolls: 1,190 small coral islands (about 200 of which are inhabited). No island's area is greater than 13 km^2 (5 square miles), and all are flat. Maldives is located in the Indian Ocean, 480 km southwest of the southern tip of India. Inhabitants are primarily Islamic seafaring people, probably descendents of people from India and Sri Lanka. Before becoming a republic in

1965, Maldives was a sultanate. Most transportation involves a boat or seaplane. Maldives has two monsoon periods: the northeast *(ruvai)* from December through March and the southwest *(ulhangu)* from April to November. The temperature is about 28° C (82° F) all year. The total area is 300 km^2 (116 square miles), and Malé is the capital. With a population of 359,008, the Maldives is one of the world's least developed countries; its gross domestic product (GDP) per capita is $3,900.

Major Languages	Ethnic Groups	Major Religions
Maldivian Divehi (official)	Sinhalese	Shafi'ite Sunni Muslim (state religion) 100%
English	Dravidian	
Arabic	Arab	
Hindi	African	
	Indian	

Dhivehi is a dialect of Sinhala, and English is spoken primarily by government officials. No religions other than Muslim are permitted, and adherence to Islam is required for citizenship. Literacy rates are 97% for both men and women.

Health Care Beliefs: Acute sick care; traditional. Attitudes about health and hygiene-related concerns are generally conservative, and until recently only limited focus was given to health promotion and disease prevention. In 2000, the Health Promotion Plan was introduced. Despite rapid population growth, family-planning programs were not effective until the 1980s, when nongovernmental programs focused on improving overall health and included birth spacing and later age of marriage. The World Health Organization (WHO) monitored the use of various contraceptive methods for 4 years in the mid-1980s, but by the 1990s the government still had not taken action to reduce the number of children born per couple. Because it is an Islamic culture, women are modest about exposure of the body during physical examinations. Health care beliefs are influenced by traditional beliefs involving evil spirits called *jinnis* that can come from the land, sea, or sky. When modern medical methods cannot adequately explain reasons for illness, jinnis are often thought to be the cause, and people resort to using various charms and spells to combat them. Some observers have identified a magico-religious system parallel to Islam known as *fanditha*, which provides a way for people to deal with actual or perceived problems.

Predominant Sick-Care Practices: Biomedical and some magico-religious. Health services are organized into a five-tier referral system that comprises the central health services, including the referral hospital, regional hospitals, atoll hospitals, atoll health centers, and island health posts. The tertiary level Indira Gandhi Memorial Hospital in Malé embodies the fifth or highest referral level. There are also two private hospitals in Malé. The fourth level is the five regional hospitals. They provide secondary level clinical services and, through public health units, implement preventive health programs to two to five atolls. The third level is the four atoll hospitals, which serve high-population atolls with difficult access to regional hospitals; they can handle obstetric and surgical emergencies. The atoll health center is the second level, with one to three centers per atoll. Doctors provide primary care and limited secondary care in attached wards, and community health workers provide preventive services. Finally, the island health post is at the first level, and family health workers provide limited primary care and preventive services. The resources in health facilities are limited at all levels, and some medications are not available. Many doctors are Indian expatriates.

Ethnic-/Race-Specific or Endemic Diseases: Endemic diseases include dengue, diarrheal diseases, and acute respiratory infections. Malaria was eradicated in 1984. Water-borne diseases (e.g., gastroenteritis, typhoid) are prevalent because of limited potable water supplies in the atolls; the freshwater table is shallow and easily contaminated by organic and human waste. About 77% of the population has reasonable access to safe drinking water. Efforts have been made to address this problem, but no sewerage plants exist in the other islands and sewerage systems are limited. There were scrub typhus outbreaks in 2002 and 2003. Like Tristan de Cunha and the Caroline Islands, Maldives has the highest prevalence for asthma in the world. People are at risk for β-thalassemia, histoplasmosis, tuberculosis, leptospirosis, measles, eye infections, salmonella, leprosy, and filariasis. Since the 1970s, WHO has carried out numerous disease-eradication projects. HIV continues to be well-controlled. UNAIDS estimates the prevalence of HIV in adults (aged 15 to 49 years) as less than 0.2%. The cumulative total of positive local cases since screening began in 1991 stood at 11 at the end of 2003. On the other hand, because of a comprehensive screening program, a cumulative total of 123 positive cases was documented among immigrant workers.

Dominance Patterns: Individual freedoms related to religion and workers' and women's rights are restricted. The legal system is based on Islamic (shari'a) law. A significant gap exists between the elite on Malé (the traditional home of the sultans) and the populations of the other islands. Ruling families control much of the government, business, and religion. Regional control over atolls is exerted by *atolu verin,* or atoll chiefs, and the *gazi,* or community religious leaders. About 80% of the households consist of a single nuclear, rather than an extended family, and the man is the head of the household. Descent is patrilineal. Women maintain their maiden names after marriage, and inheritance of property can be through both men and women. Muslim men may have as many as four wives. However, divorces are easy to obtain by men or women, and Maldives has one of the highest divorce rates in the world. According to a recent census, almost 50% of women older than 30 had been married four or more times, and half the women had been married by age 15. The status of women is surprisingly high; the country has had four sultanas (female sultans). Women do not wear veils and are not strictly secluded except in mosques and during certain public gatherings.

Birth Rites: The infant mortality rate is decreasing and is about 14 deaths per 1000 live births. The fertility rate is five children born per woman. Contraception rates, using modern methods, have increased from 10% in 1991 to 32% in 1999. Abortion is not legal. Life expectancy is 70 for men, 71 for women.

Death Rites: Autopsies are uncommon because the body must be buried intact. Cremation is not permitted. For Muslim burials, the body is wrapped in special pieces of cloth and buried without a coffin in the ground as soon as possible after death.

Food Practices and Intolerances: Only 10% of the land is arable. Food produced includes coconuts, taro, and limited fruits and vegetables such as millet, corn, sweet potatoes, and watermelons. Fish and rice are staple foods; meat and chicken are consumed primarily on special occasions. National dishes include fish soup, fish curry, and fried fish. Alcohol is not generally available in this Muslim country, but a local brew *(raa)* is made from the crown of the palm trunk. A local nut (arecanut) is commonly chewed with cloves, lime, and betel leaf after dinner. Nutritional studies have reported marginal nutritional status and marginal malnutrition because of low intakes of fat, fruits, and vegetables; this is of particular concern for children.

Child-Rearing Practices: Unmarried adults usually remain with relatives rather than live on their own. About 46% of the population is 14 or younger. Maldives has three types of schools: Koranic, Dhivehi-language, and English-language. Most students attend Koranic schools that charge a fee rather than the free government-sponsored schools. University education is unavailable, so students must go overseas.

National Childhood Immunizations: BCG at birth to 3 years; DTwP at 6, 10, and 14 weeks; OPV at birth and 8, 12, and 16 weeks; HepB at birth and 4 and 12 weeks; measles at 9 months; vitamin A at 6 months to 14 years; and TT CBAW at 15 to 49 years. The percent of the target population vaccinated, by antigen, is: BCG and DTP1 (99%); DTP3, HepB3, and Polio3 (98%); MCV (97%); TT2 plus (95%); and vitamin A (98%).

Other Characteristics: Maldives has rapid economic growth that has resulted in modernization of the infrastructure and improved social indicators. The Maldives was seriously damaged by the Asian tsunami on December 26, 2004, including damage to much of the health infrastructure and the regional and atoll hospitals.

BIBLIOGRAPHY

Central Intelligence Agency: 2006: The world factbook, Maldives. Retrieved September 21, 2006, from https://www.cia.gov/cia/publications/factbook/print/mv.html.

Country Health Profile—Maldives: Retrieved February 26, 2006, from http://w3. whosea.org/cntryhealth/maldives/malstatics.htm.

Firdous N: Prevention of thalassaemia and haemoglobinopathies in remote and isolated communities—the Maldives experience, *Ann Hum Biol.* 32(2):131–137, 2005.

Golder AM Erhardt JG, Scherbaum V, Saeed M, Biesalski HK, Furst P: Dietary intake and nutritional status of women and pre-school children in the Republic of the Maldives, *Public Health Nutr* 4(3):773, 2001.

Lim S, Tackett D: Maldives, 3rd ed. Singapore, 1999, APA Publications.

Mietz C, Stoll C: Maldives, Slovenia, 1999, Munich, Germany. Nelles Verlag.

Ministry of Health: The Maldives health report 2004, Maldives, 2004, Ministry of Health. (retrieved February 26, 2006).

Neville A: Dhivehi Raajje—a portrait of Maldives, Seoul, 2003, Seven Holidays.

Robertson AG, Dwyer DE, Leclercq MG: "Operation South East Asia Tsunami Assist": an Australian team in the Maldives, Med J Aust. 182(7):340–342, 2005.

Healthweb: Retrieved February 26, 2006, from http://www.health.gov.mv/.

UNAIDS: 2006 Maldives. Retrieved September 21, 2006, from http://www.unaids. org/en/Regions_Countries/Countries/maldives.asp.

WHO Maldives: Retrieved February 26, 2006, from http://www.who.org.mv/EN/ Index.htm.

World Health Organization (WHO): 2006: Immunization, vaccines and biologicals. Retrieved September 21, 2006, from http://www.who.int/immunization_monitor-ing/en/globalsummary/countryprofileresult.cfm?C='mdv'.

http://www.health.gov.mv/latest%20publications/ebooks/pdf/stat%20docs/HR200 4final.pdf (Retrieved March 1, 2006).

✦ MALI (REPUBLIC OF)

MAP PAGE (800)

Kathleen Slobin

Location: Mali is a landlocked country in the Sudanic belt of West Africa. Its total area is 1,240,000 km² (478,765 square miles), of which nearly 60% is desert. The capital is Bamako. Its southern borders, which parallel the meandering Senegal and Niger Rivers, are fixed by the boundaries of Guinea, the Ivory Coast, Burkina Faso, and Niger. Its northern border juts upward into the Sahara Desert, adjoining Mauritania to the northwest, Algeria to the northeast, and Senegal in the west at the Falémé River. Only 11% of Mali's total surface supports cultivation, resulting in a large variation in distribution of the population corresponding to three climate zones: the southern Sudanic, middle Sahelian, and northern Sahara. The Senegal and Niger Rivers and their flood plains support transport, commerce, fishing, cultivation, and animal husbandry.

Major Languages	Ethnic Groups	Major Religions
French (official)	Mande (Bambara,	Muslim 90%
Local languages	Malinke, Sarakole) 50%	Indigenous beliefs 9%
Bamana	Peul (Fulani) 17%	Christian 1%
Fulfulde	Voltaic 12%	
Soninke	Songhai 6%	
Songhay	Tuareg/Moor 10%	
	Other 5%	

The Republic of Mali is a multiparty democracy. It is among the poorest of developing countries, with a gross domestic product (GDP) per capita of

$1,200; 64% are living below the poverty line. About 70% of its 12.2 million people live in rural areas, and about 47% is younger than 15. About 10% is nomadic, and some 80% is engaged in farming and fishing. The many ethnic groups, tradition-based and largely subsistence economies and the wide range of urban to rural lifestyles make it difficult to generalize about cultural beliefs and practices. Although French is the language of government, other official languages include Bamana (Bambara), Bomu, Bozo, Dogoso (Dogon), Fulfulde (Fulani), Hasanya, Mamara, Maninkakan (Malinke), Soninke, Sonoy, Songhay, Tamasheq, and Xaasongaxanno. Fifty living languages are regularly used. Official estimates of religious affiliation do not adequately reflect the variation in beliefs and practices encountered. The literacy rate is 54% for men, 40% for women. Many who proclaim themselves Muslim or Christian continue to integrate indigenous rituals, meanings, and practices into their relatively new faiths.

Health Care Beliefs: Acute sick care; traditional. Health care beliefs and practices reflect the ethnic and religious diversity that facilitates medical pluralism. The traditional view of illness is associated with a lack of balance between the physical and spiritual being. Even as urban and town dwellers accept the efficacy of biomedicine for some illnesses, they tend to retain their belief in indigenous medical practices, which involve the spiritual and emotional aspects of causes of illness. Indigenous classification systems identify illness as being in one of the following categories: illnesses of God, of the bush, of ancestors, and sorcery. Illnesses of the bush are said to be caused by spirits or the wind. Illnesses of the ancestors are punishments for breaking local customs or mores. Illnesses resulting from sorcery are caused by a person's enemies, people who use curses, poisons, or charms to harm others. Illnesses of God refer to simple, short-term sicknesses that follow a natural course. The illnesses in this category, such as malaria or influenza, are most readily adapted to the physical and mechanical framework of biomedicine.

Predominant Sick-Care Practices: Biomedical and magico-religious. In Bamako, publicly funded biomedical clinics staffed by doctors, nurses, and nurse practitioners operate in proximity to Muslim religious healers and indigenous specialists. Treatment choices among urban and village residents depend more on the type and duration of illness than on the proximity of care. Typically, biomedical treatments are sought by individuals who have acute ailments attributed to natural causes. Indigenous treatments are sought by those who have an illness that persists and becomes associated with sorcery or spirit possession. Within the indigenous sector of medicine, ill people or family members may consult diviners for an initial diagnosis and then consult healers who are known for their ability to treat the diagnosed illness. The healer in turn may prescribe a complex set of remedial measures that might include a combination of herbal medicine, prayers, amulets, sacrifices, or good deeds. In this sector, physical ailments are treated as culturally significant manifestations of disorder. Treatments, in turn, are activities that restore health and support the desired unfolding of events.

M

Ethnic-/Race-Specific or Endemic Diseases: Endemic diseases include chloroquine-resistant malaria, yellow fever, cholera, syphilis, leprosy, brucellosis, onchocerciasis, trypanosomiasis, and schistosomiasis. The Joint United Nations Programme on HIV/AIDS (UNAIDS) estimates that the prevalence of human immunodeficiency virus (HIV) in adults (aged 15 to 49 years) is 1.9% and that between 96,000 and 160,000 people are living with HIV. About 16,000 children aged 0 to 14 are living with HIV, and 11,000 deaths from acquired immunodeficiency syndrome (AIDS) have been reported. The number of children orphaned because of parental AIDS is 70,000; representing 12% of all orphans in Mali.

Health-Team Relationships: Health-team relationships are organized hierarchically, with doctors maintaining diagnostic and treatment authority over nurses and technical staff. Similarly, in maternity clinics, the nurse consults with a doctor but maintains authority over technical staff. In rural areas, these arrangements vary depending on the availability of trained personnel. Biomedical practitioners may consult or work with local healers if such an arrangement is thought to be in the best interests of the patient. Furthermore, biomedical personnel may train village birth attendants or other village health aids to act as clinic liaisons, provide simple medications, and administer prescribed injections. Finally, health and illness in Mali are family affairs, and the health team typically works to establish good relationships with members of a patient's family.

Families' Role in Hospital Care: In urban areas and especially in small towns, the family is the primary caregiver in the hospital. Family members typically provide meals, monitor the patient's condition, and attend to all the patient's daily needs. The relationship between the doctor and the family is important and is characterized by a certain interdependence maintained by communication and mutual respect. Forms of interaction between health care personnel and family members are not unlike those found between indigenous healers and their clients; therapeutic relationships are facilitated by responsive, open, and negotiated forms of communication.

Dominance Patterns: Among settled agricultural groups (e.g., Bambara, Dogon), village life is typically ordered by extended families and sustained by a male hierarchy in which the oldest male is accorded the most respect. Among the nomadic groups, whose subsistence depends largely on animal husbandry (e.g., Fula [Fulani], Tuareg), male hierarchies are sustained in the smaller family groups. Village and clan hierarchies are usually ordered in accordance with descending relationships of dominance from families of the chief, or royal family; to commoners; and then to persons of caste, who typically are artisans (e.g., blacksmiths, leather workers, musicians). Men are responsible for major crop production, family economy, and making decisions. Women are responsible for food preparation, providing water and cooking fuel, gardening, and child care. Marriage and family customs generally follow the patrilineal pattern, with wives becoming members of the husband's family. Many groups also practice polygyny. Wives are subordinate to their husbands. Men have conjugal rights, paternity rights to the children, and control over their wives' labor; wives must request land and permission to work from their husband. Still, through their gardening and marketing skills, women can develop some financial independence. This pattern differs among nomadic groups (Fula and Tuareg), in which monogamy and nuclear family units tend to promote greater intimacy between husbands and wives.

Eye-Contact Practices: Variations in eye contact in public tend to be dictated by gender relationships and positions of authority. Women lower their eyes and heads while talking to a man or a stranger; however, when women work in the marketing arena, work next to men in the fields, or make a request, their eye contact is more direct. In general, modesty and respect are the rule for both men and women.

Touch Practices: Practices vary among ethnic groups. Generally, men and women do not shake hands. Young adolescent women and men may hold hands while walking down the street, but this is uncommon among adults. Certain groups (e.g., Dogon) have various comportment taboos. For example, in certain Dogon villages, menstruating women are isolated, and all women of childbearing age remove their shoes on village pathways and may not enter the blacksmith's forge. These practices are more strictly observed in villages where either the chief or most of the inhabitants observe indigenous religious practices.

Perceptions of Time: Perceptions of time are typically related to seasonal agricultural requirements. The temporal ebb and flow of the river flood planes are significant for nomadic groups. Among practicing Muslims, daily prayers break the day into five units. Furthermore, when recounting events or telling stories, time might be organized according to a birth, a death, or a national or religious holiday. In urban centers, use and perception of time are beginning to reflect European influence.

Pain Reactions: Malians tend to be stoical in their response to life's difficulties and pain. Women in the predominant ethnic groups rarely cry out during childbirth. Child rearing practices, which promote modesty, nobility, and shame as responses to self-promotion or self-display, prepare men and women to tolerate and bear adversity.

Birth Rites: The birth of a boy is usually preferred; however, girls are appreciated because they will later bear children and through marriage will strengthen the family. The fertility rate is seven children born per woman. Because all the ethnic groups are patrilineal, children are said to belong to their father. In case of divorce, the child stays with the mother until weaning or soon thereafter and then joins the father's household. Today an estimated 41% of infants are born in a maternity clinic or with the aid of a skilled birth attendant. Among village and nomadic groups, women go through childbirth alone or with the help of their mother or mother-in-law. Women's primary responsibilities are to bear and raise children. Generally the newborn stays in the confines of the birthplace, being nursed and protected by the mother. At about a week of age, the infant is baptized, given a name, and presented to the community. The infant mortality rate is 117 deaths per 1,000 live births. Indicators for children under age 5 cite a rate of 225 per 100 for boys, 216 for girls. Immediate causes of death are malaria, respiratory and diarrheal infections, and malnutrition. Life expectancy is 47 for men, 51 for women.

Death Rites: Rituals associated with death vary. Although Muslims typically wrap the body in cloth and bury it without a coffin in the ground within 24 hours of the death, many continue to follow traditional indigenous practices. Both Muslim and traditional practices include periods of mourning when relatives and community members stop work and pay their respects to the family. Some groups, such as the Dogon, are known for the elaborate ritual practices associated with the death of significant members of the community. On an appointed day about a year after such a death, the young men dress in costumes and masks to represent spirits of the bush. They enter the village and dance and escort the dead person's spirit out into the wilderness.

Food Practices and Intolerances: Many urban dwellers have adopted the European diet with fish, meat, vegetables, and rice. Rural inhabitants typically eat millet porridge, couscous, or rice with either a vegetable or fish sauce. Seasonally available vegetables such as tomatoes, carrots, okra, and onions and fruits such as mangos are also eaten. Nomadic groups rely heavily on animal milk products, although they incorporate dietary grains purchased from or traded with local farmers. For holidays and celebrations, animals (goats or sheep) may be killed and roasted for the entire community. On such occasions, millet beer is produced by women and sold to the men who drink and enjoy the added revelry. Muslims do not eat pork.

Infant-Feeding Practices: Most women nurse their infants until age 2 years. However, the 2001 Demographic and Health Survey reports that only 68% of 6- to 9-month old children receive the supplemental solid food recommended by the World Health Organization (WHO). Typically, weaning is prompted by the birth of another child. Weaning is a critical and difficult time for children because mothers have few nutritious substitutes for breast milk. The primary supplementary food is liquid millet or rice porridge. Although eggs, fish, and vegetables might be available, they are typically not offered to young children.

Child-Rearing Practices: During the first 3 years, children stay near their mother's side. Infants are wrapped on the mother's back and nursed on demand, and they learn the language and the rhythms of the household. At the second stage, from 7 to 8 years, the child plays freely among members of the extended family. Boys join their brothers and male cousins, and girls play with their sisters and begin to help their mother with daily chores. During the third stage, which lasts until puberty, children's behavior is seriously monitored to ensure the development of certain values (e.g., modesty, nobility, respect, diligence) prized by the group. At the end of this stage, boys are circumcised and girls, who are typically circumcised at a younger age, begin to menstruate. Only 75% of the children reach grade 5 in school.

National Childhood Immunizations: BCG at birth; DTwP at 6, 10, and 14 weeks; DTwPHibHep at 6, 10, and 14 weeks (in part of country);

OPV at birth and at 6, 10, and 14 weeks; HepB at 6, 10, and 14 weeks; measles at 9 months; vitamin A at 6 months; YF at 9 months; TT first contact, +1, +6 months, +1, +1 year (CBAW at 15 to 49 years). The percent of the target population vaccinated, by antigen, is: BCG (82%); DPT1 (95%); DTP3 and HepB (85%); Polio3 (84%); MCV (86%); TT2 plus (75%); and Hib3 (3%).

BIBLIOGRAPHY

Adams AM, Madhavan S, Dominique S: Women's social networks and child survival in Mali, *Soc Sci Med.* 54:165–178, 2002.

Central Intelligence Agency: 2006: The world factbook, Mali. Retrieved September 21, 2006, from https://www.cia.gov/cia/publications/factbook/print/ml.htm.

Demographic & Health Surveys: Retrieved February 25, 2006, from http://www.measuredhs.com/countries/country.cfm?ctry_id=25. 2001.

Ethnologue: Retrieved February 25, 2006, from http://www.ethnologue.com. 2005.

Slobin K: Repairing broken rules: care-seeking narratives for menstrual problems in rural Mali, *Med Anthropol Q.* 12(3):363–383, 1998.

Slobin K: Healing through the use of symbolic technologies among the Dogon of Mali, *High Plains App Anthrop.* 16 (2):136–143, 1996.

UNAIDS: 2006 Mali. Retrieved September 21, 2006, from http://www.unaids.org/en/Regions_Countries/Countries/mali.asp.

UNAIDS/UNICEF: Children on the brink. Retrieved February 25, 2006, from http://www.unicef.org/publications/index_4378.html. 2002.

UNICEF: *Enfants et femmes au Mali.* Paris, 1989, L'UNICEF aux Editions: L'Harmattan.

World Health Organization: HIV/AIDS epidemiological surveillance report for the WHO African Region: 2005 update. Retrieved February 25, 2006, from http://www.who.int/hiv/pub/epidemiology/hivinafrica2005e_web.pdf.

World Health Organization: 2006: Immunization, vaccines and biologicals. Retrieved September 21, 2006, from http://www.who.int/immunization_monitoring/en/globalsummary/countryprofileresult.cfm?C='mli'.

M

◆ MALTA (REPUBLIC OF)

MAP PAGE (798)

Charles Savona-Ventura

Location: The Maltese archipelago consists of three islands: Malta, Gozo, and Comino. It is located in the middle of the Mediterranean Sea 93 km (58 miles) south of Sicily and 288 km (179 miles) from the nearest point on the North African mainland. Together, the islands have a land area of 316 km^2 (122 square miles). The largest island of the group is Malta. Valletta, the capital, is the cultural, administrative, and commercial center of the Maltese islands. Topographically, the islands consist of a series of low hills with characteristic terraced fields and several natural harbors. The climate is Mediterranean, with mild, rainy winters and hot, dry summers. The gross domestic product (GDP) per capita is $19,900. Literacy rates are 92% for men, 94% for women.

Major Languages	**Ethnic Groups**	**Major Religions**
Maltese (official)	Maltese 98%	Roman Catholic
English (official)	Other 2%	(official) 91%
Italian (widely spoken)		Other 9%

The Maltese are descendents of ancient Carthaginians and Phoenicians, with strong Greco-Roman and Arab influences. European elements—namely Italian, Spanish, and French with traces of Anglo-Saxon origins—were assimilated. With a population of 404,039 persons in the 2005 census, the country has one of the highest population densities (more than 1265 people per km^2) in the world. In the last 10 years, 4,744 migrants have returned to Malta, most from the United Kingdom (33%), Australia (25%), Canada (9%), and the United States (13%). There has also been an influx of migrants from North Africa.

Health Care Beliefs: Active involvement; health promotion important. Over the last two decades, there has been increasing awareness of the links between lifestyle and chronic diseases. The population generally strives to follow general guidelines of health promotion. The national health sector incorporated a health-promotion agency that in the last decade has initiated national campaigns for health education related to nutrition and smoking. Other campaigns are for sexually transmitted diseases, exercise, and other specific disease awareness.

Predominant Sick-Care Practices: Biomedical and religious. The Maltese are very health conscious when they feel unwell. Their first step is usually to consult their family doctor, although they frequently consult a specialist even for relatively minor disorders. Folk medicine is no longer practiced, but religious traditions still influence health attitudes among older adults and very religious people regarding an incurable disease. Recourse is then made to increasing participation in private and public religious services and attendance at faith-healing services.

Ethnic-/Race-Specific or Endemic Disease: Dietary changes associated with a higher standard of living have contributed to making the metabolic syndrome the primary health problem of the population. Obesity (aged 55 to 64 years, men 77% and women 85%); late-onset diabetes mellitus (more than 15 years, men 12.0% and women 14.4%); hypercholesterolemia (men 72%, women 75%), and hypertension (26%) are all common conditions. Long-term complications from these conditions (e.g., coronary heart disease and stroke) cause 33% of all deaths. Neoplasms account for 23% of deaths, with lung (4% of all deaths), large bowel (3%), and breast (2%) being the most common. Endocrine-related malignancies such as endometrial cancer and breast cancer in women appear to be higher than the European average. Because of the high population density and resulting road-traffic density, accidents are an important cause of death (0.5%). Certain genetic disorders, such as thalassemia and glucose-6-phosphate dehydrogenase (G6PD) deficiency, are endemic. Communicable diseases of major public health significance include food-borne illnesses such as salmonellosis, *Campylobacter* infections, and meningococcal disease. Infections such as murine typhus (spread by rats), tick-borne typhus, leishmaniasis and brucellosis are endemic to the islands. The Joint United Nations Programme on HIV/AIDS (UNAIDS) reports that the estimated prevalence rate for human immunodeficiency virus (HIV) in adults (aged 15 to 49 years) is 0.1%, with fewer than 500 people living with HIV. Fewer than 1,000 deaths from acquired immunodeficiency syndrome (AIDS) are estimated. Reliable data on HIV cases has been collected only since June 2004. Seventeen new cases of AIDS have been reported in the last 5 years, generally transmitted by homosexuals. No local outbreaks of HIV infection have been reported in intravenous drug abusers, who, however, have high prevalence rates of hepatitis C infection.

Health-Team Relationships: The medical profession retains a dominant position over other health care professionals, although interprofessional working relationships are generally good. In state hospitals, nursing and midwifery has increasingly undertaken self-management to establish a professional niche.

Families' Role in Hospital Care: Generally, families pay close attention to their hospitalized relatives and visit them regularly. Social problems experienced by most families, compounded by restricted entry to the state's "old people's" hospice, often induces relatives to leave sick and incapacitated older individuals as hospital inpatients in the hope they will obtain early admission into the hospice.

Dominance Patterns: Malta has a typical patriarchal culture; however, the mother has near absolute control in the domestic arena, especially for education and child care issues. Legislation ensures equal opportunities for the sexes, but male dominance still remains the norm on executive boards, in top management positions, and in the civil service.

Eye-Contact Practices: It is considered polite to maintain eye contact during a conversation. The listener maintains the eye contact continuously, whereas the speaker may avert the eyes occasionally during the dialogue.

Touch Practices: The Maltese have basic Mediterranean attitudes, and both sexes are very expressive when speaking, using gestures and hand movements. Physical touching, particularly of arms and shoulders, is part of this expression. During greetings, a simple handshake is expected and may be accompanied by hand, arm, or shoulder clasping or an embrace, depending on how well the individuals know each other. Kissing both cheeks is also common, especially between women and between women and men they know (e.g., family members, close friends).

Perceptions of Time: Because of their relaxed Mediterranean attitudes, the Maltese do not consider punctuality to be extremely important, regardless of social class. In general, Maltese feel the need to look toward the future. They tend to maintain traditions but at the same time adapt to change.

Pain Reactions: Attitudes and reactions to pain are generally Mediterranean: overtly expressive.

Birth Rites: The fertility rate is 1.5 children born per woman. Pregnancy termination remains illegal. The infant mortality rate is low at 4 per 1,000 live births; congenital anomalies account for 48% of these deaths. Most births occur in hospitals with standard obstetric practices and supervision. Normal deliveries are conducted by trained midwives supervised by an obstetric specialist. Old folklore beliefs are basically extinct, although pregnant women occasionally inquire about beliefs heard from the older generation. Some women opt for alternative means of pain relief such as water births and homeopathy, but they retain specialist medical supervision. Life expectancy is 77 for men, 81 for women.

Death Rites: Attitudes toward death are generally positive because of strong Christian beliefs in an afterlife. Mourning involves demonstrative expressions of emotions by surviving family members and close friends. The funeral services include a church service followed by a burial service at the cemetery. Close relatives generally wear black or dark clothing at the time of death and for some period thereafter as a mark of respect for the deceased. Concepts of organ donations and autopsies have steadily become accepted.

Food Practices and Intolerances: The Maltese diet is traditionally Mediterranean but has become more westernized in recent years, contributing to metabolic syndrome. In recent years, a public education program has emphasized the importance of a diet lower in sugar, fats, and salt; with increased consumption of low-fat milk products and whole-grain breads and cereals.

Infant-Feeding Practices: About 54% of mothers are breastfeeding their infants on the second day of life; the remainder opt for mixed or bottle-feeding. Bottle-feeding is based on industrial preparations. Weaning foods are generally introduced early at about month 3. The concept that a large infant is a healthy one persists. Childhood obesity is an increasing problem: 19% to 24% of 10-year old children are obese.

Child-Rearing Practices: Day-to-day child rearing and discipline are generally carried out by the mother. Schooling is compulsory for all between the ages of 5 and 16 years and is provided free by the state. The church and other foundations provide alternative fee-based education facilities, which are used by about a third of the children. Children generally remain with their parents until marriage.

National Childhood Immunizations: BCG at 12 years; DT at 3.5 years; DTwP at 2, 3, and 4 months; HepB at 15, 16, and 21 months; Hib at 2, 3, and 4 months; MMR at 15 months and at 8 to 9 years; OPV at 2, 3, and 4 months and at 3.5, 16, and 26 years; and Td at 16 years. The percent of the target population vaccinated, by antigen, is: BCG (80%); DTP1 and Polio3 (94%); DTP3 (92%); HepB3 (78%); Hib3 (83%); and MCV (86%). The law requires compulsory vaccination against diphtheria, polio, tetanus, and rubella for females.

Other Characteristics: Malta scores high on the human development index. The population is still "young" by European standards; the 0-to-14 age group represents 18%, and the 65+ age group represents 13% of the population.

BIBLIOGRAPHY

Central Intelligence Agency: *2006: The world factbook*, Malta. Retrieved September 21, 2006, from https://www.cia.gov/cia/publications/factbook/print/mt.html.

Central Office of Statistics (COS): *Census of population and housing—Malta* 1995. Vol 1, Population, age, gender and citizenship. Valletta, Malta, 1997, Center of Statistics.

Department of Health Information (DHI): National Cancer Registry—cancer incidence, 1994–2003. Malta, 2005, DHI. Retrieved November 20, 2005, from http://health.gov.mt/ministry/dhi/publications/tables/Incidence tables.xls.

Department of Health Information: National Obstetric Information System [NOIS] *Malta–annual report 2004*. Valletta, Malta, 2005, DHI.

Disease Surveillance Unit (DSU): *Annual report 2003*. Valletta, Malta, 2004, DSU.

National Statistical Office (NSO): *Demographic review 2003*. Valletta, Malta, 2004, NSO.

Savona-Ventura C: Thrifty diet phenotype in a small island community: Cajanus, *Carib Food Nutr Inst Q*. 36(1):42–53, 2003.

UNAIDS: 2006 Malta. Retrieved September 21, 2006, from http://www.unaids.org/en/Regions_Countries/Countries/malta.asp.

World Health Organization: 2006: Immunization, vaccines and biologicals. Retrieved September 21, 2006, from http://www.who.int/immunization_monitoring/en/globalsummary/countryprofileresult.cfm?C='mlt'.

◆ MAURITANIA (ISLAMIC REPUBLIC OF)

MAP PAGE (800)

Ould El Joud Dahada and Bertrand Graz

Location: Covering 1,030,700 km^2 (397,850 square miles), Mauritania is one of the largest countries in Africa. The country is divided into 13 regions called *wilaya* in Arabic; every wilaya is divided into departments, or *moughataa*. The country is two thirds arid desert, and the climate is dry and hot. It is windy and dusty from February to May, and the rainy season is from June to October. The Atlantic coast is 754 km (467 miles) long and has a pleasant oceanic climate. The country is bordered in the south by Senegal (and the Senegal River separates the two countries), by Mali in the south and east, Algeria and the western Sahara in the north (presently ruled by Morocco), and Atlantic Ocean to the west. The capital city, Nouakchott, contains a fourth of the population of 3.1 million. The gross domestic product (GDP) per capita is $2,200, with 40% living below the poverty line.

Major Languages	Ethnic Groups	Major Religions
Hassaniya Arabic (official)	Mixed Maur/black 40%	Sunni Muslim
Pular	Maur 30%	100%
Soninké	Black 30%	
Wolof (official)		
French		

Nouadhibou (the economic capital), Kiffa, and Zouerate are the largest cities after Nouakchott. The principal population groups are Arabic, Tou-couleur, Soninké, and Wolof. French is widely used in government and in administration. Literacy rates are 52% for men, 32% for women.

Health Care Beliefs: Biomedical and traditional. The population relies on three kinds of care systems: modern medicine where available; traditional medicine, which primarily involves herb plants, leaves, and roots; and *marabou* (traditional healers) who cure by using prayers, amulets, and other traditional methods. Pharmacy owners prescribe medications and treat illnesses, especially for those in the lower socioeconomic classes. Private clinics primarily exist in large cities but are inaccessible for most of the population. Self-medication with over-the-counter antibiotics and other drugs is common.

Predominant Sick-Care Practices: Magico-religious, alternative and biomedical when available. The Mauritanian health system is based mainly on primary health care, with essential services and medication constituting the first level of care. The second level (the hospital) in the wilaya is almost nonexistent. The tertiary level in the capital, Nouakchott, involves two general national hospitals: the Centre Hospitalier National, and Cheikh Zayed Hospital. There is also a specialized neuropsychiatric hospital. Other medical institutions are the School of Public Health, Institute for Medical Specialization, National Institute of Research in Public Health, National Transfusion Center, and National Orthopedic Center. A medical college was scheduled to open by 2007. Somewhat similar to India and Pakistan, *unani* medicine (classic Arabic medicine) (CAM) is practiced by families of the cultural elite and used in all socioeconomic strata. Families of CAM practitioners have preserved over the centuries libraries of philosophy, poetry, and medicine in several oases of the western quarter of the Sahara desert. CAM follows a written tradition dating back to ancient Greece, based on the theory of humors and imbalance of elements. This medical system proposes very individualized treatments, chiefly comprising diet, minor surgery, and rough vegetal or mineral products, some from as far away as Syria ("gum tragacanth" from *Astragalus gummifer* Labill.) and the Greek island of Chios ("gum mastic" from *Pistacia lentiscus* L.) It is used today by large parts of the Mauritanian population.

Ethnic-/Race-Specific or Endemic Diseases: There is risk for bacterial and protozoal diarrhea, hepatitis A, and typhoid fever. There is (rarely) risk for Rift Valley fever in some locations and also for meningococcal meningitis. Compulsory reportable diseases are malaria (only in the southeastern and central regions), pertussis, diphtheria, meningitis, typhoid fever, hepatitis B, cholera, and acute flaccid paralysis. Immunization-preventable diseases are diphtheria, neonatal tetanus, tetanus, measles, poliomyelitis, pertussis, tuberculosis, and hepatitis B. The most frequently reported disease is measles (5,039 cases in 2004). The Joint United Nations Programme on HIV/AIDS (UNAIDS) reports the adult (aged 15 to

49 years) prevalence rate for human immunodeficiency virus (HIV) as 0.7% (0.4% to 2.8%). An estimated 12,000 people are living with HIV, among them 6,300 women and 1,100 children aged 0 to 14. There are 6,900 orphans from parental acquired immunodeficiency syndrome (AIDS). Fewer than 1,000 deaths from AIDS have been reported.

Health-Team relationships: Doctors and nurses are generally respected.

Families' Role in Hospital Care: Having family and friends visit during an individual's hospitalization or illness at home is important. Although the presence of so many visitors occasionally interferes with the work of medical staff members, the family's assistance is needed because there are not enough staff members to look after patients. The family assumes some responsibility for direct care, often bring home-cooked meals to patients, and take turns staying with them 24 hours a day.

Dominance Patterns: The extended family includes uncles, aunts, cousins, nephews, and nieces. Tribal and ethnic life has a great influence on individuals and organizations. Respect for older adults is the norm. In general, family decisions are made by the men, but women are involved in the discussions. Women have the same rights as men and are respected and free.

Eye-Contact Practices: Direct eye contact is maintained during discussions and consultations.

Touch Practices: Among the Touchouleurs, Sonoinkés, and Wolofs, women and men greet each other by shaking hands. Arab men are not allowed to shake the hands of women or touch them and vice versa unless they are blood relatives. Between men and between women, greetings consist of shaking hands and embracing.

Perceptions of Time: Mauritanians are sometimes casual about punctuality and are oriented to the present. Definitions of *early* and *late* are flexible.

Pain Reactions: Men tend to be stoic about pain. Women and children express pain more freely.

Birth Rites: Procreation is very important, and the fertility rate is six children born per woman. Being infertile is considered a great tragedy, and usually the woman is assumed to be the problem. Pregnant women are respected by their husband and relatives, and they generally get everything they want because people believe that if they do not, their infant may be born with an abnormality. Husbands are not present during labor and birth, although the presence of a family member (who must be a woman) for natural births or cesarean sections is common. The infant mortality rate is high at 69 deaths per 1,000 live births. Male and female circumcisions are common. About 50% of all births occur at home without modern professional attendance, which may contribute to the high maternal mortality rate (747 per 100,000 live births). Newborns are named on the 7th day after birth, and the event is celebrated by feasting. The mother has a rest period for 40 days after the birth and stays with her parents. Girls may have their ears pierced in the fist year of life. Working parents continue to collect their salaries, and working mothers usually have flexible hours and time to breastfeed. The life expectancy at birth is 51 for men, 55 for women.

Death Rites: Death rites are governed by Islam. The body is wrapped in a shroud and buried as soon as possible. Before the burial, as many people as possible pray the "death prayer," and men recite from the holy *Koran* in the home. All groups have the same death, burial, and cemetery rituals. Cremation is not allowed.

Food Practices and Intolerances: Food practices are usually limited to dishes such as red meat, fish, rice and meat, rice and fish, and couscous and meat. Those in the middle and upper classes eat a great deal of red meat, particularly lamb and sheep. Camel is preferred by Arabs and beef by the Touchouleurs, Soninké, and Wolofs. The consumption of fruit, vegetables, and salads is increasing. Mauritanians do not regularly eat out or stay in hotels; they prefer to stay with parents or friends. Food restrictions are those dictated by Islam; for example, it is forbidden to eat pork or drink alcoholic beverages.

Infant-Feeding Practices: Mothers generally breastfeed until their children are 2 years of age.

Child-Rearing Practices: Children are treated with affection, and kissing and holding children are signs of affection. School begins at 5 years with *Koran* school, and modern school follows at about 7 years of age. Children in the upper classes attend nurseries and preschools.

National Childhood Immunizations: BCG at birth; DTwP at 6, 10, and 14 weeks; OPV at birth and at 6, 10, and 14 weeks; HepB at 6, 10, and 14 weeks; measles at 9 months; and TT at first contact, +1, +6 months, +1, +1 year (14 to 45 years). The percent of the target population targeted, by antigen, is: BCG (87%); DTP1 (85%); DTP3 (71%); MCV (61%); HepB3 (42%); Polio3 (71%); and TT2 plus (34%).

M

BIBLIOGRAPHY

Central Intelligence Agency: 2006: The world factbook, Mauritania. Retrieved September 21, 2006, from https://www.cia.gov/cia/publications/factbook/print/mr.html.

Graz B: How to assess traditional healers: an observational clinical study of classical Arabic medicine in Mauritania, with comparison of prognosis and outcome, *Trop Doctor*. 35(4):217–8, 2005.

Graz B, Falquet J, Morency P: Assessment of alternative medicine through a comparison of the expected and observed progress of patients: a feasibility study of the prognosis/follow-up method. *J Altern Complement Med*. 9(5):755–761, 2003.

Office National de la Statistique: *Synthèse du profil pauvreté en Mauritanie 2000*, October 2001.

Office National de la Statistique: Retrieved May 5, 2006, from http://www.ons.mr.

UNAIDS: 2004 Report on the global AIDS epidemic. Retrieved May 5, 2006, from http://www.unaids.org/bangkok2004/GAR2004_html/GAR2004_16_en.htm.

UNAIDS: 2006 Mauritania. Retrieved September 21, 2006, from http://www.unaids.org/en/Regions_Countries/Countries/mauritania.asp.

World Health Organization: 2006: Immunization, vaccines and biologicals. Retrieved September 21, 2006, from http://www.who.int/immunization_monitoring/en/globalsummary/countryprofileresult.cfm?C='mrt'.

World Health Organization, United Nations Children's Fund and United Nations Population Fund: *Maternal mortality in 2000: estimates developed by WHO, UNICEF and UNFPA.* Geneva, 2004, WHO Department of Reproductive Health and Research.

◆ MAURITIUS (REPUBLIC OF)

MAP PAGE (801)

Carolyn M. D'Avanzo

Location: Mauritius is a small volcanic island in the Indian Ocean, surrounded by coral reefs, 855 km (531 miles) off the east coast of Madagascar. The capital is Port Louis. Its nearest neighbor is Reunion to the southwest. The total area is 1869 km² (718 square miles). About 49% of the land is arable, and 22% is covered by forests and woodland. Mauritius is a developing country with a multiethnic population of 1.2 million. It has a high population density—about 611 people per square kilometer. The gross domestic product (GDP) per capita is $13,000 with 10% below the poverty line. Literacy rates are 89% for men, 83% for women.

Major Languages	Ethnic Groups	Major Religions
English (official)	Indo-Mauritian 68%	Hindu 52%
French	Creole 27%	Christian (mostly Roman
Creole	Sino-Mauritian 3%	Catholic) 28%
Hindi	Franco-Mauritian 2%	Muslim 17%
Urdu		Other or none 3%
Bhojpuri		
Hakka		

Health Care Beliefs: Active involvement; increasing health promotion. Mental illness is feared, and people with mental disorders are marginalized. Mauritians practice acupuncture, and people often take herbs as a primary relief measure. Reiki has recently become a popular means for curing such symptoms as stress, insomnia, and hypertension. Smoking prevalence has decreased significantly, likely because of increases in the cigarette tax, health-promotion programs, and a concerted effort to decrease cigarette advertising. Measures also have been taken to improve the cardiovascular health of Mauritians (e.g., encouraging them to use soybean oil instead of coconut oil for frying). These steps have improved lipid levels and decreased disease risk. Most of the people believe in God, and some consider sickness to be God's will, which may delay treatment.

Predominant Sick-Care Practices: Biomedical; traditional; and religious. Most consult doctors; however, some consult traditional healers. It is estimated that about 94 species of plants are used in traditional medicine on the island. Health care services are free in public hospitals for everyone and are of good quality. Mauritians in low-income groups particularly benefit from these services, which are accessible to all. Mauritius has five main hospitals throughout the island, and all are well equipped; it also has some private hospitals. Private companies offer health insurance, but few Mauritians are able to afford it. For primary health care, the people first go to a community health center managed by a doctor and nurses; one is usually within a 1-mile radius.

Ethnic-/Race-Specific or Endemic Diseases: Risk for hepatitis A is quite high, and hepatitis B, cryptosporidiosis, malaria, and sickle cell anemia are concerns. Patients with sexually transmitted diseases and prison inmates have a high incidence of infection with hepatitis C virus. Bronchial asthma is an increasing problem and seems to be largely attributable to house dust mites, which are considered to be the most serious allergen on the island. Mauritians are also at risk for epidemic dropsy from oil contaminated with argemone seed and for glucose-6-phosphate dehydrogenase (G6PD) deficiency. Schistosomiasis is endemic in the districts of Pamplemousses, Port Louis, and Grand Port. β-Thalassemia is prevalent because of the gene flow from India to Mauritius. Type 2 diabetes is endemic, with high prevalence rates in all ethnic groups and a high incidence of diabetic retinopathy. Mortality from coronary heart disease is among the highest in the world. Insulin resistance syndrome has been reported in a high proportion of Mauritians with premature heart disease. The seroprevalence of cytomegalovirus infection is very high in those who donate blood: 94% of men and 100% of women. Mortality from stroke is very high. Industrialization has been accompanied by a significant increase in breast cancer incidence. In early 2006, there was an epidemic of chikungunya. The Joint United Nations Programme on HIV/AIDS (UNAIDS) estimates the prevalence rate for human immunodeficiency virus (HIV) in adults (aged 15 to 49 years) is 0.6%, with 4,100 people living with HIV, including fewer than 1,000 women. Fewer than 100 deaths from acquired immunodeficiency syndrome (AIDS) are reported.

Health-Team Relationships: Relationships are doctor driven. Doctors are respected by patients and by other members of the health care team. Doctors and nurses in the service sector have a good working relationship. Nurses provide basic care and counseling and all participate in a 3-year nursing course. In addition, the Institute of Health provides refresher courses every 2 years.

Families' Role in Hospital Care: Families do not stay in hospitals overnight. However, they visit patients, and some relatives bring food even though food is provided. Because health care is free, patients do not pay unless they are treated in a private hospital or clinic, which provide more personalized care and service. In these situations, families pay the bill, which includes drug costs. Families play a key role in providing care and taking responsibility for the relative. Responsibility for care of older family members is shared by their children.

Dominance Patterns: Mauritius is a patriarchal society. Men dominate the home and social sphere. Women's status has been evolving, and women are playing a large role in the development of the country and the family. Because of free education, boys and girls go to secondary schools and universities. Many women have high aspirations and delay marriage, mostly by choice. Gender inequality still exists, especially among those in the poorer and lower classes.

Eye-Contact Practices: In general, direct eye contact is acceptable and expected.

Touch Practices: Mauritian culture is characterized by kissing, but shaking hands is common when people do not know each other well. If people are close, embracing is perfectly acceptable. Doctors and nurses are allowed to touch patients for examination purposes; however, when a male doctor is examining a female patient, a female nurse always assists.

Perceptions of Time: In general, Mauritians are conscientious about being on time for appointments.

Pain Reactions: Mauritians of Asian origin are considered to be very sensitive to pain, whereas those of African descent seem to be more capable of enduring pain. For example, it has been reported that when people of Indian or Asian origin receive a Norplant or Minilap insert, they seem to feel much pain, whereas those of African descent (i.e., Creoles) seem to tolerate the pain better.

Birth Rites: Each ethnic group has particular rites and rituals. Indo-Mauritians participate in community bathing on days 6 and 12 after birth to celebrate. The mother bathes in water that has been boiled with different kinds of herbal leaves (a priest is normally consulted regarding the appropriate timing of this bath). Special food (seven varieties of greens) is cooked, and special spices are incorporated that cleanse the body and soul. Cumin seeds are boiled, and the mother drinks the resulting water. Mauritians' preference for boys, which was common in the past, is gradually disappearing. The fertility rate is two children born per woman. The infant mortality rate is 15 per 1,000 live births. Studies indicate that congenital cytomegalovirus infection is highly likely to be associated with mental retardation and deafness in Mauritian children. Life expectancy is 69 for men, 77 for women.

Death Rites: A funeral is a social event, so families and friends gather for a 1-night vigil under a tent erected for the event. Black coffee is served, and neighbors provide support, informal counseling, and food for the bereaved family. Burial and cremation (for Hindus) tend to be dignified, although it is acceptable for relatives to cry. The government provides some monetary allowances for funerals. Death is accepted as inevitable. Autopsies are acceptable, although organ donations are not popular.

Food Practices and Intolerances: Basic foods are rice, *chappati* (flat bread), grains, vegetables, and either seafood or meat. The food of Indo-Mauritians tends to be spicy, and curries served with *chappati* are popular. They also often prepare Chinese and Indian food as well. Creoles rely more on dishes that are not vegetable-based (e.g., beef, pork, seafood) and

M

tend to eat more tinned meat and fish. Muslims eat more beef and less lamb. Mauritians are quite health conscious, and on weekdays they often consume more soup, bread, and pasta and eat more rice on the weekend. Asians in villages often eat with their hands, but this practice is changing. At weddings, food is served in a banana leaf and eaten with the hands. Many people in urban areas eat with a fork, knife, and spoon. Recent efforts promoting the substitution of palm oil with soybean oil for frying have been effective in some parts of the population, reducing the lipid levels of those groups.

Infant-Feeding Practices: The incidence of breastfeeding has gradually decreased, and surveys indicate that fewer than 20% of infants are exclusively breastfed in the first few months. At 6 to 9 months, most infants are receiving some breast milk and complementary foods and liquids. By the age of 12 to 15 months, perhaps 10% receive at least some breast milk along with complementary foods. Therefore, many women limit breastfeeding and begin supplementing breast milk with other liquids and foods when the infant is very young. Fewer women are breastfeeding, regardless of their ethnic origin. Employed women find breastfeeding difficult to manage, and many women are joining the labor market.

Child-Rearing Practices: Child rearing involves a mixture of leniency and discipline, and spanking is allowed. Parents tend to be very loving and enjoy parenting, but at the same time they are pressured to raise their children in a disciplined way. Usually the mother is responsible for raising the children. Children normally sleep with both parents until they are 5 or 6 years old. Both parents are responsible for discipline.

National Childhood Immunizations: BCG at birth; DTwP at 3, 4, and 5 months; HepB at 3, 4, and 5 months; MMR at 1 and 6 years; OPV at 3, 4, and 5 months and at 2 and 5 years; DT at 2 and 5 years; and TT at 11 years. The percent of the target population vaccinated, by antigen, is: BCG and DTP1 (99%); DTP3, HepB3, and Polio3 (97%); MCV (98%); and TT2 plus (88%).

M

BIBLIOGRAPHY

Central Intelligence Agency: 2006: *The world factbook, Mauritius.* Retrieved September 21, 2006, from https://www.cia.gov/cia/publications/factbook/print/mp.html.

Cox HS, Williams JW, de Courten MP, Chitson P, Tuomilehto J, Zimmet PZ: Decreasing prevalence of cigarette smoking in the middle income country of Mauritius: questionnaire survey, BMJ. 321(7257):345, 2000.

Gorakshakar AC et al: β-Thalassemia gene flow from India to Mauritius, *Am J Hematol.* 65(3):263, 2000.

Khittoo G et al: Mutation analysis of a Mauritian hereditary breast cancer family reveals the BRCA 26503delTT mutation previously found to recur in different ethnic populations, *Hum Hered.* 52(1):55, 2001.

Manraj M et al: Genetic and environmental nature of the insulin resistance syndrome in Indo-Mauritian subjects with premature coronary heart disease: contribution of α3-adrenoreceptor gene polymorphism and β-blockers on triglyceride and HDL concentrations, *Diabetologia.* 44(1):115, 2001.

Pultoo A et al: Detection of cytomegalovirus in urine of hearing-impaired and mentally retarded children by PCR and cell culture, *J Comm Dis.* 32(2):101, 2000.

UNAIDS: 2006 Mauritius. Retrieved September 21, 2006, from http://www.unaids. org/en/Regions_Countries/Countries/mauritius.asp.
World Health Organization 2006: Immunization, Vaccines and Biologicals. Retrieved September 21, 2006, from http://www.who.int/immunization_monitoring/en/ globalsummary/countryprofileresult.cfm?C='mus'.

◆ MEXICO (UNITED MEXICAN STATES)

MAP PAGE (795)

Eric Dumonteil and Miriam Rubí Gamboa Léon

Location: Located between the United States and Central America, Mexico is a high plateau with mountain chains on the east and west and ocean-front lowlands. The total area is 1,972,550 km^2 (761,603 square miles). The United States is to the north, the Gulf of Mexico to the east, Belize and Guatemala to the south, and the Pacific Ocean to the west. The capital is Mexico City. The population is 107.4 million. The gross domestic product (GDP) per capita is $10,000, with 40% living below the poverty line. Literacy rates are 94% for men, 91% for women.

Major Languages	Ethnic Groups	Major Religions
Spanish 99%	Mestizo 60%	Roman Catholic 89%
Nahuatl 2%	Native American 30%	Protestant 6%
Maya 1%	White 9%	Other 5%
Other 4%	Other 1%	

Health Care Beliefs: Passive role; acute sick care only. Common beliefs include *mal de ojo* (evil eye), *empacho* (bolus of food stuck to stomach wall or blocking the intestine), *caida de mollera* (fallen fontanel), *susto* (result of a fright or a traumatic emotional experience), and *mal puesto* (hex or illness imposed by another). Health is believed to be a matter of chance or God's will. Disease conditions are influenced by hot and cold imbalances. Cold illnesses are due to the invasion of the body from the exterior and are generally incapacitating (alterations of motor and sensory functions, pain, and immobility). Hot illnesses are believed to be generated from within the body and result in irritation (skin rash, fever, and cough). It is believed that a high body temperature can be broken by using warm blankets and hot drinks. Intravenous solutions (*sueros*) are also available and may be infused at home by family members or folk healers. Illness may be caused by contagion, excessive work, cold or "air" exposure, food contamination, punishment from God, bewitchment, or transgression of moral and social rules. Spiritual diseases may be cured through *limpias* (cleaning of the soul) or *leída de la suerte* (reading of the destiny). Prayer and the use of religious relics, rosaries, and crucifixes may also be used as well as various amulets. Good health in men is part of appearing macho, which results in men seeking health care less frequently than women. Thus, men are perceived as being healthier than women or children. The severity of the patient's illness may be determined in part by pain or the appearance of blood. Some call stomachaches and headaches illnesses.

Predominant Sick Care Practices: Biomedical; magico-religious; traditional and self-medication. All focus on the cure of acute sickness and are based on Western, pre-Hispanic, African, and Catholic elements. An estimated 30,000 *parteras* (traditional midwives) and 10,000 *curandero/a* (healers) attend to 15 to 20 million patients. People of all socioeconomic and educational levels use biomedical and folk health systems, sometimes concurrently. Additional folk healers include *yerbero/a* (herbalists), and *sobador/a* (masseuses). Homeopathic and other alternative medicine and those of oriental influence—such as naturopathy and spiritism—are gaining in popularity. Because the cultural context of medical versus folk practices are fundamentally different, the two systems have historically been perceived as conflicting, and traditional healers have been marginalized within the health system. In recent years, there has been a move toward greater integration of both practices, and several attempts at legislating traditional folk medicine (through registration, licenses, training) have been made. Some biomedical practitioners are also beginning to accept and use traditional medicine. An ambitious reform of the health care system is currently being implemented to address the profound disparities in insurance coverage, public expenditures, and health status of the population. The *Seguro Popular de Salud* was launched in 2004, aimed at covering the 48 million left uninsured by previous heath care schemes. The rest of the population is covered by the *Instituto Mexicano de Seguro Social* (IMSS), which covers workers in the private sector, and the *Instituto de Seguridad y Servicios Sociales de los Trabajadores* (ISSSTE), which covers workers in the public sector. Private medicine is also available for more affluent patients. The sale of drugs—except for narcotics, barbiturates, and other addictive drugs—is uncontrolled. Advice can be obtained from pharmacists, and self-medication is widely practiced.

M

Ethnic-/Race-Specific or Endemic diseases: Endemic diseases include chloroquine-sensitive malaria, leishmaniasis, and Chagas disease; risk is lower in urban areas. Mexicans are at risk for gastroenteritis and intestinal infectious diseases, obesity, diabetes, tuberculosis, dengue fever, higher hemoglobin and hematocrit levels, and alcoholism. The Joint United Nations Programme on HIV/AIDS (UNAIDS) reports the estimated prevalence rate for human immunodeficiency virus (HIV) in adults (aged 15 to 49 years) as 0.3%, with 180,000 people living with HIV, including 42,000 women and 2,400 children. About 6,200 deaths have been attributed to acquired immunodeficiency syndrome (AIDS). HIV and AIDS principally affect men who have sex with men, with a male-female ratio of 6:1.

Health-Team Relationships: The health care system is physician driven, with a strict and vertical organization of power and duties. The patient is seen as having little capacity or right to questions. The practitioner is regarded as an outsider, which affects patient confidence. The *curandero,* or folk healer, is a member of the nuclear or extended family network and thus is able to create a special relationship with the patient, who is seen in a more integral context. This has led the government to attempt the incorporation of traditional healers into the system. Family interdependence takes precedence over independence, so self-care is not an important concept. Personal matters are discussed and handled within the family. Valued behaviors by health care practitioners are being informal and friendly, including family members in the interaction, giving careful and concrete explanations, sharing experiences, and taking time to listen. Health care practitioners of the same sex as their patients are preferred, and confidence in older practitioners is greatest.

Families' Role in Hospital Care: Family members frequently accompany hospitalized patients. The male head of household should be consulted before health care decisions are made and should be included in any counseling sessions. Culturally, a mother is not allowed the authority to give consent for her child's treatment, and family decisions supersede decisions made by health care providers.

Dominance Patterns: The family structure is patriarchal; however, there is some movement toward more democratic gender roles. The mother is in charge of running the household and decides when health care will be sought, and this behavior has been encouraged by the health system by promoting health as a domestic problem. Mothers also play an important role in self-medication. Deference is given to elders, fathers, and grandfathers. The collective needs of the family, whether extended or nuclear, take precedence over those of the individual. Some ethnic groups in the state of Oaxaca have a matriarchal structure (Tecas).

Eye-Contact Practices: In rural or periurban areas, sustained direct contact is rude, immodest, or dangerous for some. *Mal de ojo* ("evil eye") is the result of excessive admiration. Women and children are thought to be more susceptible to *mal de ojo;* therefore, children may avoid direct eye contact.

Touch Practices: Touch is used often. Touching people while complimenting them neutralizes the power of the evil eye in believers. Closeness and physical contact are valued in familiar situations. However, excessive embracing, especially between men or between father and sons, may be badly perceived. People of rural origin are more reserved and less demonstrative.

Perceptions of Time: The tendency is to focus on the present and to be relatively unconcerned about the future. The concept of time is a relaxed one, with no hurry. *Mañana* may or may not mean tomorrow.

Pain Reactions: Emotional self-restraint and stoic inhibition of strong feelings and emotional expression are seen, with an impressive tolerance to pain. In rural areas, medical care is not sought unless illness is severe. Expression of pain may be a self-help relief mechanism. Pain relief might be refused as a means for atonement. During labor the loud verbal repetition of *aye, yie, yie* requires long, slow breaths; thus, it is becoming a culturally and medically appropriate method of pain relief.

480 *Mexico (United Mexican States)*

Birth Rites: The fertility rate is 2.42 children born per woman. Beliefs about pregnancy may include sleeping flat on the back, keeping active to ensure a small baby and an easy delivery, avoiding cold air, and continuing sexual intercourse to lubricate the birth canal. Folk beliefs include *antojos* (food cravings that can cause the infant to have a characteristic such as strawberry spots if not satisfied) and *cuarentena* (40-day lying-in period during which the woman rests, stays warm, avoids bathing and exercise, and eats special foods that promote warmth). It is inappropriate for the husband to be with his wife during delivery. The woman's mother or sister may be present. About 55% of infants are born in hospitals, where there has been a 30% increase in cesareans. Traditional deliveries are popular, and 45% of both urban and rural mothers deliver with the assistance of *parteras*. Women have great confidence in *parteras* because they share the same socioeconomic characteristics and cultural values. A coin or marble, wiped with alcohol, may be strapped firmly to the infant's navel to make it attractive. The infant mortality rate is 20 deaths per 1,000 live births. Life expectancy is 73 for men, 78 for women.

Death Rites: Small children may be shielded from dying and death rituals. Family members take turns staying around the clock with the dying person in the hospital. Grief can be expressive; for example, *el ataque* consists of hyperkinetic or seizure-type behavior patterns that serve to release emotions. Death rituals include overnight mourning at the funeral home before burial. For many it may be a day of music, dancing, and rejoicing, especially after the death of a child. All Souls' Day is a major celebration of the day that souls travel home to the living and they are remembered.

Food Practices and Intolerances: Lactose intolerance is not uncommon. Prenatal vitamins are thought to be a hot food, not to be taken during pregnancy. Dietary staples such as rice, corn, and beans provide complete proteins. *Tortillas* (corn flour), beans, and *chile* (hot peppers) are the main diet of many poor families, and malnutrition is still common. Poor food and water hygiene are a source of major gastroenteritis and intestinal infectious diseases.

Infant-Feeding Practices: Colostrum may be perceived as bad milk; therefore, bottle-feeding may be used until the breasts fill. Breastfeeding is commonly practiced during the first 4 months.

Child-Rearing Practices: Birth control methods other than rhythm are not popular. There is a tendency to overprotect newborns. Children are expected to respect and obey their parents and elders, and older people often help with childraising. Older male children may discipline younger siblings. Families are more protective of girls, resulting in differences in terms of rules, with boys granted greater overall freedom.

National Childhood Immunizations: BCG at birth; DTPHibHep at 2, 4, and 6 months; DTwP at 2 and 4 years + 12 years; OPV at 2, 4, and 6 months, over 12 years old and pregnant women; MMR at 1 and 6 years; Influenza at 6–22, 7–23 and 17–23 months; MR at 13–39 years; Td >12= years; Vitamin A <4 years. The percent of the target population vaccinated, by antigen, is: BCG, and DTP1 (99%); DTP3, HepB3, Hib3, and Polio3 (98%); and MCV (96%).

Other Characteristics: The first surname is the father's, and the second is the mother's. A married woman adds "de" before the husband's surname. The 15th birthday is an important social event for girls. In many rural areas, there is a strong belief in the relationship between body and social or cosmic equilibriums.

BIBLIOGRAPHY

Castaneda Camey X, Garcia Barrios C, Romero Guerrero X et al: Caesarean sections in Mexico: are there too many? *Health Policy Plan.* 16(1):62–67, 2001.

Central Intelligence Agency: *2006: The world factbook, Mexico.* Retrieved September 21, 2006, from https://www.cia.gov/cia/publications/factbook/print/mx.html.

Gómez Dantés O, Ortiz M: Seguro popular de salud: siete perspectivas, *Salud Publica Mex.* 46(6):585–596, 2004.

Martin J: *The state of health in Mexico.* OECD Forum on Mexico: Policies to Promote Growth and Economic Development, 2004.

Nigenda, G, Mora-flores G, Aldama-Lopez S, Orozco-Nuñez E: La práctica de la medicina tradicional en América latina y el caribe: el dilema entre regulación y tolerancia, *Salud Publ Mex.* 43(1):41–51, 2001.

UNAIDS: 2006: Mexico. Retrieved September 21, 2006, from http://www.unaids.org/en/Regions_Countries/Countries/mexico.asp.

World Health Organization: 2006: Immunization, vaccines and biologicals. Retrieved September 21, 2006, from http://www.who.int/immunization_monitoring/en/globalsummary/countryprofileresult.cfm?C='mex'.

◆ MOLDOVA (REPUBLIC OF)

MAP PAGE (799)

Carolyn M. D'Avanzo

M

Location: Moldova is located in southeast Europe and occupies a territory of 33,700 km^2 (13,008 square miles). In the north, east, and south it is bordered by the Ukraine, and in the west the Prut River separates Moldova from Romania. The population is 4.4 million. The landscape is extremely varied, ranging from the hills of central and northern Moldova to the Dniester steppelands and the South Moldovan plain, or the Budzhak Steppe. Moldova's chief asset is its black soil, which covers 80% of the territory; forests cover more than 9%. The capital is Chisinau. Despite economic progress, Moldova is one of the poorest countries in Europe, with a gross domestic product (GDP) per capita of $1,800 and 80% living below the poverty line. Literacy is almost 100% for both men and women.

Major Languages	Ethnic Groups	Major Religions
Moldovan (official)	Moldavan 65%	Eastern Orthodox 98%
Russian	Romanian 14%	Jewish 1.5%
Gagauz	Ukrainian 13%	Other 0.5%
	Other 8%	

482   *Moldova (Republic of)*

The Moldovan language is very similar to Romanian; therefore, it is often referred to as Moldovan-Romanian. As a heritage from Soviet times, Russian is commonly used. Moldova has always been a multiethnic state. About 35% of the population is made up of various minorities such as Ukrainian, Russian, Gagauz, Bulgarian, and Jewish. Much smaller numbers of Belorussian, Polish, German, and Roma (Gypsy) live there. The Gagauz population is historically of Turkish origin and has Orthodox beliefs.

Health Care Beliefs: Acute sick care; traditional. The society's level of knowledge about health and disease has increased overall. It is understood that good health involves good nutrition and physical exercise. It is unlikely that anyone now believes that a person can be healed by such practices as rubbing heated coins over a diseased area; however, traditional beliefs fly in the face of current medical knowledge. For example, some girls and women are actively discouraged from sitting directly on cement or stone because they believe that their reproductive systems will be damaged by the cold radiating from those materials. In addition, a vinegar compress is still considered an effective treatment for fever. The hard economic conditions during the last years have been particularly difficult for those with mental illness; they were previously marginalized and are now neglected by the society.

Predominant Sick-Care Practices: Biomedical and religious. A network of clinics, polyclinics, dispensaries, hospitals, maternity homes, and children's dispensaries is spread widely across Moldova. The new architecture of health care at the regional level includes regional hospitals that provide complex care, district hospitals, outpatient clinics, and rural preventive outpatient clinics. Medical treatment is generally free, but the country has many private medical centers where patients pay for their treatment. Private clinics have to be licensed and adhere to professional codes, as do public facilities. Doctors are most often consulted when people are in pain. People who simply do not feel well consult a family doctor at the clinic; if they feel too sick to leave the house, they send for the doctor. The doctor asks the patient about the symptoms of their illness, does a comprehensive examination, and perhaps gives an injection to relieve pain. Alternate healers are not generally consulted, and wearing amulets for prevention of illness is not a common practice. Praying for good health is common, although people also consult a doctor.

Ethnic-/Race-Specific or Endemic Diseases: Tuberculosis is a significant problem, and rural laborers, in particular, are at high risk for chronic respiratory diseases of nontuberculous causes. Moldova has high hepatitis B endemicity and high rates of acute perinatal infections with the virus. The incidence of hepatitis C and D infections among children and pregnant women is high. The hepatitis C virus is also considered endemic in dialysis centers. Malaria imported from Azerbaijan is closely monitored. In the late 1990s, a diphtheria epidemic occurred after the disease had been almost nonexistent for 20 years; it was controlled by mass immunization. The Joint United Nations Programme on HIV/AIDS (UNAIDS) estimates the prevalence rate for human immunodeficiency virus (HIV) in adults (aged

15 to 49 years) as 1.1% to 2.6%, with 29,000 people living with HIV, including 16,000 women. No reports on the number of children affected are available. About 1,400 deaths are attributed to acquired immunodeficiency syndrome (AIDS). The first cases of HIV infection were recorded in 1987. Since 1997, HIV has been considered endemic. Of cases with documented transmission routes, most (82%) are associated with injecting drug use, followed by heterosexual sex (17%). At present, heterosexual transmission is associated with new infections almost as frequently as injecting drug use.

Health-Team Relationships: The doctor is considered the chief of the health care team and plays the dominant role in decision making. Nurses are expected to take care of patients and perform tasks such as giving injections or changing surgical dressings. Working relationships between nurses and doctors are usually good.

Families' Role in Hospital Care: Relatives or friends buy everything necessary for the treatment of a hospitalized family member, and in some hospitals this includes medications. Only close relatives can visit maternity wards. It is acceptable for patients to spend the weekend with the family and then return to the hospital.

Dominance Patterns: There are strong negative attitudes toward women in rural communities, where patriarchal traditions still dominate. Since time immemorial, the role of women has been to take care of the family, cook, and raise the children. During the last two decades, women's involvement in professional, scientific, and political life has increased significantly.

Eye-Contact Practices: It is customary to maintain direct eye contact with people while talking. During conversations with friends, not looking into another person's eyes indicates a lack of respect or sincerity. It is prohibited for people outside the family to look directly at an infant's face until the baptism ceremony because of fear of the "evil eye" (i.e., the power of a person to harm others simply by looking at them).

Touch Practices: Touch is considered acceptable in the health care field, and some women have male gynecologists. People of rural origin are more reserved and less demonstrative in their attitudes and emotions. Traditional people shake hands when meeting each other. On arrival and departure, kissing acquaintances is normal. Gestures are common during interpersonal communications.

Perceptions of Time: People strive to make their plans, visits, and appointments at a particular time; thus, punctuality is an important issue. However, in rural communities, punctuality and the concept of being on time for an appointment are relative because of more relaxed attitudes toward time. Moldavian culture tends to focus on previous times and traditions. Youths are more liberal and tend to think more about the present and future.

Pain Reactions: Women in particular tend to react to pain very emotionally, and anesthetic drugs are frequently used. Pain reactions are individual and usually judged by such parameters as facial grimaces, body position, stature, and limited movement. In rural areas, people often avoid seeking medical care unless their pain is severe.

Birth Rites: Pregnancy is considered a delicate period for a woman's health, so the family takes great care to offer pregnant women the best quality and largest quantity of food they can. The fertility rate is two children born per woman. Women are typically cared for by professionals during and after delivery. Most infants are delivered in hospitals. Until recent years, fathers and other family members were not allowed to assist in the birth. Today, the father is often present in the delivery room. The birth of a child is a time for family feasting and visits to the newborn. Moldovans tend to celebrate the birth of a son or a daughter equally, although some fathers are especially happy when a son is born. Because most Moldavans are Orthodox, the birth of a child is strongly associated with the baptism ceremony, which is both a religious and a family occasion. Parents usually decide on the infant's name according to family tradition and the calendar of religious holidays. The infant mortality rate is 28 deaths per 1,000 live births. Life expectancy is 62 for men, 70 for women.

Death Rites: The family expresses grief through crying and wailing at the moment a person dies. Family members and close friends dress in black and official suits. Depending on the religious background and traditions of the person who died, a priest might be summoned to conduct the burial service. The family offers meals out of respect to the deceased on the burial day and on the 9th and 40th day after the death. Family members continue to go to the cemetery and bring flowers to the tomb, especially on sacred days or special anniversaries. Organ donations and autopsies are acceptable with the family's approval. Moldova has no tradition of cremation. Bodies are buried in graves, usually according to the rites of the Eastern Orthodox religion.

Food Practices and Intolerances: Because most people now work during the day, most prefer that the largest meal be in the evening at home rather than at lunch. Before the Christmas and Easter holidays, dietary restrictions for religious reasons are common. The national cuisine is noted for its abundance of fruit and vegetables. Typical food includes vegetables (tomatoes, cucumbers, onions) with special Moldovan cheese, soups such as *zama* and *ciorba,* and national meals, which are mamaliga and sarmale. In rural communities, Moldovans are hurt if a guest refuses an offered glass of wine because the people have a long-standing tradition of winemaking. Meat and meat products are preferred for dinner. Meals are usually eaten at a table with a spoon, knife, and fork.

Infant-Feeding Practices: It is considered traditionally important and socially expected for women to breastfeed their babies, and most do so for at least 4 months. Differences in feeding newborns and infants primarily depend on whether the mother lives in an urban or a rural area and whether she is employed. Village women breastfeed more often and longer, and women concerned about returning to work breastfeed much less frequently and for shorter periods.

Child-Rearing Practices: In some families, fathers play the dominant role and children are brought up in relatively conservative surroundings. In families with only one parent and in multigenerational families, the grandparents usually participate freely in the child-rearing process. Children usually sleep in their own beds. It is common for children to attend kindergarten, particularly if their mothers are working. In rural communities, children may be punished severely and be involved in housekeeping and agricultural work from an early age.

National Childhood Immunizations: BCG at 3 to 5 days and at 6 to 7 years; DT at 6 to 7 years; DtaP at 2, 4, 6, and 22 to 24 months; HepB at birth and at 1 and 6 months; MMR at 12 months and at 6 to 7 years; OPV at 2, 4, 6, 22 to 24 months and at 6 to 7 years; Td at 15, 20, 25, 30, 35, 40, 50, and 60 years. The percent of the target population vaccinated, by antigen, is: BCG and MCV (97%); DTP1, DTP3, and Polio3 (98%); and HepB3 (99%). The high rate of vaccination for hepatitis B has significantly lowered morbidity in newborns.

Other Characteristics: As a result of the political and socioeconomic changes that have taken place, there is a high incidence of poverty, an exhausted health care infrastructure, and a deteriorating reproductive potential and gene pool. The country has also experienced a total decline in the volume of personal goods and services and consumption. This decline may have eventual negative long-term consequences for the health of the population. The decline in living standards and the current crisis in the public health system have led to an increase in the mortality rate. In addition, because of alcohol and tobacco use, murders, and suicides, the life expectancy has decreased, particularly for men.

BIBLIOGRAPHY

Bejan-Volc I: *Femeile în comunit˘ile rurale: tendin˘e 'i afirm˘ri*, Chissinau, Moldova, 2000.
Central Intelligence Agency: *2006: The world factbook, Moldova.* Retrieved September 21, 2006, from https://www.cia.gov/cia/publications/factbook/print/md.html.
Moldova National Study: *Gender, poverty and employment,* ILO Program, Chissinau, Moldova, 2001.
Moldova National Study: *HIV/AIDS situation and social-economical sphere,* ILO Program, Chissinau, Moldova, 2001.
Republica Moldova: *Pia˘a muncii ˘i dezvoltarea social'.* L-ul anuar economic i social, Chissinau, Moldova, 2000.
UNAIDS: 2006 Moldova. Retrieved September 21, 2006, from http://www.unaids.org/en/Regions_Countries/Countries/moldova.asp.
United Nations Development Program (UNDP): *National human development report, 1999–2000, Republic of Moldova,* UNDP Moldova, 2000, 2001.
United Nations Development Program (UNDP): *Report status of women in the Republic of Moldova,* UNDP Moldova, 1999.
World Health Organization: 2006: Immunization, vaccines and biologicals. Retrieved September 21, 2006, from http://www.who.int/immunization_monitoring/en/globalsummary/countryprofileresult.cfm?C='mda'.

♦ MONGOLIA

MAP PAGE (803)

Laurie Elit

Location: Mongolia is a landlocked country north of China and south of Russia. Mountains in the northwest, vast deserts in the south, and steppes of grass-covered plains in the central and eastern regions make up the 1,500,000 km^2 (579,000 square miles) of the country. It is divided into 20 *aimags* and two large cities. Ulaan Baatar, the capital, has a population of 673,664. The population is more than 2.8 million. Fifteen percent are nomadic, and more than 50% are dependent on agriculture. The gross domestic product (GDP) per capita is $1,900, and 36% of the population is living below the poverty line. The unemployment rate is 20%.

Major Languages	Ethnic Groups	Major Religions
Mongolian (90%)	Mongol 95%	Tibetan Buddhist 50%
Russian	Turkic 5%	Christian and Shamanism 6%
	Other 2%	Muslim 4%
		None 40%

Different ethnic groups speak with slight dialects or accents (i.e., Buryat). Since 1944, the Russian Cyrillic alphabet has been used to write the language. The most common second language is Russian, and all medical training is in Russian. The literacy rate is 98% for both men and women.

Health Care Beliefs: Acute sick care; traditional. Most Mongolians do not fully understand the health care principles of preservation of health and disease prevention. Before 1921, health practices were based exclusively on Buddhist-Tibetan traditions, with lamas as the main health practitioners.

Predominant Sick-Care Practices: Ethnomedical, biomedical, and magico-religious. The use of traditional medicines is increasing, including certain foods (wolf), acupuncture, and cupping (application of heated cups to the affected body part). Some of the traditional beliefs about healing are that drinking one's mother's urine cures many diseases, walking in cold water causes tonsillitis, applying a freshly cut dog ear to an affected area heals burns, putting a newborn puppy on the liver area cures liver cancer, fermented mare's milk is good for gut disease, and vitamin injections cure many illnesses. Currently, health care is available only for those with health insurance. The national health insurance program is based on the principle of cost sharing; the employee or self-employed individual pays a basic fee for the program, and the government pays the rest of the cost. However, many individuals are unable to participate in the insurance program because they do not have the cash to make direct payments. Children receive health care provided they are registered in their home district, even when parents are unable to afford insurance.

Ethnic-/Race-Specific or Endemic Diseases: The leading causes of adult mortality are diseases of the circulatory system; neoplasms;

accident, injury, and poisoning; and diseases of the digestive and respiratory systems. Cardiovascular disease causes 4,600 deaths annually; 30% of the population over 40 has hypertension, and rheumatic fever and rheumatic heart disease are significant problems. The rate of cancer is increasing, in particular, liver, stomach, cervical, and lung cancer. The incidence of some communicable diseases is high (i.e. viral hepatitis, tuberculosis, brucellosis, and sexually transmitted diseases). Brucellosis usually affects nomads because of the consumption of unboiled milk or homemade cheese and handling of freshly killed meat or cow dung (used for building fires). Bubonic (black) plague is seasonal and infects marmots, squirrels, and rats; it is transmitted to humans through fleabites. The estimated prevalence rate of human immunodeficiency virus (HIV) in adults (aged 15 to 49 years) is 0.01%, with fewer than 500 living with HIV, including fewer than 100 women. Deaths from acquired immunodeficiency syndrome (AIDS) are estimated as fewer than 100. However, the rate of sexually transmitted diseases was 31% among pregnant women in 2001 through 2002. This high rate makes HIV/AIDS awareness a health care priority.

Health-Team Relationships: Mongolian medicine is a mixture of Western technology, oriental practice, and folk treatment. With the transition from Soviet-styled socialism to democracy in 1990, health care expenditures dropped to half of previous levels. The health care system disintegrated, with rural areas most affected. Presently, Mongolia has 754 hospitals nationwide with 18,616 beds. Physician assistants (including midwives) treat patients at 1,200 medical stations in rural areas, and 29 *somon* (medical stations). Twelve *sum* hospitals (with consulting rooms, inpatient ward, and delivery room) are staffed by physicians. There are three *aimag* (general hospitals). This system has led to a high degree of specialization among doctors, with 49% concentrated in Ulaan Baatar. Since 1993, the government has restructured health services with support from the Asian Development Bank. A major goal was to redistribute resources from the hospital sector to primary care and prevention. In 1999, there were 233 family group practices servicing 55% of the population. These doctors have moved from hospital-based clinics to premises in their target population areas, and performance contracts specify the level of essential services to be given, such as emergency coverage. About 65% of physicians are women, and their average monthly salary is U.S. $100. In 1995, there was a reorganization of the nursing curriculum with a focus on primary health and maternal and child care. Nursing is a 2-year diploma program with opportunity for degree work. The quality of nursing care is being addressed by developing nursing care standards and education in management issues. Currently, the ratio of nurses to patients is 1:40, with ratios as high as 1:70 at night.

Families' Role in Hospital Care: Family members are expected to be supporters during illness by providing personal comfort and food. Families provide basic care for members in the hospital by bringing meals, cleaning the sheets, and delivering medications. Families are not allowed in hospital rooms in major city hospitals or in the consulting room. Patients must go to a reception area or have another patient go to the reception area to get supplies from the family. If a patient needs help getting to the bathroom or eating, he or she is dependent on hospital roommates.

Dominance Patterns: Mongolians have a profound respect for elders, and the social fabric of the country revolves around the family unit. Women have traditionally enjoyed a position of respect and relative equality, but each gender has its own role. Women are primarily responsible for the sheep, animals that are important for daily sustenance. Men are primarily responsible for horses, which are considered animals of prestige, war, and sport. Women are responsible for preparing food and caring for the children. For women, there is conflict between the desire to have children and the desire to supplement household income with higher-level jobs requiring commitment of time and energy. Women have more of the lower-paying jobs, and only a token number have higher professional and administrative positions, even though girls are three times more likely than boys to receive a higher education. Mongolia joined the Convention to Eliminate All Types of Gender Discrimination in 1981. However, surveys indicate that about a third of Mongolian women are subject to some form of domestic violence, 10% by husbands or another man living in the home. Policies are in place to ensure the economic security of Mongolian women, improve the situation of rural women, increase the representation of women at management and decision-making levels, eliminate all forms of violence against women, and ensure increased access of women to information and technology.

Eye-Contact Practices: In urban areas, it is considered polite to make eye contact when talking. In the rural areas, herders are reluctant to make eye contact with those in authority, and if a woman makes eye contact with a man, it is considered flirting.

Touch Practices: Mongolians live communally with four or more people in each room and have a very small circle of personal space. It is normal for friends of all ages and of the same sex to walk arm-in-arm or hand-in-hand. Men slap the backs of other men, and it is usual to greet one another with a handshake. Mongolians do not use outward signs of affection such as hugging or kissing, and adults never touch another adult's head.

Perceptions of Time: Immense travel distances and unreliable transportation mean that it is normal to be flexible about appointment times. Appointments can sometimes be delayed by a day, or they may happen spontaneously. Most people live in the present, so planning can be an issue. Young people, especially in urban areas, are thinking more about the future.

Pain Reactions: Older people and people from rural areas are very stoic, partly because of the limited availability of narcotics for postoperative or palliative pain. Acupuncture and herbs are often used to relieve pain, and hot mineral baths in volcanic springs are used for muscle and joint pains.

Birth Rites: About 90% of pregnant women receive some antenatal care, and 94% of deliveries take place in hospitals. The fertility rate is 2.25 children born per mother. As Mongolian women embrace modern medicine, they are also rooted in past traditions. For example, a popular antenatal belief is that two pregnant women should not give each other the traditional Mongolian greeting in which the younger woman supports the arms of the older women because this may cause the infants to switch their sex. The leading cause of maternal morbidity is anemia related to poor nutrition. Women are released from domestic work for 36 days after delivery, and they are not to wash in cold water because this is believed to lead to arthritis or edema. After delivery, a certain mushroom is eaten to increase uterine contractions (decrease postpartum bleeding). Husbands or elderly mothers provide both physical and psychological care for the new mother, but other people are expected to stay away for a month. There are traditions about gifts to bring and how to present the gifts, lest you dry up the mother's milk or make her breasts sore. A baby is not named for at least the first week of life, and some names are chosen to confuse the spirits. For example, *Enbish* means "not this one" and is a plea to the spirits to leave the baby unharmed. When a baby is sick, parents sometimes change their names to confuse the spirits. For this same reason, boys may be dressed as girls. Traditionally, children do not have their hair cut until they are 3 to 5 years old. Fears of infant death are rooted in reality; the infant mortality rate is 52 deaths per 1,000 live births. Life expectancy is 63 for men, 67 for women.

Death Rites: It is taboo to talk about death. During the dying process, patients are usually in the home and depend on the care of family. People who die in the hospital automatically have an autopsy (except Kazak Muslims). The main religion in Mongolia is Buddhism. In keeping with the religion, most bodies are buried in the traditional fashion with a lama, family, and friends present.

Food Practices and Intolerances: The Mongolian diet in rural areas is based on meat and dairy products. Tea is flavored with milk and salt. *Airag* (fermented mare's milk) is the Mongolian national drink and tastes like bubbly buttermilk. Yogurt, milk, cheese, and fermented milk are easily obtained from the milk of horses, goats, yaks, camels, and cows. Boiled mutton in flour is a favorite dish, and it is considered a great honor to be given a sheep's tail. Other meat dishes include beef, horse, and camel. All parts of the animal are eaten. With the exception of potatoes and onions, fresh vegetables and fruits must be imported and therefore are rare in the countryside. Only 30% of households can dry foods for later consumption. Mongolians consume significant amounts of alcohol. Consumption increases during the milking season, when homemade vodka distilled from fermented milk can be produced cheaply on a daily basis. In rural areas, food is usually first served to the husband and fathers, and in urban settings the women serve the children first. It is polite to accept food with the right hand, with the left hand supporting the right hand at the elbow. Most people eat with a spoon and fork. Drinks such as airag are consumed from a shared bowl.

Infant-Feeding Practices: Most infants are breastfed. It is common to use fat from a boiled sheep's tail as a comforter. At 4 months, 75% of infants are exclusively breastfed, but only 21% are still being breastfed by age 6 months. About 30% of children are weaned on *bantam,* a porridge of wheat flour and meat mixed in boiling water, 20% on rice porridge with sugar and butter, and 19% on *zutan,* a porridge of wheat flour only. Children experience protein-energy malnutrition, iodine deficiency, vitamin D and A deficiencies, and iron-deficiency anemia. Of children younger than 5, only 35% consume meat three or more times per week. As a result, 33% of children younger than 5 years of age have rickets, and 42% have anemia. Attitudes and knowledge about infant feeding were explored by the Nutritional Research Center and World Vision Mongolia. When women were asked what they thought caused bowed legs, 36% said they were related to diet, 19% said they were because a child had not been breast-fed, 17% believed they were caused by horseback riding, and 15% said they were related to sunshine. These responses demonstrate that a combination of traditional and biomedical beliefs still influence attitudes toward health and the causes of illness.

Child-Rearing Practices: The extended family lives in a *ger,* a one-room circular tent. Beds are placed around the periphery surrounding a central wood or dung-burning stove. While parents work, grandparents, relatives, and young "elder siblings" care for younger children. During the absence of parental caretakers, statistics indicate that children are at high risk for injury and death. Child rearing is strict, and fathers are usually responsible for disciple. Smacking children on the bottom is common and accepted.

National Childhood Immunizations: BCG at 5 to 7 days and at 8 years; DTwP at 2, 3, and 4 months and 2 years; DT at 8 and 15 years; DTwPHib-Hep at 2, 3, and 4 months (part of country); measles at 8 to 11 and 14 to 21 months; OPV at birth, at 2, 3, and 4 months; Hep B at birth and 2 and 8 months. The percent of the target population vaccinated, by antigen, is: BCG, DTP3, MCV, and Polio3 (99%); DTP1 (97%); HepB3 (98%); Hib3 (28%); and vitamin A (86%).

BIBLIOGRAPHY

Batjargal J, Baljmaa B, Ganzorig D, Solongo A, Tsesgee P: *Care practices for young children in Mongolia.* Ministry of Health Mongolia and UNICEF, 2000.

Janes CR, Chuluundoij O: Free markets and dead mothers: the social ecology of maternal mortality in post-socialist Mongolia, *Med Anthropol Q.* 18(2):230–257, 2004.

Kotilaninen H: Rehabilitation of the hospital infrastructure in a developing country. *World Hosp Health Serv.* 37(2):25–28, 34, 35, 2001.

Nutrition Research Center and World Vision Mongolia: Micronutrient status, coverage and knowledge, attitudes and practices in children under five and pregnant and lactating women in Bulgan, Tov and Ulaanbaatar, Mongolia. July 2001.

Surenkhorllo A, Davis AJ: Country profile: Mongolia. *Nurs Ethics.* 11(3):313–315, 2004.

UNAIDS: 2006 Mongolia. Retrieved September 21, 2006, from http://www.unaids. org/en/Regions_Countries/Countries/mongolia.asp.

World Health Organization: 2006: Immunization, vaccines and biologicals. Retrieved September 21, 2006, from http://www.who.int/immunization_monitoring/en/ globalsummary/countryprofileresult.cfm?C='mng'.

http://www.wpro.who.int/NR/rdonlyres/B7C19BC9-1450-4233-9806-7181270CEF S/0/HIV_AIDS_Asia_Pacific_Region2001.pdf (retrieved February 26, 2006).

♦ MOROCCO (KINGDOM OF)

MAP PAGE (800)

Abdulbari A. Bener

Location: Morocco is located on the northwestern coast of Africa just south of Spain, across the Strait of Gibraltar. The North Atlantic Ocean is to the west and northwest, the Mediterranean Sea to the northeast, Algeria to the east and southeast, and the western Sahara to the southwest. The total area is 453,730 km^2 (175,186 square miles); Rabat is the capital. Other major urban centers are Casablanca (the country's largest city and main seaport), Marrakech and Fes (important trade centers), and Tangier (seaport on the Strait of Gibraltar). The Atlantic coast has fertile plains, whereas the Mediterranean coast is mountainous and subject to earthquakes. Morocco has the highest mountains in North Africa. Along the Mediterranean the climate is subtropical. Mountain peaks are covered with snow most of the year. The population is 33.2 million, with 32% under 15 years of age in 2005. More than 55% live in cities. The gross domestic product (GDP) per capita is $4,200, with 19% living below the poverty line. Literacy rates are 64% for men, 39% for women.

Major Languages	Ethnic Groups	Major Religions
Arabic (official)	Arab-Berber 99.1%	Muslim (Sunni) 98.7%
Berber dialects	Non-Moroccan 0.7%	Christian 1.1%
French	Jewish 0.2%	Jewish 0.2%
Spanish		

The area was ruled by successive Moorish dynasties, Spain, and in 1912 the French, who imposed a protectorate. A protracted independence struggle ended in 1956, and Morocco became independent. About three quarters of the population are of Berber descent. Arabs constitute the bulk of inhabitants of the larger cities. The Berber languages have declined in importance. Many Berbers also speak Arabic, and French is spoken in government, diplomacy, business, and postprimary education settings. The economy is growing; this has improved education and job prospects for Morocco's youth and has raised living standards.

Health Care Beliefs: Acute sick care; traditional. The declaration of Alma-Ata has allowed Morocco to help realize improvements in primary health care, with an emphasis on prevention. The government has developed strategies for improving the health of the population and increasing the efficiency of health care. At the same time, traditional beliefs are still prevalent. For example, Moroccans believe that those with the "evil eye" (the power to harm others merely by looking at them) can affect one's health and well-being.

Predominant Sick-Care Practices: Biomedical and magical-religious. Adequate medical care is available, especially in Casablanca and Rabat.

However, not all facilities meet high-quality standards, and it is not always possible to attain specialized care or treatment. The health status of Moroccans has improved slightly over the last 20 years, with a notable decrease in morbidity and mortality from many diseases. The health system is generally well run in cities, whereas inhabitants in the countryside often have long distances to treatment centers. Cities have private as well as public hospitals that offer high-quality services. At last count, Morocco had 1 physician for every 2,174 inhabitants, and 1 hospital bed for every 1,020 people. Private-sector medical activities are carried out primarily in private hospitals and private consulting offices.

Ethnic-/Race-Specific or Endemic Diseases: Endemic diseases include hydatid cystic disease, tuberculosis, trachoma (southern Morocco), leishmaniasis, and hepatitis A. Moroccans are at risk for hepatitis E, Q fever, mycotoxicoses, malaria (in certain regions), typhoid fever, schistosomiasis, and ascaridiosis. A major health issue is that water supplies are frequently contaminated by raw sewage; there also is silting of reservoirs and oil pollution of coastal waters. The major infectious food- and water-borne diseases reported in 2004 were bacterial diarrhea and hepatitis A. Vector-borne diseases are significant April through November. The Joint United Nations Programme on HIV/AIDS (UNAIDS) estimates the prevalence rate for human immunodeficiency virus (HIV) in adults (aged 15 to 49 years) as 0.1%, with 19,000 people living with HIV, including 4,000 women. About 1,300 deaths from acquired immunodeficiency syndrome (AIDS) have been reported. The main mode of transmission is heterosexual (82%).

Families' Role in Hospital Care: Family members or close friends accompany the patient and expect to participate in care or take on a vigilant, supervisory role.

Dominance Patterns: According to the constitution, all citizens are equal, but non-Muslims and women face discrimination in traditional practices and the law. Spousal violence is common. A wife who has been abused has the right to complain to the police, but she would do so only if she were prepared to bring criminal charges against the husband. Physical abuse is legal grounds for divorce, but divorce is granted only if the woman has two witnesses to the actual abuse who will support her in court. Medical certificates of injury do not suffice in the legal system. If the court rules against the woman, she is returned to the husband's home. If a man murders his wife, the sentence is generally light, although the criminal code provides severe punishments for men convicted of rape or sexual assault of a woman or girl other than their wives. Women bear the burden of proving their innocence, however, and because of the stigma attached to loss of virginity before marriage, most assaults are not reported. Victims' families may offer men who have raped women the opportunity to marry their victims to preserve family honor. Women seeking divorce may offer their husband money to agree to the divorce (a *khol'a* divorce). The husband must agree and is allowed to specify how much will be paid, with no limit. The *Moudouwana,* a code based on

Islamic law, states that women can inherit only half as much as male heirs. When women do inherit property, male relatives may pressure them to relinquish their part. Some well-educated women pursue careers in medicine, law, and education but few make it into the upper echelons of their professions.

Touch Practices: It not unusual for men to walk hand-in-hand in public.

Pain Reactions: In hospital settings, pain relief is expected, so pain medications may be persistently requested because of the belief that an ill person must conserve energy for recovery. Outside hospital settings, pain is usually expressed privately to family members or close relatives and friends. During labor and childbirth, it is expected that women will be vocal about pain.

Birth Rites: Muslim parents usually read verses of the holy *Koran* to their infants. Bathing is discouraged for 12 to 24 hours after birth if the baby is covered with vernix caseosa. The fertility rate is 3.05 children born per woman. The infant mortality rate is 41.6 deaths per 1,000 live births. Life expectancy is 68 years for men, 73 for women.

Death Rites: Muslim beliefs may or may not discourage organ donations or transplants, but Muslim doctors usually recommend transfusions to save lives. Autopsies are uncommon because the body must be buried intact. Cremation is not permitted. For Muslim burials, the body is wrapped in special pieces of white cloth and buried without a coffin in the ground as soon after death as possible.

Food Practices and Intolerances: Pork, carrion, alcohol, and blood consumption are forbidden for Muslims. The national dish is couscous— finely ground semolina that is usually accompanied by lamb and vegetables. Sweet mint tea is the drink of choice. Although Morocco is a Muslim country, it has no general ban on alcohol. Ramadan fasting is practiced, with exemptions for sick people and children.

National Childhood Immunizations: BCG at birth; DTwP at 6, 10, and 14 weeks and at 18 months; OPV at birth, at 6, 10, and 14 weeks, and at 18 months; HepB at birth, at 6 weeks, and at 9 months; measles at 9 months; MR at 6 years; vitamin A at 6, 12, and 18 months; TT first contact, +1, +6 months, +1, +1 year. The percentage of the target population vaccinated, by antigen, is: BCG (95%); DTP1 (99%); DTP3 (98%); HepB3 (96%); MCV (97%); and Polio3 (98%).

Other Characteristics: Morocco is an illegal producer of hashish; trafficking is increasing for domestic and international drug markets. Morocco is a transit point for cocaine from South America destined for Western Europe.

M

BIBLIOGRAPHY

Central Intelligence Agency: *2006: The world factbook, Morocco.* Retrieved September 21, 2006, from https://www.cia.gov/cia/publications/factbook/print/mo.html.

Hasbi B: A single window for access to the Ministry of Health studies and research in Morocco, *East Mediterr Health J.* 8(2–3):444–446, 2002.

Hotchkiss DR, Krasovec K, El-Idrissi MD, Eckert E, Karim AM: The role of user charges and structural attributes of quality on the use of maternal health services in Morocco, *Int J Health Plann Manage*. 20(2):113–135, 2005.

Naimoli JF, Rowe AK, Lyaghfouri A, Larbi R, Lamrani LA: Effect of the Integrated Management of Childhood Illness strategy on health care quality in Morocco, *Int J Qual Health Care*, Apr.18(2):134–144, 2006.

UNAIDS: 2006 Morocco. Retrieved September 21, 2006, from http://www.unaids.org/en/Regions_Countries/Countries/morocco.asp.

World Health Organization Report: *Implementation of the global strategy for health for all by the year 2000, Second evaluation*, Eighth report on the world health situation, Vol 6, Eastern Mediterranean Region, 145–151, 1996.

World Health Organization: 2006: Immunization, vaccines, and biologicals. Retrieved September 21, 2006, from http://www.who.int/immunization_monitoring/en/globalsummary/countryprofileresult.cfm?C='mar'.

http://state.gov/www/global/human_rights/1999_hrp_report/morocco.html (retrieved on January 26, 2006).

http://travel.state.gov/morocco.html (retrieved on January 26, 2006).

http://voyage.dfait-maeci.gc.ca/destinations/report_e.asp?country=Morocco (retrieved on January 26, 2006).

◆ MOZAMBIQUE (REPUBLIC OF)

MAP PAGE (801)

Aceme Nyika

Location: Mozambique stretches along the southeastern coast of Africa, bordering the Mozambique Channel, between South Africa and Tanzania. The country has uplands in the center, high plateaus in the northwest, mountains in the west, and coastal lowlands that cover nearly half of the country. The total area is 801,590 km^2 (309,413 square miles), and the capital is Maputo. The climate is tropical to subtropical, and cyclones are common. The population is 19.7 million, with 65% living in rural areas; 43% is 14 or younger. The country has experienced civil war, severe drought, crop failure, and famine. Major migration has occurred to urban and coastal areas, resulting in pollution of surface and coastal waters. The gross domestic product (GDP) per capita is estimated at $1,300, with 70% living below the poverty line. Unemployment is 21%.

Major Languages	Ethnic Groups	Major Religions
Portuguese (official)	Indigenous tribal groups (Shangaan, Chokwe, Manyika, Sena, Makua, and others) 99%	Indigenous beliefs 50%
Indigenous dialects		Christian 30%
		Muslim 20%
	Europeans, Euro-Africans, Indians 1%	

About 9% of the people speak Portuguese, and indigenous dialects are also spoken, including Emakhuwa (26%), Chichangana (11%), Elomwe (8%), Cisean (7%), Echuwabo (6%), other Mozambican languages (32%), and other languages (2%). Literacy rates are 64% for men, 33% for women.

Health Care Beliefs: Acute sick care; passive role. It is widely believed that herbs, amulets, and charms can influence health and illness. The people also strongly believe in the existence of an invisible, internal "snake" (called *nyoka* by Tsonga and Shona speakers), described as a power or force that lives in the stomach but can move throughout the upper part of the body. This belief may be related to sorcery or witchcraft, but it also may be symbolic of the need to respect the body and protect it from impurities. Prevention efforts are urgently needed to counteract a general lack of health care knowledge and traditional beliefs regarding causes of illness. For example, in cholera-prevalent areas, people do not associate the disease with consumption of unclean water or contamination of water supplies caused by a lack of latrines or toilets. Traditional beliefs also tend to be barriers to early use of biomedical prenatal care services, thus contributing to high infant and maternal mortality rates.

Predominant Sick-Care Practices: Magico-religious; traditional; and biomedical where available. Health care is nationalized and includes a policy of primary health care. However, medical facilities are rudimentary, and many medications are not available. Some general, nonemergency services are provided in cities. Traditional healers, as well as diviner mediums known as *impandes*, have a strong role in the belief system of the people and a role in treatment of illness. Traditional healers (*curandeiros*) often use a combination of herbal and magical medicine and are a comfortable choice for many people. Individuals may seek out traditional healers because of inadequate financial resources, but the choice is also affected by cultural comfort. Because of the extreme scarcity of doctors, the government is actively seeking the assistance of traditional healers, recruited through national associations, of which there are several in southern Africa. Healers are considered to be trusted advisors and can relate to the culture in areas where educational efforts may be considered taboo. For example, healers are involved in human immunodeficiency virus (HIV) and acquired immunodeficiency syndrome (AIDS) prevention programs and receive instructions about transmission and condom use that they then bring back to the villages.

Ethnic-/Race-Specific or Endemic Diseases: Endemic diseases include cholera, schistosomiasis, helminth infections, chloroquine-resistant malaria, endomyocardial fibrosis, hepatitis A and B, and bilharzias. People are at risk for Newcastle disease virus, hepatocellular carcinoma (associated with hepatitis A and B prevalence), poliomyelitis, rabies, tuberculosis, meningococcal meningitis, typhoid fever, diphtheria, tetanus, and dietary cyanide exposure from eating cassava. A recent study in Maputo City suggested that the leading causes of death are perinatal disorders, malaria, diarrheal disease, tuberculosis, lower respiratory tract infections, road traffic accidents, anemia, cerebrovascular disease, homicides, and bacterial meningitis. HIV/AIDS is a major source of morbidity and mortality. The Joint United Nations Programme on HIV/AIDS (UNAIDS) reports the estimated prevalence rate for HIV in adults (aged 15 to 49 years) as 16.1%, with 1.8 million people living with HIV, including 960,000 women. AIDS deaths are estimated to be 140,000; and 510,000 children have lost either one or both parents to AIDS. Only 9% of those who need antiretroviral treatment receive it.

Health-Team Relationships: The doctor shortage has placed the responsibility of maternity care on traditional birth attendants, midwives, and technicians. Surgical technicians have been trained to do cesarean sections, hysterectomies, and other surgical procedures. Nurse midwives are trained to perform screenings for syphilis—a major cause of poor pregnancy outcomes—and the data indicate that this approach has already decreased perinatal mortality by about 20%. This improvement demonstrates that increasing the education of midwives in developing countries can significantly decrease maternal mortality. Studies of 6-month pediatric nurse training programs at provincial hospitals also demonstrate that additional education results in significant decreases in deaths of hospitalized children.

Families' Role in Hospital Care: Families provide food and emotional support to their hospitalized relatives, and family members take turns to enable them to assess the condition of the patient. It is not unusual for relatives to administer traditional medicines secretly to their hospitalized relatives. It is therefore important for health practitioners to be aware of the parallel traditional health care system.

Dominance Patterns: Mothers usually spend the little they earn on daily food and health care for the family. The mothers who are able to earn more have more bargaining power. Although men have the dominant role in many families, some ethnic groups are matrilineal, such as the Macua in northern Mozambique. In a matrilineal kinship system, the husband and his family cannot mistreat or reject the wife, which gives her considerable protection against abuse. However, when women are infertile, they are excluded from certain social activities and traditional ceremonies, creating a very difficult situation. Studies show that a lack of bargaining power affects women's ability to negotiate sex and results in adolescent pregnancies and illnesses from sexually transmitted diseases. Studies indicate that middle-class women have fewer sexual partners; use condoms more often, challenge gender norms, and are generally more assertive toward men. It is well known that increasing educational levels of women usually means better health for themselves and for their families.

Eye-Contact Practices: Looking directly at a person of higher social status is generally regarded as a sign of disrespect. Youths are not expected to have eye contact with adults, and women are expected to avoid eye contact with husbands and in-laws. Similarly, an ordinary person should face down when talking to community leaders such as village headmen, chiefs, or traditional healers. Such power imbalances also affect doctor-patient interactions in that health practitioners are generally regarded as educated people who are better off than ordinary citizens.

Touch Practices: A handshake is the common way of greeting, and hugging is perceived as a way of expressing deep emotions. Whereas the Mozambican people are comfortable with female relatives or friends hugging each other as a way of greeting, hugging between men is viewed as being weird and "un-African." Exceptions are close relatives and, in certain rare circumstances, such as reunion with relatives after many years of separation. Holding hands or touching other parts of the body is perceived as a romantic practice that should not occur in public but is considered abnormal if between people of the same sex. Patients may feel uncomfortable with physical examinations, especially if the examiner is of the opposite sex. Traditional healers, whom communities respect, do not perform such physical examinations on their patients.

Perceptions of Time: With the exception of working class people in urban areas, there is generally a sense of laxity about time, probably because traditionally people divided their day into three parts: morning, afternoon, and evening. The sun, rather than time, was used to demarcate the three divisions. Thus, arriving at 10:00 AM for an 8:00 AM meeting is generally regarded as being punctual because it is still in the morning.

Pain Reactions: Women can openly express pain through prolonged loud crying or wailing, whereas for men such behavior is perceived as a sign of weakness and unbecoming. It is acceptable for men to shed tears quietly to express extreme pain, but they are expected to regain their composure quickly. Consequently, men tend to endure illness for some time before seeking treatment; whether traditional or biomedical.

Birth Rites: Most infants are delivered at home by traditional birth attendants or relatives. Rural infants may be delivered onto the ground and left untouched until the placenta is delivered. It is considered important to have many children, although couples are encouraged to space births. The fertility rate is 4.62 children born per woman. Given the status of health care and prevalent diseases in Mozambique, pregnancy poses serious mortality risks. Women frequently seek contraceptive methods such as herbs, charms, or amulets from indigenous healers, although oral contraceptives, intrauterine devices, and injectable drugs are available from family planning clinics. The Macua in northern Mozambique seeking treatment for infertility visit traditional healers more frequently than they visit hospitals; their beliefs about the causes of infertility are tradition based. Therefore, almost all commit adultery in the hope of conceiving. The maternal mortality rate is about 100 times higher than that of developed countries. Adolescent maternal mortality is associated with malaria, pregnancy-induced hypertension, puerperal sepsis, and septic abortion; 75% of these deaths are considered to be avoidable. Infant mortality rates are high at 129 and 152 deaths per 1,000 live births for infants younger than 1 and younger than 5, respectively, and the deaths are frequently associated with maternal malaria and syphilis. Life expectancy is very low by any standard: 40 years for both men and women.

Death Rites: Death is viewed as an important event that draws together relatives from urban and rural areas. Even if the deceased (*mfumu*) was not popular, any signs of dislike could lead to suspicion of having caused the death through witchcraft (*mfiti*). Consequently, considerable effort is made to attend the funeral (*marilo*), and everybody, including those who cannot attend, makes a contribution in cash or kind. The deceased lies in his or her (or parents') house overnight, and then the body is prepared for burial (*kuutha mtembo*) by close relatives. After body viewing (*kuona nkhope*), the body is carried to the graveyard, where the coffin is placed in the grave (*mudzi*) and mourners throw dirt on it (*kuponya dothi*), a practice believed to symbolize the end of a process of coming to terms with the loss and to cut emotional links with the deceased. A traditional cere-mony (*m'meto*) to appease the spirit of the deceased is held within a year after burial; otherwise, the spirit is believed to cause illness, bad luck, or infertility to the relatives, as is believed to be the case with the Gamba spirits that emerged from the civil war from the 1970s to 1992. The *m'meto* ceremony is also believed to bring back the spirit of the deceased (*kuzizira*) to look after the family.

Food Practices and Intolerances: The staple food is *sadza*, a thick porridge made from maize meal that is eaten with relish commonly made from vegetables. Beef and white meat such as chicken and fish are expen-sive delicacies that are eaten on special occasions such as weddings, Christmas, and New Year holidays or to honor very special visitors. Sor-ghum, rice, potatoes, bread, ground nuts, and beans are alternative foods that are less abundant than maize. Although some communities eat cas-sava as a substitute for maize during drought periods, its consumption has gradually declined based on fears of dietary cyanide poisoning from insufficient processing.

Infant-Feeding Practices: Although breastfeeding is encouraged until the infant is 18 months old, exclusive breastfeeding is undermined by use of supplementary fluids, infant formulas, and diary milk in urban areas, or maize meal porridge in rural areas. In an effort to reduce malnutrition, the ministry of health encourages mothers to add peanut butter to the maize meal porridge.

Child-Rearing Practices: Child rearing is primarily the responsibility of mothers, while fathers are supposed to fend for their families and pro-vide overall guidance. Cultural beliefs of witchcraft and evil spirits may compromise use of medical services to the detriment of children's health. The extended family and community can also enforce discipline on chil-dren. Although the legal age of majority is 18 years, once youths get married or have children they may live independently. However, proxy con-sent for invasive medical procedures or health research with more than minimal risks, is required.

National Childhood Immunizations: BCG at birth; DTwPHep at 6, 10, and 14 weeks; OPV at 6, 10 and 14 weeks; measles at 9 months; TT 1st contact, +1, +6 months, +1, +1 year; vitamin A at 6, +6, +6, +6, +6, +6 months. The percent of the target population vaccinated, by anti-gen, is: BCG (87%); DTP1 (88%); DTP3 (72%); MCV (77%); Polio3 (70%); HepB3 (72%); TT2 plus (70%).

BIBLIOGRAPHY

Central Intelligence Agency: *2006: The world factbook, Mozambique*. Retrieved September 21, 2006, from https://www.cia.gov/cia/publications/factbook/print/mz.html.

Chapman RR: Endangering safe motherhood in Mozambique: prenatal care as pregnancy risk, *Soc Sci Med.* 57:355–374, 2003.

Granja AC, Machungo F, Gomes A, Bergstrom S: Adolescent maternal mortality in Mozambique, *J Adolesc Health*, 28(4):303, 2001.

Igreja V: 'Why are there so many drums playing until dawn?' Exploring the role of the Gamba spirits and healers in the post-war recovery period in Gorongoza, Central Mozambique, *Transcult Psychiatry*. 40(4):459–487, 2003.

Lunet N, Barros H: Use of water by breastfed children in Maputo, *J Trop Pediatr.* 49 (3):193, 2003.

Machel JZ: Unsafe sexual behaviour among schoolgirls in Mozambique: a matter of gender and class, *Reprod Health Matters.* 9(17):82, 2001.

Songane FF, Bergstron S: Quality of registration of maternal deaths in Mozambique: a community-based study in rural and urban areas, *Soc Sci Med.* 54(1):23, 2002.

UNAIDS: 2006 Mozambique. Retrieved September 21, 2006, from http://www.unaids.org/en/Regions_Countries/Countries/mozambique.asp.

World Health Organization: 2006: Immunization, vaccines and biologicals. Retrieved September 21, 2006, from http://www.who.int/immunization_monitoring/en/globalsummary/countryprofileresult.cfm?C='moz'.

◆ MYANMAR (UNION OF BURMA)

MAP PAGE (805)
Soe-Soe and Aye Mu Myint

Location: Myanmar has a total area of 671,000 km² (259,006 square miles). It shares borders with China, India, Thailand, Laos, and Bangladesh. Myanmar consists of a narrow mountain range, a plateau, a flat, fertile delta, and a long coastline stretching from the Bangladesh border in the northwest to the Malay Peninsula and Thai territory in the southeast. Burma became Myanmar in 1989 because the name Burma implies only Burman, which is just one of the many ethnic groups in the country. Myanmar has a population of 48 million; the capital is Rangoon. The gross domestic product (GDP) per capita is $1,700, with 25% living below the poverty line.

Major Languages	Ethnic Groups	Major Religions
Burmese (official)	Burman 68%	Buddhist 89%
English	Shan 9%	Christian 4%
	Karen 7%	Muslim 4%
	Rakhine 4%	Other 2%
	Mon 2%	Animist 1%
	Indian 2%	
	Chinese 3%	
	Indian 2%	
	Other 5%	

All major ethnic groups have their own language and writing. English is the second language at school. Myanmar has more than 100 minor ethnic groups. Literacy rates are 89% for men, 81% for women.

Health Care Beliefs: According to Buddhism, health is the most important gift in life. Certain sayings attest to the importance of food: "Foods are nutrients as well as medicines"; "a suitable amount is medicinal, but overdose is dangerous"; and "a bad step or a mouthful of bad food can be fatal." Nutrients are categorized as "cold" or "hot" and further subdivided into six categories according to taste: salty, bitter, sweet, sour, spicy, and phan (a combination of slightly bitter and sour). Articles on food appear each month in popular journals, explaining which foods are cold and hot and which tastes promote good health for the particular month. Food taboos are common; for example, lactating mothers are not allowed to eat red meat because of the belief that to do so will cause "wind colic" in infants. Depression is rare because of the comfort and support provided by family members, and fortune tellers are believed to have tricks that can cancel bad luck. It is rare for a person to sue for malpractice because anything that goes wrong is thought to result from a person's previous bad behavior. Suicide is uncommon, as Buddhists believe that if a person commits suicide that event will be repeated in the person's next 500 lives. Blood donation is encouraged because whatever is given will be returned in some way. People emphasize natural products. Women use a special scented plant known as *thanakha (Limonia acidissma linn)* as a cosmetic: ground with water over a specially prepared stone. *Thanakha* has a very pleasant odor, soothing effect, and protects the skin from sunburn. Plant products are used to shampoo the hair, after which coconut oil is applied.

Predominant Sick Care Practices: Biomedical and traditional practices. Traditional practices consist of remedies from plants, massages with or without plant extracts, and acupuncture. Biomedical treatment is preferred for severe illness and by urban dwellers. Minor illness is treated with the traditional medications common in almost every house. For example, a minor form of diabetes is treated by eating bitter gourd, and muscle pain and fatigue are treated by massage. Acupuncture is reserved for chronic pain. Traditional acupuncture (often done by untrained personnel) is gradually being replaced by Chinese acupuncture. Public biomedical and traditional health care services are provided by dispensaries and hospitals free of charge. In private clinics and hospitals, charges have to be paid by patients.

Ethnic-/Race-Specific or Endemic Diseases: The population has genetic risk for hemoglobin E disease, thalassemia, and to a lesser extent glucose-6-phosphate (G6PD) deficiency. Nutritional goiters are common in the mountain ranges and delta areas. Malaria is endemic in the forested mountains and border areas, and chloroquine-resistant malaria is found at the border of Thailand. People are at risk for vector-, food-, and water-borne diseases such as diarrhea, hepatitis A, polio, intestinal worms, dengue fever, and typhoid. Snake bites from vipers during rice harvesting season cause high mortality rates because of the superstition that wearing boots in the rice field annoys the spiritual guardians of the field. Blood donations are systematically screened for hepatitis B and human immunodeficiency virus (HIV). Postpartum and neonatal beriberi is common in some isolated and remote villages because of a lack of proper food during pregnancy and lactation. Liver cancer is very common in men, second only to lung cancer, and occurs at relatively early ages (i.e., age 35 to 50). This high rate may be related to high hepatitis B and C carrier rates and the prevalence of aflatoxin in street food such as ground nuts and chili, which men eat more often than women do. The incidence of uterine fibroids is high in single women. Breast and cervical cancers are the most common cancers in single and married multiparous women, respectively. The prevalence rate for HIV and acquired immunodeficiency syndrome (AIDS) in adults is 1.3%, with 360,000 people living with HIV, including 110,000 women. Deaths from AIDS are about 37,000. When the mode of transmission is known, 65% of cases are acquired heterosexually, 26% from injecting drug use, and 5% from contaminated blood. The male-to-female ratio is 3.6:1.

Health-Team Relationships: Health care is doctor-driven, with active participation of patient and family members. About 4,000 medical doctors graduate yearly from a 7-year medical course. Health assistants are allowed to measure blood pressures and inject vaccines and medications under a doctor's supervision. In remote villages, dispensaries are run by health assistants. The nursing course lasts 3 years and 6 months for midwifery, and there are four grades of technicians. There are four initiatives for endemic diseases: malaria, leprosy, tuberculosis, and trachoma. Sex is not discussed among friends, relatives, or family members. Attitudes toward virginity are strict, and out-of-wedlock pregnancy is unacceptable. Kissing or embracing in public is regarded as shameful. Even holding a woman's hand without her permission is regarded as an insult and could be punishable with 5 years of prison. After age 5, kisses or body contact with girls are prohibited, even by family members of the opposite sex. Extramarital sex is also prohibited; monogamy and loyalty to one's marriage partner are stressed. Prostitution is illegal. Arranged marriage by parents is less popular than previously, although approval of the prospective spouse by the parents is common. It is considered indecent for a woman to expose her body, so when being examined she must be covered with a thin sheet of cloth. If the doctor is a man, another woman must be present. Health education is promoted on television, radio, journals and newspapers. Sex education is provided by health personnel to adults only. Workers' clinics and hospitals are for those engaged in either governmental or private industry; however, they also can go to public dispensaries and hospitals. Social welfare personnel provide help for those who cannot afford medications, transportation, or rehabilitation. The Myanmar pharmaceutical industry produces essential medications and monovalent and polyvalent antiviper and anticobra snake venoms.

Families' Role in Hospital Care: Families stay with the patient in the hospital, perform basic care, and provide meals and clean linen. If essential medicines are not available, the family must purchase them. Both fathers and mothers discuss the health of their children and participate in decision making. It is usually the mother, however, who takes care of the children.

Dominance Patterns: Women have the same rights as men in health decisions but have more dominance regarding household economy. However, it is believed that a woman cannot become a God, and women are not allowed to be physically higher than God statues or monks.

Eye-Contact Practices: Direct eye contact between friends is the norm and is considered polite and necessary, especially when greeting someone. A confidential connection between health care personnel and patients necessitates eye contact regardless of their respective ages.

Touch Practices: Hugs and kisses for young children from family members, friends, or health personnel are common, but touch among adults, especially between opposite sexes, is not. Regardless of age or gender, touching is considered natural by health care professionals, especially to comfort and assure patients. The frequency of touching in nursing care situations increases with very sick or older patients and when needed to relax and comfort patients.

Perceptions of Time: Punctuality is not stressed, and excuses are usually accepted for lateness if it is not a life-and-death situation. People are reluctant to say "no" to requests, even though the request may involve something that is difficult to accomplish in time.

Pain Reactions: Women are freely allowed to express pain; men are expected to endure pain with less of an outward reaction.

Birth Rites: The fertility rate is two children born per woman, and the infant mortality rate is high at 62 deaths per 1,000 live births. Women in urban areas practice family planning, and contraceptive pills and injections are preferred to condoms. Hospital stays are 24 hours for multiparous and 5 days for nulliparous women because of episiotomies. In villages, women prefer to give birth at home either with traditional birth attendants or midwives. The puerperium is 45 days, during which time women do no work. The focus is on involution of the uterus, regaining abdominal muscle, and encouraging the free flow of breast milk. The mother eats rice, vegetable soups with fish or chicken, and baked, dried fish. Some villagers do not consume chicken, thinking it will cause allergies. Traditionally, the mother and infant avoid exposure to the smell of frying foods. A name is chosen after consulting an expert who uses the time and date of the infant's birth to select a name that should bring health, success, and prosperity. A family name is not compulsory, and it is also not required for a woman to change her family name after marriage. The formal name-giving ceremony usually takes place when the child is about 6 months old. Before this event, parents give the child a nickname that is often chosen before birth. Life expectancy is 58 for men, 64 for women.

Death Rites: Buddhists believe in rebirth and hope for less suffering in the next life. Those who are dying are helped to recall past good deeds, which enables them to achieve a fit mental state. Patients prefer to die at home among family members. Autopsies are permitted, and cremation is preferred, usually on the third day after death. On the seventh day after death, the family has a ceremony to announce to the person's spirit that it is free to go. Relatives, friends, and neighbors accompany the family at the funeral and ceremony. Some people donate their eyes and bodies after death for corneal transplants and human anatomy education.

Food Practices and Intolerances: Rice with curry is eaten at lunch and dinner. Breakfast is usually noodles or sticky rice. Traditional curry contains oil, onions, garlic, and ginger. People tend to prefer freshwater over seawater products. The most commonly eaten meat is chicken. Some people do not eat pork because of spiritual beliefs, and some do not eat beef because they use working cows in the fields and thus owe a debt of gratitude to them. Snacks can be sticky rice cakes, pickled tea-leaf salad, appetizers, or nuts. During ceremonies, guests are served food and drinks. Alcohol prepared from fermented rice and fermented palm juice is consumed by the men, but not by women.

Infant-Feeding Practices: Most infants are breastfed; however, breast-feeding may be delayed for several days because people believe that colostrum is bad for infants. Women know that certain foods and medications can pass into the breast milk, so nursing mothers are aware of foods that are potentially harmful. A semiliquid rice mixture is introduced when the child is 1 month old, and vegetables and fruits are gradually added at about the third month. A special pillow of broken rice grains is made for the infant so that it can adapt to the infant's head and prevent malformation.

National Childhood Immunizations: BCG at 6 weeks; DTwP at 6, 10, and 14 weeks; OPV at 6, 10, and 14 weeks; HepB at 6, 10, and 14 weeks; measles at 9 months; and TT at 1 and 2 years first antenatal contact, +1 month. The percent of the target population vaccinated, by antigen, is: BCG and DTP1 (76%); DTP3 and Polio3 (73%); HepB3 (62%); MCV (72%); TT2 plus (85%).

M

BIBLIOGRAPHY

Central Intelligence Agency: 2006: The world factbook, Burma. Retrieved September 21, 2006, from https://www.cia.gov/cia/publications/factbook/print/bm.html.

Government of the Union of Myanmar: National Health Plan, 1996–2001: Forum on health *sector* development, planning document Series-3.

Soe S, Than-Than, Khin-Ei-Han: The nephrotoxic action of Russell's viper venom, *Toxicon.* 28:461–467, 1990.

UNAIDS: 2006 Myanmar. Retrieved September 21, 2006, from http://www.unaids.org/en/Regions_Countries/Countries/myanmar.asp.

World Health Organization: 2006: Immunization, vaccines and biologicals. Retrieved September 21, 2006, from http://www.who.int/immunization_monitoring/en/globalsummary/countryprofileresult.cfm?C='mmr'.

http://who.int/countries/mmr/en/ (retrieved August 30, 2006).

✦ NAMIBIA (REPUBLIC OF)

MAP PAGE (801)

Jörg Klewer

Location: Namibia is located in the southwestern corner of Africa and covers a total area of 834,295 km² (317,827 square miles). It has been an independent democracy since 1990. Namibia is divided into 13 districts, and the capital, Windhoek, is centrally located. The population is more than two million. Namibia shares long borders with Angola in the north and Botswana in the east. The Caprivi Zipfel, a small corridor from the northeastern edge, touches Zambia and Zimbabwe. Its natural boundaries are the Kunene, Kavango, and Zambezi river systems in the north and the Orange River in the south. Namibia can be divided into four distinct regions: the Namib and Kalahari Deserts, the Central Plateau, and the northern savannah grasslands. The gross domestic product (GDP) per capita is $7,000; about 35% of the population lives on $1 and 56% on $2 per day.

Major Languages	Ethnic Groups	Major Religions
English (official)	Black 87.5%	Christian 80%–90%
Afrikaans (lingua franca)	White 6%	Indigenous 10%–20%
Oshiwambo (≥50% of population)	Mixed 6.5%	
German, indigenous		

More than 70% are of Bantu ethnicities: Owambo, Herero, Kavango, Caprivi, and Tswana and about 80,000 people are of European descent. People commonly speak several languages: more than 50% speak Oshiwambo. Indigenous languages are included in primary school: English is the medium of instruction at the secondary level. Literacy rates are 84% for both men and women.

Health Care Beliefs: Acute sick care; traditional. People in rural areas often see mental illness as something magical—spells caused by witches or ghosts. Therefore, mentally ill patients are first brought by their family to traditional healers or witches to get rid of the spell. The individual "treatment" depends on the specialty of the witch or healer. If the ill person does not improve, the family usually then brings him or her to the clinic or hospital. Sometimes traditional healers create amulets to prevent the owner from specific diseases. People in the northern regions tend to visit both healers and the public health system. In some cases, patients who are admitted to the public hospital get unofficial treatment by traditional healers, which leads to conflicts with Western-based therapies. Traditional healers use a variety of herbal mixtures that may contain toxic herbs that lead to severe intoxication. People of the northern regions believe in witches and witchcraft. These witches are normally contacted by persons who believe they are bewitched and seek countermeasures for the

witchcraft or by persons who want to put a spell on someone. Some people believe these witches can take the shapes of snakes, spiders, or black
bulls to go to other villages. Traditional beliefs such as holy fires and spiritual contacts with ancient tribal chiefs are more common in the San and
Himba people.

Predominant Sick-Care Practices: Biomedical and traditional. Because
of the shortage of doctors, Namibian nurses have taken over many duties.
The country is covered by a network of more than 280 primary health
care clinics, where one to five nurses provide vaccinations, screening
examinations, and health education. Primary health care clinics offer treatment for minor illnesses (e.g., headache, sore throat, small wounds).
Those with major problems are sent to the hospital. Indicators for health
statistics are collected and analyzed by primary health care nurses,
assisted by mobile teams that reach rural areas by off-road vehicles.
The nurses provide health education, vaccinations, and medical treatment.
The health care system is predominantly a government-operated (public)
health care system based on Western (biomedical) medicine, comparable
to the South African health care system. Regional and district hospitals
are well equipped and offer services by medical doctors in outpatient
and inpatient departments. Health care (including drugs) is nearly free of
charge with only a small obligatory fee; therefore, people primarily use
public health facilities. In urban areas, private practices and pharmacies
are available, but they are open only for patients with private health insurance. Traditional healers are widespread in the northern regions, and they
employ various techniques: traditional massage (especially for musculoskeletal problems), herbal mixtures, and parallel short incisions (1 to
2 cm) in the skin over the painful part. Policies have not yet been developed to integrate traditional healers into the health care system.

Ethnic-/Race-Specific or Endemic Diseases: Current major health
problems are human immunodeficiency virus (HIV) and acquired immunodeficiency syndrome (AIDS), sexually transmitted diseases (STDs), viral
hepatitis, tuberculosis, and malaria. Additional problems, especially in
the north, are schistosomiasis, endemic plague, vitamin deficiencies and
malnutrition, leprosy, rabies, snake bites, and diarrhea. Because of open
fires in traditional houses, respiratory tract infections and burns are frequent in children. Urban areas are prone to traffic accidents, violence
(mainly stab wounds), and alcohol abuse. In northern Namibia, especially
in the Kavango territory, an acquired form of immune thrombocytopenia
called *onyalai* is present (about 660 cases annually). Epistaxis or gastrointestinal bleeding is severe and may cause shock and death. Chronic
thrombocytopenia often ensues, and recurrent episodes of clinical bleeding are common. The causative agents are mycotoxins from contaminated
millet, sorghum, or maize. The Joint United Nations Programme on HIV/
AIDS (UNAIDS) reports the estimated prevalence rate for HIV in adults
(aged 15 to 49 years) to be 19.6%, with 230,000 living with HIV, including
130,000 women and 17,000 children aged 0 to 14. HIV prevalence
among antenatal woman ranges from about 9% in Opuwo, more than

30% in Oshakati, and more than 40% in Katima Mulilo. About 85,000 children are orphans as the result of parental AIDS. More than 26,000 deaths from AIDS have been reported. The increasing number of deaths from tuberculosis, pneumonia, and diarrhea suggests that HIV is the underlying cause in many cases.

Health-Team Relationships: Medical doctors command significant power in their relationships with nurses and patients. Patients usually prefer to be examined and treated by physicians. Patients also prefer being seen by a white instead of a black doctor because they think that white physicians are better educated. The cooperation between medical doctors and nurses is usually good. Most patients attending primary health care clinics or hospital outpatient departments expect a prescription of oral medications or injections. To fulfill these expectations, patients with no therapeutic need for pharmaceuticals get some multivitamin tablets to prevent disappointed patients from receiving unnecessary treatment at the hands of traditional healers.

Families' Role in Hospital Care: Namibian hospitals provide full service, including a hospital bed, meals, and nursing care. In pediatric wards, the mothers often stay with their children and assist the nurses in daily care. Family members are allowed to stay with patients in the wards only during visiting hours; otherwise, they stay outside the hospital. Despite regular meals of good quality, family members are usually allowed to bring in soft drinks and home-cooked meals.

Dominance Patterns: Women and men have equal rights, but Namibian families are traditionally dominated by a male patriarch. The wife has to serve and cook for her husband, maintain the house, work in the fields, and bear "enough" healthy children. Officially, only monogamy is allowed, but in the rural area of northern Namibia, polygamy is common and is legitimized by traditional weddings. Changes in family patterns are not common. Other male family members take over the patriarch's role if he dies or suffers from severe illness. In urban communities like Windhoek, these traditional roles are less fixed. Women have professional jobs and enter political positions.

Eye-Contact Practices: Eye contact is normally not avoided, even when persons in superior positions are present.

Touch Practices: Physical touching by traditional hugging or handshaking is common. Greeting a friend or relative is normally accompanied by ritualized handshaking. Physical touching is accepted in medical examinations. Holding hands in public between opposite sexes is increasingly visible in urban areas but is still uncommon in rural areas.

Perceptions of Time: Punctuality is not a major issue, even though appointments and other commitments may not be kept in a timely fashion. People without watches estimate the time by looking at the direction and intensity of the sun, or by the appearance and shape of the moon. Because of this, the small plastic bags used to hand out prescribed medications are covered with sun and moon symbols, symbolizing appropriate times for medications. Events that occurred some weeks ago, such as the last menstrual period in pregnant women, are often described by terms such as "when the full moon was over the big tree." Accordingly, health professionals need some knowledge about the lunar year and regional features.

Pain Reactions: It is expected that men should be stoic, but it is acceptable for women to be expressive about pain. Men and women, even in rural areas, express physical pain by body movements, screams, tears, and occasionally hysteria. Extensive and loud expressions of emotional pain are much more common in women.

Birth Rites: The fertility rate is three children born per woman. In traditional rural communities, pregnant women continue their daily lives as farmers until they are close to delivery. The primary health care system includes antenatal clinics, which provide regular physical examinations; health education; and free iron, folic acid, and vitamin supplements. Around the estimated time of delivery, pregnant women come to the birthing facilities at the hospitals, sometimes alone and sometimes brought by relatives. They usually stay alone around the hospital until they are near labor. In general, husbands do not enter delivery rooms. Maternity wards are well equipped and managed by qualified nurses and midwives. In cases of complicated labors, a gynecologist or surgeon is usually available to perform a cesarean section. Despite this, the infant mortality rate is very high at 48 deaths per 1,000 live births. Analgesia is not routinely used for normal labor. The number of home births is decreasing, but they still occur; and mother and child come to the postnatal clinic or hospital for follow-up care. The birth of a newborn is a happy event for the whole family and is usually celebrated with relatives and neighbors. Both girls and boys are well accepted. Because of HIV/AIDS, life expectancy has significantly decreased and is 44 for men, 42 for women.

Death Rites: Death is regarded as a natural event and is marked by celebrations. The initial reaction to the death of a relative or friend is shock and denial, followed by a period of mourning and acceptance. Some men express the loss of a loved person by cutting their hair. Because of the high number of victims during the war and the present AIDS epidemic, people have developed a fatalistic attitude, resulting in reduced emotional response and stoicism. Burial ceremonies are shorter because nearly every family is faced with the death of several members. The deceased are buried in a cemetery, especially Christians. Even if most are Christian, traditional beliefs in witchcraft as a cause of death are very much present, although officially denied. There is no discussion about organ donation because no transplant unit exists. The shortage of pathologists means that autopsies are not routinely performed. Sometimes surgeons take over requested autopsies; forensic autopsies are normally accepted.

Food Practices and Intolerances: Meat is the basic food, either game or domestic animals, normally served grilled or dried. Agriculture is widespread only in northern Namibia. Cows are expensive, so people prefer to eat goats or chickens. Meat is eaten with potatoes (boiled or fried), maize, rice, or porridge made from pumpkins. Near the seacoast, fish is varied with meat, either grilled naturally or salted and grilled. In northern Namibia, omahango (mahango), a kind of millet, is the basic vegetable: Omahango plants grow up to 3 m tall and are cultivated on every small farm. In poor families, porridge made from omahango flour is served every day. To enrich their food with protein, people in northern Namibia collect special big caterpillars from the trees and serve them fried and salted. During the rainy season from November to April, fish and frogs in the rivers are used to enrich soups and porridges. In northern Namibia, fruits such as guava, bananas, and varied palm tree fruits are cultivated and enjoyed. A traditional sweet-tasting beer named otombo is brewed by using omahango flour and brown sugar. It is easy to brew in open bowls and a major public health problem in Northern Namibia, leading to domestic violence, alcoholism, and unemployment. Because of endemic goiter, all salt in Namibia for both human and animal consumption must be iodized.

Infant-Feeding Practices: Since Namibia's independence, the Ministry of Health and Social Service has promoted breastfeeding for at least 6 months after birth. Therefore, primary health care facilities educate pregnant women on its advantages. The problem of HIV transmission during breastfeeding is recognized, and women who are HIV positive can obtain infant formula free of charge. Unfortunately, formula is not always available, so these mothers may be forced to continue breastfeeding. International companies have also started to advertise and sell industrial milk products and infant formulas. These advertisements suggest that artificial food is healthier than breastfeeding, and young parents are tempted to buy it, even if they cannot afford it. Because of formula's high cost, mothers sometimes dilute it, often with contaminated or inadequately boiled water, causing malnutrition and diarrhea. Soft drinks are increasingly given to small infants. They are more expensive than traditional food and fruits and can lead to malnutrition (kwashiorkor) and dental caries.

Child-Rearing Practices: Children are reared by their parents and relatives living nearby. Young children stay with their mothers most of the time, and their mother teaches them good behavior and right or wrong. Because of the lack of jobs, numerous Namibian males work in southern Namibia, especially in Windhoek, Swakopmund, Walvis Bay, and Oranjemund. Therefore, many children grow up without their fathers, seeing them once or twice a year. Respect for older people is traditionally important in rearing children and typically is enforced by beatings. Sometimes older children (mainly girls or grandparents) look after younger siblings or children of relatives or neighbors. At age 6 to 7 years, they are sent to school. An emerging problem is the escalating number of orphans as a result of the AIDS epidemic who grow up with their grandparents or relatives.

National Childhood Immunizations: BCG at birth; DTwP at 6, 10, and 14 weeks; OPV at birth and 6, 10, and 14 weeks and at 5 and 10 years; DT at 5 and 10 years; measles at 9 months; vitamin A at 9 months; and

TT at 15 to 49 years. The percent of the target population vaccinated, by antigen, is: BCG (95%); DTP1 (93%); DTP3 and Polio3 (86%); MCV (73%); vitamin A (64%); and TT2 plus (99%). Immunizations are offered free of charge daily at most health facilities. Vaccinations are documented in individual health passports, which are often lost or damaged, so children with unknown or unclear immunization records receive full immunizations.

BIBLIOGRAPHY

Central Intelligence Agency: *2006: The world factbook, Namibia.* Retrieved September 21, 2006, from https://www.cia.gov/cia/publications/factbook/print/wa.html.

Government of Namibia: Official homepage. Retrieved March 4, 2006, from http://www.grnnet.gov.na.

Joined United Nations Programme on HIV/AIDS (UNAIDS): *Namibia—Epidemiological fact sheet, 2004 update.* Geneva, 2004, UNAIDS.

Talvera P: *Challenging the Namibian perception of sexuality.* Windhoek, 2002, Gmasberg Macmillian Publishers.

The Namibian: Official homepage of an independent Namibian newspaper, offering a great achive with information about Namibia. Retrieved March 4, 2006, from http://www.namibian.com.na.

UNAIDS: 2006 Namibia. Retrieved September 21, 2006, from http://www.unaids.org/en/Regions_Countries/Countries/namibia.asp

World Health Organization: 2006: Immunization, vaccines and biologicals. Retrieved September 21, 2006, from http://www.who.int/immunization_monitoring/en/globalsummary/countryprofileresult.cfm?C='nam'.

◆ NAURU (REPUBLIC OF)

MAP PAGE (794)

John Dixon and Alan Sanderson

Location: Nauru is a small, oval-shaped coral atoll situated in the southwestern portion of the Pacific Ocean—just below the equator and halfway between Australia and Hawaii. It has a total area of 21 km² (8.11 square miles). Its unique, barren terrain of jagged limestone pinnacles on the central plateau is the product of 90 years of continuous phosphate strip mining. Only its very narrow fertile coastal belt is habitable. Nauru has a tropical climate tempered by cool sea breezes, although it is subject to high humidity (averaging 70% to 80%) and heavy but erratic rainfall. The population is 13,287, with a population density of 1,312 per square mile. About 40% are aged between 0 and 14 years. Nauru was settled approximately 3,000 years ago by seafaring Polynesian and Melanesian explorers and thus originated from a mixture of people from Polynesia, Micronesia, and Melanesia, although they have predominantly Polynesian characteristics. Little is known of traditional Nauruan culture, although it is known that the ancestors believed in a female deity—Eijebon—and a spirit land—an island called Buitani.

Major Languages	Ethnic Groups	Major Religions
Nauruan	Nauruan 58%	Protestant 67%
English	Other Pacific Islander 26%	Roman Catholic 33%
	Chinese 8%	
	European 8%	

The indigenous spoken language is Nauruan, a distinct Pacific Island language. Significant numbers of Nauruans are illiterate in English and have a poor command of Nauruan. Until the end of the eighteenth century, the 12 tribes that made up island society lived in isolation and generally peacefully as a kingdom. Soon after discovery in 1789, the introduction of firearms, alcohol, foreign germs, and colonial exploitation began destroying the island, its people, and their traditional culture. The Germans began Nauruan cultural deterioration when they banned traditional island dancing and eventually other cultural practices after they annexed Nauru as part of the Marshall Islands Protectorate. The cultural legacy of 50 years of Australian hegemony is addiction to Australian Rule's Football, their love of Foster's lager, and other Australian sociocultural and sporting icons. Nauru thus supports a hybrid culture in which Christian and Western customs coexist with traditional ones. They have a good spirit, which has enabled them to stand up to more than two centuries or more of fractious British, American, and German seafarers; three colonial empires; and the military might of Japan. They are hospitable, honest, jovial, and unassertive. They place high value on friendliness, kindliness, and compassion. They prefer to work together, help each other, and treat everyone as equals. The gross domestic product (GDP) per capita is $7,000.

Health Care Beliefs: Acute sick care; some health promotion. Sickness prevention and health-promotion campaigns are occasionally undertaken by the government. With the assistance of the World Health Organization (WHO) in the mid-1990s, the capacity for implementing health-promotion programs (in collaboration with nongovernmental organizations, communities, schools, and youth groups), improved. Tobacco control and substance abuse prevention policies have been developed; however, there is a general lack of media-generated health information because of the paucity of local media. It is a popularly held belief that physical bulk signifies prosperity and prestige.

Predominant Sick-Care Practices: Biomedical and traditional. Nauru General Hospital and the National Phosphate Corporation Hospital joined in 1999 to become the Republic of Nauru Hospital. This institution employs five doctors and provides a medical service and community health section with a dispensary. Currently about 50% of professional health staff are expatriates on contract, but the government plans to train more local people. The hospital provides basic routine treatments, which may be supplemented with traditional healing. Sophisticated medical services are quite restricted, however, and the government pays for

Nauruans to receive specialist treatment when required overseas, notably in Australia and New Zealand. In 2003, AusAID prepared a strategic plan, in consultation with Nauru's health authorities, to investigate the partial privatization of the island's health service.

Ethnic-/Race-Specific or Endemic Diseases: In 1962, James Neel, an American geneticist, presented a now widely accepted theory that Nauruans, along with other Micronesians, have a "thrifty gene" that enables them to store surplus sugar as fat, which predisposes them to life-threatening illnesses such as diabetes, heart disease, and strokes—known collectively as the *New World syndrome.* The population's general health is not good, and life expectancy is low given the relatively high living standards. Very few people live beyond 65 years of age. The leading causes of institutional mortality in 2003 were diabetes, respiratory system diseases, circulatory system diseases, neoplasms, transport accidents, and drownings. Alcohol consumption is a serious social problem that can lead to physical assaults and dangerous driving, making traffic accidents a cause of many deaths. Drinking, particularly kava, a bitter-tasting beverage made from the root of a pepper shrub, is an important part of social and ceremonial life. More than half the population smokes. Nauru's per capita tobacco consumption is one of the highest in the world, especially among women. Most Nauruans, who are physically large like anyone of Polynesian stock, are classified as class 1 obese (70% of men and 56% of women). Diabetes affects 40% to 45% of the population (41% of men and 42% of women aged 30 to 64). Among those older than 65 years, the prevalence rate could be as high as 55%. Type 2 diabetes (non–insulin-dependent diabetes) is found in children. Nauru remains the country with the highest prevalence of diabetes. Nauruans have a high incidence of hypertension, heart disease, and cancer. Lymphatic filariasis remains endemic, and dengue fever is a serious risk. No cases of human immunodeficiency virus (HIV) or acquired immunodeficiency syndrome (AIDS) have been reported (as of 2004), although the increasing numbers of sexually transmitted diseases (STDs) suggest that the potential for an outbreak cannot be discounted. Homosexuality is illegal.

Health-Team Relationships: Doctors dominate the health care delivery system.

Families' Role in Hospital Care: Nauruans expect to do no more than visit hospitalized sick relatives during the designated visiting hours. All medical and dental services are free for Nauruans and all government employees and their family.

Dominance Patterns: Despite their traditionally matrilineal society and their tradition of worshipping a female deity, women have a subordinate role. Although Nauruan law gives them the same freedoms and protections as men, societal pressures limit their opportunities to exercise those rights fully. This trend is likely to continue while the social system remains dominated by the island's traditional council of chiefs. Anecdotal evidence suggests that alcohol abuse leads to spasmodic physical abuse against women and, although less frequently, against children. Such abuse is treated as a serious communal matter. Nauruans do not respond well to aggressive and argumentative people; diplomacy and tact are preferable to confrontation. A friendly, unassertive, cooperative approach is most likely to achieve successful interactions.

Eye Contact Practices: Making direct eye contact is a sign of respect and caring.

Touch Practices: Physical touching is a manifestation of the Nauruans' friendliness, kindness, and compassion.

Perceptions of Time: Nauruans abide by "Pacific time," in which the past, present, and future are brought into accord by ensuring that whatever can be put off until tomorrow will be—with no guilt. Punctuality requires a degree of anticipation that is inconsistent with climatic and cultural imperatives.

Pain Reactions: Pain is to be endured stoically and silently by men but not necessarily by women.

Birth Rites: Nauruan women give birth in hospitals free of charge. Births of all children are celebrated. The fertility rate is 3.5 children born per woman. The infant mortality rate is 10.52 deaths per 1,000 live births, and life expectancy is 58 years for men, 65 for women.

Death Rites: Christian beliefs about death are common. Autopsies are acceptable, but organ donations are irrelevant because organ transplant operations cannot be performed.

Food Practices and Intolerances: Because of environmental degradation, the supply of fresh food and water is limited. Only a small amount of fresh food is available, primarily fish (tainted with cadmium), which is eaten raw, especially by children; and occasionally chicken, beef, pork, or a few locally grown fruits or vegetables. The islander diet is dominated by processed, imported foods. Grisly turkey tails, mutton flaps, ice cream, and candy have become status symbols that are associated with affluence. This readily available junk food has become a staple part of the diet, and as a result, weight gain is widespread. Nauru has periodic droughts and limited natural freshwater resources. Roof storage tanks collect rain water, but people must depend on a single, aging desalination plant and supplements of imported water.

Infant-Feeding Practices: Nauruan mothers prefer to breastfeed their babies if possible, but no data have been collected regarding frequency or duration.

Child-Rearing Practices: Nauruan mothers have the dominant child-caring and -rearing responsibilities, although traditionally they were communal (tribal) responsibilities.

National Childhood Immunizations: BCG at 4 weeks; DTwP at 2, 4, 6, and 18 months; HepB at birth and at 1 and 6 months; measles at 9 and 12 months; OPV at 2, 4, 6, and 18 months and at 5 years; and Td at 5 years. The percent of the target population vaccinated, by antigen, is: BCG, DTP1 (90%); DTP3, HepB3, MCV, and Polio3 (80%).

Other Characteristics: Environmental degradation has turned the majority (90%) of central Nauru into a wasteland. Nauruans accept that the source of their wealth—phosphate—has destroyed their land and is killing them. Ecologic rehabilitation is a government priority, but little has been done, likely because of the projected cost: $230 million over 20 years. Nauru also lies downwind of the French nuclear test sites in the Pacific. Since 1888, Nauru has been exploited by the Germans, British, Australians, New Zealanders, Japanese, and, more recently, the Nauruans themselves. Its people, culture, forest, soil, and ultimately subsoil have been stripped or shipped away at the whim of colonial powers. The mining of 1,000 years of bird droppings has been lucrative; however, the valuable but finite phosphate reserves are virtually exhausted. Nauru's legacy is a standard of living that is among the best in the Third World. Nauruans pay no taxes, live in government-subsidized housing, and get free health care and education. They have a penchant for a sedentary lifestyle, simple but well-equipped traditional houses, and luxury cars. They also have a very uncertain economic future, generally poor health, and an unenviable natural environment. In recent years, they have been willing to support this lifestyle not only by accepting refugees seeking asylum in Australia (for payment), but also by accepting dubious Russian bank deposits in its off-shore banking operations—for a fee.

BIBLIOGRAPHY

McDonald CN, Gowdy JM. *Paradise for Sale: a parable of nature.* Berkeley, CA, 2000, University of California Press.

World Health Organization: 2006: Immunization, vaccines and biologicals. Retrieved September 21, 2006, from http://www.who.int/immunization_monitoring/en/globalsummary/countryprofileresult.cfm?C='nru'.

http//www.cdc.gov/tobacco/who/nauru.html (retrieved January 10, 2006).

http//www.earth.nwu.edu/people/emile/nauru.html (retrieved January 10, 2006).

http//www.ethnologue.com/show_country.asp?name=Nauru (retrieved January 10, 2006).

http//www.tbc.gov.bc.ca/cwgames/country/nauru/nauru.html (retrieved January 10, 2006).

http//www.sidsnetpacific.org/BPOANAR/nauru-pdf. (retrieved January 10, 2006).

N

◆ NEPAL (KINGDOM OF)

MAP PAGE (804)

Narbada Thapa

Location: Nepal is a landlocked country in southern Asia with a diverse, multilingual, multireligious, and multiethnic population of 28.2 million. It is situated between China in the north and India in the south, east, and west. The total area is 140,800 km^2 (53,363 square miles). Two thirds of the country is covered by hills and mountains, including Mount Everest, the highest peak in the world (8,848 m). More than 90% of the population lives in rural areas and depends on agriculture. The capital is Kathmandu.

Because of the difficult terrain, transport and communication are sparse or nonexistent in most areas. Tourism, especially trekking and mountaineering, have recently increased overall prosperity, but the gross domestic product (GDP) per capita is still low at $1,500, and 31% of the population lives below the poverty line.

Major Languages	Ethic Groups	Major Religions
Nepali 47.8%	Chhetri 15.5%	Hindu 80.6%
Maithali 12.1%	Brahmin-Hill 12.5%	Buddhist 10.7%
Bhoipuri 7.4%	Magar 7%	Islam 4.2%
Tharu 5.8%	Tharu 6.6%	Kirati 3.6%
Tamang 5.1%	Tamang 5.5%	Others 0.9%
Newari 3.6%	Newar 5.4%	
Magar 3.3%	Muslim 4.2%	
Others (≥35 languages)	Kami 3.9%	
	Yadav 3.9%	
	Others (≥50 castes, or ethnic, groups) 35.5%	

Nepal has more than 60 castes, or ethnic groups, who speak more than 40 languages. Ethnic groups can be classified into two broad categories: (1) the Indo-Aryans, or Indo-Nepalese; and (2) the Tibeto-Mongoloids, or Tibeto-Nepalese. Tibeto-Mongoloids, which include Sherpas, Tamang, Rai, Limbu, Magars, and Kiratis, live primarily in the northeastern part of the country. The bulk of the Hill and Terai (low land) groups include Indo-Aryans such as the Chhetri, Brahmin, Tharus, and Danuars. Literacy rates are 62% for men, 35% for women.

Health Care Beliefs: Acute sick care; traditional. Particularly in rural Nepal, illness is believed to be caused by purposeful intervention of an agent such as a supernatural being (deity, god), a non-human entity (ghost, ancestor, evil spirit), or a human being (witch, sorcerer). Sick people are thought of as victims—the objects of aggression or punishment directed specifically against them or their family. People who believe that the cause of their illness is naturalistic in origin seek biomedical or ayurvedic treatments from various sources such as a pharmacist, grocer, hospital, clinic, or health care provider, or rely on home remedies such as herbal preparations. People who believe that the cause of their illness is the wrath of a god, the influence of an evil spirit, sorcery, or breech of a taboo, seek treatment involving witchcraft and magic, pray, perform rituals to please the god or deity and priest, and use charms and amulets. Spiritual practices include praying, singing hymns, cupping, and rubbing or burning the skin with a heated spoon. Beliefs in the effects of "hot" and "cold" foods are also common. Mental illness is thought to be the result of sins in a past life.

Predominant Sick-Care Practices: Biomedical; magical-religious; and traditional practices. Geography and altitude influence the types of health problems and the availability of health care. Basic health services are provided by 84 hospitals, 188 primary health care centers, 698 health posts, and 3,129 sub-health posts throughout the country. Health care treatments include indigenous, Western, and ayurvedic medicine. More than 70% use traditional methods (involving faith or spiritual healers, priests, and home remedies) before seeking biomedical treatment. Ayurvedic medicine and natural therapies have become popular in recent years.

Ethnic-/Race-Specific or Endemic Diseases: Chloroquine-resistant malaria and kalazar are endemic, but there is no risk of these illnesses in urban and hilly regions. The patterns of diseases vary according to the geographic setting and socioeconomic conditions rather than ethnicity or race. Nepalese are at risk for cholera, Japanese encephalitis, leprosy, diarrhea, nutritional deficiencies, pneumonia, tuberculosis, and hepatitis. Common causes of death among children are respiratory tract infections, diarrhea, and malnutrition. The first case of acquired immunodeficiency syndrome (AIDS) in Nepal was reported in 1988. The Joint United Nations Programme on HIV/AIDS (UNAIDS) reports the prevalence rate of human immunodeficiency virus (HIV) in adults (aged 15 to 49 years) to be 0.5%, with 75,000 people living with HIV, including 16,000 women and fewer than 930 children aged 0 to 14. About 5,100 deaths are attributed to AIDS. Men in younger age groups are most affected. Nepal is currently classified as experiencing a "concentrated" epidemic, particularly among injecting drug users and female sex workers.

Health-Team Relationships: Most doctors are men, and nurses are primarily women. People and patients pay more respect to doctors than nurses. Although nurses are highly qualified, doctors' dominance over nurses continues in hospital settings. Paramedics and community health workers are also important providers of health services on the community level. Generally, attitudes toward all health providers are positive. In most settings, people are reluctant to receive care from a person of the opposite sex.

Families' Role in Hospital Care: People live together in extended family units. If one member gets ill, other members of the family take care of them. Families stay with hospitalized relatives, helping them eat and perform hygiene tasks as well as providing psychological support. They also purchase medications, take specimens to the laboratory if necessary, pay hospital bills, and do anything else that is necessary. Providing care for ill family members is considered an act of love and respect and is done with a sense of responsibility.

Dominance Patterns: The family unit is important, but gender inequities in the society remain. Because Nepal has a patriarchal society, young women move to the home of their in-laws after marriage, where they immediately assume responsibility for many chores and are low in the family hierarchy. Men are more powerful and the decision makers in most families, except in the Tibeto-Mongoloid ethnic group. In certain special situations, such as the selection of a daughter-in-law, pregnancy, childbirth, and care of newborns, mothers-in-law and older women are most influential. Sons are responsible for looking after their parents in their old age.

Eye-Contact Practices: Looking into a person's eyes during a conversation, especially of a senior citizen or woman, is considered disrespectful and impolite. It is believed that some individuals have the ability to cast a spell on another by just looking at their faces, foreheads, palms, or body in general. When individuals cast this "evil eye," the subject faces misfortune and will become ill. A witch can injure others by the power of her eyes; she may destroy others with a curse or make them ill. Witches are generally believed to be women.

Touch Practices: Men are not allowed to touch women unless they have a specific reason for doing so. Only a mother, sister, daughter, or wife can be touched by a male family member. The head is considered the place of God and is not to be touched by another unless necessary. Older adults can touch a younger person's head to extend good wishes. Spiritual healers touch the forehead or other parts of the body of an ill person during the process of diagnosis and treatment; a practice that is considered acceptable. Handshaking is uncommon between men and women. Dress tends to be traditional, and a woman who immodestly exposes her body is culturally unacceptable.

Perceptions of Time: Traditionally, punctuality is not considered important. More recently, perceptions have been changing, and punctuality is becoming more important and appreciated. Time is very important during rituals such as birth, death, and marriage, when timing is strictly followed according to a priest's calculations. Nepalese people live between the past and present and are trying to establish a better future.

Pain Reactions: People generally have a high tolerance for pain and discomfort. Men and rural people are more stoic than people from urban areas. Women from rural areas do not express pain, even during childbirth. People remain quiet and even smile when experiencing pain, which can cause health practitioners to underestimate the severity of the problem and delay treatment.

Birth Rites: The fertility rate is four children born per woman. To ward off evil spirits and ensure a safe pregnancy and birth, the woman wears a protective band around her neck. During his wife's pregnancy, a husband is not allowed to slaughter an animal, and a pregnant woman does not eat spicy food. Pregnancy before marriage is unacceptable and is a sensitive issue. For numerous social and cultural reasons, many women get abortions from untrained persons or quack healers, and these women frequently become septic. To provide safe abortion services, the government introduced the "Legal Right for Safe Abortion and National Safe Abortion Policy" in 2002. More than 80% of deliveries take place at home and are attended by untrained people. The infant mortality rate is very high at 65 deaths per 1,000 live births. In rural areas, many women give birth alone in animal sheds. Males, unmarried girls, and children are not allowed to be in an area where childbirth is taking place. The period of childbirth and menstruation is considered a "polluted period" for the women, so no one is allowed to touch them because of issues related to the deities and gods. People believe that if a deity or god becomes angry, the mother and infant may develop health problems. Therefore, the mother is isolated for 7 to 11 days after birth in a separate room that is kept warm and draft free. The mother and newborn sit in the sun each day and have oil massages with hot mustard oil that is often cooked with fenugreek-seed *(methi)* and trachysperous ammi *(jwano)*, a spice believed to have healing powers. Male and female infants are given equal care. Special foods given to the mother include meat, rice, mustard oil, cumin, soup with trachysperous ammi *(jwano)* (believed to increase the mother's milk production), sugar candy, and butter. Methi and jwano are also used in curries. Women reduce their salt intake for 6 to 10 days because salt is believed to cause swelling and infections. Green spinach, pumpkins, and apple consumption is also restricted for 2 to 3 months after delivery because they are considered "cold" food that can cause diarrhea in children as they drink their mother's milk. Food restrictions are not as strict among the Tibeto-Mongoloid ethnic group.

Death Rites: People believe God decides the timing of birth and death for all. Most older people try to do good deeds to ensure a place in heaven or to increase their wealth and decrease their suffering in the next life. Death at home is preferred. The body is washed and wrapped with a new, special cotton cloth. If the dead person is a married woman, she is dressed as a bride. Relatives and friends express their grief; they are present when death is expected and afterwards as well. Autopsies are uncommon. In most cases, the body is cremated immediately. The son and wife of the deceased are isolated for 13 days and eat plain food they cook themselves. Salt, meat and meat products, vegetables, beans and grains, and spices are restricted. Rituals are performed at 13 days, 45 days, 3 months, 6 months, and every year after the death to keep the dead person's soul at peace. The family offers meals and household goods through a priest out of respect for the dead person. The mourning ceremony is different in Sherpa and Lama ethnic groups. Some express grief through singing sad songs. Organ donation is considered a holy work: donation of the eyes after death, for example, is believed to reduce the sins of the person, allowing entrance into heaven.

N

Food Practices and Intolerances: The staple foods are rice, chapatti, corn, dal (lentils), beans, green vegetables, meat, and fish. People eat three times a day—lunch, tiffin, and dinner—and consume meat or fish once or twice a week. Traditionally, people eat with their hands. Elders and male members of the family eat first, and the daughter-in-law eats last. In mountain areas, potatoes and barley are staples.

Infant-Feeding Practices: Most women breastfeed exclusively for 3 to 6 months and then introduce supplementary foods. Weaning foods are introduced at the age of 5 months to daughters and the age of 6 months to sons. Infant feedings are usually supplemented by porridge prepared at home (a mixed flour of grain and pulses). After a weaning ceremony, the child is allowed to eat normal adult foods. Cow's milk is commonly used. More than 50% of the children in Nepal are malnourished.

Child-Rearing Practices: Child rearing is undertaken primarily by the grandmothers and elder siblings. Sons are preferred. Infants up to 6 months old are massaged in oil, often mustard oil, and placed in the sun several times a day. The oil is believed to make the child strong and prevent air from going into the body. This practice is based on the belief that cool air passing through the body of the mother and new-born could make them sick with diseases thought to be caused by cold-ness, such as pneumonia, diarrhea, abdominal pain and distension, dysentery, and edema. To keep the shape of the infant's head round, a pillow of mustard seed is made and molded to the infant's head. Because of limited access to health services and lack of awareness, most women do not use maternal and pediatric health clinics, resulting in high maternal mortality rates (539 per 100,000 live births). With 38.6 neonatal deaths per 1,000 live births, Nepal has the third highest neonatal mortality rate in the world. Children go to school at the age of 3 to 5 years, but education for girls has a low priority, particularly in rural areas.

National Childhood Immunizations: BCG at birth or at first contact; DTwP at 6, 10, and 14 weeks; DTPHep at 6, 10, and 14 weeks; OPV at 6, 10, and 14 weeks; measles at 9 months (up to 36 months); HepB at 6, 10, and 14 weeks; vitamin A at 6 months; and TT at 15 to 44 years ×3, one each pregnancy. The percent of the target population vaccinated, by antigen, is: BCG (87%); DTP1 (81%); DTP3 (75%); HepB3 (41%); MCV (74%); Polio3 (78%); TT2 plus (40%); and vitamin A (95%). Because of the difficult geographic conditions, coverage is still not uniform within the country, with some districts achieving 100% coverage and others far behind.

BIBLIOGRAPHY

Central Bureau of Statistics: Nepal in figures 2002. Kathmandu, 2002, National Planning Commission Secretariats, 2002.

Central Intelligence Agency: *2006: The world factbook,* Nepal. Retrieved September 21, 2006, from https://www.cia.gov/cia/publications/factbook/print/np.html.

Department of Health Services: *Annual report 2003/2004,* Kathmandu, Nepal, 2004, Department of Health Services, Ministry of Health.

Jones CM: The meaning of being an elder in Nepal, *Nurs Sci Q.* 5(4):171, 1992.

NCASC, Ministry of Health: *National estimates of HIV infections Nepal 2003.* NCASC, HMG Nepal. March 2004.

Thapa N et al: Infant death rates and animal-shed delivery in remote rural areas of Nepal, *Soc Sci Med.* 51:1447–1456, 2001.

UNICEF: Nepal statistics. Retrieved May 15, 2006, from http://www.unicef.org/info-bycountry/Nepal_statistics.html.

UNAIDS: 2006 Nepal. Retrieved September 21, 2006, from http://www.unaids.org/en/Regions_Countries/Countries/nepal.asp.

World Health Organization: 2006: Immunization, vaccines and biologicals. Retrieved September 21, 2006, from http://www.who.int/immunization_monitoring/en/globalsummary/countryprofileresult.cfm?C='npl'.

◆ NETHERLANDS (KINGDOM OF THE)

MAP PAGE (798)

Frits van Merode and Emily Brounts-Hendrickx

Location: The Netherlands is situated in the northwestern part of Europe at the North Sea. Because of the warm gulf, the climate is mild. Most of the country is flat, and a substantial part is gained from the sea and protected by dikes: 60% of the Dutch live below sea level. The western part is also known as Holland. It has large ports (including Rotterdam, the largest port in the world) and an elaborate infrastructure into the continent (especially Germany). Schiphol is the third largest airport of Western Europe. The capital is Amsterdam. The Netherlands is one of the smallest countries in the world with a total area of 37,330 km^2 (14,413 square miles). The population is 16.4 million. In the past, the Netherlands had colonies: Indonesia, New Guinea, Surinam (Dutch Guyana), and the six Caribbean Islands, of which Curacao is the largest, located north of Venezuela. The Caribbean Islands are independent in their domestic affairs but belong to the Kingdom of the Netherlands. The Netherlands has large groups originating from these former colonies. The gross domestic product (GDP) per capita is $30,500.

Major Languages	Ethnic Groups	Major Religions
Dutch (official)	Dutch 96%	Roman Catholic 34%
Frisian	Moroccan, Turk, Other 4%	Protestant 25%
		Muslim 3%
		Other 2%

Dutch is spoken by almost everyone; most speak English as a second language. Literacy rates are 99% for both men and women. Protestants live primarily in the northern and western parts of the Netherlands; Catholics live in the south. Immigrants from northern Africa (especially Morocco) and Turkey adhere to Islam. A large part of the Dutch population does not actively practice religion.

Health Care Beliefs: Active role; prevention important. Prevention is one of the cornerstones of Dutch health care. All municipalities have a legal obligation to have a policy for prevention and hygiene. Often the tasks resulting from this obligation are outsourced to a municipal or regional community health service (Gemeentelijke Gezondheidsdienst, or GGD). Aside from the numerous national prevention programs (e.g., eating practices, smoking cessation, hygiene), health is largely considered an individual responsibility. Individuals also are becoming increasingly assertive about what they want from health care providers, an attitude that is not always appreciated by providers because they feel that they are being thrust into negotiation situations.

Predominant Sick-Care Practices: Biomedical and limited alternative practices. A small proportion (7% in 2004) of the population seeks help from homeopathic and alternative medical practitioners. Some private insurance companies reimburse these nonstandard practices up to a certain amount of Euros. General practitioners and dentists provide general care. Only with a referral from a general practitioner can patients access medical specialists, who almost always have their practices in hospitals. Costs of health care were 8.4% of GNP in 2004. This percentage has not changed much in the last years. If the cost of care outside the health care sector (e.g., social care) were also counted, the total cost of care increased from 10.5% to 12.6% of GNP from 2000 to 2003. Costs for nursing and care are 24% of total health care expenditures, and about 25% of these costs relate to psychological disorders, primarily dementia. About 75% of nursing and care costs are spent for women, whereas their share in total health care is only 59%, a result of their higher life expectancy.

Ethnic-/Race-Specific or Endemic Diseases: Infectious diseases and accidents, back and neck problems, and contact eczema have the highest incidence. The main causes of death are cardiovascular diseases and cancer. The number of deaths from cardiovascular diseases dropped from 45% in 1980 to 33% in 2003. The number of cancer deaths remained almost the same in this period (27% in 1980, 28% in 2003). The number of deaths by injuries (e.g., traffic accidents) is fairly low compared with that of other European countries. Lung cancer is a major cause of cancer deaths in women. The incidence has greatly increased compared with other European countries. Illness prevalence (more than 1,000,000 cases per year) is the highest for anxiety and hearing disorders and back and neck complaints. The Joint United Nations Programme on HIV/AIDS (UNAIDS) estimates the prevalence rate for human immunodeficiency virus (HIV) in adults (aged 15 to 49 years) to be 0.2%, with 18,000 people living with HIV, including 5,900 women and 48 children aged 0 to 15. The number of people who have died from acquired immunodeficiency syndrome (AIDS) has dropped from 522 in 1995 to 87 in 2003.

Health-Team Relationships: The doctor has a dominant position in Dutch health care. Nurses are becoming more important as process managers, a change that was taking place especially in the 1990s. In addition, during the 1990s, hospitals changed their organizational structures in a way that integrated doctors more into hospital management. Most hospitals have implemented a structure that resembles a divisional organization, in which each division has a doctor as the medical manager. The position of nurses has become more central in the health care system through the introduction of specialized nursing (e.g., diabetes nursing, asthma nursing). In most hospitals, nurses work in teams involving a mixture of patient-centered and task-oriented nursing.

Families' Role in Hospital Care: Families do not play a role in hospital care; however, some hospitals are experimenting with training the families of patients to assume certain care roles after discharge. The goal of hospitals is to shorten the length of stay; therefore, the role of families in providing care outside the hospital is becoming more important. This "informal" care is an important part of care and is stimulated by a nursing shortage and increase in demand for care as the Dutch population grows older.

Dominance Patterns: Men and women are relatively equal in the Netherlands.

Eye-Contact Practices: During conversations, direct eye contact is essential.

Touch Practices: Some touching is acceptable, but most people are conservative about touching others.

Perceptions of Time: Punctuality is highly valued, and it is expected that a person will never be late (not even 5 minutes) for an appointment. Even for informal visits (e.g., with friends), it is customary to make an appointment. Even if a person has an invitation to "drop by," it is expected that the person will confirm the appointment at least several hours before the visit. It is important to arrive exactly on time because it is also considered impolite to arrive too early (even a few minutes).

Pain Reactions: The reaction of individuals toward pain is moderate—neither stoic nor expressive. Some pain is considered natural; for example, during childbirth, and analgesics are neither expected nor required. However, the term *unbearable pain* is used in discussions about euthanasia.

Birth Rites: Many consider a home birth with the assistance of midwives to be the supreme choice; therefore, it is encouraged. However, because of a shortage of midwives, the demand for home births is greater than the number of midwives. The infant mortality rate is 5 deaths per 1,000 live births. Many cities have "open birth centers" with delivery rooms that can be rented. These centers do not have to be connected to a hospital. The father is expected to support the mother during the delivery. It is becoming quite usual for couples who are not married but are living together to have a child. Of the total of 194,007 babies born in 2004, 130,978 were born to married couples. The age at which women have their first child is increasing (26 years in 1950 versus 29 in 2004), although this trend seems to have reached a plateau. The mean age of mothers having a child was 31 years in 2004. The fertility rate is 1.66 children born per woman, and overall fertility rates are decreasing. Life expectancy is 77 for men, 81 for women.

Death Rites: Euthanasia is allowed under strict conditions. The person must have a medical problem, the euthanasia must be conducted by a doctor, peer consultation must be involved, and a report must be submitted by the practicing doctor that can be checked by the Ministry of Justice. It is expected that close family remain with dying relatives. The Netherlands has a national organ donation register of all Dutch people that indicates whether they are willing to have their organs donated to another person or, alternately, for scientific study. However, in many situations, the immediate family must also give permission to use the organs. It is difficult for doctors and nurses to talk with families about organ donation immediately after they have lost a loved one, so the country still has a significant shortage of donor organs.

Food Practices and Intolerances: Breakfast often consists of a combination of yogurt products, bread, coffee or tea, cereal, cheese, and juice. People have sandwiches for lunch. The main meal is in the early evening. Potatoes, rice, or pasta with meat or meatballs is the main meal (about 5:00 or 6:00 PM). Young people are adapting to the American way of eating, with no strict times for meals and more frequent consumption of snack or fast foods, a particular problem for children in secondary school. It is unacceptable to use the hands for other than small sandwiches, small cakes, and biscuits.

Infant-Feeding Practices: Breastfeeding is becoming more popular.

Child-Rearing Practices: Children begin school when they are 4 years old. They do not sleep with their parents. Children are taught to be assertive. Parents are neither too permissive nor too strict.

National Childhood Immunizations: DTaPHibIPV at 2, 3, 4, and 11 months; DTIPV at 4 and 9 years; aP at 4 years; HepB at 2, 4, and 11 months (children with at least one parent from a country with prevalence ≥2%); MenC_conj at 14 months; and MMR at 14 months and 9 years. The percentage of the target population vaccinated, by antigen, is: Polio3, DPT1, and DPT3 (98%); Hib3 (97%); and MCV (96%).

BIBLIOGRAPHY

Centraal Bureau voor de Statistie: http://statline.cbs.nl/StatWeb (retrieved March 14, 2006).

Isken LD, ed: Rijksvaccinatieprogramma samengevat. In: *Volksgezondheid Toekomst Verkenning, Nationaal Kompas Volksgezondheid.* Bilthoven: RIVM. Amsterdam, 2006.

Rijkers GT, Geelen S, Sanders EAM: Pneumococcen conjugaatvaccins, Staatstoezicht op de Volksgezondheid. *Inf Bull.* 8(3):47, 1997.

UNAIDS: 2006 Netherlands. Retrieved September 21, 2006, from http://www.unaids.org/en/Regions_Countries/Countries/netherlands.asp.

Van de Laar MJW, Op de Coul ELM, eds: HIV and sexually transmitted infections in the Netherlands in 2003. In: *RIVM Report 441100020/2004 An update: November 2004.*

World Health Organization: 2006: Immunization, vaccines and biologicals. Retrieved September 21, 2006, from nhttp://www.who.int/immunization_monitoring/en/globalsummary/countryprofileresult.cfm?C=".

http://www.nationaalkompas.nl> Preventie\ Van ziekten en aandoeningen\Infectieziekten/Rijksvaccinatieprogramma, (retrieved January 20, 2005).

http://www.nationaalkompas.nl> Preventie\Van ziekten en aandoeningen\Infectieziekten\Rijksvaccinatieprogramma, 20 januari 2005; (retrieved March 14, 2006).

N

◆ NEW ZEALAND/AOTEAROA

MAP PAGE (794)

Lynne S. Giddings

Location: Located in the South Pacific, Aotearoa New Zealand is approximately 2,012 km (1,200 miles) east of Australia. New Zealand consists primarily of two islands: North Island and South Island, separated by Cook Strait with a total area of 268,680 km^2 (103,738 square miles). The capital is Wellington. Climatic conditions range from semitropical in the north to cool temperate in the south, with glaciers in the southwest. New Zealand has volcanic activity (e.g., volcanoes, hot springs, mud pools), predominantly in the North Island. A mountainous chain stretches along the spine of the North and South Islands, and abundant pastoral plains support the mainly agricultural economy. Geographic isolation has created a natural biological border so that many worldwide diseases are not present. New Zealand has no snakes or dangerous carnivores except for a mildly poisonous native spider—the katipo. The population of Aotearoa/New Zealand is more than four million. The gross domestic product (GDP) per capita is $25,200. Literacy rates are almost 100% for both men and women.

Major Languages	Ethnic Groups	Major Religions
English (official)	European 75%	Christian 81%
Maori (official)	Maori 15%	Hindu, Confucian 1%
	Pacific Islander 5%	Other 18%
	Asian 4.6%	
	Other 0.5%	

Maori, the Tangata Whenua (People of the Land) of New Zealand, were the first people to settle in the land. In 1840 a treaty was established, Te Tiriti O Waitangi, with the British Crown. This founding document forms the bicultural basis for the government's approach to issues concerning health. Numerous waves of immigration have come since 1840: Scots, English, Irish, Chinese, Dutch, Pasifika, and recently Asian immigrants and refugees from around the world. Sport is an important focus for cultural identity, with the most popular being water sports (swimming, canoeing, rowing and yachting), mountaineering, skiing, netball, squash, cricket, and rugby.

Health Care Beliefs: Active role; holistic; health promotion important. Although the health care system is primarily based on the biomedical model, alternative therapies and holistic practices are popular and include acupuncture, osteopathy, homeopathy, naturopathy, and indigenous (Maori) herbal remedies.

Predominant Sick-Care Beliefs: Health care is largely government funded and hospital based. There are, however, private and voluntary organizations working in the community to provide specialized assistance. Since the 1970s, care and treatment of mental illness are largely community based, and the range of services includes supported accommodation, individual community support, cultural services, medical and multidisciplinary treatments, and 24-hour crisis services. Antidiscrimination programs and the political work of the consumer movement supplement the community focus.

Ethnic-/Race-Specific or Endemic Diseases: The major causes of death are malignant neoplasms, ischemic heart disease, and cerebrovascular disease. The Maori and Pasifika populations have an increased incidence of diabetes (three to five times higher than the norm), asthma (one and a half times higher), heart disease, and smoking-related diseases. Smoking causes at least 22% of all cancer deaths and is the single greatest preventable cause of early death. It is estimated that 20% to 25% of the overall population smoke. However, approximately 45% of Maori men smoke, 57% of Maori women smoke, and 12% of young Maori (ages 10 to 15 years) smoke regularly. The Joint United Nations Programme on HIV/AIDS (UNAIDS) estimates the prevalence rate for human immunodeficiency virus (HIV) in adults (aged 15 to 49 years) to be 0.1%, with 1,400 people living with HIV. Most infections (85%) occur in men.

Health-Team Relationships: The medical profession dominates the health care system, and people are successfully challenging the patriarchal structure. The system includes indigenous health services (often *marae-*, or tribal-based *iwi* buildings and land, which have a strong spiritual and cultural dimension), independent midwives (the preferred childbirth practitioner), consumer advocates (addressing patient rights and mental health issues), and independent nurse practitioners (with prescribing rights).

Families' Role in Hospital Care: Family involvement in the care of a hospitalized relative is encouraged and supported. Visiting hours are extended, and special arrangements can be made for family and significant others to stay overnight with a patient. *Whanau* (family) rooms are available in most hospitals, providing accommodations and acknowledging the special needs of patients and their extended families.

Dominance Patterns: Domestic violence, and older adult, child, and sexual abuse have been a focus of concern since the early 1990s. However, reliable population-based rates of family violence are not yet available. Since the emancipation of women in 1893, gender inequality has been a contentious issue. Inequalities between genders still exist in relation to salaries, promotions, and child-rearing practices. Although women are represented at the highest level in New Zealand (e.g., prime minister, governor general, chief justice), gender inequalities continue to affect all levels within society. For example, currently the average wages for women in public service can be as much as $41,000 less than the wages of their male colleagues. These gender differences are compounded by various forms of prejudice, including racism and heterosexism.

Eye-Contact Practices: Some groups maintain eye contact (e.g., Europeans), whereas others (e.g., Maori, Pasifika) consider it polite to avert their gaze.

Touch Practices: It is difficult to generalize cultural interpersonal practices in New Zealand because of the effects of European colonization and cultural mixing over time. However, a diverse range of practices exist, ranging from reserved English and European practices with limited touching and a focus on the nuclear family, to Maori *marae*-based living, with its more open expressions of intimacy and focus on the extended family (*whanau* and *hapu*).

Perceptions of Time: Modern European perceptions of time predominate.

Pain Reactions: Pain reactions vary according to gender and cultural characteristics. Some groups can be stereotyped as more stoic (e.g., Pasifikas and men).

Birth Rites: The fertility rate is 1.79 children born per woman. Traditionally, childbirth has taken place in hospitals and is monitored by doctors and obstetricians. More recently, women have been choosing home births under the guidance of midwives. The infant mortality rate is 5.7 deaths per 1,000 live births. For people who identify themselves as Maori, the connection with the land, or *whenua,* is strong. For many Maoris, an infant's connection to the land is confirmed through the burial of the placenta, which is also called *whenua,* soon after birth. Life expectancy is 76 for men, 82 for women.

Death Rites: Many families of European origin leave the body at a funeral home, and burial or cremation follows a religious or secular service. More recently, because of the influence of Maori funeral practices, New Zealand European *(Pakeha)* families are asking for their loved ones to be returned home so that family and friends can mourn together until burial or cremation. Maori funeral practices involve a *tangi* or *tangihanga* mourning that is held on the *marae* for 3 days and 3 nights. This period is a time of farewell speeches, tears, and mourning as extended family members and friends attend to the body before burial.

Food Practices and Intolerances: Availability of nourishing food (e.g., seafood *[kaimoana],* lamb, beef, a wide variety of vegetables and fruit including kiwi) and a high incidence of physical activity (two of every three people are active during their leisure time) contribute to a generally healthy population. However, abundant dairy and meat products have also contributed to high rates of heart disease, diabetes, and the increasing incidence of obesity. Fast food, a recent phenomenon, is exacerbating this situation.

Infant-Feeding Practices: From 1974 to 1993 onward, a trend toward breastfeeding has been increasing; 80% to 90% of women are breastfeeding on discharge from the hospital.

National Childhood Immunizations: DTaPHib at 15 months; DTaPIPV at 6 weeks, at 3 and 5 months, and at 4 years; Hib-HepB at 6 weeks and 3 months; HIB at 15 months; HepB at 5 months; MMR at 15 months and 4 years; IPV at 11 years; and Td at 11 years. The percent of the target population vaccinated, by antigen, is: DTP1 (92%); DTP3, Polio3 (89%); HepB3 (87%); Hib3 (80%); and MCV (82%).

Acknowledgments: The author acknowledges the help of librarians Donna Jarvis and Andrew South, Akoranga Library, AUT, Auckland, New Zealand.

BIBLIOGRAPHY

Bateman New Zealand encyclopedia, 6th ed: Auckland, NZ, 2005, Bateman.

Davis P, Ashton T: *Health and public policy in New Zealand.* Auckland, NZ, 2001, Oxford University Press.

Davis P, Dew K: *Health and society in Aotearoa New Zealand,* 2nd ed. Auckland, NZ, 2005, Oxford University Press.

Maori to English translation. Retrieved February 6, 2006, from http://www.classys-isters.co.nz/Maori-dictionary.html.

Ministry of Health, New Zealand: Retrieved February 6, 2006, from http://www.moh.govt.nz.

Statistics New Zealand: *New Zealand official yearbook 2000. Wellington, NZ, 2000,* Author.

Statistics New Zealand: Includes NZ Yearbook. Retrieved February 6, 2006, from http://www.stats.govt.nz.

UNAIDS: 2006 New Zealand: Retrieved September 21, 2006, from http://www.unaids.org/en/Regions_Countries/Countries/new_zealand.asp.

UNICEF: New Zealand. Retrieved February 6, 2006, from http://www.unicef.org.nz/.

Wepa D, ed: *Cultural safety in Aotearoa New Zealand.* Auckland, NZ, 2005, Pearson Education New Zealand.

World Health Organization: Epidemiological fact sheets on Oceania, November 2005. Geneva. Retrieved February 6, 2006, from http://www.unaids.org/en/Regions_Countries/Regions/Oceania.asp.

World Health Organization: 2006: Immunization, vaccines and biologicals. Retrieved September 21, 2006, from http://www.who.int/immunization_monitoring/en/globalsummary/countryprofileresult.cfm?C='nzl'.

◆ NICARAGUA (REPUBLIC OF)

MAP PAGE (795)

Jean Macq

Location: Nicaragua is in Central America, bordered on the north by Honduras and on the south by Costa Rica. The Caribbean Sea lies to the east and the Pacific Ocean to the west. The total area is 129,494 km^2 (49,998 square miles). About 62% of the population of 5.5 million is concentrated in the Pacific region, the location of the capital, Managua. The central region has approximately 33% of the country's population, and the Atlantic region has the remaining 6%. The gross domestic product (GDP) per capita is $2,900, with 50% living below the poverty line. Literacy rates are 67% for men, 68% for women.

Major Languages	Ethnic Groups	Major Religions
Spanish (national)	Mestizo 69%	Roman Catholic 95%
	White 17%	Protestant 5%
	Black 9%	
	Amerindian 5%	

Many Nicaraguans are becoming involved in Evangelical churces; so the 5% figure for Protestant worship may be a conservative estimate. The indigenous and Creole populations (mainly in the Atlantic region) speak Miskito (or other indigenous languages), Creole English, or both.

Health Care Beliefs: Acute sick care; passive role. Preventive services offered for women focus on family planning, prenatal care, childbirth, the puerperium, and timely detection of cervical and breast cancer (offered in urban areas). For adolescents, prevention of drug addiction and of unwanted pregnancies or pregnancy at a young age is stressed. Most seek health care for treatment of symptoms. Mental illness is understood, and yet treatment through the public health system is generally inadequate because health resources and training concentrate more on other types of illness. In urban areas, people have no widely practiced traditional rituals for curing illness; however, prayer is common among the majority Catholic population.

Predominant Sick-Care Practices: Biomedical and traditional. Western health care is provided through the national public health system. Clinics and hospitals are contracted by the Social Security Institute for formal-sector workers (5% of the population), nongovernmental and church-sponsored programs, and the private sector. The Ministry of Health continues to be the main provider of services for the population. The Ministry's health center is the most common source of outpatient care, accounting for three fourths of all services provided in the public sector. Because of the lack of drugs in public health facilities, people frequently use private pharmacies that are often allied with private medical practices *(consultorio)*. Although community-level health posts exist, they are little used because of the lack of personnel and insufficient drugs. Access to services, mainly drugs and diagnostic facilities, has become strongly related to ability to pay. Nicaragua's indigenous population and Anglo-speaking groups on the Atlantic Coast are more likely to seek health care from indigenous healers *(curanderos)*, especially for illnesses believed to be mental or spiritual in origin. Herbs and other locally grown plants are used for their medicinal qualities, although the trend is toward Western practices. Immunization of infants has contributed to great reductions in infant and childhood mortality.

Ethnic-/Race-Specific or Endemic Diseases: Poverty determines who has special health needs. About 60% of the rural population lives below the poverty line, and 25% of this population lives more than a 2-hour walk from a health center. Rural families are therefore more likely to become ill but less likely to seek medical attention. Life expectancy is lower in rural areas than in urban areas. The causes of death in infants and children younger than 5 years are common diseases of poverty (e.g., acute diarrheal disease, respiratory infections), whereas the major causes of death in adults are diseases of the affluent such as cancer, hypertension, diabetes, and cardiovascular problems. Only two thirds of the population has access to safe drinking water, a situation that increases the high incidence of diarrheal diseases. The population contracts two water-related diseases carried by mosquitoes: malaria and dengue fever. Both are on the increase. Agricultural workers who work on large farms have significant health risks. The fairly uncontrolled use of pesticides in agriculture makes acute pesticide poisoning the major health problem among workers. The World Health Organization (WHO) estimated the prevalence rate for human immunodeficiency virus (HIV) and acquired immunodeficiency syndrome (AIDS) as 0.2%, although the incidences appear to be increasing slightly (4 new cases per 100,000 in 2003 and 8 in 2005). Although accurate figures are difficult to determine, there may be 7,300 people living with HIV, including 1,700 women and fewer than 100 children aged 0 to 15. The male-to-female ratio is 4:1, and 65% of transmission is heterosexual.

Health-Team Relationships: The Ministry of Health oversees Nicaragua's public health services. In recent years the Ministry has decentralized operations, delegating functions to integrated local health care systems (Sistema Local de Atencion Integral a la Salud, or SILAIS). Allocation of medical personnel has become a major problem. Medical doctors often have dual practices because of low public salaries, and there is a shortage of nurses. Doctors generally control the operations of hospitals and clinics, but doctors and nurses generally have good working relationships. Patients tend to prefer speaking directly with doctors (and mainly with clinical specialists when possible) about their ailments. In rural areas, doctors often have a revered status.

Families' Role in Hospital Care: Practices vary. Hospitals in Managua generally restrict family visits and the types of items visitors bring to patients. In other areas, particularly rural areas, policies are more lenient, and it is not uncommon for family members to bring food and other supplies. In some maternity wards, female family members are permitted to stay with the new mother.

Dominance Patterns: Some argue that Nicaragua has a patriarchal society, whereas others think that it is matriarchal. The Sandinista revolution drew women into public life in new ways and spawned a women's movement in the country that resulted in gender equality that was ensured in the national constitution. Still, many traditional values and customs are still practiced. Traditional values include the notion that a woman's place is in the home and her role is to raise her children. Traditionally, men have had the freedom to have extramarital affairs and leave the home chores to their women. Also, traditionally, women have been the caregivers.

Eye-Contact Practices: Eye contact is not avoided. Flirting is common.

Touch Practices: Touching is acceptable. People often kiss on the cheek when they are introduced to a stranger. Men may touch each other (with a hand on the shoulder) while talking. Women may hold hands. Nicaraguans, even those who work together, often shake hands when they greet each other.

Perceptions of Time: Punctuality is not a major issue. People operate on "tiempo nica," meaning they come to events whenever they decide to, which is usually not at the posted time. Meetings tend not to start on time. Nicaraguans live in the present, although many yearn for what they recall as "the better times" (the previous era) and hope for better times in the future.

Pain Reactions: Nicaraguans tend to react to pain quietly. At times of death, family and friends gather for wakes and may cry together.

Birth Rites: The fertility rate is five children born per woman, and 25% of women begin having children while they are still adolescents. Nicaraguan families are following a worldwide trend toward having children in a health facility, especially hospitals in urban areas. Cesarean section is a frequent practice, and indications for it are often questionable. If the birth takes place at home, a trained person is likely to be in attendance. Only 20% of births take place without a trained attendant, and nearly 50% take place in a health care institution. The infant mortality rate is 28 deaths per 1,000 live births. Specific ethnic or religious practices are allowed at birth as long as they do no harm to mother or child. For the most part, mothers are allowed to eat what they like before, during, and after the birth. Newborns are normally breastfed within an hour after birth. However, mothers must be constantly convinced that it is more beneficial to give the newborn the nutrient-rich colostrum than to wait several days for breast milk. Although Nicaragua's macho culture still slightly favors the birth of a son, this preference does not seem to affect parents' decisions about educating their daughters. Life expectancy is 68 for men, 73 for women.

Death Rites: Family members are present at death, and rituals are predominantly governed by Catholic religious ceremonies. In some rural areas, newborn infants are not named until at least a week after birth because of the fear that the infant may die. Similarly, registration of newborns may be delayed to prevent unnecessary effort (e.g., a trip to the health center) and fees in case the infant dies soon after birth. Organ donation is acceptable but not generally possible because the technology is not available. Autopsies are rare. However, a "verbal autopsy" is a method often used by health organizations trying to understand the causes of maternal death in order to develop strategies to lower the rate. When a woman dies before, during, or after childbirth, the verbal autopsy consists of a series of structured interviews with people who were familiar with the situation and have insight into the specific circumstances surrounding the woman's death.

Food Practices and Intolerances: Basic staples of the diet are rice mixed with beans *(gallo pinto)*, corn tortillas, and chicken. Black coffee sweetened with sugar is the most popular beverage, and children begin consuming it at a young age. Rural families consider animals such as pigs, goats, cows, and chickens to be assets. Thus, they are more likely to sell them or use them for bartering than to consume them. The general diet of poor families is based on carbohydrates such as rice, potato, cassava, and other root vegetables (e.g., *quequisque.*) Fresh fruit and vegetables are abundant and low priced when they are in season, and many rural families grow their own. The two greatest barriers to a good diet are income (regardless of food available) and education. Low educational levels are associated with poor diets, even when nutritious foods are available and affordable. The need for mothers to work outside the home and commute long distances has been leading to more reliance on ready-made foods. Families of all income brackets commonly consume

processed foods such as noodles, Magi soup, bread, cookies, and crack-
ers. Wealthier families also consume imported soft drinks, snack foods,
and gourmet items.

Infant-Feeding Practices: Nicaraguan mothers understand the importance of breastfeeding, and almost without exception, their infants begin
their lives nurtured by breast milk. However, only one third of mothers
breastfeed exclusively for the first 3 months. Many mothers erroneously
believe that because of the country's warm climate the infant needs additional fluids, so they provide water, juice, teas, thin gruels, or even infant
formula in addition to breast milk. By the time the infants are 4 months
old, about 50% are already receiving cereal-based gruels in addition to
breast milk. In many cases, mothers who would normally continue to
breastfeed exclusively must return to work; therefore, babies are often
fed poor substitutes while the mother is away. The diets for children are
often lacking in sufficient fruits and vegetables, especially those rich in
vitamin A. Because many of these foods are not expensive and readily
available, the main barrier to a nutritious diet is lack of understanding.
The high prevalence of chronic undernutrition in children is most often a
combination of food shortage (either because of low production or low
purchasing power), repeated illness, and poor feeding practices.

Child-Rearing Practices: Children are valued, and child-rearing practices tend to be permissive. Infants generally sleep with their parents. Children are raised in large families, and many members of the extended
family take an active part in raising them and providing support to the parents. Grandparents are especially valued in this regard. Children in poor
families, who constitute the majority of the Nicaraguan population, are
expected to help with household chores at a young age. When not in
school, these children are also likely to work in the informal labor market,
either with their parents or independently. This is true in rural families and
urban families alike.

National Childhood Immunizations: BCG at birth; DTwP at 18 months;
DTwPHibHep at 2, 4, and 6 months; OPV at 2, 4, 6, and 12 months and
2 to 3 years; MR at 6 to 39 years, Td at 6, 10, 12, and 14 years; vitamin
A at 6 months and at 1, 2, 3, 4, and 6 years. The percent of the target
population vaccinated, by antigen, is: BCG (94%); DTP1 (95%); DTP3,
HepB3, and Hib3 (86%); MCV (96%); Polio3 (87%); and vitamin A (98%).

BIBLIOGRAPHY

Ministerio de Salud of Nicaragua: Retrieved February 6, 2006, from http://www.
    minsa.gob.ni/vigepi/html/boletin/2005/editorial46.htm, 2005.
Pan American Health Organization: Information on Nicaragua. Retrieved April 4,
    2006, from http://paho.org.
World Health Organization: 2006: Immunization, vaccines and biologicals. Retrieved
    September 21, 2006, from http://www.who.int/immunization_monitoring/en/
    globalsummary/countryprofileresult.cfm?C='nic'.
http://centralamerica.com/nicaragua/info/general.html (retrieved April 4, 2006).
http://www.lanoticia.com.ni (retrieved April 4, 2006).
http://www.laprensa.com.ni (retrieved March 20, 2006).

http://library.thinkquest.org/17749/health.html (retrieved April 4, 2006).
http://wwsw.nuevodiario.ni (retrieved March 15, 2006).

◆ NIGER (REPUBLIC OF)

MAP PAGE (800)

Conerly Casey

Location: Niger is bordered by Algeria and Libya to the north, Chad to the east, Mali to the West, Nigeria to the south, and Benin and Burkina Faso to the southwest. The total area is 1,267,000 km² (489,189 square miles). The north of Niger has volcanic mountains plunging to the east into the Tenere, a vast area of sand dunes, and to the west into fossil valleys, once teeming with animal and plant life. Part of the Tenere is a transitional zone between the Sahara Desert and the Sahel, a low-lying plateau crossed by the Niger River. Four fifths is desert, populated by nomadic pastoralists in the narrow fertile belt south of the Niger River. The population is more than 13 million, and the capital is Niamey. In 2004, drought, an infestation of locusts, and chronic food shortages resulted in a third of the population starving. Niger is ill equipped to handle a public health crisis of such magnitude. It is one of the poorest countries of the world, with a gross domestic product (GDP) per capita of $900 and 63% living below the poverty line. Literacy rates are 26% for men, 10% for women.

Major Languages	Ethnic Groups	Major Religions
French (official)	Hausa 56%	Islam 85%
Hausa	Songhai and Zarma 22%	Christian 15%
Zarma (Dyerma, Djerma, Songhai, Songhay)	Fulani 8.5%	
Fulfulde (Fula, Peul, Fulani)	Tuareg 8%	
Tamajaq (Tamacheq, Tamachek, Tamajeq)	Kanuri 4.3%	
Kanuri (Kanouri, Manga, Dagara)	Toubous 1.2%	
Dazaga (Dasa, Toubou, Tebu)		

Niger's nomadic Fulani and Tuareg are pastoralists, herding the few animals that survived the recent drought through the northern and central parts of the country. In the western and central areas, small villages of Songhai and Zarma farmers appear interspersed with fields of millet and guinea corn. Songhai and Zarma are considered "cousins" who, for centuries, have used the insults of "joking relationships" to forge friendships and cultural similarities, although their social histories are quite different.

Current use of the term *Hausa* extends beyond ethnicity to describe cultural and language communities on both sides of the Niger-Nigeria border. Most Hausa are farmers and traders, living in the south-central part of Niger, close to the border with Nigeria. Hausa and Fulani intermarry and maintain "joking relationships" while trading animal and agricultural products. The Kanuri live in the eastern part of Niger and Nigeria, often in villages with Hausa. Although most Nigeriennes self-identify as Muslim, people may use Islamic and Christian beliefs and practices along with those of their traditional religions.

Health Care Beliefs: Acute sick care; traditional holistic, religious, and biomedical. Although communities in Niger have distinctive health beliefs based on gender, descent, class, ethnicity, religion, and region, there are a number of similarities. For most, Islam is an integral part of health beliefs about the causes of illnesses and appropriate treatments for them. Submission to the will of Allah is marked by patience; accepting illness with a quiet confidence. The concept of balance in all aspects of one's life, whether physical, social, psychological, or spiritual, is critical to Nigerienne health beliefs, with biomedical metaphors such as "killing" or "eradicating" disease, counter to traditional, holistic, homeopathic ones. Nigeriennes report witchcraft, sorcery, and spirit possession as the most common disease causes. The psychological, social, and spiritual bases for illnesses are as important as the physical, so that an understanding of historical and contemporary conflicts among people is a vital aspect of health care. Depending on the community, cultural and linguistic taboos are associated with the consumption of certain foods, sex, and punishments for breaking taboos.

Predominant Sick-Care Practices: Traditional holistic; religious; and biomedical when available. Primary health care and medical practices are based on the sequential or concurrent use of traditional, holistic, religious, and biomedical beliefs and practices. Traditional, holistic, and religious practices include the use of herbal medicines, appeals to spirits and sorcerers for interventions, and Islamic treatments of religious prayers and the recitation of Qur'anic verses. Although the government has a system of primary health care services, surveys indicate that it is frequently not well used because of the high costs of medications (29%), service charges (19%), easy access to traditional healers (39%), and the difficulty of getting transportation to a health care facility (30%). Respondents also complain about the unfriendly attitudes of health care workers (4%) and wasting time at government facilities (8%).

Ethnic-/Race-Specific or Endemic Diseases: Endemic diseases include malaria, typhoid, cholera, shigellosis, measles, hepatitis A and B, schistosomiasis, dracunculiasis, onchocerciasis, and meningitis. People are at risk for leprosy, tuberculosis, enteric fever, yellow fever, tetanus, and pertussis. Malaria alone is responsible for 30% of outpatient consultations and 50% of deaths in children under 5 years. Severe malnutrition is common during the "rainy season" (June through August) when grain stocks are low and the fall harvest has yet to begin. Increased vulnerability to endemic diseases from malnutrition is further compounded by a lack of safe water and poor sanitation, which also varies by season. Meningococcal meningitis outbreaks tend to occur in the winter harmattan or "windy season" (December through March) and in the hot, still "dry season" (April through June), with cholera outbreaks toward the beginning of the "rainy season" (June through September). Malaria incidence peaks in August and September. The Joint United Nations Programme on HIV/AIDS (UNAIDS) estimates the prevalence rate for human immunodeficiency virus (HIV) and acquired immunodeficiency syndrome (AIDS) in adults (aged 15 to 49 years) to be 1.1%, with 79,000 people living with HIV, including 8,900 children aged 0 to 14. About 46,000 children are orphans because of parental AIDS, and 7,600 deaths are attributed to AIDS.

Health-Team Relationships: In the diverse communities of Niger, there are disagreements about the appropriateness and efficacy of traditional, holistic, religious, and biomedical approaches to health care. Most Nigeriennes find comfort in approaches that link the present, past, and future, forging a sense of communal completeness and balance. Nigeriennes may associate biomedically trained health teams with the violence of colonization, worrying that doctors or nurses may judge them as inferior or that doctors will become angry if they acknowledge using nonbiomedical treatments. In such cases, patients may be reluctant to divulge information about their use of herbal medicines (many of which have strong purgative and psychotropic effects) or other practices that impact their health status.

Dominance Patterns: With the exception of Tuareg, who are Muslim and matrilineal, the majority of Nigeriennes are Muslim and patrilineal, with the eldest man as head of the extended family and the father as head of household, making all final decisions. Muslim Hausa women of fertile ages may practice partial seclusion, staying inside their compounds, away from nonrelated men, unless they have permission from their fathers or husbands to visit relatives or to seek health care. In polygamous households, wives have some autonomy in early decisions about health care for themselves and their children, with the first wife having authority to make decisions that impact the other wives and their children, particularly if the husband is away from home. Dominance patterns are most clear when there is disagreement in the household about the type of health care appropriate for each family member—whether, for instance, the family should seek traditional, holistic, religious, or biomedical care or in relation to specific issues such as family size.

Pain Reactions: Nigerienne Muslims accept pain as the will of Allah, minimizing their emotional expressions. Although cancer patients report severe pain, oral preparations of strong opioids are generally not available.

Birth Rites: The fertility rate is seven children born per woman. There is a high prevalence (50%) of food and nonfood pica in pregnant women, with nonfood pica significantly greater. The maternal mortality rate is very high: 1,200 per 100,000 live births. The infant mortality rate is also very high: 118 deaths per 1,000 live births. Among Muslims, shouting or crying during birth may be considered a lack of faith in Allah, so mothers tend to be quiet. Traditional first-time mothers often give birth in their parents' house, in a sqatting position, with their mother or a traditional birth attendant assisting the delivery. After birth, mothers observe a 40-day period of rest and extremely hot baths, and they consume a drink high in potassium. The placenta is buried in or near the house with the maternal side facing the sky. Life expectancy is 44 for both men and women.

Death Rites: Muslim doctors may recommend transfusions to save lives, but organ donations and transplants are rare. Deceased Muslims must be buried intact, so autopsies are uncommon and cremation is forbidden. The bodies are wrapped in special pieces of white cloth and buried without a coffin as soon as possible after death. There is a mourning period, with certain days for condolences and the sharing of food and company. Life is considered a gift from Allah, with death a predestined part of Allah's plan. Muslims tend not to cry or weep in public because such behavior is considered a lack of faith in the will of Allah. Yet the smooth, tranquil face of faithful acceptance may mask the depth of grief and the range of feelings that emerge with the loss of a relative or friend.

Infant-Feeding Practices: Many Nigeriennes believe that breastfeeding weakens the mother, so infants are quickly weaned if the mother discovers she is pregnant again. A popular weaning food is millet flour and water.

Child-Rearing Practices: The first-born children of Muslim families may be sent to live with grandparents or an older female relative for an unspecified period. Surrogate parents receive financial assistance for the care they provide, but they assume all other responsibilities. Muslims have taboos about speaking the names of first-born children. Children attend Qur'anic school. They also may attend primary school, or the Islamiyya school, which has a broader curriculum, along with Qur'anic school in the afternoons and evenings. To instill religious prohibitions, respect, deference, and good manners, Muslim children are taught to control or restrain their consumption of food, their amount of sleep, excessive talking, and emotional expressions. Muslim boys are circumcised, and female circumcision and excision are widespread within some groups. Niger has one of the highest rates of child mortality in the world, with 259 deaths per 1,000 children.

National Childhood Immunizations: BCG at birth; DTwP at 6, 10, and 14 weeks; OPV at birth and 6, 10, and 14 weeks; measles at 9 months; vitamin A at 6 months; YF at 9 months; and TT at first contact, +1 month, +6 months, +1, and +1 year. The percent of the target population vaccinated, by antigen, is: BCG (93%); DTP1 (97%); DTP3 and Polio3 (89%); MCV (83%); vitamin A (63%); YF (65%); and TT2 plus (54%).

BIBLIOGRAPHY

Central Intelligence Agency: *2006: The world factbook, Niger.* Retrieved September 21, 2006, from https://www.cia.gov/cia/publications/factbook/print/ng.html.

Chawla M, Ellis RP: The impact of financing and quality changes on health care demand in Niger, *Health Pol Plann.* 15(1):76, 2000.

Katung PY: Socio-economic factors responsible for poor utilization of the primary health care services in a rural community in *Niger, Niger J Med.* 10(1):28, 2001.

Masquelier A: *Prayer has spoiled everything: possession, power, and identity in an Islamic town of Niger,* Durham, NC, 2001, Duke University Press.

Rassmussen S: *Healing in community: medicine, contested terrains, and cultural encounters among the Tuareg.* Westport, Conn, 2001, Bergin and Garvey.

Stoller P: Stranger in the village of the sick: a memoir of cancer, sorcery, and healing. Boston, 2004, Beacon Press.

Tectonidis M: Crisis in Niger—outpatient care for severe acute malnutrition, *N Engl J Med.* 354:3, 2006.

Wasunna A: Towards redirecting the female circumcision debate: legal, ethical and cultural considerations, *McGill J Med.* 5:104–110, 2000.

UNAIDS: 2006 Niger. Retrieved September 21, 2006, from http://www.unaids.org/en/Regions_Countries/Countries/niger.asp.

World Health Organization: 2006: Immunization, vaccines and biologicals. Retrieved September 21, 2006, from http://www.who.int/immunization_monitoring/en/globalsummary/countryprofileresult.cfm?C='ner'.

World Health Organization: Niger: communicable diseases risk assessment, July 2005. Retrieved March 20, 2006, from http://www.who.int/entity/diseasecontrol_emergencies/guidelines/Niger_risk_assessment.pdf.

◆ NIGERIA (FEDERAL REPUBLIC OF)

MAP PAGE (800)

Adebowale A. Adeyemo

Location: Nigeria is located in West Africa, bordered on the west by Benin, on the north by Niger, and on the east by Cameroon. The country occupies a total area of 923,768 km^2 (356,667 square miles), and the vegetation ranges from mangrove forest on the coast to desert in the far north. Nigeria is Africa's most populous nation with rapid population growth: 86 million in 1991 and 132 million in 2006. The population is split equally between rural and urban areas. Abuja is the capital. The population is quite young, with nearly 50% under age 18. The gross domestic product (GDP) per capita is $1,400, and 60% live below the poverty line. Literacy rates are 76% for men, 61% for women.

Major Languages	Ethnic Groups	Major Religions
English (official)	Hausa, Fulani 20%	Muslim 50%
Hausa	Yoruba 21%	Christian 40%
Yoruba	Ibo 18%	Indigenous beliefs 10%
Ibo	Ijaw, Kanuri, Ibibio,	
Fulani	Tiv 10%	
	Other groups 31%	

Nigeria has more than 380 distinct ethnic groups. The major groups include the Edo, Efik, Fulani, Hausa, Igbo, Ijaw, Kanuri, Tiv, Urhobo, and

Yoruba. The three largest ethnic groups are the Hausa-Fulani in the north, the Yoruba in the west, and the Igbo in the east. However, many other ethnic groups exist, and Nigeria has entire states in which none of the three largest ethnic groups constitute a majority or even a significant minority. Nigeria came into being as a nation-state in 1914, when the British colonial administration merged the North and South Protectorates and the colony of Lagos into one administrative unit; it became a republic in 1963. For most of Nigeria's history since independence, it has been under military rule. Nigeria returned to democratic rule in May 1999.

Health Care Beliefs: Active participation; health promotion important. Health promotion activities often involve either general issues (such as personal cleanliness, good nutrition, and environmental hygiene) or specific taboos (such as the belief that pregnant women should not walk in the hot sun or their fetus might develop congenital malformations). Immunization of children and pregnant women, exclusive breastfeeding, and growth monitoring of children are practiced with varying degrees of success. Mental illness is widely feared and is usually blamed on evil spirits, demons, ghosts, the gods, or human agents of such spirits (such as wizards and witches). Because of this belief, it is probable that indigenous healers treat more patients with mental illnesses, although an increasing proportion is treated in modern hospitals. Indigenous treatment of mental illness often involves the patient's living with the healers in their compound. Divinations are carried out to ascertain the source of the illness, after which treatment with herbal preparations is often accompanied by rituals and sacrifices. Patients go home when it is believed they are again in their "right mind." Because mental illness is believed to be potentially hereditary, members of families with persons who are mentally ill often find it difficult to find spouses. Others do not want to risk having affected children, thereby stigmatizing their own extended families. Religion and indigenous medicine are closely interwoven. Illness is believed to be caused by four sources: natural, supernatural, mystical, and hereditary. A wide variety of treatment methods may be used, including herbal preparations that are drunk, inhaled, rubbed into scarification marks, or used as an enema; divination aids (such as stones and bells); and rituals and sacrifices.

Predominant Sick-Care Practices: Traditional; biomedical; and magical-religious. Nigeria has a three-tiered health care system comprising primary, secondary, and tertiary care. The primary care system is meant to be the first point of contact for an ill person (in addition to providing such services as immunization, health education, and promotion). Secondary health care comprises general hospitals with radiology and surgery, intended to treat sick people who cannot be treated at the primary care level. Tertiary health care comprises the specialist and university teaching hospitals that provide the most sophisticated care available, mainly through referrals from the lower levels. In addition to these levels, some patent medicine vendors, or "chemists," officially sell nonprescription, over-the-counter drugs and often serve as major sources of health care delivery. In reality, people use both official and unofficial sources of health care delivery. Unofficial sources include indigenous healers, diviners, fortunetellers, herbalists, bone setters, and traditional birth attendants or midwives. These categories are not exclusive, and a particular healer may assume two or more of these roles. Some indigenous health practitioners are specialists in specific areas such as mental illness or circumcision. Indigenous healers have considerable status and are increasingly organized, having fairs and sponsoring television advertising. People also have turned to religious or spiritual sources, usually in Pentecostal churches, where the belief in miraculous healing for all who have faith is a basic tenet. Many people often seek health care from multiple sources.

Ethnic-/Race-Specific or Endemic Diseases: Among children, malaria, respiratory tract infections, diarrhea, vaccine-preventable diseases (especially measles and tetanus), and malnutrition are major causes of illness and death. Sickle cell anemia is the single most common serious hereditary disorder. Burkitt's lymphoma and leukemia are the most common cancers among children. Among adults, aside from malaria and other infections, hypertension is probably the most common noncommunicable disease. In addition, pregnancy-related complications related to infection and bleeding cause considerable morbidity among women, whereas accidental injuries are a major problem for men. The most common cancers are cervical and breast among women and prostate and liver among men. The Joint United Nations Programme on HIV/AIDS (UNAIDS) estimates the prevalence rate of human immunodeficiency virus (HIV) to be 5.4%, but it could range from a low of 3.6% to a high of 8.0%. The north-central and south-south zones have twice the HIV prevalence of the southwest zone. Between 2.4 and 5.4 million people are living with HIV (810,000 to 2.4 million of them women), with only 31,694 receiving antiretroviral therapy. About 240,000 children aged 0 to 14 are living with HIV, and there are 930,000 orphans aged 0 to 17 as a result of AIDS. Deaths from AIDS are estimated at 220,000.

Health-Team Relationships: The health team is led by a doctor. Doctors and nurses often have a good working relationship, although it varies from place to place and is often worse in the larger hospitals. Patients' attitudes toward doctors and nurses are usually positive, although many patients complain that their health care providers do not spend enough time with them. This attitude is hardly surprising considering the heavy caseload that doctors and nurses routinely carry, which greatly limits the amount of attention any one patient can have. Medical practice is still more paternalistic than it is in Europe and America.

Families' Role in Hospital Care: Families often accompany patients to clinics and emergency facilities, especially on their first visit. Families are often expected to stay with admitted patients, not necessarily on the ward but somewhere on the hospital premises. Because hospital fees are unaffordable for most and no health insurance exists, families contribute funds to pay for hospital bills. They also provide food in some cases.

Dominance Patterns: Even in a few communities with matrilineal lines of inheritance, men still dominate, even during times of illness, when

538 *Nigeria (Federal Republic of)*

decisions about seeking health care and treatment are usually made by the household head. Some people have to wait for days to obtain care because they are waiting for the head of the household to return home and grant permission to go to a hospital. In female-headed households, however, these traditional patterns are no longer followed.

Eye-Contact Practices: Eye contact is common and is not avoided because of status or gender. However, age is greatly respected, so younger people may avoid direct eye contact with an older adult. In some places, no one (with a few exceptions) is expected to make direct eye contact with a traditional ruler.

Touch Practices: Physical touching is acceptable, but public displays of affection are unusual. Children touch each other during play and hold hands. Men may shake or touch hands but are unlikely to walk down the street holding hands. Women may hug one another, especially after a long separation.

Perceptions of Time: Time is flexible, and people do not often get to appointments on time. This is considered normal for social occasions; a person may say an event starts at 10:00 for 10:30 AM, meaning the occasion will actually start at 10:30 AM. For official or business appointments, punctuality is important, although it may be impossible to be on time because of the poor infrastructure (poor roads, poor transportation systems, bad phone networks). The culture throughout Nigeria values past traditions, and these are invoked in discussions of almost all issues. However, there is a dynamic tension between looking backward to tradition and looking forward to "modernization."

Pain Reactions: Pain reactions vary. For example, the Fulani (in the north) and the Igbo (in the east) are generally perceived to be stoic, whereas the Yoruba (in the west) are usually very expressive. However, men are expected to tolerate pain better and be more stoic in the face of severe pain than are women. Children are allowed to express pain but are often admonished to learn to be more tolerant of it.

Birth Rites: The fertility rate is 5.49 children born per woman. In many instances, the mother is confined indoors for a varying period after birth, often for 40 days. During this period, she has hot baths once or twice a day, breastfeeds the infant, and does little else. Relatives usually help to perform the usual household chores, and grandmothers are expected to help the mother take care of the family and chores. A naming ceremony usually takes place on the seventh or eighth day of life; with some ethnic groups, this may be as late as 3 months. A son may be celebrated more than a daughter, but it is probably more accurate to say the birth of the first-born son is celebrated more than other births. With urbanization and changes in lifestyle, many of these customs are breaking down. For example, few women are still completely confined for 40 days before resuming their normal activities. The mortality rate of children younger than 5 is currently 183 per 1,000, and the infant mortality rate is about 103 per 1,000. Life expectancy is 47 for men, 48 for women.

Death Rites: Death means the person assumes another existence and becomes one of the ancestors who watch over the living and can be consulted in times of difficulty. Some believe in reincarnation, often in two very different contexts. In one context, a child born shortly after the death of a grandparent of the same sex is often considered to be the reincarnation of the deceased relative and therefore may be named after the person. In the second, some dead children are believed to reincarnate and be born again to the same woman, only to die again at about the same age. The death of an older person (who is thought to have lived a long and full life) is often celebrated with elaborate ceremonies. If death occurs at home, family members usually take responsibility for preparing the corpse for burial. Among Muslim families, burial usually takes place the same day (before sunset), and autopsy and organ donation are generally prohibited. However, many non-Muslims also prohibit autopsies. Some also believe that whatever information is obtained during an autopsy is not of any practical use because it does not bring the dead person back to life.

Food Practices and Intolerances: Food practices vary, but staple foods include roots and tubers (e.g., yams, cassava, cocoyam), grains and cereals (e.g., millet, guinea corn, maize, rice), and legumes. Palm and peanut oils are often used for cooking soups and stews that contain tomatoes, peppers, or other vegetables and meat or fish. Villages often keep chickens and goats. The items available may vary. For example, in the north where cattle are kept, milk is available and more likely to be consumed than it is in the south. In coastal areas seafood (e.g., crabs, shrimps, other shellfish) is a significant part of the diet. Traditionally, food is eaten with the fingers, but in urban areas and among the more educated, the use of cutlery is more common. It is believed that some foods, such as pounded yams, are best eaten with the fingers, regardless of the time and place.

Infant-Feeding Practices: Breastfeeding is universal, and it is a major social issue if a woman does not breastfeed her child at all. Even if the mother dies during delivery, a wet nurse may be used if the child lives. However, water or herbal preparations may also be given to the infant in addition to breast milk. Women traditionally breastfeed for at least 2 years; this period is only shortened by a new pregnancy, which would be considered shameful because Nigerians often consider it taboo for breastfeeding women to have sexual intercourse. They also consider it taboo for a pregnant woman to breastfeed, so a woman who gets pregnant must stop breastfeeding. Weaning and introduction of food take place at about 4 to 6 months, and by the second year of life, most children are eating from the family pot.

Child-Rearing Practices: Child-rearing practices vary from place to place but overall is more strict than permissive. Children are expected to be well disciplined, show good manners, be quiet, and be respectful and obedient to adults. Child rearing is considered a task for the whole family, including the parents, grandparents, uncles, and aunts, although bad behavior is usually blamed on the mother. Older children (especially girls) help care for the younger ones. Children learn household and other chores as they grow older. Boys may be spared from performing any household chores in traditional societies.

National Childhood Immunizations: BCG at birth, DTP1 at 6 weeks, DPT2 at 10 weeks, DPT3 at 14 weeks, OPV0 at birth, OPV1 at 6 weeks, OPV2 at 10 weeks, OPV3 at 14 weeks, and measles at 9 months. The percentage of the target population vaccinated, by antigen, is: BCG (48%); DPT 1, 2, 3 (25%), and measles (35%).

Other Characteristics: Nigeria is rich in both agricultural products and mineral resources. Nigeria is the sixth largest producer of crude oil in the world and earns several billion U.S. dollars annually; however, these earnings have not translated to a healthy national economy because of decades of mismanagement and corruption by successive military regimes. This has deprived the health and education sectors of much needed support and funding.

BIBLIOGRAPHY

Central Intelligence Agency: *2006: The world factbook, Nigeria.* Retrieved September 21, 2006, from https://www.cia.gov/cia/publications/factbook/print/ni.html.

Jegede AS: *African Culture and Health.* Lagos: Stirling-Horden Publishers (Nigeria) Limited: 1998.

National Population Commission: Macro International. *Nigeria demographic and health survey 1999.* Federal Government of Nigeria.

UNAIDS: 2006 Nigeria. Retrieved September 21, 2006, from http://www.unaids.org/en/Regions_Countries/Countries/nigeria.asp.

World Health Organization: 2005 World health report. Retrieved March 31, 2006, http://www.who.int/whr/2005/annex/annexe7_en.pdf.

◆ NORWAY (KINGDOM OF)

MAP PAGE (798)

Lars Lien

N

Location: Norway occupies the western part of the Scandinavian Peninsula in northwestern Europe and extends approximately 483 km (300 miles) above the Arctic Circle. It consists of 385,155 km^2 (148,693 square miles), including Svalbard and Jan Mayen. More than two thirds of the country is uninhabitable because of glaciers, mountains, moors, and rivers. The capital is Oslo. The population is 4.6 million. Norway is a constitutional monarchy. The gross domestic product (GDP) per capita is $42,300. Literacy rates are 100% for both men and women.

Major Languages	Ethnic Groups	Major Religions
Norwegian (official)	Norwegian 91%	Evangelical Lutheran
Lapp- and Finnish-	Lappish (Sami) 1%	(state church) 86%
speaking minorities	Immigrant groups	Roman Catholic, other
Other languages spoken	8%	Protestant 3%
by minority groups		Other 11%

Health Care Beliefs: Active participation; health promotion important. Norwegians are actively involved in health care, and illness prevention and health promotion are valued. Health promotion is emphasized, particularly in prenatal and child care (children 18 years and younger), and pregnant women, children, and adolescents receive regular physical examinations to ensure wellness. Being clean, resting, exercising, eating healthy food, and taking cod liver oil are believed to improve health, so these practices are followed by a large percentage of the population. People tend to consider their health good, even if they have one or more diseases. Although mental illness has been socially stigmatized, this problem is slowly decreasing as people become more accepting of counseling and drug therapies for various mental health complaints.

Predominant Sick-Care Practices: Biomedical; with some alternative practices. The biomedical model dominates the health care system, and Norwegians consult doctors for health care. A primary care practitioner plan was introduced in 2001, and all citizens are being encouraged to choose a general practitioner, who refers them to specialists as necessary. Alternative health care practices such as acupuncture, homeopathy, chiropractic, and naturopathy may be sought for some health care problems. Use of homeopathic medicine and holistic approaches such as acupuncture are increasing. The country has a nationalized health and social care service that is financed through indirect taxation. Those using the system pay a minimum fee for doctor visits, tests, and prescription medication. A hospital stay is entirely covered without fee. Older adults and those with disabilities account for 45% of all expenditures in health and social care. The basic tenets of the system are equity, equality, and solidarity for all residents.

Ethnic-/Race-Specific or Endemic Diseases: The geographic differences in life expectancy are increasing, especially in the capitol of Oslo, where there is a large health divide between the rich western part of the city and the poor eastern inner city. Much of the disparities are due to a high proportion of immigrants settling in poor urban areas. Immigrants have an impact on the health care system because they experience more mental health problems and lifestyle-related diseases such as coronary heart disease and diabetes than Norwegians. For example, only 1% of Norwegians between the ages of 45 and 66 have diabetes compared with 9% of immigrants. From Pakistan alone, 19% have diabetes. Although lifestyle-related heart and cardiovascular diseases are decreasing, cancer, musculoskeletal ailments, and respiratory diseases are increasing and are the most common causes of long-term sick leave and disability. Cardiovascular deaths, however, still accounted for 364 deaths per 100,000 persons in 2004; cancer accounted for 235, respiratory diseases for 86, infections for 13, endocrine disorders for 20, mental health-related for 28, AIDS for 0.4, and violent deaths for 45 (of which suicides account for 11 per 100,000 persons). Human immunodeficiency virus (HIV) testing is systematically done for blood donations, pregnant women, and patients with sexually transmitted diseases. By the end of

2005, 3,046 HIV cases had been reported. The number of new cases was 205 in 2002, 238 in 2003, 251 in 2004, and 219 in 2005. The number of acquired immunodeficiency syndrome (AIDS) deaths has decreased from 49 in 2003 to 30 in 2005. The Joint United Nations Programme on HIV/AIDS (UNAIDS) estimates the prevalence rate of HIV in adults (aged 15 to 49 years) to be 0.1%. About two thirds of those infected have been infected outside of Norway.

Health-Team Relationships: In the formal sense, the doctor has more power and influence during the admission, treatment, and discharge of patients. However, doctors and nurses often collaborate and discuss patients and tests, medications, and further exploration of health problems. Working relationships are usually good, but questions about leadership roles in various situations that occur in hospital wards and units create occasional tension in the working relationship. Patients are generally open and direct in their relationship with nurses, whereas they tend to adopt a more formal and detached attitude toward doctors. Patients are granted essential health assistance from specialists, the right to a medical examination within 30 days, the right to a second opinion, and the right to choose their hospital. Norwegians want to be given options and have a role in decision making. New patient rights legislation makes it easier for patients to influence their treatments, participate more actively, be provided with information, and access their medical records on request. The new law also has rules for handling patient complaints and provisions for patient representatives and those that govern special rights for children.

Families' Role in Hospital Care: Norway is divided into five health regions. Hospital services are organized so that each has three types of hospitals: district, central, and regional. The district hospitals are small and designed to meet the requirements of the local community with respect to internal medicine, surgery, obstetrics, x-ray, and laboratory. Central hospitals are larger, with more than 200 beds. They provide a much broader range of services and are intended to meet the needs of areas beyond the local hospital. Regional hospitals cover much wider areas and have highly specialized functions and services. The nursing and medical staffs provide all care in hospitals. The rights of children in hospitals are protected by regulations based on Norwegian legislation, which addresses teaching, housing of parents (with one allowed to remain at all times), and the economic rights of parents. Children are usually placed in rooms with other children, parents often stay overnight, and friends and siblings are allowed and encouraged to visit. Provisions are made for children to continue their education when they are ill for long periods.

Dominance Patterns: Norwegians have a passion for equality in society and in the relationship between the sexes. However, the female partner continues to do most of the domestic work in families. Norwegians usually take time to make a decision, and matters tend to be debated at length.

Families usually share the decision-making responsibilities, child rearing, and other household duties to some degree. When a partner is ill, the other partner assumes household duties as necessary and cares for the ill partner. However, as a general rule, women have the primary responsibility for caring for sick relatives. Treatment of men and women is considered to be fairly equal in the workplace, but discrimination still occurs; women may receive lower wages than men for the same job, or men may receive preferential treatment during hiring.

Eye-Contact Practices: Direct eye contact is usually preferable and acceptable.

Touch Practices: The Norwegian culture accepts touching, especially in familiar settings, and younger people are the mostly likely to have the most contact. Although touching between individuals of the same or opposite sex is accepted, it is considered more acceptable for women to touch other women than for men to touch other men.

Perceptions of Time: Norwegians are both present and future oriented, although many have the attitude that if things are going well today, they do not have to worry about tomorrow. People tend to be punctual, with a 5- to 10-minute deviation. Being more than 10 minutes late is regarded as inconsiderate.

Pain Reactions: Individuals are traditionally expected to react with stoicism to pain, and extremely emotional expressions of discomfort are not the norm. However, health professionals provide pain relief as necessary, monitor pain in hospitalized patients, and encourage attitudes promoting the admission of pain and expectation of pain relief.

Birth Rites: The fertility rate is 1.78 children born per mother. The infant mortality rate is among the lowest in the world (3.67 deaths per 1,000 live births). Many mothers attend prenatal birth preparation courses, and natural childbirth is common. Most births take place in hospitals, and the father is encouraged to be in the delivery room to support the mother. Rooming in is common (i.e., having the infant stay in the hospital room with the mother at all times). To allow the new mother to rest, infants may be taken to the nursery at night if the mother desires. The gender differences in life expectancy are decreasing because of more similar health risk behaviors. Life expectancy is 78 for men, 82 for women.

Death Rites: Most Norwegians die in health care institutions rather than at home. The closest family members are usually with the dying person because they believe no one should die alone. A religious ceremony accompanies most cremations or burials, and family and friends are present to comfort the family of the deceased. Organ donations and autopsies are considered acceptable.

Food Practices and Intolerances: Breakfast may consist of a combination of yogurt products, bread, coffee or tea, cereal, cheese, salami, and juice, and people generally have a sandwich for lunch. The main meal is eaten in the early evening. Potatoes with meat or meatballs and boiled or fried fish are traditional food staples. Rice, spaghetti, and pizza are becoming more popular, especially among young people. Great quantities of milk are also consumed. When the main meal is eaten at midday or early afternoon, another light meal is eaten between 8:00 and 10:00 pm. It is unacceptable to use the hands unless eating small sandwiches, small cakes, or biscuits.

Infant-Feeding Practices: Breastfeeding is encouraged and common. In 1999, 92% of Norwegian mothers were breastfeeding 1 month after the birth of the infant; 80% were breastfeeding 6 months after birth.

Child-Rearing Practices: Child-rearing practices are quite permissive, although when discipline is necessary, it is shared by both parents. Children are allowed to participate in decision making and generally have a great deal of autonomy. Children do not begin school until they are 6 years of age.

National Childhood Immunizations: BCG at 13 to 15 years; DTaPHibIPV at 3, 5, and 11 to 12 months; DTaPIPV at 7 years; IPV at 6 to 8 and 14 years; MMR at 15 months and 12 to 13 years; HepB at birth and 1 and 6 months; and Td at 11 years. The percent of the target population vaccinated, by antigen, is: DTP1 (97%); DTP3 and Polio3 (91%); Hib3 (93%); and MCV (90%).

BIBLIOGRAPHY

Dybendal KE, Skiri H: Clear geographical differences in life expectancy between areas in *Oslo, Samfunnspeilet.* 6:18–27, 2006.

Kumar BN, Holmboe-Ottesen G, Lien N, Wandel M: Ethnic differences in body mass index and associated factors of adolescents from minorities in Oslo, Norway: a cross-sectional study, *Public Health Nutr.* 7(8):999–1008, 2005.

Lien L: Financial and organisational reforms in the health sector; implications for the financing and management of mental health care services, *Health Policy* 63 (1):73–80, 2003.

Lien L, Claussen B, Hauff E, Thoresen M, Bjertness E: Bodily pain and associated mental distress among immigrant adolescents: a population-based cross-sectional study, *Eur Child Adolesc Psychiatry.* 14(7):371–375, 2005.

Nortvedt L, Kase BF: Children's rights in Norwegian hospitals—are children and parents satisfied? *Tidsskr Nor Laegeforen.* 4(120):469–471, 2001.

Tronstad KR: *Immigration and immigrants 2005.* Statistical analysis 66, Statistics Norway, 2005.

UNAIDS: 2006 Norway: Retrieved September 21, 2006, from http://www.unaids.org/en/Regions_Countries/Countries/norway.asp.

Vikan ST: An uneven process towards equality, *Samfunnsspeilet.* 4:13–25, 2001.

World Health Organization: 2006: Immunization, vaccines and biologicals. Retrieved September 21, 2006, from http://www.who.int/immunization_monitoring/en/globalsummary/countryprofileresult.cfm?C='nor'.

www.msis.no: Rate of infectious diseases (retrieved March 2, 2006).

www.fhi.no/tema/vaksine/dekning: Rates of vaccine coverage (retrieved March 2, 2006).

www.ssb.no/døde: Death rates and life expectancy (retrieved March 2, 2006).

www.ssb.no/befolkning: Population structure (retrieved March 2, 2006).

N

✦ OMAN (SULTANATE OF)

MAP PAGE (802)

Euan M. Scrimgeour

Location: The Sultanate of Oman is located on the southeast corner of the Arabian Peninsula. The capital is Muscat. Oman is a primarily hot and dry country with a narrow coastal plain and a wide arid plateau, which is largely desert. The total area is 212,460 km^2 (82,031 square miles). It is mountainous to the north and south. Most of the deep valleys in the north have adequate water resources and are fertile, with numerous isolated small villages. The district of Salalah on the south coast is the only part of the Arabian Peninsula affected by the Indian summer monsoon (June to August), when it is relatively cool and rainy. Frankincense trees thrive in this region. The population is more than three million (including 577,293 non-nationals). The gross domestic product (GDP) per capita is $13,250. Literacy rates are 83% for men, 67% for women.

Major Languages	Ethnic Groups	Major Religions
Arabic	Omani Arab 75%	Ibadhi Muslim
Swahili	East African Arab	Sunni Muslim
Baluchi (Urdu)	15%	Shiaa Muslim (all Muslim
Persian	Baluchi 9%	groups account for 75%)
Malayalam, Hindi	Lawati 1%	Other or none 25%
English	Indian	
	Other	

Ibadi Muslims follow an early fundamentalist sect of Islam. Most Omanis speak Arabic, but many understand English. The tribal hill people of southern Dhofar Province have a seminomadic, tribal lifestyle and speak a distinct Arab language, Jabali. Many Dhofari women (and many rural Omani women) still wear masks covering their nose, cheeks, and mouth. Until 1958 Oman had a coastal enclave, Gwadar, Baluchistan, and large numbers of Baluchis have settled in Oman. Until 1964, Oman administered Zanzibar; after its independence, many thousands of Swahili-speaking, ethnic Omani Arabs migrated to Oman. Today many members of the latter group occupy important roles in many professions (e.g., banking, commerce, oil production, medicine). Most (70%) Indian expatriates working in Oman are from Kerala, speak Malayalam, and are Christian. Fewer Pakistani, Sri Lankan, Filipino, and various European nationalities are employed. Although Omanis are devout and pray five times a day, they permit non-Muslims to practice their own religions. Until 30 years ago, Oman was one of the most isolated and backward countries in the Middle East, with only 5 km of surfaced road. Today Oman is one of the most advanced and progressive countries in the region, although it retains much of its traditional customs and way of life. Oman has decreed that Omanization is to be strongly promoted. Thus, within the past 5 to 10 years, numerous expatriates (e.g., Indians, Pakistanis) who

O

have unskilled or semiskilled labor jobs have been replaced by Omanis. The policy has now been extended to shopkeepers and businessmen and is having a greater impact on white-collar workers, teachers, and academic staff.

Health Care Beliefs: Active participation with emphasis on health promotion. Omanis believe that ill health is an inevitable part of life, not divine retribution. The overriding characteristic of all patients and their families is acceptance of Allah's will. Disease prevention is strongly promoted by the Ministry of Health.

Predominant Sick-Care Practices: Biomedical and traditional. Oman has an excellent health care system, with countrywide primary health care clinics and modern regional hospitals. Muscat has two well-equipped and staffed tertiary referral hospitals. In the past, patients traditionally consulted village healers for herbal remedies and skin cautery over affected areas. Many Omanis continue to seek this treatment before (and even after) receiving modern medical care. Many Indians working in Oman seek traditional, a yurvedic medical treatment. When a patient is admitted to a hospital, the family provides strong support. As a rule, very elderly, incapacitated patients are cared for in their own homes, in accordance with religious teaching. Long-term geriatric hospitals are not available. Patients do not accept amputations easily because they believe the body should be intact at the time of death.

Ethnic-/Race-Specific or Endemic Diseases: Health care is essentially free, but all expatriates and their employers must pay for treatment. Adults have a high prevalence of diabetes mellitus, hypertension, and atherosclerotic arterial disease (causing strokes and myocardial infarction). Among children, acute respiratory tract infections and gastroenteritis are common. Malaria is now rare, and the incidences of tuberculosis, brucellosis (which is largely restricted to the Salalah region), and sexually transmitted disease are decreasing. A single focus of schistosomiasis persists in permanent lakes and streams in the Salalah district. The Joint United Nations Programme on HIV/AIDS (UNAIDS) continues to report a low human immunodeficiency virus (HIV) prevalence rate for Oman (<0.2%). As of April 2006, about 1,570 persons were infected with HIV; UNAIDS reports the total number of acquired immunodeficiency syndrome (AIDS) cases as 601. Infected persons who are not Omanis are advised that they cannot receive long-term treatment in Oman and must be repatriated to their countries of origin. Where the mode of transmission is known, HIV is primarily contracted by heterosexual contact (65%). Increasingly, antiretroviral treatment is provided free of charge for adults and children. HIV-positive mothers are discouraged from breastfeeding their infants.

Health-Team Relationships: When the first modern hospitals were built in the 1970s, they were staffed almost entirely by foreign doctors and nurses. A few senior doctors were Omanis from Zanzibar who had graduated in the United Kingdom. The first graduates from the medical school of the Sultan Qaboos University have gradually filled junior posts and now consultant posts. Nurses have been recruited from the Philippines, India, and Malaysia, with Europeans and some foreign-trained Omanis occupying senior posts.

Omanis are now being trained locally as nurses. The medical teams are doctor driven, but the team spirit is strong, and nurses are held in high esteem. Patients and their families are invariably pleasant and grateful for medical care, and medical litigation is almost unknown.

Families' Role in Hospital Care: A family member stays with seriously ill patients. Families do not help patients with personal care or eating tasks (unless the patient is a child). Families have a role in decision making about invasive procedures (e.g., lumbar puncture) or surgical operations. A patient's illness must be explained in detail to the family because sometimes a senior family member forbids an operation even when a patient agrees to it. It is not uncommon in these situations for the family to remove the patient from the hospital against medical advice and seek an opinion in another hospital or even overseas, often in India or Jordan.

Dominance Patterns: Oman is essentially a male-dominated society, particularly in rural areas. In urban, more Westernized families, men and women are more equal. Arranged marriages are customary, but today they are usually conducted with the agreement of both parties.

Eye-Contact Practices: Women tend to avoid eye contact with men they do not know, and in general eye contact is indirect between strangers. Men usually avoid looking directly at women, especially if the women are alone. When women wear the traditional face mask, however (which covers the nose and mouth but leaves most of the face uncovered), they tend to have more confidence in eye contact with strangers.

Touch Practices: Handshaking is restricted between individuals of the opposite sex. Men do not shake hands with women, although women may shake each other's hands. Men may greet good male friends or relatives with an embrace and a kiss on both cheeks.

Perceptions of Time: In traditional desert tribal life and in early times in coastal towns, Omanis had a relaxed attitude when conducting their affairs. Time was not dictated by the clock and was marked by the timing of the five daily prayers, which changed during the lunar cycle. As a result, patience was an attribute that was encouraged and valued. Today Omanis have adjusted to the rapid pace of modern life and the need to be punctual and conscientious in their work commitments. As a rule, Omanis are punctual for appointments.

Pain Reactions: Most patients are relatively stoic in response to pain. They rely implicitly on Allah and are prepared to withstand considerable discomfort and pain without complaint; however, the administration of analgesics, including opiates, is routine when required.

Birth Rites: Most women go to antenatal clinics. About 40% of infants in rural and 90% in urban areas are born in hospitals. Abortion is not permitted other than in exceptional medical situations. There is usually strong opposition by husbands to cesarean sections and what is perceived as a disfiguring scar. During birth, the mother or mother-in-law of the woman must be present. The birth of a son is usually greeted with extra enthusiasm, and all boys are circumcised. Birth spacing (a gap of 2 years) is the national policy to limit family size. The total fertility rate is estimated at 5.77 children born per woman. The infant mortality rate is 19 deaths per 1,000 live births. About 43% of the population is younger than 15 years. Life expectancy is 71 for men, 76 for women.

Death Rites: When a Muslim dies, the body is washed, wrapped in special cloth, and buried without a coffin in the ground. When a patient dies in the hospital, the family removes the body immediately for a private burial. Autopsy is almost invariably refused. Both cadaver and living donor organ transplantations (e.g., renal, bone marrow) are acceptable; however, patients go out of the country for liver or other major organ transplants.

Food Practices and Intolerances: Pork is forbidden for Muslims, and all meat must be *halal* (slaughtered incorporating Islamic rites). During the holy month of Ramadan, Muslims fast during daylight hours. Unless given special permission, patients are not permitted to swallow any medication that contains nutrients or fluid or receive injections. Food is eaten only with the right hand. Muslims are not permitted to drink alcohol; however, alcohol is available in larger hotels and in licensed restaurants for expatriates (also permitted to have alcohol at home).

Infant-Feeding Practices: Most infants are breastfed (except by HIV-positive mothers); a practice strongly promoted by the Ministry of Health. As a result, gastroenteritis in infants is unusual. Weaning starts at 6 to 8 months, and most mothers stop breastfeeding at 2 years.

Child-Rearing Practices: Both parents help raise the children, frequently with the help of grandparents or other relatives. Discipline tends to be quite permissive, but when it is required, both parents are involved. Spanking and other forms of physical punishment are generally discouraged.

National Childhood Immunizations: BCG at birth; OPV1 at birth, 6 weeks, and 3 months; OPV2 at 5 months; OPV3 at 7 months; OPV booster at 18 months; HBV-1 at birth; Penta-I at 6 weeks; Penta II at 3 months; Penta III at 5 months; Penta IV at 18 months; measles at 12 and 18 months. (In addition, 200,000 units of vitamin A are given at 7, 12, and 18 months) The percent of the target population vaccinated exceeds 98%.

Other Characteristics: Omanis are renowned for their friendly and tolerant attitude toward foreigners. Almost all wear traditional dress: embroidered caps or turbans and white robes or dishdasha for men, head scarves and the black *abeiya* ("ankle-length cloak") for women. As noted, many rural women still wear the Omani face mask. Permission must always be obtained before photographing any Omani, including a child; as a rule, women do not agree to be photographed. Foreign women are expected to dress modestly but are not required to wear a head covering. All forms of communication, including magazines, films, television, and videos, are strictly censored, and any material deemed morally offensive is banned.

BIBLIOGRAPHY

Central Intelligence Agency: *2006: The world factbook, Oman*. Retrieved September 21, 2006 from https://www.cia.gov/cia/publications/factbook/print/mu.html.

Gordon FL, Walker J, Ham A, Maxwell V: *Arabian peninsula*, Melbourne, 2004, Lonely Planet Publications.

Scrimgeour EM, Mehta FL, Suleiman AJM: Infectious and tropical diseases in Oman: an epidemiological review. *Am J Trop Med Hygiene* 61:920-925, 1999.
UNAIDS: 2006 Oman. Retrieved September 21, 2006, from http://www.unaids.org/en/Regions_Countries/Countries/oman.asp.
Vine P: *The heritage of Oman.* London, 1995, Immel Publishing.

◆ PAKISTAN (ISLAMIC REPUBLIC OF)

MAP PAGE (804)

Shehzad Parviz

Location: Located in South Asia, Pakistan borders India in the east, China in the northeast, and Iran in the southwest; Afghanistan abuts its western and northern edges. The Arabian Sea is Pakistan's southern border. Pakistan's Hindu Kush and Himalayan Mountains contain the second highest peak in the world. Pakistan has desert lands in the east and areas of alluvial plains along the Indus River. The capital is Islamabad; 34% of the population lives in urban areas. The total area is 796,096 km^2 (307,361 square miles); the estimated population is 165.8 million. The gross domestic product (GDP) per capita is $2,400, with 32% living below the poverty line. Literacy rates are 66% for men, 42% for women.

Major Languages	Ethnic Groups	Major Religions
Punjabi	Punjabi 66%	Sunni Muslim 77%
Sindhi	Sindhi 13%	Shi'a Muslim 20%
Pashtu	Pashtun 9%	Other 3%
Balochi	Balochi, Other 12%	
Urdu (national language)		
English (official language), Other		

Health Care Beliefs: Acute sick care; traditional. People believe that health and sickness are provided by God. Sickness may be attributed to some evil deed done in the past or to sorcery. Mentally ill people are considered by some to be possessed by an evil spirit, or *gin*. Mental illness is stigmatized; therefore, those who are affected might not seek care. Doctors and family members avoid telling patients about a grave diagnosis such as cancer so they will not become depressed. If someone gets ill, is cured, or has a child, it is common to donate money called *sadiqa* to the poor or needy to obtain good wishes and inhibit evil spirits. Some may sacrifice goat or sheep and distribute the meat to the poor. Women may believe that reproductive tract infections are caused by "melting bones," consuming foods that are "hot," poor personal hygiene, or procedures such as dilatation and curettage. They do not generally perceive sexually transmitted diseases as the cause of reproductive problems.

Predominant Sick-Care Practices: Allopathic, homeopathic, and indigenous methods. Some people use all three methods concurrently. Pakistan has many modern private hospitals, and government hospitals provide free or subsidized care. People prefer to go to private hospitals or doctors if they can afford to do so. Among those who are sick, about two thirds in urban areas and one third in rural areas consult private doctors; fewer than one sixth use government health facilities. It is common for doctors to overprescribe antimicrobials, vitamins, minerals, and injections. Sexual health problems are rarely discussed with other family members or elders, in accordance with social norms. Many would not clean wounds from a dog bite, and only a few would apply an antiseptic or water; instead, many would use red chilies, calcium carbonate, herbal medicine, or ground tobacco or would perform a ritual. Injections and intravenous fluids are considered more effective than oral medication.

Ethnic-/Race-Specific or Endemic Diseases: Endemic diseases include chloroquine-resistant malaria, tuberculosis, acute respiratory tract infections, bacillary dysentery, typhoid fever, amoebiasis, and rabies. Diarrhea is the chief cause of death of children. Almost two thirds of children under age 5 have mild to moderate protein-energy malnutrition. The Joint United Nations Programme on HIV/AIDS (UNAIDS) estimates the prevalence rate of human immunodeficiency virus (HIV) in adults (aged 15 to 49 years) to be 0.1%, with 85,000 persons living with HIV, including 14,000 women. Most frequently infected are individuals aged 20 to 44 years, mostly men (5:1 ratio). About 3,000 deaths from acquired immunodeficiency syndrome (AIDS) have been reported. The vast majority of detected infections have been found among injecting drug users. Knowledge regarding HIV or AIDS and sexually transmitted diseases is poor among high-risk groups.

Health-Team Relationships: Criticizing a person of higher status or rank is unacceptable. Men traditionally fill positions of authority; therefore, female health care workers are under the authority of male doctors and hospital administrators. Nursing has not been perceived as a preferred occupation, and there are more doctors than nurses with a ratio of 6:1. Traditional practitioners are called *hakims*.

Families' Role in Hospital Care: Hospitals supply meals, but they are usually of substandard quality. In government hospitals, patients who do not have needed medicines must buy them from an outside pharmacy or simply not take them. Female wards in hospitals are separated from male wards, and opposite-sex adult relatives are usually not allowed to stay overnight.

Dominance Patterns: Women are expected to be obedient to men and are discouraged from making decisions. In some places, it is preferable that women stay in their homes and go out only if they are completely covered and unrecognizable. Women have access to higher education. Most medical schools have more women than men, although most opt not to practice after graduation because of family obligations. Women feel they have limited control over their lives, exemplified by young marriages, high expectations for newlywed women to conceive, and poor access to contraceptives. Women frequently express a strong preference for sons, primarily for economic reasons, reflecting women's subordinate position in society and the low economic value placed on women's work. Most women wear a soft cloth called a *dupulta* around the neck or over the head; they almost always wear traditional clothes, whereas men may opt for Western clothes. Mortality statistics are higher for women than men, perhaps because men receive preferential treatment. Domestic violence against women is common, and in cases of infertility, the female partner is subject to contempt, abuse, and exploitation.

Eye-Contact Practices: A peripheral gaze or no eye contact may be preferred during male-female interactions. The eyes remain down as a sign of obedience during interactions with older adults or persons in a superior position.

Touch Practices: At times, patients are reluctant to expose body parts to health care practitioners of the opposite sex. Members of the opposite sex do not shake hands or embrace another person unless the person is a close family member. Women embrace and kiss on the cheek when greeting other women; men shake hands and embrace.

Birth Rites: The fertility rate is four children born per woman. Infant mortality rates are 71 deaths per 1,000 live births, and about one fourth of births are attended by trained health personnel called *dai*. A *tawiz*, an amulet containing verses from the Koran, is placed around the neck or shoulder of the infant. After 1 month of age, the infant's head is shaved because birth hair is considered unclean. The head shaving is accompanied by a family function known as *haqiqa*, during which a goat or sheep is sacrificed. Life expectancy is 62 for men, 64 for women.

Death Rites: Organ donations or transplants are very uncommon. However, Muslims believe that blood transfusions are acceptable. All family members congregate when a relative is dying. Death is usually ascribed to fate determined by God. A holy Imam does not have to be present; however, Muslims recite, "There is no God but God, and Muhammad is his messenger." When the person dies, others recite the following: "We all belong to God, and to him shall we return." According to Islamic tradition, family members must wash the body before the funeral. Autopsies are uncommon because the body must be buried intact, and cremation is not permitted. For Muslim burial, the body is wrapped in special pieces of cloth and buried without a coffin in the ground.

P

Food Practices and Intolerances: Food practices vary. For example, Pashtuns and Balochis are meat lovers but also eat a special kind of bread called tandoori roti that is made in a furnace. The Punjabi staple diet consists of lentils, rice, and bread known as chapatti. Food tends to be spicy, and the diet is high in fat. Spicy chicken is very popular. Milk tea is consumed every day at work and during the evening. *Kahwa*, a yellow tea without milk, is preferred in the morning during winter. Consumption of alcohol, pork, carrion, and blood is forbidden to Muslims. Ramadan fasting is practiced by all except those who are sick or traveling. The mean daily intake of calories and micronutrients is lower for rural than urban children.

Infant-Feeding Practices: Breastfeeding is recommended by Islam, and women may breastfeed for up to 2 years, although this practice is declining. More than half of the women who breastfeed do so for longer than 1 year. Two thirds of mothers do not give their infants colostrum. Most women provide supplemental bottle-feedings by 5 months; the most common reason is worry about insufficient breast milk. Mothers who are illiterate, poor, or have had girls may stop breastfeeding sooner. Weaning is usually initiated between 3 and 4 months of age, and weaning foods are usually rice, cereals, eggs, and later fruit and vegetables.

Child Rearing Practices: Some associate dehydration, malnutrition, marasmus, and inevitable death with spirits and close contact with "unclean" women: those who are menstruating or did not take a ritual bath after sexual intercourse. The most traditional Pakistanis may wrap their infants in cow dung to give them the strength and warmth needed for growth. Some mothers do not associate a lack of growth with lack of food. A sick child is a reflection of the mother's carelessness and social disgrace; therefore, the family of the sick child may be ostracized. The high fat content in the buffalo milk that is fed to some infants makes it hard to digest. Each Muslim boy and girl is taught the Koran at a young age and to read it completely at least once.

National Childhood Immunizations: BCG at birth; DTwP at 6, 10, and 14 weeks; OPV at birth and at 6, 10, and 14 weeks; hepatitis B at 6, 10, and 14 weeks; measles at 9 months; and TT at first contact and at +1, +6 months, +1, and +1 year. The percentage of the target population vaccinated, by antigen, is: BCG (82%); DPT1 (84%); DTP3 (72%); HepB3 (73%); Polio3 (77%); MCV (78%); TT2 plus (57%).

Other Characteristics: People with medical emergencies in cities with ambulances usually do not use them. This practice is not only a result of poor accessibility, but it also results from cultural barriers and an inability to recognize the danger signs of true emergencies.

BIBLIOGRAPHY

Afsar HA, Mahmood MA, Barney N, Ali S, Kadir MM, Bilgrami M: Community knowledge, attitude and practices regarding sexually transmitted infections in a rural district of Pakistan, *J Pak Med Assoc.* 56(1 suppl 1):S50–S54, 2006.

Bhatti LI, Fikree FF: Health-seeking behavior of Karachi women with reproductive tract infections, *Soc Sci Med.* 54(1):105–117, 2002.

Central Intelligence Agency: *2006: The World factbook, Pakistan.* Retrieved September 21, 2006, from https://www.cia.gov/cia/publications/factbook/print/pk.html.

Parviz S, Luby S, Wilde H: Post-exposure treatment of rabies in Pakistan, *Clin Infect Dis.* 27(4):751–756, 1998.

Raglow GJ, Luby SP, Nabi N: Therapeutic injections in Pakistan: from the patients' perspective, *Trop Med Int Health.* 6(1):69–75, 2001.

Sarwar T: Infant feeding practices of Pakistani mothers in England and Pakistan. *J Hum Nutr Diet.* 15(6):419–28, 2002 Dec.

Shaikh MA: Domestic violence against women–perspective from Pakistan, *J Pak Med Assoc.* 50(9):312–314, 2000.

Statistic Division: The government of Pakistan. Retrieved May 14, 2006, from http://www.statpak.gov.pk/.

UNAIDS: 2006 Pakistan. Retrieved September 21, 2006, from http://www.unaids.org/en/Regions_Countries/Countries/pakistan.asp.

Winkvist A, Akhtar HZ: God should give daughters to rich families only: attitudes towards childbearing among low-income women in Punjab, Pakistan, *Soc Sci Med.* 51(1):73–81, 2000.

World Health Organization: Country Profile. Pakistan. Retrieved May 14, 2006, from http://www.who.int/countries/pak/en/.

World Health Organization: 2006: Immunization, vaccines and biologicals. Retrieved September 21, 2006, from http://www.who.int/immunization_monitoring/en/globalsummary/countryprofileresult.cfm?C='pak'.

http://www.int/countries/pak/en/ (retrieved September 1, 2006).

◆ PANAMA (REPUBLIC OF)

MAP PAGE (795)

Carolyn M. D'Avanzo

Location: Panama is situated between the Caribbean Sea on the north, Colombia on the east, the Pacific Ocean on the south, and Costa Rica on the west. The total area is 75,517 km^2 (29,157 square miles). From east to west, the country is divided by the Cordillera Central, with elevations of more than 3000 m, and from north to south by the Panama Canal, which is 80 km long and stretches from the Caribbean Sea to the Pacific Ocean. Panama City, the capital, is on the Pacific Coast. The country is divided into nine provinces and five Amerindian territories. The climate is tropical. Panama has two seasons: a dry season from December to April and a rainy season from May to December. The population is 3.2 million. The gross domestic product (GDP) per capita is $7,200, with 37% living below the poverty line. Literacy rates are 93% for men, 92% for women.

Major Languages	Ethnic Groups	Major Religions
Spanish (official)	Mestizo 70%	Roman Catholic
English	Amerindian, mixed (West Indian) 14%	(official) 85%
	White 10%	Protestant 15%
	Amerindian 6%	

The Amerindian population is bilingual (speaking both Spanish and indigenous languages). Illiteracy is primarily restricted to Amerindians (with the exception of the Kunas) and very poor people. Some Amerindians and Afro-Panamanians practice their own indigenous religions. Witchcraft practitioners and those who perform magic rituals are disseminated among the population. The population consists mainly of Hispano-Amerindians and Afro-Panamanians. The Amerindian population consists of six groups: Kuna in the San Blas Islands and Darien; Embera and Wounaan in Darien (the Colombian frontier); Ngöbe-Buglé in the three western provinces; and the Bokotas, Teribes, and Bri Bri in Bocas del Toro (the Costa Rican frontier).

Health Care Beliefs: Acute sick care; increasing efforts in the area of disease prevention. The Ministry of Health and some doctors' associations are very active in the promotion of healthy lifestyles, and prevention is a part of medical services. Inhabitants of urban areas are open to prevention campaigns; lifestyle problems are generally related to poverty. In rural areas, the concepts of prevention are less understood, although prevention of childhood diseases and hygienic delivery of infants are becoming increasingly accepted. Other programs, such as reproductive and sexual health, birth control, and cancer prevention for women, meet some resistance. Amerindians generally do not attend health programs for economic or cultural reasons (beliefs or language barriers) and because of what they consider to be the dominating attitude of doctors and nurses. Some of the Embera and Wounaan groups believe that illness can be drawn out with heated coins, but this belief is disappearing with migration from the countryside and the extension of services by the Ministry of Health. Mental illness is generally feared but accepted, probably because of the influence of African and Amerindian beliefs. People with mental illness who are not dangerous live with their relatives. The members of the upper class are the least accepting of those with mental illness.

Predominant Sick-Care Practices: Biomedical and traditional. Western health care is offered through the national public health system, an employment-linked prepaid health and retirement plan called Seguro Social, and through a high, fee-for-service private urban sector. Medical services of the Ministry of Health cover the entire country, with hospitals, health centers and polyclinic centers, and health subcenters. Public and private highly specialized hospitals are located in Panama City. The government pays 80% to 100% of hospital costs, depending on the family's income. Amerindians have their own healers, but they also use Western medical services, primarily after a community member has had a positive experience with the Western health service. Relationships between healers and doctors often conflict, primarily because of the rejection of indigenous beliefs among doctors. Self-medication, excluding antibiotics, is common. Herbs and other locally grown plants are widely used for their medicinal qualities and are sold in the open markets.

Ethnic-/Race-Specific or Endemic Diseases: The principal causes of death are cancer (primarily prostate and gastric cancer among men and cervical cancer among women), violence (automobile accidents, aggression, and suicide), ischemic heart disease, cerebrovascular diseases, diabetes mellitus, chronic pulmonary illnesses, human immunodeficiency virus (HIV) and acquired immunodeficiency syndrome (AIDS), other heart illnesses, prenatal illnesses, and pneumonia. Afro-Panamanians are usually afflicted with sickle cell disease; diabetes and cardiovascular diseases particularly affect Afro-Panamanian women older than 40. Amerindian communities have all the diseases common among the poor: respiratory tract infections, diarrhea, and other infectious diseases in children younger than 5 years, with high mortality rates; complications of pregnancy and high maternal mortality among women; and tuberculosis in both sexes. Life expectancy is almost 15 years lower in Amerindians. The Joint United Nations Programme on HIV/AIDS (UNAIDS) estimates the prevalence rate for HIV in adults (aged 15 to 49 years) to be 0.9%, with 17,000 people living with HIV, including 4,300 women. Fewer than 1,000 deaths from AIDS have been reported. The primary mode of transmission is heterosexual.

Health Team Relationships: Health team relationships depend on many different factors: the type of service provided (with hospitals being more hierarchical than health centers), the style of the head of the team, the number of years of close work, and the academic preparation and professional experience of each member of the team. The term *doctor* is used to express respect or affection, and nurses are addressed by *miss*. In public practice as in private, attitudes toward doctors and nurses are generally trusting. People are generally unassertive toward doctors and, although to a lesser degree, toward nurses. If they do not trust a doctor or nurse at one health service, they go to another health service. Individuals who feel they have received poor treatment have the right to a "people's defender" (a lawyer named by the government for defense of human rights).

Families' Role in Hospital Care: Since 1980, families have been staying with their hospitalized children in the Child Hospital of Panama, but food from the outside is prohibited. The hospital has special facilities for mothers from rural areas, and all parents have access to the library to read about their child's illness. In other hospitals, families stay only when patients have special needs, but they can bring the patients food and, in some situations, medications. Ngobe families and a special rural group of Hispano-Amerindian people with strong Spanish traditions move near the hospital when a family member is ill to care for the person until recovery or death.

Dominance Patterns: Men dominate Panamanian culture, but work for legal equity between men and women has been in process since 1995. Health maintenance and care of the ill are the responsibilities of women, who take care of every member of the family. Women have access to all sorts of services and can choose what they prefer for themselves or for family members. In the median and upper classes, male dominance is apparent only if the costs of services are too high or during very important decision making. In the lower classes, control of the economic resources of the family is in the hands of men, and they make the decisions regarding women's sexual and reproductive health.

Eye-Contact Practices: Eye contact is generally maintained in all but two situations, the most important one involving eye contact with a newborn. Mothers, worried about women with the "evil eye" (i.e., the power to harm the newborn through her gaze), try to avoid interacting with these women until they can arrange a witch ceremony to combat the curse. The other situation involves interactions with Ngobe people, who think that pregnant women should avoid eye contact with men, although this belief does not tend to be as relevant during interactions with health practitioners.

Touch Practices: Physical touching is acceptable, but men prefer that only male doctors examine them for sexually related diseases. Women say that they prefer female doctors for sexually related examinations, although they often change their minds after having a respectable and positive experience with a male doctor. It is always best to examine patients of the opposite sex in the presence of a nurse or other doctor, particularly if the examination involves the genitalia. Use of touch is used to make personal or social contact in urban areas. Men greet each other by shaking hands or an embrace, and kissing one cheek is common between women, or men and women, as an initial greeting. In rural or indigenous areas, touch is used only between members of the same family.

Perceptions of Time: Punctuality is an issue for people who interact with public or private health services. People may arrive nearly 2 hours before appointments, but the doctors may consider being behind schedule as a sign that they are successful. Panamanian culture is very reality based, and people tend to live in the present. Focus on the past is limited to older adults and academics, and a focus on the future is often associated with those in politics or who are wealthy.

Pain Reactions: Reactions to pain depend on culture and education. Stoicism seems to characterize Amerindian and rural people, whereas those with high levels of education may cry calmly and discreetly. Very expressive reactions are the norm among Afro-Panamanian or Hispano-Panamanian people, and shouting, screaming, and gesticulating are not uncommon.

Birth Rites: In urban areas, almost all deliveries involve professional assistance, whereas in rural areas, the coverage can be about half (particularly in Amerindian territories). The poor coverage of Amerindian territories can be attributed to their long distance from any health care center, language barriers, the high cost of transportation, preferences for delivery in a vertical position (assisted by the husband or mother), and the tradition of burying the placenta. Infant mortality is 16 deaths per 1,000 live births. The Ministry of Health has an active program of family planning in its centers, including contraceptives and intrauterine devices at minimal cost. This program is facing opposition from the Catholic Church and from men, particularly in poor and rural communities. The fertility rate is 2.68 children born per woman. Life expectancy is 73 for men, 78 for women.

Death Rites: Death is perceived as a significant loss, even when the person is older. All family members are usually present at a relative's death, and the death ceremony (which is familiar and religious) is a social event in the community. When a person is dying in the hospital, staff members allow the family to visit, and the parents can stay with the person until the priest or the pastor arrives. Rural and Amerindian people prefer to take deceased family members home themselves because of transportation costs and to perform their own ceremonies. Organ donations and autopsies are not usually acceptable. Acceptance depends on the educational level of the family; the decision of whether to allow the procedure to be performed is made by all adult family members.

Food Practices and Intolerances: The basic diet and preferred foods are related to the social and economic status of families as well as their ethnic background. In the upper classes, families adopt the typical Western diet or the cultural diet of the ethnic group to which they belong. Hispano-Panamanian families commonly eat rice with meat and beans. Ngobe families eat rice with beans and occasionally chicken, but from July to September, they eat only once a day. Panamanians' favorite foods are traditional ones, but people enjoy soft drinks such as Coke and Pepsi. It is unusual to eat with the hands.

Infant-Feeding Practices: Breastfeeding is considered a common cultural practice among Amerindian and rural families and a healthy choice in urban areas. The Ministry of Health promotes breastfeeding through the health services, and bottle-feeding is prohibited in maternity hospitals. In rural areas, infants are breastfed until they are a year old and occasionally until they are 2 years old. In urban areas, the ability to breastfeed often depends on the working needs of the mother. The Work Code allows 3 months for breastfeeding and then 1 hour of work time until the infant is 6 months old. Mothers gradually introduce solid foods as their infants grow and develop during the first year. In the Amerindian population, infants between 8 months and a year (who have their first teeth) eat what the family is eating.

Child-Rearing Practices: Child-rearing practices are very permissive, although parents and grandparents may spank children when they consider it necessary. Generally, the father is the head of the family, but discipline is the responsibility of both parents. Until age 1 to 2 years, children sleep with their parents or (if they are in the upper class) with a "nana." They then sleep with their brothers or sisters or alone. In very poor families, houses have only one room, so these separations are impossible.

National Childhood Immunizations: BCG and HepB at birth; DTwP at 4 to 5 years; DTwPHib at 18 months; DTwPHibHep at 2, 4, and 6 months; OPV at birth, 2, 4, 6, and 18 months and at 4 to 5 years; MMR at 12 months and at 4 to 5 years; influenza before age 2 and after age 60 years; Td at 6 years ×2; vitamin A at 6 to 11, 12, 18, 24, 30, and 36 months; and YF 1 year. The percent of the target population vaccinated, by antigen, is: BCG and MCV (99%); DTP1 (95%); and DTP3, HepB3, and Hib3 (85%).

BIBLIOGRAPHY

Central Intelligence Agency: *2006: The world factbook*, Panama. Retrieved September 21, 2006, from https://www.cia.gov/cia/publications/factbook/print/pm.html.

Contralorí de la República de Panamá: *Dirección de Estadística y Censo*: Panamá en Cifras, 2001, Panama.

Rudolf G: *Panama's poor—victims, agents and historymakers*, Tampa, 1999, University Press of Florida.

UNAIDS: 2006 Panama. Retrieved September 21, 2006, from http://www.unaids.org/en/Regions_Countries/Countries/panama.asp.

World Health Organization: 2006: Immunization, vaccines and biologicals. Retrieved September 21, 2006, from http://www.who.int/immunization_monitoring/en/globalsummary/countryprofileresult.cfm?C='pan'.

✦ PAPUA NEW GUINEA (INDEPENDENT STATE OF)

MAP PAGE (794)

Franklin H.G. Bridgewater

Location: Papua New Guinea is in the South Pacific and comprises the mainland and approximately 600 offshore islands, with a total area of 461,690 km² (178,259 square miles). The mainland constitutes the eastern portion of the island of New Guinea; Irian Jaya, a province of Indonesia, constitutes the western portion. From the border with Indonesia, Papua New Guinea reaches east. The capital is Port Moresby. The population is 5.6 million. The gross domestic product (GDP) per capita is $2,600, with 37% living below the poverty line. The island has one of the largest unspoiled rain forests in the world. The mainland is thickly forested, with dense jungle and relatively unexplored mountains. The climate is temperate in the highlands and tropical in the coastal lowlands and islands.

Major Languages	Ethnic Groups	Major Religions
Pidgin English	Papuan 95%	Indigenous beliefs (animist,
English (official)	Other (Negrito,	pantheist) 34%
Motu	Micronesian,	Roman Catholic 22%
Other	Melanesian,	Lutheran 16%
	Polynesian) 5%	Other Christian 28%

As a result of isolation caused by the rugged terrain, diverse tribes and language groups evolved. More than 700 different languages and dialects have been recorded. Pidgin English developed as a common means of communication. It primarily derives from English but incorporates elements of German, Malay, Motu (a language of the Port Moresby area), and other local words; it has a limited vocabulary. English is spoken by only 1% to 2% of the population. Literacy rates are 71% for men, 58% for women. Some have advocated for a division of the population into two major groups, Papuan and Melanesian. Others suggest smaller groupings such as Papuans (from the south of the mainland), Highlanders, New Guineans (from the north of the mainland), and Islanders. The latter suggestion is more in line with the country. This variability in culture and physical characteristics makes it impossible to produce cultural statements that apply to all of Papua New Guinea. Perhaps the most consistent tenet is the importance of land and the manner in which it is held.

Health Care Beliefs: Traditional; both active and passive involvement. People have a widespread belief that evil spirits are a reality and inhabit some jungle and forested areas. Illness may be attributed to personal actions that have offended these spirits or to the work of a sorcerer acting at the behest of a hostile individual. Basically, the people have no precise differentiation between mental and physical illness. Some people simply accept an illness because of an underlying belief that there is no cause for it. They may say that investigations into its cause will *kamap nating* ("come-up with nothing"). Most health promotion is carried out at the village level by direct personal contact or in small groups with the use of basic illustrative posters. Some additional teaching occurs at hospital clinics and in schools.

Predominant Sick-Care Practices: Biomedical and magical-religious. In the towns and larger centers, most people accept modern health care practices. However, even those who are avowed Christians may follow traditional practices to treat illness, which involve animist and pantheist practices. In some cultures, particular individuals assume a healer's role and may receive payment, whereas in others, relatives may accept this responsibility. Certain leaves and botanical preparations are thought to have curative qualities. Placating the aggrieved spirits is common to promote healing. Traditions vary from region to region, and some from the Lufa, Daru, Kwikila, Samarai, and Rigo subprovinces have been documented.

Ethnic-/Race-Specific or Endemic Disease: Malaria (including chloroquine-resistant forms) is endemic in the lowlands and coastal areas. People are also at risk for tuberculosis and leprosy. In addition, pig-bel (enteritis necroticans), a severe form of gastroenteritis, is encountered in the highlands; it is caused by a specific bacterium. It is associated with pig feasts, an important cultural feature of the region. A person with pig-bel may need surgery, but immunizations against the organism are now common in the highlands. Anemia affects all age groups and is associated with chronic malaria and worm infestation. Kuru, a spongiform encephalopathy, affects the Kuku Kuku, a small group in the Fore area. Its relationship to the local practice of cannibalism has been investigated; the disease first appeared early in the twentieth century and stopped appearing in the youngest age group in 1964; thereafter, it progressively ceased affecting older age groups. Kuru, like bovine spongiform encephalopathy (BSE, or "mad cow disease") in Europe, may have been transmitted to humans through the food chain. Sexually transmitted diseases are common, particularly in urban areas. The Joint United Nations Programme on HIV/AIDS (UNAIDS) reports the prevalence rate for human immunodeficiency virus (HIV) in adults (aged 15 to 49 years) to be 1.8%, with 60,000 people living with HIV, including 34,000 women. About 3,300 deaths have been attributed to acquired immunodeficiency syndrome (AIDS). The trend in the annually reported number of AIDS cases has continued to rise more sharply each year since the mid-1990s.

Health-Team Relationships: Government aid posts, staffed by people trained in first aid and basic hygiene, are scattered throughout the country. Subprovincial and provincial centers have more advanced health care and education because of the hospitals and more highly trained personnel, but access to these facilities may be limited by weather, transportation, and finances. Health care relationships between members of the opposite sex are definitely reserved. AusAID, the Australian Government's overseas aid program, has significantly supported the Papua New Guinea government with providing health care in numerous areas. The provision of aid by personnel on military deployments highlights certain features. Although overtly beneficial, such aid creates dependence and may denigrate local workers, invite abuse of the system by local practitioners, create an undesirable secondary economy, and develop unrealistic expectations.

Families' Role in Hospital Care: Families consider it a duty and an obligation to provide companionship and care, including provision of food and firewood. These practices have economic and social implications. Hospital budgets are constrained, so additional food is needed for patients. Extra help is always needed and may be used for performing basic nursing tasks. Some may have unjustified concerns that care provided by an outsider (someone other than a tribal member, or *wantok* ["one-talk"], that is, a person who speaks the same language), may be prejudiced in some way and provide substandard or even harmful care or treatment.

Dominance Patterns: Male dominance and individuality are important to some. Condom use to prevent the spread of HIV/AIDS is a challenge for health care professionals because it is important to obtain the husband's approval for use of contraceptives. Polygamy is practiced in some areas. In rural areas, women are responsible for growing and preparing food and tending children and animals. Pigs are highly valued, so piglets are breastfed if necessary. Girls may be married by the age of 14 years.

Touch Practices: The sight of young men and women holding hands with members of the same sex is common and simply indicates valued companionship. Grooming a friend in various ways, such as combing hair or removing lice, may occupy a considerable amount of time. Children, particularly if they are white, may be patted or stroked incessantly by young and old and male and female indigenous Papua New Guineans.

Time Perception: Generally, little effort is made to adhere to a strict schedule, and events are often allowed to happen at their own rate. A request to follow a set program rigidly may lead to intense frustration and create animosity.

Birth Rites: The fertility rate is 3.88 children born per woman. About two thirds of women receive some antenatal care. Most births are supervised only by a local tribal midwife or older female family member. A delivery that becomes complicated usually eventually enters the health care system but often at a late stage, a practice associated with high infant mortality (50 deaths per 1,000 live births). Almost all infants are breastfed. In remote areas dominated by traditional practices, infants with physical anomalies may be left to die, unattended and unfed. Life expectancy is 63 for men, 68 for women.

Death Rites: Death rites, including different forms of burial, vary enormously between regions. Women in some cultural groups are expected to express grief; however, men are not. Traditionally, when Highlander women experience the death of a husband, they amputate a finger just above the first knuckle as a sign of their sorrow. These wounds often heal well. Illness and death can be the provocative event that begins a "payback" for previous misdeeds. Those held responsible for the death are required to recompense the aggrieved party in some way. Such paybacks may initiate a conflict that continues for a long period. An extreme example occurred in the Highlands in 1972. An islander doctor and the driver of a vehicle involved in an accident in which a child was killed stopped to give help and were immediately stoned to death by local villagers. Historically, amputated body parts have been valued and buried. It is assumed that the deceased will be buried in the same plot and will be able to use the appendages again in the next life. Organ donations are not performed, but if they were available they would likely conflict with traditional beliefs.

Food Practices and Intolerances: Sweet potatoes (kaukau) are eaten as the staple food in the highlands, and sago palm (*saksak*, which is almost pure starch) is eaten in the lowlands. Taro, bananas, and greens are common. Dietary iodine deficiency was a cause of endemic goiter in the highlands, but widespread use of iodine supplementation by injection provided the initial solution to this problem. Pig feasts are a social highlight and may be used to celebrate significant social occasions. The consumption of large amounts of poorly cooked, contaminated pork that has been passed for several days from person to person and area to area as a gift (according to tradition) is responsible for the previously mentioned outbreaks of pig-bel. People know certain plants can cause them to become intoxicated and that alcoholic beverages can be produced in numerous ways (*hom-bru*, or "home-brew"). Intoxication can be a serious, socially disruptive problem and often results in public brawls and domestic violence. More and more automobile accident fatalities are being associated with alcohol, and alcohol consumption is associated with a large and growing health problem. Perhaps the most common recreational drug is betel nut (*buai*), which is chewed with mustard and lime, producing characteristic red saliva. Some have proposed an association between this habit and oral cancer.

Infant-Feeding Practices: The current birth rate is 29.36 births/1000 (2006 est.). Breastfeeding may continue until a child is 4 or 5 years old

P

and may help prevent pregnancy. In the past, when breastfeeding was replaced by bottle-feeding, it was frequently associated with an infant's failure to thrive because of an inadequate understanding about formula preparation and hygiene. Legislation was introduced, and prescriptions are now required for infant formula.

Child-Rearing Practices: Significant differences in child rearing are apparent among various groups, and changes are occurring throughout the country. Previously, during tribal fighting in some areas, warriors were banned from having conjugal relationships. The lack of tribal fighting has made this restriction obsolete, resulting in an increase in young siblings within a family grouping. Discipline for young children is generally verbal, but they may receive an occasional slap. At a young age, girls assume responsibility for siblings. Boys have a longer period without such responsibilities. Parents often encourage secondary education for sons but not for daughters. The parents may be concerned about their daughter's safety in an area other than her home, or they might believe that females simply do not need such an education. The practice of demanding a "bride price" is still common and creates significant difficulties.

National Childhood Immunizations: BCG at birth; DTwP at 1, 2, and 3 months; OPV at birth and at 1, 2, and 3 months; HepB at birth and at 1 and 3 months; measles at 6 and 9 months; vitamin A at 6 and 12 months; TT at first and second contact, next pregnancy, and 7 and 13 years; and pig-bel at 1, 2, 3, and 4 months and during the first and last year of community schooling. The percent of the target population vaccinated, by antigen, is: BCG (73%); DTP1 (80%); DTP3 (61%); MCV (60%); Polio3 (50%); and TT2 plus (10%).

BIBLIOGRAPHY

Bridgewater F, Harris M, Rahdon R, Bohnstedt S: Provision of emergency surgical care in a unique geopolitical setting, *Aust N Z J Surg.* 71:606–609, 2001.

Central Intelligence Agency: *2006: The world factbook, Papua New Guinea.* Retrieved September 21, 2006, from https://www.cia.gov/cia/publications/factbook/print/pp.html.

Mueller I, Namuigi P, Kundi J, Ivivi R, Tandrapah T, Bjorge S, et al: Epidemic malaria in the highlands of Papua New Guinea, *Am J Trop Med Hyg.* 72(5):554–560, 2005.

Neuhaus S, Bridgewater F, Kilcullen D: Military medical ethics: issues for 21st century operations, *Aust Defence Force J.* 151:49–58, 2001.

Poka H, Duke T: In search of pigbel: gone or just forgotten in the highlands of Papua New Guinea? *Papua N Guinea Med J.* 46(3-4):135–142, 2003.

Reade MC: Medical assistance to civilians during peacekeeping operations: wielding the double-edged sword, *Med J Aust.* 173: 586–589, 2000.

UNAIDS: 2006 Papua New Guinea. Retrieved September 21, 2006, from http://www.unaids.org/en/Regions_Countries/Countries/papua_new_guinea.asp.

van Amstel H, van der Geest S: Doctors and retribution: the hospitalisation of compensation claims in the Highlands of Papua New Guinea, *Soc Sci Med.* 59 (10):2087–2094, 2004.

World Health Organization: 2006: Immunization, vaccines and biologicals. Retrieved September 21, 2006, from http://www.who.int/immunization_monitoring/en/globalsummary/countryprofileresult.cfm?C='png'.

P

http://www.ausaid.gov.au/country/papua.cfm (retrieved April 17, 2006).
http://coombs.anu.edu.au/SpecialProj/PNG/Index.htm (last revised August 16, 2005, retrieved April 17, 2006).
http://www.defence.gov.au/publications/dfj/index.cfm (retrieved April 17, 2006).
http://www.who.int/GlobalAtlas/predefinedReports/EFS2004/EFS_PDFs/EFS2004_PG.pdf (retrieved April 17, 2006).

◆ PARAGUAY (REPUBLIC OF)

MAP PAGE (797)

Richard G. Bribiescas

Location: Paraguay is a landlocked South American nation with a total area of 406,752 km^2 (157,006 square miles). Brazil and Bolivia border the country to the north and Argentina and Uruguay to the east and south. The eastern departments are characterized by subtropical woodland, whereas the Chaco region to the north is sparsely populated and consists primarily of dry scrub land. The gross domestic product (GDP) per capita is $4,900. Most people live near the two major cities of Asuncion (the capital) and Cuidad del Este. The western Chaco region represents 60% of the land area but only has 3% of the population.

Major Languages	Ethnic Groups	Major Religions
Spanish (official)	Mestizo (mixed Spanish	Roman Catholic 90%
Guarani (official)	and Indian) 95%	Protestant 5%
	Whites, Amerindians 5%	Other or none 5%

Paraguay is one of the few Latin American nations to adopt an indigenous language as an official language. Spanish is taught in school and is the predominant language in urban areas, whereas Guarani is the language of choice in rural communities. The population is 6.5 million, with 32% living below the poverty line. Isolated communities of Amerindians with limited European influence live in the eastern departments of Canindeyú and Alto Paraná and the northern regions of the Gran Chaco. Major indigenous groups include the Ache, Ayoreo, Chiripa, Guarani, Lengua, and Maká. About 5% of the population consists of Protestants, including several Mennonite colonies. Literacy rates are 95% for men, 93% for women.

Health Care Beliefs: Acute sick care; traditional; Western-based. Health care beliefs reflect the differences among the various communities. Many people, especially those in the rural areas, either believe in some aspects of or practice *yuyos* (pronounced "YOO yohs"), a form of herbal and spiritual home medicine. The practice derives from indigenous medical beliefs, mainly from the Guarani, Maká, and Chiripa peoples. The use of yuyos is quite complex and involves not only the use of an herb for the particular ailment but also interactions with spiritual aspects of the herb.

Predominant Sick-Care Practices: Biomedical and indigenous. Sick-care practices vary widely among communities and are driven primarily by socioeconomic status. Although much of the population is familiar with or practices yuyos, traditional Western-based medicine is widely accepted and desired by those who can afford it. Indigenous healers and yuyos are especially prevalent among the Ayoreo peoples of the Chaco and the Guarani, Chiripa, and Maká communities in eastern and central Paraguay. Among nonindigenous Paraguayans, the use of yuyos is more prevalent in rural areas, although it may simply be a result of lack of access to contemporary Western medical resources.

Ethnic-/Race-Specific or Endemic Diseases: Malaria was endemic in 2002, with most cases being reported in the provinces of Alto Paraná, Caaguazu, and Canindeyú. In 2000, an epidemic of Dengue fever was caused by the Dengue virus-1. An outbreak of Dengue virus-2 was also reported in 2001 but was quickly controlled. Chagas disease, a previously serious health concern, has been large curtailed, but surveillance remains to be fully implemented. The Maka and Chamacoco communities have the highest rates of tuberculosis: 10 times higher than the rest of the population. A recent investigation of Ache Amerindians in eastern Paraguay suggested that tuberculosis risk and prevalence has increased dramatically within this population. The top 10 causes of death among all Paraguayans in 2002 were cerebrovascular disease (11%), ischemic heart disease (10%), perinatal conditions (9%), lower respiratory infections (6%), diabetes mellitus (6%), violence (4%), diarrheal diseases (3%), tuberculosis (3%), hypertension (2%), and traffic accidents (2%). Diarrhea and related causes account for the largest proportion of deaths in children under age 5. Among neonates, prematurity (37%) and birth asphyxia (29%) accounted for the top causes of death. Accidents and violence have become increasing concerns. Drug trafficking and armed assaults are also becoming more common. Automobile accidents are more frequent and severe because of the opening of new asphalt roads, the growing number of large vehicles such as logging trucks on the road, and poor traffic control. The Joint United Nations Programme on HIV/AIDS (UNAIDS) reports the overall prevalence of human immunodeficiency virus (HIV) to be 0.4%, with about 13,000 adults (aged 15 to 49 years) living with HIV, including 3,500 women. Total deaths from acquired immunodeficiency syndrome (AIDS) are fewer than 500. The prevalence of HIV among sex workers was 3.14% in 2005. Between 2000 and 2003, HIV/AIDS mortality among children under age 5 was less than 1%.

Health-Team Relationships: As of 2002, Paraguay had 11 doctors and 17 nurses per 10,000 people. The issue of doctor-nurse relationships is somewhat irrelevant in most areas. However, the doctor predominantly controls the relationship. Although nurses offer some basic care, doctors dictate the strategy of treatment.

Families' Role in Hospital Care: Family care and attention in hospitals are crucial, especially in rural areas. Food and basic necessities such as sheets, blankets, and pillows are often unavailable and are provided by the family or, in some cases, by relief workers, such as religious missionaries. In urban hospitals, it is more likely for these basic necessities to be provided, but only after the family or patient has demonstrated the ability to pay for services.

Dominance Patterns: Men in Amerindian and non-Amerindian communities have a dominant role in social and political matters. Nonetheless, women's influence in social and familial situations varies among cultures. For example, in indigenous communities such as the Ache, women play a significant role in political and social matters and are likely to play a central role in guiding their family's health care practices.

Eye-Contact Practices: Paraguayans have no social taboos against direct eye contact, although younger women may be more reluctant to maintain eye contact with an unknown man.

Touch Practices: Shaking hands is a common form of greeting, especially between men. Women do not usually shake hands, although it is not uncommon to do so. Some indigenous groups do not shake hands with others in their community but understand that it is the norm among Paraguayans of European descent.

Perceptions of Time: Most communities understand the importance of punctuality, although practical factors, such as the availability of transportation, child care, or the freedom to leave a job, may make some seem chronically tardy. The tradition of the afternoon siesta, which involves returning home for a meal and a rest between approximately 3:00 and 6:00 PM, can affect the ability to set appointment times, especially in urban areas where commuter traffic is a constant problem.

Pain Reactions: Pain reactions are not especially stoic or expressive compared with those of Americans or Europeans.

Birth Rites: About 36% of deliveries are performed by trained medical personnel. Infant mortality rates are 33 deaths per 1,000 for males, 26 for females. Birthing practices vary widely, especially among indigenous groups. For example, an Ache father is never present during a birth; instead, he may be out hunting or getting food for his wife and new infant. Newborns are given an Ache name based on a special aspect of the mother's diet during her pregnancy. For example, the name *Chachugi* may be given if the mother ate an unusual amount of wild boar *(chachu)* meat. Similar customs are evident in other tribes as well. The fertility rate is 3.9 children born per woman. The Paraguayan government ranks among the lowest in national spending per person on family planning ($0.01 per person). Education level is positively associated with contraceptive use. Among rural women using contraceptives, *yuyos,* a form of traditional herbal remedy care, was the most common form of birth control (88%). Older women or those who already have children are most likely to use yuyos, as are rural women, compared with those with more education in urban areas. Although yuyos are widely known and accepted, their contraceptive efficacy remains to be clinically demonstrated. Life expectancy is 73 for men, 78 for women.

Death Rites: Most death rites follow Roman Catholic practices. Family members are often present and play an active role in funeral planning. Autopsies are uncommon, so families should be approached with sensitivity and care when an autopsy is necessary. Although the official doctrine of the Catholic Church understands the need for autopsies, Paraguayan Catholics may be fearful about an autopsy of a loved one. Similarly, organ transplantation is relatively new to Paraguay, although cardiac and renal transplants are becoming more common. The availability of transplants is extremely limited and restricted to the most modern urban hospitals. Death rites of indigenous groups vary widely. For example, the body of a deceased Ache may be bound at the wrists and ankles with twine from vines and buried in a fetal position in a simple grave with many possessions—such as knives, glasses, cups, and clothing.

Food Practices and Intolerances: Manioc (mandioca), a starchy root, is eaten at most meals. It is typically served peeled and boiled, although it may be fried or made into flour to make traditional bagel-like breads known as *chipa*. Meats such as roasted chicken, boiled beef, and pork are also common fare. In general, traditional Paraguayan food is not heavily spiced. Use of eating implements is common in all but the poorest communities, who cannot afford them. Dried and ground leaves of the yerba mate plant are used extensively to make warm tea known as *mate,* or cold tea known as or *te tade.* Mate with sugar and other spices added is known as *cocido.* Mate is usually consumed socially throughout the day, drunk from a communal cup known as a *bombea* and a filtered straw, the *wompa.* The cup is passed from person to person. When people decide they have had enough, they simply say "gracias" when the wompa is offered to them again. Mate has a slight stimulant affect, similar to but distinct from caffeine. Although some have proposed that mate has beneficial health effects, some studies have linked mate consumption with esophageal cancer, although the heat of the drink, not its ingredients, seems to be the most risky aspect.

Infant-Feeding Practices: Breastfeeding is a common practice in rural and urban settings. No customs that would seem unusual to Westerners are practiced. Virtually all Ache infants are weaned by around 3 years.

Child-Rearing Practices: In urban areas, children are raised in typical Western fashion. Depending on socioeconomic status, mothers breastfeed discretely in public; poorer mothers often nurse a child in public to keep a job such as selling chipas or mate on the street. In rural regions, breastfeeding is discrete and common.

National Childhood Immunizations: BCG at birth; DTwP at 18 months and 4 years; DTwPHibHep at 2, 4, and 6 months; HepB at contact, +1, + 6 months (high-risk groups); Td CBAW first contact, +1, +6 months, +1, +1 year; OPV at 2, 4, 6, and 18 months and at 4 years; MMR at 1 and 4 years; and YFV younger than 1 year along endemic borders. The percent of the target population vaccinated, by antigen, is: BCG (82%); DTP1 (91%); DTP3, HepB3, and Hib3 (76%); MCV (89%); TT2 plus (93%); and Polio3 (75%).

Other Characteristics: When arriving at a person's home, it is considered rude to knock on the door. The common practice is to clap the hands loudly two or three times. About 39% of the population (59% urban, 7% rural) has access to drinking water services, with "access" being defined as being within 200 m of a water source; 32% (22% urban, 44% rural) has access to sanitation services. Urban systems include basic latrines and septic tanks, whereas rural facilities include mostly latrines.

BIBLIOGRAPHY

Bull SS, Melian M: Contraception and culture: the use of yuyos in Paraguay. *Health Care Women Int.* 19:49–60, 1998.

Castellsague X, Munoz N, De Stefani E, Victora CG, Castelletto R, Rolon PA: Influence of mate drinking, hot beverages and diet on esophageal cancer risk in South America. *Int J Cancer.* 88:658–664, 2000.

Center for HIV Information. Retrieved September 22, 2006, from http://hivinsite. ucsf.edu/global?page=cr05-pa-00.

Central Intelligence Agency: *2006: The world factbook, Paraguay.* Retrieved September 21, 2006, from https://www.cia.gov/cia/publications/factbook/print/pa.html.

Country Profiles: Paraguay. *Epidemiol Bull.* 25(2):12–15, 2004.

Russell KL, Carcamo C, Watts DM, et al: Emerging genetic diversity of HIV-1 in South America, *AIDS.* 14:1785–1791, 2003.

Santiago-Delpin EA, Garcia VD: Organ transplantation in Latin America, *Clin Transplant.* 115:22, 2000.

Pan American Health Organization: Retrieved September 23, 2006, from http://www.paho.org/English/DD/AIS/cp_600.htm.

UNAIDS: 2006 Paraguay. Retrieved September 21, 2006, from http://www.unaids.org/en/Regions_Countries/Countries/paraguay.asp.

World Health Organization: 2006: Immunization, vaccines and biologicals. Retrieved September 21, 2006, from http://www.who.int/immunization_monitoring/en/globalsummary/countryprofileresult.cfm?C='pry'.

World Health Organization: Paraguay. Retrieved September 23, 2006, from http://www.who.int/countries/pry/en/.

World Health Statistics: Retrieved September 24, 2006, from http://www.who.int/entity/healthinfo/statistics/bodgbddeathdalyestimates.xls.

◆ PERU (REPUBLIC OF)

MAP PAGE (797)

Haq Nawaz and Devon L. Graham

Location: Peru is located on the western coast of South America and is the continent's third largest country in land area and fourth largest in population. It covers a total area of 1,285,222 km^2 (496,225 square miles). The country is divided into geographic regions—the Pacific Coast, Andes Mountains, and Amazon lowlands—and 23 departamentos (provinces). The capital, Lima, is on the central Pacific coast. The rugged Andes Mountains run the length of the country. The eastern third is covered by largely intact Amazon rain forest. The climate varies by the region. Coastal areas are arid and mild, the Andes are temperate to frigid, and the Amazon lowlands are typically warm and humid.

Major Languages	Ethnic Groups	Major Religions
Spanish (official)	Amerindian 45%	Roman Catholic (official)
Quechua (official)	Mestizo (European,	80%
Aymara	Amerindian) 37%	Protestant 7%
Other native	White 15%	Other non-Christian 13%
languages	Other (Japanese,	
	Chinese, Black) 3%	

The population is estimated as 28.3 million. About 74% live in urban areas, with the Lima-Callao metropolitan area home to almost one third of the population. The lowest population density is in the Amazon lowlands. White and Mestizo populations are concentrated along the coast and in highland urban areas. Pure Amerindian populations predominate in the southern Andean highlands, on the eastern slopes of the Andes, and in the Amazon lowlands. Quechua and Aymara are widely spoken among the Amerindian population of the highlands, and various dialects are spoken among Amazonian tribes. Peru has a rich upper class (predominantly of European background) and a poor lower class (primarily Amerindian and Mestizo). There is a small middle class. About 54% live below the poverty line. The gross domestic product (GDP) per capita is estimated at $5,900. Literacy rates are 94% for men, 82% for women. Catholicism in the highlands has been heavily influenced by Amerindian beliefs dating from the Inca Empire. In the Amazon lowlands, rural people often meld Catholicism with traditional animist beliefs. Only about 15% of declared Catholics attend church regularly.

Health Care Beliefs: Acute sick care; traditional. In urban areas, most people have a basic understanding of disease and its causes. In remote and the poorest urban areas, many people have a limited education, and folklore and native concepts of disease are prevalent. Many consider illness to be a direct result of witchcraft, whereas others may believe it to be caused by "hot" and "cold" imbalances. In one study about mothers' beliefs about children's diarrhea, most thought that diarrhea was caused by ingesting "cold" food, with consequent invasion of the body by "cold" elements. Milk was withheld as a treatment. Similarly, a survey conducted by the authors revealed that only 34% of the people in some Amazon villages believe that mosquitoes cause malaria. About 47% of people in the survey reported using alternative health care, and about 73% strongly believed that it was effective.

Predominant Sick-Care Practices: Biomedical; alternative; and magical-religious. Magico-religious practices are most prevalent in areas with high numbers of Amerindians. Modern medicine may be combined or supplanted by traditional practices. Many communities have curanderos, shamans, or brujos who are consulted in cases of illness or misfortune.

Curanderos can be men or women and function primarily as herbalists, using a wide range of plant species to treat an equally wide range of medical conditions. Many rural people maintain small medicinal plant gardens for home treatment of common conditions, and most rural people (and many urban ones) are familiar with the medicinal uses of various plants. Shamans (exclusively men) combine herbal medicine with magico-spiritual beliefs and practices and are consulted for particularly serious cases and for cases in which evil spirits or influences may be involved. Shamans practice what would be considered in Western European culture to be white magic. In contrast, *brujos* ("warlocks") and *brujas* ("witches") practice black magic and are consulted for the purposes of casting harmful spells or curses on perceived enemies. Brujos and brujas are rarely publicly acknowledged and maintain a low profile. Curanderos and shamans are well known and respected. Peru has several systems of health care. Branches of the military and police each have their own independent hospital or clinic system to attend to their employees and their families. The EsSalud hospital system is the social security and insurance health system, with participants (or their employers) making monthly payments into the system. Numerous private hospitals and clinics cater primarily to the middle and upper classes. Most of the population is served by the public health system operated by the Peruvian Ministry of Health; previously a fee-based system. In 2002, a new system of medical care was instituted for Peruvians with no other medical coverage. Participants must register with the public health system, which requires a background check to ensure that they do not have any other health coverage; medications and most procedures are free. Public hospitals are located in larger urban centers, and areas outside these cities have a network of small hospitals (with one or two doctors) or health posts (*puestos de salud*— operated by a doctor or nurse). Most communities have a health promoter (*promotor de salud*), an unpaid member of the community who receives some medical and public health training. The health promoter is responsible for assisting during vaccination campaigns, promoting sanitary practices, and reporting contagious disease outbreaks. Many people, particularly those in rural areas, are reluctant to go to clinics or hospitals when they are ill. Rural people (other than schoolchildren) rarely benefit from any form of health coverage and consequently must pay for consultations and medications. Although cost is one deterrent, clinics and hospitals are difficult to access and often are many hours or even days of travel away from home. Conditions such as epilepsy may be thought of as the result of a curse or actions of evil spirits. Most medications, including antibiotics, are available without a prescription at pharmacies. However, people from the lower economic classes may still find them unaffordable.

Ethnic-/Race-Specific or Endemic Diseases: Malaria and dengue fever are prevalent, and tuberculosis is a major public health problem. Diseases linked to poor hygiene and infections are common and include yellow fever, diphtheria, salmonella, and typhoid fever. Incidence of malaria varies with the terrain and local environment and is higher in the tropical northern coast and lowland Amazon jungle. The prevalence of cholera is greater in rural and jungle areas. Yellow fever is endemic in some areas of rain forest. The indigenous population in rural areas has higher rates of infectious diseases and lack many amenities, such as safe drinking water–(available to the urban population), which partially explains their poorer health. At the end of August 2006, the Peruvian Ministry of Health (MOH) reported an official 26,025 cases of human immunodeficiency virus (HIV) and 18,712 cases of acquired immunodeficiency syndrome (AIDS). Underreporting is a serious problem, however, and as of 2005, the Joint United Nations Programme on HIV/AIDS (UNAIDS) estimated that 93,000 (56,000 to 150,000) Peruvians were living with HIV, including 26,000 women, and that 5,000 (3,400 to 8,500) people had died of AIDS. About 1,200 to 1,500 new cases of AIDS are diagnosed by the MOH each year, 34% of which are women. Between 70% and 75 % of those infected live in Lima. The prevalence of HIV in adults (aged 15 to 49 years) is officially 0.6% but might be higher. The male-to-female ratio is 6:2. About 96% of HIV is acquired via sexual transmission. Since 2004, the program Trata-mientos Antri-Retrovirales de Gran Accion (TARGA) has been providing free antiretroviral treatment to eligible patients.

Health-Team Relationships: Peruvians are conscious of status and title. Most people (other than close friends and family) with an advanced degree or position are addressed by their title or position as a sign of respect and recognition. The term *doctor* is used (with or without the surname) when addressing medical doctors. Likewise, *enfermera* and *technico* are used to address nurses and laboratory technicians. The health care system has a clear hierarchy of responsibility and authority.

Families' Role in Hospital Care: Although larger hospitals provide food, smaller clinics and hospitals might not have this capability, so family members are responsible for providing food for patients. One or more family members will often stay for part of the day, although they may stay all day and night with relatives who have critical or terminal conditions. Families are generally involved in decisions concerning medical procedures, and the extended family may come together to raise money to pay for expensive treatments. Patients and families are generally deferential to medical personnel, and prevention of—or interference with—medical examinations and procedures is rare.

Dominance Patterns: Families are male dominated, although women may play a strong role in maintaining finances and determining activities. Older, more established families are the most likely to have a strong male leader. Young couples often live with the wife's family until they establish a household of their own. Likewise, aging parents generally live with the family of one of their children. Godparents are expected to be involved in important aspects of the lives of godchildren (e.g., higher education, marriage, illness) and are usually friends (or relatives) of the family. Children are given the surnames of their fathers' and mothers' families, with the mothers' surname last. The second surname is often not used in daily life but is given on all documents and used for formal occasions. Women are active in all levels of politics, and even in small, remote communities, they may be elected to positions such as village chief. Women are also becoming more involved in business, education, and medicine, and near parity has been achieved in medical school admissions. Women are poorly represented in the military.

Eye-Contact Practices: Direct eye contact is common within and between sexes and among social classes.

Touch Practices: Men and women typically greet female acquaintances by touching cheeks on one or both sides of the face. Lip contact with the other person's cheek is common but not necessary. Men greet other men with a handshake, and men and women also use a handshake for greeting women with whom they are not familiar. Greetings in a professional relationship generally include a handshake. Amerindians of the Peruvian highlands are generally more reserved in social settings than urban people or Amerindians of the Amazon lowlands. Touching during conversations is common.

Perceptions of Time: Among rural people, time is relative to other events, rather than being a discrete entity. Rural people are very aware of what day it is and what important events occur on which days (thanks to the medium of radio and to the elementary schools that are present in all but the smallest communities), but there is little urgency (or, in most cases, need) to initiate or complete tasks by certain times or dates. Urban people are necessarily more time conscious. Punctuality is expected of employees of lower status but not necessarily for higher-ranking individuals. One measure of social standing or importance of position is how long people will wait for you.

Pain Reactions: Pain may be expressed vocally and through facial expressions; however, rural people, whether adults or children, are often stoic. Often the health care provider may have to ask direct questions about whether a patient has pain. Men seem to be expected to bear pain better than women, and women seem to be more vocal about their pain.

Birth Rites: Births usually occur at home, particularly among the lower classes. The maternal mortality rate in 2001 was 185 per 10,000 live births, whereas in rural areas it may have been more than double. A midwife generally assists the expectant mother, and female relatives may help as well. Fathers are not usually present. Hospital deliveries are increasingly common in urban areas and among the upper classes. In some remote areas, a priest visits only once a year, so he baptizes all the infants born since his last visit and gives a mass for those who have died. In rural areas, parents take little or no time off from their normal schedule after a birth. In urban areas, working women continue to work well into their pregnancies and generally take some time off after delivery. Births of both boys and girls are celebrated. The fertility rate is 2.51 children born per mother; rates are higher in rural areas (i.e., 3.6). Government programs encourage family planning, and in 2000 more than 50% of women of childbearing age reported using modern contraceptive

P

methods. Tubal ligations are common among rural women but are generally performed only after a woman has had five to eight children. Few men obtain vasectomies, and condom use is not widespread except among younger educated people. Respiratory tract and intestinal infectious diseases are the most common causes of death in infants. The infant mortality rate has been decreasing steadily and is 32 deaths per 1,000 live births. There is a large disparity between urban (28 in 1,000) and rural (60 in 1,000) infant mortality. Life expectancy is 68 for men, 72 for women.

Death Rites: Death rites are class dependent. In smaller communities, most community members join the funeral procession and interment rituals. In the highlands and Pacific coastal areas, elaborate tombstones and mausoleums are common, even for relatively poor families. Graves are visited at least annually to place flowers and religious items. In the Amazon lowlands, the dead are buried in simple graves in small cemeteries located away from villages because of fears about ghosts. Graves are marked with a simple wooden cross. Coffins are used in urban areas and are elaborate among the higher social classes. Poor families may rent coffins for processional purposes, and in rural areas, poorer people may simply wrap the body in a blanket or sheet. Burial is usually the day after death, and relatives have a wake, or *vela* ("candle"), the night before the funeral. In urban areas, it is common for poorer families to have a procession with one or two musicians and family members carrying religious images and a collection box. Donations from passersby and area businesses are used to defray funeral expenses. Embalming and cremations are rare and practiced only by some of the upper class. Autopsies and organ donation occur only in larger urban centers.

Food Practices and Intolerances: Rural people usually eat two meals per day, whereas urban people eat three meals daily. Most meals are prepared and eaten at home, although those in the urban middle and upper classes eat out regularly. It is common to use the hands to consume fruit, fish (i.e., to remove bones), and various other food items. Rural people working away from home may take a prepared lunch wrapped in a large leaf, and the meal is typically eaten with the fingers. Washing hands before eating is uncommon for rural people unless their hands are heavily soiled. On the coast, large amounts of fish and seafood are consumed, and various irrigated crops are widely available, including vegetables and grains and starches, such as rice, corn, and potatoes. Processed and "fast" foods are widely available in urban areas. In the mountainous highlands, dietary staples are corn, potatoes (many varieties), and indigenous grains such as *quinoa* and *kiwicha*. Meat protein in the mountains comes in part from *cuy* (guinea pig) and llama. In mountain and coastal regions, domesticated animals (e.g., cattle, pigs, sheep, chickens, turkeys) are also raised, and some dairy industry is active. In the Amazon lowlands, fish is consumed at most meals, and fish allergies are common. Basic starches include *manioc* (yuca) and *platano* (plantains) and some rice and corn. Few vegetables are cultivated or consumed, and almost no dairy products are consumed in other than larger urban areas. Native and introduced fruit trees of many species are commonly planted around homes and villages, and children often consume fruit. A wide variety of wild game is also eaten in the Amazon lowlands, including monkey, peccary (wild pig), deer, paca (a large nocturnal rodent), and wild birds. Chickens, ducks, and pigs are commonly raised in the Amazon, whereas cattle and water buffalo are rare. Indigenous alcoholic beverages are prepared and consumed in all parts of the country. In the coastal area and highlands, the common alcoholic beverage is *chicha*, prepared from fermented germinated corn kernels. In the Amazon lowlands, *masatto* is prepared from cooked and chewed manioc root. *Aguardiente*, or firewater, distilled from sugar cane juice, is widely available in the Pacific and Amazon lowlands. Children in rural areas often drink lightly fermented *chicha* or *masatto*. Alcoholism is a problem among the poorer classes and occurs in rural and urban areas. Smoking of processed or crude tobacco is widespread, but most people do not smoke large quantities daily or on a regular basis. In the highlands, it is common to chew coca leaves for their mild stimulant effects to combat fatigue and the effects of altitude, and use of the coca leaf is not considered drug abuse. In the Amazon lowlands, consumption of the *ayahuasca* hallucinogenic drink (prepared from banisteropsis vines, psychotria leaves, and other plant additives) for medical, magical, and spiritual purposes is likewise an accepted practice. Peru has an increasing problem in larger urban areas with abuse of hard drugs (cocaine, heroine, various designer drugs).

Infant-Feeding Practices: Breastfeeding in public is accepted and common in rural areas, although less so in urban centers. Infant formula is available only in urban areas, and most rural people do not have access to it or cannot afford it. In urban areas, middle-class families often feed their children formula to indicate their superior social status. The period of exclusive breastfeeding is usually short, and supplementation with solids and other foods begins at a relatively young age. In 2004, among infants under 6 months, 64% were exclusively breastfed and 28% were given formula. About 81% of children aged 6 and 9 months received both breastfeeding and solid food, and 43% were formula fed. Obesity in infants or children is considered a sign of health. Chronic malnutrition is prevalent and is attributable to inadequate food intake, poor food preparation, the presence of intestinal parasites, and frequent illnesses.

Child-Rearing Practices: Physical discipline is rare, and children are expected to help with household chores at a young age, particularly in rural areas. By the age of 8 to 10 years, boys assist their fathers with clearing fields, fishing, and care of domestic animals, and girls help with cooking, caring for younger siblings, and other domestic chores. Older sisters routinely care for younger siblings, and all members of extended families (and even entire villages) are involved in child rearing. In the Amazon lowlands, children play in canoes and in the water and learn to swim at a young age. It is common to see toddlers in canoes being paddled around by slightly older siblings. Grandparents typically live with the family of one of their children and help to keep an eye on grandchildren. Upper-class families often hire a nursemaid or nanny. Middle- and upper-class children are generally enrolled in private or parochial schools. Peruvian law dictates that all children attend 6 years of school, but children in rural areas and from poorer families often miss school because no school is nearby or they need to help support the family. Children who are homeless (because either both parents have died or their families are too poor to support them) are found in the larger cities. These children support themselves by begging or doing odd jobs for spare change. Except among the middle and upper classes, children share a single room with their siblings or parents. In rural areas, sleeping arrangements are often a mattress or mat on the floor. In areas with malaria, government programs provide each family with a large mosquito net under which most family members sleep.

National Childhood Immunizations: BCG at birth; DT at 3 and 4 months; DTwP at 3 months; DTwPHibHep at 2 and 4 months; HepB at birth; HIB at 3 months; MMR at 1 year; MR CBAW (16 to 20 years), first contact; OPV at 2, 3, and 4 months; TdCBAW first contact, $+1$, $+6$ months, $+1$, $+2$ years; and YF at 1 year. The percent of the target population vaccinated, by antigen, is: BCG (91%); DTP1 (95%); DTP3, HepB3, and Polio3 (87%); Hib3 (91%); and MCV (89%). Vaccinations for hepatitis B are administered only in areas where it is endemic (e.g., Rio Pastaza, Rio Napo area).

Acknowledgment: We thank Javier Cairo, M.D., for help in updating statistics.

BIBLIOGRAPHY

Background Note: Peru. U.S. Department of State. Bureau of Western Hemisphere Affairs, December 2005. Retrieved January 25, 2006, from http://www.state.gov/r/pa/ei/bgn/35762.htm.

Central Intelligence Agency: *2006: The world factbook, Peru.* Retrieved September 21, 2006, from https://www.cia.gov/cia/publications/factbook/print/pe.html.

Instituto Nacional de Estadística e Informática del Perú: Retrieved January 25, 2006, from http://www.inei.gob.pe/.

Nawaz H, Rahman MA, Graham D, Katz DL, Jekel JF: Health risk behaviors and health perceptions in the Peruvian Amazon, *Am J Trop Med Hyg.* 65(3):252–256, 2001.

UNAIDS: 2004 report on the global AIDS epidemic, July 2004. Retrieved January 26, 2006, from http://www.unaids.org/bangkok2004/report.html.

UNAIDS: 2006 Peru. Retrieved September 21, 2006, from http://www.unaids.org/en/Regions_Countries/Countries/peru.asp.

World Health Organization: 2006: Immunization, vaccines and biologicals. Retrieved September 21, 2006. from http://www.who.int/immunization_monitoring/en/globalsummary/countryprofileresult.cfm?C='per'.

P

◆ PHILIPPINES (REPUBLIC OF THE)

MAP PAGE (805)

Hélène Carabin and (Consultant: Mushfiqur R. Tarafder)

Location: An archipelago 500 miles off the southeast coast of Asia, the Philippines consists of approximately 7107 volcanic islands, of which 880 are inhabited. The total area is 300,000 km² (115,830 square miles). The larger islands—Luzon in the north, Visayas in the central region, and Mindanao in the south—are crossed with mountain ranges. Only about 7% of the islands are larger than 1 square mile. Its boundaries are the Luzon Strait to the north, Philippine Sea to the east, Celebes Sea to the south, Sulu Sea to the southwest, and the South China Sea to the west. Luzon and Mindanao account for 66% of the land area; the capital is Manila. The population is 89.4 million. The gross domestic product (GDP) per capita is $5,100, and 40% live below the poverty line.

Major Languages	Ethnic Groups	Major Religions
Pilipino (i.e., Tagalog, official)	Christian Malay 91%	Roman Catholic 83%
English (official)	Muslim Malay (Moro) 4%	Protestant 9%
Other	Chinese 2%	Muslim Malay (Moro) 4%
	Other (upland tribal) 3%	Buddhist, Other 3%

Eleven languages and 87 dialects are indigenous in the archipelago. Dialects such as Tagalog, Cebuano, Ilocano, Hiligaynon, Bicolano, Waray-Waray, Pampangan, and Pangasian are still the native languages for much of the population. Literacy rates are 93% for both men and women. The Philippines is one of the most disaster-prone areas on earth, with floods, earthquakes, volcanic eruptions, typhoons, tsunamis, and landslides all being significant problems. After centuries of intermarriage, Filipinos have become a blend of Chinese, Malay, Spanish (Mestizos), Negrito, and American. The Roman Catholic Church's influence on the government remains strong.

Health Care Beliefs: Crisis health care; passive role. Mental illness is highly stigmatized and is usually believed to be rooted in witchcraft or demonic possession. For example, people with the "evil eye" can curse another person with their eyes or mouth. If orthodox medical therapies are unsuccessful, illness may be attributed to forces of nature, dwarfs, spells, sins, or past misdeeds.

Predominant Sick-Care Practices: Biomedical; magical-religious; and traditional. Both modern medicine and traditional systems are used. People in urban areas rely on professional providers, whereas the traditional magico-religious system (most common in remote areas) relies on home remedies and is based on taboos set by supernatural forces. A sense of fatalism stems from beliefs that ghosts and spirits control life and death. Usurping the powers of the gods is believed to have a cause-and-effect relationship to subsequent misfortunes. Many individuals alternate between the two systems, using a combination of home remedies, professional providers, and traditional healers. Poverty has made mainstream health care unaffordable for most people, and mainstream health care is used as a last resort. Alternative therapies—herbal, unapproved medications, consultation with an *albularyo* or a *hilot* (village healer), faith healing, and prayer—are the norm outside major cities. *Albylaryos,* or medicos, lack formal education and are the primary dispensers of health care. *Hilots* are midwives and chiropractic and massage practitioners. It is believed that individuals born by breech delivery are destined to become hilots. Because fees are thought to decrease their powers, albylaryos and hilots are paid with goods or services. The health care system is considered adequate in urban and minimal in rural areas. Improvements in public- and private-sector health programs are attempting to fill in the gaps in health care delivery. Some employees receive medical and dental benefits from their employers. Private insurance is available for those who can afford it, and many people choose private-pay systems. Some government-sponsored hospitals charge minimal fees, and public assistance programs are a safety net for the poor.

Ethnic-/Race-Specific or Endemic Diseases: Chloroquine-sensitive and chloroquine-resistant malaria and tuberculosis are still considered endemic in some rural areas. Vitamin A deficiency is a common cause of childhood blindness, and there are dengue hemorrhagic fever outbreaks every few years. Schistosomiasis, an infectious disease transmitted by amphibious snails, is endemic in the regions of the Visayas and Mindanao and is thought to be reemerging in areas of northern Luzon. Infectious diseases continue to be the leading cause of morbidity and mortality. The top four leading causes of morbidity are pneumonia, diarrhea, bronchitis or bronchiolitis, and influenza; tuberculosis is the sixth leading cause and measles the 10th. Other significant infectious diseases include chickenpox, typhoid, and paratyphoid fever. Significant noninfectious disease morbidity is attributed to hypertension and heart disease. The leading causes of mortality, in descending order, are heart disease, vascular system diseases, cancer, pneumonia, accidents, cancer, tuberculosis (all forms), chronic obstructive pulmonary disease, congenital malformations, diabetes mellitus, and nephritis and nephritic syndrome. The Joint United Nations Programme on HIV/AIDS (UNAIDS) reports the estimated prevalence rate of human immunodeficiency virus (HIV) in adults (aged 15 to 49 years) is less than 0.1%, with 12,000 people living with HIV, including 3,400 women and 100 children aged 0 to 15 years. Most infections are transmitted heterosexually. An active sex industry and a considerable population of intravenous drug users have prompted a national prevention and control program for HIV and other sexually transmitted diseases.

Health-Team Relationships: Respect for authority and the belief that a professional's time is valuable dictate that a health problem must be serious or it is not mentioned. Nurses do not question a doctor's order. Rather than give a "no" answer to a question, patients may remain silent or respond with a hesitant "yes." An intermediary may be used for confrontational situations. Nurses and doctors have migrated to the United States for training and work experience, and many have become permanent residents. At last count, the Philippines had approximately 739,000 health professionals, including 95,000 doctors. About 1,700 hospitals with 85,000 beds are concentrated in urban areas.

Families' Role in Hospital Care: Loyalty is a social imperative, so children generally feel an obligation to parents who are ill. Because loyalty to the extended family comes first, often several members of the family help each other care for loved ones. Because of the close family bonds, care is also traditionally provided for more distant extended family members as well. People cling to traditional values, particularly in rural areas. The family is central to Filipinos' identity, and kinship ties are central to friendships and relationships.

Dominance Patterns: The interests of the family are considered before individual needs. The oldest child is educated through the family's efforts; therefore, that child is expected to continue to "sacrifice" for the next sibling and so on. Protection against outsiders, dependency, harmony, and reciprocity of obligation are group values. Women in the Philippines have always enjoyed greater equality with men than in most other parts of Southeast Asia, with unquestioned rights to legal equality and inheritance. It is common for women to be appointed to important positions in business and government, although most such positions continue to be held by men. Women traditionally control the family finances and yet are generally submissive and have tolerated a double standard of sexual conduct. In rural areas, wives usually stay at home to take care of the children. When the children are grown, the wife then helps the husband earn their livelihood.

Eye-Contact Practices: Some fear eye contact; however, if it is established, it is important to return and maintain it.

Touch Practices: Touch is considered a friendly gesture, especially between friends of the same sex. It is not unusual to see girls walking together arm in arm. In some parts of the country, it is believed that an "evil eye" curse that has been placed on a child can be neutralized by putting a bit of saliva on the finger and making the sign of the cross on the child's forehead while giving a compliment.

Perceptions of Time: Filipinos have a relaxed sense of time. Time generally moves ahead slowly, and they have the attitude that "We'll get there when we get there." Being an hour late for appointments is considered perfectly acceptable. Life is lived from day to day.

Pain Reactions: Pain is endured for as long as possible. High thresholds of pain are expected, especially if a cure is financially out of reach. People also may seem stoic if they believe pain is the will of God and that God will give them the strength to bear it.

Birth Rites: Filipino women are modest. They often delay or neglect receiving prenatal care and Pap tests to avoid being examined by male doctors. Millions of poor women have little or no access to adequate family planning or reproductive health care. About 20 million women are in their childbearing years, and their greatest health risks are related to pregnancy and childbirth. Department of Health studies indicate that more Filipino mothers die from pregnancy and childbirth than from any other cause because of hemorrhaging, hypertension, and abortive outcomes. The fertility rate is 3.5 children born per woman. USAID is targeting poor Filipinas to reduce birth rates. It is believed daily bathing and shampooing during pregnancy results in a clean baby and that sexual intercourse may harm the woman and the infant. In the past, women were encouraged to stay in bed for a week or longer after birth, and bathing or showering were prohibited. These practices are now obsolete, and restricted activities are now the norm. In rural areas, new mothers take a special bath with warm water and herbal leaves at some point after birth. After the bath, regardless of the room temperature, the new mother wears warm clothing and keeps covered with blankets if necessary to keep warm. The infant mortality rate is 23 deaths per 1,000 live births. Life expectancy is 67 for men, 73 for women.

Death Rites: Frequently, patients are not told about a poor prognosis because relatives prefer not to add to the person's suffering. Family members who die are kept for 1 week in the family home. Religious ceremonies are held nightly, and family and friends have a feast on the ninth day after the burial. The Organ Donation Act of 1991 promotes transplantation of organs.

Food Practices and Intolerances: Rice is the staple food. Preferred foods are a mixture of fish, vegetables, and native fruits. Malnutrition is a continuing problem. In a recent report from the World Health Organization, 31%, 31%, and 6% of children under age 5 were underweight, stunted, and wasted, respectively. Targeted food assistance for preschoolers and lactating mothers has improved these numbers. In the late 1980s, consumption of milk tripled, and fats and oils nearly doubled, which are believed to be contributing to increases in cardiovascular diseases.

Infant-Feeding Practices: Breastfeeding is common until 2 years of age, although the percentage of breastfed babies has decreased. Infants are usually fed on demand if the mother is not working outside the home, and scheduled feedings are unusual. Even breastfed infants begin receiving solid foods such as mashed cooked rice and fruits such as bananas when they have teeth, or as young as 4 months.

Child-Rearing Practices: Infants are not usually separated from their mothers, and until they are toddlers they sleep with their parents in cribs in the parents' room. Disposable diapers are used by those who can afford them; washable diapers are usually used for the first year. Infants are toilet trained at a young age without diapers, and they learn quickly not to urinate on themselves. Children stay with parents until they are married, regardless of their age. Parents have the responsibility to send their children to school, and older children are obligated to help their parents or younger siblings.

National Childhood Immunizations: BCG at birth; DTwP at 6, 10, and 14 weeks; OPV at 6, 10, and 14 weeks; Hep B at 6, 10, and 14 weeks; measles at 9 months; vitamin A at 6, 12, 18, 24, 30, and 36 months; and TT at first contact during pregnancy, +4 weeks, +6 months, +1, +1 year. The percent of the target population vaccinated, by antigen, is: BCG (91%); DTP1 (90%); DTP3 (79%); HepB3 (44%); MCV and Polio3 (80%); TT2 plus (46%); and vitamin A (88%).

Other Characteristics: Filipinos are hospitable and tend to value shared, rather than private, possessions or property. A bond between two people may be formed on the basis of *utang na loob*, a predominantly rural concept. For example, it is assumed that when a gift is given, it will be repaid; some debts (such as obligations to parents) can never be fully repaid, so the obligation lasts for generations. Gifts may result in long-term dependencies in which the giver and the debtor feel free to request other favors over time.

BIBLIOGRAPHY

Central Intelligence Agency: *2006: The world factbook, Philippines.* Retrieved September 21, 2006, from https://www.cia.gov/cia/publications/factbook/print/rp.html.

Department of Health Republic of the Philippines: Field Health Services Information System (FHSIS) updates, 2002. Retrieved on March 13, 2006, from http://www.doh.gov.ph/data_stat/html/healthstatus.htm.

Department of Health Republic of the Philippines: Health statistics. Retrieved on March 13, 2006, from http://www.doh.gov.ph/data_stat/html.

Department of Health Republic of the Philippines: Ten leading causes of mortality by sex, 2002. Retrieved on March 10, 2006, from http://www.doh.gov.ph/data_stat/html/mortality.htm.

Republic of the Philippines National Statistics Office: The Philippines in figures, 2005. Retrieved March 10, 2006, from http://www.census.gov.ph/data/publications/PIF2005.pdf.

UNAIDS: 2006 Philippines. Retrieved September 21, 2006, from http://www.unaids.org/en/Regions_Countries/Countries/philippines.asp.

United Nations Development Program: Human development reports—Philippines. Retrieved March 10, 2006, from http://hdr.undp.org/statistics/data/countries.cfm?c=PHL.

World Health Organization: 2006: Immunization, vaccines and biologicals. Retrieved September 21, 2006, from http://www.who.int/immunization_monitoring/en/globalsummary/countryprofileresult.cfm?C='phl'.

World Health Organization Regional Office for the Western Pacific: Malaria annual data, 2003. Retrieved March 10, 2006, from http://www.wpro.who.int/sites/mvp/data/malaria/mal_2003.htm.

P

◆ POLAND (REPUBLIC OF)

MAP PAGE (798)

Pawel Stefanoff

Location: Poland is a north-central European country with an opening to the Baltic Sea. Most of the country consists of broad plains, except for the Carpathian and Sudetan Mountains in the south and uplands, mostly in the southeast. Poland borders Russia, Lithuania, Belarus, and Ukraine on the east; Slovakia and the Czech Republic on the south, and Germany on the west. The total area is 322,577 km^2 (124,547 square miles), and the capital is Warsaw. The population is 38.5 million. The gross domestic product (GDP) per capita is $13,300, with 17% living below the poverty line. Literacy is almost 100% for both men and women.

Major Languages	Ethnic Groups	Major Religions
Polish	Polish 97%	Roman Catholic 90%
	German, Ukrainian,	Russian Orthodox,
	Belarussian 2%	Protestant, Other 10%
	Other 1%	

Poland also has smaller numbers of Lithuanians, Jews, and Gypsies (Roma).

Health Care Beliefs: Active role; prevention important. Most Poles believe health is the most important human value; therefore, an increasing number of people are taking care of their own health by such steps as daily physical exercise, low-fat diets, and more involvement in sports during holidays. Healthy living is promoted by the mass media. The quality of care for people with mental disorders has improved, and people with less serious mental impairments are being integrated into the workforce. Society's level of knowledge about health and disease has increased. In addition, there is a greater interest in the benefits of alternative medical practices, primarily in more affluent groups who can afford these treatments.

Predominant Sick-Care Practices: Primarily biomedical with some traditional. Poland has a public health care system with free basic and specialist care for everyone. Despite free and unlimited access to public health care, about 25% of the population use private health care services. Alternative medicine in the form of bioenergy and herbal therapies, acupressure, and massage are popular. According to surveys, most of the people (95%) who consult folk medicine practitioners say they simultaneously consult practitioners in the public health care system. Wearing amulets to prevent illness is no longer common practice, whereas praying for better health is typical because most Poles are Christians.

Ethnic-/Race-Specific or Endemic Diseases: The highest mortality rates are from diseases of the circulatory system and cancer. Endemic

P

diseases specific for Poland include tick-borne encephalitis in the northeast and south, toxoplasmosis primarily in the eastern part of the country, and *Trichinella* infections in wild boars, transferred to humans when hunters consume the meat. Hepatitis A is classified as a low-endemic disease, but countries neighboring Poland to the east have high endemicity and constitute a potential risk as sources of imported outbreaks. Some vaccine-preventable diseases—such as mumps, rubella, varicella. and meningococcal disease (predominantly type B)—are still not well controlled and occur among children. Measles is almost eradicated (cases mostly among immigrants from the east). There is a decreasing trend in tuberculosis incidence, from 16,653 cases in 1994 (43 per 100,000) to 9,493 cases in 2004 (25 per 100,000). The highest incidence is in the over 65 age group. The most prevalent is the pulmonary form of tuberculosis, diagnosed in more than 90% of reported cases. Poland has a more severe epidemic of human immunodeficiency virus (HIV) than many other central European countries, driven by injecting drug users. Among HIV cases with a known route of transmission, about 82% are infected through injecting drug use. The Joint United Nations Programme on HIV/AIDS (UNAIDS) estimates the prevalence rate of HIV in adults (aged 15 to 49 years) to be 0.1%, and 25,000 people are living with HIV, including 7,500 women. Fewer than 1,000 deaths are attributed to acquired immunodeficiency syndrome (AIDS).

Health-Team Relationships: Doctors are dominant in the health care system. In some situations, the dominance takes the form of autocratic, superior-subordinate relationships, but in others, the dominance of doctors is considered natural by nurses because of doctors' superior knowledge and level of responsibility. However, nurses are not submissive; they foster the partnership relationships necessary for care of patients. Patient-doctor interactions tend to be more formal, whereas patient-nurse relationships are more informal, natural, and unceremonious.

Families' Role in Hospital Care: Polish hospitals have removed strict visitation rules. In many hospitals, families are allowed to visit their relatives just after the morning doctors' rounds, and visits in the afternoon are now common. The meals served in hospitals are usually sufficient, but families may bring snacks, mineral water, and juice.

Dominance Patterns: The matter of who dominates male-female relationships involves Polish history and tradition. For ages, women have played an important role in the family life of Poles, and men have respected their role. Men, on the other hand, provided for the entire family and played an important role in professional, scientific, and political life. These relationships began to change in the second half of the nineteenth century, when women began to claim their rights to study and to work. The twentieth century was the time of women's emancipation as women increased their active participation in professional and political life. Today many women have important, even dominant, roles. Men and women are generally considered partners and tend to cooperate.

Eye-Contact Practices: Most people avoid extended periods of direct eye contact when standing close to someone. Male-female eye contact follows the pattern of most Western societies, where direct eye contact usually means attentiveness, interest, and attention.

Touch Practices: Touch is socially acceptable within limits of propriety and depends on age and gender, the range and character of the relationship, and the situation in which it occurs. Touching between members of the same sex is generally more socially acceptable than it is between members of the opposite sex. Doctors and nurses have historically used touch to communicate empathy. Shaking hands is common during greetings and during Roman Catholic religious services.

Perceptions of Time: People consider punctuality to be important, although the importance varies with the location. Rural people tend to be more relaxed about time, whereas people living in large cities who have professional jobs are more bound to strict time schedules. Tradition is valued, which is reflected in preserved cultural objects, historical buildings, and other monuments of national identity. A distinctive characteristic of Poles is their hospitality and enjoyment of traditional celebrations, especially religious feasts such as Christmas and Easter. Differences in orientation to the present, future, or past reflect a person's age and life experience. Young people primarily live in the present and future. Older adults, as is true in most cultures, tend to focus on past memories because thoughts of the future may conjure images of loss of independence and death.

Pain Reactions: Poles usually have high levels of pain tolerance, and differences can be attributed to gender, educational level, and past and current experiences of pain (i.e., frequency, duration, cause, intensity). Pain is assessed by evaluating facial expressions, body position, and movement. Poles usually use modern medicine for pain relief, and all citizens, regardless of their formal rights, are entitled to pain relief.

Birth Rites: Most children are born in hospitals, and fathers are often present in the delivery rooms. Perinatal care has greatly improved in recent years. Infant mortality has decreased from 19 per 1,000 live births in 1990 to 7 in 2006. In most Polish families, the birth of a child evolves into a family festivity involving visits to the newborn and gifts. Mothers avoid certain foods when they are breastfeeding (e.g., beans, peas, cabbage) but consume vegetable and fruit juices in the postpartum period. Boys and girls are equally valued, although fathers are especially happy when a son is born. The fertility rate is 1.25 children born per woman. Because most Poles are Roman Catholic, the baptism ceremony is an important event. Life expectancy is 71 for men, 80 for women.

Death Rites: The traditions in many regions of Poland determine patterns of behavior for those who are dying and those who are providing companionships for the dying. Those who are dying must be reconciled with their enemies and God. They bid farewell to friends and family members, reveal inheritances, and fulfill life obligations. Until recently, most people died at home, but today most die in hospitals because Poles are more concerned about prolonging life whenever possible. A "good death" is thought to be a painless death that occurs during sleep or suddenly at an older age and one that does not involve equipment artificially sustaining life. Those in the process of dying are in the presence of their family and friends. Most people support the transplantation of human organs from cadavers. Bodies are buried in the ground, usually according to the rites of Roman Catholicism. Cremation is possible in a few cemeteries and is becoming increasingly popular.

Food Practices and Intolerances: Poles consume large amounts of animal fats and sugars, although recent trends show this is decreasing. There is a tendency to consume more vegetables, but consumption of fruits, milk, and milk products remains low, and Poles tend to prefer white flour products. Eating habits include irregular meal schedules, no breakfast, heavy dinners, and hasty meal consumption. Typical foods include potatoes, soups, sauerkraut stew, sausage, and *piernik* (cake with honey). Poles are fond of spices such as horseradish, garlic, and mushrooms. About 90% of meals are eaten at home. During the last decade, eating outside the home has become increasingly popular.

Infant-Feeding Practices: In the 1960s and 1970s, bottle-fed infants were the norm, but during the 1990s breastfeeding was actively promoted. About 50% of women breastfeed their children for 6 weeks, and most continue for 14 weeks. Better educated and rural women are more likely to breastfeed and to do so for longer periods. Breastfeeding is a commonly accepted and socially expected behavior as evidenced by the associations for the support of breastfeeding and the national promotion programs.

Child-Rearing Practices: Various birth planning methods are used; abortion is allowed only in exceptional situations. Children are usually brought up in nuclear families in which decisions about upbringing are made by both parents. In multigeneration families, the grandmother plays an important role in caring for the children. Crèche, nursery school, and others are popular, and parents rely on these places for their children to learn negotiation, proper behaviors, and necessary educational tasks. Upbringing and education of children and youth are considerably influenced by the mass media, primarily television and the Internet.

National Childhood Immunizations: BCG at birth; DTPw at 6 to 8 weeks, 3 to 4, 5, and 16 to 18 months; DTPa at 6 years; and Td at 14 and 19 years; IPV at 3 to 4, 5, and 16 to 18 months; OPV at 6 years; HepB at birth and at 2 and 6 to 7 months; MMR at 13 to 14 months and 12 years; Hib at 2, 4, and 12 to 15 months (free only for high-risk groups). The percent of the target population vaccinated, by antigen, is: BCG (94%); DTP1, DTP3, and Polio3 (99%); HepB3 and MCV (98%).

P

BIBLIOGRAPHY

Central Intelligence Agency: *2006: The world factbook, Poland.* Retrieved September 21, 2006, from https://www.cia.gov/cia/publications/factbook/print/pl.html.

Central Statistical Office: *Demographic yearbook of Poland,* 2005, Warsaw, 2005, Central Statistical Office.

Central Statistical Office: *Healthcare in households in 2003.* Warsaw, 2004, Central Statistical Office.

Central Statistical Office: *Health of Poland's population in 2004.* Warsaw, 2005, Central Statistical Office.

Kaweczynska-Butrym Z: *Family-health-disease: concepts and practice of family nursing,* 1st ed. Lublin, 2001, Czelej.

National Institute of Hygiene and Chief Sanitary Inspectorate: Infectious diseases and poisonings in Poland in 2004. Official annual bulletin published by National Institute of Hygiene and Chief Sanitary Inspectorate, Warsaw, Poland, 2005. Retrieved April 10, 2006, from http://www.pzh.gov.pl/epimeld/index_a.html#04.

UNAIDS: 2006 Poland. Retrieved September 21, 2006, from http://www.unaids.org/en/Regions_Countries/Countries/poland.asp.

World Health Organization: 2006: Immunization, vaccines and biologicals. Retrieved September 21, 2006, from http://www.who.int/immunization_monitoring/en/globalsummary/countryprofileresult.cfm?C='pol'.

◆ PORTUGAL (PORTUGUESE REPUBLIC)

MAP PAGE (798)

Félix Neto, Ana Veríssimo Ferreira, and Maria da Conceição Pinio

Location: Portugal is located in the southwestern part of Europe in the Iberian Peninsula and has a total area of 90,000 km^2 (34,749 square miles). The capital is Lisbon. It is mountainous in the north and flat in the south and is crossed by three major rivers that originate in Spain. Portugal also has two small archipelagos of volcanic origin: the Azores and Madeira. The winters are usually cold and wet, the summers hot and dry. The population is 10.5 million. The population is getting older, with 1.7 million pensioners. The gross domestic product (GDP) per capita is $19,300, and 19% are living below the poverty level. Literacy rates are 96% for men, 91% for women.

Major Language	Ethnic Groups	Major Religions

Portuguese	Hetergeneous:
	Mediterranean stock on
	    mainland and in Azores
	On the Madeira Islands;
	    also African ($\leq$100,000)
	    Indians, Eastern
	    Europeans, and Chinese
		Roman Catholic 96%
		Protestant 1%
		Other 3%

For decades, Portugal has been a country of emigration. Gypsy (Roma) communities, although in small numbers, have long been a presence in Portuguese society. The presence of ethnic minorities has increased in recent years, with immigrants from Africa, Brazil, India, East European countries, and China. Portugal has been a democracy since 1974 and a member of the European Union since 1985. Portugal cooperates with all African countries where Portuguese is the official tongue (CPLP), and since 2000 it has cooperated with the most recent country of the world, Timor Leste, through education, agriculture, and basic sanitation because Timor Leste's official tongue is Portuguese. Portugal has experienced a major decrease in religious practices, particularly in the cities, although there are many Roman Catholic churches as well as Hindu, Muslim, and Jewish temples.

Health Care Beliefs: Traditional and Western; active role. In rural areas, people use a significant amount of tradition-based medicine. It is common for older people to use homemade infusions and syrups in addition to biomedical care. The use of alternative medicines and natural treatments is increasing. Many ill people choose to have treatment from an *endireita*, a type of faith healer (without formal training) because they believe these people have special powers. Many believe in divine intervention for the cure of disease. Faith in healing by Our Lady of Fátima is strong; promises are made to go to Fátima on foot and light candles to the saint. Religion-based limitations on health care are rare. Most Portuguese seek health care at health centers and hospitals.

Predominant Sick-Care Practices: Biomedical. Most people have a compulsory health card which verifies that they can access treatment. Health care is free for children younger than 13 and for retired people. Others pay a fee for consultations (2€ in the health centers and 7€ for emergency service in hospitals). Foreign citizens living legally in Portugal may access health care and medicine. Problems related to health tend to aggravate socioeconomic situations, enhancing poverty and social exclusion. The numbers of handicapped people have been increasing. The concept of individualism is growing, which tends to exclude those in the society not socially, culturally, or economically fortunate. Therefore, mental illness is increasing and is frequently stigmatized. Drug addiction appears to be a major problem in incarcerated individuals (65% are or were addicted). The least favored populations live in social situations that facilitate isolation rather than social and cultural integration. Poverty, unemployment, immigration, conflicts, violence (particularly in cities), lack of shelter and social supports, drug abuse, and the lack of social networks are major factors for stress, mental illness, and subsequent poor health. Attention is being given to the youth of the country, particularly in the area of sexuality, through programs of counseling and guidance.

Ethnic-/Race-Specific or Endemic Diseases: Cardiovascular diseases are responsible for about 40% of all deaths. Lifestyle factors such as minimal daily physical activity, time pressures and stress, unbalanced eating habits, cigarette smoking, and negative sociocultural factors are strong predictors of cardiovascular risk. Diabetes is a growing problem; between 400,000 and 500,000 diabetics live in Portugal. Rheumatic illnesses are frequent, which appears to be related to lifestyle issues as well as to the increasing longevity of the population. Major causes of death result from illnesses of the circulatory system (38%) and malignant tumors (21%). Tuberculosis is one of the most frequent infectious diseases. Treatment is free, but the course of treatment requires long-term adherence. Portugal has a relatively low incidence of human immunodeficiency virus (HIV) and acquired immunodeficiency syndrome (AIDS). The Joint United Nations Programme on HIV/AIDS (UNAIDS) estimates the prevalence rate for HIV in adults (aged 15 to 49 years) to be 0.4%; 32,000 people are living with HIV, including 1,300 women and 500 children aged 0 to 15 years. Fewer than 1,000 deaths from AIDS have been reported. Considerable stigma is associated with having HIV. Reporting is obligatory as of 2005. Antiretroviral therapy has been free since 1987 and is distributed by hospitals.

Health-Team Relationships: Nurses and medical doctors work together in a hierarchical relationship; doctors are dominant. Doctors and nurses have separate tasks, with doctors responsible for treating patients and nurses providing daily caring functions. Formally, the relationships are good, and communication tends to be cooperative. Patients tend to communicate more freely with nurses. Trends in nursing education have progressed toward higher educational standards and increased specialization.

Families' Role in Hospital Care: Involvement of the family is limited, although the family's role is expanding to include participation in decision making and provision of care, particularly in the specialties of oncology and pediatrics. When patients are admitted, most hospitals allow a family member to remain for the day to help with meals and comfort measures. Families and visitors also bring flowers, food (cakes, fruit, water, and juices) and night clothes. Hospitalized children receive assistance from educators and school support services, especially when they are hospitalized for long periods.

Dominance Patterns: The family structure is patriarchal; however, a movement toward more equal gender roles is taking place and is influencing young couples, particularly in major cities. The mother is traditionally in charge of running the household and deciding when health care practitioners should be consulted. Deference is given to older adults, parents, and grandparents, especially in more traditional areas of the country.

Eye-Contact Practices: Direct eye contact is an important part of communication. It is generally believed that looking others directly in the eyes is a sign of honesty. *Piscar de olhos,* or eye blinking, is considered a seduction strategy.

Touch Practices: The Portuguese consider touch to be socially acceptable. In health care, touch is frequently used as a form of nonverbal communication, especially to reassure patients. Shaking hands is common between both men and women. Women may greet each other with a kiss on the cheek, as may men and women who are friends. Friends may give each other two light slaps on the back at the time of the handshake.

Perceptions of Time: The Portuguese tend to live in the present, but they consider past traditions and habits to be important as well.

Pain Reactions: Except in small rural areas, public expressions of pain are unusual.

Birth Rites: The fertility rate is 1.47 children born per woman. Most births (98%) occur in hospitals with doctors in attendance. In rural areas, midwives still have a major role in delivering babies. Portugal has no established, organized system of medical and nursing support for home birth. Birth control is used by most of the population. There is great pressure to teach sex education in schools as a prevention strategy for sexually transmitted diseases and also to reduce the number of adolescent mothers. Since 2000, fewer children have been born as a result of lower fertility rates, older marriages, and older ages of parents. At the same time, the number of children born outside marriages is increasing (31,766 in 2004), about 80% to parents who live together. Portugal has the second highest rate of adolescent mothers in Western Europe. Portugal has a very restrictive abortion law, and abortion is permitted only if the pregnancy causes a risk of death for the mother, in cases of fetal malformation, or when pregnancy results from rape. It is estimated that about 20,000 illegal abortions occur yearly. Because of complications of these abortions, 5,000 women are admitted to hospitals each year and about 100 women have died over the past 20 years. The "day after" pill is used mostly by adolescents and by adult women who want to prevent pregnancy. The infant mortality rate is 5 deaths per 1,000 live births. Life expectancy is 74 for men, 81 for women.

Death Rites: Widows are expected to remain unmarried for at least 1 year and to wear black clothing for the rest of their lives unless they marry again. Bodies are buried. Cremation is not accepted by the general population and is uncommon. Most people have a Roman Catholic funeral, with a mass and funeral procession. Organ donation is not done, and euthanasia is not authorized.

Food Practices and Intolerances: Most Portuguese have a Mediterranean diet that is high in fish, vegetables, fruit, and olive oil. Fast food is becoming more common in major cities and among young people. Consumption of alcohol is higher in rural areas and is increasing among young people in the major cities. In the last few years, red wine, which is believed to have cardiovascular benefits, has been largely replaced by beer and imported spirits. The cuisine of Portugal is varied in all regions of the mainland and on the islands. One of the most typical dishes is Cozido à Portuguesa, which is made with several kinds of meat boiled with vegetables. Obesity is increasing, both in adults and children; however, the number of vegetarians is also increasing, especially among young and ill people.

588   *Portugal (Portuguese Republic)*

Infant-Feeding Practices: Most infants are breastfed during the first 3 months after birth. At around month 4, mothers progressively introduce soup, meat, and vegetables and then add fish at about 8 months. Between 1 and 2 years, all foods are introduced.

Child-Rearing Practices: Children are expected to respect and obey their parents and older adults, and the older adults often help with child rearing. Families are usually more protective of girls.

National Childhood Immunizations: BCG at birth; DTwP at 5 to 6 years; DTwPHib at 2, 4, 6, and 18 months; OPV at 2, 4, and 6 months and at 5 to 6 years; HepB at birth and at 2 and 6 months; IPV at 2, 4, and 6 months and at 5 to 6 years; MMR at 15 months and at 5 to 6 years; Td at 10 to 13 years. The percent of the target population vaccinated, by antigen, is: BCG (89%); DTP1 and HepB3 (94%); and DTP3, Hib3, MCV, and Polio3 (93%). Vaccines for meningitis and hepatitis are free. Technicians from The Ministry of Health regularly visit schools for verification and compulsory updating of vaccines.

Other Characteristics: Tourism is important to Portugal, with its good weather, social activities, restaurants, bars, and dancing clubs, which are open late at night in every town in the country. *Fado* is the typical music of Lisbon, which "comes from the Portuguese soul," a genuine part of Portuguese culture. Themes such as love-hatred, solitude, and *saudade* (the feeling of missing someone, a word that exists only in the Portuguese language) are the essence of Fado. Because it is unique, it is always a surprise for tourists visiting Lisbon. New generations of Fado singers have taken this art form all over the world.

BIBLIOGRAPHY

Destaque—Informações à comunicação social: Estatísticas demográficas 2004. INE. Retrieved February 9, 2006, from http://www.ine.pt.

Dia Mundial da Sida: Estatísticas de saúde 2004/2010. Vol I. Prioridades; Vol II, Orientações Estratégicas. Retrieved February 9, 2006, from http://www.dgsaude.min-edu.pt/pms/.

IDT: Relatório Anual 2004: a situação do país em matéria de drogas e toxicodependências, Vol I. Retrieved January 20, 2006, from http://www.drogas.pt.

INE: As pessoas/The people. Análise/analysis. *Anuário Estatístico de Portugal/statistical yearbook of Portugal.* Retrieved February 9, 2006, from http://www.ine.pt.

Neto F: *Psicologia intercultural.* Lisboa, 2002, Universidade Aberta.

Portal da Saúde: Programa Nacional de Vacinação em vigor desde 1 de Janeiro de 2006. Retrieved February 18, 2006, from http://www.portaldasaude.pt.

UNAIDS: 2006 Portugal: Retrieved September 21, 2006, from http://www.unaids.org/en/Regions_Countries/Countries/portugal.asp.

World Health Organization: Portugal. Retrieved February 26, 2006, from http://www.who.int/countries/port/_en/index.html.

World Health Organization: 2006: Immunization, vaccines and biologicals. Retrieved September 21, 2006, from http://www.who.int/immunization_monitoring/en/globalsummary/countryprofileresult.cfm?C='prt'.

◆ QATAR (STATE OF)

MAP PAGE (802)

Nigel John Shanks

Location: Qatar is situated halfway along the west coast of the Arabian Gulf. Together with numerous islands and reefs, the country covers a total area of 11,437 km^2 (4416 square miles), with 700 km of coastline. The population is 8.8 million. The topography consists of flat, rocky surfaces at or below sea level. The Jebel Dukhan in the west has some spectacular limestone outcrops and sand dunes that reach a height of 60 m near the inland sea. Qatar has a moderate desert climate with long, hot, humid summers and short, mild winters with some rainfall. The sovereign state of Qatar became independent in 1971 and is one of the Gulf Cooperative Council (GCC) states along with Saudi Arabia, Kuwait, Oman, the United Arab Emirates, and Bahrain. The gross domestic product (GDP) per capita is $27,400. Literacy rates are 89% for both men and women.

Major Languages	Ethnic Groups	Major Religions
Arabic (official)	Arab 40%	Sunni Muslim 95%
English	Pakistani 18%	Other 5%
Hindi	East Indian 18%	
Urdu	Iranian 10%	
	Other 14%	

The people of Qatar are the descendents of ancient Arabians. Qataris have strong historical and family ties to the other Gulf Arab states because of the migratory nature and freedom of movement of the Bedouin tribes. Qatar also has families of Persian origin. Most (60%) of the inhabitants live in the capital of Doha, but large numbers also live in the towns and villages of Wakrah, Dukhan, Umm Said, Al Khor, and Madinat Shamal. The population distribution is 88% urban and 12% rural, and 25% of the population is Qatari. The remainder are foreign nationals with residency status; the vast majority are Arab, Pakistani, Indian, and Iranian. All official documents must be completed in Arabic, but English is widely spoken, particularly in business and health care arenas. Qatar is an Islamic state, and most have orthodox beliefs. Islamic law *(Shari'a)* is the main form of legislation.

Health Care Beliefs: Active role; Western and traditional. Belief in traditional or Koranic healing practices persists, usually in conjunction with conventional medicine. Traditional practices range from the recitation of healing verses from the Koran, to anointing patients with special oils, to cauterizing certain body parts (thus many older Qataris have cautery scars). The traditional approach is dying out. Recently, numerous complementary medical clinics (e.g., chiropractic, massage, reflexology) have been established.

Predominant Sick-Care Practices: Biomedical; alternative; and religious. Health care is available to residents and visitors at government health centers. For a small fee (100QR, about U.S.$27), residents can purchase an annually renewable health card and register at the nearest primary health care center. Treatment and prescriptions are heavily subsidized. Provision of all health care is under the auspices of the newly formed National Health Authority, charged with providing specialty health services, establishing and organizing hospitals and health centers, and declaring quarantines. The Hamad Medical Corporation is the main provider for government hospitals. The Hamad Hospital, the main hospital in Doha, offers a full range of medical specialties. In addition to government hospitals, Qatar has private hospitals and clinics. Qatar Petroleum, the state oil and gas company, and its subsidiaries are also mandated to provide primary health care for their employees and dependants. The vast majority of health care services are in the public health care system.

Ethnic-/Race-Specific or Endemic Diseases: Infectious diseases are less of a concern primarily because of extensive immunization programs. Obesity and diabetes mellitus are becoming more common, as are hypertension and heart disease. The traditional diet of rice, fish, and small amounts of red meat has changed to one that is higher in animal fat and sugar because of the advent of a plethora of Western fast-food outlets and importation of preserved foods. Asthma is common. Injuries from automobile accidents are a major problem; seat belt legislation was introduced in February 2002. Non-Qatari residents are required to be screened and test negative for hepatitis (B and C), tuberculosis, and HIV infection before obtaining full residency status. Qatar has a limited amount of natural fresh water, so people are becoming more dependent on desalination facilities. There is limited information on the human immunodeficiency virus/acquired immunodeficiency syndrome (HIV/AIDS) and sexually transmitted diseases. The Annual Health Report 2005 estimates the prevalence rate for HIV/AIDS is 0.0018%.

Health-Team Relationships: Relationships among different health care professionals tend to be collaborative. The roles of doctors and nurses are clearly defined in hospitals. The health team has a true hierarchy, with the doctor at the top and the nurse at the bottom. The nurse is not allowed to do anything unless instructed to do so—not even change dressings after operations.

Families' Role in Hospital Care: Families and patients have a right to, and expect, a high level of health care. Patients generally have at least one relative with them during their hospital stay. Families may be very demanding of health care professionals to ensure that the patient receives care and attention. Gifts of sweets and chocolates are common and may lead to conflicts with dietary restrictions. Families also expect to be allowed to spend as much time, whenever they like, visiting a patient. These frequent visits can lead to conflicts between hospital routines and family desires.

Dominance Patterns: Qatar has a patriarchal culture, and family is the top priority. Polygamy is common among men, who are largely regarded as providers and protectors. Families tend to be large and extended because polygamous relationships tend to be complex. Tribal ties are still strong. Important decisions relating to family life are always made by the father. When a boy reaches the age of 7 years, he is entrusted to the care of his father, who accompanies him everywhere; thus, the bonds between father and son are strong. Women play an increasingly important role, and many work in professions such as teaching and medicine. Women always cover their head with a scarf, generally wear a veil, and are usually accompanied by a male relative when they go out. Recently, women have experienced more personal freedom. Traditional restrictive practices are no longer the norm as they are in Saudi Arabia.

Eye-Contact Practices: Men maintain eye contact with other men during conversation. Eye contact between men and women is brief and limited.

Touch Practices: Touching between men and women is discouraged. Kissing, shaking hands, and holding hands are quite acceptable among males.

Perceptions of Time: Qataris live for today and do not dwell on the past. They tend not to think of the future because it is ordained by Allah.

Pain Reactions: Reactions to pain are varied and can be stoic or vocal. It is more acceptable for women to express pain. Medical practitioners are reluctant to provide adequate pain medications; for example, intravenous opiates for severe pain are rarely given to those with traumatic injuries. Qatar has no hospice movement, and pain relief is generally inadequate.

Birth Rites: Large families are encouraged through the provision of state benefits for each child and a desire to increase the population. The fertility rate is 2.81 children born per woman. The population growth rate estimate for 2003 was 3.6%. Qataris generally prefer to have boys, particularly as their first-born child. The infant mortality rate is 18 deaths per 1,000 live births. After birth, Qatari women tend to stay with their mothers for up to 40 days to recover, allowing the grandmother to care for the infant. Life expectancy is 71 for men, 77 for women.

Death Rites: Death or a poor prognosis is generally only discussed with male members of the family. Islamic regulations *(Fatwah)* state that life support can be discontinued when certain conditions are met and that organ donations are acceptable; however, family desires are the ultimate deciding factor. When a death has occurred, male members of the family are not expected to show their grief, whereas women can be very vocal. Religious beliefs dictate that the soul moves on to a better place after death, which can be a great comfort to the family. Autopsies are uncommon because of the religious mandate that the body must be buried intact. Interment is carried out usually within 1 day after death, and the body is buried wrapped in special shrouds without a coffin in the ground. Cremation is not permitted. Condolences are received by family members, with separate venues for men and women.

Food Practices and Intolerances: The traditional diet is fish and rice, with a small amount of red meat. All types of ethnic and international foods are available, however. Food is good and inexpensive, and multinational fast-food chains are found all over the country. Many large hotels have

Q

world-class restaurants and are licensed to serve alcohol. Pork, blood, and carrion consumption is forbidden for Muslims, so these foods are not imported into the country. Fasting during the holy month of Ramadan is mandatory for all adults but not for children or for those who are sick, although it is common for hospitalized adults to fast between sunrise and sunset. Eating, drinking, and smoking in public during Ramadan is forbidden. It is acceptable to eat with the fingers, but only the right hand can be used because the left is considered unclean.

Infant-Feeding Practices: Breastfeeding is the usual practice and may continue for 1 year, depending on the mother's health and quantity of milk.

Child-Rearing Practices: Child rearing tends to be permissive, and discipline is usually inconsistent. Infants often sleep with mothers until they are 1 or 2 years of age. Child rearing is often the responsibility of older female siblings or domestic servants. Qatar places great emphasis on the importance of education, offering girls and boys equal opportunities. Primary education is compulsory for all children, and education is provided free from the primary to the university level by the state. The state provides textbooks, transportation, sports clothes, and equipment at all levels. There are more than 200 schools. Qatar is currently experiencing a transition to a modern world-class education system. Sports have always played a pivotal role in the social lives of Qatar's residents. Participation of young people in sports is encouraged. More emphasis is placed on male activities, especially soccer, and men and women are segregated during sport and fitness activities; however, women are taking a more active role in fitness than in the past.

National Childhood Immunizations: BCG at birth; OPV at 2, 4, 6, and 18 months and at 4 to 6 years; HepB at birth, +6 to 8 weeks, + 5 months after second visit; DTwPHiBHep at 2, 4, and 6 months; MMR at 1 year and at 4 to 6 years; and DT at 4 to 6 years; Pneum_conj at 2, 4, 6, and 18 months; Td at 13 to 16 years; varicella at 1 year; and TT at 1 and 6 months. The percent of the target population vaccinated, by antigen, is: BCG, DTP1, and MCV (99%); DTP3, HepB3, and Hib3 (97%); and Polio3 (98%).

Other Characteristics: Restrictions for those who are not nationals are less severe than in some other Arab countries; for example, women are allowed to drive and go out alone. Female Qataris are allowed to vote and hold high office. Alcohol is available from a syndicate for expatriates with a liquor license, and it is also served in some hotels in Doha. The recent discovery and development of large natural gas reserves have given Qatar a substantial income, and it currently has the fastest growing economy in the world.

Q

BIBLIOGRAPHY

Al-Shahiri MZ, Kinchin-White J: Continous quality improvement. A proposal for Arabian Gulf Medical Associations, Saudi Med J. 21(1):135, 2000.

Central Intelligence Agency: 2006: The world factbook, Qatar. Retrieved September 21, 2006, from https://www.cia.gov/cia/publications/factbook/print/qa.html.

Gehani AA et al: Myocardial infarction with normal coronary angiography compared with severe coronary artery disease without myocardial infarction: the crucial role of smoking, *J Cardiovasc Risk.* 8(1):1, 2001.

Helmi I, Hussein A, Ahmed AH: Abdominal trauma due to road traffic accidents in Qatar, *Injury.* 32(2):105, 2001.

McGivern SA: Patient satisfaction with quality of care in a hospital system in Qatar, *J Healthc Qual.* 21(1):28, 1999.

Shanks NJ, Papworth G: Environmental factors and heat stroke, *Occup Med.* 51(1):45, 2001.

World Health Organization: 2006: Immunization, vaccines and biologicals. Retrieved September 21, 2006, from http://www.who.int/immunization_monitoring/en/globalsummary/countryprofileresult.cfm?C='qat'.

World Health Organization: *June 2000, Epidemiological fact sheets by country,* Geneva. Retrieved March 1, 2002, from http://www.unaids.org/hivaidsinfo/statistics/june00/fact_sheets/index.html.

◆ ROMANIA

MAP PAGE (798)

Mary G. Schaal and Emil Doru Steopan

Location: Romania is in southeastern Europe, bordering the Black Sea, Hungary, Moldova, Yugoslavia, Bulgaria, and Ukraine. The total area is 237,500 km^2 (91,699 square miles), and the capital is Bucharest. The highest peak of the Carpathian Mountains is 244 m (8,346 feet). The climate is temperate, with cold, cloudy winters and frequent snow and fog, and sunny summers with frequent showers and thunderstorms. The population is 22.3 million. The gross domestic product (GDP) per capita is $8,200, and 25% live below the poverty line.

Major Languages	Ethnic Groups	Major Religions
Romanian (official)	Romanian 89.5%	Eastern Orthodox
Hungarian	Hungarian 6.6%	87%
German	Serb, Croat,	Roman Catholic 6%
	Russian, Turkish,	(including 3%
	Roma (Gypsy),	Uniate)
	German, Ukrainian	Protestant 7%
	2.5%	

Romanian is a Romance language derived primarily from Latin. Minority languages include Hungarian, German, Turkish, Serbo-Croatian, and Romani (the language of the Roma, or Gypsy, population). English and French are taught in many schools and are the most common second languages spoken. The literacy rate is almost 100% for both men and women. Before 1989, the educational system heavily emphasized practical and technical studies. In recent years, however, management, business, and social sciences have become more popular.

R

Health Care Beliefs: Passive role; acute sick care, but health promotion considered important. Health-promotion practices encourage prenatal and child care in particular. The health care system addresses acute problems and tertiary care; however, rehabilitation is not emphasized. During the communist regime, people were given lectures on health care and medical treatment. Courses were organized to teach older people and women about symptoms of frequent diseases and ways to cure them. These efforts have improved the health care knowledge of the general population. In rural areas, older people may use herbs in teas, lotions, or potions to treat illness, but it is not the predominant practice. A few people in the country are known as healers by the power of God, and they use their hands (bioenergy), herbs, and prayers to cure various diseases. Most healers are deeply religious and encourage people to have faith. They are usually consulted by people with terminal illnesses. Some older Gypsy women called *ghicitoare* ("fortunetellers") serve as healers, although Gypsies use biomedical services as well.

Predominant Sick-Care Practices: Biomedical; coexisting holistic, folk, and Western medical practices. Health promotion and illness prevention do not predominate; the focus is on care for those who are ill. Romanians prefer medical treatment for their diseases, even in rural and remote areas. Generally, the doctor is highly respected and trusted. Although medical technology is not updated, Romania has hospitals and centers where people can receive health care, especially in the major cities. Romanians are beginning to consider regular examinations for disease prevention. National health care services are paid by employers and employees through salary deductions. In addition, private services are available for those who can afford them. Hospitalization is usually free, but often patients must pay for medications. The house doctor can prescribe a limited amount of medication free of charge. A wider range of facilities and services are available for children and older adults.

Ethnic-/Race-Specific or Endemic Diseases: Industrial pollution continues to influence health. Diseases of the respiratory system are the leading cause of morbidity in adults in both inpatient and outpatient settings, followed by diseases of the circulatory, digestive, and genitourinary systems, and neoplasms. Circulatory-system diseases, particularly cerebrovascular and ischemic heart problems, are the leading causes of mortality, followed by neoplasms, digestive- and respiratory-system disorders, and diabetes mellitus. According to the World Health Organization (WHO), Romania probably has the highest number of human immunodeficiency virus (HIV) infections in the subregion of central and southeastern Europe. In 1989 Romania experienced a major nosocomial HIV epidemic in children, the result of thousands of children receiving blood transfusions. Whereas discrepancies in reporting have prevented an accurate assessment, the estimated number of individuals living with HIV is probably between 5,500 and 14,000. The Joint United Nations Programme on

HIV/AIDS (UNAIDS) reports the prevalence rate for HIV in adults (aged 15 to 49 years) as being less than 0.1%, and government officials and doctors frequently deny that HIV/acquired immunodeficiency syndrome (AIDS) is of any significance.

Health-Team Relationships: The doctor is the primary authority in hospital settings, and nurses are subordinate. Nurses are given more respect if they are the only health care professionals in the setting. Doctors and nurses practice primarily in hospitals, all of which are public. Some new and well-equipped private clinics are being established, and the best doctors practice in them after their work in the public arena. Recently, social workers and psychologists have been included on the medical teams of hospitals. Nursing education is provided by *scoala postliceala sanitara* ("post high schools") and takes 3 years. Schools can be public or private. National examinations are held after graduation for licensing and specialization (e.g., pediatrics, psychiatry, gynecology, surgery, public health). More recently, a 4-year nursing program at the University of Medicine and Pharmacy has been offered. Beginning in 2005, specialty education is offered at the master's and Ph.D. levels.

Families' Role in Hospital Care: Families rally around people who are sick and play an important role in their care. Family members are expected to stay with patients, provide food, and assist with basic hygiene tasks, although the nurses and cleaning women help as well. It is expected that friends will visit hospitalized patients.

Dominance Patterns: The principle of gender equality is new and has not yet been embraced by a significant percentage of the population. Women do not have an important role in decision-making processes, although there are many well-educated and professionally trained women. Women's nongovernmental organizations play an important role in increasing public awareness about the role of women in political and social life.

Eye-Contact Practices: Direct, sustained eye contact is the norm. It is customary to maintain eye contact with other people while talking. Avoiding eye contact during conversations with friends portrays a lack of respect or insincerity.

Touch Practices: Two kisses on the check for greetings and farewells are common. Touch is an important part of nonverbal communication.

Perceptions of Time: Time schedules are followed more precisely in urban areas than in rural regions. Punctuality has not been an important value, although perceptions have been changing. Romanians try to focus on a better future, although it is hard for them to ignore the difficulties of the present and forget the sacrifices of the past. Romanians live primarily between the past and the present as they try to establish a future-oriented view.

Pain Reactions: Romanians typically have a high tolerance for pain and discomfort. Some are communicative about their pain, and others are stoic. Some prefer injections for pain relief. Women are not expected to cry out in pain during labor; loud verbal expressions in response to pain are considered shameful.

Birth Rites: The infant mortality rate is 26 deaths per 1,000 live births and is among the highest in Europe. The fertility rate is 1.37 children born per woman. Romanian women deliver in hospitals, and localized anesthesia is generally not offered. Pregnancy is considered a delicate period, and the family takes great care to offer the woman the best quality and quantity of food they can. Women are typically cared for by professionals during and after delivery. Women are treated for the infections they are likely to contract because of poor sanitation conditions at maternity hospitals. Women usually go home after the first or second day after the delivery unless they have problems requiring special treatment. New mothers rely on an older woman, often the mother or mother-in-law, to care for her during the first 2 weeks at home. Mothers are encouraged to breastfeed and eat food that increases milk production. The family tries to ensure that the mother is emotionally stable because they believe that erratic emotions can spoil milk production. Infants must be named within the first 2 weeks and registered in the family register of city population. Visitors, both friends and family, are expected to visit the family of the newborn and bring gifts, clothes, or money. The mother's family of origin customarily buys most of the clothes and the crib for the infant. Parents usually decide on the name, but occasionally grandparents name them after themselves or with other names they prefer. This naming tradition is more common in rural areas, where the traditional family predominates. Mothers who have a job during their pregnancy get a 1-year leave. The employer pays 50% of her salary during this period. Many women take a shorter leave, especially those who work in the private sector, because they do not want to lose their full salary. Abortion and contraceptives are legal. Life expectancy is 68 for men, 75 for women.

Death Rites: Relatives and friends expend considerable effort to be present when a person is near death, when the family starts expressing their grief through crying and wailing. Family members and close friends of the deceased dress in black and official suits. Family members expect visits from relatives, friends, and neighbors. The body is buried within 48 hours. If the deceased was a young woman, she is dressed in a white bridal dress. If a young man dies, he is dressed in a bridegroom suit. The whole family and close relatives are in mourning at least 40 days. Autopsies are not routinely performed. Most people die at home and are embalmed and prepared for viewing at home. If a person is ill and dies in a hospital, the embalming and preparation of the body occurs there. In either situation, the body is dressed in nice clothes, and it lies in state in the home, usually in the living room. Often a few personal effects of the deceased are placed in the coffin, such as jewelry, shaving implements, watches, glasses, writing implements, and cigarettes, and these items are eventually buried with the deceased. The family offers meals as a sign of respect on the day of the burial, the 40th day after burial, on the 6-month anniversary, and on the 1-year anniversary of the death. The meal marking the 1-year anniversary ends the period of mourning. Few families continue to offer meals for very close family members after a year. Family members do, however, continue to go to the cemetery and take flowers to the tomb, especially on sacred days, special anniversaries, birthdays, or special days for each family.

Food Practices and Intolerances: Traditionally, the largest meal is lunch. Supper in the evening includes meat and vegetables, rice, pasta, or beans, and the meat and vegetables are well cooked. During the last 10 years, with the transition in the economy, people began working for the entire day and thus prefer the largest meal in the evening. Popular foods include *mititei* ("seasoned grilled meatballs") and *mamaliga* ("a corn-meal porridge served in many different ways"). Wine and a plum brandy called *tuica* are popular beverages, and *placinta* (turnovers) are a typical dessert.

Infant-Feeding Practices: Breastfeeding is typical; most women recognize that it is healthy. Women do not breastfeed in public. If breastfeeding is impossible for medical reasons, or the mother simply chooses not to, formula is available.

Child-Rearing Practices: Child rearing is not specifically strict or permissive. Parents try to educate their children in a traditional way, but often children respond more to peer influence and ignore traditional values. Young adults often live with or receive financial support from their parents because of limited financial resources and increasing rates of unemployment. Grandparents may supervise children when parents work, telling them stories, playing with them, and accompanying them to and from school. Even when in difficult situations, parents still try to sacrifice so that their children can be educated. Education in Romania is free and compulsory for children between the ages of 7 and 14, and most children choose to stay in school after age 14. The education of girls is considered much more important so that they will not be subject to family slavery. Unfortunately, social disruption during the postcommunist era has made education more difficult because some village schools were destroyed, and many teachers left for more profitable occupations. Children who are likely to receive an inadequate education include Gypsies (Roma), children of illegal migrants in cities, and children without families. Unfortunately, drug abuse is a growing problem of youth because of easy access to drugs and their doubts about the future.

National Childhood Immunizations: BCG at birth; DT at 7 and 14 years; DTwP at 4, 12, and 30 to 35 months; DTwPHep at 2 and 6, months; DTwPIPV at 2, 4, 6, and 12 months in part of the country; HepA in high-risk areas; HepB at birth (HepB is given at birth alone and at 2 and 6 months in combination with DTP and at 18 years); rubella at 14 years; MMR at 12 to 15 months and at 7 years; OPV at 2, 4, 6, and 12 months and 9 years; Td every 10 years. The percent of the target population vaccinated, by antigen, is: HepB3 and BCG (99%); DPT1 (98%); DPT3, MCV, and Polio3 (97%).

BIBLIOGRAPHY

Central Intelligence Agency: 2006: *The world factbook, Romania.* Retrieved September 21, 2006, from https://www.cia.gov/cia/publications/factbook/print/ro.html.

Public Health Ministry of Romania, 2004: *Romania Public Health.* Retrieved September 22, 2006 from http://www.photius.com/countries/romania/society/romania_society_public_health.html

UNAIDS: 2006 Romania. Retrieved September 21, 2006, from http://www.unaids.org/en/Regions_Countries/Countries/romania.asp.

UNICEF: Retrieved August 29, 2006, from http://www.unicef.org/romania/health_nutritions_hivaids.html.

World Health Organization: *Health care systems in transition Romania.* Copenhagen, 1996, WHO. Available at: http://www.who.int/countries/rou/en/ (retrieved July 12, 2006).

World Health Organization: Retrieved August 29, 2006, from http://www.who.int/hiv/countries/en/.

World Health Organization: 2006: Immunization, vaccines and biologicals. Retrieved September 21, 2006, from http://www.who.int/immunization_monitoring/en/globalsummary/countryprofileresult.cfm?C='rou'.

◆ RUSSIA (RUSSIAN FEDERATION)

MAP PAGE (799)

Gennadij G. Knyazev, Helena R. Slobodskaya, and Tatiana I. Ryabichenko

Location: Massive disintegration of the former Soviet Union's Communist Party and territory occurred in 1992. Declarations of independence by the republics of Latvia, Estonia, and Lithuania were followed rapidly by declarations of other republics. Russia extends from the western Black and Baltic Seas to the Pacific Ocean and has a total area of 17,075,200 km^2 (6,592,745 square miles). The population is 142.9 million, and the capital is Moscow. Its vast areas of plains and plateaus are punctuated by low mountain ranges. The climate varies from arctic severity during the winter to subtropical heat during the summer. The gross domestic product (GDP) per capita is $11,100, with 18% living below the poverty line.

Major Languages	Ethnic Groups	Major Religions
Russian	Russian 80%	Russian Orthodox
Other (English, Tatar,	Tatar 4%	Muslim
German, Ukrainian)	Ukrainian 2%	Other
	Chuvash, Bashkir 1%	
	Other 13%	

R

About 98% of the population speaks Russian, 5% English. Literacy is almost 100% for both men and women. Most emigrants from the former Soviet Union speak Russian, and it is uncommon to overhear Ukrainian, Belarussian, Uzbek, or Armenian in Russian cities. On the other hand, in several republics inside Russia, local languages may dominate, especially in rural areas, namely, Bashkortostan, Tatarstan, Chechnya, Evenkia, the Jewish Autonomic Republic, the Republic of Tuva, Buryatia, the Chuvash Republic, the Kabardino-Balkarian Republic, Mari El, Sakha, and Udmurt.

Health Care Beliefs: Acute sick care; passive role; increasing efforts toward prevention. Medical information and advice about healthy food and the need for exercise frequently appears in the mass media, although some of it is of dubious quality. Cigarette advertisements always include the health ministry's declaration that smoking is unhealthy. Oriental traditional medicine such as Chinese medicine is popular. In Soviet times, schizophrenia was the primary diagnosed mental disorder, and the same is true today. Psychotherapy is an emerging field of uncertain quality. It is becoming popular among the wealthy, but most patients have illnesses of a psychosomatic nature. Fear of mental illness is widespread, not only because of prejudice and fear of being ridiculed but also because of the punitive characteristics of psychiatry in the former Soviet Union. Superstitions about the magical healing properties of some drugs or objects are widespread.

Predominant Sick-Care Practices: Biomedical; alternative and magical-religious. Most people, especially those in the cities, go to outpatient clinics that are generally free. Drugs such as analgesics are not free. These clinics provide only a limited number of services, and the quality is generally not very good. Numerous private clinics have emerged recently, and services are better in these clinics, but they are expensive. Even in the state clinics, serious surgical operations are not free; they are expensive and unaffordable for many people. Indigenous healers are rare in cities but still popular in rural areas, especially in the northern territories, where shamans practice among aboriginal people. Many charlatans have recently appeared in cities. They pretend to have extrasensory powers or to be magicians with the ability to heal.

Ethnic-/Race-Specific or Endemic Diseases: For many years, opisthorchiasis foci have existed in the northern Ob River region and in the Kama and Vyatka river basins. Natural foci of tick-borne encephalitis exist in Siberia, the Far East, and the Ural region and during the last years has spread to the European part of Russia. Tuberculosis incidence is increasing. Hepatitis delta virus genotypes I and II co-circulate in the endemic area of Yakutia. In Siberia, the prevalence of hepatitis B virus infection is very high. Biliary pathology in the far northern population is related to ethnic and geographic factors. Viliuisk encephalomyelitis seems to be endemic among the native populations of Yakutia. More cases of hemorrhagic fever with renal syndrome, tick-borne encephalitis, Crimean

R

hemorrhagic fever, and West Nile fever (with a high proportion in urban populations) are being registered annually. An increase in the epizootic activity of the natural foci of plague is noted despite the absence of morbidity among humans. Outbreaks of tularemia are linked not only with the increased activity of natural foci but also with reduced immunization coverage in endemic regions. The main causes of death are cardiovascular diseases (58%), malignant tumors (18%), traumas and poisoning (13%), and, according to autopsy findings, alcohol-associated lesions of different organs (9%). Russia, among the Eastern European countries, has the most alarming increase in human immunodeficiency virus (HIV), despite the relatively low reported prevalence rate. The Joint United Nations Programme on HIV/AIDS (UNAIDS) estimates the prevalence rate for HIV in adults (aged 15 to 49) to be between 0.6% and 1.9%, with 560,000 to 1,600,000 living with HIV, including 110,000 to 370,000 women. Of the 89 regions, 88 have reported HIV cases, but the epidemic is distributed unevenly across the country, with more than half of all infections being reported in just 10 regions. The prevalence in St. Petersburg has increased 100-fold. The epidemic is relatively young, with most individuals infected between 1999 and 2002. The proportion of people living with HIV or acquired immunodeficiency syndrome (AIDS) needing treatment is therefore still low but is likely to increase dramatically over the next 5 years. Deaths from AIDS are estimated at 22,000 to 56,000. The Russian Federation has a concentrated HIV epidemic disproportionately affecting vulnerable populations; injecting drug users constitute 87% of registered cases.

Health-Team Relationships: Doctors dominate. Patients' attitudes toward doctors and nurses are dubious.

Families' Role in Hospital Care: Family members generally do not stay with patients in the hospital. The exceptions are mothers of hospitalized infants and relatives of those who are seriously ill and whose complete care cannot be provided by the hospital. Even if family members do not stay, they usually come as often as possible to assist the patients and bring them food.

Dominance Patterns: Men dominate politics and business, but many women are health care professionals and school teachers. In the family, the father traditionally dominates, although this pattern is changing. More than 20% of households are headed by women.

Eye-Contact Practices: Eye contact is not avoided, and gender differences are not great.

Touch Practices: Touch practices vary, but physical touching is not generally common. Three kisses on the cheek for greetings and farewells is now an exotic practice in Russia. Kisses on the cheek are still common among Orthodox believers greeting each other during the religious holidays, especially during Easter, the main Orthodox holy day. Generally, only men shake hands.

Perceptions of Time: Punctuality is not terribly important. Some people are punctual, but being late to appointments or breaking promises is common and generally not a problem. Traditions have changed several times during the last century and are still changing today. After the dissolution of the former Soviet Union, some older Russian traditions were revived. Older adults mainly focus on past traditions (i.e., traditions from Soviet times); middle-aged and young people tend to look to the future.

Pain Reactions: Expressions of pain are acceptable for women and children, but men are expected to be stoic.

Birth Rites: The fertility rate is 1.28 children born per woman. Most births occur in maternity hospitals with the assistance of a midwife who is under the supervision of a doctor. The infant mortality rate is 15 deaths per 1,000 live births. After birth, the woman is placed in a ward with others, and the newborn goes to the nursery with other newborns. If no complications are involved, the mother and the infant stay in the hospital about 5 days and go home under the observation of the child clinic. New changes in obstetric care include wards where the mother and infant can stay together, shorter stays, and provisions for fathers to be present in the delivery room. The sex of the newborn makes no difference to modern Russian parents; any preferences are individual. Life expectancy is 60 for men, 74 for women.

Death Rites: The death of a family member is usually considered a tragedy. As a rule, all family members, colleagues, and friends try to attend the funeral. Organ donations and autopsies are acceptable.

Food Practices and Intolerances: Meat or fish with potato garnish is the prevalent dish. Bread and sausage, eggs, and milk products are usual for breakfast. A type of ravioli and boiled buckwheat are among favorite Russian foods. Cabbage, sauerkraut, carrots, and beets are staple vegetables in winter, whereas in the summer, apples, local berries, cucumbers, tomatoes, and salads are added to the diet. Recently, a vast range of fruits and vegetables have become available, but most are too expensive to be widely purchased; bananas and oranges are the most popular. It is unacceptable to eat with the hands. According to government regulations, alcoholic beverages (including beer) can be sold to adults only; however, alcohol consumption and binge drinking have been increasing.

Infant-Feeding Practices: Breastfeeding is the usual practice, especially during the first 6 months, but bottle-feeding is increasingly popular. Infant feeding in most areas is not culture specific and tends to be based on the recommendations of the child health clinics.

Child-Rearing Practices: Permissiveness predominates, and children do not usually have strict rules. The mother is responsible for most of the discipline. Children are generally loved, and parents are often overly concerned about a child's success in school. Children are not expected to be quiet and obedient and are not discouraged from pursuing independent activities or confrontations. Traditional gender roles usually apply, especially for boys.

National Childhood Immunizations: BCG at birth (3–7 days) and 7 and 14 years; DTwP at 3, 4.5, 6, and 18 months; OPV at 3, 4.5, 6, 18, and 20 months and at 14 years; MMR at 12 months and 6 years; HepB at birth (first 12 hours) and 1 and 6 months; measles at 12 months and 6 years; MM at 12 months and 6 years; rubella at 12 months and 6 and 13 years; Td at 14 years; mumps at 12 months and 6 years. The percent of the target population vaccinated, by antigen, is: BCG and HepB3 (97%); DTP1, DTP3, and Polio 3 (98%); and MCV (99%).

BIBLIOGRAPHY

All-Russian population census: 2002: Retrieved March 14, 2006, from http://www.perepis2002.ru/index.

Central Intelligence Agency: 2006: *The world factbook, Russia.* Retrieved September 21, 2006, from https://www.cia.gov/cia/publications/factbook/print/rs.html.

Kalichman SC, Kelly JA, Sikkema KJ, Koslov AP, Shaboltas A, and Granskaya J: The emerging AIDS crisis in Russia: review of enabling factors and prevention needs, *Int J STD AIDS.* 11(2):71–75, 2000.

Khazova TG, Iastrebov VK: Combined focus of tick-borne encephalitis, tick-borne rickettsiosis and tularemia in the habitat of *Haemaphysalis concinna* in south central Siberia, *Zh Mikrobiol Epidemiol Immunobiol.* 1:78–80, 2001.

Malyutina S, Bobak M, Kurilovitch S, Ryizova E, Nikitin Y, and Marmot M: Alcohol consumption and binge drinking in Novosibirsk, Russia, 1985–95, *Addiction.* 96 (7):987–995, 2001.

Onishchenko GG: Infectious diseases in natural reservoirs: epidemic situation and morbidity in the Russian Federation and prophylactic measures, *Zh Mikrobiol Epidemiol Immunobiol.* 3:22–28, 2001.

Takashima I, Hayasaka D, Goto A, Kariwa H, and Mizutani T: Epidemiology of tick-borne encephalitis (TBE) and phylogenetic analysis of TBE viruses in Japan and Far Eastern Russia, *Jpn J Infect Dis.* 54(1):1–11, 2001.

UNAIDS: 2006 Russian Federation. Retrieved September 21, 2006, from http://www.unaids.org/en/Regions_Countries/Countries/russian_federation.asp.

World Health Organization: 2006: Immunization, vaccines and biologicals. Retrieved September 21, 2006, from http://www.who.int/immunization_monitoring/en/globalsummary/countryprofileresult.cfm?C='rus'

Zairat'iants OV: Analysis of fatal outcomes according to the Moscow pathology service data (1996–2000), *Arkh Patol.* 63(4):9–13, 2001.

◆ RWANDA (RWANDESE REPUBLIC)

MAP PAGE (801)

Kizito Bishikwabo Nsarhaza and Michel Carael

Location: Rwanda is located in central Africa to the east of the Democratic Republic of Congo. It has a rugged landscape with high hills and deep valleys. The principal geographic feature is the Virunga Mountains, which run north of Lake Kivu and include Rwanda's highest point, Volcan Karisimbi. In addition to the capital city, Kigali, other major towns include Butare, Gisenyi, and Ruhengeri. The country has a total area of 26,340 km² (10,170 square miles), with a population of 8.6 million. With more than 300 persons per square kilometer, Rwanda is the most densely populated country in

Africa, with an annual growth rate of about 2.4%. About 18% of the population is living in urban areas. About 60% of the population lives below the poverty line; the gross domestic product (GDP) per capita is $1,500. Literacy rates are 76% for men, 65% for women.

Major Languages	Ethnic Groups*	Major Religions
Kinyarwanda (official)	Hutu 84%	Roman Catholic 57%
French (official)	Tutsi 15%	Protestant 26%
English (official)	Twa (pygmy) 1%	Adventist 11%
		Muslim 5%
		Indigenous beliefs and none 1%

*Estimations were made 40 years ago. No estimation has been available since the genocide in 1994.

Since its independence, ethnic violence has led to large-scale massacres. At the end of the 1980s, extremist Hutu leaders (both national and local), exploited intergroup tensions and generalized poverty to justify dictatorship. This policy culminated in 1994 with the elimination of more than 800,000 Tutsi and moderate Hutu opponents. Following the genocide, two million people became refugees in neighboring countries.

Health Care Beliefs: Primary health care through health promotion is an important aspect of health programs and interventions. However, because of the synergy of malnutrition and infectious diseases, and the lack of coverage of health interventions, life expectancy has declined. Most illnesses are believed to be caused by the breakdown of one of the hundreds of social taboos, such as lack of respect for parents or ancestors, failures to observe rituals, or sexual abstinence at particular events. If the disease persists, suspicion of poisoning or cursing will always prevail. In rural areas, people wear amulets or get scarification for protection.

Predominant Sick-Care Practices: Biomedical; traditional; and magical-religious. The population consults doctors or traditional healers depending on numerous factors: the practitioners' location (urban or rural), cost of treatment, cultural beliefs, and type of illness. Often healers prepare medications at the healing site, using fluids to treat health, love, and illness issues. Because of the 1994 Tutsi genocide, mental illness has become an important aspect of health care seeking and requires psychosocial programs for large refugee populations that aim to strengthen community structures. The centerpiece of the mental health system of Rwanda is the neuropsychiatric Hospital of Ndera, which plays a key role in decentralization of mental services and their integration with primary health care services. Effort has been made to integrate traditional medicine into the modern health system.

Ethnic-/Race-Specific or Endemic Diseases: Endemic diseases are not associated with any particular minority group, and biological differences among ethnic groups have not been identified. Major illnesses affecting the country are malnutrition (lack of protein and calories), diarrhea, respiratory infections, human immunodeficiency virus (HIV)/acquired immunodeficiency syndrome (AIDS), tuberculosis, malaria, and shigellosis. Hospitalized older adults occupy 18% of available beds. Their disease pattern is different from that of younger patients, placing heavier demands on medical resources. The Joint United Nations Programme on HIV/AIDS (UNAIDS) estimates the prevalence rate for HIV in adults (aged 15 to 49 years) to be 3.1%, with 190,000 people living with HIV, including 27,000 children aged 0 to 14. The number of children aged 0 to 17 who are orphans as a result of AIDS is about 210,000. HIV trends show a decline in urban rates, but an increase in rural rates, where the majority live.

Health-Team Relationships: Although health-team relationships are doctor driven, the dominance of doctors does not impede good working relationships. Patients' attitudes toward doctors and nurses are characterized by submission. When accessible, health professionals are expected to have the knowledge and ability to cure serious illnesses.

Families' Role in Hospital Care: Community and family ties are very strong. Families assist their hospitalized relatives; they tend to stay with patients and bring them food. This sign of solidarity has been accentuated by the exacerbated conflict among ethnic groups. Patients prefer to eat food brought by relatives rather than hospital food.

Dominance Patterns: Absolute patriarchal authority is common. Children, even when married, are dependent on their parents; the parent's support contributes to their overall wellness. In turn, respect, veneration, and assistance to parents are the norm. In general, Rwandan culture is male dominated. Men and women have separate conjugal roles (e.g., wife doing housework and crop cultivation, husband doing gardening) and joint conjugal roles (e.g., wife and husband disciplining children). Some decisions and their implementation can involve extended families or community members (e.g., taking care of elderly, those with disabilities, orphans). Women have an important role in cooking and taking care of older family members, children, and ill family members. A woman never challenges her husband in public. Despite subordination in all aspects, however, women's remarks and even criticisms are encouraged in private and in close family settings.

Eye-Contact Practices: Eye contact is usually avoided as a sign of respect, not only between members of the opposite sex but also among generations. A youth never looks directly into the eyes of an older adult and usually bows when talking to the father. These practices are also expected from women during interactions with their husbands.

Perceptions of Time: In rural settings, seasons and daily sun cycles are the main reference for time, and moments are often defined in terms of events. People are patient; they tend to consider it normal for people to be late to appointments; however, educated people tend to be less patient and are more easily irritated by a lack of punctuality, leading to a dual perception of punctuality in the culture. During official activities, people make efforts to be prompt. During unofficial activities, time has little meaning; for example, discussions may be extended with little regard for their length.

Pain Reactions: Stoicism is encouraged because expressions of pain are considered a sign of weakness. Calmness and serenity are praised, but the calmness is not passive. People are encouraged to stay calm and stoic when facing adversity and to concentrate their energy on preparing a response.

Birth Rites: For life to be worthwhile and meaningful, it is believed to be essential to have children. Therefore, contraception use is low, and the fertility rate is 5.4 children born per woman. In rural traditional settings, childbirth takes place in a banana plantation, where women are assisted by female relatives such as the mother-in-law. Difficult deliveries are blamed on infractions of social rules, offenses against the ancestors, or bad spirits seeking vengeance against the woman by impeding the birth. Offerings or animal sacrifices may be used to correct these situations. In urban settings, most women give birth in maternity hospitals, and they are often accompanied by female relatives. Men do not traditionally witness childbirth because it is considered a secret activity in which only women participate. After delivery, women are not expected to do any work in the household and are considered impure until they are ready for sexual intercourse (usually 1 or 2 weeks after delivery). The prevalence of infants with low birth weight is estimated to be 9%. The maternal mortality rate is 1,400 per 100,000 live births, and the infant mortality rate is 90 deaths per 1,000 live births. Efforts are being made through traditional birth attendants to educate at-risk women to give birth in health centers. Life expectancy is 44 for men, 47 for women.

Death Rites: The body is exposed for viewing for no more than 3 days, and people visit the family. All family members are expected to attend the bereavement ritual. Men are separated from the women, and each group grieves in specific ways.

Food Practices and Intolerances: Basic food is composed of cassava, beans, potatoes, and cassava leaves, and beans are the favorite food. Beans are often combined with other foods such as corn or meat. Cultural practices limit people's consumption of certain foods. For example, lamb is not a common food, and women are not allowed to eat certain parts of chickens. Some foods are thought to have magical powers to facilitate pregnancy or the delivery of an infant. On average, rural inhabitants eat two meals per day, and the main meal is eaten in the evening. Main meals differ according to altitude. In zones with a tropical climate, the diet comprises four main foods: beans, sweet potatoes, cassava, and bananas, with the first two providing 50% of the total energy supply. At high altitudes, the main foods are pulses (beans), cereals (maize), and potatoes; protein intakes are very low. Vitamin A deficiency is also prevalent. The percentage of children with moderate or severe stunting is around 40%. It is the usual practice to eat with the hands. Families that have adopted Western culture use a knife and spoon and eat from individual rather than collective plates.

R

Infant-Feeding Practices: Maternal milk *(amashereka)* is generally given to infants; breastfeeding is nearly universal, with a median duration of 3 years (less in urban areas). There are no postpartum sexual taboos limiting breastfeeding as in other Great Lakes cultures. Breastfeeding is suspended when the mother is sick or in the case of a subsequent pregnancy because these situations are believed to provoke diarrhea in the infant. Birth intervals are more than 2 years because of prolonged postpartum amenorrhea. Children are not fed with solid food until they start crawling.

Child-Rearing Practices: Child discipline is a role of all the men in the community (e.g., fathers, uncles, grandfathers), although final decisions rest with the parents. Because children spend most of their time with their mothers, however, the mother's influence is profound. Children sleep with parents until they start eating solid food, and they are treated tenderly. Children are expected to be respectful to their parents all their lives. Children usually stay with their mothers while they do household chores (e.g., cultivation, fetch water, prepare meals) and accompany them to social activities such as wedding ceremonies. Later, they are regularly sent to spend time with their relatives. Sharing, strict respect, generosity, the importance of giving gifts, and a sense of community are taught. Because of the synergy between malnutrition and infectious diseases, including HIV, the overall child mortality rate is estimated to be around 200 per 1,000, one of the highest in Africa.

National Childhood Immunizations: BCG at birth; DTwPhIBHep at 6, 10, and 14 weeks; OPV at birth, at 6, 10, and 14 weeks; measles at 9 months; TT at first contact, +1, +6 months, +1, +1 year. The percent of the target population vaccinated, by antigen, is: BCG (86%); DTP1 (94%); DTP3, HepB3, and Hib3 (89%); MCV (84%); Polio3 (89%); and TT2 plus (76%).

BIBLIOGRAPHY

Columbia Encyclopedia: Rwanda. Retrieved November 22, 2005, from www.bartleby. com/65/rw/Rwanda.html.

De Jong JP, Scholte WF, Koeter MW, and Hart AA: The prevalence of mental health problems in Rwandan and Burundese refugee camps, *Acta Psychiatr Scand.* 102(3):171, 2000.

Rahlenbeck S, Hakizimana C: Deliveries at a district hospital in Rwanda, 1997–2000, *Int J Gynaecol Obstet.* 76(3):325–328, 2002.

UNAIDS: 2006 Rwanda: Retrieved September 21, 2006, from http://www.unaids. org/en/Regions_Countries/Countries/rwanda.asp.

UNICEF: Retrieved September 1, 2006, from http://www.unicef.org/infobycountry/ rwanda_statistics.html.

World Bank: World Development Indicators database, Retrieved August 2005 from http://devdata.worldbank.org/external/CPProfile.asp?PTYPE=CP&CCODE=RWA.

World Health Organization: 2006: Immunization, vaccines and biologicals. Retrieved September 21, 2006, from http://www.who.int/immunization_monitoring/en/ globalsummary/countryprofileresult.cfm?C='rwa'.

R

◆ SAMOA (INDEPENDENT STATE OF)

MAP PAGE (794)

Tolu Muliaina

Location: Samoa is a small island nation in the southwest Pacific to the east of Wallis and Futuna, west of American Samoa, and northeast of Tonga and the Fiji Islands. Widely known as Western Samoa until 1997, in 1962 it was the first Pacific Island to gain political independence from New Zealand. Samoa has a tropical climate with a year-round average temperature of 28 °C. December through April is the warmest and wettest time of the year, and May through November is generally cooler and drier as the result of the southeast trades. The four inhabited islands are Savaii, Upolu, Apolima, and Manono, and four rocky islets northeast of Upolu are also inhabited. The total area is 2,849 km^2 (1,100 square miles). Samoa is blessed with a natural unspoiled environment. Upolu is the second largest island and was the fastest to be "transformed." It is the center of administration, commerce, education, health, and entertainment, and is the site of the capital, Apia, the only urban area. The population is 176,908. Samoa has a young population; 41% was in the 1- to 14-age group in 2001. About 22% resides in the Apia urban area; the remaining 78% is rural. The population is mostly of Polynesian origin, but there are also small percentages of German-Samoan, Chinese-Samoan, and other European-Samoan descent. The gross domestic product (GDP) per capita is $5,600. Literacy rates are almost 100% for both men and women.

Major Languages	**Ethnic Groups**	**Major Religions**
Samoan (official)	Samoan 92%	Christian 99.7%
English (official)	Euronesian 7%	Other or none 0.3%
	European 1%	

Samoa had a complex polytheistic religion, that differentiated between non-human (*Atua*) and human (*Aitu*), and incorporated elements of ancestor worship before European contact. Even today, religion is deeply rooted in the culture as reflected in the country's motto, "Samoa is founded on God." Most Samoans are committed Christians of different denominations. Mainstream churches are Methodist, Roman Catholic, Congregational, and various other small but fast growing churches such as Baptist, Seventh Day Adventist, Latter Day Saints, Jehovah Witnesses, and Bahai. The growth of the last has raised concern and has been the center of much debate among the mainstream churches. Sunday is a special day of absolute rest and prayer. Everyone is expected to attend morning and afternoon services and are expected not to engage in usual daily activities outdoors other than preparing the Sunday meal. Going for picnics is not encouraged, and in some villages, use of beaches for picnics is restricted for visitors and villagers alike. Although Samoan is the first

S

language, English is widely spoken in urban areas, and Samoan is spoken in the villages.

Health Care Beliefs: Acute sick care; passive role. Samoans practice some form of traditional healing, even with the introduction of modern medicine. Many people, particularly the "older" generation, hold firmly to the values of traditional medicine. Modern medicine and treatment provided by hospitals sometimes conflict with traditional healing methods. Because most Samoans are Christians, their health beliefs often attribute poor health to divine will. Despite the growing influence and efficacy of modern medicine, many retain traditional medical beliefs and practices. In rural areas, patients first go to traditional healers, then to the hospital. Sometimes they go to both at the same time. The health system is struggling to inform patients and the public about the causes and effects of noncommunicable diseases such as obesity, diabetes, and hypertension. Although small and ineffective at times, the health care system through its Komiti Tumama program, managed mainly by nurses, provides community basic health services and continuing education in biology, sociobehavioral, and cultural factors that influence patient-provider partnerships in managing chronic diseases.

Predominant Sick-Care Practices: Biomedical and traditional. Most seek acute and chronic care for illnesses at the government hospital in Apia, four other district hospitals, and several health centers. A growing private sector also provides medical services. Many consult traditional healers, although it is difficult to estimate the number of people using such services. There are various forms of traditional healers: the *faatosaga* (midwife), those who *fofo* (massage newborns), *fofo gau* (orthopedists), *fofo aitu* (spirit healers who banish trouble), and *taulasea* (herbalists). The government's health care system is in the midst of a major review and modernization of curative, emergency, and preventive services. The changing patterns of morbidity from childhood infectious diseases to adult noncommunicable diseases such as diabetes and hypertension have been recognized, and are leading to renewed emphasis on preventive medical services and public health primary and secondary prevention activities.

Ethnic-/Race-Specific or Endemic Diseases: One of the difficult issues facing Samoa is the emergence of adult noncommunicable diseases such as diabetes and hypertension. Modern Samoans have a high prevalence of these conditions because of their high proportion of overweight adults. Management of the diseases linked to obesity requires cooperation and knowledge sharing between patients and health care providers. Despite the decrease in childhood infection rates, filariasis remains a problem, although the health department has preventive teams who visit villages and focus on vector control and treating infected individuals. The Joint United Nations Programme on HIV/AIDS (UNAIDS) has no estimated prevalence rates for human immunodeficiency virus (HIV) and acquired immunodeficiency syndrome (AIDS). Nine cases of HIV infection had been reported up to 1998, with seven deaths from AIDS reported since 1993. Transmission appears to be primarily heterosexual. Recent data on HIV indicate that four new cases were diagnosed in 1996. Life expectancy is 68 for men, 74 for women.

Families' Role in Hospital Care: The family is the core of Samoan society. Under normal circumstances, at least one family member attends to all the patient's daily needs: washing, bathing, conversation, linen changes, and monitoring the patient's conditions. Because hospital food is not always appealing, families provide home-cooked meals that are often shared with other patients and sometimes with nursing staff. Providing bouquets of flowers is also a frequent gesture.

Pain Reactions: Research among Samoan migrants in California has suggested a tendency toward stoicism in the face of pain, although this has not been studied in the Samoan archipelago.

Food Patterns: Evidence from a number of sources confirms that before European contact, Samoans, like other Pacific island societies, enjoyed balanced and nutritious diets that consisted of root crops (*taro, taamu,* bananas, breadfruit, coconuts, fresh fish, wild edible greens/ferns from the forest, and *niu* (young coconut juice) or water. In the past, working on the farm, fishing, and taking part in other household activities or village sports fostered good relationships in villages and also kept many people fit and healthy. Today many people work in offices rather than outdoors. They rely heavily on automobiles instead of walking. Many people have acquired tastes for imported, processed nutrient-inferior but convenient food and drinks: rice, flour, canned fish and beef, frozen fatty meat, carbonated drinks, and alcoholic beverages. These preferences are encouraged by modern convenient eating outlets (e.g., McDonald's) around Apia. Some view these changes as expected as Samoa integrates into the world economy—that globalization, modernization, and development are the costs of becoming a consumer society. There are, however, serious health implications, with lifestyle diseases such as obesity, high blood pressure, heart disease, and diabetes claiming many lives. The costs of managing these lifestyle diseases also consume money that could have been committed to other priority areas within the health sector.

Infant-Feeding Practices: Many women breastfeed, and the weaning period varies significantly. For some time, efforts have been made by health personnel to educate mothers on the value of breastfeeding. Many mothers, however, do not breastfeed longer than a year for many reasons. In the past, mothers were encouraged to feed infants with mashed local food: taro, fish, greens, and water. With the availability of store-purchased baby foods, however, mothers are attracted to the convenience and comfort of this new lifestyle. The fertility rate is 2.94 children born per woman. The infant mortality rate is 27 deaths per 1,000 live births. Life expectancy is 68 for men, 74 for women.

Child-Rearing Practices: Child rearing is indulgent and lenient during infancy and early childhood. Mothers provide the primary care of children, but other females, especially older siblings and other relatives, also participate. As children become older, they are expected to learn to be obedient to parents, older siblings, and older village members. Fathers teach their sons how to cook, farm, fish, and perform other outdoor activities. Mothers do the same with their daughters. From early youth, children are socialized to work cooperatively and to view responsibility toward the *nuu* (village) as equally important as responsibilities to their *aiga* (family). An adult who is thought not to have met his or her obligation to either is seen as a disgrace to the *aiga*. These values are so ingrained, particularly among rural Samoans, that years of residence in Apia or abroad does not extinguish feelings of linkage and obligation to one's *aiga*, *lotu* (church), and *nuu*. However, the breakdown and weakening of family values have been on the rise in recent years. Single parenting is common and is considered a worrisome trend.

National Childhood Immunizations: BCG at birth; DTwP at 6, 10, and 14 weeks; OPV at 6, 10, and 14 weeks and at 5 years; HepB at birth and at 6 and 14 weeks; MR (measles) at 12 months; DT at 5 years; and TT antenatal at 7 and 8 months and 6 weeks postpartum. The percent of the target population vaccinated, by antigen, is: BCG and DTP1 (86%); DTP3 (64%); HepB3 (60%); MCV (57%); and Polio3 (73%).

BIBLIOGRAPHY

Central Intelligence Agency: *2006: The world factbook, Samoa*, Retrieved September 21, 2006, from https://www.cia.gov/cia/publications/factbook/print/ws.html.

Government of Samoa: *Antenatal STI clinic survey.* Apia, 2000, Ministry of Health in collaboration with the World Health Organization.

Government of Samoa: *Statement of economic strategy 2001-2001: partnership for a prosperous Samoa.* Apia, 2000, Treasury Department.

Government of Samoa: *Strategy for the development of Samoa.* Apia, 2002-2004, The Pacific Islands: an Encyclopedia.

Muliaina T: 2005. Migration and remittances: serious threats to food production in Samoa. *Just Change.* Wellington, 2005, Dev-Zone.

UNAIDS: 2006: Samoa. Retrieved September 21, 2006, from http://www.unaids.org/en/Regions_Countries/Countries/samoa.asp.

World Health Organization: 2006: Immunization, vaccines and biologicals. Retrieved September 21, 2006, from http://www.who.int/immunization_monitoring/en/globalsummary/countryprofileresult.cfm?C='wsm'.

http://hivinsite.ucsf.edu/global?page=cr04-ws-00 (retrieved March 16, 2006).

http://www.prb.org/TemplateTop.cfm?Section=PRB_Country_Profiles&template=/customsource/countryprofile/countryprofiledisplay.cfm&Country=447 (retrieved February 16, 2006).

http://www.samoa.co.uk/music&culture.html (retrieved March 16, 2006).

http://www.who.int/csr/don/archive/country/wsm/en/ (retrieved March 16, 2006).

◆ SAUDI ARABIA (KINGDOM OF)

MAP PAGE (802)

Abdulbari A. Bener

S

Location: The Kingdom of Saudi Arabia, 1,960,582 km², (758,981 square miles) occupies most of the Arabian Peninsula. The Red Sea and the Gulf of Aqaba are on the west; the Persian Gulf is on the east. A mountain range spans the length of the western coastline, and east of the mountains is a massive plateau—the Rub Al Khali (the Empty Quarter)—which contains the world's largest sand desert. Saudi Arabia borders Iraq, Jordan, Kuwait, Oman, Qatar, the United Arab Emirates, and Yemen. Almost all is semidesert and desert with oases; half is uninhabitable desert. The southwest has mountains as high as 3,000 m; it is the greenest and freshest climate in the entire country. There are no rivers or lakes. Saudi Arabia has a harsh, dry desert climate with great temperature extremes. Natural hazards include severe sand and electrical storms and flash flooding.

Major Languages	**Ethnic Groups**	**Major Religions**
Arabic (official)	Arab 90%	Muslim (official) 96%
	Afro-Asian 10%	Other 4%

The population of more than 27 million includes 5.8 million expatriate workers. Literacy rates are 85% for men, 71% for women. Most people live near the larger cities, such as the capital, Riyadh, with a small number of nomadic Bedouin tribes; 90% are ethnic Arabs, descendants of indigenous tribes that still maintain strong tribal affiliations. Arabia has been inhabited for thousand of years by nomadic Semitic tribes. The legislature is the Sharia, which is considered the law of God. The vast majority is Sunni Muslim (82%), but Shiite Muslims (14%) live on the east coast. With two of the most sacred sites in Islam (Mecca and Medina) within its borders, Saudi Arabia considers itself the birthplace and heart of Islam. There are extreme differences between rich and poor, and these differences are found in both urban and rural areas. Much development has taken place in the last 20 years because of growing profits from the oil industry. Saudi Arabia is the largest oil exporter in the world. The gross domestic product (GDP) per capita is $12,800.

Health Care Beliefs: Acute sick care; Koranic medicine; passive role. In Islam, people believe that "there is no disease that Allah has created except that He also has created its remedy, except for one ailment, namely old age." Even though advanced medical care is available, some (particularly nomadic tribes) still favor traditional Koranic medicine. According to a common traditional view, illness is not necessarily related to human behavior but is caused by spiritual agents such as *jinn*, the "evil eye" (the power of a person to harm others merely by looking at them), or the will of Allah. Prevention and treatment of disease are therefore based on appealing to the spiritual agent responsible by using methods such as prayer to Allah, votive offerings, or amulets to ward off the evil eye. Local practitioners specialize in various treatments, such as exorcism for mental illness, setting broken bones, herbal remedies, and cauterization. Consultations with untrained healers are decreasing as access to more effective health care and health education becomes available. Many believe that intrusive procedures such as injections and intravenous fluids are more effective than noninvasive ones. Nomadic tribes and people in remote areas often seek treatment only when they are in the terminal stages of an illness.

Predominant Sick-Care Practices: Biomedical and traditional healing. The health care sector has expanded rapidly, with $448 million allocated to construction and renovation of health facilities in 2005. Saudi Arabia boasts the finest medical services in the Arab World, with numerous hospitals and primary health care centers throughout the country. Good access and effective care have been reported for immunization, maternal child health care, and control of epidemic diseases.

Saudi Arabia has 330 hospitals with a capacity of about 50,000 beds, nearly 1,800 health care centers, and almost 800 private clinics. Advanced surgical procedures such as open-heart surgery and organ transplants are routinely performed. The Saudi government is the largest provider of health care services, accounting for more than 70% of health needs; and health care is free to all citizens. State-of-the-art care is available in the major cities (Riyadh, Dharan, and Jeddah) in the main hospitals affiliated with the Ministry of Defense and Aviation, the National Guard, and universities. The private sector is small, but participation is being encouraged in the provision of services, the financing of construction, management of facilities, and the production of pharmaceuticals. The treatment and rehabilitation of the mentally and physically handicapped have become a priority of the mental health and social services system.

Ethnic-/Race-Specific or Endemic Diseases: Major leading causes of morbidity include diabetes, gastrointestinal diseases, tuberculosis and other respiratory ailments, ophthalmologic conditions, cardiovascular diseases, and malaria. About 24% of adults are afflicted by type 2 diabetes, the leading cause of stroke, cardiovascular disease, blindness, kidney failure, and limb amputation. Costs of diabetic care are greater than $13 billion annually. Diabetes in Saudi Arabia is usually non–insulin dependent, and its clinical symptoms are different from those in the West. For example, patients can tolerate extremely high blood sugar levels (more than 10 times normal) and have minimal symptoms. However, the long-term consequences of the disease (e.g., peripheral vascular problems, retinopathy, renal and heart disease) are the same. Respiratory ailments are also very common as a result of the high incidence of cigarette smoking. Hepatitis is endemic throughout the Arabian Peninsula, and 80% of the indigenous population has markers for hepatitis B infection. Antimalaria control measures started in 1948 have eradicated malaria transmission in northern and eastern regions, but malaria is endemic in the Tohama Valley and Jazan regions; a control program was applied in these regions only recently. Bilharzia (schistosomiasis) is a continuing but minor problem in Jizan, Al-Bahah, Asir, Najran, Medina, Al-Jawf, Hail, and Taif. Eliminating infestations of the bilharzia parasite and preventing reinfestation are continuing challenges. Cases of leishmaniasis, both cutaneous and visceral, have occurred in almost every province along with expansion of agricultural lands, which provide breeding grounds for disease-carrying sand flies. Trachoma is considered one of the main causes of blindness, despite programs to combat the disease. Asthma is exceedingly common and tends to be seasonal, developing when the pollen count from certain grasses is high. Leprosy is decreasing. Obesity and heart disease are endemic because of changes in dietary and lifestyle habits. Poor dental hygiene is common and results in dental caries; adverse sequelae of frequent consumption of carbonated soft drinks. As of the beginning of 2004, the number of human immunodeficiency virus (HIV) infections since the epidemic began was estimated at 2,460 cases. The Joint United Nations Programme on HIV/AIDS (UNAIDS) reports HIV prevalence in adults (aged 15–49 years) as <0.2%. The main mode of transmission appears to be heterosexual, with most of the cases among male expatriates, who are usually returned to their homelands.

Health-Team Relationships: Most doctors are now Saudi nationals and tend to be well respected by their patients. Doctors are the dominant force in the health team. Most nurses are expatriates, mostly from the Philippines. Nursing is not a respected profession, and they are thought of as servants. Efforts are being made to rectify this situation through the establishment of schools of nursing to educate Saudi nationals in the science of nursing. Saudi Arabians are no longer obligated to travel abroad to obtain specialized medical treatment. Sophisticated surgical procedures are routinely performed in various Saudi hospitals to the highest international standards.

Families' Role in Hospital Care: Most patients have an attendant or sitter with them for the duration of their stay to ensure optimum care and attention. Sitters may be family members but are usually servants. Family members are often demanding because they want to ensure that patients receive proper care and attention. Gifts of sweets and chocolates are common, and families expect to be able to visit for as long as and whenever they desire. These frequent visits can conflict with dietary restrictions and hospital routines.

Dominance Patterns: The culture is patriarchal, and the oldest male family member makes all important decisions. The Saudi mother is revered, and most sons seek their mothers' opinion on family issues. Women are primarily confined to the home to run the household, and they are not expected to play a prominent role in the family; this is generally perceived as a protective measure. However, younger Saudi women are now acquiring positions in teaching and medicine in increasing numbers. Women are usually not allowed to give consent for medical procedures; husbands or brothers give consent for them. In emergency situations, a woman can give consent so long as her signature is witnessed by two men who are Saudi nationals. Although polygamy is allowed for men, it is quite uncommon.

Eye-Contact Practices: Eye contact among men is expected during conversation and is a sign of honesty and integrity. Eye contact between men and women is discouraged, and if it occurs, it is expected to be brief. Women can make direct eye contact only with other women and family members.

Touch Practices: Touching between men and women is forbidden except among family members. It is acceptable and quite common for

S

men to kiss one another on the cheek and to hold hands in public. Greetings and handshakes among men may be prolonged.

Pain Reactions: Reactions to pain are individual rather than specific to Saudi culture. Pain is expressed verbally and nonverbally and with emotion. Pain-relieving medications are demanded frequently and must be provided immediately. Bedouins tend to be more stoic than city dwellers.

Perceptions of Time: *Inshallah,* or "as Allah wills," is the norm. Inshallah can mean anything from "immediately" to "never." The concept may be used as a euphemism for "no." Time has little meaning in any situation other than business, and social rituals continue while appointments go by unheeded. It is common for people to arrive for hospital appointments late or on the wrong day.

Birth Rites: Large families are the norm and are encouraged by family pressure and state child benefits. The fertility rate is four children born per woman. The overwhelming preference is for male children, particularly for the firstborn. Husbands can divorce women if they do not bear sons. Childlessness is pitied, and infertility is considered a condition that must be rectified. Most Saudi women prefer a doctor rather than a midwife for the birth. Celebrations and congratulations are effusive but are delayed for up to 3 months after birth. Women are considered unclean after birth and may be sequestered in their home or, more commonly, in their mother's home for up to 40 days. The infant mortality rate is 13 deaths per 1,000 live births (down from 51 in 2001). Life expectancy is 74 for men, 78 for women.

Death Rites: It is believed that only Allah knows the true prognosis for a patient, so confronting a patient with a grave prognosis shatters hope and can create mistrust. Islamic regulations *(Fatwah)* state that life support can be discontinued if certain conditions are met. Transplantation of human organs is completely acceptable; however, the desires of the family are considered the most important factor. Death is usually discussed only with male family members. After death, the body must be washed ceremonially (possibly by a family member), after which no non-Muslim is allowed to touch the body. Interment is usually carried out within 1 day, and the body is buried in the ground wrapped in a shroud without a coffin. Cremation is not allowed, and autopsies are rare because the body must be buried intact. When a family member dies, male family members are expected to repress any outward signs of grief. Women are frequently very vocal, wailing and ululating. Men and women receive condolences in separate venues for up to 3 days after death.

Food Practices and Intolerances: The traditional diet is rice, chicken, fish, and a small amount of red meat. Dates and *laban* (buttermilk) are common snacks. All types of ethnic, international, and fast foods are available in towns and cities. The standard and variety of cuisine are among the best in the world. It is acceptable to eat with the fingers of the right hand, particularly at communal feasts. Pork, blood, carrion, and alcohol consumption is forbidden, so they are not imported into the country. Fasting between sunset and sundown is mandatory during the holy month of

Ramadan for all people other than pregnant women, breastfeeding mothers, children, and the ill, although some hospitalized patients choose to fast anyway. Eating, drinking, and smoking are forbidden in public places during Ramadan.

Infant-Feeding Practices: Breastfeeding is the preferred method; it is acceptable in public and may continue for 18 months to 2 years. However, many mothers actually employ "wet nurses," and thereafter the care of the children is transferred to either an older female sibling or a maid. Infants who are not breastfed are generally fed with premixed formulas or dried Nido milk. A random cross-sectional survey conducted in the Kingdom between 2000 and 2001 reported that partial breastfeeding was the dominant mode of infant feeding for 66% of the mothers who breastfed their infants. Exclusive breastfeeding was the next most common for 27% of mothers. Exclusive bottle-feeding was the least common (7%).

Child-Rearing Practices: Child rearing tends to be permissive. Discipline is inconsistent and is largely the responsibility of the female members of the family. Care is often the responsibility of older female siblings or servants. Families are generally large, and several families live in the same housing compound. Children today spend many hours watching television; creating widespread childhood obesity and exercise-shy children. Education is free for all, but boys and girls are educated separately. Boys are raised in the female section of the household until they are 10 years of age; then they are transferred to the male part of the household. Parenting is largely the responsibility of the father from this point on. Discipline is strict and firmly enforced. Girls are considered adults by the age of 12 or at puberty. Although it has been outlawed, circumcision of girls still occurs on occasion, and it remains fairly common among Sudanese expatriate workers' families.

National Childhood Immunizations: BCG at birth; DTwP at 4 to 6 years; DTwPHib at 18 months; DTwPHibHep at 2, 4, and 6 months; HepB at birth; MMR at 1 and 4 to 6 years; OPV at 2, 4, 6, and 18 months and at 4 to 6 years. The percent of the target population vaccinated, by antigen, is: BCG, DTP3, HepB3, Hib, MCV, and Polio3 (96%); DTP1 (97%). Child allowances are paid only after proof of completion of childhood vaccinations. Also, 54% of pregnant women have a tetanus vaccination before their delivery.

BIBLIOGRAPHY

Al-Ahmadi H, Roland M: Quality of primary health care in Saudi Arabia: a comprehensive review, *Int J Qual Health Care.* 17(4):331–346, 2005.

Central Intelligence Agency: 2006: *The world factbook, Saudi Arabia.* Retrieved September 21, 2006, from https://www.cia.gov/cia/publications/factbook/print/sa.html.

Health Statistical Year Book, 2003: Riyadh, Kingdom of Saudi Arabia.

Ogbeide DO, Siddiqui S, Al Khalifa IM, Karim A: Breast feeding in a Saudi Arabian community: profile of parents and influencing factors, *Saudi Med J.* 25(5):580–584, 2004.

S

World Health Organization: 2006: Immunization, vaccines and biologicals. Retrieved September 21, 2006, from http://www.who.int/immunization_monitoring/en/globalsummary/countryprofileresult.cfm?C='sau'.

http://www.emro.who.int/emrinfo/index.asp (retrieved January 15, 2006).

http://www.espicom.com/web.nsf/structure/med_bksmaudi (retrieved January 3, 2006).

http://www.hejleh.com/countries/saudi.html (retrieved January 3, 2006).

http://www.infoplease.com/ipa/A0107947.html (retrieved January 15, 2006).

◆ SENEGAL (REPUBLIC OF)

MAP PAGE (800)

Stephen E. Hawes

Location: Senegal is the westernmost country on the African continent, lying on the Atlantic coast. Mauritania is to the north, Mali is to the east, and Guinea and Guinea-Bissau are to the south. Senegal encircles the Gambia on three sides. The northern border is formed by the Senegal River, and other rivers include the Gambia and Casamance. The capital, Dakar, is a sprawling city of 2.5 million; it lies on the Cap-Vert peninsula, the westernmost point on the African continent. Senegal is a developing country comprising a rural population that lives by subsistence farming and a large urban population that are nearly equal in proportion. Much of Senegal is characterized by low, rolling plains, with foothills in the southeast and rainy (June to October) and dry seasons. The total area is 196,190 km^2 (75,749 square miles), and the population is 12 million. The gross domestic product (GDP) per capita is $1,800, with about 54% living below the poverty line.

Major Languages	Ethnic Groups	Major Religions
French (official)	Wolof 43%	Muslim 94%
Wolof	Pular 24%	Christian 5%
Pulaar	Serer 15%	Indigenous beliefs (1%)
Diola	Diola 4%	
Mandinka	Mandinka, Soninke, European, Lebanese 4%	

The Wolofs are the most represented ethnic group and make up the majority of the population in all regions. More than 50 distinct languages are spoken, but 80% speak Wolof. Literacy rates are 50% for men, 31% for women.

Health Care Beliefs: Traditional and biomedical with some prevention. Both traditional healing and modern medical treatments are available in urban areas, but fewer than 40% have access. Preventive medicine and health promotion, especially with respect to infectious diseases, is

Senegal (Republic of)   **617**

increasing. The Joint United Nations Programme on HIV/AIDS (UNAIDS) and the Senegalese Ministry of Health have sponsored mass media interventions, targeted information campaigns, promotion of volunteer human immunodeficiency virus (HIV) counseling and testing, and research to help slow the spread of HIV/AIDS. Other health programs are being conducted, such as child survival programs (nutritionally focused), prevention of malaria during pregnancy, and promotion of oral rehydration therapy for the treatment of diarrheal disease in children. Male circumcision is nearly universal and usually takes place between the ages of 5 and 7. Female genital circumcision was recently outlawed but is still common in some ethnic groups, mostly in rural areas.

Predominant Sick-Care Practices: Acute sick care and traditional healing. People often attempt other methods before they seek modern medical treatment; about 90% of the population has used the services of around 5,500 traditional healers. Traditional practitioners are generally more accessible, affordable, and culturally accepted. Health centers are usually located in cities, and so rural inhabitants might be hours from the nearest clinic. There is a large disparity in the quality and extent of health services between urban and rural regions. Access to medicine is limited also by an inadequate supply of drugs, and even critical drugs are often missing in health centers and private pharmacies. Expense is another barrier to access, especially in rural Senegal. Self-medication is a common practice, and the illegal sale of drugs is common. Traditional herbal remedies are still commonplace, especially in rural Senegal. Mystical medicine, performed by healers, often combines both the physiologic and psychological aspects of treatment. A Senegalese who is seeking cure for sickness often pursues multiple traditional methods of therapy, including amulets (*gris-gris*), herbal teas or potions, spirit divination, holy water, and Koranic readings in addition to, or before, seeking Western therapy. Immunizations against vaccine-preventable diseases are becoming more common, despite fears that vaccines diminish fertility. Cancer screening is rare, even for the highly educated. Dentistry is available in urban areas but is most often for treatment of dental problems. Most Senegalese use dental chewing sticks (*socc*) for teeth cleaning. Senegal has good office-based psychiatric services but no inpatient facility.

Ethnic-/Race-Specific or Endemic Diseases: Senegal suffers from health problems that can be attributed to extreme poverty, with almost 25% of the population suffering from malnutrition. There is a high rate of infectious and parasitic diseases. Endemic diseases include West Nile virus; trachoma; bilharziasis; goiter (which is regional); hepatitis A, B, and C; schistosomiasis (resistant to, or tolerant of, praziquantel); and intestinal parasites (amebiasis). Chloroquine-resistant malaria is mesoendemic, particularly during the rainy season, and is the primary cause of disease morbidity. People are at risk for yellow fever, onchocerciasis (which is regional), chanchroid, tuberculosis, measles, borreliosis, cholera, typhoid fever, and meningitis. Cholera outbreaks are a recurring hazard during the rainy season in much of Senegal, and recent outbreaks of yellow fever, chikungunya fever, and meningococcal infections have been reported. Schistosomiasis was recently introduced during building of the Diama dam on the Senegal River. As a result of early mobilization, Senegal is considered one of the success stories of HIV/AIDS prevention. UNAIDS estimates the prevalence rate for HIV in adults (aged 15 to 49 years) to be 0.9%, with 61,000 people living with HIV, including 33,000 women and 5,000 children aged 0 to 14 years. Deaths from acquired immunodeficiency syndrome (AIDS) are estimated at 5,200; and there are 25,000 orphans due to parental AIDS. This low prevalence is attributed to strong political leadership, early involvement of religious leaders, and a comprehensive strategic approach; including systematic testing of the blood supply, registration and medical monitoring of commercial sex workers, and promotion of condom use. Free or low-cost antiretroviral therapy is available to most people who need it.

Health-Team Relationships: Senegal lacks health care facilities and trained personnel. Only 40% of the population has access to health services. There are 17 regional hospitals, with 7 located in Dakar; 52 district health centers (Centre de Santé); and 900 health posts (Poste de Santé). In addition, there are two university hospitals and numerous private clinics. Senegal's rates of doctors, health workers, and birth attendants per population are far below the standards set by the World Health Organization, and training and education are lacking. Relationships between doctors and nurses are very hierarchical, with doctors dominating interactions. Public hospitals do not meet Western standards, but private clinics are considered to be at the level of small European hospitals and approaching American community hospital standards. Outside Dakar, facilities and trained personnel are limited.

Families' Role in Hospital Care: Families and neighbors share responsibilities for patient care, including meals, when a family member or neighbor is hospitalized. All hospitals have areas where families set up and cook meals for sick family members.

Dominance Patterns: Customs relative to family life and women are consistent with Islamic culture. Respect for elders is of great importance. Male-female relationships are usually initiated by men. Marriage usually follows traditional Islamic custom with an overlay of ethnic practices and is an elaborate celebration. Polygamy is still common, and it is usually regarded as a sign of wealth to have up to four wives, the maximum allowed by Islamic law. Wives usually live together in the husband's compound, and the first wife holds the senior position. In rural areas, co-wives may share a common living room and visit their husband's room on a rotational basis. Although men marry at a somewhat later age, most women marry between the ages of 14 to 20 (20 to 30 in urban areas). Marriage is primarily an arrangement between two families, not between individuals, especially when it is a case of a second or third wife, although today the couple to be wed is usually consulted and their wishes respected. Although there is a general principle that women should be obedient to men, women have a degree of choice in negotiating their status and authority within the family. Husbands are generally responsible for bring-ing food, building houses, repairing fences, and similar tasks. The father teaches his sons how to farm and sends them to circumcision camps. Sons take care of their parents financially and materially, and fathers arrange marriages for their children in consultation with his parents. Wives are responsible for all domestic chores and the education of children. Women guide daughters about whom they should marry.

Eye-Contact Practices: It is considered impolite to look at older people directly because to do so is a sign of disrespect. Children should not look into their parents' eyes. Direct eye contact is much less common than in other parts of the world.

Touch Practices: Greetings are an essential aspect of Senegalese culture, the importance of which cannot be overemphasized. It is important to shake everyone's hand, even the youngest child. Elders are generally greeted first. Senegalese do not use their left hand in eating, handing out things (especially money), or greeting people. If one has to use the left hand (if the right hand is wet or dirty, for example), the person apologizes for doing so. The Wolof expression *baal ma camon* means "excuse my left hand" and is used for this purpose. People shake hands as often as they see each other during dif-ferent times of the day. Women, especially in villages, are not normally expected to shake hands when greeting. Also, physical affection for a loved one or emotion in general is not openly shown in public.

Perceptions of Time: The pace of life is relaxed, and there is a greater emphasis on relationships rather than on how many tasks one can accom-plish in a day. In rural areas, it is considered safer to stay at home after dusk because evil sprits and wild animals are most active at this time.

Pain Reactions: Senegalese culture tends to emphasize control of emo-tions. Showing pain is synonymous with weakness, especially for adult men, who should never cry in public. It is acceptable for women to express their emotions when they are in physical or emotional pain, for example, when mourning the loss of a loved one.

Birth Rites: Having children is considered very important in Senegalese life. The fertility rate is 4.38 children born per woman; and the infant mor-tality rate is very high at 53 deaths per 1,000 births. About half of all births are attended by a skilled birth attendant; in rural areas, the maternal grandmother often acts as midwife. Especially in rural areas, women want many children. Knowledge of contraception is near universal, but less than 20% of women use birth control (2% in rural areas). A great deal of mys-tery surrounds pregnancy and childbirth. Senegalese believe that talking about the pregnancy could endanger the life of the baby. After a baby is born, numerous ritual precautions are taken. Among some ethnic groups, a fire burns continuously in the house for the first week, during which time the mother remains indoors. One week after the infant's birth, a ceremony takes place to reveal the child's name. Children are usually named by the father's side of the family after relatives or friends. It is customary in many communities to sacrifice an animal when a newborn child is given a name. Life expectancy is 58 for men, 61 for women.

S

Death Rites: Muslim doctors may recommend transfusions to save lives. Autopsies are uncommon because the body must be buried intact. The body is wrapped in special pieces of cloth and buried without a coffin in the ground as soon as possible after death. Cremations are not permitted. As on other ceremonial occasions, some Islamic rituals are superimposed on traditional ethnic practices; no less so when a death occurs. Burial of the body must occur within 6 hours if at all possible or the following morning if death occurs late in the day. Arrangements are made by family elders or respected members of the community, especially those versed in Islamic ritual. The body is washed following a special rite, perfumed, and wrapped in a percale cloth. Then the body is taken to the mosque for prayers, or it remains in the compound until the burial. It is customary to sacrifice an animal during funerals. The widow must remain in seclusion for 4½ months, when special prayers are said. In certain ethnic groups, the practice of *levirate,* in which a man is obligated to take as his wife the widow of a deceased brother, is common. Similarly, *sororat,* in which a woman marries the spouse of her deceased sister, is also practiced.

Food Practices and Intolerances: The vast majority of the population is Muslim, so pork, carrion, blood, and alcohol consumption are generally forbidden. Rice and millet are the major staple food crops. The rural population relies mainly on staple foods such as millet and sorghum, often served with dried fish and sauces. However, the urban population relies more on imported grains such as rice and on fresh fish and meat. A rice and fish dish (*tiéboudienne*) is the most common midday meal. Food tends to be spicy. Ramadan fasting is practiced, with exemptions for the sick and certain other individuals. At the Muslim Feast of the Lamb (*Tabaski*), a whole sheep is slaughtered and grilled for family and friends. Traditional-style meals are generally served with participants seated on floor mats in a circle around the food, which is served in one or two large bowls, one of which usually contains rice. Food is normally eaten with the right hand and is taken from the part of the bowl in front of the person. Meals are often large in quantity and geared to feed large families.

Infant-Feeding Practices: Most women in rural areas breastfeed their children, and the median age at weaning is about 24 months, the age prescribed by Islamic canon.

Child-Rearing Practices: About 44% of the population is 14 years of age or younger. In urban areas, education of children, including girls, is widely accepted. However, formal education is less common in rural areas. Although many children attend elementary school, only 21% of school age children attend middle school. Mothers and members of the community traditionally raise children; the father is in charge of religious education. Daughters often stay with the mother as they grow older, and sons spend more time with fathers. About 14% of all children born in Senegal die before their fifth birthday.

National Childhood Immunizations: BCG at birth; DTwP at 6, 10, and 14 weeks; DTwPHibHep at 10 and 14 weeks; DTwPHibHep at 6 weeks (from July 2005); HepB at 6, 10, and 14 weeks; OPV at birth and 6, 10, and 14 weeks; measles at 9 months; YFV at 9 months; and TT for pregnant women, +1, +6 months, +1, +1 year. The percent of the target population vaccinated, by antigen, is: BCG and DTP1 (95%); DTP3 (87%); HepB3 (54%); MCV (57%); Polio3 (87%); and TT2 plus (85%).

Other Characteristics: Senegal remains one of the most stable democracies in Africa. Commercial sex is legal (since the 1960s) and is carefully monitored. Prostitutes get free condoms and mandatory medical examinations, including testing for sexually transmitted infections.

BIBLIOGRAPHY

Africa Consultants International: Retrieved September 1, 2006, from http://www.lclark.edu/~nicole/SENEGAL/HOME.HTM.

Central Intelligence Agency: 2006: *The world factbook, Senegal.* Retrieved September 21, 2006, from https://www.cia.gov/cia/publications/factbook/print/sg.html.

Centre Africain de l'Entrepreneuriat Feminin (CAEF): Interviews with Dr. Papa Salif Sow and Macoumba Toure, Dakar, Senegal, July 21, 2001, 2006, Muslim Women and Development Action Research Project, Senegal, 2001.

Fatou S: Fundamentalisms, globalization and women's human rights in Senegal. *Gender and Development,* 11:69–76, 2003.

Seybold D: Choosing therapies: a Senegalese woman's experience with infertility, *Health Care Women Int.* 23:540–549, 2002.

UNAIDS: 2006 Senegal. Retrieved September 21, 2006, from http://www.unaids.org/en/Regions_Countries/Countries/senegal.asp.

USAID Health Profile: Senegal. Retrieved September 1, 2006, from http://www.usaid.gov/locations/sub-saharan_africa/countries/senegal/.

U.S. Department of State: Country reports on human rights practices—Senegal. Released by the Bureau of Democracy, Human Rights, and Labor, 2002. Retrieved September 1, 2006, from http://www.state.gov/g/drl/rls/hrrpt/2001/af/8400.htm.

World Health Organization: 2006: Immunization, vaccines and biologicals. Retrieved September 21, 2006, from http://www.who.int/immunization_monitoring/en/globalsummary/countryprofileresult.cfm?C='sen'.

◆ SERBIA (REPUBLIC OF)

MAP PAGE (798)

Snezana Bosnjak, Draga Plecas, and Ana Jovicevic Bekic

Location: The Republic of Serbia is located in southeastern Europe on the Balkan Peninsula; the capital is Belgrade. It borders Hungary on the north, Croatia and Bosnia-Herzegovina on the west, Montenegro and Albania on the southwest, and Macedonia and Bulgaria on the southeast. Serbia is mainly flat, but its central and southern areas consist of highlands and mountains. Serbia includes two autonomous provinces: (1) Vojvodina and (2) Kosovo and Metohija. Kosovo and Metohija have been governed by the United Nations Interim Administration Mission in Kosovo

S

(UNMIK) since June 1999 under the authority of the UN Security Council Resolution 1244. The total area is 88,361 km^2 (34,116 square miles) and the population is 9.4 million. The gross domestic product (GDP) per capita is $4,400, with 30% living below the poverty line. Literacy rates are 99% for men, 94% for women.

Major Languages	Ethnic Groups	Major Religions
Serbian (primary)	Serb 66%	Christian Orthodox (Serbs)
Albanian	Albanian 17%	Muslim (Albanians)
Hungarian	Hungarian 4%	Roman Catholic (Albanians
	Other 14%	and Hungarians)

Health Care Beliefs: Western; traditional; active and passive roles. People generally believe in biomedical care. The health care system is organized on three levels: the first (primary) has a well-developed network of outpatient services and primary health care centers providing services to residents of their respective municipalities. The secondary level includes general hospitals and health care centers. The third, the tertiary level, includes clinics and clinical centers. There is also a network of public health institutions and a private sector, but services are not covered by state insurance. Prevention of infectious disease is well organized and functions adequately. However, health care measures for the prevention of chronic and noncommunicable diseases are insufficient and poorly implemented because of the lack of national policies and the inadequate, low health care budget. Programs for cancer prevention, early detection, and public education on cancer are organized mainly by oncologic institutions, institutes of public health, medical faculties, and cancer societies on their own or in coordination with one another.

Predominant Sick-Care Practices: Biomedical and traditional. All Serbians are a part of a national health care system. Private practice exists as well. In Kosovo and Metohija, the ethnic Albanian population has set up a parallel health care system. The resident population of the province occasionally uses the state and the parallel systems, although no official data exist on the latter.

Ethnic-/Race-Specific or Endemic Diseases: The five most commonly diagnosed diseases are acute respiratory tract infections, hypertension, diseases of the skeleton and connective tissue, neurotic and personality disorders, and acute bronchitis. So-called endemic nephropathy (idiopathic tubulointerstitial nephropathy) is an endemic disease. The leading causes of death are circulatory diseases (62% of deaths), malignancies (19%), and respiratory diseases (4%). The Programme for acquired immunodeficiency syndrome (AIDS) prevention and control was adopted in 1995. In the past 3 to 4 years, the incidence of AIDS is 5 to 9 cases per million; and the mortality rate has fallen from greater than 8 in 1995 to fewer than 4 in 2000. However, cases are most likely underreported given that the last report from Kosovo and Metohija is from 1997. Of the 860 AIDS cases reported so far, most have been in intravenous drug users (413), followed by heterosexuals (164); homosexuals, bisexuals (122), and mother-to-child transmission (7). No accurate statistics are available for the Kosovo and Metohija region. Life expectancy is 70 for men, 74 for women.

Health-Team Relationships: Communication and cooperation between doctors and nurses are usually good, although nurses are subordinate. Generally, patients communicate more openly with nurses. Recently, nurses have been making greater and more active contributions to the health team, especially those on multidisciplinary palliative care teams. Practitioners treating people with cancer, AIDS, and other chronic debilitating diseases are also beginning to include social workers, psychologists, psychiatrists, and hospital chaplains on their health care teams.

Families' Role in Hospital Care: Family and friends are important because they support hospitalized relatives. They visit patients very frequently and bring them food, sweets, and clothes. Mothers stay with hospitalized infants and young children when possible.

Dominance Patterns: In urban, educated populations, there are few differences between men and women in terms of dominance. In rural populations, however, men are more dominant, and infant boys are more appreciated than infant girls. In Kosovo and Metohija (and other Muslim populations), men are totally dominant.

Eye-Contact Practices: Direct eye contact is acceptable.

Touch Practices: Physical touching is acceptable, but in the Muslim population in Kosovo and Metohija, medical services staffed by non-Muslim and non-Albanian practitioners are considered unacceptable.

Perceptions of Time: Serbians are generally punctual.

Pain Reactions: It is common for Serbians to accept and tolerate suffering. Individuals react to pain with a reasonable level of stoicism. Patients report pain reluctantly because they do not want to be considered weak or complainers. They also refuse to take pain medications, especially opioids, for chronic pain, because of fears about addiction or because they believe pain is necessary for salvation. Cancer patients are reluctant to take morphine for pain control because of its strong association with death and dying, and taking it is considered a sign of weakness and a "last resort."

Birth Rites: Serbia has a national program for prenatal health that includes pregnancy confirmations, laboratory tests, blood pressure and weight monitoring, obstetric examinations, health-behavior counseling, and ultrasounds. It is recommended that every pregnant woman visit a maternal care clinic at least four times during her pregnancy and 6 weeks after delivery. The fertility rate is 1.78 children born per woman. Antenatal classes that offer psychophysical preparation for childbirth are available. Nearly all deliveries are attended by a health care team that includes an obstetrician and a midwife. Child mortality is 17 deaths per 1,000 for boys and 13 for girls. The proportion of hospital visits has consistently been in the high 90th percentiles, with the constant exception of Kosovo and Metohija (77% in 1990). Almost all births take place in one of the

S

74 maternity wards across the country, and some take place in one of the 12 outpatient maternity wards. In Kosovo and Metohija, as well as in the rural populations of Serbia, the birth of a son is celebrated more than the birth of a daughter. Birth rates are decreasing. Life expectancy is 71 for men, 76 for women.

Death Rites: Serbians generally focus on the quantity of life rather than its quality. Dying is not easily accepted and is perceived tragically. However, occasionally death provides relief from suffering and pain (e.g., for patients with cancer). Family members and close friends of a dying person are usually present. After the person dies, visits from all relatives, friends, and neighbors are expected. Family members and close friends of the deceased dress in black and are in mourning for at least 40 days after the death. Organ donations are acceptable but rare. Autopsies are performed if they are medically necessary but usually require verbal consent from the family.

Food Practices and Intolerances: Diet varies according to region and religion. In the northern and central part of Serbia, the typical diet consists of milk and dairy products (e.g., soft cheese), vegetables, legumes, wheat and corn flour products, fruit, and meat (primarily pork, especially in Vojvodina). Fish is eaten occasionally. In Kosovo province and among Muslim people, pork is excluded (mutton and beef are consumed).

Infant-Feeding Practices: Breastfeeding has never been completely abandoned and is always the first choice. Bottle-feeding is used when a mother is unable to breastfeed and to supplement breast milk.

Child-Rearing Practices: Child-rearing practices are permissive but vary with the educational level of the parents, location of the family, ethnicity, and religion. Children in Muslim communities in urban or rural settings must attend religious classes at local mosques during weekends.

National Childhood Immunizations: BCG at birth; DTwP at 8, 16, and 20 weeks and at 18 months; OPV at 8, 14, and 20 weeks, at 18 months, and at 7 and 14 years; HepB at 8 and 14 weks and 12 months; MMR at 1 and 12 years; DT at 7 years; Td at 14 years; and TT at 18 years. The percent of the target population vaccinated, by antigen, is: BCG (98% in 2000; 93% in Kosovo and Metohija province); DTP3 (95% in 2000; 89% in Kosovo and Metohija province); OPV3 (98% in 2000; 89% in Kosovo and Metohija province); and MMR (91% in 2000; 84% in Kosovo and Metohija province).

BIBLIOGRAPHY

Bosnjak S, Miliæeviæ N, Lakiæeviæ J: 2006: Palliative care in Serbia and Montenegro: where are we now? *Arch Oncol. 2006;* 141:8–10.

Central Intelligence Agency: 2006: *The world factbook, Serbia,* Retrieved September 21, 2006, from https://www.cia.gov/cia/publications/factbook/print/rb.html.

Federal Republic of Yugoslavia: National report on follow-up to the World Summit for Children. 2001, Government of FR Yugoslavia.

Savezni Zavod za Statistiku: Stanovnistvo i prirodno kretanje stanovnistva SR Jugoslavije u 20. I na pragu 21. veka, saopstenje 035, str. 15, Beograd 2002.

World Health Organization: 2006: Immunization, vaccines and biologicals. Retrieved September 21, 2006, from http://www.who.int/immunization_monitoring/en/globalsummary/countryprofileresult.cfm?C='scg'.

S

Janković S, Vlajinac H, Bjegović V, Marinković J, Šipetić-Grujičić S, Marković-Denić L, Kocev N, Šantrić-Milićević M, Terzić-Šupić Z, Maksimović N, Laaser U: *The burden of disease and injury in Serbia*. Belgrade, 2003, Ministry of Health of the Republic of Serbia.

http://www.pallcare.belgrade2005.org.yu/ Data on Serbia from the website of the European Conference on Palliative Care (retrieved August 20, 2006).

✦ SEYCHELLES (REPUBLIC OF)

MAP PAGE (801)

Conrad Shamlaye and Heather Shamlaye

Location: A group of 115 islands scattered in the western Indian Ocean, east of Kenya and northeast of Madagascar, forms the Seychelles. The total area is 455 km² (176 square miles). The population of 81,541 is found mainly on the three granitic islands of Mahé, Praslin, and La Digue. The capital is Victoria. Many of the islands are uninhabited coral atolls. The islands were all uninhabited until the latter part of the eighteenth century, when French settlers and African slaves colonized them. Later coming under British rule, the population grew with European settlers, liberated African slaves from the eastern coast of Africa, and Indian and Chinese immigrants. French and African cultural influences remain strong. The climate is tropical marine: a cooler season during the southeast monsoon from late May to September, a warmer season during the northwest monsoon from March to May. Water supply is dependent on catchment of rainwater. Seychelles is outside of the cyclone belt. Literacy is fairly high: about 92% for both men and women. About 92% of the population speaks Creole, 5% speak English, and 3% speak various other languages. The gross domestic product (GDP) per capita is $7,800.

Major Languages	Ethnic Groups	Major Religions
Seychellois Creole (official)	Seychellois 100%	Roman Catholic 90%
English (official)		Protestant 8%
French (official)		Other, none 2%

The population is predominantly of African origin, but intermarriage among Africans, Europeans, Indians, and Chinese has occurred. The Seychellois are proud of their unique national identity, and ethnic origin is not considered relevant. Small communities of Bahai's, Muslims, and Hindus have been established. Seychelles is classified as a middle-income country. Literacy rates are 91% for men, 92% for women. With most professionals training outside the country, frequent travel by all sectors of the population, regular contact with tourists, and universal access to communications such as the Internet, the Seychelles is open to international influences.

S

Health Care Beliefs: Active and passive roles. As a result of health education and promotion efforts, the concept of illness and disease are generally
based on scientific understanding. Some older people retain beliefs that illness may arise from the evil intentions of others. There is a long tradition
of using herbal home remedies for minor ailments and for boosting health.
Consulting herbalists, usually in addition to, rather than as an alternative to
a doctor, is not unusual. There is growing interest in legalizing and regulating
herbalists as a means of promoting potentially useful natural therapies, and
discarding incorrect magical practices, but progress in this regard has been
hampered by the past association of herbalism with witchcraft: practitioners
were consulted frequently to cause harm to others or to seek protection
from evil. Illnesses such as epilepsy or mental disorders are not stigmatized. On the contrary, there is increasing awareness of the rights and needs
of disabled, elderly, and other potentially vulnerable groups.

Predominant Sick-Care Practices: Biomedical; traditional; and alternative. People readily turn to doctors and the biomedical health system.
Because of the policy of decentralizing health care services, community
health centers are found throughout the main populated islands, and there
is a high level of use. Health care is provided free at the point of use to all
citizens. Services include those in the predominantly government-funded
modern health care system of health centers staffed by multidisciplinary
teams, and a central referral hospital offering specialist services. The
number of individual private medical and dental practitioners is growing,
as is the number of complementary health practitioners.

Ethnic-/Race-Specific or Endemic Diseases: Changes in lifestyle
have resulted in an epidemiologic transition whereby cardiovascular diseases now account for more than a third of all mortalities. Cancers are
the second largest cause. Childhood infectious diseases have mostly disappeared. In early 2006, there was an epidemic of chikungunya (4,650
reported cases). With the assistance of the World Health Organization
(WHO), a public health campaign was launched that focused on education
and reduction of mosquitos by destroying breeding sites, which led to a
rapid decline. Although there are no significant water-borne infections, diseases such as chikungunya (most recently) and dengue fever (in the past)
reflect the susceptibility of the country to insect-borne infections that
might be introduced from neighboring countries. Cases of leptospirosis,
often arising from occupational exposure, reflect endemic infection in
rats, which are the main reservoirs. In general, the health awareness of
the people is high, and there are no particular ethnic or cultural differences in people's utilization of health care services. Awareness is increasing that men need to be targeted by specific preventive programs
because of the increasing prevalence of cardiovascular diseases as well
as excessive alcohol consumption. The Joint United Nations Programme
on HIV/AIDS (UNAIDS) has no reported prevalence rate for HIV. According
to Seychelles statistics, there were 18 cases per 10,000 people at the
end of 2005. UNAIDS has noted that despite the apparent low prevalence,
the epidemic is progressing. Data from laboratory-based HIV surveillance

indicate that the number of infected persons is increasing. Factors that might be contributing to the steady increase in cases are the common practice of nonregular or multiple sexual partners and high rates of unprotected sex, as evidenced by high numbers of sexually transmitted infections, teenage pregnancies, and abortions.

Health-Team Relationships: A large proportion of doctors and dentists are non-nationals (Indians, Cubans, Africans, and Europeans) on 2-year contracts. Difficulties in communication sometimes arise because of doctors who do not speak Creole and have to use nurses or nursing assistants as interpreters. Most patients expect to engage in a dialogue with their doctors to receive explanation and advice. They expect a thorough consultation and complain when they feel they have not been adequately examined. Community health teams are usually led by a nurse-manager who is well accepted by the community, and in the hospital setting there is shared leadership between doctor and nurse. Emphasis is on professional team building, and there is good collaboration with social services, schools, and community organizations. Health professionals are expected to be aware of, and responsive to, the needs of their patients and families. Doctors and nurses carry out home visits, both for individual patient care and as a means of getting to know the patient's social setting.

Families' Role in Hospital Care: The Seychellois are quite dependent on service providers (e.g., health care, social services, housing) and tend to expect early referrals to specialists and hospitalization. As a result, there is an increasing trend toward hospital-based care and use of laboratory and radiologic diagnostic facilities. Waiting lists for operations are generally measured in weeks. Apart from the case of young children and the terminally ill, family members are not encouraged to remain with the patient overnight. As a rule, family members do not take part in the care of patients in the hospital, and all meals are provided.

Dominance Patterns: The society is matriarchal in the sense that women head many households and succeed in housing, feeding, clothing, and bringing up their children with little help from the children's fathers. Consequently, many children are given their mother's surname. Although it is becoming more common for men to share in household duties, many working women still passively accept that men, even unemployed men, expect women to see to all child care and domestic chores.

Eye-Contact Practices: Eye contact is normal in conversation, and avoidance of eye contact is considered impolite or a sign of falseness. Patients expect to make eye contact with service providers of both genders.

Touch Practices: Greetings usually involve shaking hands and, among friends and relatives (male to female and female to female), kissing on both cheeks. Generally, there are no barriers to physical examination, although the presence of a nurse is compulsory when a doctor carries out an intimate examination.

Perceptions of Time: People are time conscious, and they expect to be seen on time and to have services provided courteously and efficiently.

Patients frequently arrive well before their appointment time and complain if they have to wait too long.

Pain Reactions: Patients are generally quite stoic about enduring pain, and older persons in particular may delay seeking medical attention. Early ambulation is common after surgical operations. However, there is often a prolonged feeling of disability if individuals are unable to resume work after surgery or even from illnesses such as high blood pressure and diabetes.

Birth Rites: Children are highly valued. Nearly all deliveries occur in hospitals, and home deliveries are not considered acceptable. The infant mortality rate is 15.4 deaths per 1,000 live births. An increasing number of fathers are present at the birth. There are no particular birth rites and no gender preferences. The fertility rate is 1.74 children born per woman (replacement level for Seychelles), and three of four births occur outside marriage. Women tend to take on most responsibilities for child rearing, and the father is frequently absent. Life expectancy is 67 for men, 78 for women.

Death Rites: Extended families are still common, although there is growing pressure for the government to provide residence and care for the elderly. Dying at home is becoming less common as hospitalization and care in institutions increase. Families strongly feel the need for patients to be attended by a priest before death. No particular death rites are favored. Church funerals are attended not only by immediate family and friends but also by distant relatives and acquaintances. Postmortem medical examinations are generally accepted if the relatives are approached with sensitivity. Organ donations are not sought, and there are no legal provisions for it.

Food Practices and Intolerances: The Seychellois diet, like many other aspects of the culture, is in a state of transition. Consumption of fish is common, usually highly spiced and eaten with rice and vegetables. Root crops such as cassava and sweet potatoes are consumed, although perhaps less frequently than in the past. Eggs, fresh and processed meat, pasta, and potatoes are increasing parts of the diet, and fast-food outlets are becoming more common. The consumption of carbonated soft drinks is alarmingly high, especially by children.

Infant-Feeding Practices: Breastfeeding rates are high in the first few weeks but drop rapidly after the completion of maternity leave (12 weeks). Some women believe that when a woman resumes sexual relations she should stop breastfeeding because sperm will enter the breast milk and harm the baby.

Child-Rearing Practices: Childrearing practices are generally permissive, but beating children, especially boys, to discipline them is widely practiced, especially by fathers and stepfathers. Corporal punishment is no longer permitted in schools. Both parents and teachers frequently shout at children. Girls are still generally expected to do more housework than boys.

National Childhood Immunizations: BCG birth and 6 years; DT at 6 years; DTwP at 3, 4, 5, and 18 months; OPV at 3, 4, 5, 18 months and at 6 and 15 years; HepB at 3, 4, and 9 months; MMR at 15 months and 6 years; YF at 12 months; TT 15 and after 25 years. The percent of the target population vaccinated, by antigen, is: BCG, DTP1, DTP3, HepB3, MCV, and Polio3 (99%).

BIBLIOGRAPHY

Central Intelligence Agency: 2006: *The world factbook, Seychelles.* Retrieved September 21, 2006, from https://www.cia.gov/cia/publications/factbook/print/se.html.

Government of Seychelles (Ministry of Health): *Annual reports,* 2005.

Government of Seychelles (National Statistics Bureau): *Statistical Bulletin* August 2006.

Government of Seychelles (Ministry of Health): *National strategy for the prevention and control of HIV/AIDS and STIs, 2005.*

Govinden P, Henderson J, Rizvi Z, Seth V, Shamlaye H: Maternal and child health in Seychelles, *Seychelles Med Dent J* 7(1), 20–27, 2004.

Shamlaye C, Shamlaye H, Brewer R: Health in Seychelles: an overview, *Seychelles Med Dent J.* 7(1):13–20, 2004.

UNAIDS: 2006: Seychelles. Retrieved September 21, 2006, from http://www.unaids.org/en/Regions_Countries/Countries/seychelles.asp.

World Health Organization: 2006: Immunization, vaccines and biologicals. Retrieved September 21, 2006, from http://www.who.int/immunization_monitoring/en/globalsummary/countryprofileresult.cfm?C='syc'.

◆ SIERRA LEONE (REPUBLIC OF)

MAP PAGE (800)

Carolyn M. D'Avanzo

Location: Sierra Leone is located on the western side of the African continent, bordered on the north and east by Guinea and on the southeast by Liberia. The remaining third of its border is formed by the Atlantic Ocean, with a heavily indented coastline of mangrove swamps and beautiful sandy beaches. The total area is 71,740 km^2 (27,699 square miles), and the capital is Freetown. Ten years of civil war has resulted in tens of thousands of deaths and displacement of two million people. The social, educational, and health infrastructures of the country have been badly damaged. The population is made up of 20 native African tribes and is estimated at more than six million people, with 45% aged 0 to 14 years. The gross domestic product (GDP) per capita is $800, with 68% living below the poverty line. Literacy rates are 40% for men, 21% for women.

Major Languages	Ethnic Groups	Major Religions
Mende	Mende 30%	Muslim 60%
Temne	Temne 30%	Indigenous beliefs 30%
Krio (English-based)	Creole 10%	Christian 10%
Limba	Other 30%	

S

Health Care Beliefs: Acute sick care; traditional; passive role. People have little or no scientific concept of disease causation, and illnesses are blamed on enemies, witchcraft, or displeased ancestors. Charms are often worn to keep evil spirits away. Disease prevention is rarely practiced. Patients tend to prefer injections rather than tablets, and rectal suppositories are frequently unacceptable. Health-promotion programs are usually based on focused group discussions complemented by traditional dancing and role playing, mainly involving women. Mental illnesses are regarded with suspicion and kept secret and are not considered in the domain of Western medicine. Practitioners with special spiritual powers are consulted to exorcise the devil causing the illness.

Predominant Sick-Care Practices: Biomedical; traditional; magical-religious. Sick care practices depend on availability of services: 90% of the urban and 20% of the rural population has access to health care. Predominant practices in rural areas involve traditional healers and herbalists. Traditional birth attendants are trained in basic aseptic techniques and safe practices. Extensive, itchy skin rashes are believed to be caused by evil spells, so patients expect to be scrubbed vigorously and shown desquamated skin debris as evidence of removal of the offending cause. Even in urban areas, Western medicine is often abandoned in favor of traditional methods if the illness is prolonged or complicated.

Ethnic-/Race-Specific or Endemic Diseases: Malaria is endemic, accounting for significant morbidity and mortality, especially among children. Most infections are chloroquine sensitive, but the prevalence of resistant infections is increasing. Onchocerciasis is endemic in the north, and schistosomiasis is endemic in the east of the country. Other frequently encountered diseases include hepatitis A and B, bacterial and protozoal diarrhea, typhoid fever, Lassa fever, and yellow fever in some locations. Hypertension is common in urban areas, with a prevalence of about 25% in the capital and 14% in rural communities. Diabetes is virtually nonexistent in rural villages. Ten years of civil war have created a large internally displaced population susceptible to malnutrition, tuberculosis, HIV/AIDS, and diarrheal diseases. The Joint United Nations Programme on HIV/AIDS (UNAIDS) estimates the prevalence rate for human immunodeficiency virus (HIV) in adults (aged 15 to 49 years) to be 1.6%, with 48,000 people living with HIV, including 26,000 women and 5,200 children aged 0 to 14. About 31,000 children aged 0 to 17 are orphans as a result of parental deaths from acquired immunodeficiency syndrome (AIDS). Deaths from AIDS are reportedly about 4,600. All these statistics may be underestimated because of inadequate reporting, but the information available indicates a steadily worsening epidemic.

Health-Team Relationships: The doctor is head of the health team in planning activities and hospital settings. However, district clinics are administered by community health officers, who are high school graduates with 3 years of paramedical training from a college. In urban areas, doctors' clinics are complemented by practices run by dispensers, who are essentially nurse practitioners with an additional 3 years of training in pharmaceuticals and basic clinical skills. Nurses play supporting roles in hospitals and clinics. Patients tend to be subservient to their healers and readily accept their decisions.

Families' Role in Hospital Care: Families and friends provide much support for those who are ill, particularly during hospitalizations. They provide food and medications, help with hygiene tasks, and offer moral support. Family members stay with the patients most of the day and frequently spend the night, often sleeping on the floor.

Dominance Patterns: Sierra Leone has a male-dominated society. Traditionally, men have been the primary breadwinners, but this is changing, especially in urban settings. Women are still expected to fulfill traditional duties such as looking after the home and children and, in rural areas, working on the farms. However, women have attained prominent positions such as supreme court judge, chief medical officer, commissioner of income tax, and university professor. Politics is firmly in the male domain, and few women have made inroads into this arena.

Eye-Contact Practices: Direct eye contact in some situations is considered rude or defiant, particularly when children or subordinates are being cautioned or reprimanded, because they are expected to look down. Eye contact among equals is common and expected.

Touch Practices: Touching is common and in many instances may be considered intimate by Western standards. Handshaking is part of the greeting process. Touching of the arms, backs, or even thighs is common during conversation and has no sexual connotation. Men often hold hands with other men, and women readily embrace each other. Patients are unsatisfied if their doctors do not touch or examine them.

Perceptions of Time: Punctuality is not taken seriously. The expression "African time" is used to mean "later than scheduled." Clinic appointments are impractical, and patients are served on a first-come, first-served basis. Sierra Leoneans live in the past, remembering the time when the country was known as the "Athens of West Africa" and had the first high school, university, railway, and television network in the subregion. Ten years of civil war destroyed most of the country's infrastructure and left many despondent and pessimistic about the future.

Pain Reactions: Sierra Leoneans have a high pain tolerance, although this varies by tribe. For example, Fullah women are known to give birth with no assistance and in silence; they get up and begin moving about within a matter of hours after birth. Otherwise, pain is occasionally expressed through dramatic facial and vocal expressions.

Birth Rites: About 70% of all deliveries take place in the home, and the infant mortality rate is incredibly high at 160 deaths per 1,000 live births. Traditional birth attendants deliver most infants born in villages, but obstetric services are available in towns. Mothers usually lie on their backs but may squat. The buttocks of girls and limbs of boys and girls are "molded" to ensure a perfect figure when they grow up. In some cultures,

S

people bury the placenta or a piece of the umbilical cord and plant a fruit tree at the spot, thereby relating the birth to the universe. The tree becomes known as the child's tree; fruits from the tree are sold, and the money is used to buy things for the child. The naming ceremony is on the seventh day for girls and the ninth for boys. During the naming ceremony, an older female family member takes the infant out of the house for the first time. Piercing of girls' ears and circumcision of boys take place soon after birth. The fertility rate is six children born per woman. Life expectancy is 38 for men, 42 for women.

Death Rites: In some cases, the family begins preparing for death long before a patient dies. Families have been known to withdraw financial support for medication once it is clear that a patient is going to die and start saving instead for the funeral. When the patient dies, family members congregate at the home of the deceased and openly grieve. For Muslims, burial takes place the same day. The body is laid in a room in the house, and prayers are said for several hours. Men and women segregate in different rooms, and women usually do not attend the burial ceremony. Christians spread funeral activities out over several days or even weeks. Family and friends visit the deceased person's home daily to say prayers and commiserate with close family members. The night before the funeral is the wake, when prayers are recited and religious songs are sung. Tributes are delivered well into the early hours of the morning. Food and drinks, including alcohol, are served. On the day of the funeral, the family has a "laying out" ceremony. The body is laid out in the house or a public place for a final public viewing and then taken to the church for the funeral service. After the burial, family and friends return to the house for refreshments. Further commemorations take place on the 7th and 40th days after death and on the 1st, 5th, and 10th anniversaries. During these occasions, black-eyed peas are cooked, some of which are on a table with a glass of water for the dead person. Autopsies are uncommon because of family reluctance to grant permission. Often an order from the coroner is required.

Food Practices and Intolerances: The staple food is rice, which is eaten every day. In rural areas in particular, tuberous plants such as yams, cassava, and sweet potatoes are eaten. Fermented cassava cooked into a thick paste called *foofoo* is also popular. Several varieties of green leaves are cooked with palm oil mixed with onions, pepper, meat, or fish as a sauce (*palava* sauce) for rice and *foofoo*. Traditionally, one main meal is eaten each day either in the morning or evening. Food is cooked by the women after they return from the farm or market. More Westernized sections of society have three meals each day. Food is eaten either with a spoon or by hand. Forks and knives are used by the elite. Fruits are plentiful and eaten when in season. Food taboos are common during pregnancy and involve primarily protein-rich foods, especially chicken and eggs. Pregnant women are discouraged from eating pepper and ginger because they might cause the infant to be haughty or have a bad temper. Some groups believe that fish causes worms in children,

S

and children are discouraged from drinking coconut milk because it is believed that it will make them less intelligent.

Infant-Feeding Practices: In some tribes in Sierra Leone, colostrum is discarded, but prolonged breastfeeding is the norm. Bottle-feeding is actively discouraged. Mothers start introducing foods at 4 to 6 months but continue to breastfeed for up to 2 years. A government program to manufacture and distribute a weaning food (*Bennimix*) based on locally grown, protein-rich beniseed has been very successful. Breastfeeding also is used as a means of contraception and for child spacing. In addition, some nursing mothers move away from their husbands and stay with their mothers for several months after delivery. Forced feeding of infants is practiced by many groups and occasionally leads to death by aspiration.

Child-Rearing Practices: Children's upbringing is strict and authoritarian, and although discipline is enforced by both parents, the mother is usually the enforcer. Relatives and any older members of the community also enforce discipline. Children do not talk back to parents or adults. Corporal punishment is common in school and in the home. Children are expected to help with domestic chores and develop housekeeping skills at an early age. Girls must learn to cook and look after younger siblings. In poorer communities, children, even those who attend school, are expected to contribute to the household income by helping to sell wares. Female circumcision is widespread but is limited primarily to the clitoris. This is part of a more detailed initiation process involving tutorials in child rearing and other domestic practices that takes place around puberty. Boys are circumcised at a young age, usually during the first year after birth. Uncircumcised boys are ridiculed by their peers. The education arena has no gender discrimination. Most primary schools are coeducational, but the older and more traditional secondary schools are segregated by sex. Children grow up with great respect and reverence for their parents, characteristics that are maintained throughout life as they care for and support their aging parents in later years.

National Childhood Immunization: BCG at birth; DTwP at 6, 10, and 14 weeks; OPV birth and 6, 10, and 14 weeks; measles at 9 months; vitamin A at 6 and 9 months; YF at 9 months; and TT at first contact, +1, +6 months, +1, and +1 year. The percent of the target population vaccinated, by antigen is: BCG (82%); DTP1 (77%); DTP3 and Poliio3 (64%); and MCV (67%). After the civil war, surveys revealed that only 25% of infants were fully immunized, and only 17% of mothers completed the three doses of TT required to prevent neonatal tetanus in their infants.

BIBLIOGRAPHY

Central Intelligence Agency: 2006: *The world factbook, Sierra Leone. Retrieved September 21, 2006, from https://www.cia.gov/cia/publications/factbook/print/sl.html.*

Lisk DR, Gooding EC: Doctors' knowledge, attitude, and practice in the management of hypertension in a developing country. *Ethnicity Dis.* 10, 2000.

Lisk DR, Pabs-Garnon E: Pregnancy associated hypertension in urban Sierra Leonean Africans, *Ethnicity Dis.* 10, 2000.

Lisk DR, Williams DEM, Slattery J: Blood pressure and hypertension in rural and urban Sierra Leoneans, *Ethnicity Dis.* 9:254–253, 1999.

Williams DEM, Lisk DR: A high prevalence of hypertension in rural Sierra Leoneans, *W Afr J Med.* 17:85–90, 1998.

UNAIDS: 2006 Sierra Leone. Retrieved September 21, 2006, from http://www.unaids.org/en/Regions_Countries/Countries/sierraleone.asp.

World Health Organization: 2006: Immunization, vaccines and biologicals. Retrieved September 21, 2006, from http://www.who.int/immunization_monitoring/en/globalsummary/countryprofileresult.cfm?C='sle'.

◆ SINGAPORE (REPUBLIC OF)

MAP PAGE (805)

Carolyn M. D'Avanzo

Location: A small island nation off the southeast coast of Malaysia, Singapore is one of the most densely populated areas in the world, with a total area of only 659.9 km^2 (254.7 square miles) and a population of approximately 4.5 million. It is a leading economic power with one of the world's largest ports. Its boundaries are the Johor Straight to the north, the Pacific Ocean to the east, the Straight of Malacca to the southwest (separating Singapore from Sumatra), and the Indian Ocean to the west. Singapore has a lowland central plateau with a few hills and has hot, humid, tropical, and rainy weather with two distinct monsoon seasons. The gross domestic product (GDP) per capita is $28,100, and its economic power has contributed to high standards in health, education, and housing. Most people live in the capital city of Singapore on the main island. Literacy rates are 97% for men, 89% for women.

Major Languages	Ethnic Groups	Major Religions
Chinese (official)	Chinese 77%	Chinese: mainly Buddhist, atheist, and Christian
Malay (official)	Malay 14%	Malays: mainly Muslim
Tamil (official)	Indian 8%	Minority religions: Christian, Hindu, Sikh, Tao, Confucian
English (official)	Others 1%	

Health Care Beliefs: Passive role; fatalistic belief that life and death are beyond their control. Muslims have beliefs based on the four pillars of Islam: fasting, fitrah, pilgrimage to Mecca, and prayer five times a day. Muslims fear mental illness but believe in health promotion. The government health services actively promote preventive medicine and since the 1990s has had a program dedicated to prevention: the National Health Lifestyle Campaign.

Predominant Sick Care Practices: Biomedical; traditional; magical-religious. Muslims use holy water, pray, and go to Mecca. Hindus use amulets to ward off illness. Singapore has a dual system of health care delivery: a public system managed by the government and a private system of general practitioners and private hospitals. Eighty percent of primary care services are provided by doctors in private practice. Eighty percent of hospital care is provided by the public sector. The system stresses personal responsibility, and employees must contribute 6% to 8% of their monthly salary to a tax-deductible individual account. Self-employed individuals are also required to contribute. An endowment fund serves as a safety net for those who are poor. Although only 8% of the population is over age 65, this percentage is expected to increase substantially by 2030, which will undoubtedly increase overall costs.

Ethnic-/Race-Specific or Endemic Diseases: High-level medical services, safe water, and sanitation have increased overall health indicators for Singaporeans. Endemic diseases include hepatitis B, typhus, melioidosis, and dengue hemorrhagic fever. Antimicrobial drug resistance is a significant problem. Singaporeans are at risk for hand, foot, and mouth disease. Leading causes of morbidity are the noncommunicable diseases: cancer, coronary heart disease, stroke, diabetes, hypertension, and injuries. Cancer and cardiovascular diseases account for about 62% of the total causes of death. The joint United Nations Programme on HIV/AIDS (UNAIDS) estimates that the prevalence rate for HIV in adults (aged 15 to 59 years) is 0.3%, with 5,500 people living with human immunodeficiency virus (HIV), including 1,500 women. Deaths from acquired immunodeficiency syndrome (AIDS) are estimated as fewer than 100.

Health-Team Relationships: Doctors have good relationships with nurses, and patients' attitudes toward doctors and nurses are also good. In general, doctors are held in high esteem and expected to know the cause of an illness just from a quick examination that does not involve a thorough history or physical examination. Patients also expect to receive several medications (e.g., vitamins, antibiotics) after each visit and feel cheated if they do not. They also expect to feel well soon after the visit, usually by the next day. Because of conflicts with this attitude, doctors must take time to explain medical practice so that patients will accept advice and comply with treatments. A large segment of primary medical care is also provided by Chinese doctors *(sinseh)*, who treat with traditional herbs.

Families' Role in Hospital Care: Parents may stay overnight with their hospitalized children, and it is common to bring food to the hospital.

Dominance Patterns: Males are dominant. Parents may defer to the oldest son or daughter as they become older and unable to handle their affairs without assistance.

Touch Practices: The head is considered sacred, and it is considered offensive to pat a child on the head or to hit another person in the

S

head. Reaching over a patient's head to pass something to another person is rude, involving one of the pillars of Islam called *fitrah*. Malay custom does not allow touching between men and women, particularly in public.

Perceptions of Time: Malays are generally on time; other ethnic groups' attitudes toward time vary.

Pain Reactions: The Chinese tend to be more stoic about pain than other groups. Indians and Malays seem to have lower pain thresholds.

Birth Rites: The fertility rate is one child born per woman. Malays celebrate a son more than a daughter because the son's role is to protect the mother. Most Malay mothers breastfeed their infants, occasionally until they are 3 years old. The infant mortality rate is 2.3 deaths per 1,000 live births. Life expectancy is 79 for men, 84 for women.

Death Rites: The 1992 Medical Therapy, Education, and Research Act allows donation of organs and tissues from deceased persons for transplantation. Organ donation is encouraged by the government and well accepted by the Chinese; however, Malay Muslims are generally against the practice. Autopsies are done primarily for forensic rather than medical reasons.

Food Practices and Intolerances: In general, Malays eat at home, and the Chinese eat out. Favorite foods include seafood, sweet potato fritters, banana fritters, curry puffs, and all kinds of sweets. Malays and Indians use their hands to eat except in public, when they use forks.

Infant-Feeding Practices: Infant feeding practices vary, but the government is encouraging breastfeeding.

Child-Rearing Practices: Strict child rearing is the rule, and both parents are responsible for discipline. Young children usually sleep with their parents.

National Childhood Immunizations: BCG at birth; DTwP at 3, 4, and 5 months; OPV at 3, 4, and 5 months, after age 6 and 11 years; HepB at birth and at 1 and 5 to 6 months; MMR at 15 months and after age 11 years; Td after age 6 and 11 years. The percent of the target population vaccinated, by antigen, is: BCG (98%); and DTP1, DTP3, HepB3, MCV, and Polio3 (96%).

Other Characteristics: Some friction exists among the various ethnic groups. However, the government actively promotes community cohesion and a sense of being a Singaporean first and foremost.

BIBLIOGRAPHY

Central Intelligence Agency: 2006: *The world factbook, Singapore.* Retrieved September 21, 2006, from https://www.cia.gov/cia/publications/factbook/print/sn.html.

UNAIDS: 2006: Singapore. Retrieved September 21, 2006, from http://www.unaids.org/en/Regions_Countries/Countries/singapore.asp.

World Health Organization: 2006: Immunization, vaccines and biologicals. Retrieved September 21, 2006, from http://www.who.int/immunization_monitoring/en/globalsummary/countryprofileresult.cfm?C'sgp'.

✦ SLOVAK REPUBLIC

MAP PAGE (798)

Peter Ciznar and Scott J.N. McNabb

Location: The Slovak Republic (Slovakia) is an interior country situated in east central Europe. The capital is Bratislava. It was formerly part of Czechoslovakia. Slovakia's topography is characterized by fertile low-lands, hills, and snow-capped mountains (the High Tatras). The Danube River flows through the western tip of the country. The total area is 49,035 km^2 (18,932 square miles). The official language is Slovak, but in the southern parts many people communicate in Hungarian. The population is 5.4 million, and the gross domestic product (GDP) per capita is $16,100. Literacy rates are high: almost 100% for both men and women.

Major Languages	Ethnic Groups	Major Religions
Slovak	Slovak 85%	Roman Catholic 70%
Hungarian	Hungarian 10%	Evangelical 7%
	Romany 2%	Greek Catholic 4%
	Czech 1%	Calvinistic 2%
	Ruthenian, Ukrainian, Russian, German, Polish, Other 2%	Nondenominational or atheist 17%

Health Care Beliefs: Active role; health promotion encouraged. Exercise, a healthy diet, and rest are believed to promote and protect health. By law, children 18 years and younger visit doctors regularly, and regular examinations during pregnancy are obligatory. Fear of mental illness is slowly decreasing, and it is no longer acceptable to "imprison" individuals with mental illness so that they cannot participate in public life. People attempt to integrate those with mental illness into society if possible. Slovakia has special "protected shops" in which individuals with relatively minor disabilities can work safely.

Predominant Sick-Care Practices: Biomedical; natural and alternative therapies. The old state system is being actively transformed to a privatized one. Sick care is primarily biomedical, but use of some alternative therapies has increased in recent years. The status of doctors is honored, although many feel unappreciated because of their low wages. Health care is provided in hospitals and ambulatory care sites, and primary, secondary, and tertiary care is available. Primary care is provided by three types of doctors: general practitioners for adults, general pediatricians for children and young people, and gynecologists for women. Maternity and infant care is free. There is a small charge for treatment at clinics for children over 3 and adults, regardless of medical insurance. Health care insurance is obligatory, but the state covers insurance for children, retirees and the unemployed. When people are ill, they generally seek out doctors first, but some also consult natural healers, particularly if the recommended medical treatment is unsuccessful. Alternative therapies such as acupuncture, homeopathy, and natural healing are also well accepted.

Ethnic-/Race-Specific or Endemic Diseases: The major causes of deaths for adults are heart and circulatory diseases (55%), malignant neoplasms (22%), respiratory diseases (7%), injuries and poisoning (7%), and gastrointestinal tract diseases (4%). Increases in cancer and cardiovascular diseases such as hypertension are believed to be caused by factors such as chronic stress, frustration, and apathy in the population. Oxidative stress is also blamed because of people's high consumption of nicotine and alcohol and low intake of antioxidants. Children primarily have respiratory and gastrointestinal diseases and urinary infections. Most deaths of children are from injuries, followed by neoplasms and congenital abnormalities. The Joint United Nations Programme on HIV/AIDS (UNAIDS) estimates the prevalence rate for human immunodeficiency virus (HIV) in adults (aged 15 to 49 years) to be 0.1%, with fewer than 500 people living with HIV, including fewer than 100 children aged 0 to 15. HIV tests are obligatory for those giving blood and during pregnancy, and they can be requested without charge. By the end of 2004, Slovak authorities had reported a cumulative total of 216 HIV cases (39 with acquired immunodeficiency syndrome (AIDS), including 26 who died). In 2004, 15 new HIV and 2 new AIDS cases were reported as well as 3 AIDS deaths. Slovakia has relatively low prevalence and a stable epidemic. HIV is primarily transmitted by men who have sex with men. Well-designed prevention programs are given credit for the low incidence among injecting drug users.

Health-Team Relationships: The health team is doctor driven. Nurses are expected to take care of health maintenance tasks such as giving injections and prescribed medications and fulfilling treatment tasks. Under Slovak law, nurses have little power and are not allowed to make independent decisions. The working relationship between doctors and nurses is usually good, but tensions inevitably arise because medicine is such a demanding occupation.

Families' Role in Hospital Care: The medical and nursing staff members provide all hospital care. Visiting hours are quite liberal, and some wards allow small children to visit. The rights of children in hospitals are protected by Slovak law, which addresses issues such as teaching, housing of parents, information communication, and the economic rights of parents. Parents are allowed to stay with children in the hospital, and friends and relatives are allowed to visit.

Dominance Patterns: Men were previously in control of all decision making, but this has changed in the family and in society. However, men still have higher salaries and better jobs. In the home, women still do most of the domestic work, care for the children, and are the primary caregivers for sick relatives. Women are becoming increasingly more career oriented and more likely to expect that household and other obligations should be shared.

Eye-Contact Practices: Long-lasting, direct eye contact is unacceptable and often regarded as hostile during interactions with strangers. It is customary to make direct eye contact during conversations with well-known individuals.

Touch Practices: Touching is acceptable, and it is common to give a person a hug in the street or shake hands when meeting a friend or acquaintance. Men are less expressive with other men than women are with other women.

Perceptions of Time: Punctuality is valued, but being 5 minutes late is usually not a concern. People live in the present and future, but because of the country's history of war and conflict, they often have concerns about what the future holds.

Pain Reactions: People react to pain very differently, ranging from being stoic to very expressive. However, even Slovaks with severe injuries tend to stay relatively calm, and health professionals expect patients to endure pain without unnecessary outward expressions of emotion. Crying out loud during labor and delivery is acceptable.

Birth Rites: The fertility rate is 1.33 children born per woman. Many mothers, especially those from middle-class backgrounds, attend prenatal birth preparation courses. Most infants are born in hospitals, and when conditions are appropriate, the father is admitted to the delivery room. The mother has a choice of delivery options such as a natural birth with no anesthesia or birth with epidural anesthesia. Hospitals are attempting to accommodate a range of birth positions and styles such as standing or births underwater. The infant mortality rate is 7.26 deaths per 1,000 live births. Some hospitals allow the infant to stay in the mother's room ("rooming-in") on the second or third day if there are no complications and the mother requests it. Many hospitals do not have enough space, and staff members are often unwilling to conform to new methods. Therefore, most mothers and babies are separated except during feedings, which take place six times a day. This procedure is gradually changing as the positive benefits of rooming in are becoming more evident. Mothers and infants usually leave the hospital on the fifth day after birth or the ninth if a cesarean section was performed. Life expectancy is 71 for men, 79 for women.

Death Rites: Most people die in health care institutions, and the closest family members usually stay with the dying person. In cities, funeral providers have all-inclusive services, including cleaning and dressing the body, a coffin, and a ceremony accompanying cremation or burial in the ground. In the countryside, it is still common to display the body in an open coffin at home, particularly if the person was a Roman Catholic. This practice allows friends and relatives to have a last personal visit in the home, after which they accompany the coffin in the hearse on the person's journey to the cemetery. Organ donations and autopsies are acceptable.

Food Practices and Intolerances: Most people eat three times a day. Breakfast usually consists of a combination of bread, butter, jam, yogurt,

S

salami, cheese, and tea, milk, or coffee. Traditional food staples are potatoes, rice, and pasta, combined with pork, beef, and poultry (that is stewed or roasted). Vegetables and fruit (including tropical fruits) are available most of the year. A typical traditional meal is gnocchi with *brynza* (sheep cheese) and bacon topping and potato pancakes with sauerkraut. Pizza, hot dogs, and sandwiches with various fillings are the favorite among young people in particular.

Infant-Feeding Practices: Breastfeeding is typical, and women are encouraged to breastfeed as long as possible, but for at least 3 to 4 months. Because mothers understand that breast milk is the best and the only natural food for babies, Slovakia has several women's clubs providing breastfeeding support. These groups are led primarily by doctors and mothers with breastfeeding experience. Although breastfeeding in public is frowned on, it is not unusual to see a 20-month-old child being breastfed. If breastfeeding is impossible for medical reasons, formula is available. In Slovak culture, the image of a woman breastfeeding her infant is considered a pure and wonderful expression of womanhood.

Child-Rearing Practices: Child-rearing practices are quite permissive and loving. However, children are expected to obey rules and have good manners. Parents usually supervise their children, try to support them mentally and financially, and help them when they are ready to become independent. Both parents are responsible for discipline. Physical punishment is unacceptable, but an occasional smack on the bottom is considered a part of raising a child. Small children often sleep in a room with their parents. The maternity leave by law is 3 years, and many mothers stay at home with their babies for the entire time. Fathers and mothers are both allowed maternity leave. According to the law, employers cannot eliminate the job of a person who is on maternity leave or refuse to allow the person to return to work after the leave.

National Childhood Immunizations: BCG at 3 days and 10 years; DT at 9, 15 to 19 weeks, 9 to 13 months, 2 and 15 years (children with contraindication of pertussis component vaccine); DTwP at 2 and 5 years; DTwPHiblpv at 9, 15 to 19 weeks, and 9 to 13 months; HepA at 2 years (gypsy children living in bad hygienic conditions); HepB at 9, 15 to 19 weeks, and 9 to 13 months; MMR at 14 months and 11 years; Td at 13 years. Vaccinations are free and required. The percent of the target population vaccinated, by antigen, is: DTP1, DTP3, HepB3, Hib3, and Polio3 (99%); BCG and MCV (98%).

BIBLIOGRAPHY

Central Intelligence Agency: 2006: *The world factbook, Slovakia.* Retrieved September 21, 2006, from https://www.cia.gov/cia/publications/factbook/print/lo.html.

The Statistics Office of the Slovak Republic: *Slovak census 2001*, Bratislava, Slovakia, 2001, Statistics Office.

The statistics yearbook of the government office of the Slovak Republic, Bratislava, 2000.

UNAIDS: 2006: Slovakia. Retrieved September 21, 2006, from http://www.unaids.org/en/Regions_Countries/Countries/slovakia.asp.

S

World Health Organization: 2006: Immunization, vaccines and biologicals. Retrieved September 21, 2006, from http://www.who.int/immunization_monitoring/en/globalsummary/countryprofileresult.cfm?V='svk'.
http://www,geaktg,giv,sj/ (retrieved March 3, 2006).
http://www.uvzsr.sk/ (retrieved March 3, 2006).

♦ SLOVENIA (REPUBLIC OF)

MAP PAGE (798)

Marija Bohinc and Miro Gradisar

Location: Slovenia is in the southeastern part of Europe; it was part of Yugoslavia until June 1991, when it declared independence. Slovenia is 230 km from Vienna, Austria; 240 km from Budapest, Hungary; and 460 km from Milan, Italy. The capital is Ljubljana. Slovenia is a green place in the heart of Europe. It is largely mountainous, and forests cover almost half of the land. The landscape is very diverse, with mountains, hills, villages, spas, and the sea. The total area is 20,256 km^2 (7,820 square miles), and the population is more than two million. Slovenia acceded to the European Union and the North Atlantic Treaty Organization (NATO) in 2004. The gross domestic product (GDP) per capita is $21,600. Literacy rates are nearly 100% for both men and women.

Major Languages	Ethnic Groups	Major Religions
Slovenian (official)	Slovene 88%	Roman Catholic 58%
Serbo-Croatian	Croat 3%	Christian Othodox 2%
English	Serb 2%	Muslim 2%
German	Bosniak 1%	Other Christian 1%
Italian	Other 6%	Unaffiliated 4%
		Other or unspecified 23%
		None 10%

In addition to Slovenian most of the population also speaks Serbo-Croatian.

Health Care Beliefs: Active role; health promotion important. Family and health are reported as the most important values for Slovenes. A national program was developed for promotion of healthy lifestyles and the prevention and early detection of diseases. The health-promotion initiative is organized to promote healthy nutrition, exercise, smoking cessation, and lower rates of alcohol and drug consumption. An important initiative is improvement of people's tolerance for and acceptance of those with mental disorders, and promotion of their integration into the community. Care for those who are homeless and unemployed is the domain of other health-promotion programs and self-help groups. People with minor disabilities can live, study, and work in the community.

Predominant Sick-Care Practices: Biomedical and alternative therapies. The state system focuses on an active approach and individual
responsibility for health. Doctors are trusted and appreciated for their
knowledge, but they played a more paternal role in the past. Today
patients are more insistent about being included in decision making
because they are informed about their rights. Medical knowledge, expertise, technology, and practice are excellent, and primary health care takes
place in health care centers. Secondary care is provided by general hospitals and outpatient clinics; tertiary care by clinics and institutes. The vast
majority of people are insured, so they have access to health care centers
and emergency wards. Maternal infant care, preventive programs for
scholars, and a portion of care for older adults are free. When people
are ill, they first visit a doctor in a primary health care center; 80% solicit
care at this level. Private health care is also developing, involving general
doctors, private community nurses, and dentists. Community nurses are
respected, valued, and considered an asset to the system. In addition to
biomedical care, the use of alternative therapies is common, especially
when standard medical treatment is not successful. Homeopathy, bioenergy, acupuncture, and natural healing methods are alternative treatment
options.

Ethnic-/Race-Specific or Endemic Diseases: The major causes of
death are cardiovascular diseases (39%), cancer (26%), injuries/poisoning
(8%), and gastrointestinal diseases (7%). Increases in the incidence of cancer, cardiovascular disease, hypertension, high cholesterol, and diabetes
are attributed to unhealthy lifestyles: excessive alcohol consumption,
smoking, poor nutrition, and stress. Children primarily have respiratory,
gastrointestinal, and urinary diseases. Prenatal mortality is very low and
comparable to rates of Scandinavian countries. The Joint United Nations
Programme on HIV/AIDS (UNAIDS) estimates the prevalence rate for
human immunodeficiency virus (HIV) in adults (aged 15 to 49 years) to
be less than 0.1%, with fewer than 500 people living with HIV. Fewer than
100 deaths are attributed to acquired immunodeficiency syndrome (AIDS).
By the end of 2004, Slovak authorities had reported a cumulative total of
216 HIV cases, and 39 of these individuals had developed AIDS, including
26 who had died. The low death rate is attributed to good access to health
care. Slovenian statistics indicated 128 AIDS cases as of 2006: 112 men
and 16 women. HIV is predominantly transmitted by men who have sex
with men. Well-designed national programs are thought to have contributed to low prevalence among injecting drug users and to the low incidence
in the noninjecting population. HIV tests are obligatory for anyone giving
blood, and these tests can be requested without cost. Special programs
address prevention of sexually transmitted infections.

Health Team Relationships: The leader of the health team is the doctor,
and the leader of the nursing team is the registered nurse. Slovenian
nurses are becoming more independent and autonomous. Efforts to
increase the academic level of nursing to the bachelor of science degree
are strong, and professional development is significant. Nurses can make

independent decisions, and legislation for nursing practice is in process. It is expected that the relationship between doctors and nurses will be more synergistic in the future—more of a partnership and collaboration, although current relationships are generally quite good between the professions.

Families' Role in Hospital Care: Visiting hours in hospitals are very flexible and liberal. Relatives can visit almost any time during regular hours and beyond scheduled visiting hours with a doctor's permission. The rights of patients are in accordance with the 1994 Declaration of the Rights of Patients in Amsterdam, and with the country's health care laws. All patients receive information outlining their health care rights.

Dominance Patterns: In most cases, men have the highest positions, receive better salaries, and have access to better jobs. Most women are employed, and many are pursuing careers. They have as much education as men, and as times are changing, more are moving into high-level managerial and leadership positions in all areas of public life. In the home, women still have the major responsibility for cooking, housekeeping, and taking care of children and sick relatives. In younger families, the division of work is more balanced, and couples usually do not live with their parents.

Eye-Contact Practices: Long-lasting, direct eye contact is not always acceptable. It is more common during conversational situations among people who know each other well.

Touch Practices: Touching is acceptable among friends or relatives. When people meet, it is common to shake hands.

Perceptions of Time: Being on time is becoming more important. Popular proverbs say "to be on time is a nice habit" and "time is golden." It is very common, especially for older people, to be at least 5 or more minutes late for appointments. Younger people are more oriented to the future.

Pain Reactions: Slovenes react very differently to pain. Reactions range from calm to serious, anxious, fearful, and powerless. It is not unusual for individuals to cry out and express their feelings.

Birth Rites: Many mothers and fathers, especially those from the upper and middle classes, attend prenatal birth preparation courses. Most infants are born in hospitals with excellent facilities, and fathers are allowed to be present during delivery. Mothers can choose to have delivery without drugs or to have epidural anesthesia. Hospitals are attempting to accommodate options such as underwater births or births in the standing position. Most hospitals promote rooming-in (infant and mother in the same room) from the first day. If the mother desires, the infant may be kept in the nursery. Some hospitals are specifically considered "baby-friendly hospitals." Mothers and infants usually stay until the third day after normal deliveries; births by cesarean section usually require a 7-day stay. The infant mortality rate is 4 deaths per 1,000 live births. Breastfeeding is promoted. Legally, maternity leave is 1 year, which can be extended after premature deliveries. Both parents are allowed to take a paid maternity

S

leave, and the employer cannot refuse to take the parents back when the leave is over. The fertility rate is 1.25 children born per woman. Life expectancy is 73 for men, 80 for women.

Death Rites: Nearly 50% of all people die in hospitals. The rest die in nursing homes, their own homes, or at the homes of family members. In cities, funeral facilities provide all services, including cleaning and dressing the body, coffin selection, and cremation or burial with an accompanying service or ceremony. In the countryside, it is common to display the body in a place other than the home—often a special hall in the village. Relatives and friends come to say good-bye, bring flowers, light candles, and pray for the deceased. The priest usually leads Roman Catholic funerals. Organ donations and autopsies are acceptable with the permission of the deceased or an accountable person.

Food Practices and Intolerances: More eduated people tend to have healthier nutritional patterns. They eat more black bread, fish, and chicken and less pork and beef compared with those who have only an elementary school education. For this reason, the Ministry of Health initiated a program to promote healthy nutrition from 2005 through 2010. Women tend to have healthier habits than men. According to population studies, women are more likely to have breakfast (only 50% of the total population have breakfast every day). Breakfast usually consists of bread, milk, coffee, jam, honey, yogurt, cheese, eggs, margarine or butter, and tea. Traditional foods include vegetable soups, potatoes, rice, pasta with meat, and salads. Vegetables and fruit are available throughout the year. The typical Sunday meal is beef soup, cooked beef with roasted potatoes, green salad, and fruit. Fast food is becoming popular, especially among young people, who eat all types of pizza, hot dogs, and sandwiches.

Infant-Feeding Practices: Breastfeeding is valued and considered a good investment in the health of the child. Women are encouraged to breastfeed for as long as possible but at least for 3 or 4 months. If breastfeeding is not possible for medical reasons, formula can be prepared at home. In health care centers on the primary level of the national health care system, each community has a dispensary for infants and preschool children. Slovenia has prevention and health-promotion programs for disease prevention, immunizations, and counseling, all of which are supervised by pediatricians, registered nurses, and—in the home—community nurses.

Child-Rearing Practices: Child rearing is caring, loving, and permissive. Physical punishment is not allowed. Parents attempt to take good care of their children and support them financially, emotionally, and socially. They help children become independent so that they can finish secondary school and college or begin working and become independent. Most children have separate rooms for sleeping.

National Childhood Immunizations: BCG at birth; DTPaPHibIPV at 4.5, 6, and 18 months; MMR at 1 and 6 years; Td at 9 years; and TT at 18 years. The percent of the target population vaccinated, by antigen, is: DTP1 (92%); DTP3, Hib3, and Polio3 (96%); and MCV (94%). Hepatitis B is given in the first year of elementary school. Vaccinations are free of cost. Parents can refuse to have children vaccinated but are held responsible.

BIBLIOGRAPHY

Albreht T, Cesen M, Hindle D, et al: Health care systems in transition—Slovenia. In: Jakubowski E, ed: European Observatory on Health Care System. Copenhagen, 2002, World Health Organization 4–7.

Bohinc M, Cibic D: Country profile: Slovenia. *Nursing Ethics.* 12(3)317–322, 2005.

Central Intelligence Agency: 2006: *The world factbook, Slovenia.* Retrieved September 21, 2006, from https://www.cia.gov/cia/publications/factbook/print/si.html.Council of Europe, Kalcina L, MocnikV, eds: Patients' rights: Informacijsko dokumentacijski center Sveta Evrope (IDC SE) pri NUK v Ljubljani) 2005.

Health Statistical Report Review: Slovenia 2001, Zdrav Var, 2001 (special issue). Retrieved August 15, 2006, from www.si.gov.si/ivz.

Ministry for Health: The Health Care Reforma. Ljubljana, July 2003. Retrieved August 15, 2006 from http:// www.gov.si.

Ministry for Health: *Nacionalni program prehranske politike od 2005–2010.* Ljubljana, 2005, National Program of Nutrition Policy, 2005-2010.

National Program of Health Care of Republic Slovenia: *The health for all to 2004,* Official Report for Republic Slovenia, No 49, pp 6650–6678, 2002:6.

Prijavljeni primeri: AIDSA in okužb s HIV v Sloveniji do 30.6. 2006. Retrieved August 14, 2006 from http: //www.izv.si/javne-datoteke/1056. AIDScHIV: Klavs I, Kastelic Z, eds).

Statistical Office of the Republic of Slovenia: Retrieved August 14, 2006, from http:// www.stat.si/eng/index.asp. http://www.stat.si/eng/tema-demografsko-prebivalstvo.asp.

UNAIDS: 2006 Slovenia. Retrieved September 21, 2006, from http://www.unaids. org/en/Regions_Countries/Countries/slovenia.asp.

World Health Organization: 2006: Immunization, vaccines and biologicals. Retrieved September 21, 2006, from http://www.who.int/immunization_monitoring/en/ globalsummary/countryprofileresult.cfm?C='svn'.

http://www.observatory.dk (retrieved August 15, 2006).

◆ SOLOMON ISLANDS

MAP PAGE (794)

John Connell

Location: The Solomon Islands is an archipelago in the South Pacific, east of Papua New Guinea and about 1,200 miles northeast of Australia. About 93% of the people are Melanesian, and about 85 indigenous languages are spoken. The total area is 28,000 km^2 (10,900 square miles), mainly consisting of forested high islands and some low atolls, with 10 main large and rugged volcanic islands. The climate is tropical, with few extremes of temperature or weather. However, the islands are vulnerable to occasional typhoons, earthquakes, and tidal waves. The population is 552,438 and is primarily rural. The capital is Honiara. From 1999 to 2003, the country experienced a major political crisis, centered on

S

conflict between the people of the two islands of Malaita and Guadalcanal. This was resolved through external intervention, which weakened the ability to deliver health services, led to the emigration of some doctors, and reduced overall health status. The gross domestic product (GDP) per capita is $1,700.

Major Languages	**Ethnic Groups**	**Major Religions**
Melanesian Pijin	Melanesian 93%	Anglican 34%
English	Polynesian 4%	Roman Catholic 19%
	Micronesian, European,	Other Protestant 43%
	Chinese 3%	Traditional beliefs 4%

Pijin is spoken throughout the country, and some English is spoken by most.

Health Care Beliefs: Active role; health promotion encouraged. Modern medical care is sought for most illness and injuries; however, traditional healers are also active and prescribe various herbs and other traditional medications. Biomedical and traditional beliefs are often combined. For serious illnesses such as malaria, drugs are better than traditional medications or healers. Malaria poses a great risk to Solomon Islanders, and studies indicate that chloroquine resistance is about 25%. Hospitals and pharmacies are only found in population centers and mission facilities. The nearest reliable medical facilities are in New Zealand or Australia.

Predominant Sick-Care Practices: Biomedical and traditional. The Solomon Islands has targeted prevention activities aimed at addressing the more serious problems faced by residents, notably malaria and the growing extent of noncommunicable diseases. The incidence of malaria is the highest in the Asia-Pacific region. The government has implemented policies for prevention that focus on early diagnosis and treatment at a health center, reduction of vector-human contact through use of insecticide-impregnated bed nets, and provision of chemoprophylaxis for pregnant women. However, protection against mosquitoes is poor during evenings, when mosquitoes are most active. Selective primary care activity mobile unit teams may visit villages annually to seek out those who have malaria and provide chloroquine and primaquine treatments. Gains made after the 5-year National Malaria Control Policy that started in 1993 were lost during the political crisis.

Ethnic-/Race-Specific or Endemic Diseases: Chloroquine-resistant falciparum malaria is hyperendemic. Other endemic diseases include human T-lymphotropic virus type 1 (HTLV-1), hepatitis A and B, gonorrhea, and vitamin A deficiency. Solomon Islanders are at risk for hepatitis A, C, and G; helminthic infections; diarrheal diseases; typhoid fever; and injuries from accidents. A resurgence of yaws that occurred in the 1990s appears to have been counteracted. Biotoxin poisoning from tropical fish and shellfish can occur. Other leading causes of morbidity include tuberculosis, eye infections, and sexually transmitted diseases (STDs). Almost half of the gonorrhea infections are penicillin resistant. The country has national guidelines for prevention and treatment of this and other STDs; however, clinics do not collect data properly, serologic testing for syphilis is low (28%), fewer than 50% of the clinics have personnel who understand the national guidelines, and contact tracing is rarely performed. A high male: female notification ratio (3.6:1) for gonorrhea has been detected. Overall attention to public health fundamentals regarding prevention and treatment is not optimal. Infectious diseases remain the major causes of morbidity and mortality, but noninfectious diseases, particularly cancer, diabetes, and hypertension, are putting increased demands on the system. Alcohol abuse and high levels of oral cancer from betel nut chewing are not unusual, and domestic violence is now a critical problem. The number of skilled health care workers is inadequate. The incidence of human immunodeficiency virus (HIV) and acquired immunodeficiency syndrome (AIDS) is increasing but remains low. No prevalence rates have been reported from the Joint United Nations Programme on HIV/AIDS (UNAIDS); however, a post–political crisis increase in prostitution may worsen STD and HIV levels.

Health-Team Relationships: To improve educational opportunities for nurses, the Ministry of Health has implemented five post-basic nursing certificate courses for health workers using distance education modules. This program is proving to be highly successful for increasing skills and knowledge, but the ratio of health care workers to population is relatively low, and medical staff is highly concentrated in population centers.

Families Role in Hospital Care: Families are important as a source of support and food, as hospital services are usually overstretched. At least one family member usually accompanies a sick patient. About 80% of deaths occur outside hospitals.

Dominance Patterns: There are significant ethnic differences between the black-skinned people of the western Solomon Islands, the lighter-skinned people of the eastern islands, and the Polynesians of most outer islands, and also between the matrilineal groups of the west and the more patrilineal societies in the east and center. However, these differences are largely incidental other than for land tenure and inheritance. Solomon Islands remains a male-dominated society, evident in access to education, politics, economic power, employment, and even health care. Women tend to have domestic responsibilities and are the main subsistence agriculturalists.

Birth Rates: The population growth rate of about 3% is one of the highest in the world and has raised concerns. The fertility rate is four children born per mother. The country has a shortage of agricultural land, limited places in schools, and health services that cannot keep up with the increasing demands of more people. Although some want smaller families, meager health resources and medical infrastructure, culture, and religion are hampering efforts to provide family planning services. The infant mortality rate is 21 deaths per 1,000 births. Life expectancy is 70 for men, 76 for women.

Food Intolerances and Practices: The overall prevalence of malnutrition in children may be as high as 28%, and malnourished children have been found to be at higher risk for malarial treatment failure. Vitamin A

S

deficiency is common and a major cause of morbidity, mortality, and blindness (xerophthalmia) in children.

Child-Rearing Practices: About 42% of the population is 14 years of age or younger. Some 85% of births are attended by a skilled health worker.

National Childhood Immunizations: BCG at birth; DTaP at 2, 4, and 6 months; OPV at 2, 4, and 6 months, and at 5 years; HepB at birth and at 2 and 4 months; measles at 9 months; TT at 5, 24, and 28 years; vitamin A for underweight infants and children. The percent of the target population vaccinated, by antigen, is: BCG (84%); DTP1 (82%); DTP3 (80%); HepB3 and MCV (72%); and Polio3 (75%). Coverage rates have fallen significantly since the political crisis.

BIBLIOGRAPHY

Carroll K, Malefoasi G: Comparison of outcomes from a district tuberculosis control programme in the Pacific: before and after the implementation of DOTS, *Trop Doct.* 34(1):11, 2004.

Central Intelligence Agency: 2006: *The world factbook, Solomon Islands.* Retrieved September 21, 2006, from https://www.cia.gov/cia/publications/factbook/print/bp.html.

Kenyon M, Chevalier C, Gagahe V, Sisiolo R: The community in the classroom: designing a distance education community health course for nurses in the Solomon Islands, *Pac Health Dialog.* 7(2):76, 2000.

Kuschel, R, Takiika A, Angiki K: Alcohol and drug use in Honiara, Solomon Islands. In: Marsella A, Austin A, Grant B, eds, *Social change and psychosocial adaptation in the Pacific Islands.* St. Louis, 2005, Springer.

Lucas RE: A survey to gather sexually transmitted disease epidemiological and management data in the Solomon Islands, *Trop Doct.* 30(2):97, 2000.

Lumukana R, Temalesi K: Smoking and chewing habits of oral cancer patients in the Solomon Islands, *Pac Health Dialog.* 10(1):13, 2003.

Over M, Bakote'e B, Velayudhan R, Wilikai P, Graves PM: Impregnated nets or ddt residual spraying? Field effectiveness of malaria prevention techniques in Solomon Islands 1993–1999, *Am J Trop Med Hyg.* 71(2 suppl):1, 2004.

Solomon Islands: *Human development report. 2002.* Building a Nation, Honiara.

World Health Organization: 2006: Immunization, vaccines and biologicals. Retrieved September 21, 2006, from http://www.who.int/immunization_monitoring/en/globalsummary/countryprofileresult.cfm?C='slb'.

http://www.healthfax.org.au/pacific.htm (retrieved June 10, 2006).

http://www.wpro.who.int (retrieved June 10, 2006).

◆ SOMALIA

MAP PAGE (800)

Helen D. Rodd

S

Location: Somalia is in Eastern Africa and has a strategic location on the Horn of Africa. It shares boundaries with Djibouti, Ethiopia, and Kenya, and its extensive 3000-km coastline borders the Gulf of Aden and the Indian

Ocean. It is 637,567 km² (246,165 square miles), and the terrain is mostly flat with a more mountainous region in the north. The capital city, Mogadishu, is located in the south. Since the late 1980s, Somalia has been ravaged by civil war, factional fighting, droughts, and famine. It is one of the world's poorest and least developed countries, with a gross domestic product (GDP) per capita of $600. Although no official data on poverty rates or unemployment are available, there are very few skilled laborers: 71% of workers are employed in agriculture.

Major Languages	Ethnic Groups	Major Religions
Somali	Somali 85%	Sunni Muslim 97%
Arabic	Bantu groups 5%	Other 3%
English	Arab, Other 10%	
Italian		

Accurate population statistics are difficult to obtain because many Somalis are nomadic, and many have fled the country. However, the population is estimated at 8.8 million, including about 1 million refugees living in neighboring countries. Thousands of asylum seekers have resettled in Europe or the United States. The Somali language did not adopt a uniform orthography until 1973: about 50% of men and 26% of women are literate.

Health-Care Beliefs: Passive role; active sick care; traditional. Numerous illnesses are attributed to the presence of angry spirits within a person. To appease these spirits, people may hold healing ceremonies, which may last 1 or 2 days and involve eating special foods, reading the Koran, and burning incense. Mental health problems are generally not acknowledged. An individual is either considered "well" or "mad," and Somalis have little understanding of mental illness. Psychological problems attributed to posttraumatic stress disorder and chewing *khat* (a leaf with hallucinogenic properties) are becoming more prevalent.

Predominant Sick Care Practices: Magical-religious; herbal; biomedical where available. Traditional medicine is widely practiced. Common practices include applying heated sticks to the skin ("fire burning") and blood letting. People often remove primary canine tooth buds (*ilkodacowo,* or "fox teeth") from infants because it is believed that these teeth are the cause of many childhood ailments. The use of herbs and natural remedies provides a valuable adjunct to biomedical practices. Most Somalis have had some experience with Western medicine, although they invariably only seek curative, not preventive, treatments. Many humanitarian and nongovernmental organizations are currently active and work under the framework of the voluntary Somalia Aid Coordination Body. These groups are striving to implement primary health care programs but are continually threatened by the highly unstable situation.

Ethnic-/Race-Specific or Endemic Diseases: Somalis are at very high risk for bacterial and protozoal diarrhea, hepatitis A and E, and typhoid fever. Malaria and dengue fever are high risks in some locations, and schistosomiasis and rabies exist in some. Somalia has one of the highest incidences of tuberculosis in the world, and cholera is endemic in most areas. The major causes of death in childhood are respiratory infections, malaria, and diarrhea-related sequelae. Sporadic outbreaks of measles also contribute to high infant mortality. HIV statistics are not available for all of Somalia; however, baseline data obtained for northwest Somalia found the prevalence to be close to 1%. This is consistent with the Joint United Nations Programme on HIV/AIDS (UNAIDS) data that estimate the prevalence rate for human immunodeficiency virus (HIV) in adults (aged 15 to 49 years) as 0.9%. About 44,000 people are living with HIV, including 23,000 women and 1,500 to 13,000 children aged 0 to 14. Deaths from acquired immunodeficiency syndrome (AIDS) are estimated as 2,000–8,000, and the number of orphans 0–17 as a result of parental AIDS is 11,000–45,000.

Health-Team Relationships: Health care professionals in primary and secondary care settings are held in high regard. Nurses and auxiliary staff play an important role in service provision, particularly in rural areas. However, service provision in the main hospitals is predominantly headed by doctors. Many overseas agencies are involved in providing medical training within the local communities. The United Nations Children's Fund (UNICEF) in particular has a major role in designing and implementing new health policies.

Families' Role in Hospital Care: The family must assume a significant role in caring for a relative during a hospital admission. A patient depends entirely on relatives to provide their food while they are in the hospital.

Dominance Patterns: Women have high status in the Somali family structure. The wife and mother is the head of the family unit and takes a major role in child rearing and keeping the family accounts. It is common for people to live with their extended family or jointly with another family; however, as in many Islamic cultures, men and women are separated in most other aspects of life.

Eye-Contact Practices: Direct eye contact is considered extremely rude and is avoided by traditional Somalis.

Touch Practices: Physical contact between men and women is unacceptable unless it is among family members.

Perceptions of Time: Punctuality is not very important in Somali life. It is expected that individuals may be too early or, more commonly, too late for an appointment.

Pain Reactions: It is difficult to generalize about pain thresholds and reactions to pain. However, the Somali do not like to show any sign of weakness, which is particularly evident during childbirth, when women are extremely stoic.

Birth Rites: Somali culture is extremely supportive of expectant or new mothers. The fertility rate is seven children born per woman, and the overall population growth rate is 2.85%. After childbirth, new mothers remain at home and are cared for by female relatives and friends for 40 days (a period known as *afatanbah*). During this time, many special customs are observed. The mother is given special food and wears

S

earrings made from string passed through a clove of garlic. The newborn infant is welcomed into the community, and neonatal care includes warm water baths, sesame oil massages, and passive stretching of the infant's limbs. An herb called *malmal* is usually applied to the umbilicus for the first 7 days of life. In addition, the baby wears a bracelet made from malmal to ward off evil spirits. At the end of the 40 days, a celebratory family gathering is held at a friend or relative's house to mark the first time the mother and infant have left their home since the birth. All boys and girls are circumcised. Boys are usually circumcised before 5 years, and a traditional doctor, hospital nurse, or hospital doctor performs the procedure. The most common form of female circumcision is infibulation, and a female member of the family usually performs the procedure on infants or young girls. During childbirth, the mother's genital infibulation is opened and after birth is usually reinstated. Most women consider circumcision to be expected and desirable. The infant mortality rate is high at 115 deaths per 1,000 live births. Life expectancy is 47 for men, 50 for women.

Death Rites: When a person is about to die, relatives and friends gather to read special passages from the Koran and pray. After death, a male or female sheik attends the corpse, which is washed, perfumed, and wrapped in white cloth. The body is then taken to a mosque or directly to a grave prepared by the next of kin, where additional prayers are recited. The body is finally laid to rest facing Mecca. Somali believe that after death, a person's soul passes into *barzakh*—the transition between the two worlds—until the day of judgment; when the soul and body will be reunited.

Food Practices and Intolerances: The food that Somali Muslims are allowed to eat (*halal* food) includes fish, grain, fruits, and vegetables. Conversely, haram food is forbidden and includes anything from an animal that eats another animal and is therefore unclean (e.g., a pig). Furthermore, even animals that are considered clean must be killed in a certain way to be halal. During Ramadan (during the ninth month of the lunar calendar), people pray, fast, and refrain from drinking during daylight hours. Rice is the staple component of the diet and is usually mixed with meat (called *isku-dhexkaris*). Vegetables are more commonly available in southern Somalia, whereas the nomadic northern Somali consume more milk and meat. Extreme food shortages throughout Somalia continue to affect the nutritional status of the population, and malnutrition is a chronic problem in all areas.

Infant-Feeding Practices: Children are commonly breastfed until they are 2 years of age, but supplementation with animal milk (usually with a cup) is common in early infancy. At the age of 6 months, the child receives a mixture of rice and cow's milk before the introduction of solid foods.

Child-Rearing Practices: Children usually sleep with their parents until the age of 2 years. Toilet training begins at a young age, as diapers are not usually used. The infant is held over a small basin on the mother's lap for toilet training.

S

652 *South Africa (Republic of)*

National Childhood Immunizations: BCG at birth; DTwP at 6, 10, and 14 weeks; measles at 9 months; OPV at birth, 6, 10, and 14 weeks; TT first contact, +1 month, +6 months, +1 year, + 1 year; vitamin A at 6 to 59 months. The percent of the target population vaccinated, by antigen, is: BCG and DTP1 (50%); DTP3 (30%); and MCV (40%).

BIBLIOGRAPHY

Central Intelligence Agency: 2006: *The world factbook, Somalia.* Retrieved September 21, 2006, from https://www.cia.gov/cia/publications/factbook/print/so.html.

Harborview Medical Centre: Ethnic medicine guide, 1996. Retrieved March 30, 2006, from http://www.ethnomed.org/ethnomed/cultures/Somali.html.

Rodd HD, Davidson LE: "Ilko-Dacowo": canine enucleation and dental sequelae in Somali children, *Int J Paed Dentistry.* 10:290, 2000.

UNAIDS: 2006 Somalia. Retrieved September 21, 2006, from http://www.unaids.org/en/Regions_Countries/Countries/somalia.asp.

United Nations Children's Fund: 2004: Somalia basic datasheet, Retrieved March 30, 2006, from http://www.unicef.org/somalia/factfig/basic.html.

World Health Organization: 2006: Immunization, vaccines and biologicals. Retrieved September 21, 2006, from http://www.who.int/immunization_monitoring/en/globalsummary/countryprofileresult.cfm?C='som'.

◆ SOUTH AFRICA (REPUBLIC OF)

MAP PAGE (801)

Hester Klopper

Location: The Republic of South Africa occupies the southernmost part of the African continent and has a total area of 1,219,090 km² (470,691 square miles). It has common boundaries with Zimbabwe, Botswana, Namibia, Mozambique, Swaziland, and Lesotho. To the west, south, and east, it borders on the Atlantic and southern Indian Oceans. The landscape is characterized by bush, veld, deserts, and forests on the majestic mountain peaks and wide, unspoiled beaches and coastal wetlands. The capital is Pretoria. The gross domestic product (GDP) per capita is $12,000, with 27% unemployment and 50% living below the poverty line.

Major Languages	Ethnic Groups	Major Religions
English	African 77%	Christian 80%
Afrikaans	White 11%	Jewish, Muslim, Hindu,
IsiZulu	Coloured 9%	other 20%
IsiXhosa	Indian, Asian 3%	
Sepedi		

The population is 44.4 million and consists of the Nguni people (two thirds of the population), the Sotho-Tswana people (southern, northern, and western Sotho), the Tsonga, the Venda, Afrikaners, English,

Coloureds, Indians, and immigrants from the rest of Africa, Europe, and Asia. A few members of the Khoi and the San also remain. South Africa's constitution mentions 11 official languages: English, Afrikaans, IsiZulu, Sepedi, IsiNdebele, IsiXhosa, Sesotho, Setswana, SiSwati, Tshivenda, and Xitsonga. Literacy rates are 87% for men, 86% for women. Freedom of worship is guaranteed by the constitution, and the official policy is not to interfere with religious practices.

Health Care Beliefs: Passive and active roles; traditional; alternative; folk. Health care beliefs are part of the complex phenomenon of medical pluralism—the coexistence of different ways of perceiving, explaining, and treating illness. Two broad groups of health care delivery can be identified: (1) the system comprising allopathic, modern, and Western medicine and (2) the complementary system comprising traditional, alternative, and folk medicine. Although the allopathic system is dominant, South Africans strongly support traditional healers, who tend to share the same sociocultural values as their communities, including beliefs about the origins, significance, and treatment of ill health. In the traditional (rural) societies, ill health and other forms of misfortune are often blamed on social causes (bad relationships or witchcraft) or on supernatural causes (gods and ancestors), and traditional healers play a significant role. The healer focuses on the indigenous supernatural paradigm, historical legitimacy, sacred roles, tribal interest, and holistic treatment. Natural and supernatural explanations of disease are often compatible, as illustrated by the following story. A qualified nursing professor's mother had become ill. She discussed the illness with a social anthropology professor who was a good friend. It was evident that the nurse thought the origin of the illness might be witchcraft. The professor found it surprising that someone with scientific training would still believe in witches. "I know that the illness is a viral infection," said the nurse, "but I also need to know who sent the virus" (Boonzaaier, 1998). Mental disorders in particular are often considered by the African community to be supernatural and influenced by the ancestors.

Predominant Sick-Care Practices: Biomedical and magical-religious. Almost 50% consult a traditional healer before practitioners of Western medicine, or they consult them concurrently. As a result, many people receive a mixture of both forms of treatments. Treatments used by traditional healers may include ashes, amulets, and holy water. Since 1994, the government has made a concerted effort to integrate the two systems. Health care is financed through two systems: the private and public health sectors. The private health sector is a crucial part of the current health care system. The private sector provides care (primarily curative) to only 20% of the population. Private health care delivery is heavily concentrated in the densely populated wealthier urban areas and contributes little to alleviate the desperate shortages of resources in rural areas. Patients attending private health services need to pay for the service either as private patients in cash or through their medical plan. By April 1999, 168 private medical plans were registered in terms provided by the Medical Schemes Act, 1967 (Act 72 of 1967), established February 1, 1999. The intention was to make affordable health care more accessible. The ANC Health Plan intends to ensure health services for all South Africans, primarily through the achievements of equitable social and economic development. The funding of health care, especially for the poor, will continue to come from general tax revenues. Free health care is provided in the public sector for children younger than 6, pregnant or nursing mothers, older adults, people with disabilities, and certain people who are chronically ill. Preventive and health-promotion activities, school health services, antenatal and delivery services, contraception, nutritional support, curative care for public health problems, and community-based care are also provided free in the public sector.

Ethnic-/Race-Specific or Endemic Diseases: The most common communicable diseases are tuberculosis (TB) , malaria, measles, and sexually transmitted diseases. Malaria is endemic in the low-altitude areas of Northern Province, Mpumalanga, and northeastern KwaZulu-Natal. The highest risk area is a strip of about 100 km along the Zimbabwe, Mozambique, and Swaziland border. The disease should therefore be considered a regional, not a country-specific, problem. TB has been a problem in South Africa for more than 200 years. The epidemic is increasing by 20% per year, an increase resulting from the increasing poverty and decreasing social status of the population. A complicating factor is that TB is often not cured after the first attempt at treatment. Human immunodeficiency virus (HIV) and acquired immunodeficiency syndrome (AIDS) are also complicating the disease; 40% to 50% of TB cases are associated with HIV infection. Cancer, cardiovascular diseases, and strokes are thought of as diseases of the white man, although the incidence of myocardial infarctions in the Indian population is continuously increasing. HIV is a major health risk. The Joint United Nations Programme on HIV/AIDS (UNAIDS) reports the prevalence rate in adults (aged 15 to 49 years) is 18.8% (16.8% to 20.7%), and 5.5 million persons are living with HIV, including 3.1 million women and 240,000 children aged 0 to 14. Deaths from AIDS are estimated as 320,000 and an estimated 1.2 million children have been orphaned by AIDS.

Health-Team Relationships: Health personnel are considered the cornerstone for the realization of the Department of Health's vision. The main objectives are to integrate staff members and allocate them equally between urban and underserved areas. General practitioners play an important role in providing health care services. With the government's focus on primary health care, nursing professionals are playing a more important role because they are the frontline service providers. Other members of the health team include pharmacists and physical and occupational therapists. Nursing professionals and doctors work as close teams in all disciplines of health care delivery.

Families' Role in Hospital Care: All hospitals—state and private—allow visitors during visiting hours. Family members are encouraged to assist when possible with the care of the patient, and many stay overnight to care for sick children. Because of financial constraints in state hospitals, families are more likely to provide bedding and food.

Dominance Patterns: In most African households, the father is the head of the family, and usually the primary decision maker. In the Western (mostly white) households, men and women tend to have more equal relationships, and both help make decisions. Most of the women of South Africa contribute to its economic growth.

Eye-Contact Practices: In most of the African cultures, it is an insult to make direct eye contact. Guests and friends are usually greeted with a handshake, but family members are greeted with a kiss.

Touch Practices: Touch practices differ from culture to culture. In most African cultures, touching is common practice. In the more Western cultures, touching among family members (but not with others) is common. Children are frequently hugged and kissed. Nursing professionals often make physical contact with their patients to show they care; however, the doctor's role is such that limited physical contact occurs.

Perceptions of Time: Punctuality is not highly valued; people operate according to what is often referred to as "Africa time." This lack of timeliness often causes friction in the business world. Health care practitioners simply expect patients to be late. Many primary health care nurses and doctors meet with patients who do not have an appointment. Patients simply show up, get in line, and wait their turn. When patients obtain a sick note from a doctor, they are not penalized for taking a day off from work.

Pain Reactions: Patients are given the opportunity to discuss and describe their pain experiences. Analgesics are the primary treatment for pain relief, but lately more people have been using alternative therapies such as reflexology, aromatherapy, massage, and psychotherapy. In some hospitals, pain assessment forms are used to ensure effective pain management.

Birth Rites: The fertility rate is 2.2 children born per woman. Most infants of rural African women are born at home with the assistance of an older woman (often referred to as a midwife, although she has no formal training), and pain is not eased with any medication. The infants of women of the Western cultures are born primarily in a hospital with the assistance of a trained midwife. If patients choose one of the luxurious private hospitals for birth, they are able to have a medical doctor who is very often (in at least 70% of the cases) an obstetrician. Of the patients choosing private hospitals, 50% of the infants are born by cesarean section, often at the request of a mother who wants a planned delivery. After birth in the hospital, rooming-in is common (i.e., keeping the infant and mother together in the same room). "Kangaroo care" is used, and breastfeeding is usually the feeding method of choice. The overall infant mortality rate is high at 61 deaths per 1,000 live births. Life expectancy is 43 for men, 42 for women.

Death Rites: In the Western cultures, most sick people die in a hospital setting, and family members are usually very involved in the patient's care. The funeral or cremation usually takes place within 4 to 7 days after

S

death. Occasionally a memorial service is held in addition to the funeral or cremation service. In the African cultures, the body is dressed in clothing provided by the family and the body lies in state in the house of a family member, usually in the living room. Family and friends of the deceased come and visit during a 2- or 3-day period. Visitation is followed by a service that precedes the burial. It is customary for all family and friends of the deceased to attend the funeral service and pay their last respects. After the service and burial ceremony, family and friends join in celebrating that the deceased is "saved." It is not uncommon to slaughter a cow, 3 sheep, and 20 chickens for a funeral because most relatives or friends of the deceased person and the person's family participate in the celebration.

Food Practices and Intolerances: People from urban communities usually eat three times a day and may have the main course either at lunch or in the evening. The South African diet includes a wide variety of vegetables, fruits, fish, and meat such as chicken, beef, sheep, and pork. Because the diet is high in red meat, white men have a high incidence of high cholesterol and heart disease. The urban population also eats too many refined grains and breads. The rural South African's staple food is unrefined corn with seasonal vegetables if they are available. An estimated 55% to 60% of all South Africans are overweight, either because of the wrong diet or from overeating.

Infant-Feeding Practices: Breastfeeding is the standard practice, and most women are aware of its benefits. If for any reason a mother cannot or chooses not to breastfeed, formula is available. For white women, breastfeeding is a private affair. However, African women feed on demand, even in public.

Child-Rearing Practices: Child rearing practices have tended to be very strict; children are seen but not heard. Child rearing is the primary responsibility of the parents but is shared by the teachers at school. Children are now taught to express their opinions freely and to think critically in school. South Africa strongly supports the United Nations Convention on the Rights of the Child by banning corporal punishment in schools. Single-parent families are relatively common. Because many African mothers work in the cities, their children are often left in the care of grandparents in rural areas. The mother or father visits about every 3 months, depending on the travel distance. Working mothers are now granted 4 months of paid maternity leave, and fathers receive 5 days of paternity leave.

National Childhood Immunizations: BCG at birth; DT at 5 years; DTwP at 18 months; DTwPHib at 6, 10, and 14 weeks; OPV at birth, 6, 10, and 14 weeks, at 18 months, and at 5 years; HepB at 6, 10, and 14 weeks; measles at 9 and 18 months; TT antenatal and trauma; vitamin A at 0 to 5, 6 to 11, 12 to 60 months and postpartum women. The percent of the target population vaccinated, by antigen, is: BCG (97%); DTP1 (99%); DTP3 (93%); HepB3 and Hib3 (92%); MCV (81%); Polio3 (94%); TT2 plus (61%); and vitamin A (66%).

BIBLIOGRAPHY

Center for Health Policy: *A national health service and the future of the private sector-the case for a national health insurance, 1991,* JHB, University of the Witwatersrand.

Central Intelligence Agency: 2006: *The world factbook, South Africa.* Retrieved September 21, 2006 from https://www.cia.gov/cia/publications/factbook/print/sf.html

Dennill K, King L & Swanepoel T: Aspects of primary health care, Johannesburg, South Africa, *1995,* Halfway House: Southern Book Publishers.

Government Communication and Information System: *South Africa yearbook, 2002/2003,* Pretoria, South Africa.

UNAIDS: 2006 South Africa. Retrieved September 21, 2006, from http://www.unaids.org/en/Regions_Countries/Countries/south_africa.asp.

World Health Organization: 2006: Immunization, vaccines and biologicals. Retrieved September 21, 2006, from http://www.who.int/immunization_monitoring/en/globalsummary/countryprofileresult.cfm?C='zaf'.

◆ SPAIN (KINGDOM OF)

MAP PAGE (798)

Joaquín Tomás-Sábado and Montserrat Antonín Martin

Location: Spain is situated in southwest Europe and occupies most of the Iberian Peninsula. The capital is Madrid. Separated from France (and the rest of Europe) by the Pyrenees Mountains, its eastern and southeast coasts are bordered by the Mediterranean Sea, and those in the southwest and north are met by the Atlantic Ocean. Spain also includes two island regions: the Balearic Islands in the Mediterranean Sea and the Canary Islands in the Atlantic Ocean. With a total area of 504,790 km² (194,884 square miles), Spain is the second largest country of the European Union (EU). The population is more than 44 million, of which more than 8% are foreign immigrants, mainly from Morocco, Ecuador, Romania, and Columbia. Spain is part of the EU and the North Atlantic Treaty Organization (NATO).

Major Languages	Ethnic Groups	Major Religions
Castilian Spanish (official)	Spanish 73%	Roman Catholic 99%
Catalan (official)	Catalan 16%	Other (Islam and
Galician (official)	Galician 8%	Protestant) 1%
Basque (official)	Basque, Other 3%	

Spain has four official languages: Castilian Spanish (73%), Catalan (16%), Galician (8%), and Basque (3%). There is great diversity among the Spanish people. During a large part of its history, the territory was ruled by other civilizations, such as the Romans and the Arabs, and each group left its mark in terms of culture, art, and landscape. The gross

S

domestic product (GDP) per capita is $25,500. Literacy rates are 99% for men, 97% for women.

Health Care Beliefs: Active role; minimal use of folk remedies; health promotion important. In the early part of the century, such practices as cupping and folk remedies for warts were common, but these have mostly given way to modern medicine, in which interdisciplinary health care teams play a key role. It is difficult to know how many people consult folk healers and believe in their precepts. Some people combine this practice with that offered by institutional centers. People attempt to resolve physical health complaints as well as psychological, personal, social, and financial problems.

Predominant Sick-Care Practices: Biomedical primarily. The health care system is centralized and socialized and provides equal access for all at both primary care and hospital levels. Each autonomous community draws up its own plans for maintaining and protecting health. In general, citizens adhere to a Western medical-model belief system and are more likely to use the modern medical system than alternative approaches.

Ethnic-/Race-Specific or Endemic Diseases: The disease profile of Spain mirrors that of developed countries. Cardiovascular disease is the major cause of death (34%), followed by tumors (26%) and respiratory diseases (11%). Traffic accidents are the main cause of death among young people aged 15 to 34. Human immunodeficiency virus (HIV) and acquired immunodeficiency syndrome (AIDS) and substance abuse are increasing problems. The country is undergoing an immigration crisis as thousands of North Africans, Central Americans, and Eastern Europeans immigrate for a better life. The immigration is changing infectious diseases rates and places a great burden on the public health system. The Joint United Nations Programme on HIV/AIDS (UNAIDS) estimates the prevalence rate for HIV in adults (aged 15 to 49 years) to be 0.6%, with 140,000 people living with HIV, including 32,000 women. Deaths from AIDS are estimated at 2,000.

Health-Team Relationships: Emphasis among health professionals is on teamwork, and doctors and nurses work cooperatively. The nurse is transitioning from a dependent to a more independent role, but nurses still must practice under a doctor's supervision. Friendliness, patience, efficacy, and professionalism distinguish their respective roles. In selected areas, the qualities of nurse practitioners are highly valued by patients. Communication between nurses and patients is usually better than that between patients and doctors.

Families' Role in Hospital Care: Hospitals encourage the patient and family to collaborate in care. Some children continue their schooling while in the hospital. In most instances, families are expected to stay with relatives and provide much of their personal care. Family members take turns staying with patients, who are seldom left alone. As dual-career households increase, families are finding it harder to care for the growing population of older adults. Some families hire extra assistance because placing a loved one in a nursing home is still very difficult for them.

Dominance Patterns: Spain has an ethnically diverse society, with notable differences among its regions in food, music, and traditions. During the last 40 years, Spain has undergone great political, social, and economic changes, which have influenced the role of women. According to the Spanish constitution, women have equal rights; they are represented in all areas of employment and hold many elected offices. As a result, the relationship between men and women parallels that of the rest of Europe. Although rural areas may still have traces of the more traditional male-dominant pattern, the younger generation of women is experiencing more equality.

Perceptions of Time: Although Spaniards have a reputation for having a casual attitude about time, the exigencies of modern society have made punctuality more important. Banks, stores, factories, and other establishments open on time, and public transportation tends to be reliable. Nonetheless, the Spanish people have a casual attitude about being on time for personal visits, dates, and similar appointments.

Pain Reactions: Some Spaniards are very stoic and do not admit they are in pain unless it is extreme, whereas some are extremely vocal. Hospice care is emerging as people begin to realize that patients need proper and adequate pain control. Most hospitals have pain units and palliative care teams.

Birth Rites: Both birth and infant mortality rates are decreasing, and the age at which women are first becoming pregnant is increasing. Spain's birth rate is the lowest in Europe; the fertility rate is 1.28 children born per woman. The infant mortality rate is 4.37 deaths per 1,000 live births. Births usually take place in the hospital, and fathers may witness a delivery if there are no complications. The contraceptive methods used, in decreasing order of popularity, are condoms, birth control pills, intrauterine devices, diaphragms, and biological rhythm (which is used by religious couples who do not approve of other contraceptive methods). In general terms, the Spanish population has undergone a process similar to that of other European countries. High birth and mortality rates have changed to low birth and mortality rates. Life expectancy is 76 for men, 83 for women.

Death Rites: The family has a wake for 24 hours. Except in some rural areas, the custom of keeping vigil over the deceased's body at home has practically disappeared, and funeral homes have become widespread. Although most bodies are buried, about 20% are cremated, and this practice is becoming more common. Most funerals include a Catholic mass.

Food Practices and Intolerances: The notable differences in climate and lifestyle mean that each region maintains the typical dishes of the area. In general, Spanish food is characterized by the combination of fresh produce (with olive oil as the main condiment), vegetables, abundant fruit and garden produce, cheese, fish, meat, bread, and moderate wine consumption. Spices and hot seasonings are infrequently used.

Child-Rearing Practices: In the past, infant care was primarily the job of the women, but today the responsibility is beginning to be shared by the father. Education about sex role differences begins early. Students must pass a competitive qualifying examination to enter their desired field of education.

S

National Childhood Immunizations: DT at 4 to 6 years; DTaP at 4 to 6 years; DTaPHibIPV at 2, 4, 6, and 15 to 18 months; HepB at birth and 1 and 6 months (or 2, 4, and 6 months); MenC_conj at 2, 4, and 6 months; MMR at 12 to 15 months and at 3 to 6 years; and Td 14 to 16 years. The percentage of the target population vaccinated, by antigen, is: DTP1 (98%); DTP3 and Hib3 (96%); HepB3, MCV2, and Polio3 (97%).

Other Characteristics: Spaniards have been called the "night owls of Europe" because they like to stay up late, partly because of the great weather and partly because they like to have a good time. The Roman Catholic Church plays a major role in the social life of Spain. Religious festivals are common throughout the country and offer an opportunity for major and minor celebrations throughout the year. Given the notable cultural diversity among the different regions, the typical stereotypes about Spanish people rarely reflect today's society.

BIBLIOGRAPHY

Artazcoz L, Moya C, Vanaclocha H, Pont P: Adult health. *Gac Sanit* 18(1): 56–68, 2004.

Borrell C, Benach J: Health differences in Catalonia, Barcelona, 2003, Mediterrania.

Central Intelligence Agency: *2006: The world factbook, Spain.* Retrieved September 21, 2006, from https://www.cia.gov/cia/publications/factbook/print/sp.html.

Espino A, Duaigües S, Montenegro Q, Viló L: Mortality records in a health district. *Aten Primaria* 36(8): 466, 2005.

Falcó A: Nursing care following the values and ethical principles of the profession, *Enfermeria Clin.* 15(5):287–290, 2005.

Guillen M, Vidiella A: Forecasting Spanish natural life expectancy, *Risk Anal.* 25(5): 1161–1170, 2005.

Lete I, Martinez M.: Reproductive health: some data and reflections, *Gac Sanit.* 18(1): 170–174, 2004.

Spector RE, Muñoz MJ: *The cultures of health,* Madrid, 2003, Pearson Educacion.

Spanish Ministry of Health and Consumer: Retrieved February 13, 2006, from http://www.msc.es/en/ciudadanos/proteccionSalud/infancia/.

UNAIDS: 2006 Spain. Retrieved September 21, 2006, from http://www.unaids.org/en/Regions_Countries/Countries/spain.asp.

World Health Organization: 2006: Immunization, vaccines and biologicals. Retrieved September 21, 2006, from http://www.who.int/immunization_monitoring/en/globalsummary/countryprofileresult.cfm?C='esp'.

◆ SRI LANKA (DEMOCRATIC SOCIALIST REPUBLIC OF)

MAP PAGE (804)

K.A.L.A. Kuruppuarachchi

S

Location: Sri Lanka is tropical island just off the southeastern tip of the Indian subcontinent. It has a total area of approximately 62,705 km^2 (24,204 square miles). The central hilly area has mountains and plains and a mean temperature ranging from 14° C to 24° C, whereas the low-country plains and coastal areas are between 26° C and 28° C. Sri Lanka has traditionally been an agricultural country, and Ceylon tea, grown in the central hills, is world famous. The estimated population is 20.2 million, with the greatest population density in the capital city of Colombo. The majority of the people are Sinhalese. The other significant ethnic groups include the Tamils, Moors, and Burghers.

Major Languages	Ethnic Groups	Major Religions
Sinhala	Sinhalese 74%	Buddhist 70%
Tamil	Tamil 18%	Hindu 15%
	Moor 7%	Christian 8%
	Burgher, Malay, Veddah 1%	Muslim 7%

The Sinhalese speak Sinhala, whereas the Tamils and most Moors speak Tamil. Schoolchildren are encouraged to learn Sinhala and Tamil. Importance is also placed on English, knowledge of which is highly beneficial for social mobility and employment. The literacy rate is 95% for men, 90% for women. Buddhism is practiced by most Sinhalese, Hinduism by most Tamils, Islam by the Moors, and Christianity by some in each of these groups. Since the outbreak of hostilities between the government and Tamil separatists in the 1980s, several hundred thousand Tamil civilians have fled the island, and more than 200,000 have sought refuge in the West. The gross domestic product (GDP) per capita is $4,300, with 25% living below the poverty line.

Health Care Beliefs: Active and passive roles; traditional. The majority believe that ill health has physical origins. However, some people, particularly those in rural areas, attribute it to supernatural or astrological influences. *Bodhi poojas*—pouring water on the bo tree, which is considered sacred—and visiting fortune tellers are common.

Predominant Sick-Care Practices: Biomedical; alternative; magical-religious. Western medicine is freely accessible through the state health sector and has replaced traditional and indigenous practices. However, some people with chronic, debilitating diseases or mental illness rely on indigenous magico-religious rituals such as wearing enchanted threads or amulets, applying oils, and performing *thovil* (an exorcism ceremony). Trained and untrained ayurvedic practitioners have learned the art from their predecessors. Homeopathy and acupuncture are also practiced. Herbal preparations are widely used as complementary medicine. Western practitioners should be aware of potential drug interactions, enzyme induction, and hepatotoxicity associated with these herbal preparations. Many people resort to both Western and complementary medicine when the illness is long lasting.

Ethnic-/Race-Specific or Endemic Diseases: Malaria is endemic in certain provinces. Other infectious diseases include Japanese encephalitis, dengue hemorrhagic fever, and leptospirosis. Mass vaccination has eradicated polio. Diarrheal diseases, acute respiratory infections, filaria-sis, tuberculosis, and leprosy are common concerns. The morbidity and mortality associated with snakebites are significant; traditional healers place a particular stone over the site of the bite in the belief that it will remove the venom. Prevention of rabies is another important task. It is compulsory to report many of the communicable diseases, and the coun-try supports public health programs for control. Alcohol-, tobacco-, and cannabis-related disorders are emerging health care issues. Suicide and deliberate self-injury rates have been alarming in the last few years and are particularly high among Buddhists, although Buddhism discourages suicide. Rapid socioeconomic change over the last few decades may have contributed to these increased numbers. Depressive disorders and mental health problems are increasing, and it has been estimated that nearly 400,000 Sri Lankans suffer from serious mental illnesses. The Joint United Nations Programme on HIV/AIDS (UNAIDS) estimates the preva-lence rate for HIV in adults (15–49) is <0.1%, with 5,000 living with HIV, including fewer than 1,000 women. Fewer than 500 deaths have been reported attributable to acquired immunodeficiency syndrome (AIDS). Sri Lanka is classified as a low-level epidemic country. Most infections are acquired heterosexually.

Health-Team Relationships: Doctors are highly regarded, and most health care services revolve around them. However, a multidisciplinary approach to health care is becoming more popular in all areas, including mental health, although it is greatly hindered by the lack of trained personnel.

Families' Role in Hospital Care: The extended family members take turns staying with patients, and bathe and feed them. They are also involved in decision making and long-term care if the patient has a chronic illness. The involvement of the family is helpful, especially for patients with mental illnesses, because community care for these individuals is not well developed. Women played a major role in caring for the sick and elderly in the past. As a result of urbanization and economic needs, many women now seek employment. As a result, many have the expanded role of wage earner and looking after children, the infirm, and the elderly. The elderly population is increasing, and dementia is a major concern.

Dominance Patterns: Men are usually dominant, especially in rural areas. Children usually have the father's surname. Women play a central role in the home; they are respected and revered by children and are the primary caretakers. Women traditionally wear sarees. The workforce has a considerable number of women in every sector, and women are in some managerial positions. Unfortunately, violence against women and domestic violence are on the increase.

Eye-Contact Practices: Direct eye contact is common, regardless of sex. In rural settings, it is still common for young women to avoid eye con-tact because of shyness.

Touch Practices: Touching is common among friends of the same sex who are talking. When greeting one another, Sri Lankans place their palms together in front of their chest, as if praying, and say *ayubowan,* or "long life." However, greetings in professional situations may be limited to a handshake.

Perceptions of Time: Punctuality is emphasized from childhood, and most ceremonies are performed at specific times designated as *naketh,* usually determined by astrologers. Many Sri Lankans are relaxed about time during other activities. They are proud to talk about the country's previous prosperity and history.

Pain Reactions: Pain is expressed verbally by most. Many weep, which is thought to resolve the bereavement process. Mental distress is expressed verbally and by somatization (where the mental anguish is expressed in bodily symptoms such as burning pain in the head or abdomen).

Birth Rites: The fertility rate is 1.84 children born per woman. Most births occur in hospitals. The time of the birth is considered important, and horoscopes are developed based on it. Many believe the time of birth determines various aspects of the future, including education, employment, and marriage. Birth is a celebratory time for family and friends, and the mother and child are cared for by family members, especially by grandmothers. The mother is fed a broth prepared with rice and chilies. Children of both sexes are equally valued, although certain families may prefer boys. The infant mortality rate is 14 deaths per 1,000 live births. Life expectancy is 71 for men, and 76 for women.

Death Rites: Those who are dying are helped to recall their past good deeds so they will be in a sound state of mind at the time of death, which facilitates a better rebirth. When grieving, many Sri Lankans weep. Buddhists have priests chant *pirith,* or religious songs. Funerals vary according to religious rituals and rites. Family and friends attend the burial or cremation ceremony. Some families have burial plots in their ancestral lands, but most bury their family members in public cemeteries. The body is carried in a wooden casket, and some Sri Lankans play a special drum rhythm during the procession. The funeral procession walks on white cloth or sand that has been placed on the ground. Flower wreaths are common. On the seventh day and various intervals afterward, priests are offered food in the belief that it will help the deceased person during rebirth. Autopsies are generally acceptable, and Buddhism encourages organ donations.

Food Practices and Intolerances: Rice is the staple food and is eaten with curries of vegetables, fish, or meat. The food is spicy and hot, and coconut milk is used liberally in the curries. *Kiribath,* or milk rice, is a traditional specialty made with coconut milk and cooked for celebrations such as the New Year. Most Sri Lankans eat with their right hand. Fast food is becoming more popular as a result of Western influence and urbanization; along with sedentary and stressful lifestyles, these changed eating patterns are contributing to increases in the rates of diabetes, hypertension, and coronary artery disease along with sedentary and stressful lifestyles.

S

Infant-Feeding Practices: Breastfeeding is popular and may continue for 2 to 5 years. Most mothers are aware of its benefits.

Child-Rearing Practices: Children are generally raised in extended families who display tendencies toward overinvolvement and overprotection. Children have a religious upbringing and learn traditional values. Parents, older adults, and teachers are respected and honored with betel leaves on special occasions. An event of cultural significance with many elaborate customs is when a young girl attains menarche. The girl is usually kept in a room, and minimal contact with males is allowed. Certain dietary restrictions are placed; for example, no fried foods are allowed. At a predetermined auspicious time, she is taken out of the room by the mother and bathed in water containing scented flowers, followed by a celebration with friends and relatives during which the girl is given gifts to mark the event of her reaching womanhood.

National Childhood Immunizations: BCG at birth; DT at 5 years; DTwP at 2, 4, 6, and 18 months; OPV at 2, 4, 6, and 18 months and 5 years; HepB at 2, 4 and 6 months; JapEnc at 12, 13 and 24 months-part of country (children below age of 10 years in high risk areas, in 18 districts); MR at 3 years; Rubella at 8 years; Td at 12 years; TT pregnant women, + 6 weeks × 2, 6 weeks apart in first pregnancy, × 3 in subsequent pregnancies; Vitamin A +9, +18 months, +5, +9, +12 years. The percent of the target population vaccinated, by antigen, is: BCG, DTP1 (98%); DTP3, Polio3 (97%); HepB3 (85%); MCV (96%); TT2 plus (65%).

BIBLIOGRAPHY

Central Intelligence Agency: *2006: The world factbook, Sri Lanka.* Retrieved September 21, 2006, from https://www.cia.gov/cia/publications/factbook/print/ce.html.

Department of Health Services: *Annual health bulletin, Sri Lanka,* 2002, Department of Health Services.

Kuruppuarachchi KALA, Rajakaruna RR: Psychiatry in Sri Lanka, *Psychiatric Bull.* 23:686–688, 1999.

Kurruppu L: *Psychiatry in Sri Lanka.* In: De Sousa A, De Sousa D, eds. *Psychiatry in Asia* Mumbai, 2005, Vikas Medical Publishers, pp 197–212.

World Health Organization, Regional Office for South-East Asia: *Suicide prevention: emerging from darkness, 2001.* WHO.

World Health Organization, Sri Lanka: *WHO country cooperation strategy 2006–2011.* The Democratic Socialist Republic of Sri Lanka, 2006.

UNAIDS: 2006 Sri Lanka. Retrieved September 21, 2006, from http://www.unaids.org/en/Regions_Countries/Countries/sri_lanka.asp.

United Nations Development Program: Human and income poverty: developing countries. Retrieved October 15, 2006, from http://hdr.undp.org/statistics/data/indicators.cfm?x=25&y=1&z=1.

World Health Organization: 2006: Immunization, vaccines and biologicals. Retrieved September 21, 2006, from http://www.who.int/immunization_monitoring/en/globalsummary/countryprofileresult.cfm?C='lka'.

http://www.who.int/countries/1ka/en/ (retrieved August 27, 2006).

◆ SUDAN (REPUBLIC OF THE)

MAP PAGE (800)

Samir Shaheen

Location: Sudan lies in the northeastern part of Africa and is bordered on the west by Chad and Central African Republic; on the south by Congo, Uganda, and Kenya; on the east by Ethiopia and Eritrea; and on the north by Libya and Egypt. Sudan is the largest country in Africa, with a total area of 2,505,810 km^2 (967,495 square miles). The capital is Khartoum. The population is 36.2 million, and is expected to be 40.5 million by 2010. About 64% are rural or nomadic, and 45% are between 6 and 45 years of age. The gross domestic product (GDP) per capita is $2,100, with 40% living below the poverty line.

Major Languages	Ethnic Groups	Major Religions
Arabic	Black 52%	Sunni Muslim 70%
English	Arab 39%	Indigenous beliefs 25%
Tribal dialects	Beja 6%	Christian 5%
	Other 3%	

More than 100 languages are spoken in Sudan. They are being replaced by Arabic, the language of trade and government. Commonly spoken are Dinka, Nuer, Triggering, Fur, and Nubian. Literacy rates are 51% and 54% for men in the northern and southern states, respectively, and they are 49% and 52% for women in the northern and southern states, respectfully.

Health Care Beliefs: Traditional; active role; health promotion important. Health centers have health promotion and prevention units, and societies have been established for health promotion. These groups also help poorer patients with their finances. Mental illness is feared, and many believe it is the result of demonic possession. Most people in remote villages and slums of large towns and cities consult a holy man, or *Faki*, before they consult a doctor. A surprising number of educated people also consult Fakis. The number of traditional healers far outnumbers psychiatrists and psychologists. Treatment of patients with mental illness can be appalling. Patients are kept in solitary confinement, given only bread and water, and may be beaten in an attempt to drive out the demons or evil spirits thought to possess them. Some patients develop scurvy, and they are eventually brought to the hospital because scurvy prevents their wounds from healing. Traditional healers and psychiatrists collaborate by referring patients to one another. Traditional healers are not only consulted for psychiatric problems but also for organic diseases. A form of traditional treatment is *zar*, commonly practiced in urban and rural areas in northern Sudan and Ethiopia, where it probably originated. Zar is the name of a demon, or *jinni*, that is believed to cause many changes in physical and psychological health or welfare: it can cause illness, pregnancy or

S

birth, or death. These invisible beings are believed to number 88 and are divided into two equal groups. Forty-four are controlled by a chief called Warrar, the other 44 by another chief called Mama. In the Sudan, the Zar Mama is more influential; he is often mentioned and called on during chants of the Zar ceremonies. During these ceremonies, the targeted patient goes into a trance under the influence of chants, burning incense, and the sound of drums. The songs are thought to appease the jinni or demon possessing the person. During these trances and dances, the patient is free to indulge in activities that are normally taboo; for example, women are allowed to smoke and drink. The person may express suppressed needs- perhaps therapeutic. A woman may be dressed in a man's attire to symbolize certain idolized figures. Probably because of the influence of white men during British colonization of the country, patients dress in European attire and smoke a pipe. The resulting figure is known as a *khawaga,* a term used for any white man. Another figure that may be seen is the *Arabi,* or Arab. Those under the influence of the Arabi dress in the fashion of the Beja tribes (the Fuzzy Wuzzy of Kipling) of eastern Sudan. In contrast, men may dress as women during the ceremonies.

Predominant Sick-Care Practices: Biomedical and magico-religious. In remote rural areas, where health services are poor or unavailable, patients still use traditional healers. In many rural areas, fractures and orthopedic problems (particularly low back pain) are treated by Baseers (bone setters). Treatments given by traditional healers often include herbal medicines (such as henna for treatment of hepatitis), scarification, and cauterization. In Muslim communities, patients are treated with recitations from the *Koran* over the affected body part, and the healer usually spits over the body part as well. This practice is common for treating headaches. Verses from the *Koran* may be written on a piece of wood, and the writings are washed with water that is given to the patient to drink or rub on the affected area. Or the verses may be written on paper, which is burned and inhaled. The smoke practice is commonly used when a disease is believed to have been caused by someone with the "evil eye" (i.e., the power to harm others merely by looking at them) or possession by a jinni. Sorcery is practiced in both Muslim and non-Muslim communities. The Faki, or holy man, in Muslim communities, and other sorcerers in non-Muslim areas, are called on to reverse the effects of witchcraft. Verses from the *Koran* and mysterious symbols are worn on amulets as protection against the evil eye. Belief in evil spirits and sorcery is common, and in the Nuba Mountains, the *kujur* performs rituals to rid the patient of evil spirits. Roots of certain plants are often used to treat snake and scorpion bites in rural areas and are used as protective amulets. In urban areas, where modern medical facilities are available and people are more educated, people usually consult doctors. In the past, medical care was free, but at present there is a fee-for-service system. Recently a health insurance system was introduced in which the government or private companies cover costs. Most government employees and many farmers now have coverage.

S

Ethnic-/Race-Specific or Endemic Diseases: Malaria, tuberculosis, leprosy, cutaneous and visceral leishmaniasis, and schistosomiasis are the major endemic diseases. An ethnically related disease is kala-azar. Evidence shows that under similar exposure conditions, individuals from the tribes of southern Sudan and the Nuba Mountains are more suscepti-ble to kala-azar than individuals from tribes of the northern Sudan. Sickle cell anemia is more common in the Messeyria tribes of Kordofan, and goi-ter is common in the west. The Beja tribes of the Red Sea hills are partic-ularly susceptible to tuberculosis. In northern Sudan, diseases of affluence such as heart disease and diabetes are becoming important health pro-blems. The Joint United Nations Programme on HIV/AIDS (UNAIDS) esti-mates the prevalence rate for human immunodeficiency virus (HIV) in adults (aged 15 to 49 years) to be 1.6%, with 320,000 living with HIV, including 180,000 women and 30,000 children (aged 0 to 14). Deaths from acquired immunodeficiency syndrome (AIDS) are reportedly around 34,000.

Health-Team Relationships: Overall, doctors are dominant. In rural areas the midwife is highly respected and quite influential. Doctors and their assistants are highly regarded by the community. A commonly used name for a doctor is *hakeem* (Arabic for "the wise").

Families' Role in Hospital Care: Family and friends play an important role in supporting patients in hospital and home, staying with them and, until recently, providing food. They also donate blood if needed. Mothers can stay with sick children. Among the Masalit tribes of western Sudan, those with a disease such as leprosy, which carries a stigma in many com-munities, are accepted and cared for by the family in a separate hut in the family's housing compound. Their clothes are washed, and their meals are prepared. In areas where leprosy is rare, the stigma is stronger; many people leave their families and are never heard from again.

Dominance Patterns: Generally speaking, men are dominant. With the recent increase in education for women, greater economic independence and emancipation have been evident in urban areas. Relationships between men and women are changing significantly, reflected in the enhanced role of women in social and economic fields. Women now have senior positions in both public and private sectors.

Eye-Contact Practices: In certain situations, direct eye contact is pro-hibited. For example, conservative women do not have direct eye contact with unknown men or with holy men.

Touch Practices: The handshake is a common greeting. In some Muslim factions, women are not allowed to shake hands with men other than their husbands or first-degree relatives.

Perceptions of Time: In areas of traditional agriculture, the timing of events is related to the cycles of agricultural activities (e.g., harvest time, the rainy season, the flooding of the Nile). In urban areas, perceptions of time are similar to those in modern industrial societies. During the current difficult chapter in the nation's history, people often reminisce about the "good old days."

S

Pain Reactions: People in rural areas appear to have a high pain tolerance. The younger generation, particularly in urban societies, are more
responsive to pain.

Birth Rites: The infant mortality rate is high at 61 per 1,000 live births,
and the fertility rate is 4.72 children born per woman. In rural areas, traditional birth attendants assist with births. In larger towns and cities, trained
midwives assist. After birth, the mother is confined to the house for about
40 days. In northern Sudan, she is taken with the infant to the Nile River,
where part of the child's body is washed with water, a habit dating from
the time when the population in this area was Christian. This may also have
been practiced in the ancient kingdoms of Nubia. During the 40 days, the
woman cannot be visited by anyone who has seen a dead body or who has
been to a cemetery. In rural areas, the confined woman wears a *masha-
hara,* which is a collection of beads and figures of humans and various animals believed to ward off the evil eye and spirits. Immediately after birth, a
male relative recites verses from the *Koran* to the infant. Every newborn
Muslim is named Mohamed or Fatima (after the prophet Mohamed and
his daughter) at birth, depending on the sex. On the seventh day after
birth, infants are given a permanent name and a ram is sacrificed. Boys
are preferred. Among the Nilotic tribe of the Dinka of southern Sudan,
where clans are traced through the male lineage, it is important for men
to marry and produce a male child to maintain the lineage link. If no son
is born, they face oblivion after death. The birth of a girl is celebrated
because she brings her family wealth when she marries. Dinka women
stay in their mother's house for the birth of their children and remain in
the hut for 5 days. Their mothers care for them and cut the umbilical cord.
The placenta is placed in a skin and washed and is later buried by both
women outside the house. The father sacrifices a bull or sheep, and the
blood is spilled outside the hut. The grandmother dips her finger in the
blood and smears it on the infant's forehead, neck, and chest; some is
smeared on the mother as well. Some foods are taboo during pregnancy
and during nursing, including antelope, buffalo, and certain types of fish.
If these rules are broken, it is believed that the child will die. Nuba women
give birth in their house; the umbilical cord is cut with a fragment of millet
stalk, and the placenta is buried inside the hut. Traditionally, the first-born
male is named Kuku, the second Kafi, the third Tia, and the fourth with the
female name Tutu. The first-born female is named Kaka, the second Toto,
the third Kash, and the fourth Kiki. Maternal deaths have decreased from
556 per 100,000 in 1990 to 509 in 1999. It is hoped that maternal
deaths will be reduced further by 2015 to 127 per 100,000. Life expectancy is 58 for men, 60 for women.

Death Rites: In the hot climate of the Sudan, the body is buried as quickly
as possible. Women wail and lament, mentioning the virtues of the
deceased. Muslims wash the body with water in a ritual dictated by Islam.
The body is then dabbed with perfumes and wrapped in new white cloth
before it is finally buried after a short prayer. Inside the grave the body
is laid on its right side with the face toward Mecca. Only men are allowed

S

to attend the burial. Women wail and may throw sand on their uncovered heads, a sign of intense mourning. Mourning continues for 3 days, during which time friends and relatives visit. The Dinka—the main Nilotic tribe of southern Sudan—dig a grave outside the hut and the body is buried in a fetal position with skins placed over and beneath it. Among the Nuba of Kordufan, the family graves are shaped like a funnel. A 6- to 8-foot long shaft expands in its lower part into a space that is 3 feet high and 8 feet long. A couple of men are lowered in the grave to receive the body. Hoes, broken spears, and knives are buried with the corpse. The spirit of the deceased is believed to stay in the grave with the body and leave occasionally to visit the village and appear to relatives in dreams. Many of these rituals (but perhaps not all) are still practiced by the Dinka and Nuba tribes in their homelands. Those who have been displaced from their tribal areas seem to have abandoned these practices and follow either Christian or Muslum practices.

Food Practices and Intolerances: The diet consists of vegetables, meat, bread, thin bread *(kissra)*, and porridge made from sorghum, millet, or wheat. People living near the Nile and its tributaries or on the shores of the Red Sea eat fish. Poor people may not have meat except during festivities such as the Eid al-Adha festival, when Muslims are required to sacrifice an animal, usually a sheep. A popular affordable dish consists of beans with sesame oil, eaten with wheat bread, usually for breakfast and as an evening meal. *Aseeda,* a type of thick porridge made from sorghum or millet, is eaten with milk or stewed meat and vegetables. In some tribes, certain items of food are taboo; for example, the Beja tribes of eastern Sudan do not eat fish or eggs. Most eat with their hands.

Infant-Feeding Practices: Most women breastfeed for 2 years according to the teachings of Islam. Nursing is supplemented by bottle-feeding if the mother feels she does not have enough milk. In urban communities, bottle-feeding is becoming fashionable and is increasing.

Child Rearing Practices: Child rearing is strict, and the father is responsible for most discipline. It is common for children to sleep with their parents. Deaths of children under 5 years are approximately 68 per 1,000.

National Childhood Immunizations: BCG at birth and first contact; DTwP at 6, 10, and 14 weeks; OPV at 6, 10, and 14 weeks; measles at 9 months; HepB at 6, 10 and 14 weeks; TT at first contact, +1, +6 months, +1, + 1 year. The percent of the target population vaccinated, by antigen, is: BCG (51%); DTP1 (79%); DTP3, Polio3 (55%); MCV (59%); TT2 plus (41%).

BIBLIOGRAPHY

Central Intelligence Agency: *2006: The world factbook, Sudan.* Retrieved September 21, 2006, from https://www.cia.gov/cia/publications/factbook/print/su.html.

Eltom A, Eltom M, Idris M, Gebre-Medhin M: Thyroid function in the newborn in relation to maternal thyroid status during labour in a mild iodine deficiency endemic area in Sudan, *Clin Endocrinol.* 55:485, 2001.

EPI: Monthly joint club of the Federal Ministry of Health, primary health care, EPI, Report. January 2006.

S

Federal Ministry of Health: *Annual health statistical report of the Federal Ministry of Health,* Republic of Sudan, 2003.

Sadig AGMM: *Personal comunication,* 2006.

UNAIDS: 2006 Sudan. Retrieved September 21, 2006, from http://www.unaids.org/en/Regions_Countries/Countries/sudan.asp.

World Health Organization: 2006: Immunization, vaccines and biologicals. Retrieved September 21, 2006, from http://www.who.int/immunization_monitoring/en/globalsummary/countryprofileresult.cfm?C='sdn'.

Zijlstra EE, el-Hassan AM: Leishmaniasis in Sudan: visceral leishmaniasis, *Trans R Soc Trop Med Hyg.* 95(suppl 1):27, 2001.

http://www.africanlanguages.com/ (retrieved January, 2, 2006).

http://www.globalhealthreporting.org/ (retrieved January 10, 2006).

http://www.hivinsite.ucsf.edu/global (retrieved January 10, 2006).

http://www.who.int/countries/sdn/en/ (retrieved August 27, 2006).

✦ SURINAME (REPUBLIC OF)

MAP PAGE (797)

Carol Vlassoff, Dawn Bichel, and Monique Essed-Fernandes

Location: The Republic of Suriname is situated on the northeast coast of South America and is bordered by Guyana on the west, French Guiana on the east, Brazil on the south, and the Atlantic Ocean on the north. The country has a total area of 163,820 km^2 (63,250 square miles) and consists of narrow coastal plain with swamps, rolling hills, and tropical rainforest. The population is estimated to be 492,829. The capital city is Paramaribo, distinguished by its fine (although deteriorating) wooden architecture dating from the Dutch period. The interior of Suriname covers about 85% of the total, and much is untouched and sparsely populated, consisting of dense flora and fauna. About 83% of the population lives in or around Paramaribo or in the coastal towns (the districts of Wanica, Commewijne, Saramacaa, Coronie, and Nickerie). The remainder is primarily Carib and Arawak Indians and Maroons, who are descendants of slaves who escaped to the hinterland in the seventeenth century.

Major Languages	Ethnic Groups	Major Religions
Dutch (official)	Hindustani (East	Hindu 20%
English	Indian) 27%	Christian 41%
Sranan Tongo	Creole (Black, mixed) 31%	Muslim 14%
(Surinamese)	Javanese 15%	Indigenous beliefs
Hindustani	Maroon 15%	4%
Javanese	Amerindian 2%	Unknown 16%
Indigenous	Chinese 2%	
languages	European, Other 3%	

Dutch is the national language, and Sranan Tongo (Surinamese) is also widely spoken. Suriname has been influenced by many cultures, and yet little racial tension exists among the different groups. Surinamese of all backgrounds pride themselves on their ability to get along with one another. The gross domestic product (GDP) per capita is $4,100, with 70% living below the poverty line. Literacy rates are 92% for men, 84% for women.

Health Care Beliefs: Both traditional and modern beliefs; somewhat active role with increasing prevention activities. Governmental and non-governmental organizations (NGOs), development assistance agencies, and international organizations support the formal health care sector, especially its health-promotion aspects. Local NGOs and development agencies promote and host health days to increase awareness about water and sanitation, safe motherhood, and mental health. Mental illnesses are highly stigmatized and attributed to supernatural causes. Illnesses such as epilepsy are thought by many to come from a spirit or person with the "evil eye" (the ability to harm others merely by looking at them). Hence, people with such illnesses tend to consult traditional healers rather than medical professionals. Nonetheless, Paramaribo has one psychiatric institution that, despite limited resources, has established programs to encourage those with mental illness to visit the institution for inpatient and outpatient care. Beliefs about mystical origins of disease are starting to change as a result of health promotion and public education.

Predominant Sick-Care Practices: Biomedical; traditional healing; and magico-religious. Medical services are provided through public and private hospitals in the two major cities: Paramaribo and Nieuw Nickerie. Primary health care is delivered through polyclinics of the Regional Health Services in the coastal area (including urban areas) and through the Medical Mission in the hinterland. Although both are non-governmental organizations (NGOs), they now obtain most of the funding for their activities from the Surinamese government. Suriname has four types of health insurance: (1) free care for the poor and near poor, financed through the Ministry of Social Affairs; (2) co-financed health insurance for government workers provided through the State Health Insurance Foundation; (3) free care for the approximately 40,000 people in the interior, administered through the Medical Mission; and (4) privately financed health care for about 70,000 people who use either out-of-pocket funds or private (individual) and company (collective) insurance policies. About 8% to 18% pay for their own medical care. People who do not have a health card and do not want to pay for treatment may consult traditional healers. Healers charge less for services and medications and will take delayed payments or payment in kind. Others consult healers when they have a disease they think cannot be cured by a doctor or one that has been induced by black magic or an evil spirit. Occasionally, people consult both to determine which treatment works best. This use of two health systems can sometimes lead to problems because the combination of medications can interact dangerously and cause adverse reactions. Most physicians are aware of the use of traditional treatment. Sometimes it is difficult to diagnose and

S

treat these patients because of lack of information about other remedies they have already tried or are trying.

Ethnic-/Race-Specific or Endemic Diseases: The top 10 causes of death in decreasing order of importance are cardiovascular disease, accidents and injuries, cancer, perinatal conditions, diabetes, human immunodeficiency virus (HIV) and acquired immunodeficiency syndrome (AIDS), gastrointestinal disorders, urinary tract disorders, acute respiratory tract infections, and chronic respiratory diseases. Because malaria occurs in the interior, the Maroons are mainly affected by this severe and recurring illness. Data collected on dengue fever and leptospirosis indicate that highest rates are among the Hindus and Creoles. Malnutrition is most common among the Maroons and Creoles. Cardiovascular disease is the main cause of death for adults older than 40. Preliminary results of a survey of different ethnic groups show that the prevalence of hypertension is significantly higher among Creoles and people of mixed origin compared with those of Asian origin. The prevalence of diabetes is slightly higher among the Hindustanis compared with the Javanese and Creoles. More than 70% of people do not participate in regular physical activity, and people with lower incomes and less education are more at risk for disease. The Joint United Nations Programme on HIV/AIDS (UNAIDS) estimates the prevalence rate of HIV in adults (aged 15 to 49 years) to be 1.9%, with 5,200 people living with HIV, including 1,400 women and fewer than 100 children aged 0 to 14. Fewer than 500 deaths from AIDS have been reported. Epidemiologic surveillance is not being conducted systematically or in a standardized manner.

Health-Team Relationships: The health care system is doctor driven, and doctors have a higher social status than nurses. However, doctors and nurses generally have good relationships. Patients consider doctors to be responsible for diagnosis and treatment and therefore to have a more important role. Nurses are seen as liaisons between doctors and patients. Rural health facilities rely more on nurses because they are more accepted and thought to play an important role. Doctors visit the villages once a month and provide guidance to nurses when needed, but the nurses and health assistants diagnose and treat patients.

Families' Role in Hospital Care: Families and friends of hospitalized patients can visit twice a day but are not allowed to stay overnight. Although it is not required for them to do so, family members frequently bring clean towels, sheets, and pillows because of the low standards of cleanliness in some hospitals.

Dominance Patterns: Men are generally dominant and are often in higher and more powerful positions. Many women stay at home caring for children while the men earn money for the family. Women are expected to be subservient to men. Men are more dominant in public life than in the home, but attitudes and roles are changing as women, particularly of the younger generation, obtain more education and higher positions in the workforce and society. Creole households are often headed by women, who provide for their children and make all the decisions for the family.

The Creole hierarchy's origins derive from Suriname's history of slavery. The men were forced to leave their families to work on plantations, leaving the women to make all decisions. In the interior, most village leaders are men, and they make all the decisions for their families and their village. Polygamy is an accepted practice among the Maroons, but recently changing economic patterns and lifestyles—and the increasing incidence of HIV—are making it less acceptable.

Eye-Contact Practices: People usually make direct eye contact during conversations with acquaintances. Eye contact with strangers is usually avoided.

Touch Practices: Physical touching is acceptable but not common in public, except during greetings. Professionals greet each other with a handshake. Friends of the opposite sex and female friends often greet each other with three kisses alternating on each cheek, and male friends greet each other with a handshake or pat on the back. Compared with other Caribbean countries, society is reasonably tolerant about homosexuality, although it is not openly discussed or expressed.

Perceptions of Time: Punctuality is not a priority, and many people joke about their tardiness and attribute it to being on "Suriname time." Tardiness is sometimes blamed on the limited infrastructure, poor roads, and heavy traffic, but most Surinamese are tardy because they are expected to be. The importance of punctuality is increasing, especially for business meetings and other important appointments, such as medical visits. The people of Suriname have lived somewhat isolated from the world, especially the older generation. Isolated rural areas also seem to be more traditional than populated coastal areas. Poverty is forcing some people to live on a day-to-day basis; this is also a health issue because it is hard to convince people to take medications for future health, especially those with chronic diseases. Doctors have to relate medical issues to life today, being careful not to make patients worry about the future.

Pain Reactions: Pain reactions vary among individuals and cultures.

Birth Rites: The infant mortality rate is 23 deaths per 1,000 live births; the fertility rate is 2.32 children born per woman. About 95% of women in the coastal area go to a hospital to give birth. Women are the responsibility of an obstetrician or family practitioner, but the midwife delivers the infant. Midwives employed by the hospital must have a degree in nursing. Some women do not consult doctors and prefer to have midwives during pregnancy; some even give birth at home. Doctors deliver infants during a medical emergency. A family member is allowed to be present; pain control is not generally used. In the absence of maternal leave legislation, government and some private companies entitle women to a maternity leave: 6 weeks before and 6 weeks after birth. Most pregnant women in rural areas are monitored and delivered by a health assistant. Some mothers who live in the interior also prefer going to a traditional midwife. If a problem occurs the patient is airlifted to a Medical Mission hospital, and if additional problems develop, she is transported to a hospital in Paramaribo. Women have many rituals after the birth. Many tie their stomachs with string or bandages to help reduce its size. Some take herbal baths or steams to heal wounds and tighten the vagina, practices common among the Maroon, Javanese, and Creole cultures. Although abortion is illegal, it is widely provided by qualified doctors, although counseling before and after is not included in most services. The percentage of adolescent deliveries is increasing. Contraceptive use, although relatively high (40% to 50%) among women aged 15 to 44, is only 23% for married or in-union girls aged 15 to 19. An estimated 60% of first-time pregnancies among girls 15 to 19 years old are unplanned, and an estimated 8,000 to 10,000 pregnancies end in abortion yearly. Life expectancy is 67 for men, 72 for women.

Death Rites: Most deaths occur at home. The body is then taken to a mortuary to be prepared for subsequent rituals. Christians may cremate the body, and the deceased person must be baptized to be buried at the cemetery. In the Muslim culture, which includes many ethnicities, the bodies are buried within 24 hours after death. Ceremonies of mourning are held on the 7th, 40th, one hundredth, and one thousandth day after the funeral. Muslims bury the deceased; they do not cremate. The Hindu death ceremony takes place as soon as possible after death, usually the same day, and the body is cremated. The Maroon death ceremony involves praying to ancestors, and the funeral can take place any time from a few days to a few months after death, even longer if the deceased was the tribal chief. Women, children, whites, and men in Western clothes are not allowed to go the burial site. Wives are not permitted to be present at the funeral of a deceased husband, and they must go into a mourning period involving many restrictions, such as isolation. The Maroons believe in reincarnation and that the soul stays with the body after death. It is only after a period of mourning that the soul can move to the world of the dead. The Amerindians also have traditional celebrations of death. When a person in the Awarak tribe dies, family members sit around the body until the day of the funeral. In the Carib tribe, a ceremony takes place immediately after death, and people gather at the home to prepare the body and commemorate the deceased with prayer, song, and dance. Organ donations and autopsies are uncommon. People do not like to tamper with the dead; however, bodies and organs can be donated to the medical department at the academic hospital for student doctor training.

Food Practices and Intolerances: The Surinamese diet is as rich and varied as the ethnic makeup of the country. Rice is the main staple and is of very high quality. Cassava, sweet potatoes, plantains, and hot red peppers are commonly used. The enormous selection of tropical fruits is seasonal and can be expensive, and yet the fruits are well liked by everyone. Surinamese typically eat three meals a day. Most use a fork and spoon, but it is also quite common for people to eat with their hands. Religious beliefs and traditional ceremonies play an important role in diet. Most Hindus do not eat beef; many are also vegetarian or eat only vegetarian once a week. Most Muslims do not eat pork and are forbidden to drink alcohol.

Infant-Feeding Practices: Women usually breastfeed during the first weeks after birth. However, they typically do not exclusively breastfeed for more than 1 to 2 months, at which time they begin to bottle-feed as well. It is usually working women who combine formula and breastfeeding. In the last few years, more mothers have become aware of breastfeeding as a healthy practice through educational campaigns promoting safe motherhood. Most women breastfeed (although not exclusively) for about a year; some members of some ethnic groups offer the breast for 3 or 4 years regardless of whether they still have milk to comfort their children.

Child-Rearing Practices: Child rearing practices vary from family to family, and some families are stricter than others. Both parents discipline. For the most part, children are expected to be quiet and obedient and are punished if they are not. Some children sleep with their parents for comfort or because no other bed is available.

National Childhood Immunizations: DT at 2, 4, 6, 18 months and at 5 and 15 years; DTwP at 18 months and 5 years; DTwPHibHep at 2, 4, and 6 months; MMR at 1 and 5 years; OPV at 2, 4, 6, 18 months and at 5 and 15 years; Td at 12 years, YF 1 year for high-risk part of country; and YF 10 years. The percent of the target population vaccinated, by antigen, is: DTP1 (92%); DTP3 (85%); MCV (86%); Polio3 (84%); and YFV (97%). Immunization services are available at health posts only on scheduled days of the month because of a lack of functional cold-chain equipment (the ability to keep vaccines refrigerated) at all facilities, poor accessibility in remote interior areas, and lack of qualified staff members.

Other Characteristics: The health sector has a shrinking financial base, insufficient investment in and poor maintenance of facilities and equipment, and too few drugs and reagents. Many trained public health professionals, medical specialists, and registered nurses are leaving. There is a shortage of qualified teachers, classrooms, and teaching materials; low wages, especially in the public sector; and increasing poverty among single-parent families, the majority of which are headed by women. Child labor, malnutrition, sexual abuse, and youth prostitution are reported to be increasing.

BIBLIOGRAPHY

Bureau of Public Health, Department of Epidemiology: *Epidemiology data 2000– 2001,* Paramaribo, Suriname, 2001, Bureau of Public Health.

Central Intelligence Agency: *2006: The world factbook, Suriname.* Retrieved September 21, 2006, from https://www.cia.gov/cia/publications/factbook/print/ns.html.

Pan American Health Organization (PAHO): Health in the Americas, 2002 edition, Washington, DC, 2001, PAHO.

PAHO: Vol II, Werkgelegenheids- en Onderwijskarakteristieken, November 2005. Suriname MDG Baseline Report, 2005.

Terborg J, Ramdas S, Eiloof D: *Report on 10 years Program of Action of the International Conference on Population and Development (ICPD) in Suriname 1994– 2004,* ProHealth, MOH, and UNFPA, December 2005.

van Eer MY, Eersal MGM, Vreden SGS, and Stehouwer C: *Ethnic differences in cardiovascular risk factors in Suriname,* Paramaribo, Suriname, 2000, unpublished manuscript.

S

Zevende Algemene Volks- en Woningtelling in Suriname, Landelijke Resultaten Vol I, Demografische en Sociale karakteristieken, ABS/Censuskantoor, Augustus 05.
UNAIDS: 2006 Suriname. Retrieved September 21, 2006, from http://www.unaids.org/en/Regions_Countries/Countries/suriname.asp.
World Health Organization: 2006: Immunization, vaccines and biologicals. Retrieved September 21, 2006, from http://www.who.int/immunization_monitoring/en/globalsummary/countryprofileresult.cfm?C='sur'.

◆ SWAZILAND (KINGDOM OF)

MAP PAGE (801)

Aaron G. Buseh

Location: The Kingdom of Swaziland is a small country located in southern Africa. Swaziland is bordered by the Republic of South Africa to the north, southeast, and west and Mozambique to the east. Swaziland is landlocked, with diverse geographic terrain that comprises lower altitude and mountainous elevations. The capital is Mbabane. The geographic diversity leads to a range of climatic zones and characteristics. The climate is mostly temperate. The total area is 17,400 km² (6703 square miles). The population is 1.1 million, 60% of whom are under age 21. About three fourths of the population live in rural areas, and only one fourth live in urban settings. The gross domestic product (GDP) per capita is $5,893, with 69% living below the poverty line. Unemployment is reported to be about 34%.

Major Languages	Ethnic Groups	Major Religions
Siswati	Swazi 90%	Christian 60%
English	Zulu 2%	Indigenous beliefs 40%
	European 3%	
	Other 5%	

Unlike other sub-Saharan African countries, Swaziland is ruled by a king (King Mswati). It is a country rich in traditional cultural ceremonies. Two main rituals and ceremonies are the Umhlanga dance (reed dance) and the Incwala ceremony (first fruits). Historically, authentic ceremonial dress has been worn during these special occasions. Many Swazis, especially women, wear a distinctive national dress, known as the *emahiya*, in their everyday lives. The emahiya is regularly worn with different accessories and head dresses, depending on the status and age of the individual, as well as the occasion. Other Swazis, especially young people and business professionals, have adopted Western-style clothing. The literacy rate is 83% for men, 81% for women.

Health Care Beliefs: Traditional healing practices coexist with modern health care delivery. During illness, people often consult both a traditional healer and modern health care practitioner. Swaziland has numerous indigenous healers, including *sangomas, inyangas,* faith healers, throat scratchers, and traditional birth attendants, all of whom attribute illness to supernatural forces, violations of indigenous rules, the environment, or the influence of ancestors. The health care system naturally attibutes most causes of morbidity and mortality to infectious and communicable diseases. Therefore, disease prevention and health promotion activities are actively encouraged by nongovernmental organizations (NGOs) and various governmental health institutions. This is especially important because of the high prevalence of human immunodeficiency virus (HIV). Mental illness is poorly understood and carries an enormous burden of social stigma at family, community, and health institutional levels. Mentally ill people are feared; in some instances, they are mistreated and left to fend for themselves. Understanding these interrelated beliefs, attitudes, and practices from a holistic Swazi approach is critical for the provision of health care.

Predominant Sick-Care Practices: Biomedical and traditional. Modern biomedical health care delivery is not accessible to all Swazi people, especially in rural areas. As a result, the first tier of accessing health care for most is the traditional healer. Traditional healers treat their clients within the environment where they live, sometimes with direct involvement of the family. They use a holistic approach to address health needs, such as the use of herbs, plants, and animal products; magico-religious or spiritual resouces; and consultations with ancestral spirits to prevent and treat diseases. They can be grouped into a variety of practitioners: traditional birth attendants (TBAs), herbalists, bonesetters, and mental healers. Because most Swazis still attribute their illnesses to supernatural forces, they first consult indigenous healers. If healers cannot provide a cure, they then resort to doctors and nurses. If they still do not improve, they pray to their ancestors for intervention. One practice involves heating the tip of a cow's horn or neck of a bottle and holding it over an incision to draw out impurities. Another involves inducing vomiting and diarrhea or taking steam baths to rid the body of toxins. The biomedical model uses scientific principles to diagnose, intervene, and evaluate outcomes. Such interventions include primary prevention methods such as immunizations, pharmaceuticals, and surgical procedures. Although traditional healers do not follow the scientific approach, they also seek to protect individuals from diseases, evil spirits, or the wrath of ancestral spirits. Just as Western-trained practitioners follow certain standards of care, so do the traditional healers. Precise rituals and ceremonial acts are used to protect or treat clients; preparation and training are critical for both groups. Whereas the modern practitioner undergoes rigourous academic training, traditional healers perceive themselves as being "called" to be a healer. The knowledge and skills that make them an experienced healer are based on observations of other healers in practice, and knowledge that is handed down from one generation to the next. Increasingly, traditional healers recognize that some health conditions such as malaria, tuberculosis, cholera, and other infectious diseases are beyond their abilities, and they acknowledge that modern medical treatment may be more appropriate.

Ethnic-/Race-Specific or Endemic Diseases: Endemic diseases are tuberculosis; pneumonia and bronchitis; and malnutrition in the form of kwashiorkor, infantile diarrhea, and dysentery. Recent outbreaks of cholera (contained) and malaria in the Lowveld occur during the summer months. Enteric fever and advanced periodontal disease are prevalent. Schistosomiasis (bilharzia) is also endemic. Bilharzia is caused by flatworms, which use snails in swamps as an intermediate host before the parasite is transmitted to humans. The disease affects the urinary-genital, gastrointestinal, and hepatic systems in humans; it is known in siSwati as *umtfundzangati,* translated as "blood in the urine." Because of better treatment and prevention efforts, the incidence of leprosy is decreasing. Swaziland has been hard hit by the HIV epidemic. According to the Joint United Nations Programme on HIV/AIDS (UNAIDS), the prevalence rate for HIV in adults (aged 15 to 49 years) is very high at 34%, with 220,000 people living with HIV, including 120,000 women and 15,000 children aged 0 to 15 years. One in three people aged 15 to 49 is infected. About 16,000 deaths are attributed to acquired immunodeficiency syndrome (AIDS). An estimated 63,000 children aged 0 to 17 are orphans because of parental AIDS. These rates are extremely high for a country with a population of approximately one million people.

Health-Team Relationships: There is a critical shortage of health care professionals, and this shortage undermines the public health system's capacity to delivery healthcare. This is especially crucial at a time when the system is attempting to expand the administration of antiretroviral medications to HIV and AIDS patients. A cadre of health care workers developed by the Ministry of Health (Rural Health Motivators [RHM]) may be critical in easing this professional shortage. They are community health workers recruited from their local communities, usually selected by the chief. RHMs are usually older women of community status who have undergone a 10-week training program where they are taught to recognize common conditions and administer home-based care. Strengthening this program and linking it with the formal health sytems structures will be important. Health teams tend to be doctor-driven in hospitals and nurse-driven in community clinics. Doctors and nurses have good working relationships as they work together for the common good. Most patients understand the different roles of doctors, nurses, and nurses' aids and are cooperative when dealing with members of the health system.

Families' Role in Hospital Care: The role of the patient's family is vital because of the serious shortage of nurses and doctors. Families often stay to care for relatives, and they also bring food. They are part of the network of informal caregivers in health care settings.

Dominance Patterns: Men dominate Swazi culture, although when people are ill, women have a more prominent role in making decisions about health care. Swaziland is a polygamous society, and men may marry several women. Marriage involves a payment or dowry for each wife; this payment is known as *lobola* and usually entails giving cattle to the bride's parents. Monogamous marriages, modeled on Western traditions, are becoming increasingly common among young and educated Swazis; but even within a marriage based on Western customs, Swazis are proud of their cultural heritage and traditions, and weddings reflect a blend of both cultures.

Eye-Contact Practices: Women and men avoid direct eye contact, as do people speaking with elders or others of a higher status.

Touch Practices: Physical touching between men and women in public is unacceptable.

Perceptions of Time: Life has a relaxed pace, and punctuality is often not important, particularly in rural areas. People who are late are said to be operating on "African time." The country values past traditions and celebrates them with public holidays and ceremonies, which contributes to a strong national identity. Many of the celebrations are in honor of the king.

Pain Reactions: People believe that pain and sickness are private and should be hidden from the general public.

Birth Rites: The infant mortality rate is very high at 108 deaths per 1,000 live births, and the fertility rate is 3.8 children born per woman. There are many beliefs that govern behavior. For example, a pregnant woman does not linger in a doorway because she believes it could make her birth more difficult. Some believe a child will be born lazy if a pregnant woman lies down for any length of time during the day, and she does not expose her stomach to anyone. The mother tends to avoid eating liver and eggs because it is believed they can cause a child to be born without hair. Traditional birth attendants, untrained in modern birthing procedures, assist in about 20% of deliveries. When a child is born, some traditionalists do not bathe the children in water but rather use only an herbal solution because it will protect the child from evil. The mother eats large amounts of boiled chicken and sour porridge, and she stays secluded in a room for 3 months after the birth. She may abstain from sexual relations for up to 6 months. Mothers in rural areas cover their heads in public until the child's fontanelles close. Births of sons have traditionally been celebrated more than daughters. If available in a health care setting, modern family planning and birth control services can be accessed for a small fee. With the onset of HIV/AIDS, men are offered condoms, sometimes for no cost, but use is more common in urban areas. Life expectancy is 36 for men, 39 for women. The progress made toward improvement in life expectancy in the latter half of the twentieth century was reversed by the HIV epidemic.

Death Rites: Many Swazis believe that death has supernatural causes. Neither organ donation nor autopsies are culturally acceptable. Some traditionalists take the body to the *kraal* (an enclosure for cattle) to inform the ancestors that a person has died. A night vigil is held, and early in the morning the person is buried in a coffin with a straw mat and blanket.

S

Food Practices and Intolerances: In rural areas, people eat primarily corn porridge, wild and cultivated vegetables, peanuts, chicken, eggs, milk, sour milk, avocados, and a little fruit. In the urban and semiurban areas, people tend to eat more of a Western-style diet comprising primarily fast food. Schoolchildren are eating more junk food, which is frequently sold close to schools. In rural areas, it is common to use the hands for eating; people in urban areas use a spoon. At home, older adults are served food first, and then others are served according to their status, with children served last.

Infant-Feeding Practices: National policies support an intensive program that monitors and promotes growth in children and works to eliminate stunted growth caused by malnutrition. Although rural mothers quickly return to agricultural work, they breastfeed their babies exclusively, without supplemental foods, for as long as possible. Urban mothers also return to work soon after birth to supplement their families' incomes; about 45% of these mothers express their breast milk and feed it to the infant with a bottle for the first 3 months. Others use a combination of expressed milk and soft foods, which are introduced at 6 to 8 weeks, a practice that can slow the infant's growth. Despite the commercial promotion of infant formula, the culture supports breastfeeding as an optimal source of nutrients for infants.

Child-Rearing Practices: Children sleep in their parents' bed until the age of 4 years. Discipline is the responsibility of the oldest woman in the home. Child-rearing practices are very strict, especially in rural areas. Children are expected to be quiet and obedient. Because mothers must supplement family incomes soon after giving birth, women in the community band together to care for each other's children.

National Childhood Immunizations: BCG at birth; DT at 5 years; DtaP at 18 months; DTaPHep at 6, 10, and 14 weeks; measles at 9 and 18 months; OPV at birth and 6, 10, and 14 weeks, 18 months, and 5 years; TT CBAW and first contact pregnancy, +4 weeks, +6 months, +1, +1 year; vitamin A at 6, 12, 18, 24, 30, and 36 months; YF at first contact + 10 years. The percent of the target population vaccinated, by antigen is: BCG (84%); DPT1 (94%); DPT3 and TT2 plus (83%); HepB3 (78%); MCV (70%); Polio3 (82%); and vitamin A (54%).

BIBLIOGRAPHY

Bruce JC: Marrying modern health practices and technology with traditional practices: issues for the African continent, *Int Nursing Rev.* 49:171–167, 2002.

Buseh AG, Glass LK., McElmurry BJ: Cultural and gender issues related to HIV/AIDS prevention in rural Swaziland: a focus group analysis. *Health Care Women Int.* 23:173–184, 2002.

Central Intelligence Agency: 2006: *The world factbook, Swaziland.* Retrieved September 21, 2006 from https://www.cia.gov/cia/publications/factbook/print/wz.html.

UNAIDS: 2006 Swaziland. Retrieved September 21, 2006, from http://www.unaids.org/en/Regions_Countries/Countries/swaziland.asp.World Bank: World development report 2005: A better investment climate for everyone. Washington, DC, 2004, World Bank.

S

HRH Gobal Resource Center (World Health Organization). The world health report 2006: *Working together for health.* (retrieved August 28, 2006). Retrieved August 1, 2007 from http://www,hrhresourcecenter.org/node/91.

World Health Organization: 2006: Immunization, vaccines and biologicals. Retrieved September 21, 2006, from http://www.who.int/immunization_monitoring/en/globalsummary/countryprofileresult.cfm?C='swz'.

◆ SWEDEN (KINGDOM OF)

MAP PAGE (798)

Ulrike Kylberg

Location: This northern European country is located in eastern Scandinavia along the Baltic Sea. The capital is Stockholm. Sweden is a land of many lakes, and half of it is covered by forests. Its northern boundary extends into the Arctic Circle. The total area is 449,964 km^2 (173,731 square miles). The country is divided into three regions: Götaland in the south, with large fields of corn, industries, a strong economy, and major universities; Svealand in the central region, with its strong cultural roots, traditions, industries, and mountains; and Norrland, an area of large forests, vast expanses, mountains, and Nordic tundra. Sweden's population is greater than nine million: the gross domestic product (GDP) per capita is $30,000. Literacy rates are almost 100% for both men and women.

Major Languages	Ethnic Groups	Major Religions
Swedish (official)	Swedish 80%	Evangelical Lutheran
Samish (Lapps)	Lapp (Sami) 4%	80%
	Finnish 2%	Roman Catholic 5%
	Foreign-born or first-generation immigrants (Balkan, Middle East, African from Somalia, Croatia, Chile, Afghan Kurd) 14%	Islam 4%
		Other or none 11%

Health Care Beliefs: Active role; health promotion important. Health promotion is organized by law for all inhabitants. It particularly emphasizes prenatal and child care, adolescent health promotion and occupational health. More recently, emphasis has also been on women's health care (including cardiovascular), care for older adults, and health care for immigrants. The Swedish government has established health-promotion programs focused on smoking, obesity, and stress. About 90% of Swedish women are employed and working outside the home, and higher stress levels resulting from managing both work and home are leading to serious stress-related illnesses. People are expected to be responsible for their

S

own health; however, many social services are available to assist them. A biomedical focus is dominant, and many medications are used as treatment. More recently, paramedical professionals, including physiotherapist, osteopaths and acupuncturists are becoming increasingly accepted by doctors, particularly for the treatment of pain. Basic health care is provided for a small fee, and hospital care costs are based on patients' incomes. The focus of care is on health facilities rather than on community and family settings. During the 1990s, Sweden changed from a relatively homogeneous society to a multiethnic society. Many immigrants come with socioeconomic problems and both noncommunicable and communicable illnesses, straining the system and increasing health care costs.

Predominant Sick-Care Practices: Biomedical. Biomedical treatment dominates, and is offered by the Swedish national health care system and partly financed by income tax. Most companies offer health care services to their employees. There are more alternatives today in health care: daily life health care (egenvård), alternative health care and the biomedical system. Many problems are solved in daily life by consulting pharmaceutical professionals or by searching Internet health care sites. It is common for Swedes to consult with alternative medical professionals such as physiotherapists, chiropractors, acupuncturists, and massage therapists. However, most people still consider biomedical care to be primary, and consult doctors and nurses. The health care system is divided into two systems. The basic system is for health treatment and social welfare, and the other system is for health and social support. The professional health care system is divided into a primary sector on the community level with general practitioners and specialized nurses. There is also an institutional and specialized sector on the regional and national level. Sweden also has some hospices and a few private hospitals.

Ethnic-/Race-Specific or Endemic Diseases: The rates for osteoporosis are the highest in Europe among older men and women. Sjögren-Larsson syndrome is frequently diagnosed in women. Causes of death are mainly related to old age; however, cardiovascular diseases and cancer dominate. The Sámi, an indigenous people, have lived in the northern part of the country for many hundreds of years. Despite some outside influences to which the Sámi have been exposed, they and their culture have retained their distinctiveness. Today they are represented in government, and they have full rights to practice their culture in daily life. Most Sámi are settled in "villages," although a few still migrate during the year with their reindeer herds. One of Sweden's biggest challenges is multiresistent tuberculosis coming to Sweden in infected immigrants from the countries of the former Soviet Union. The incidence of human immunodeficiency virus (HIV) is about 323 cases per year, and most of those are "imported" by immigrants who become infected before they enter Sweden. HIV testing is systematically done for blood donors, pregnant women, and patients with sexually transmitted diseases. The Joint United Nations Programme on HIV/AIDS (UNAIDS) reports the prevalence rate of HIV in adults (aged 15 to 49 years) to be 0.2%, with 8,000 people living with

HIV, including 2,500 women and fewer than 100 children aged 0 to 15 years. Deaths from acquired immunodeficiency syndrome (AIDS) are fewer than 100.

Health-Team Relationships: Receptionist nurses who are contacted by telephone are the first point of contact in the health care system. The doctor has an authoritarian role and is not questioned. Although patients are expected to say what they think, health professionals do not encourage such outspokenness. Patients expect to help make decisions when planning medical treatment and nursing care. The Swedish welfare program is facing a reconstruction with focus on cost-effectiveness, quality assurance, and evidence-based medicine as well as nursing and patient satisfaction. More people are opting for care in the home, and the concepts of hospices and palliative care are growing in popularity.

Families' Role in Hospital Care: The staff meets all the patients' needs; however, the family can assist if they like. Flexible visiting hours are encouraged. Stipends are paid to individuals who provide care for a sick family member at home.

Dominance Patterns: Sweden has an egalitarian society; however, women are usually responsible for household chores and purchasing and preparing food. A never-ending debate exists about equality and relationships to minority ethnic groups, such as Sweden's relationships with the European community relative to migration of workers from former Eastern bloc countries.

Eye-Contact Practices: It is customary to maintain eye contact during conversations.

Touch Practices: Touching is uncommon, even in health care environments (other than during examinations).

Perceptions of Time: Northern Swedes are not as time conscious as southern Swedes from large cities. People are generally expected to be 15 to 30 minutes late. Swedes are present and future oriented, and they plan for important future events.

Pain Reactions: Nonexpressive and expressive reactions to pain are both acceptable. When in pain, Swedes may contract the muscles of their faces or bodies and verbally express their discomfort. Immediate pain relief is expected.

Birth Rites: Sweden has one of the lowest maternal and infant mortality rates in the world, the result of targeted health-promotion programs for pregnant women and newborns.

The infant mortality rate is 2.76 deaths per 1,000 live births. Women can choose any position in which to give birth—even underwater. ABC-Clinics provide many choices for delivery, including births that include the participation of the father and siblings. For example, the father may cut the umbilical cord, after which the infant is placed on the mother's abdomen, and the family is left alone for several hours. Rooming-in (keeping the infant and mother in the same room) is common. The total fertility rate is 1.66 children born per woman. Life expectancy is 78 for men, 83 for women.

S

684 Sweden (Kingdom of)

Death Rites: Subdued or public expressions of grief are both acceptable. A dying person is not left alone, and family members stay at the bedside. After death, bodies are placed in a coffin. Before the closure of the coffin in the mortuary, the family is allowed to say a final farewell.

Food Practices and Intolerances: Breakfast often consists of coffee or tea and a sandwich of cheese or ham, cereal, or porridge. A large meal is eaten at lunch or dinner, but fast food usually dominates lunch. Meatballs with potatoes and gravy are popular. Coffee breaks may include a sandwich at midmorning and sweets at midafternoon. Fish, meat, and bananas are common.

Infant-Feeding Practices: Breastfeeding is preferred and encouraged and continues for about 1 year. Other foods are introduced at 4 or 5 months.

Child-Rearing Practices: Children are raised in a permissive but safe environment. School starts at age 6. Nurses from government-sponsored daycare centers supervise preschool children. Both parents are responsible for caring for children when they are not in school.

National Childhood Immunizations: BCG at 6 months (in high-risk groups); DTaP at 10 years; DTaPHibHeplpv at 3, 5, and 12 months; DTaPHibIPV at 3, 5, and 12 months; MMR at 18 months and 12 years; and IPV at 5 to 6 years. The percent of the target population vaccinated, by antigen, is: BCG (16%); DTP1, DTP3, and Polio3 (99%); Hib3 (98%); and MCV (94%).

BIBLIOGRAPHY

Central Intelligence Agency: *2006: The world factbook, Sweden.* Retrieved September 21, 2006, from https://www.cia.gov/cia/publications/factbook/print/sw.html.

Ekdahl K, ed: *The Sigtuna report: combating infectious diseases in the Baltic Sea and Barents regions.* Solna, 2000, Swedish Institute for Infections Disease Control (SMI).

Ministry of Agriculture, Food and Consumer Affairs. *The Sámi—an indigenous people in Sweden.* Stockholm, 2005, Ministry of Agriculture, Food and Consumer Affairs.

National Board of Health and Welfare: *The national public health report 2005.* Stockholm 2005, National Board of Health and Welfare.

National Board of Health and Welfare: *The national social health report 2006.* Stockholm 2006, the National Board of Health and Welfare.

Red Cross, Noak's Ark, 2005. Retrieved June 15, 2006, from http://www.noaksark.redcross.se/hivaids/statistik.htm.

Robine J-M, Jagger C, Michel J: Trends in life expectancies. In: Robine J-M, Jagger C, Mathers CD et al, eds: *Determining health expectancies.* Chichester, 2003, Wiley.

Svenska Smittskyddsinstitutet (SMI): 2005. Retrieved June 19, 2006, from http://www.smittskyddsinstitutet.se.

UNAIDS: 2006 Sweden. Retrieved September 21, 2006, from http://www.unaids.org/en/Regions_Countries/Countries/sweden.asp.

World Health Organization (WHO): *The European health report 2002.* Copenhagen, 2002, WHO.

World Health Organization: 2006: Immunization, vaccines and biologicals. Retrieved September 21, 2006, from http://www.who.int/immunization_monitoring/en/globalsummary/countryprofileresult.cfm?C='swe'.

http://www.ssi.dk/euvac/vaccinations/sweden.html (retrieved June 19, 2006).
http://en.wikipedia.org/wiki/Demographics_of_Sweden (retrieved June 15, 2006).
http://en.wikipedia.org/wiki/List_of_countries_by_infant_mortality_rate   (retrieved June 15, 2006).

◆ SWITZERLAND (SWISS CONFEDERATION)

MAP PAGE (798)

Matthias Bopp

Location: Switzerland is a landlocked nation in central Europe. It is characterized by a rugged landscape that includes glaciers, lakes, and a large plateau between the Alps and the Jura, where most people reside. The Alps consists of a high mountain chain traversing the country from southwest to southeast. The Jura is a low mountain range in the northwest. Italy is to the south, France to the west, Germany to the north, and Austria and Liechtenstein to the east. The climate is temperate—in the south sometimes even Mediterranean—but it varies with the altitude. Switzerland has cold, cloudy, rainy or snowy winters and cool to warm, cloudy, humid summers with occasional showers. The capital is Bern. The total area is 41,290 km^2 (15,938 square miles). The elevated sea level—generally more than 400 m (1300 feet)—and the scarceness of plains do not support much agriculture; less than 10% of the surface is arable land. Dairy farming is important. The population is 7.5 million, and the gross domestic product (GDP) per capita is $34,087. Literacy rates are almost 100% for both men and women. Life expectancy is 79 for men, 84 for women.

Major Languages	Ethnic Groups	Major Religions
German (official) (64%)	Swiss[a] 73%	Roman Catholic 42%
French (official) (20%)	Italian 6%	Protestant 35%
Italian (official) (6%)	Ex-Yugoslavian 5%	Muslim 4%
Romansch (0.5%)	Other European 12%	Other or not
	Other 4%	reported 8%
		No affiliation 11%

Swiss is a term that is restricted to Swiss nationals born in Switzerland and not having a second nationality. In case of inconsistency, foreign ethnic groups are defined by nationality rather than by country of birth. Linguistic and religious partitions of the country do not coincide geographically, nor are they substantial for differences in economic growth or wealth. In the last decades, the characterization of regions by their religious traditions has lost much of its importance, the more so

S

because a majority of the population does not attend religious services. Foreign nationals amount to 21% of the total population: 634,000 Swiss nationals live abroad (71% having a second nationality): 11% in the United States and 6% in Canada.

Health Care Beliefs: Active role; health promotion important. Biomedical health care is predominant, but complementary alternative methods (e.g., homeopathic, Chinese) are not uncommon. Traditional naturopathy is marginal. Health is largely considered an individual responsibility: legislation prefers health-promotion efforts rather than prescriptions and regulations. Free choice of health care and health insurance providers is considered important. Each of the 26 cantons (states) has its own government, fully responsible for education and health care. Despite the absence of a national health policy, the Federal Office of Public Health has promoted some prevention programs and health care campaigns for the prevention of significant issues such as human immunodeficiency virus (HIV) and acquired immunodeficiency syndrome (AIDS).

Predominant Sick-Care Practices: Biomedical and predominantly complementary; alternative practices. Most Swiss seek biomedical care first, but alternative practices may also be used as complementary care. Massage therapy, acupuncture, and homeopathic and herbal treatments are adjuncts to standard medical care. Good biomedical care is available throughout Switzerland. Patients have direct access to primary care, specialist physicians, and emergency departments. Managed care schemes (health maintenance organizations [HMOs], and preferred provider organizations [PPOs]) cover only 6% of the insured. Health insurance has been mandatory since 1996 and is offered for per capita contribution payments varying by company and geographic area. Generally, 10% of costs up to an eligible upper annual limit (300 to 2,500 Swiss Francs) have to be paid out of pocket. Because insurance rates exceed the financial resources of some people, every third person is eligible for subsidies. Treatments and medications not included in the standard list of reimbursable state-provided health care benefits (e.g., dentists or alternative medicine) also must be paid out of pocket or covered by private health care insurance.

Ethnic-/Race-Specific or Endemic Diseases: The main causes of death are cardiovascular disease (almost 40%; predominantly coronary heart disease), and cancer (25%). In line with the overlapping cultural influences, Swiss death rates for most causes of death vary between Western and Southern European figures. Notable exceptions are cerebrovascular diseases (lowest death rates worldwide) and suicide rates (traditionally elevated). The incidence of breast and prostate cancers is fairly high. In the French-speaking part of the country, cardiovascular mortality is lower than in the German speaking part, but alcohol-related mortality is higher. The prevalence of certain infectious diseases such as tuberculosis and hepatitis is higher in immigrants from the Balkans. The Joint United Nations Programme on HIV/AIDS (UNAIDS) estimates the prevalence rate for human immunodeficiency virus (HIV) in adults (aged 15 to

49 years) is 0.4%, with 17,000 living with HIV, including 5,900 women and 100 children aged 0 to 15. The estimated incidence of acquired immunodeficiency syndrome (AIDS) is fewer than 300 cases per year. The number of newly diagnosed infections varies between 700 and 800 yearly. The annual number of deaths attributed to AIDS peaked in 1994 (662 cases) but has decreased since then and is now fewer than 100. Having significantly decreased after 1995, the incidence of AIDS may be slightly increasing since 2002, particularly among homosexual men and those having heterosexual contacts with persons originating from high-prevalence countries.

Health-Team Relationships: In the last decades, the organization, role, and status of nursing have changed considerably. There has been a transition from the disadvantages of "functional" care and team nursing (where many individuals accomplished pieces of the nursing care for a patient) to promotion of "primary nursing" practice (where a primary nurse is responsible for overseeing each patient's care). This patient-centered approach provides better organization of patient needs and treatment. The primary nurse is responsible for assessment of resources needed, evaluation of the need for nursing care, agreement on what is to be accomplished, and determination of whether the goals of nursing care have been accomplished, both during and after hospitalization. Professional nursing is part of a multidisciplinary team consisting of nurses, physicians (for medical diagnostics and therapy), and other health professionals. The physician is still considered the head of the health care team, but the work of all members of the team is increasingly collaborative. The costs of health care in 2004 were 51.7 billion Swiss Francs (41.6 billion U.S. dollars), or 11.6% of the GNP, a proportion exceeded only by the United States. There are more than 426,000 persons employed in the health and social services sector (317,000 full-time equivalents [FTE], 2004), with 123,000 FTE in hospitals and 88,000 in long-term care facilities. Most hospitals are managed by a canton (state), a district (regional sublevel of a canton), or a city. Privately managed hospitals total about 17% of hospital beds and 12% of the employed.

Families' Role in Hospital Care: Families do not play a role in hospital care but are involved in treatment decisions. However, as hospitals attempt to reduce the length of stay to reduce costs, the role of families in providing care outside the hospital, such as home and ambulatory care, is becoming more important.

Dominance Patterns: Men and women are becoming increasingly equal in Switzerland, but most women living with a partner are engaged only in a part-time occupation. Care of aged parents is still managed by daughters rather than sons.

Eye-Contact Practices: During conversations, direct eye contact is essential.

Touch Practices: Touching and hugging are becoming increasingly popular, particularly for the younger generation. Handshaking is customary in official contacts and business relations as well as in health care.

S

Perceptions of Time: The Swiss are known for their punctuality. Even for informal visits (e.g., with friends), it is customary to make an appointment. Arriving too early or more than a quarter of an hour too late is considered impolite.

Pain Reactions: The reaction of individuals toward pain is moderate—neither stoical nor expressive. There is strong support for the concept of palliative care and adequate pain relief.

Birth Rites: The infant mortality rate is 4 deaths per 1,000 live births. More than 95% of all deliveries occur in hospitals attended by obstetricians and midwives, and generally fathers are present. The proportion of deliveries by cesarean section is close to 30%. The birth rate is decreasing: the fertility rate is 1.4 children born per woman. The age at which women have their first child is rapidly increasing. The mean age of mothers having a child is now 30.4 years. Having a child without being married is still rather exceptional (13% of all births). Breastfeeding rates were recently reported to be more than 80% at 3 months and more than 60% at 6 months. The median duration was 31 weeks, substantially more than 9 years before. The duration of breastfeeding was longer if the delivery occurred in a baby-friendly hospital and with increasing age or socioeconomic status of the mother. In a former study, duration of breastfeeding was shorter if the mother was employed and longer if the mother originated from Africa, Asia, the Middle East, or Latin America.

Death Rites: About 33% of deaths occur in hospitals, 33% in nursing homes, and 33% in the home. In the hospital, end-of-life decisions are usually discussed and made together by physicians, patients, and family members. Frequently, close family members remain with dying relatives. Cremation or burial is usually accompanied by religious services. Assisted suicide is not punishable in Switzerland. Euthanasia organizations have a long tradition, and it is estimated that they are involved in about every fifth suicide of elderly persons. Organ donations must have the explicit permission of the deceased person or the immediate family; resulting in a significant shortage of donor organs.

Food Practices and Intolerances: Swiss cuisine has Italian, German, and French influences. Breakfast usually includes coffee, milk products, and cereals. Cheese is an important part of the diet; fondues of Emmenthaler and Gruyère cheese as well as raclette are common dinners. Pasta and rice are as common as potatoes. A popular potato dish is *roesti* (a kind of shredded and fried potatoes). Perch and trout from the many lakes are plentiful, and Swiss chocolate is known worldwide. Meals have tended to be hearty and to include filling soups, but lighter meals with many vegetables and salads have recently become more popular.

National Childhood Immunizations: DTaPHibIPV at 2, 4, 6, and 15 to 24 months; DTaPIPV at 4 to 7 years; HepB at 11 to 15 years, +1, +6 months; MenC_conj 12 months and 11 to 15 years; MMR at 12 and 15 to 24 months; Pneumo_conj at 2, 4, and 12 months; and varicella at 11 to 15 years (adolescents without anamnesis). The percent of the target population vaccinated, by antigen, is: DTP1 (98%); DTP3 and Polio3 (95%); Hib3 (91%); and MCV (82%).

BIBLIOGRAPHY

Central Intelligence Agency: *2006: The world factbook, Switzerland.* Retrieved September 21, 2006, from https://www.cia.gov/cia/publications/factbook/print/sz.html.

Highlights on health in Switzerland, 2005: http://www.euro.who.int/document/e88386.pdf (retrieved June 14, 2006).

HIV and AIDS: Epidemiology in Switzerland. Retrieved June 14, 2006, from http://www.bag.admin.ch/hiv_aids/01033/01143/index.html?lang=de.

Kocher G, Oggier W, eds: *Gesundheitswesen Schweiz 2004–2006.* Eine aktuelle Übersicht. Bern, Göttingen, Toronto, Seattle, 2004, Hans Huber.

Merten S, Dratva J, Ackermann-Liebrich U: Do baby-friendly hospitals influence breastfeeding duration on a national level, *Pediatrics.* 116:e702–e708, 2005.

Swiss Federal Statistical Office: http://www.bfs.admin.ch (retrieved June 14, 2006).

Swiss Federal Office of Public Health: Retrieved June 14, 2006, from http://www.bag.admin.ch.

Swiss Federal Office for Professional Education and Technology: Retrieved June 14, 2006, from http://www.bbt.admin.ch.

UNAIDS: 2006 Switzerland. Retrieved September 21, 2006, from http://www.unaids.org/en/Regions_Countries/Countries/switzerland.asp.

van der Heide A, Dellens L, Faisst K, et al. End-of-life decision-making in six European countries: descriptive study, *Lancet.* 362(9381):345–350, 2003.

World Health Organization: 2006: Immunization, vaccines and biologicals. Retrieved September 21, 2006, from http://www.who.int/immunization_monitoring/en/globalsummary/countryprofileresult.cfm?C='che'.

http://www.euro.who.int/countryinformation/CtryInfoRes?language=English&Country=SWI (retrieved June 14, 2006).

◆ SYRIA (SYRIAN ARAB REPUBLIC)

MAP PAGE (802)

Kenneth D. Ward

Location: Syria is bordered on the north by Turkey, on the east by Iraq, on the south by Jordan, and on the west by Lebanon and the Mediterranean Sea. The republic has a total area of 185,180 km² (71,498 square miles). The population is estimated at 18.8 million; in addition, about 40,000 people live in the Golan Heights. About 37% of the population is under 15 years, and 3% is older than 65. The gross domestic product (GDP) per capita is $3,900, and 20% are living below the poverty line.

Major Languages	Ethnic Groups	Major Religions
Arabic (official)	Arab 90%	Islam 90%
French	Kurdish, Armenian,	Christian 10%
English	Other 10%	

S

Syria is the only Arabian country that uses the Arabic language for university instruction in almost all sciences, including medicine and nursing. Tremendous efforts have been made in the past few years to translate textbooks into Arabic. Syrian society is composed of different cohesive groups characterized by their distinct linguistic and religious characteristics. About 40% of Sunni Muslims are urban dwellers; of those, 80% live in the five largest cities. Alawis (Shia Muslims who believe in divine incarnation and the divinity of Ali) are poor and live in rural areas. About 90% of the inhabitants of Jabal Al Arab are Druze, whereas Jews and Armenians are primarily urban traders. The cultural differences between groups extend beyond religious beliefs and rituals to differences in clothing, household architecture, etiquette, and agricultural practices. Kurds are believed to constitute 9% of the population, and most of them came from Turkey between 1924 and 1938. They speak their own language, Kirmanji. Numerous Armenians live in Syrian cities and towns. They speak their own language and are the largest unassimilated group, maintaining their own schools and newspapers. Other small ethnic groups are Turkomans, Circassians, Syrianics, and Assyrians. Literacy rates are 90% for men, 64% for women.

Health Care Beliefs: Traditional and modern; passive role. Most citizens (80%) who live in the five major cities tend to consult health care professionals first, although they usually use more traditional therapies as a last resort when health care professionals cannot cure them. The use of drugs for other than therapeutic reasons is strictly forbidden. However, Syrians do smoke cigarettes, despite strong warnings by some Islamic scholars; this is the unhealthiest behavior among Syrians. Water-pipe smoking is traditional and widely practiced. Suicide is not a serious social problem, as is true in all Arab nations. Islam forbids suicide, and strong family support helps prevent suicide attempts.

Predominant Sick-Care Practices: Biomedical, indigenous and magical-religious. People from rural areas usually consult indigenous and other traditional healers such as those who use the *Koran* (the holy Islamic book) for healing. People with infertility problems generally seek medical advice from a doctor and a religious person *(shykh)* for amulets. Shykhs use traditional cures such as "closing the back" of a woman in which a female healer rubs the women's pelvis with olive oil and places suction cups on her back. Some indigenous female healers also massage the abdomen around the ovaries and use vaginal herbal suppositories. The most prevalent practice is massaging children with warm olive oil. Traditional health practices are the domain of women, and some female healers are known in their communities for their skill in treating injuries and curing some disorders. In families, women assume responsibility for nutrition and treatment of illness. People's beliefs in the efficacy of traditional healers often prevent or postpone medical attention. The health system is based on primary health care that is delivered at three levels: village, district, and provisional. In 2003, Syria had 76 public hospitals, 364 private hospitals, and 1,124 public primary health centers (821 rural, 303 urban). The total number of beds in hospitals was 21,817 (70% of which were in public sector hospitals). Syria, which has a socialist government, provides free medical care to all citizens and imposes limits on charges by private hospitals.

Ethnic-/Race-Specific or Endemic Diseases: The incidence of malaria and tuberculosis (TB) has decreased. However, gastrointestinal and parasitic diseases are endemic, particularly in rural areas. In the Damascus area, hepatitis E is endemic, and cutaneous leishmaniasis has been endemic in Aleppo for generations. Syrians are at risk for ascariasis (which often has the symptoms of biliary disease) and echinococcosis. In 2003 through 2004, the World Health Organization (WHO) reported 13 cases of malaria and 4,820 cases of TB. The Joint United Nations Programme on HIV/AIDS (UNAIDS) reports the prevalence rate of human immunodeficiency virus (HIV) in adults (aged 15 to 49 years) as less than 0.2%. The first case of acquired immunodeficiency syndrome (AIDS) was reported in 1987. In 1997 through 2000, when transmission was known, 73% of cases were acquired heterosexually, 8% were in men who had sex with men, 8% were injecting drug users, 8% were from infected blood, and 4% were from mother-to-child transmission.

Health-Team Relationships: Doctors are dominant. They tend to discount nurses' knowledge and expertise; therefore, patients seldom rely on nurses for health education. This ideology is embedded in the social structure because the deans and educators in schools of nursing are doctors. Doctors' representation of nursing on national committees and councils continues to be the norm in some nursing programs. Nurse-doctor interactions are very limited and occur only during rounds (in the morning and evening) or when a nurse needs to call a doctor about a patient. In 2003 Syria had 24,473 doctors, 14,917 dentists, 10,809 pharmacists, and 32,229 qualified nurses and midwives. About 77% of doctors and 94% of dentists are employed in the private sector.

Families' Role in Hospital Care: Many close relatives accompany patients during an admission to mitigate their uncertainties and worries and occasionally answer questions. Relatives tend to prepare nutritious food such as meat, vegetables, and rice for patients. Nurses rely on the patients' companions for basic nursing tasks such as assistance with bathing, eating, walking, and changing clothes. Close relatives who stay most of the day show hospitality to visitors by serving them coffee, candy, or fruit. Visitors often do not comply with the visiting hours and policies set by health institutions, and hospitals use special security personnel to control visitors who interfere with routine and emergency care. Visitors tend to come in groups during the day, and although well intentioned, occasionally keep patients from getting enough rest and sleep.

Dominance Patterns: In a male-dominated society such as Syria, men are valued more than women are, particularly because they carry on the family name and care for parents in their old age. The father is usually

S

the head of the family and its breadwinner, whereas the mother plays the major role in raising children and maintaining the house. However, many educated women have jobs in health care, education, and private and public institutions. Grandmothers care for children whose mothers work outside the home. Older people in extended families are highly valued, so educated women may have difficulties obtaining health care for their children if they live in an extended-family household. Older women usually have more authority than the mother regarding decisions about the children's health and nutrition and health expenditures.

Eye-Contact Practices: Body language is particularly important. A lowered gaze and shyness are the preferred behaviors for women during their interactions with men. In addition, it is inappropriate for children to make direct eye contact with their parents, grandparents, or older people. People of the same sex from the Middle East are likely to stand quite close to each other, but those of the opposite sex keep a wider distance.

Touch Practices: Arabs behave conservatively in public and keep their feelings private. Displays of affection between spouses (kissing, cuddling, and hugging) are considered rude and extremely inappropriate in public areas. It is unacceptable for men and women to shake hands with strangers of the opposite sex. As a rule, health professionals treat patients who are the same sex unless too few professionals are available. Islam prohibits touching between males and females except during an emergency or when no competent health professional of the same sex is available.

Perceptions of Time: Punctuality is not of great importance. Arabs typically begin their meetings with "small talk" about family and health and usually serve tea or coffee before getting down to business. They tend to live more in the past and present and focus less on the future. Arabs think ahead and have plans for the future, but they are reluctant to overwhelm themselves with thoughts of accomplishing the tasks.

Pain Reactions: The cultural beliefs of Syrians play a major role in their expression of pain because they believe their suffering will be counted on the Day of Judgment. They tend to attribute wellness and illness to God's will, so they often pray to cope with stressful experiences. Patients may not request a pain assessment or medication because they want to be considered "good" patients (i.e., patients who do not complain). Health care professionals do not expect patients to ask much of them. Men are particularly reluctant to mention their pain because it would be considered weakness unless a health care professional asked about it. Men who endure pain and do not complain are considered more masculine, so it is more acceptable for women to mention pain and ask for analgesics.

Birth Rites: When a woman gives birth, relatives, friends, and neighbors visit and give her gifts, which are usually items for the infant. The fertility rate is 3.4 children born per woman. Most families believe that mothers should stay home for the first 40 days. During this time, she is cared for by her mother and sisters and occasionally by her husband's family. Circumcision is the norm for boys because it is part of the culture and considered necessary for cleanliness reasons. Most families prefer to circumcise their male infants during the first week of age, but others postpone it for many years. Despite discouragement from the medical community, most families still use *kohl,* a charcoal-like powder, to dilate the pupils of female infants' eyes. Swaddling infants with a blanket and rope is still very common and is used to strengthen the muscles, prevent scoliosis, and prevent movements that might frighten them during the night. Infants are usually kept in a crib close to their mother. The infant mortality rate is 29 deaths per 1,000 live births. During the postpartum period, the mother is not allowed to perform religious rituals (e.g., pray, fast during Ramadan) or to have sexual relations until she is completely free of postpartum discharge. The mother is encouraged to consume special drinks such as water with boiled cinnamon sticks and boiled hilbah seeds because it is believed this accelerates discharge and increases milk production. Life expectancy is 69 for men, 72 for women.

Death Rites: Donation of human organs is allowed according to two specific Islamic rules: when "necessities overrule prohibition" and when there is a "choice of the lesser of the two evils if both cannot be avoided." In other words, organ donation that can save a life is more important than preserving the integrity of the body of the donor. Autopsy is permissible if it is conducted for the right purpose, such as to determine the cause of a suspicious death, and for educational purposes. It is preferred to bury the dead body quickly in the same place (i.e., same country) where the person died, even if the death occurred far from the place of birth. Most people prefer burying the body at home. After death, the body is washed and wrapped with white cloth and taken to the mosque for prayer; it then goes to the cemetery and is buried in the ground without a coffin. Relatives go back to the home and accept condolences for 3 days. Cremation is forbidden.

Food Practices and Intolerances: Pork and alcohol are strictly prohibited in Islam, although less observant Muslims do not follow these proscriptions. Muslims fast during the month of Ramadan each year. They consume no food or drink and abstain from sexual intercourse between sunrise and sunset. People who are ill and older adults who cannot tolerate fasting do not have to do so. A popular dish is Middle Eastern shish kebabs, which are pieces of lamb or marinated chicken that are speared on a wooden stick and cooked over a charcoal fire with tomatoes and onions. *Tabbouleh* is a Syrian salad of bulgur (wheat crumbles) mixed with flat-leaf parsley, fresh mint, green onion, diced tomato, lemon juice, olive oil, and salt. Eggplant dip *(baba ghannooj)* is baked (mashed eggplant blended with onion, garlic, lemon juice, oil, and salt). *Lahme bel ajin* is small balls of dough that are rolled out and filled with a mixture of finely chopped lamb, pine nuts, chopped onion, and green pepper, and

S

served with labani *(yogurt).* Hummus is a dip or spread of finely mashed, cooked chickpeas that are mixed with tahini, olive oil, salt, parsley, garlic, and hot peppers. Popular desserts include baklava, Turkish delights, and qatayef.

Infant-Feeding Practices: Breastfeeding is the norm. Working women, primarily those in urban cities, bottle-feed and then leave their infants with a close relative during the day. In rural areas, women usually follow the advice of health care professionals and breastfeed. Infants are introduced to solid food as young as 9 months. Infants are given starchy foods, primarily potatoes, at younger than 6 months. Anemia in young children is a serious problem because of the practice of giving them bread soaked in tea.

Child-Rearing Practices: Children usually sleep in their parents' room for up to 3 or 4 years. Because of housing and financial constraints, it may be impossible to separate young girls and boys, although it is preferable. Mothers are more responsible for discipline and tend to use less physical forms of punishment than fathers. Older people in the extended family live in their older son's (or daughter's if they have no sons) home their entire lives—with respect and dignity. Older adults might assume some responsibility for disciplining their grandchildren even when the mother thinks that it interferes with her methods. Discipline of children is highly emphasized because unacceptable and inappropriate behaviors affect the reputation and honor of the family.

National Childhood Immunizations: BCG at birth; DTwP at 18 months; DTwPHib at 3, 4, and 5 months; OPV at birth and 3, 4, 5, and 18 months and at 6 years; HepB at birth and at 3 and 10 months; measles at 10 months; vitamin A at 10 months and after birth; DT at 6 years; Td at 12 years; TT at first contact, +1, +6 months, +1, +1 year; MenACWY at 6 years (in high-risk groups). The percent of the target population vaccinated, by antigen, is: MCV (98%); BCG, Polio3, DTP1, DTP3, HepB3, and Hib3 (99%).

BIBLIOGRAPHY

Central Intelligence Agency: *2006: The world factbook, Syria.* Retrieved September 21, 2006, from https://www.cia.gov/cia/publications/factbook/print/sy.html.

UNAIDS 2006 Syria. Retrieved September 21, 2006, from http://www.unaids.org/en/Regions_Countries/Countries/syrian_arab_republic.asp.

World Health Organization: 2006: Immunization, vaccines and biologicals. Retrieved September 21, 2006, from http://www.who.int/immunization_monitoring/en/globalsummary/countryprofileresult.cfm?C='syr'.

World Population Prospects: The 2004 revision, New York, 2005, United Nations.

http://www.arab.net/cuisine/ ABC of Arab Cuisine (retrieved February 24, 2006).

http://www.emro.who.int/emrinfo/index.asp?Ctry=syr WHO EMRO – Country Profiles, (retrieved February 23, 2006).

http://www.emro.who.int/rbm/epidemiology-2004.htm WHO EMRO. Roll Back Malaria (retrieved February 23, 2006).

S

◆ TAIWAN (THE REPUBLIC OF CHINA) T

MAP PAGE (803)

Hsiu-Chin Chen and Fu-Jin Shih

Location: Taiwan is made up of one large and several smaller islands in a chain of mountainous islands in the Western Pacific off the southeast coast of mainland China. Taiwan is separated from China by the Taiwan Strait. The island of Taiwan has an oblong shape and a total area of 35980 km^2 (13,892 square miles). Taiwan's population is more than 23 million, and the capital is Taipei. Taiwan has a growing economy; the gross domestic product (GDP) per capita is $27,600, with 0.9% living below the poverty line.

Major Languages	Ethnic Groups	Major Religions
Mandarin (official) Han languages include Taiwanese and Hakka, which are spoken mainly by those whose ancestors immigrated from China's Fujian and Guangdong Provinces	Han people (Southern Fujianese and Hakka) 98% 12 Major indigenous people, including the Amis, Atayal, Bunun, Kavalan, Paiwan, Pinuyumayan, Rukai, Saisiyat, Thao, Truku, Tsou, and Yami 2%	Taoism, Buddhism, and Yi Guan Dao 85% Protestant 4.7% Catholicism and Lord of Universe Church 4.4% Other 5.9%

Twenty-five religions are recognized by the government of Taiwan. Literacy rates are 96% for both men and women.

Health Care Beliefs: Active role and traditional. Chinese philosophies and religions such as Confucianism, Taoism, and Buddhism strongly influence the implementation of self-care and health behaviors. In Confucianism, harmony with others, a lack of self-centeredness, respect for parents and elderly, and loyalty to family are the main teachings. Chinese people are convinced that a satisfactory social life and a happy and peaceful mood promote one's health and prevent illness. *Tao,* or path, is the major concept of Taoism. Taoism emphasizes that human beings should live harmoniously with nature, that is, with Tao. *Yin* and *Yang*, expanded by Taoism, have a great impact on health behavior and beliefs. Disease is caused by an upset in the balance of Yin and Yang; for instance, food is classified as one or the other. If a pregnant woman has a Yin condition, she needs to consume Yang food. Buddha is a powerful religious symbol, important to maintain, protect, and restore health. Buddhism teaches *Inn* and *Ko* (cause and effect) to encourage people to do good and right and to receive good in return. In general, Taiwan's people view the holistic concept of health as the harmonic and integral interrelationship between humans and their environments. Self-care, diet therapy, herbal remedies, and exercise are valued as health practices. Religious activities such as prayer, taking *Fu* water for curing diseases, and temple ceremonies are essential components for patients and their families when dealing with the physical and psychological distress resulting from illness.

Predominant Sick-Care Practices: Biomedical; traditional; Taiwan's people value traditional Chinese medicine (TCM) as well as Western medicine. TCM includes herbal treatment, acupuncture, diet therapy, moxibustion, and folk therapies such as massage for stimulating circulation and relaxing muscles. Physicians practicing TCM use four methods to make a diagnosis: they listen to a description of symptoms, observe the patient's appearance, palpate the rhythm and strength of the pulse, and check the color and texture of the tongue. Action has been taken in recent years to make Western medicine more available and appealing. Modern hospitals with Western medicine are the primary sites for biomedical care practices.

Ethnic-/Race-Specific or Endemic Diseases: Changes in lifestyle, serious air pollution, industrial development, and the fast growth of urban traffic have a major impact on health care needs. The five leading causes of death are cancer, heart disease, cerebrovascular disease, diabetes, and accidents. Communicable diseases such as enterovirus and severe acute respiratory syndrome (SARS) were severe illnesses in 2001 and 2003. By the end of 2005, 2,446 cases of acquired immunodeficiency syndrome (AIDS) and 10,709 persons infected with human immunodeficiency virus (HIV) (including foreigners) had been reported. Since Taiwan implemented a hepatitis immunization program, the rate of hepatitis B carriers among 6-year-olds decreased from 11% to 2%. The cases of hepatitis A decreased from 258 in 2001 to 160 in 2003; 204 cases were reported in 2004.

Health-Team Relationships: Doctors head the medical team, but there are cooperative relationships among medical personnel. At the end of 2003, there were 183,103 individuals involved in health care, including 32,390 physicians, 4,266 doctors of Chinese medicine, 64,478 registered professional nurses, and 30,793 registered nurses. Medical institutions provide 136,331 beds, with an average of almost 60 beds per 10,000 people. The government launched the National Health Insurance (NHI) program in 1995 to provide universal coverage for medical care. By 2004, more than 90% of Taiwan's people were covered by the NHI.

Families' Role in Hospital Care: Family caregivers have a pivotal role in providing care to family members who are ill. The extent of care provided shows the closeness and commitment of family members. Spouses often must change their job schedules, reduce their working hours, or leave their jobs to undertake caregiver responsibilities. With rapid economic growth, a large number of women in the workforce, and a change

T

from extended to nuclear families, more elders are being cared for by health care institutions such as nursing homes rather than by family members.

Pain Reactions: Several strategies for pain management have been practiced in Taiwan, including massage, hot or cold packing, water therapy such as hot-spring baths (spa), mediation with music, yoga, acupressure, acupuncture, and transcutaneous electric stimulation. Although it is believed that "living without the sense of pain" is a human right, most health professionals and the public hesitate in applying conservative pain-control medications and the use of opioid drugs. Furthermore, most of Taiwan's physicians—and patients with cancer; display inadequate knowledge and negative attitudes toward the optimal use of analgesics and opioid medications. The barriers for using optimal cancer pain management (CPM) include physician-related problems such as inadequate guidance provided from pain specialists, inadequate knowledge of practicing CPM and pain assessment, and also inadequate education of patients.

Birth Rites: A population policy of "more are just right" was approved to increase the low birth rate. Fathers are encouraged to stay with mothers during pre-labor, labor, and the postpartum period. It is common for women to take a month off after delivery for the purpose of rest and nutritional support; this is taken at home or in a professional health institute. Daytime or 24-hour babysitting services are available for working women without childcare support. When a baby is 1 month old, families like to share their happiness with relatives and close friends by providing food while they receive baby gifts in return. The infant mortality rate is six deaths per 1,000 live births, and the fertility rate is 1.57 children born per woman. Life expectancy is 75 for men, 80 for women.

Death Rites: Dying at home is traditional in Chinese culture, thereby helping the spirit of the deceased reunite with forebears. Different religious believers have their own preferred funeral rituals, and the oldest son usually consults with the elders in the family about arrangements. Wearing black, white, or dark blue clothes is appropriate for mourning. Most families delegate funeral arrangements to a professional funeral company and worship services. The mourners usually prepare money in a white envelope for the grieving family. The deceased is buried in a coffin or cremated and then put in a tomb or temple. Families pay respects to the deceased by visiting the tomb at the Pure Brightness Festival on April 5th annually.

Food Practices or Intolerances: Various sorts of high-quality foods—including meat, seafood, vegetables, and fruit—are available year round. The staple food is rice. People are gradually changing from a salty and oily diet to low-salt, low-sugar, and high-fiber foods. Some restrictions on eating habits, rooted in traditional Chinese culture, are practiced to avoid bad luck. For instance, a person hitting the bowl while eating will become a beggar, and putting chopsticks in a standing position in a rice bowl will be followed by evil. According to the perspective of traditional Chinese medicine, the essence of a human body can be cold to mild to hot. In each season, a person needs to take foods and herbs based on his or her body nature for the purpose of maintaining a balanced internal environment and obtaining well-being. Some foods are contraindicated while taking Chinese herbs. For example, bananas should not be eaten when a bone is fractured, and wine, cigarettes, and eggplant should not be consumed when a person has lung disease.

Infant-Feeding Practices: More bottle-feeding than breastfeeding is practiced. The Taiwan government has been promoting hospitals to become "friendly maternal-fetal hospitals" for promoting better quality and quantity of breastfeeding since 1998. Because of this effort, Taiwan's pregnant women have a more positive attitude and a higher level of social support for breastfeeding. Additional food or drink is not recommended for infants younger than 6 months old because they have immature digestive functions and the potential for developing diseases such as asthma and allergy. Taiwan's caregivers like to hug, kiss, and talk to their infants.

National Childhood Immunizations: BCG, HepBIG, HepB, DPT, oral polio, MMR, Hib, Japanese encephalitis, and varicella are routine. The percent of the target population vaccinated, by antigen, is: Polio (94%) (the highest rate in the world); DPT (94%) (the highest rate in the Pan-Pacific region and the fifth highest worldwide); and MMR (90%).

BIBLIOGRAPHY

Anonymous: Constrictions of eating habits in traditional Chinese culture. Retrieved March 8, 2006 from http://content.edu.tw/junior/co_tw/ch_yl/city/citch3.htm.

Bureau of Health Promotion, Department of Health, Taiwan: Breastfeeding education— historical review and contemporary status in Taiwan, 2005. Retrieved March 8, 2006, from http://www.bhp.doh.gov.tw/breastfeeding/index05-2.htm.

Centers for Disease Control: Taiwan. Retrieved March 8, 2006, from http://www.cdc.gov.tw/index_info_info.asp?data_id=1446.

Central Intelligence Agency: 2006: *The world factbook, Taiwan.* Retrieved September 21, 2006, from https://www.cia.gov/cia/publications/factbook/print/tw.html.

Chen YC: Chinese values, health and nursing, *J Adv Nurs.* 36(2):270–273, 2001.

Department of Health: Executive Yuan, Taiwan. Retrieved March 8, 2006 from http://www.doh.gov.tw.

Ger L, Ho S, Wang J: Physician's knowledge and attitudes toward the use of analgesics for cancer pain management: a survey of two medical centers in Taiwan, *J Pain Sympt Manage.* 20(5):335–344, 2000.

Huang HC, Wang SW, Chen CH: Body image, maternal-fetal attachment, and choice of infant feeding method: a study in Taiwan, *Birth.* 31(3):183–188, 2004.

Ministry of Interior, Taiwan, Republic, of China: Crude birth rates, crude death rates and natural increase rates by locality, Taiwan area, 2004. Retrieved March 1, 2006, from http://www.doh.gov.tw/statistic/data/biostatistic/93/Table3.xls.

Public Health: Taiwan yearbook 2005. Retrieved February 24, 2006, from http://www.gio.gov.tw/taiwan-website/5-gp/yearbook/p250.html.

Tang ST: Meanings of dying at home for Chinese patients in Taiwan with terminal cancer, *Cancer Nurs.* 23(5):367–370, 2000.

Tzeng HM, Yin CY: Demands for religious care in the Taiwanese health system, *Nurs Ethics.* 13(2):163–179, 2006.

UNAIDS: 2006 Taiwan. Retrieved September 21, 2006, from http://www.unaids.org/en/Regions_Countries/Countries/taiwan.asp.

World Health Organization: http://www.who.int/hiv/countries/en/. (retrieved September 1, 2006).

◆ TAJIKISTAN (REPUBLIC OF)

MAP PAGE (799)

Joshua E. Abrams

Location: This southeast central Asian country is more than 90% mountain-ous, and glaciers are the source of its rivers. Tajikistan is bordered by Kyr-gyzstan to the northeast, China to the east, Afghanistan to the south and southwest, and Uzbekistan to the north and northwest. The total area is 143,100 km^2 (55,251 square miles). The capital is Dushanbe. Tajikistan has hot summers and mild winters, and the country is prone to earthquakes. The climate is semiarid to polar in the Pamir Mountains. The country became an independent state during the dissolution of the former Soviet Union and has been experiencing profound political and economic changes. Since 1991 the country has had three changes in government and a 5-year civil war. The population is 7.3 million, and the gross domestic product (GDP) per capita is $1,200 (one of the lowest among the 15 former Soviet repub-lics). About 64% live below the poverty line. Approximately 52% are younger than 19 years. Literacy rates are almost 100% for both men and women.

Major Languages	Ethnic Groups	Major Religions
Tajik (official)	Tajik 79.9%	Sunni Muslim 85%
Russian (widely used in	Uzbek 15.3%	Shi'a Muslim 5%
government and business)	Russian 1.1%	Other, none 10%
Uzbek	Kyrgyz 1.1%	
Shugni (Pamiri is the	Other 2.6%	
predominant language in		
Gorno-Badakhshan		
Autonomous Province)		

Health Care Beliefs: Traditional; biomedical when available. Because of difficulties in accessing appropriate biomedical care, people are forced to rely on herbal and traditional methods. The use of traditional healing methods is very common, particularly in rural areas and among large families. Acquiring medication is difficult. There is no guaranteed supply of standard basic medicines to the socially vulnerable. Government-run pharmacies stock only 26% of basic medicine supply inventories, and regional hospitals stock 37%. Private pharmacies stock more—66%—but are also more expensive.

Predominant Sick-Care Practices: Traditional; biomedical when available. The medical infrastructure is significantly below Western standards. Medical equipment and medications are scarce, and many doctors have left the country because of the unsettled social and political climate. Those who have stayed often increase their meager incomes by expecting bonuses or informal payments for providing medical treatment or care. Others have moved out of the health care sector to higher paying jobs in other areas. The Republic inherited the Soviet system of health care in which doctors and other health care workers were poorly paid, and most were specialists. The years of civil war that followed independence in 1991 continue to leave economic and political pressures that have made reform difficult. Endemic corruption constrains the effectiveness of reforms, and the departure of skilled professionals during and after the war has left a "brain drain" that also adversely affects the country's potential. It is estimated that more than 80% of Tajikistan's health care facilities are substandard. Most have no running water or central heating and experience power shortages during the winter months. The percentage of the adult population with access to health services in 2001 was 22%. The doctor-to-patient ratio declined drastically after the civil war. The worst doctor-patient ratios are in rural areas, where 30% of the people live 1.5 hours or more from the nearest hospital. A master plan for complete reform of the health care system was adopted in 2002. The plan calls for a shift to primary care, with family doctors rather than specialists forming the cornerstone of the system. The Ministry of Health has estimated that a minimum of 4,000 trained general practitioners are needed to meet the needs of Tajikistan's population, and is cooperating with international organizations on a program to retrain specialists as family doctors. As of 2006, however, only 400 family doctors had been trained in what is still considered a "pilot" project. Emphasis remains on retraining specialists rather than on institutionalized family medicine curricula for medical students, although the government is working on a plan eventually to introduce formal courses in medical schools. Efforts are also being made to correct the uneven distribution of personnel so that rural citizens will have better health care access. Efforts are also being made to restore essential hospital services.

Ethnic-/Race-Specific or Endemic Diseases: The most common causes of death are infections, parasitic diseases, circulatory and respiratory disorders, tumors, and accidents. In 2003, about 85% of all deaths were caused by noncommunicable diseases, approximately 3% attributed to external causes, about 4% to communicable diseases, and about 8% to ill-defined conditions. Immunity as a whole is low, and the country has experienced breakdowns in disease surveillance and health care services. Shortages of qualified medical personnel, products, and resources, combined with increased migration, add to the problem. Serious health threats continue to come from the water supply, 41% of which by 2003 had pathogenic organisms and toxic chemicals from environmental pollution. About 48% of the population uses water from sources of questionable sanitary-epidemiologic quality. Overall, the country has threats of significant disease outbreaks because of population shifts and the breakdown in immunizations. Hepatitis A and E (non-A and non-B) are hyperendemic. Endemic diseases include hepatitis B, resurgent tuberculosis (TB), and falciparum malaria. Civil war, the mass return of refugees from Afghanistan, and the interruption of antimalarial control measures are responsible for the large increase in malaria cases and the significant outbreak in the mid-1990s. Hepatitis B rates have been very high, and TB has been increasing. Despite an 80% reduction in malaria cases since 1997, when 30,000 cases were reported, malaria remains a serious problem. The risk is highest in the country's low-altitude, primarily agricultural areas, particularly the southern Khatlon region where it is mesoendemic, and parts of the northern Sughd region. In June 1997, the country had a major outbreak of typhoid fever in the Dushanbe area and in the south from polluted municipal water. The typhoid strain was resistant to multiple drugs and resulted in 95 deaths; reported cases of typhoid remain high. The risk for cholera and other water-borne illnesses is also high, mostly because of inadequate sanitation. Mass diphtheria vaccination occurred in 1996, with very few cases reported since then; in 2005 only two cases were confirmed. The country has had major epidemics of multidrug-resistant strains of salmonella and a high prevalence of micronutrient deficiency among children and young women, notably iron deficiency and anemia. Tajikistan is hyperendemic for acute enteric diseases in children. *Shigella* infections accounted for 32%, enterovirus diarrhea 12%, and *Escherichia* infections 9%. Tajikistan has been certified by the World Health Organization (WHO) as a polio-free country since 2002. The Tajik government reported an increase in infectious diseases transmitted from domestic animals to people in 2006. The excessive use of pesticides, which pollute the environment and enter water sources, is also a health hazard. The Joint United Nations Programme on HIV/AIDS (UNAIDS) estimates the HIV prevalence rate in adults (aged 15 to 49 years) to be between 0.1% and 1.7% and that 4,900 people are living with human immunodeficiency virus (HIV), including fewer than 500 women and fewer than 400 children aged 0 to 15 years. Acquired immunodeficiency syndrome (AIDS) deaths are fewer than 100. The actual prevalence of HIV and AIDS in Tajikistan is unknown because of a continued lack of testing facilities, despite the creation of AIDS centers in Dushanbe and in all regional capitals. HIV testing is mandatory for blood donors, for those at risk for HIV infection, and for foreign residents. Among the HIV cases with known routes of transmission, about 86% are through injecting drug use, reflective of the increased numbers of heroin users.

Health-Team Relationships: Historically, nurses have not been allowed to perform to their full capacities. Although doctors are the head of the health care team, they outnumber nurses in most clinics and usually

T

perform tasks more suitable for nurses. As part of the Tajik government's master plan to reform medical care, more effort is being made to increase nursing capacity according to Western standards. As of 2005, 412 new nurses have been trained. More significantly, four medical colleges in Tajikistan now provide institutionalized nursing programs, with 700 new nurses graduating in 2006.

Birth Rites: The infant mortality rate has improved somewhat since the early 2000s but remains unacceptably high at 106 deaths per 1,000 live births. Factors contributing to infant mortality are family poverty; inadequate nutrition for nursing mothers, infants, and children; lack of medicines or access to medical professionals; and a lack of safe drinking water. Only 50% of the population is reported as having access to clean drinking water. Environmental pollution is believed to be increasing the incidence of birth defects and maternal and child mortality. The fertility rate is four children born per woman. The WHO compiled maternal mortality statistics for 2000 only, but they indicate the very high ratio of 100 deaths per 100,000 live births. Official Tajik statistics for 2002 cite 51 deaths per 100,000 live births. Unattended home deliveries are estimated by the United Nations Development Program (UNDP) as 41% of the national total and up to 80% in some, primarily rural, regions. About 50% of women suffer from anemia during their pregnancies. Life expectancy has decreased: 62 for men, 68 for women.

Infant-Feeding Practices: Anemia prevention-control programs have been established that include education, oral supplementation for high-risk groups, and fortification of wheat flour with iron and other micronutrients. The goal of this program, which is supported by the United Nations Children's Fund (UNICEF) and the International Nutrition Foundation, is to reduce iron-deficiency anemia in young children and women of childbearing age. Recognition of the importance of breastfeeding appears to be high and is emphasized by the international community and the government.

Child-Rearing Practices: According to studies, most school children have diets with insufficient calories, protein, carbohydrates, and fats. Acute malnutrition has steadily decreased since 1999. According to government sources, just less than 5% of children aged 6 to 59 months currently suffer from acute malnutrition, although at least 6% remain at risk. Chronic malnutrition rates have remained steady since the late 1990s, with more than 30% of Tajik children affected. In some parts of the country, the chronic malnutrition rates have worsened. Basic education rates have been declining since the 1990s, although some improvements have been seen in the 2000s. Literacy rates are high, and the total secondary school enrollment rate in the 2000s is 76%. Total secondary school enrollment in 2001 improved to 79%. More boys than girls continue to be enrolled in school, and many girls do not complete their secondary education.

National Childhood Immunizations: BCG at 3 to 5 days; HepB at birth and at 2 and 4 months; DTwP at 2, 3, 4, and at 16 to 23 months; DT at

6 years; OPV at birth and 2, 3, 4, and 12 months; measles at 12 months and 6 years; vitamin A at 6 to 59 months ×2. The percent of the target population vaccinated, by antigen, is: BCG (97%); DTP1 (87%); DTP3 (82%); MCV (89%); Polio3 (84%); and HepB3 (81%).

BIBLIOGRAPHY

Aliev, S, Shodmonov P, Babakhanova N, Schmoll O: *Rapid assessment of drinking-water quality in the Republic of Tajikistan: country report, UNICEF,* Dushanbe, 2006, UNICEF.

Avesta News Agency: Number of typhoid, malaria cases goes down as dysentery epidemic ramps up in Tajikistan. Retrieved July 19, 2006, from www.avesta.tj.

Babaev GJ, Fattoev FS, Mirzoev AR, Aminjanov RM, and Khamraliev FM: Poverty reduction strategy paper, Dushanbe, 2002, Government of the Republic of Tajikistan.

Central Intelligence Agency: *2006: The world factbook, Tajikistan.* Retrieved September 21, 2006, from https://www.cia.gov/cia/publications/factbook/print/ti.html.

Government of the Republic of Tajikistan: Poverty reduction strategy paper—first progress report. Dushanbe, March 2004, Government of the Republic of Tajikistan.

Rebholz CE, Michel AJ, Maselli DA, Saipphudin K, and Wyss K: Frequency of malaria and glucose-6-phosphate dehydrogenase deficiency in Tajikistan, *Malaria J.* 5:51, 2006.

Saifuddinov SR, Sheraliev I. Sh, Khakimov FR, and Mirsaidoba MU: Health and Health Care in the Republic of Tajikistan in 2005, *Centre of Medical Statistics and Information,* Ministry of Health of the Republic of Tajikistan, Dushanbe, 2006.

Pisarejeva N: 90% of traditional healers in Dushanbe Provide illegal services, Avesta News Agency. Retrieved July 19, 2006, from www.avesta.tj.

UNAIDS: 2006 Tajikistan. Retrieved September 21, 2006, from http://www.unaids.org/en/Regions_Countries/Countries/tajikistan.asp.

World Health Organization: 2006: Immunization, vaccines and biologicals. Retrieved September 21, 2006, from http://www.who.int/immunization_monitoring/en/globalsummary/countryprofileresult.cfm?C='taj'.

World Health Organization: http://www.who.int/countries/tjk/en/. (retrieved September 1, 2006).

World Health Organization Regional Office for Europe: Highlights on health, Tajikistan 2005. Retrieved July 19, 2006, from http://www.euro.who.int/eprise/main/who/progs/chhtjk/home.

http://www.malariajournal.com/content/5/1/51 (retrieved July 19, 2006).

◆ TANZANIA (UNITED REPUBLIC OF)

MAP PAGE (801)

Gemma Burford (Consultants: Mohamed Yunus Rafiq and Lesikar Ole Ngila)

Location: The United Republic of Tanzania is located in eastern Africa on the Indian Ocean, and incorporates the islands of Zanzibar, Pemba, and Mafia in addition to the mainland. The total area is 945,090 km² (364,900 square miles). The capital is Dar es Salaam. The climate is

T

hot and humid on the coast, arid in the central area, and temperate in the northern highlands. The population is 38 million. The gross domestic product (GDP) per capita is $700, and about 36% live below the poverty line.

Major Languages	Ethnic Groups	Major Religions
Swahili (official and primary language)	Black African 99%	Christian 45%
English	Arab <1%	Muslim 35%
Indigenous (e.g., Maasai, Sukuma)	Indian, Pakistani <1%	Indigenous religions (animist traditions) and others (e.g., Sikh, Hindu, and Bahá'i) 20%
Other minority languages (Punjabi, Arabic)	European <1%	

Tanzania has 120 separate ethnic groups, or tribes, representing five linguistic families; by far, the largest family is Bantu (95%). Many tribes have become assimilated into the national culture, but others (particularly Maasai) have retained a distinct ethnic identity. Swahili is spoken by 99% of the population, and English is spoken (in secondary education and some official settings) by approximately 6%. Literacy rates are 86% for men, 71% for women.

Health Care Beliefs: Traditional; indigenous; passive role. In Swahili, health *(afya)* is associated with a physique that would be regarded in most industrialized countries as slightly overweight. Smooth, shiny skin is also an indicator of good health. Most ethnic groups have some traditional beliefs in social causes (e.g., witchcraft, sorcery, the "evil eye" [the belief a person can harm others by looking at them], possession, angry ancestral spirits) for at least some illnesses. These beliefs are more prominent in rural than in urban areas, are less common among those with a formal education, and are less prevalent among Christians and Muslims than among followers of traditional religions. Mental illness is usually attributed to possession by demons or spirits and may be treated by private or public exorcism. Those with mental illness are stigmatized almost everywhere. Minor ailments such as coughs and diarrhea are usually thought to have natural causes or simply be "the work of God." Some of the Bantu believe in the concept of vital force, a force that can be weakened by illness, wounds, disappointments, and suffering. Disease prevention involves observing dietary restrictions, using mosquito nets, and avoiding major climate changes when possible. Rural Maasai believe that all food should be consumed with plant preparations, such as acacia-bark tea, to strengthen the body and prevent disease. Some of these preparations have been shown to contain cholesterol-reducing substances. Injections are often considered superior to oral medication. Brightly colored capsules are considered more effective than white tablets, and antibiotics are overused.

Predominant Sick-Care Practices: Traditional; magical-religious; biomedical where available. It is not unusual for an illness to be treated simultaneously or in succession by biomedical and traditional methods. The principal factors influencing health care decisions are practical ones, such as cost and distance, although cultural factors and experience also play a role. The introduction of user fees for health and education in the 1980s led to the near collapse of government health facilities in some areas. As a result, traditional health services and the private clinic sector have expanded. Tanzania has a continuum of traditional health practitioners ranging from herbalists, who rely entirely on natural products, to spiritualists practicing symbolic healing. A few specialize in bone setting or mental health practice. In cities, practitioners may dispense their own herbal tablets; in rural areas, they often provide amulets to be attached to children's wrists and bring blessings. Self-treatment for chronic illnesses is formalized among Maasai, who have holistic forest retreats involving song, dance, prayer, the use of plant-based medications, and the consumption of meat. Although a few villages still have no formal health care facilities, most have at least one health post or dispensary staffed by a nurse or medical assistant. Tanzania has about 100 district-level hospitals, 17 regional hospitals, and 4 specialist referral centers serving the whole country. The official attitude toward traditional health care is one of cautious acceptance, and the Ministry of Health licenses only herbalists who do not practice ritualism. Integration of traditional and biomedical approaches remains an ideal rather than a reality, with notable exceptions. The regional hospital in Tanga has allocated a whole floor to the Tanga AIDS Working Group, which has so far treated more than 5,000 patients with human immunodeficiency virus (HIV) or acquired immunodeficiency syndrome (AIDS) using herbs prescribed by local healers. The herbs are claimed to alleviate opportunistic infections, improve appetite, and increase longevity.

Ethnic-/Race-Specific or Endemic Diseases: Chloroquine-resistant malaria is endemic, although risk varies with altitude and climate, as is also true for Rift Valley fever and plague. Other common causes of morbidity and mortality are bacterial diarrhea, hepatitis A, and typhoid fever. Thirty-two percent of the population has no access to safe water, causing risk for typhoid and cholera. Trypanosomiasis and schistosomiasis are endemic in some areas. Bilharzia, onchocerciasis, tuberculosis, yellow fever, leprosy, and lymphatic filariasis also may occur. The Joint United Nations Programme on HIV/AIDS (UNAIDS) estimates the prevalence rate of HIV in adults (aged 15 to 49 years) to be 6.5%, with about 1.4 million people living with HIV, including 710,000 women and 110,000 children aged 0 to 14. More than a million children aged 0 to 17 are orphans as a result of parental AIDS, and total deaths from AIDS are between 110,000 and 180,000. Of the 263,000 people estimated to need antiretroviral therapy in 2004, only 8,300 were actually receiving it by 2005.

Health Team Relationships: Within the health team, doctors (generally men) tend to be superior to nurses (who are almost always women), and some patients prefer to see a doctor.

T

Families' Role in Hospital Care: Family members usually remain near the patient's bedside and provide assistance with hygiene, nutrition, and surveillance. If the family considers a treatment to be ineffective, they may try to supplement it with herbal medications or ask for an early discharge, but usually the doctor's authority is respected.

Dominance Patterns: In almost every aspect of public life, men are dominant. Many people think the sexes have different but complementary roles and that women wield considerable power in their own sphere, which includes treating minor ailments in children. Regardless, men's public roles tend to be valued more than women's private roles. Domestic violence is widespread, especially in areas where alcohol consumption is high. Because the family is emphasized more than the individual, language that reflects group ownership rather than individual ownership tends to be used. Age is an important factor, especially in ethnic groups with a tradition of formal age grades. Health professionals from the younger generation are often thought to lack wisdom or experience and may be ignored in favor of older relatives.

Eye-Contact Practices: Eye contact is acceptable in almost all settings, although in some rural areas, mothers of small children may be afraid of strangers "putting the evil eye" on their infants.

Touch Practices: The acceptability of touch depends on many factors, including ethnic group, gender, religion, relative ages of the people involved, and social setting. Even handshakes are unacceptable in certain circumstances (e.g., between a Muslim woman and an unrelated man). Health professionals should consult with the patient and family before beginning any health intervention that could be regarded as improper or disrespectful.

Perceptions of Time: In Swahili, the system of time keeping is based on sunrise and sunset (6:00 AM and 6:00 PM, respectively), not midday and midnight as in the West. Thus, "hour 1" in the morning is 7:00 AM. In general, unplanned events and interactions play a greater role in daily life than schedules. If someone meets a friend or relative while on the way to another appointment, avoiding a conversation to avoid being late is considered rude. Plans for the future are almost always qualified by the phrase "God willing."

Pain Reactions: Many ethnic groups were warrior tribes fighting for land or other resources. The men of these societies were trained from early childhood to face pain without flinching. This attitude still persists, as reflected in the Swahili proverb "A man does not cry for nothing." Crying and screaming are acceptable for women in some cultures, but they are expected to be stoic in others.

Birth Rites: Infant mortality rates are high at 96 deaths per 1,000 live births, and the fertility rate is five children born per woman. Pregnant women usually abstain from sexual intercourse and respect certain dietary taboos, such as not eating eggs and fish heads (a practice of the Bantu). The Maasai believe that women should not be given rich food during the last 3 months of pregnancy because it makes the fetus grow too quickly and causes a difficult delivery. Nurse-midwives, traditional birth attendants, female relatives, or all of these assist at births. In some tribes, the umbilical cord is smeared with cow dung or herbal preparations. The new mother may live with the infant at her mother's house for several months. She also may stay at home and be assisted by older female relatives. She is usually given rich food, such as beef, chicken, or mutton, and confined indoors for 2 to 6 months to regain strength and protect the infant from illness and sorcery. In most areas, sons are preferred. Children are regarded as wealth and as an investment for the future, so large families are preferred. Life expectancy is 45 for men, 47 for women.

Death Rites: Family members are present at the death of a relative in almost all situations, and death rites depend on religious affiliation. Muslims are buried on the day of death, wherever possible. Most people prefer to die at home rather than in a hospital and to be buried in their home territory. Rural funerals are often elaborate celebrations lasting up to 3 days, and all the deceased person's relatives and friends are expected to attend. Among Bantu peoples, the death of young adults may bring about accusations of witchcraft or sorcery. Autopsies and organ donations are not practiced.

Food Practices and Intolerances: Food is eaten with the fingers or a spoon. The main staple is *ugali,* a stiff corn porridge that is usually served with beans, meat or fish stew, or green leafy vegetables. Rice and plantains are also popular. Bananas, mangoes, and many other tropical fruits are commonly eaten. Modern foods such as carbonated soft drinks, white bread, and doughnuts are becoming more popular, especially in towns. Very few pastoralists now subsist on milk, blood, and meat; their staple diet is usually boiled corn supplemented with milk, yogurt, and wild fruits, and meat is eaten on ceremonial occasions only. Fish, insects, and wild game are taboo for Maasai. In many areas, alcohol is traditionally consumed only by older adults, and it is rarely used in the predominantly Islamic coastal regions. Muslims follow dietary restrictions in accordance with their religion, namely eating only *halal* meat and avoiding pork.

Infant-Feeding Practices: Children may be breastfed for as long as 3 to 4 years, but weaning with soft corn soup, semolina, or millet porridge usually begins at 3 to 4 months. Crushed fruit and honey are often provided as well. In rural areas, mild plant-based medicines may be mixed with food to treat childhood illnesses.

Child-Rearing Practices: During the preschool years, female relatives and neighbors help with child care. Child rearing is strict, and children are taught to work hard, respect elders, listen and obey without argument, and learn by rote. In Islamic societies, boys are circumcised as infants; those who practice indigenous religions often perform the procedure during puberty. Female genital mutilation is officially illegal but is still common in the Arusha and Dodoma regions (with 81% and 68% of girls, respectively, being circumcised).

National Childhood Immunizations: BCG at birth; DTwPHep at 4, 8, and 12 weeks; measles at 9 months; OPV at 4, 8, and 12 weeks; vitamin

T

A at 9, 15, and 21 months; TT first contact, +1, +6 months, +1, +1 year. The percent of the target population vaccinated, by antigen, is: BCG, Polio3, and MCV (91%); DTP1(95%); and DTP3, HepB3, and TT2 plus (90%).

Other Characteristics: Swahili greeting rituals (e.g., asking for news of family members, discussing recent events in the person's life) occur before any other verbal interactions, even during professional consultations.

Acknowledgments: The author would like to acknowledge the kind assistance of Gerard Bodeker, chairman of the Global Initiative for Traditional Systems of Health, University of Oxford, Oxford, England.

BIBLIOGRAPHY

Burford G, Rafiki MY, Ole Ngila L: The forest retreat of orpul: a holistic system of health care practised by the Maasai tribe of East Africa, *J Altern Complem Med.* 7(5):547–551, 2001.

Burford G, Bodeker G, Kabatesi D, Gemmill B, Rukangira E: Traditional medicine and HIV/AIDS in Africa: a report from the International Conference on Medicinal Plants, Traditional Medicine, and Local Communities in Africa, *J Altern Complem Med.* 6(5):457–472, 2000.

Central Intelligence Agency: 2006: *The world factbook, Tanzania.* Retrieved September 21, 2006, from https://www.cia.gov/cia/publications/factbook/print/tz.html.

Chhabra SC, Mahunnah RLA, Mshiu EN: Plants used in traditional medicine in eastern Tanzania, parts I-VI, *J Ethnopharmacol.* 21(1987), 25(1989), 28(1990), 29(1990), 33(1991) and 39, 1993.

Johnsen N: The forest of medicines: Maasai medical practice and the anthropological representation of African therapy, *Folk.* 38:53–82, 1996.

Ministry of Health. Retrieved March 6, 2006, from http://www.tanzania.go.tz/health.htm.

UNAIDS: 2006 Tanzania. Retrieved September 21, 2006, from http://www.unaids.org/en/Regions_Countries/Countries/tanzania.asp.

United Nations Children's Fund: Statistics—Tanzania. Retrieved March 6, 2006, from http://www.unicef.org/infobycountry/tanzania_statistics.html.

World Health Organization: 2006: Immunization, vaccines and biologicals. Retrieved September 21, 2006, from http://www.who.int/immunization_monitoring/en/globalsummary/countryprofileresult.cfm?C='tan'.

World Health Organization: Tanzania. Retrieved March 6, 2006, from http://www.who.int/3by5/support/june2005_tza.pdf, 2005.

◆ THAILAND (KINGDOM OF)

MAP PAGE (805)

Jitra Waikagul

Location: Thailand (formerly "Siam") is located in Southeast Asia. It borders Myanmar on the northwest, Laos on the northeast, Cambodia on the southeast, and Malaysia on the south. The total area is 514,000 km^2 (198,456 square miles); the capital is Bangkok. The northwest is hilly to mountainous with some forests. The northeastern plains, the poorest part of the country, are arid, and the central plains are fertile. The south borders on the Gulf of Siam and the Andaman Sea. The population is more than 64.6 million. The gross domestic product (GDP) per capita is $8,300; 10% are living below the poverty line.

Major Languages	Ethnic Groups	Major Religions
Thai	Thai 75%	Buddhist 94%
Chinese	Chinese 14%	Islam 4%
English	Other 11%	Hindu, Christian 2%

Thai and different Chinese dialects (e.g., Toei Chiew, Mandarin, Cantonese) are spoken; some English, Lao, Burmese, and Malay are also spoken. By far, most Thai people are Buddhist, but Muslims are predominant in the south. All religions have the patronage of the king. The literacy rate is 95% for men, 91% for women.

Health Care Beliefs: Traditional and modern; active involvement. Thais and Chinese go to temples often for meditation, "merit making," or if they or a family member is ill. If children are frequently sick or otherwise "difficult," they are given to a monk, as a representative of Buddha, for a specified period of time or until the monk thinks it is no longer necessary. The Ministry of Public Health runs regular and well-publicized health promotion and illness prevention campaigns throughout the country.

Predominant Sick-Care Practices: Biomedical; traditional; and magical-religious. People use a mix of modern medicine and traditional Thai, Chinese herbal, and magical practices, such as using blessed amulets from monks that are believed to protect the wearers from bad luck and disease. If a serious illness strikes, however, the vast majority of people go to the nearest modern medical facility. The health care system is composed of a huge network of government district, provincial, and tertiary care centers that are crowded and have too little money. The country has an excellent private medical sector, although it is unaffordable for most of the Thai population. A new system that offers care to all registered inhabitants, whether they are rich or poor, for 30 Thai baht ($0.70 US) per clinic visit (including medications) was inaugurated during the last general election. It is now rapidly making the government health sector dysfunctional, and the health sector will have to be revised in the near future.

Ethnic-/Race-Specific or Endemic Diseases: There is high degree of risk for bacterial diarrhea, hepatitis A, dengue fever, malaria, Japanese encephalitis, and plague in some locations. Rabies and leptospirosis also pose significant risk. In addition to infectious diseases, liver cancer (mostly due to chronic hepatitis B), nasopharyngeal carcinoma, and other cancers are now becoming major problems. The Joint United Nations Programme on HIV/AIDS (UNAIDS) reports the prevalence rate for HIV in adults (aged 15 to 49 years) to be 1.4%, with 580,000 people living with human immunodeficiency virus (HIV), including 220,000 women and 16,000 children aged 0 to 14 years. About 21,000 deaths are attributed to acquired immunodeficiency syndrome (AIDS). The government expects

T

nearly 50,000 new AIDS cases per year for the next several years. Where the mode of transmission is known, 88% are believed to be have been infected heterosexually. Critical populations that need treatment interventions and services, particularly injecting drug users and migrant and mobile populations, continue to be marginalized. Thailand has increased access to antiretroviral treatment to roughly half the number of people who need it.

Health-Team Relationships: Doctors have high status in Thai society. Nurses are highly regarded as well and are usually very industrious and capable; they are often addressed by the same title as doctors *(Khun Moh)*. A significant difference exists between health care facilities in rural areas compared with those in large cities. The number of health care personnel in rural Thailand is still insufficient, although everybody works hard and team relationships are casual and congenial. In Bangkok, health-team relationships are more formal, and practitioners have clearly defined tasks. Licensing of foreign nurses, dentists, and doctors requires passing a qualifying examination, which requires fluency in spoken and written Thai.

Families' Role in Hospital Care: In rural government facilities, families may be in charge of the patient's hygiene and food. In cities such as Bangkok and in private hospitals, nurses take care of all needs. At least one family member remains with the patient at all times, and most private hospitals provide an extra bed in the room for a family member or trusted servant.

Dominance Patterns: Officially, men are the heads of families, and sons are still considered more important than daughters. However, women usually rule behind the scenes. They basically run the family and have their names on most property deeds.

Touch Practices: The head of the body is considered sacred, but it is acceptable to pat a child on the head. Reaching over a patient's body to pass something is considered impolite, and stepping over a patient who is lying on the floor also is considered rude. Male doctors should not touch female patients without a nurse or another person present, preferably a woman. The usual greeting is the *wai*—folding the hands in front of the upper chest and face. Shaking hands and other forms of social touching while talking are uncommon between Thais and foreigners but are acceptable. Pointing the feet at another person is unacceptable.

Perceptions of Time: The Thai are rather casual about punctuality and are oriented to the present. Immediate gratification is preferred to delayed rewards. Past events are usually forgiven and forgotten quickly. The political enemies of today become the partners of tomorrow if it is beneficial.

Pain Reactions: Although Thais try not to express pain loudly, each person has an individual pain threshold.

Birth Rites: The infant mortality rate is 19.5 deaths per 1,000 live births; and the fertility rate is 1.64 children born per woman. Thais believe that after childbirth a new mother needs "fire." She is expected to sit near a fire, drink hot water and tea, and keep warm regardless of the ambient temperature because doing so keeps her healthy and gives her strength. These customs are now rapidly disappearing, particularly in cities. A rest period of 1 month after giving birth is common, and oily food is avoided. In the north and northeast, it is believed that the wrists of infants must be bound with a string to prevent them from losing their soul. Other traditional practices such as giving birth at home and burying the placenta are rapidly disappearing. Life expectancy is 70 for men, 75 for women.

Death Rites: The dead are kept at home or in a temple from 3 days to many months, depending on the financial and social background of the family. After this period, the bodies are usually cremated, but many Chinese-Thai families still bury their dead. During the mourning period, the monks have daily prayer sessions to which all can come to pay their respects. No religious or other customs prohibit organ donations or autopsies.

Food Practices and Intolerances: Rice is a staple. In the morning and late at night, rice gruel is the favorite food. Food is important and available everywhere at almost any time. Fish sauce, seafood, pork, and chicken are the main staples; many do not eat beef. The primary utensils are spoons, forks, and chopsticks. Most Thais eat with a spoon in the right and a fork in the left hand, a practice that is acceptable even in the upper class. Many farmers still eat most food with their hands.

Infant-Feeding Practices: During the first month, breastfeeding is common, but children are bottle-fed at young ages because their mothers have to return to work. In rural areas, cooked banana with mashed rice is a favorite substitute infant food and is introduced at a very young age in addition to breastfeeding.

Child-Rearing Practices: Child-rearing practices vary greatly between Bangkok and rural areas. Although small, middle-class families are emerging, the vast majority still live with extended family; grandparents, especially grandmothers, play an important role in child rearing. Many families who work in towns leave their small children at their parents' rural homes and only see them during holidays. Seniority plays an important role in daily life, and children are taught to be deferential to elders. In general, children are given much space, and child rearing is fairly permissive.

National Childhood Immunizations: BCG at birth; DTwPHep at 2, 4, and 6 months in 13 provinces; OPV at 2, 4, and 6 months; MMR at grade 1; HepB at birth and at 2 and 6 months; JapEnc at 12 to 18 months and 2 to 2.5 years (in endemic areas); HIB at 2, 4, and 6, months (not part of EPI); measles at 9 to 12 months; Td schoolchildren grade 6 and pregnant women first contact, +1, +6 months; TT pregnant women first visit, +1, +6 months, +10, +10 years. Optional vaccinations include Hep A and rabies (not part of EPI). The percent of the target population vaccinated, by antigen, is: BCG and DTP1 (99%); DTP3 and Polio3 (98%); and HepB3 and MCV (96%).

Other Characteristics: Thai and Chinese patients tend to expect medication when consulting a doctor. If symptoms do not improve within a

T

day, patients often visit another doctor and ask for new medication. Thai doctors tend to prescribe too many medications, a practice that may result from patient expectations and a traditional Chinese practice in which doctors did not charge for their services but did charge for medications. It is not uncommon, even in excellent hospitals, to be given a prescription for an antibiotic (usually the latest on the market), one or two analgesics, a decongestant, a multivitamin, and a nighttime sedative to treat a common cold.

BIBLIOGRAPHY

Asia-Pacific Development Center on Disability [Online]. Retrieved December 19, 2005, from http://www.apcdproject.org/countryprofile/thailand/thailand.html.

Central Intelligence Agency: *2006: The world factbook, Thailand*. Retrieved September 21, 2006, from https://www.cia.gov/cia/publications/factbook/print/th.html.

Department of Pediatrics. Mahidol University. Retrieved December 19, 2005, from http://www.ped.si.mahidol.ac.th/cpg2.php/.

Dhamcharee V, Romyanan O, Ninlagarn T: Genetic counseling for thalassemia in Thailand: problems and solutions, *Southeast Asian J Top Med Public Health*. 32(2):413, 2001.

Triteeraprapab S, Kanjanopas K, Porksakorn C, Sai-Ngam A, Yentakam S, Loymak S: Lymphatic filariasis caused by Brugia malayi in an endemic area of Narathiwat Province, southern Thailand, *J Med Assoc Thailand*. 84(suppl 1):182–188, 2001.

UNAIDS: 2006 Thailand. Retrieved September 21, 2006, from http://www.unaids.org/en/Regions_Countries/Countries/thailand.asp.

UNAIDS: Retrieved December 22, 2005, from /www.unaids.org/EN/Geographical+Area/by+country/Thailand.asp.

van-Griensven F, Supawitkul S, Kilmarx PH, Limpakarnjanarat K, Young NL, Manopaiboon C, Mock PA, Korattana S, Mastro TD: Rapid assessment of sexual behavior, drug use, human immunodeficiency virus, and sexually transmitted diseases in northern Thai youth using audio-computer-assisted self-interviewing and noninvasive specimen collection, *Pediatrics*. 108(1):13, 2001.

World Health Organization: 2006: Immunization, vaccines and biologicals. Retrieved September 21, 2006, from http://www.who.int/immunization_monitoring/en/globalsummary/countryprofileresult.cfm?C='tha'.

◆ TIMOR-LESTE

MAP PAGE (794)

Franklin H.G. Bridgewater

Location: Timor Island is the largest and easternmost of the Lesser Sunda Islands of Southeast Asia. The capital is Diu. Timor Island is 470 km long (278 miles) and 110 km wide (68 miles) and has a rugged, mountainous spine. The western portion is part of Indonesia, and the eastern half is the Democratic Republic of Timor Leste. Timor Leste includes the enclave of Oecussi-Ambeno and the islands of Atau'ro and Jaco. The land area is about 19,000 km^2 (7,334 square miles). The temperature ranges between 19° and 34° C (66° to 93° F), with high humidity; the hotter, wetter time is usually from November to May. The higher altitude (more than 600 m) areas are usually cooler and wetter, and the northern coastal area may dry significantly from April to May. The population is about 800,000. The Antoni-Meto live in the northwest, the Tetum-Balu in the central and eastern areas, the Bunak in the southern and central areas, and the Helong in the southwest areas. Smaller cultural groupings include the Baikenu, Fatuluku, Kemak, Tokodede, Makkassae, Idate, Galoli, and Mambai. Although it is impossible to produce cultural statements that are consistent throughout Timor Leste, the most consistent tenet would be the importance of land and the manner in which it is held. Livestock are also highly valued. The gross domestic product (GDP) per capita is $400, with 40% living below the poverty line.

Major Languages	Ethnic Groups (Indigenous)	Major Religions
Portuguese, Tetum: official	Antoni-Meto	Roman Catholic 90%
Indonesian and English: working languages	Tetum-Balu Bunak Helong	Protestant, Muslim, Hindu, Buddhist, Animist 10%

There are twelve mutually unintelligible indigenous languages with 35 dialects and subdialects. Those educated before 1975 tend to speak Portuguese. Bahasa Indonesian was the official language during the Indonesian occupancy from 1976 to 1999, and those educated during that period speak Bahasa or Tetum. At that time, the Catholic Church replaced Portuguese as the ecclesiastical language with Tetum, which is the first language of some 23% of the population. This aligned the Church more closely with the people and presents a major task in ongoing education. This alignment also influences future "governality" and improvement in general health status. The indigenous groups hold animistic beliefs; demonstrated in superstition and reverence for the spirits of those dead, manifested through stones, animals, water sources, and other objects. Spirits may be either benevolent or malevolent. The Catholic faith is widespread across the eastern half of the island. During the Indonesian occupation, if a person had no religious alliance, this implied to the authorities that they were Communist.

Health Care Beliefs: Biomedical; magical-religious; traditional. There is a widespread belief that evil spirits inhabit some jungle and forested areas. Illness is often attributed to personal actions that offended such spirits or the work of a sorcerer *(buan)* acting at the behest of a hostile third party. There is no precise differentiation between mental and physical illness. It can be accepted that an illness may have no particular cause; this attitude of resignation does not lend itself to diligent inquiry or effective prevention efforts.

Predominant Sick-Care Practices: Acute sick care; health promotion important. In the towns and larger centers, there is wide acceptance of

Timor-Leste

modern health care delivery. In some cultures, healers receive payment, but in other areas relatives accept this responsibility. Placation of aggrieved spirits is often invoked by a sorcerer to achieve healing. Certain leaves and botanical preparations are thought to have curative qualities. Elements of traditional practices from India, Malaysia, and China may be encountered. Seasonal activities, such as crop planting and harvesting, may take priority over medical attention. There is often reluctance to leave the local area to have more expert care at a distant facility.

Ethnic-/Race-Specific or Endemic Diseases: The common presenting symptoms are fever, diarrhea, and vomiting. Malaria is endemic (in areas lower than 2000 m) and a risk (predominantly from *Plasmodium falciparum*). It exists throughout the year in the entire country, and drug- resistant forms have been reported. Dengue fever, another mosquito-borne illness, is prevalent in both village and urban areas. It may be associated with a severe acute illness ("break-bone fever") and occasional serious complications such as a hemorrhagic tendency. Incidence peaks February through March. No prophylactic or therapeutic drugs are available, so preventive behavior is critical. In September 1999, a refugee group in Darwin, Australia, was screened for tuberculosis. A point prevalence of 542 per 100,000 for smear-positive and 2,060 per 100,000 for culture-positive cases was demonstrated. Drug resistance and human immunodeficiency virus (HIV) co-infection were low. Rural practitioners suggest higher rates of both the incidence and resistance. Currently more than 8,000 active cases are recognized. Local cultural factors frequently result in inadequate treatment with the development of resistant strains. Leprosy is endemic and a high incidence is reported; there is no control program. Pockets of yaws have been noted around Aileu, Bobonaro, Los Palos, and Viqueque. The recent economic recovery has resulted in a larger number of motorized vehicles being driven by those with little experience on inadequate roads in an almost unregulated manner. Road fatalities are common. Anemia occurs in all age groups and is associated with chronic malaria, worm infestation, and poor nutrition. Anemia during pregnancy is particularly hazardous. Chewing betel nut is common; areca nut use is regarded as an independent risk factor in oral carcinoma; in contrast, it may have therapeutic value for schizophrenia. No mental health services existed before 1999. AusAid has funded a program to ensure attention to mental health, and interactions with traditional practitioners will be particularly challenging. They might not freely exchange "privileged spiritual knowledge" or cooperate in treatment with a system seen as competitive and destructive. Sexually transmitted diseases are common. Social disruption combined with ignorance and promiscuity are factors conducive to high incidence of and particular concern for HIV and acquired immunodeficiency syndrome (AIDS). Between October 1999 and January 2000, a French military medicosurgical unit did HIV serologic testing on 1,285 residents (both male and female adults aged 15 to 49 years). No serum sample was positive, suggesting that the prevalence rates of HIV and AIDS might be low. Many of the foreigners working in Timor Leste are from countries with high endemic rates of HIV-1 infection, and there is concern that an HIV-1 epidemic like that seen in Cambodia after the 1992 United Nations (UN) mission could occur. A National HIV/AIDS Awareness Campaign was launched in April 2002. The need for condom use presents a challenge.

Health-Team Relationships: During the campaign of terror that followed the UN-organized referendum in 1999, nearly four fifths of all hospital and health care facilities were damaged or destroyed. In 2000, the Australian Government committed A$150 million for reconstruction and development, and in December of the same year, international donors agreed to provide US$520 million. Revenue from oil and gas resources in the Timor Gap is seen as a critical future source of national income. AusAID has significantly supported the government in providing health care. There has been concern that nongovernmental organizations (NGOs) have not been sufficiently incorporated into the process of reconstruction. A number of countries have provided military personnel who have been involved in humanitarian assistance tasks and projects. Dili National Hospital, the main referral center, has 228 beds and provides medical, surgical, pediatric, and obstetric care. Peripheral referral hospitals are at Baucau, Suai, and Maliana. Future development is planned for Oecussi and Ainaro (Maubisse). Smaller community health centers (levels 1 to 4) support health posts and mobile clinics. Access may be severely limited by terrain, weather, transport, and finances. The average walking time to a health facility is more than an hour. Aerial medical evacuation, presently provided under UN aegis, will be progressively more stringently controlled.

Families' Role in Hospital Care: Almost everyone considers it both a duty and obligation to provide companionship and care to their children and family members. Hospital budgets are constrained but may provide for the patient and one attendant. Patients are not charged for care, but there is little effort from patients' attendants to contribute to hospital maintenance. There may be unjustified concern that care provided by someone other than a tribal member speaking the same language might be prejudiced or harmful.

Dominance Patterns: Male dominance is observed in many settings. Boys may be favored in the matter of food distribution and educational opportunities. Women are responsible for food, children, and tending animals, and this society has been described as matriarchal with land tenure passing through the daughter. The practice of the prospective groom providing a dowry is common, which generally means that the groom is rather older than the bride. Marriage for girls is at an early age, previously 12 but now 14, with pregnancy soon following. Polygamy is occasionally encountered. About 26% of parliamentary members are women, and women in general earn about 86% of male earnings.

Touch Practices: The head and hair on the head have special significance, and in adults they are sacred and should not be touched. Holding hands with members of the same sex is common and an indicator of a valued companionship. Handshaking is not traditional but is accepted

T

and performed limply. In the context of an animistic environment, objects should not be moved with the feet because to do so is deemed disrespectful; the act of removing any natural object from its surroundings should be duly and respectfully considered.

Perceptions of Time: Generally, little attempt is made to adhere to a strict timetable. Events are often allowed to happen at their own inherent rate, and long -term planning does not occur. A requirement to follow a set program rigidly may lead to intense frustration.

Birth Rites: About 5% to 10% of women receive some antenatal care. Most births are attended by a local tribal midwife or an older female family member. Trained midwives are present at no more than one fifth of births. A complicated delivery usually enters the health care system at a late stage. The maternal mortality rate is 890 per 100,000—double the rate for Indonesia. The infant mortality rate is high at 125 deaths per 1,000 live births. Naming may be delayed until survival is assured, and the family name may come from either parent. Ineffective, usually herbal, traditional birth-control techniques exist. During the Indonesian occupation, the policy of "Javanization" saw a concerted effort to limit indigenous population growth. The most effective and simplest method was the use of agents such as Depo-Provera, still available over-the-counter from village stores. The complications of this drug are not understood, and there are no legislative controls. The Roman Catholic Church is against widespread contraception, and obtaining a husband's approval before initiation of contraception is considered important. Abortions may be done for unwanted pregnancies, and complications from criminal abortions are rarely seen. Life expectancy is 48 for men, 50 for women.

Death Rites: Practices, including forms of burial, vary enormously from one region to another. Catholic traditions, such as the attendance of priests and wearing of black clothes, have been adopted in urban settings. In remote areas, more traditional burial rites persist, which may involve smoking and drying the corpse before burial and not using a coffin. Women in some cultural groups are expected to express grief with overt displays of tears and weeping (and occasional gentle self-flagellation); however, men are not expected to express themselves thus. Historically, amputated body parts were valued and retained to be buried in anticipation that the owner would have them available again in the next life. Organ donation is not possible given the medical facilities, but conflict with traditional beliefs could be anticipated.

Food Practices and Intolerances: Rice and corn are eaten as staple foods. There is a developing preference for polished rice, with its dietary inadequacies. Chickens, pigs, dogs, goats, and buffalo are common, but meat is not often included in the diet. The practice of milking goats and cattle is not usual, but eggs may be consumed. Sheep and horses are evident in some localities, and fish is abundant in coastal areas. Many vegetables and fruits are available: tubers, carrots, beans, pumpkins, green leaves, pawpaw, bananas, breadfruit, pineapple, and limes. Chile and ginger are used as condiments. Malnutrition is common; 80% of infants are affected, and significant numbers show stunting or wasting. Dietary iodine and vitamin A deficiencies are both seen. Iodized salt is now mandatory, and vitamin A is given to children as part of a government-supported NGO program. Domestic animals are generally unrestrained and cohabit with the family. Food is often prepared, cooked, and eaten in the area frequented by animals. Worm infestation is consequently common, and infestation with the pork tapeworm *(Taenia solium)* with associated cysticercosis is widespread. Alcoholic beverages are freely available and intoxication frequently observed. This is often allied to road trauma and longer-term consequences with liver disease. Associated domestic violence is not tolerated by the extended family. Alcoholic beverages can be produced from native plants *(nipa)*.

Infant-Feeding Practices: Breastfeeding is usual and may continue until the child is 4 or 5 years old or more; this practice may have some pregnancy-control value. Bottle-feeding is frequently associated with failure to thrive because of insufficient hygiene and an inadequate understanding of milk formulation.

Child-Rearing Practices: A stillborn infant is accorded no status, but any sign of life brings significance to the event. Multiple births and infants with physical anomalies are accepted without discrimination. Male children may be preferred over female. Circumcision is not customary. Parents are firm with older children, and corporal punishment may be given for disobedience. Older siblings carry some responsibility for younger ones. Destruction of many schools in 1999 has meant that schooling is now limited. It is not compulsory and usually costs about US$15 per month; about 10% of children attend.

National Childhood Immunizations: BCG at birth; DTwP at 6,10, and 14 weeks; measles at 9 months; OPV/Sabin at birth and at 6,10, and 14 weeks; TT first contact pregnancy, +1, +6 months; +1, +1 year; and vitamin A at 6 to 36 months. The percent of the target population vaccinated, by antigen, is: BCG (72%); DTP1 (65%); DTP3 and Polio3 (57%); and MCV (55%).

Acknowledgments: Drs. Jyothi Natarajan and Cecilia Muñoa and the staff at Maliana Hospital, Bobonaro District, Timor Leste, together with Warrant Officer (Gr. 2) John McDade of Deploying Forces Support Unit, Randwick Barracks, Sydney, NSW, Australia, were important personal sources of information.

BIBLIOGRAPHY

Australian Government: AusAid—country programs. Country brief—East Timor. Retrieved April 17, 2006, from http://www.ausaid.gov.au/country/country.cfm? CountryID=911&Region=EastAsia.

Central Intelligence Agency: *2006: The world factbook, East Timor.* Retrieved September 21, 2006, from https://www.cia.gov/cia/publications/factbook/print/tt.html.

Davis R, Icke G: Division of Laboratory Medicine, Royal Perth Hospital, Perth, Western Australia. Malaria: an on-line resource. Retrieved April 17, 2006, from http://www.rph.wa.gov.au/malaria/html.

Ethnologue report for East Timor. Languages of Timor Lorosae. Retrieved April 17, 2006, from http://www.ethnologue.com.

Kelly PM, Scott L, Krause VL: Tuberculosis in East Timorese refugees: implications for health care needs in East Timor, Int J Tuberc Lung Dis. 6(11):980–987, 2002.

Kuruppuarachchi K, Williams S: Betel use and schizophrenia, Br J Psychiatry. 182:455, 2003.

McAuliffe AV, Grootjans J, Fisher JE: Hasten slowly: a needs analysis for nurse and village health worker education in East Timor, Int Nursing Rev. 49(1):47–53, 2002.

Neuhaus S, Bridgewater FH: Medical aspects of complex emergencies: the challenges of military health support to civilian populations, Austral Defence Force J. 172:56-72, 2007

Patrick I. East Timor emerging from conflict: the role of local NGOs and international assistance, Disasters. 21(1):48–66, 2001.

United Nations: National HIV/AIDS awareness programme launched. Retrieved April 17, 2006, from http://www.un.org/peace/etimor/DB/db030402.htm.

Warnakulasuriya S, Trivedy C, Peters T: Areca nut use: an independent risk factor for oral cancer: the health problem is under-recognised. BMJ. 324(7341):799-800, 2002.

Wikipedia Contributors. East Timor, Wikipedia, The Free Encyclopedia. Retrieved April 17, 2006, from http://en.wikipedia.org/wiki/East_Timor.

World Health Organization: Leprosy. Retrieved April 17, 2006, from http://www.who.int/lep/Reports/wer8034.pdf.

World Health Organization: East Timor. Retrieved April 17, 2006, from http://www.who.int/countries/tls/en/.

World Health Organization: 2006: Immunization, vaccines and biologicals. Retrieved September 21, 2006, from shttp://www.who.int/immunization_monitoring/en/globalsummary/countryprofileresult.cfm?C='tl'.

World Health Organization: Human Development Indicators: United Nations; 2003. WHO Immunization surveillance, assessment and monitoring. Retrieved April 17, 2006, from http://www.who.int/immunization_monitoring/en/.

Zwi A, Silove D: Hearing the voices: mental health services in East Timor, Lancet. 360(suppl):s45–s46, 2002.

www.un.org/Depts/Cartographic/map/profile/timoreg.pdf.

◆ TOGO (TOGOLESE REPUBLIC)

MAP PAGE (800)

Adama Dodji Gbadoé and Edoh Azankpé

Location: Togo, in West Africa, has a total area of 56,600 km^2 (21,848 square miles) and is one of the smallest and poorest countries in Africa. It is bordered on the west by the Republic of Ghana, on the north by the Republic of Burkina Faso, and on the east by the Republic of Benin. The Atlantic Ocean is to the south. Togo is divided into two zones by a long chain of mountains. The north has a tropical, humid climate, with only one rainy season from May to October, and one dry and very hot season, from November to April characterized by the dry and dusty harmattan wind. The south has two dry seasons (from November to March and July to August) and two rainy seasons (from March to July and September to October). Little rain falls, especially in the south, so forests are found only on mountains and adjacent to rivers. The plains are part savannah and part woodlands. Rich soils cover only 20% of the total. The capital is Lomé. The southern part of the country is more populated, and about 75% of the people live in rural areas. The population is 5.5 million. The gross domestic product (GDP) per capita is $1,700, with 32% living below the poverty line.

Major Languages	Ethnic Groups	Major Religions
French (official)	South: Adja/Ewe 44%	Christian 51%
Ewe and Mina (south)	Akposso/Akebou 4%	Animist 27%
Kotokoli-Tem and Kabye	Ana/Ife 3%	Muslim 11%
(north)	North: Kabye/Tem 30%	Other 11%
	Para-Gourma/Akan 14%	
	Foreign 5%	

Togolese people believe deeply in God and divinities, and traditional Togolese believe that there is a greatest god (God) who can be reached through small gods (divinities). These divinities are venerated in ceremonies, rituals, and prayers to ancestors. The gods most adored are *Vaudou Sakpaè*, god of the earth, who expresses himself through smallpox, chickenpox, or measles; *Hèbiesso*, god of rain and justice, who expresses himself through thunderclaps and by killing thieves whenever he is asked for justice; *Legba*, the protector god against enemies and bad spirits; *Mami-wata* (siren), the sea or ocean goddess who is the expression of wealth; and *Gnigblin*, the god of the forest and alliance, who is expressed by the rainbow. Togo has 40 local languages. In addition to major languages, there are Tchokossi, Moba, Bassar, Ana, Akposso, Adja, and Fon. Other than French, only Ewe and Kabyè are acknowledged as national languages. English is studied as a second language and is being used increasingly. Literacy rates are 75% for men, 47% for women.

Health Care Beliefs: Because the Togolese believe that mental illness is induced by another person or a spirit, such people are kept as part of society. Families take charge of their family members and bring them to traditional healers or pastors for treatment. Ceremonies, amulets, scarifications, prayers, and potions of all sorts are treatments. It is rare to confine these patients to an institution such as a psychiatric hospital, and only one psychiatric hospital is available. Priority for prevention and health education is given to infectious and contagious disease programs such as those for human immunodeficiency virus (HIV) and acquired immunodeficiency syndrome (AIDS), tuberculosis, leprosy, malaria, acute respiratory tract infections, and diarrheal diseases. Togo also has prevention programs for noninfectious diseases such as sickle cell disease, which affects 16% of the population. Prevention efforts are adversely affected by traditional beliefs and lack of information. For example, 10% to 20% of people think that malaria is caused by the sun, fieldwork, or eating

too much *cacahuets* or palm oil. To prevent anemia, people treat themselves with beets or infusions of red herbs (because they are the color
of blood), although they do not contain the iron, folic acid, or B_{12} vitamins
that are normally recommended.

Predominant Sick-Care Practices: Equipment in public hospitals is
poor. Togo has no social health insurance system, and hospitals are over-
flowing with patients who could be treated in peripheral health units. With
such an influx of patients, nursing performance is affected. People go
to hospitals rather than to health units because they believe that they
can get better care, referrals from peripheral health units are difficult,
and there are not enough ambulances to transfer them because of long
distances between facilities. About 31% use home remedies, and more
than 25% resort to traditional medicine by consulting indigenous healers.
Traditional medicine involving herbs is legalized, and there is a research
team at the University of Lomé that is studying the healing abilities
of plants. Numerous Togolese also pray or perform rituals for gods.
Patients usually consult a pastor, priest, traditional healer, or fetish priest
before going to a modern health center. Spiritual and medical treatments
are often combined, and the doctor is unaware of it. It is common for
priests or prayer groups to be in hospitals during the day after a doctor
has left and for traditional healers and fetish priests to be at hospitals
at night.

Ethnic-/Race-Specific or Endemic Diseases: Some diseases are
specific to the northern part of the country, such as onchocerciasis, which
is endemic. Cerebrospinal meningococcal meningitis is endemic in the dry
season. Schistosomiasis, cholera, goiter, malaria, and childhood illnesses
such as mumps are endemic throughout the country. Because of immunizations; pertussis, diphtheria, tetanus, and poliomyelitis are becoming
rare. Goiter affects primarily the districts of Wawa, Kozah, Doufelgou,
Binah, and Amou. The National Service of Nutrition recommends consumption of iodized salt to compensate for iodine deficiencies. Malaria
is the primary cause of mortality. It is endemic all year, with a recurrence
at the end of rainy seasons, so every person may have four to six attacks
per year. *Plasmodium falciparum* is the most common (98% of cases),
whereas *P. malariae* and *P. ovale* are diagnosed in 2% of cases. Severe
malaria especially affects children aged 6 months to 6 years and pregnant
women. Malaria hinders the economic development of the country, but
most people do not like using impregnated mosquito nets (it makes them
feel hot or like they are suffocating). Nutritional diseases such as kwashiorkor and marasmus are common. The Joint United Nations Programme
on HIV/AIDS (UNAIDS) estimates the prevalence of HIV in adults (aged
15 to 49 years) to be 3.3%, with 110,000 people living with HIV, including
61,000 women and 9,700 children aged 0 to 14 years. About 9,100 have
died of AIDS, and 88,000 children (aged 0 to 17 years) are orphans as a
result of parental AIDS. The government has adopted blood screening,
access to antiretroviral treatment, nondiscriminatory policies, and promotion of condom use (only 1.6% use condoms). The principal modes of

transmission (>90%) are heterosexual and mother-to-child transmission during pregnancy. Only 5 health centers of 100 provide health services to prevent infants from being infected, and only 8 of 100 infected children benefit from free medical care.

Health-Team Relationships: Nurses have approximately 7 fewer years of school attendance and training than doctors, so they often feel inferior. Paradoxically, this creates good relationships within the medical staff. Relationships between patients and health teams in public health centers are not so conflicting as in private ones.

Dominance Patterns: Socially and officially, children belong to the father in this patriarchal society. Mothers are the first educators of the children. In most ethnic groups, the widow is automatically "given" (married) to a brother of her deceased husband so that she can have someone to support her and take responsibility for her children's education. More than 80% of working women are in agriculture, especially in rural areas. In urban areas, it is common to find women at many levels in public administration, private enterprise, or the trade sector. Togo is called the country of *Nana Benz*; women who were part of the cloth trade in the West African subregion became so rich that they were the first to own Mercedes Benz cars in West Africa. Today, a *Nana Benz* means a rich woman.

Families' Role in Hospital Care: The health care system has too few nurses and "sick-nurses." Families have an important role in the care of patients because they are often asked to monitor intravenous fluids, provide food, and bathe the hospitalized person. The family finds someone to remain with the hospitalized family member at all times.

Eye-Contact Practices: It is considered improper and impolite, especially for children, to look directly into the eyes of an older adult.

Touch Practices: Most widows and widowers do not shake hands with persons other than other widows and widowers. Children do not initiate a handshake when greeting an older adult because it is impolite. In some areas, men do not deliberately touch the wife of another man because it is regarded as adultery; if this occurs, the woman must be cleansed by rituals or she may become ill.

Perceptions of Time: People do not place much importance on punctuality, especially those who are less well educated. Lateness has become so common that people are not worried when they are not on time. It is common to hear people say that an event will start "on African time," meaning later than the scheduled time.

Pain Reactions: In public health centers, where care is less expensive, patients seem to be more stoic and talk little about their pain because they do not want to annoy doctors. In private centers, patients are more demanding and may ask for morphine, which is not yet used in the hospitals. The pain of newborn infants is not considered. In general, the more someone is able to bear pain, the more the person is appreciated and considered courageous. In some ethnic groups (e.g., Peuhls), stoicism is a proof of virility. Young people ready to be engaged are invited to flog one another; whoever expresses pain is considered weak and ineligible for marriage until the ritual can be completed with no outbursts.

Birth Rites: Pregnant women are treated with consideration because pregnancy is considered a sacred time. Mothers prepare spiritually by asking divinities what to do to make the delivery easier. Some pregnant women wear amulets that protect the infant from witchcraft or that will promote an easy birth. More than 50% of deliveries occur in the home attended by traditional "obstetricians." Because health centers are far from homes, especially in rural areas, some organizations provide training for birth practitioners. Simple naming ceremonies are held for a single infant born with the head coming out first. A ritual is performed after a prayer to the ancestors, and then a name is given to the infant. Usually a second name (for Christians and Muslims) is chosen, even if the family members are not believers. After the ceremony, the infant can be taken outside at any time. As for twins, they are considered divines, expressing hope as well as fear, and they also represent animals such as monkeys or buffalos according to geographic area. During or after the naming ceremony, families of twins organize a very expensive event to integrate them into society; they are almost venerated. No member of the family of twins is allowed to eat or kill the animal the twins represent, because legend says the twins will die. Special ceremonies also are performed for infants born legs first, and they are given special names. Every male infant is circumcised. The infant mortality rate is 61 deaths per 1,000 live births. The mortality rate for children younger than 5 years is 146 per 1,000, and 5.4 children are born per woman. The maternal mortality rate is 478 deaths per 100,000 live births. Life expectancy is 55 for men, 59 for women.

Death Rites: Every death is thought to be provoked spiritually by an enemy or angry gods, even if clinically proven to be caused by other factors. So, instead of an autopsy, people consult an oracle or a necromancer *(Xoyoyo)* to know "the real" cause of the death and how the deceased must be buried. Rites and sacrifices are performed to calm down the angry god or to allow the spirit of the deceased to chase the murderer. Older adults are not considered dead; they are thought to be in another world (Awlimé). Dead twins are symbolized by statuettes and are maintained as living beings. Togolese believe that dead people can see and judge acts of others, so no one wants to offend them. Organ donations and autopsies are not practiced because they are considered an offense to the dead person. Widowers and widows are supposed to protect themselves from being carried away by their late husbands or wives by putting pieces of charcoal in their meals or by using special herbs (such as *ahamè*). A widow has more restrictions than a widower; she must shave her head, wear dark clothing, stay in her room at night, and wear a dark cloth rope around the waist.

Food Practices and Intolerances: In the city, the largest meal is lunch. Most poor people eat only once a day, at noon. Vegetables and meat are always well cooked. Basic foods differ according to areas, but some foods—such as pounded yam or cassava, ayimolu or watsé (a meal made of rice and beans), and rice (mostly imported)—are consumed throughout the country. Rice is the main meal during festivities. Some meals such as *gari* (made out of cassava), ademè, fétri (vegetables), and akoumé (which is made of corn) are especially popular in the south. Cereals such as sorghum or millet are eaten in the north. Certain meals, such as beans combined with vegetable oil and gari, are rich in protein and used in hospitals for malnourished children, although people consider this to be food for poor people. Mothers incorrectly think that pasta is a nutrient-rich food. Most Togolese eat with their hands.

Infant-Feeding Practices: Until the last 12 years, because of Western influences and advertising about cow's milk formulas, women, especially those with a Western education, substituted bottle-feeding for breast-feeding or reduced the duration of breastfeeding to 3 months at the longest. Today, exclusive breastfeeding is practiced for about 6 months. From the seventh month to 2 years of age, cereal and solid foods are added.

Children-Rearing Practices: It is rare for children to have their own room; most sleep with their parents. Respect for adults, politeness, and obedience are the essential virtues taught. Children who call older adults by their names are considered to have bad manners.

National Childhood Immunizations: BCG at birth; DTwP at 6, 10, and 14 weeks; OPV at birth and 6, 10, and 14 weeks; measles at 9 months; vitamin A at birth to 59 months; YF at 9 months; and TT pregnant women first contact, +1, +6 months, +1 +1 year. The percent of the target population vaccinated, by antigen, is: BCG (91%); DTP1 (83%); Polio3 and DTP3 (71%); MCV (70%); and TT2 plus (61%).

BIBLIOGRAPHY

Central Intelligence Agency: 2006: The world factbook, Togo. Retrieved September 21, 2006, from https://www.cia.gov/cia/publications/factbook/print/to.html.

Gbadoé AD, Dogba A, Segbena AY, Nyadanu M, Atakouma Y, Kusiaku K, Vovor A, Assimade JK: Priapism in sickle cell anemia in Togo: prevalence and knowledge of this complication, *Hemoglobin*. 25:355–361, 2001.

Gbadoé AD: *L'utilisation des structures de soins par les enfants de 0 à 5 ans au Togo. Résultats de la première phase d'une enquête menée dans la région des Plateaux* [Mémoire de DES de Pédiatrie], p 74, Lomé, Togo, 1993, Université du Bénin.

Togo-presse: Our nation, Lomé, Wednesday, 7th December 2005.

UNAIDS: 2006 Togo. Retrieved September 21, 2006, from http://www.unaids.org/en/Regions_Countries/Countries/togo.asp.

UNFPA/Direction de la Planification de la Population: Principaux indicateurs démographiques du TOGO, Lomé, Juillet 2003.

United Nations Department of Economic and Social Affairs Population Division: *Population and HIV/AIDS 2005.* United Nations Publications, New York, NY.

World Health Organization: 2006: Immunization, vaccines and biologicals. Retrieved September 21, 2006, from http://www.who.int/immunization_monitoring/en/globalsummary/countryprofileresult.cfm?C='tgo'.

T

◆ TONGA (KINGDOM OF)

MAP PAGE (794)

Barbara Burns McGrath and Mavae Nofomuli Aho-Redmond

Location: The Kingdom of Tonga (the Friendly Islands) is a archipelago of 169 islands (36 inhabited) in the South Pacific Ocean, about two thirds of the way from Hawaii to New Zealand. The islands cover a total area of 748 km^2 (289 square miles) and are divided into three main groups: Tongatapu, Hapai, and Vava'u. The population is 112,422. Two thirds of the people live on the largest island, Tongatapu, where the capital, Nuku'alofa, is located. It is ethnically a very homogeneous society, with non-Polynesians numbering only in the hundreds. Tongan oral traditions hold that Tongans originated from Pulotu—an island that is northwest of Tonga. Tonga was first settled some 3,000 years ago by a pottery-making people (the Lapita people), who entered through Vanuatu and Fiji. They were originally from Taiwan and the southeastern coast of China and are the ancestors to all Polynesians. The government is a hereditary constitutional monarchy. Despite a long history of European contact, Tonga is the only island group in the Pacific to avoid colonization. Tonga became a British protectorate in 1900 but declared its independence in 1970 and joined the Commonwealth of Nations, followed by membership in the United Nations in 1999. A pro-democracy movement began in the 1970s and 1980s and continues as a challenge to the traditional electoral and political system. The gross domestic product (GDP) per capita is $4,218. Remittances from abroad were estimated at 55% of the GDP in 2004. The number of Tongans living overseas (in the United States, New Zealand, Australia) is about equal to the number living in Tonga.

Major Languages	Ethnic Groups	Major Religions
Tongan (official)	Polynesian	The Free Wesleyan
English (official)	About 300	Church of Tonga
	Europeans	Roman Catholic
		Free Church of Tonga
		Anglican
		Seventh Day Adventist

Tongan and English are used in schools; most Tongans speak English as their second language. There are three main levels of Tongan language: Tu'i (language of the King and the Royal family; it is also the language used to address God), Hou'eiki (language of the chiefs and nobles), and Tu'a (language of the commoners). Much of the social life is structured around the church, and ministers have great influence. Sunday is considered a day of rest and prayer with many restrictions. Education is free and mandatory, resulting in a literacy rate of 98% for both men and women. The government operates most primary schools: churches sponsor most secondary schools.

Health Care Beliefs: Contemporary health care beliefs reflect a syncretism of Christian and traditional beliefs that were predominant before the arrival of missionaries in the nineteenth century. In the past, Polynesian gods were consulted and appeased; today a belief in a single benevolent God is virtually universal. Belief in spirits is widespread, and their presence is felt in cemeteries but also in places such as open fields and abandoned gardens. They often visit in dreams to give advice or to warn of some impending misfortune. The concepts of *mana* and *tapu* are central to an understanding of health and illness in Tonga. *Mana* refers to the degree to which objects and persons are endowed with supernatural powers. Having mana offers some protection against misfortune and bad luck and is the force that allows healers to act as a vessel for the healing power of God. Tapu is sacred and expresses a connection with the gods. It also describes the forbidden and prohibited (the English word *taboo* is derived from the Tongan *tapu*). Breaking a tapu or misusing mana may result in misfortune or illness through the agency of supernatural forces.

Predominant Sick-Care Practices: Biomedical and traditional; prevention efforts. Both traditional and Western beliefs and practices coexist. One may receive care from traditional healers (*faito'o faka* Tonga) who prescribe herbal cures, set bones, and use therapeutic massage, or from physicians and registered nurses who practice in hospitals and clinics. The special power of *faito'o faka-Tonga* can be transferred to an apprentice through the cultural practice of *fanofano'i*. There are 4 hospitals, 14 health centers, and 34 maternal health clinics. Health promotion is valued, with active programs. Health care that is provided at a government facility is free for all citizens. Individuals with conditions requiring resources beyond Tonga's means or needing complicated medical procedures are most often transferred to New Zealand. About 200 healers on Tongatapu treat a variety of illnesses, both "natural," such as stomach ache or skin infection, and those caused by spirits. Decisions determining which type of practitioner to consult are based on a number of factors, including whether the illness is thought to be "Western" (e.g., cancer) or indigenous (e.g., fallen fontanel); past experience; or pragmatic concerns, such as ease of transportation to the site of care. There are also strong proponents of traditional methods, especially if they are used in a complementary manner.

Ethnic-/Race-Specific or Endemic Diseases: There are no official death certificates for many Tongans and there may be misclassification of the actual causes of death. Diseases of the circulatory and respiratory systems; neoplasms; and endocrine, nutritional, and metabolic conditions are prevalent. Although communicable diseases have largely been brought under control, obesity, diabetes and cardiovascular diseases have increased to epidemic proportions. Leading causes of morbidity are acute respiratory infections, influenza, bronchopneumonia, and diarrhea.

The prevalence of type 2 diabetes more than doubled from 7% to 15% in the last 25 years, and as many as 80% remain undiagnosed and untreated. The Joint United Nations Programme on HIV/AIDS (UNAIDS) has very little information on human immunodeficiency virus (HIV) in Tonga. The first case was detected in 1992; in 2004, 14 infections had been reported, most in men. The primary mode of transmission is heterosexual.

Families' Role in Hospital Care: It is important to understand the role of each person in the family before communicating extensively with any one individual or groups of individuals. Close relatives visit, help with personal care and bathing, and bring food. It is common for at least one close relative to stay 24 hours a day, sleeping on a mat next to the bed. Family members have a voice in decisions about procedures, including surgery and referrals, and may bring traditional medicines with or without the physician's or nurse's knowledge. Tongans prefer to care for older people at home, but this is sometimes difficult in urban families who work outside the home.

Dominance Patterns: Tonga is a mixture of Western and Tongan cultures and has retained much of its Polynesian culture. The beloved Queen Salote, who ruled until 1965, often described core Tongan values as *faka'apa'apa* (respect), *loto to* (humility, willing heart), *mamahi'i me'a* (loyalty), and *tauhi vaha'a* (keep up good relations). Respect for traditional authority and customs endures, and the lifestyle is conservative. Gender differences originate from *anga fakatonga* ("the Tongan way"). It is not customary for women to freely associate with men unless they are chaperoned, and women do not usually leave their homes alone. Tonga has a highly stratified and status-conscious society. Lower-status persons are expected to demonstrate respect and to be unquestioningly obedient to those of higher status. The proper way to show respect in Tonga is by sitting on crossed legs and clasping the hands on the lap. Although caste is not as rigid and elaborate as it was in the past, Tonga still has two clearly defined social classes: the nobles and the commoners. The royal family and the 33 hereditary nobles and their families are the highest ranking people. All other Tongans are commoners. Nobles cannot marry commoners unless they want to risk losing their royal titles, and a commoner who marries a noble can never attain noble status.

Eye-Contact Practices: Body language or direct eye contact is common between sexes and among social classes. Raising the eyebrows is a way to say "yes" in answer to a question.

Touch Practices: Touching between men and women who do not know each other is unacceptable; some women may not even want to shake hands. Men and woman alike greet those they know extremely well with an embrace or kiss on either cheek *(fe'iloaki)*, a sign of affection. Men usually greet each other verbally or by shaking hands. Greetings during professional and formal interactions are limited to a handshake and verbal exchanges.

Perceptions of Time: Tongans are generally very punctual to work, school, or church because it is disrespectful to arrive late. However, it is common to be less prompt with other more casual functions. There is a expression, *taimi fakaTonga,* or Tongan time, that is familiar within all Tongan households. *Taimi faka-Tonga* is basically governed according to social relations so that individuals are punctual or late according to what it will take to maintain good social relations.

Pain Reactions: Although some gender differences in pain reactions exist, both sexes tend to be stoic.

Birth Rites: The infant mortality rate is 17 per 1,000 live births, and the fertility rate is three children born per woman (higher in rural families). More than 99% of pregnant women attend antenatal clinics, and 98% deliver in a health facility. Neither fathers nor any male members of the family are usually allowed to be present during childbirth, although close female relatives are usually present. During the time when there were home births, according to Tongan tradition, a messenger (usually the husband) was sent to retrieve a midwife when the delivery was imminent. It was believed that if the first person the messenger met was female, the child would be a girl and vice versa. After the birth, family members play an active role as primary caregivers. For the first 10 days, the mother's diet includes only yams and hot coconut milk *(veifua).* Immediately after childbirth, the mother and infant are painted with turmeric *(enga)* and oil, and the mother does not leave the house or bathe for 5 days. Each day for 2 or 3 months the mother and child are given a sponge bath and repainted with turmeric, which are thought to keep them warm and help the mother produce plentiful milk. The practice of burying the umbilical cord and the placenta *(fonua)* and of marking the burial spot is still the custom. The mother's placenta is the child's first *fonua* (land-nourishing environment), the land-people is the child's second *fonua,* and the grave is the final *fonua* for a person. All these places (placenta, land-people, grave) are called *fonua* in Tonga. Usually the cords are buried in mounds just outside the door of the house, so that those who visit their home can stand on it. It is believed that if many people stand on it, the child will happily stay within the home and will not stray. The *tope,* a long lock of hair worn by small boys over the temple is cut off at puberty; and the boy's hair is cut in the style of an adult male. Male circumcision (modern procedure) and supercision (traditional procedure) are common and usually take place at age 6 to 12 years.

Death Rites: Funeral rituals, or *putu,* are points of pride in Tongan culture and are held up as evidence that "ancient Tonga" is still alive and viable. These are elaborate and important social events. The length of the ritual period varies from 1 to 10 days (for royalty it can last a year). As soon as a person dies (commoner or chief), he or she is treated with the same respect given to a chief. During the funeral, chiefly language is used in addressing the deceased. They are respected because they have become an ancestor, a status of respect. Death ideally occurs at home, surrounded by close family. Typically, he or she will remain in bed or on a mat on the floor. A piece of *ngatu* or cloth may be hung up to separate the space where the person lies from the rest of the house. Only specific

T

relatives are allowed near the dying person. Personal care is performed by women, usually daughters and other female relatives who are of the same or higher rank. Expressions of strong emotions and physical contact such as touching are avoided. It is thought that it will be more difficult for the person to leave if those around are very sad or having a hard time. After death, the body will be washed with water, and the skin will be rubbed with coconut oil, powder, and perfume. The rituals begin with the 'āpō, or wake, in the home. Everyone who has a connection to the person will come by to pay respects. The body is on display or the casket is open, allowing people to kiss the deceased on the cheek and to say goodbye. An 'āpō is considered to be a chance to say goodbye to the deceased as he/or she embarks on the final voyage or journey. Although some relatives are inside the house, keeping watch over the body and welcoming mourners, others are outside preparing and serving food and drinks. The main activity outside is the gift exchange. Koloa—wealth or valuables—are ritually presented and may include very finely woven mats and bark cloth. These will be redistributed during the following days. Until recently, the body was wrapped in tapa cloth and put in the earth; however, coffins are becoming more common. During the mourning period, friends and relatives will wear black clothing covered by a ta'ovala, a woven mat wrapped around the waist. Some relatives wear a very large one extending from under the arms to the ground. The size and appearance of one's ta'ovala indicate how one is related to the deceased and signifies respect. It is also a symbol for the fonua-land-people. Wearing the ta'ovala is similar to wrapping the fonua around the waist. Graves are distinctive, with shaped mounds of white sand that are then decorated by women. These decorations have altered with cultural change and prevailing taste, so that, in addition to more traditional crushed coral and woven flowers, one finds beer bottles or plastic syringes carefully arranged on the grave. After burial, the head of the household invites the entire community to a feast and announces how long the mourning period is to be. The time of mourning is marked by special clothing, ta'ovala putu, a mat wrapped around the waist, and prohibitions against sporting games, dances, music, and beating tapa in the village.

Food Practices and Intolerances: The diet consists of root crops and cassava (manihot esculenta), yams (Dioscorea alata), taro (Colocasia esculenta), taro root, plantains (Musa paradisiaca), breadfruit, coconut products, fresh fruit, pork, chicken, corned beef, and fish. Elaborate feasts are used to commemorate all important events. The introduction of a Western diet has taken a toll on the health of Tongans. Imported foods are easily available but are low in nutrition (e.g., white bread, mutton flaps, imported chicken parts, Spam). Public health programs have increased awareness of healthy food choices and the importance of physical activity. The late king took the lead in this campaign, and when his health allowed, was often seen riding a bicycle as a role model for others. Kava, called 'ava in Samoa, is widely drunk throughout most of the Polynesian Islands. Kava is made from the dried root of the piper methysticum plant, a member of the pepper family. Its use as a ceremonial drink before the start and conclusion of important meetings and functions goes back centuries. In the past, the kava ceremony consisted of individuals drinking the substance and then chasing the taste with sugarcane. Today, the kava ceremony is the same, but hard candies or sodas are substitutes for the sugarcane. There are a variety of purposes for kava: medical, religious, political, cultural, and social. It is one of the best ways to bring families and groups together to talk about important topics. Tongans use kava for headaches, pulmonary pains, gonorrhea, blackwater fever, tuberculosis, leprosy, cancer, asthma, stomach upsets, and insomnia. Kava also helps to minimize the risk of infections.

Infant-Feeding Practices: It is estimated that about 74% of mothers currently breastfeed their infants; however, a large proportion of mothers also give additional foods and drinks to infants because they are not confident they have enough milk or that their infants are satiated. Bottle-feeding is also common. Boiled water, orange, or *lesi* (pawpaw) juice is usually given within the first 2 months. Before the fourth month, mothers introduce papaw and bananas as the most common first foods. Older infants are also given imported infant foods.

Child-Rearing Practices: Everyone is expected to contribute to the well-being of the extended family, and words used to describe relatives express the social ties between them. Most cousins are called the same name as brother and sister. There are separate words for older and younger siblings, a practice that signifies that brother-sister and elder-younger relations are culturally significant. Maternal aunts, maternal uncles, and paternal uncles may also be referred to as *parents*. Paternal aunts are not referred to as a parent because they have a special status and are called *mehekitanga*. All older people may be called *grandparents* by younger members. Parents are generally willing to share their children with other family members through the practice of formal or informal adoption, and children are frequently shifted from one household to another. Children are effectively reared by the entire family and may have several places they call home. Women have the most involvement in child rearing. Infants and young children sleep with their parents. Discipline is usually the father's duty. Most parents expect their children to be obedient and live according to their culture.

National Childhood Immunizations: BCG at birth; DTwP at 6, 10, 14 weeks, 18 months, and 5 to 6 years; DTwPHib at 6, 10, and 14 weeks; OPV at 6, 10, and 14 weeks; HepB at birth and at 6 and 14 weeks; MR 1 year and 18 months; TT first contact, 4 weeks, 6 months, and at 5 and 6 years. The percent of the target population vaccinated, by antigen, is 99% for all.

Other Characteristics: The head of the body is *tapu* in Tongan culture, so one should never unexpectedly touch any part of another person's head. Children are taught not to touch the head of their father or to eat his leftovers. Traditional clothing is modest. There are fewer restrictions on men than on women, but men wear a shirt at all times in public except at the beach. Women usually cover their shoulders and chests completely and their legs at least to the knees. Until recently, a woman who wore pants or a short skirt in public risked being considered disreputable (also true for visitors). Cleanliness and presentable dress indicates respect for oneself and others, an important concept conveyed in everyday behavior, particularly for those in superior positions.

BIBLIOGRAPHY

Australian Bureau of Statistics: http://www.abs.gov.au/ (retrieved March 24, 2006).

Evans M, Sinclair RC, Fusimalohi C, and Liava'a V: Globalization, diet, and health: an example from Tonga, *Bull WHO*. 79(9):856–862, 2001.

Filihia M: Men are from Maama, women are from Pulotu: female status in Tongan society, *J Polynes Soc*. 110:377–390, 2001.

Halavatau V et al: Tongatapu infant feeding survey. *SPC Technical Paper No 217*, Noumea, New Caledonia, 2000.

Ka'ili TO: Tauhi va: nurturing Tongan sociospatial ties in Maui and beyond, *Contemp Pacif*. 17:3–114, 2005.

Lockwood VS: *Globalization and culture change in the Pacific Islands*, Upper Saddle River, NJ, 2004, Pearson Education.

McGrath BB: Swimming from island to island: healing practice in Tonga, *Med Anthropol Quart*. 13(4):483–505, 1999.

Statistics New Zealand: Tongan People in New Zealand. Retrieved March 24, 2006, from http://www.stats.govt.nz/analytical-reports/pacific-profiles/tongan/default.htm.

UNAIDS: 2006 Tonga. Retrieved September 21, 2006, from http://www.unaids.org/en/Regions_Countries/Countries/tonga.asp.

World Health Organization: 2006: Immunization, vaccines and biologicals. Retrieved September 21, 2006, from http://www.who.int/immunization_monitoring/en/globalsummary/countryprofileresult.cfm?C='ton'.

World Health Organization: Tonga. Retrieved March 17, 2005, from http://www.who.int/countries/ton/en/.

◆ TUNISIA (REPUBLIC OF)

MAP PAGE (800)

Nissaf Bouafif Ben Alaya and Afif Ben Salah

Location: Located in the Mediterranean basin between Algeria in the west and Libya in the southeast, Tunisia is part of North Africa. The size of the population is 10.1 million, and the total area is 185,000 km² (71,410 square miles). The capital is Tunis. The climate is very different in the north above the Atlas chain of mountains (where it is cold) and the south (the continental area), which is characterized by desert and oasis. The central region and east coast are temperate. Tunisia is primarily an agricultural country. The gross domestic product (GDP) per capita is $8,300, with about 7% below the poverty line. The literacy rate is 83% for men, 65% for women.

Major Languages	Ethnic Groups	Major Religions
Arabic (official)	Arab-Berber 98%	Sunni Muslim 98%
French	European 1%	Christian 1%
	Jewish 1%	Jewish 1%

Arabic is typically used for administrative communication (in letters and for laws), but French is the language used in universities. More recently, English has taken on a more important role in education. In secondary schools, English is required for international scientific communication. Local Arabic is spoken in families. The Berber language is still used in some areas of southern Tunisia, where a few Berber tribes still live in the hilly area of Tataouine. Because of its geographic location and invasions throughout the centuries, the Tunisian population is a mixture of Berbers (the original ethnic group), Arabs, Turks, and Europeans. Although Sunnite Islam is the major religion, Christianity and Judaism are freely practiced and respected.

Health Care Beliefs: Traditional; passive role. Since achieving independence, five schools of medicine were built, leading to strong promotion of modern medicine. However, traditional medicine is an important asset in the health care arena, particularly among people in rural areas and lower social classes. When the health care system cannot cure a person, the people may believe an illness has a supernatural origin and therefore needs traditional treatment. It is also common to use herbs to treat illnesses or perform rituals to protect against the "evil eye" (i.e., the ability to harm others by looking at them).

Predominant Sick-Care Practices: Biomedical and magical-religious. Tunisia has a decentralized health care system in which primary care constitutes the major component. Traditional medicine also plays a role, particularly with the less educated. Although health care accessibility is considered universal, it may take several consultations to diagnose diseases such as visceral leishmaniasis because of a lack of continuity in care related to the high turnover of doctors and inadequate access to health care in remote rural areas. A patient may have up to six consultations at different levels of the health care system (e.g., primary, emergency, private doctor) and receive symptom-related treatments such as aspirin, paracetamol, antibiotics, and iron. Parents who are not literate take their children to traditional healers and often receive a diagnosis of splenomegaly *(jilf)*. Splenomegaly is a common diagnosis in traditional culture, and healers prescribe herb recipes for treatment. When a diagnosis of splenomegaly is established by the healer, the community usually consults the pediatric medical specialist of the region who is known to be able to cure this disease. Therefore, the path to treatment may involve the simultaneous use of traditional and modern medical systems.

Ethnic-/Race-Specific or Endemic Diseases: The country has experienced a shift from infectious diseases and malnutrition to cancer, atherosclerosis, diabetes, and accident-related deaths. However, infectious and emerging diseases are still serious health problems. There is intermediate risk for bacterial diarrhea and hepatitis A. In addition, there may be a significant risk for vector-borne diseases in some locations during the transmitting season, generally, April through November. Leishmaniasis and tuberculosis also may be causes of morbidity. The major causes of mortality are cardiovascular disease, tumors, accidents, gastroenteric disease, infectious, hormonal and genitourinary tract diseases, and unspecified causes. The Joint United Nations Programme on HIV/AIDS (UNAIDS) reports the prevalence rate for human immunodeficiency virus (HIV) in adults (aged 15 to 49 years) to be 0.1%, with 8,700 people living with HIV, including 1,900 women. Fewer than 100 deaths from acquired immunodeficiency syndrome (AIDS) have been reported. The route for transmission has been primarily through heterosexual contact and intravenous drug use.

Health-Team Relationships: Doctors play the key role in case management of patients, particularly for specialized care. In the primary health care setting, however, nurses are responsible for most of the preventive programs such as immunizations, water, and food hygiene; therefore, nurses tend to have more influence on the community. Practitioners work together as a team, sharing roles and responsibilities according to their strengths. In addition, nurses maintain a global focus on quality health care and patient satisfaction.

Families' Role in Hospital Care: The family plays a key role in supporting its members when they are ill. Hospitalization is an important event because historically it was linked to serious conditions that generally led to death. Despite the evolution of the health care system and improvements in quality of care in hospitals and private clinics, the family continues to help to care for hospitalized patients. They may decorate the room, bring blankets, and feed patients, especially women who are about to give birth. In private clinics, pregnant women usually are accompanied by their mothers for the entire stay. In public hospitals, which have a limited number of beds, one family member usually visits the patient every day, brings food, and helps with personal and hygiene tasks.

Dominance Patterns: Historically, men have been more dominant in the culture. Since the country's independence in 1956, however, conditions for women have improved and have resulted in greater literacy, liberal abortion laws, and effective integration of women into the workforce. Today, women are well represented in various professions, including medicine. The Tunisian government has a Ministry of Women's Affairs that influences social, cultural, and political life. Women play a key role in family health, particularly during pregnancies or childbirth or when children are ill.

Eye-Contact Practices: Rural people avoid direct eye contact during interactions with parents or grandparents out of respect and obedience. This behavior is changing in urban and educated families, where people use direct eye contact to be more convincing.

Touch Practices: Physical touching is part of Tunisian culture and denotes sympathy. During events such as religious feasts or marriages, women kiss each other when they first meet. Men may also kiss each other when greeting after a long separation. Men and women commonly shake hands. In the context of medical care, women consult male gynecologists, and breast palpations are considered routine procedures in urban areas. In rural areas, women sometimes prefer to have female doctors for such intimate procedures.

Perceptions of Time: Time is not money, so punctuality is not a major issue. Delays of hours are not considered a problem, even when an appointment was made. People may not even make a phone call to apologize when they are late. With the increased use of mobile phones, this behavior may be changing.

Pain Reactions: In urban areas where communities have more medical amenities, pain is not tolerated. People in pain often consult doctors quickly, even when the pain is caused by factors such as stress or menstrual bleeding. In rural areas, people tend to be more tolerant of pain and ultimately consult a traditional healer or barber to perform scarification procedures to remove the pain.

Birth Rites: Tunisia has a relatively young population, and family planning programs have reduced the birth rate. Both sexes are equally welcomed during the first pregnancy. After the first pregnancy, parents prefer that the next child be one of the opposite sex; they become particularly sad if they never have a son. The fertility rate is 1.74 children born per woman. When a child is born, the family meets and slaughters a lamb for a meal. Each person brings a present for the newborn, such as new clothes or money. The infant mortality rate is 24 deaths per 1,000 births. Maternal mortality is still a public health problem in rural areas, where midwives, rather than doctors, continue to be consulted. Hemorrhage, hypertension, and infections remain the major causes of maternal mortality. Life expectancy is 73 for men, 77 for women.

Death Rites: Although a sad event, death is accepted and believed to be God's will, which is a source of comfort for the family. Family members disseminate the news of a relative's death quickly so that they can congregate and console one another. Autopsies are performed when the cause of the death is suspicious. Organ donations are encouraged by Tunisian law, and people are free to donate their organs after death, a preference they can write on their identification card.

Food Practices and Intolerances: Food habits vary, but couscous is the most famous dish in the country. Originally a traditional Berber food, couscous is made by most families at home with wheat. In the central region, it is often cooked with lamb and in the coastal region, with chicken or fish. Olive oil and fresh vegetables are also very popular among all social groups. Even though the country's calorie intake has not increased significantly during the last 20 years, the types of food they consume are beginning to change and signal a dietary transition. Consumption of sugar has increased significantly, as has consumption of meat and fat.

T

Infant-Feeding Practices: Breastfeeding is the cornerstone of the Tunisian primary health care strategy for the prevention of diarrheal diseases and other infections. In 2000, the prevalence of breastfeeding was 95%, and the mean duration was 12.4 months. The mean for exclusive breastfeeding is 3 months. Early termination is attributed to a new pregnancy (32%), insufficient milk production (32%), and illness of the child (10%). Subsequent pregnancies are a well-documented reason for cessation of breastfeeding and highlight inadequate contraceptive practices, which are important at the individual and community levels. Insufficient milk production is thought to shorten the period of amenorrhea associated with breastfeeding and is associated with stressful lifestyles—a biocultural phenomenon.

Child-Rearing Practices: In urban areas, women usually work outside the home, and children from the age of 3 to 6 months are cared for in special facilities *(crèches),* which are either public or private. In rural areas, child rearing is the responsibility of women. Children are transported on their mother's backs, even when they go to work in the field. They also sleep near their mothers. Discipline is usually the responsibility of both parents in urban areas but is mainly the responsibility of the father in rural and less wealthy communities. Grandparents may play a key role in rearing children if both parents are employed outside the home or when a large family lives in the same dwelling (a practice common in rural areas).

National Childhood Immunizations: BCG at birth and 6 years; DTwP at 3, 4, 5, and 18 months; OPV at 3, 4, and 5 months and at 6, 12, and 18 years; HepB at 3, 4, and 9 months; Hib at 3, 4, and 5 months; measles at 15 months and 6 years; MR at 12 years; Td at 6, 12, and 18 years, CBAW. The percent of the target population vaccinated, by antigen, is: BCG, Polio3, Hib3, DTP1, and DTP2 (97%); HepB3 (96%); and MCV (95%). This program eradicated polyomyelitis and controlled measles.

BIBLIOGRAPHY

Ben Salah A, Najah M, Marzouki M, Ducic S: The determinants of the duration of breastfeeding in semi-rural Tunisia, *EMR Health Serv J.* 6:28–31, 1989.

Central Intelligence Agency: 2006: The world factbook, Tunisia. Retrieved September 21, 2006, from https://www.cia.gov/cia/publications/factbook/print/ts.html.

Direction de soins de santé de base, Ministère de la santé publique. *Rapport annuel,* 2004.

Direction de soins de santé de base, Ministère de la santé publique. *Enquête MICS2,* 2000.

Institut National de las statistique: *Annuaire Statistique de la Tunisie,* Décembre 2000.

Ministère de la santé publique: Office Nationale de la famille et de la population.

Mongalgi Bouguerra L, Ben Alaya N, Trabelsi S, Zouari B. For better promotion of breastfeeding, *Tunisie Médicale.* 2004;82(5):438–445.

UNAIDS 2006 Tunisia: Retrieved September 21, 2006, from http://www.unaids.org/en/Regions_Countries/Countries/tunisia.asp.

World Health Organization: 2006: Immunization, vaccines and biologicals. Retrieved September 21, 2006, from http://www.who.int/immunization_monitoring/en/globalsummary/countryprofileresult.cfm?C='tun'.

◆ TURKEY (REPUBLIC OF)   **T**

MAP PAGE (798)

Nurgün Platin

Location: Turkey is a southeastern European country at the northeastern end of the Mediterranean Sea. The Black Sea is to the north, the Aegean Sea is to the west. The total area is 780,580 km^2 (301,382 square miles). The capital is Ankara. A narrow coastal plain surrounds Anatolia, an inland plateau that becomes increasingly rugged as it progresses eastward. Although the coastal areas have milder climates, the inland Anatolian plateau experiences extremes, with hot summers and cold winters with limited rainfall. The population is 70.4 million. The gross domestic product (GDP) per capita is $8,200, and about 20% live below the poverty line. Literacy rates are 94% for men, 79% for women.

Major Languages	Ethnic Groups	Major Religions
Turkish	Turkish 82%	Muslim 99%
Kurdish	Kurdish 18%	Other 1%
Arabic		

Health Care Beliefs: Passive role; acute sick care only. Health promotion is demonstrated but practiced little. People accept treatment passively. Some may postpone elective medical treatment during the month of Ramadan or fasting. Families often believe in the "evil eye." Mothers may fasten an evil eye pin on the shoulder of a child's clothing for protection.

Predominant Sick-Care Practices: Biomedical; alternative; magical-religious. Biomedical treatment is valued, but the Turkish also consult various alternative medical and health care practitioners. Use of herbal teas, chiropractors, and folk medicine is fairly common. Particularly in rural areas, "the evil eye" (a curse from someone who looks at a child maliciously) is believed to cause childhood illnesses.

Ethnic-/Race-Specific or Endemic Diseases: Endemic diseases include chloroquine-sensitive malaria in the southeastern region, β-thalassemia on the Mediterranean coast and in the southeastern region, and goiter in the northern Black Sea area. Hepatitis A and tuberculosis are becoming more common. Information on human immunodeficiency virus (HIV) and acquired immunodeficiency syndrome (AIDS) is limited. The United Nations Children's Fund (UNICEF) and the Joint United Nations Programme on HIV/AIDS (UNAIDS) report that the prevalence rate for HIV in adults (aged 15 to 49 years) is less than 0.2%, with fewer than 2,000 people living with HIV. From 1985 through 2004, Turkish authorities had reported a cumulative total of 1,922 HIV cases; they also reported that 551 had developed AIDS and that 63 had died of AIDS. Where mode of transmission is known, about 50% are transmitted heterosexually, and about one third of new cases are in women. UNAIDS recently reported that both the incidence and

T

prevalence of HIV/AIDS in Turkey are low and stable. Stigmatization and discrimination against people with HIV are widespread, making it difficult to reach and provide targeted interventions to vulnerable groups. It is estimated that only 9% of those infected are receiving antiretroviral therapy.

Health-Team Relationships: Patients do not question doctors. Most doctors are men and have absolute authority. They are expected to use good judgment. Consent forms are generally not used, and information is not freely shared with patients. Information is often shared more freely with family members, and medical decisions are made in conjunction with families. Patients often address health professionals by title rather than by name. Professional dialogue between doctors and nurses is weak. Almost all nurses are women, and they are not considered powerful by the health team. Women, especially those in rural areas, may prefer a nurse midwife or a female doctor for obstetric and gynecologic examinations, family-planning treatments, or counseling.

Families' Role in Hospital Care: A family member usually stays with the patient day and night and is expected to help with personal and therapeutic care.

Dominance Patterns: Men generally make most major decisions, and they are traditionally accepted as the leader of the family. Women are passive and perceived as having a lower status, with variations between urban and rural areas. Rural women pass through four stages: young bride (ages 15 to 30) with low status; middle age (ages 30 to 45) with medium status; mature (ages 45 to 65) with highest status; and finally old (age 65 and older), when women are respected the most but are not powerful. Women are the quietly dominant decision makers in their homes, especially when health care decisions must be made; however, husbands are responsible for official business such as filling out insurance forms for a hospital visit. Increasing numbers of women work outside the home. Parents expect to be cared for by their children in their old age.

Eye-Contact Practices: Traditional groups consider sustained eye contact with authority figures to be impolite and disrespectful.

Touch Practices: Unlike in social settings, no physical contact occurs during greetings among health care professionals and patients. However, patting a patient on the back is a sign of support. In social settings, kissing once on both cheeks and shaking hands are customary greetings.

Perceptions of Time: The Turkish have a relaxed attitude toward time. People are more oriented to the present and near future.

Pain Reactions: Tolerating pain and not verbalizing it are common. Pain is considered a part of life and is not loudly discussed.

Birth Rites: The infant mortality rate is 40 deaths per 1,000 live births. Most births are attended by qualified personnel in health institutions. The fertility rate is two children born per woman. A prone position on a flat surface and the kneeling position (which is used in some rural areas) are the most common delivery positions. Fathers are not present during childbirth, nor are relatives. Relatives and neighbors help with housework and infant care for 40 days after birth, during which the mother is considered to be vulnerable to infection. Life expectancy is 70 for men, 75 for women.

Death Rites: The deceased are buried as soon as possible—the same day or the day after death. The time of burial depends on the amount of paperwork involved or the arrival time of close relatives. For Muslim burials, the body is wrapped in special pieces of cloth and buried without a coffin in the ground. A religious person *(imam)* recites a short prayer during the burial ceremony, and additional prayers are recited at home or the local mosque on the 7th, 40th, and 52nd days after the burial. Although this practice follows Islamic rituals, these gatherings for prayer provide a lot of support for the family. Live-organ donations are becoming relatively common, but cadaver donations are uncommon because people prefer that the body be buried intact. For the same reason, autopsies are uncommon. Cremations are not permitted.

Food Practices and Intolerances: People near the Black Sea coast consume a great deal of black cabbage. Pork is a forbidden food for Muslims. Fresh fruits and vegetables are favorites, and legumes, vegetables, and bread are food staples. Red meat and poultry are consumed throughout the country, whereas fish and seafood are primarily eaten in coastal areas and in large cities. Breakfast and dinner are the main meals in rural, and dinner is the main meal in urban areas. One month of fasting during Ramadan is practiced by all, except for children and those who are sick. Tea is the most commonly consumed beverage.

Infant-Feeding Practices: About 97% of infants are partially breastfed. Only 44% are exclusively breastfed in the first 2 months. By the age of 2 to 3 months, only 16% are breastfed, and by 4 to 5 months, only 11% are. A mother's ability to continue breastfeeding depends heavily on whether she is working outside of the home. Plain and fresh yogurt, fresh fruit juices, fruit purees, vegetable soups, and soups with grains are introduced at 3 months. Multivitamins are started at the end of the first month, especially for infants born in the winter. Boys are breastfed longer because of the belief that breastfeeding makes them stronger. According to studies, less educated mothers breastfeed longer than well-educated mothers. The use of commercial infant food is more common in urban areas.

Child-Rearing Practices: The mother is the primary caregiver for children, but the paternal grandmother also has an important influence. Mother and child relationships are strong. Discipline is strict, and obedience and respect are valued; however, these attitudes are changing. Parents are more permissive with boys, whereas girls are taught to become productive, hard workers. Girls start helping with household chores when they begin school. Girls socialize with girls, and boys socialize with boys. Mothers are more protective of their sons than their daughters.

National Childhood Immunizations: BCG at 8 weeks and 6 years; measles at 9 months and 6 years; OPV at 8, 12, and 16 weeks and at 16 months; DTwP at 8, 12, and 16 weeks and at 16 months; TT at first contact,

+1, +6 months, +1, +1 year; Td at 6 and 14 years; HepB at birth and 36 weeks; and HepB at 12 weeks and high-risk groups. The percent of the target population vaccinated, by antigen, is: BCG (88%); DTP1 (86%); DTP3 and Polio3 (85%); HepB3 (77%); MCV (81%); and TT2 plus (41%).

BIBLIOGRAPHY

Central Intelligence Agency: *2006: The world factbook, Turkey.* Retrieved September 21, 2006, from https://www.cia.gov/cia/publications/factbook/print/tu.html.

Temel Saglik Hizmetleri Genel Mudurlugu: 2004 Yili Ilk Alti Aylik Geribildirim Degerlendirmesi, Tablo 23. Bildirilen AIDS Vaka ve Tasiyicilarinin Yillara Gore Dagilimi, Turkiye, 01 Ekim 1985 – 30 Haziran 2004. Retrieved March 4, 2006, from http://www.saglik.gov.tr/extras/istatistikler/geribildirim_haziran/tablo23-24-25.htm.

Turkey Demographic and Health Survey (TDHS): 2003: Antenatal care and delivery assistance, 2003. Retrieved March 4, 2006, from http://www.hips.hacettepe.edu.tr/tnsa2003/data/English/chapter10.pdf.

Turkey Demographic and Health Survey (TDHS): 2003: Infant feeding practices and children's and women's nutritional status. Retrieved March 4, 2006, from http://www.hips.hacettepe.edu.tr/tnsa2003/data/English/chapter12.pdf.

UNAIDS: 2006 Turkey. Retrieved September 21, 2006, from http://www.unaids.org/en/Regions_Countries/Countries/turkey.asp.

World Health Organization: 2006: Immunization, vaccines and biologicals. Retrieved September 21, 2006, from http://www.who.int/immunization_monitoring/en/globalsummary/countryprofileresult.cfm?C='tur'.

◆ TURKMENISTAN

MAP PAGE (799)

Jason Anderson

Location: Once part of the Persian Empire, Turkmenistan became an independent republic in 1991 with the dissolution of the Soviet Union. This earthquake-prone country is located in southwestern central Asia, with Kazakhstan to the north, Uzbekistan to the north and east, Iran to the south, Afghanistan to the southeast, and the Caspian Sea to the west. The terrain is flat to rolling sandy desert, with dunes rising to mountains in the south, and low mountains along the Iranian border. The great Garagum Desert occupies 80% of the country. The climate is subtropical desert. The total area is 488,100 km^2 (188,456 square miles). The capital, Ashgabat, is located in the southern center of the country. The population is more than five million. The gross domestic product (GDP) per capita is $8,000, with 58% living below the poverty line.

Major Languages	Ethnic Groups	Major Religions
Turkmen (official)	Turkmen 85%	Muslim (mostly Sunni) 89%
Russian	Uzbek 5%	Eastern Orthodox 9%
Uzbek	Russian 4%	Unknown 2%
English	Other 6%	

Turkmen is spoken by about 80% of the population. Russian was the official language before the 1992 constitution and is still often used in official communications. During the Soviet era, many Turkmen parents, especially of the educated ruling class, spoke to their children only in Russian so as to ease assimilation into the governing culture and maximize opportunities for advancement. Hence many educated Turkmen, schooled in Russian, have only recently mastered the now-emphasized Turkmen language. Literacy rates are 99% for men, 98% for women. Many who profess to be Muslim are not active adherents. Prayer at mosques is not widespread. There has been a correspondent rise in official references to Islamic traditions with the government's emphasis on Turkmen nationalism, but the government maintains a primarily secular attitude.

Health Care Beliefs: Passive role; acute sick care only. Because it is currently difficult to receive adequate health care, particularly in rural areas, healers who use prayers and herbs are common. In some areas, healers may provide the only care available. People needing serious attention and procedures almost always go to the capital for better care.

Predominant Sick-Care Practices: Traditional; biomedical where available. The Soviet free health care system is still in place, with its emphasis on specialist rather than primary care. In the early 1990s, supply shortages and poorly trained doctors led to inadequate levels of care, leading to the highest infant mortality rates and lowest life expectancy in central Asia. One study found that because 70% of the obstetricians and gynecologists in Dashowuz Province lacked adequate surgical training, 50% of their patients died. In 1996, only 15% of maternity clinics had piped-in water. In 1999 the Republic had 13,800 doctors (36 per 10,000 people), and 40,600 other medical personnel (107 per 100,000). Present medical care is far below Western European and North American standards. The country has private and public doctors and public hospitals, but modern technologies and medical supplies such as disposable needles, oral rehydration salts for children, vaccines, anesthetics, and antibiotics may be in short supply or unavailable. Sanitation is generally lacking. In addition, ground water supplies have become considerably polluted from excessive pesticide use, and pesticides have also contaminated the dust that blows across the region. Health care is more readily available in urban areas than in rural areas, but treatment is frequently primitive. The state maintains control over the system and proudly declares free health care and education as evidence of the nation's prosperity. However, statutory sickness benefit programs have been instituted and involve an employment-based strategy that restricts coverage to those who are formally employed. The programs are funded by employer and employee contributions. At the same time, it is widely (unofficially) known that one must pay for quality care; families often need to pay for complex operations that otherwise would not be available

T

under the official "availability" of care. This includes dispensation of better and more effective medicines, available only to those who can pay for them.

Ethnic-/Race-Specific or Endemic Diseases: The most common causes of death are cardiovascular diseases, cancer, respiratory diseases, and accidents. Poor diet, polluted drinking water, and industrial wastes and pesticides cause many health problems, especially in the areas near the Amu Darya and Aral Sea. Endemic diseases include malaria, tuberculosis, poliomyelitis, typhoid, and hepatitis A. The people (especially children and women of childbearing age) are at risk for anemia, leishmaniasis, and cryptosporidiosis. In 2004, the incidence rate for tuberculosis was 65 per 100,000 people. Turkmenistan is at risk for polio as a result of its close links with Afghanistan, one of the six remaining polio-endemic countries. Traffic accidents are a major source of injury for drivers, passengers, and pedestrians. Sexually transmitted infections (STIs) such as syphilis, gonorrhea, and hepatitis B are increasing. The Joint United Nations Programme on HIV/AIDS (UNAIDS) estimates the prevalence rate of human immunodeficiency virus (HIV) in adults (aged 15 to 49 years) is less than 0.1%, with fewer than 500 people living with HIV. A leading at-risk population is thought to be injecting drug users. A National Programme on HIV/AIDS and STI Prevention was inducted in 2005 to provide informational resources and to combat the expected increase of acquired immunodeficiency syndrome (AIDS).

Dominance Patterns: Since the nation's independence and the government's sustained emphasis on Turkmen nationalism, large numbers of ethnic Russians have left, in many cases leaving professions of high technical competency and responsibility, which were then filled by ethnic Turkmen. Ethnic Turkmen have also filled new jobs, with exceptions made for experienced veterans in military and engineering positions. The pervasiveness of the Russian language in daily life is little changed. Although all public and holiday ceremonies are conducted in Turkmen, the vast majority of the elite and the intelligentsia attended Russian schools, completed higher education in Russian, and speak Russian by choice. Turkmen have traditionally been divided into territorial groups similar to tribes or clans (*halk* or *taipa*). In the past, tribes were differentiated by their dialects, carpet patterns, clothing, and headgear. Tribal identity still affects social relationships (such as in arranged marriages). In urban and rural settings, community elders retain the greatest influence and are sources of wisdom and spirituality. Women have (though infrequently) become influential leaders in the system. Families still tend to be closely knit, and it is common for sons to remain with their parents after marriage. As in other areas of Central Asia, older parents are cared for at home by grown children and remain sources of guidance, if not always of authority. Although labor is divided into male and female tasks and women do not usually actively participate in politics, women generally do not wear veils and are not kept in seclusion. Economic necessity has forced many women into the workforce, disrupting traditional Muslim values, and many have professional careers. In some conservative households, however, the daughter-in-law is not permitted to speak in the presence of the father-in-law, much less directly to him, and will wear a scarf over her mouth in the presence of visitors. The observance of custom depends on the family.

Birth Rates: Childbirth often occurs at home, especially with the lack of facilities in rural areas, and even poorly equipped hospitals in the few cities that have them. The infant mortality rate is high at 73 deaths per 1,000 live births; Tajikistan is the only country in the region with a higher rate. The maternal mortality rate from 2000 was 31 per 100,000 live births, very high for the region. As of 2006, the fertility rate was 3.37 births per woman. Women in their childbearing years, and children, seem to have the worst health and are the most susceptible to disease compared with other groups in the society. Cultural norms among Turkmen tend to prize male children more than female children, and stories circulate about informal "expectations" that the first child will be a son and of girl infants being smothered "accidentally." Life expectancy is 58 for men, 65 for women—the lowest in central Asia.

Child-Rearing Practices: About 35% of the population is 14 years or younger. Education is compulsory through the eighth grade. Educational practices persist from the Soviet system, such as rote learning and memorizing massive amounts of data, and required curricula include exaltation of the country's president and advancement of Turkmen nationalism. The advent of Turkish schools in different cities and a university in the capital have improved opportunities for capable students, although the Turkish institutions enroll only males and, except for scholarship opportunities, are not free of charge.

National Childhood Immunizations: BCG at birth and 6 to 7 and 15 years; DTwP at 2, 3, 4, and 18 months; DT at 6 years; HepB at birth and at 2 and 4 months; HepA at birth and at 2, 3, 4, and 18 months; OPV at birth and 2, 3, 4, and 18 months; measles at 12 to 15 months and at 6 years; and Td at 15 and 25 years. The percent of the target population vaccinated, by antigen, is: BCG (99%); DTP1 and Polio3 (98%); DTP3 and MCV (97%); and HepB3 (96%).

Other Characteristics: In Turkmen society, marriage is an important event and is often arranged by matchmakers *(sawcholar)*. The ceremony includes a bride price *(galyng)* that may be excessive. Most couples freely consent to the arrangement, and divorce is relatively rare. The tradition of boys kidnapping girls to claim them as brides is also practiced among more conservative families and communities. In addition, reports continue of girls being killed by family members for suspected or admitted premarital sex, so-called honor killings, which occur in many areas of central and south Asia. Turkmenistan is a limited illegal cultivator of opium poppies, mostly for domestic consumption; the country has a weak government eradication program.

U

BIBLIOGRAPHY

Central Intelligence Agency: *2006: The world factbook, Turkmenistan.* Retrieved September 21, 2006, from https://www.cia.gov/cia/publications/factbook/print/tx.html.

Dixon J: A global perspective on statutory Social Security programs for the sick, *J Health Soc Pol.* 13(3):17, 2001.

Foreign & Commonwealth Office of the UK. Endemic diseases. Retrieved July 12, 2006, from http://www.fco.gov.uk/travel.

O'Hara SL, Wiggs B, Mamedov B, Davidson G, and Hubbard R: Exposure to airborne dust contaminated with pesticide in the Aral Sea region, *Lancet.* 355(9204):627, 2000.

Polio Eradication: At-risk for polio. Retrieved July 13, 2006, from http://www.polioeradication.org/features/countryprofiles/TKM5.asp.

Small I, van der Meer J, Upshur RE: Acting on an environmental health disaster: the case of the Aral Sea, *Environ Health Perspect.* 109(6):547, 2001.

Strelkova MV, Eliseev LN, Ponirovsky EN, Dergacheva TI, Annacharyeva DK, Erokhin PI, and Evans DA: Mixed leishmanial infections in *Rhombomys opimus*: a key to the persistence of Leishmania major from one transmission season to the UNAIDS: 2006 Turkmenistan. Retrieved September 21, 2006, from http://www.unaids.org/en/Regions_Countries/Countries/turkmenistan.asp

UNICEF: HIV program info. Retrieved July 14, 2006, from http://www.unicef.org/turkmenistan/hiv_aids_3782.html.

World Health Organization: 2006: Immunization, vaccines and biologicals. Retrieved September 21, 2006, from mhttp://www.who.int/immunization_monitoring/en/globalsummary/countryprofileresult.cfm?C='tk'.

World Health Organization. TB incidence: WHO TB reports. Retrieved July 13, 2006, from http://www.who.int/GlobalAtlas/predefinedReports/TB/PDF_Files/TM_2004_Brief.pdf.

http://www.who.int/countries/tkm/en World Health Organization country data. (retrieved July 3, 2006).

◆ UGANDA (REPUBLIC OF)

MAP PAGE (801)

Francis Bajunirwe

Location: Uganda is located in the eastern part of the African continent and has a total area of 241,038 km^2 (94,322 square miles). The capital is Kampala. Uganda has Kenya as its neighbor to the east, Tanzania to the south, Rwanda to the southwest, Democratic Republic of Congo to the west, and Sudan to the north. It is a landlocked country with many mountains, fertile valleys, forests, grasslands, lakes, and rivers. The river Nile, the longest in Africa, has its source in Uganda at Lake Victoria, the largest freshwater lake in Africa. The population is 28.1 million, with about 50% aged 0 to 14 years. The gross domestic product (GDP) per capita is $1,800; about 35% live below the poverty line.

Major Languages	**Ethnic Groups**	**Major Religions**
English (official)	Baganda 17%	Roman Catholic 42%
Swahili	Banyankore 10%	Protestant 36%
Luganda	Basoga 9%	Islam 12%
Ateso	Iteso 7%	Pentecostal 4.6%
Luo	Bakiga 7%	Seventh Day Adventist 1.5%
	Langi 6%	Traditional 1%
	Acholi 5%	Others 2.9%
	Bagisu 5%	
	Lugbara 5%	
	Others 29%	

Uganda has three major ethnic groups—Bantu, Luo, and Nilo-Hamites— who collectively speak more than 32 languages with more than 50 dialects. English is the official language and it is widely spoken, especially in urban areas and schools. Swahili is spoken mainly in urban centers and by members of security organizations such as the army, police, and prisons. Literacy rates are 80% for men, 60% for women.

Health Care Beliefs: Traditional and modern; active role. Prevention and health promotion are widely promoted by the government as its main strategies for disease control. The use of abstinence, behavior change— including faithfulness to a single partner and condom use—have been emphasized in the control of human immunodeficiency virus (HIV). This so called "ABC strategy" has been partly credited for the declines observed in incidence. Parents have also been encouraged to adopt family planning methods so they can have the ideal number of children for their circumstances, but this tends to be disregarded in most rural areas. Mental illness is feared and stigmatized, and potential suitors may not want to marry individuals from families with members who are mentally ill. The provision of psychiatric services has improved, and outreach programs have helped families cope. The relatives of those who are mentally ill often do not want to see the affected family member, and some may even wish that the person were dead. In some tribal communities, people wear amulets to protect themselves from harm or cure illness, especially illness "sent" by those who are envious. The society is in transition, but some still wear amulets under their clothes because exposing them may elicit criticism. One traditional practice is making cuts on the body area that has pain, putting a small animal horn (from goats or antelopes) on the cut, and sucking blood through it. The horn is believed to have special powers to remove disease. Herbs are also rubbed in the wound.

Predominant Sick-Care Practices: Biomedical and magical-religious. In cities, sick people generally seek modern medical treatment in government hospitals or health units, and those who are relatively well off seek care at private clinics. Most people in rural areas seek treatment from traditional healers or obtain herbal medicine before biomedical treatment.

Some use herbal treatments and biomedicine concurrently and may also consult with church leaders, witch doctors, or soothsayers.

Ethnic-/Race-Specific or Endemic Diseases: There is a very high degree of risk for water-borne diseases such as bacterial diarrhea, hepatitis A, and typhoid fever. Falciparum malaria affects the majority of the population, and people often buy modern medicine from private clinics or government health centers. Most who go to private clinics, especially in rural areas and the poor in cities, get less than the required dosage of malaria medicine because of limited resources. Therefore, recurrent malaria is common and can cause death. Because of economic constraints, when many people in the same family are sick, they share medications (even a single dose), so none of them receive enough. The government has attempted to control malaria by training lay persons in recognizing and treating malaria in the home. Other strategies include providing mosquito nets cheaply and spraying houses in areas where epidemics are common. Kaposi's sarcoma, a cancer associated with the human herpesvirus-8, accounts for a large proportion of the reported cases of cancer. In addition, acquired immunodeficiency syndrome (AIDS)-associated Burkitt's lymphoma is also endemic. Others include sleeping sickness (*Trypanosoma brucei* gambiense and T. *brucei* rhodesiense), onchocerciasis (in the Rukungiri district), lymphatic filariasis, nonfilarial elephantiasis (in Mt. Elgon), dracunculiasis, schistosomiasis, tuberculosis, *Shigella* infections, dengue fever, and endomyocardial fibrosis. Meningococcal disease occurs as small epidemics in a few places in the dry season, mostly in the northeast. Colds are a major cause of morbidity in infants. The minority Pygmies of western Uganda still live in the forests and have no exposure to modern health facilities. In most cases, they use local herbs to treat themselves. With government prohibitions on the use of forests, most of these people have no land, are malnourished, and have no access to health care or resources. Vigorous and constant campaigns against HIV/AIDS have been launched by the government, service organizations, and church organizations. According to the Joint United Nations Programme on HIV/AIDS (UNAIDS), the prevalence rate for HIV in adults (aged 15 to 49 years) is very high at 6.7%, with one million people living with HIV, including 520,000 women and 110,000 children aged 0 to 15 years. There are also one million orphans as a result of parental AIDS. About 91,000 deaths are attributed to AIDS.

Health-Team Relationships: Doctors are usually consulted for complicated cases. Most doctors and nurses are stationed in urban areas, leading to a huge disparity in the distribution of health care workers. Nurses and doctors work collectively as a team, and they are generally overworked (with 1 nurse per 7,000 and 1 doctor per 23,000 people). Generally, their professional working relationships are good. Patients' attitudes toward doctors and nurses are positive. Medical work is mystifying, however, and visiting a clinic is still a fearful experience for many people. Doctors are highly respected but are also feared, which may explain why many people, especially those from rural areas, prefer to visit clinics as a last resort. Health personnel seldom give complete explanations to patients about their medical conditions or treatments, primarily because of the heavy workload.

Families' Role in Hospital Care: When a sick relative is admitted, family members stay with the patient and take complete care of him or her until discharge. For example, they ensure that the patient receives and takes medicine. They provide food and drinks, bathe the patient, wash clothes, and even notify medical personnel when the patient's condition is questionable.

Dominance Patterns: Ugandan culture favors men. In times of illness, women cater to their male relatives. When married women are sick, their sisters or mothers have traditionally left their homes to take care of them; however, the culture is changing, especially in urban areas. Today, many husbands care for their sick wives.

Eye-Contact Practices: Eye contact is used for communication. For example, a twinkle of the eye can be used to warn someone not to say anything when asked a question. If an adult or close relative winks an eye to a child, it may imply that the child should go away. Lovers and young people in particular use eye contact to convey loving messages, especially when they do not want other people to suspect their love affair. Young people are considered rude if they look directly into the eyes of an adult. Eye contact between young men and women is discouraged, and women who make unrestrained eye contact with men are taken to be harlots. Older women, however, can look directly into the eyes of a mature man. It is as if at a certain age a woman acquires the same status as a mature and responsible man. Her advice is sought and is taken seriously. She therefore has the confidence and cultural support to look directly into the eyes of a man without being ridiculed.

Touch Practices: Depending on a person's geographic area, physical touching may or may not be acceptable. For example, the Bakiga greeting involves embracing others regardless of sex or age, but not if they are strangers. In other cultures, it is not culturally acceptable to touch others, especially members of the opposite sex or strangers.

Perceptions of Time: Punctuality is not an issue in Uganda's traditional cultural settings. People do not make appointments because they are generally allowed to visit others without telling them first. Two exceptions are visits by many people at once and appointments at hospitals or health units. Those who come first are served first. Even when a person makes an appointment to see a doctor at a certain time, the doctor may not see the patient at the agreed on time. Procedures are gradually changing, and some people make appointments and adhere to the arranged times.

Pain Reactions: During childbirth, women from central Uganda are free to shout and cry, whereas women in other areas may face the wrath of other women if they do so. Occasionally pain, especially from a medical procedure, is appreciated, because people think a medical procedure that inflicts pain is more effective. Women and children enduring pain from the loss of a loved one normally express it by crying, whereas men are expected to be more reserved. On the whole, men rarely show that they are in pain. Culture dictates that men are supposed to be strong and brave so that they can protect the women, children, and older adults.

Birth Rites: The infant mortality rate is high at 66 deaths per 1,000 live births. During and after birth, various rituals are performed in some rural areas, whereas in others and in cities, generally nothing is done. Mothers bathe immediately after giving birth and are given the best food the family can afford. The traditional culture still favors and celebrates a son's birth more than a daughter's. In most homes with no sons, a man is allowed to marry another wife to have a son, but this practice is gradually changing. The contraceptive prevalence rate stands at 15%. This low contraception rate may explain why Uganda is a country with one of the highest fertility rates in Africa: 7 children born per woman. Life expectancy is 52 for men, 54 for women.

Death Rites: Especially in the central and eastern parts of the country, certain customs are followed after death. When a woman dies and leaves behind young children, someone is appointed to take the place of the mother. When a man dies, a male relative is appointed to take care of the family. Death is feared and believed in traditional communities to be caused by someone. Family and community divisions may develop, and occasionally suspected families are attacked and ostracized. Those in strong Christian homes believe God allows death and that everyone dies at their predetermined time. If a person has been at home and sick for some time, relatives are likely to be close. After learning of a family death, all close relatives and friends are informed either through radio announcements or by messengers. All close relatives participate in the burial arrangements in some way. Organ donations are uncommon, and few people agree to autopsies because it is believed that removing body organs may cause bewitchment of the dead person's family. Others do not approve of autopsy, a result of cultural beliefs about tampering with dead people. In most circumstances, there are not enough medical personnel to perform autopsies, except for medico-legal reasons.

Food Practices and Intolerances: In the past, certain foods were eaten only by certain sexes, although men were allowed to eat most foods. Banyankole women were not allowed to eat chicken, the tongue of any animal, or goat meat. It was believed that if a woman ate a cow's tongue, she would become the main spokesperson for her family and leave the man in an inferior position. These practices are not common today. People in the north mostly consume millet, *posho* ("cornmeal"), meat, and beans as their staple foods. People from the western part consume mostly millet, bananas (locally called *matooke*), meat, beans, Irish potatoes, and milk. Those in the central part usually include matooke in every meal. People may use their hands or a fork, spoon, and knife while eating; however, in rural areas, most people still use their hands. Typically, the family gathers around and eats from the same dish.

Infant-Feeding Practices: Most mothers breastfeed their children, with the exception of a few employed and busy mothers who work far away from their homes. These mothers bottle-feed during the day and breast-feed after office hours. Most mothers believe that as long as they are breastfeeding, they cannot become pregnant; so breastfeeding is also used as a family planning method.

Child-Rearing Practices: Child rearing may be permissive or strict, depending on whether people live in a rural or urban area. Mothers in rural areas have a significant role in looking after their children, but extended relatives such as grandparents also take part. They help feed the children and take care of them when their mothers are working. In rural areas, anyone looking after the children can discipline them when they do something wrong. In urban areas, child rearing is more complex because no extended family members are available. Parents hire maids to look after the children when they are not at home. In these situations, parents are responsible for most of the disciplining. Most parents, even in rural areas, do not sleep with their children in the same bed. They may sleep in the same room until the children can be alone in their rooms or huts, or share accommodations with older siblings.

National Childhood Immunizations: BCG at birth; DTwPHibHep at 6, 10, and 14 weeks; measles at 9 months; OPV at birth and at 6, 10, and 14 weeks; TT in pregnant women first contact and +1, +6 months +1, +1 year; vitamin A at 6, 12, 18, 24, 30, 36, and 42 months (total 10 doses). The percent of the target population vaccinated, by antigen, is: BCG and DTP1 (99%); DTP3, HepB3, and Hib3 (87%); MCV (91%); Polio3 (86%); and TT2 plus (53%).

BIBLIOGRAPHY

Central Intelligence Agency: *2006: The world factbook, Uganda.* Retrieved September 21, 2006, from https://www.cia.gov/cia/publications/factbook/print/ug.html.

Kater V: Health education in Jinja, Uganda, *IMAGE: J Nurs Sch* 28(2):161, 1996.

Ministry of Health: Uganda HIV/AIDS Sero-Behavioural Survey 2004-2905. Preliminary Report. *Ministry of Health,* Kampala, Uganda, 2005.

UNAIDS: 2004: *Report on the global AIDS epidemic,* Uganda Country Report.

UNAIDS: 2006 Uganda: Retrieved September 21, 2006, from http://www.unaids.org/en/Regions_Countries/Countries/uganda.asp.

World Health Organization: 2006: Immunization, vaccines and biologicals. Retrieved September 21, 2006, from http://www.who.int/immunization_monitoring/en/globalsummary/countryprofileresult.cfm?C='uga'.

◆ UKRAINE

MAP PAGE (799)

Igor Y. Galaychuk

Location: Ukraine is located in southeastern Europe, and it shares borders with Moldova and Romania (on the southwest); Hungary, Slovakia, and Poland (on the west); Belarus (on the north); and Russia (on the east). To the south, Ukraine's borders are defined by the Black Sea and the Sea of Azov. Ukraine has a total area of 603,700 km^2 (233,100 square miles). After Russia, it is the second largest country on the European continent. The country has large areas with arable black soil, as well as the Carpathian and Crimean mountain chains. The Dnieper (Dnipro) and Dniester are the major rivers. The population is about 46.9 million. Kiev is the capital city and is located on the Dnieper River. Chernobyl, where the nuclear power-plant disaster occurred in 1986, is located 100 km north of Kiev. Ukraine regained its independence in 1991 with the dissolution of the former Soviet Union. Literacy rates are almost 100% for both men and women. The gross domestic product (GDP) per capita is $7,200, and about 29% live below the poverty line.

Major Languages	Ethnic Groups	Major Religions
Ukrainian	Ukrainian 73%	Orthodox 76%
Russian	Russian 22%	Ukrainian Catholic (Uniate) 14%
	Jewish 1%	Jewish 2%
	Other 4%	Baptist, Mennonite, Protestant, Muslim 8%

Health Care Beliefs: Traditional; modern; acute sick care. The population realizes that diseases can be prevented. However, smoking, alcohol abuse by young and middle-age people, hard manual labor in rural areas, and stress connected with the economic crisis of the society are the background against which many mental and somatic diseases have emerged. Lately, so-called "healers" and extrasensory practitioners have expanded their practices, and patients who have not received proper qualified help in legal medical institutions consult these healers as a last resort.

Predominant Sick-Care Practices: Biomedical; traditional. Ukraine has a state system of health promotion. The treatment and disease prevention service is established in hospitals that are divided into comprehensive (province, city, and district) and specialized facilities, such as pediatric, communicable disease, oncology, endocrinology, ophthalmology, and maternity. Other facilities include outpatient clinics, polyclinics for adults and children, women's clinics and maternity welfare centers, and village outpatient clinics. Doctors also provide health services in patients' homes. Ukraine has urgent-care clinics as well. Physicians (e.g., therapists, cardiologists, general surgeons, traumatologists, pediatricians) may be called to the home of a sick person to provide medical consultations. If necessary, patients are admitted to the hospital. Sanatoriums and health resorts (e.g., general health resorts, children's sanatoriums) are popular for treatment. Another popular facility is the balneological hospital— a resort where patients can be treated with mineral water, silt, salt, and other natural items. In Ukraine, natural resources are used extensively for treatment (e.g., mineral and spring waters for drinking and bathing, therapeutic mud and wax baths for skin, radon and oxygen baths, salt-mine air). Because of the current economic crisis, the financing of health promotion has been reduced dramatically, causing the closure of small hospitals in rural areas and a subsequent lack of care for these populations.

Ethnic-/Race-Specific or Endemic Diseases: The major illnesses are cardiovascular diseases (e.g., high blood pressure, ischemia, cerebrovascular diseases), infections and parasites, trauma, mental illness, malignancies, and tuberculosis. Cardiovascular diseases are the major causes of mortality, followed by malignant diseases, trauma, infectious diseases, tuberculosis, and mental disorders. Thyroid disease, caused by a lack of iodine in soil and water, is endemic in western Ukraine. The first case of human immunodeficiency virus (HIV) was registered in 1987, but by 1995 infections were reaching epidemic proportions. The Joint United Nations Programme on HIV/AIDS (UNAIDS) reports that the adult (aged 15 to 49 years) prevalence rate for HIV is 1.4%, with 410,000 people living with HIV, including 200,000 women. Deaths from acquired immunodeficiency syndrome (AIDS) are estimated at 22,000. There are no estimates for children or for AIDS orphans. The majority do not have access to antiretroviral therapy. Almost all pregnant women are tested for HIV; more than 91% of women who delivered infants in recent years received prophylaxis to prevent vertical transmission.

Health-Team Relationships: Doctors are in a dominant position relative to nurses. Nurses generally carry out doctors' orders, and occasionally conflicts arise when nurses do not perform as expected. The relationships between the patient and the doctor and patient and nurse often involve "gifts" (bribes) from the patient.

Families' Role in Hospital Care: Most patients do not have medical insurance, and the state provides only a little medication. Patients have to buy most of their medications, bandages, and other supplies in drugstores. Today, people can buy any type of medicine, but they are very expensive and difficult to afford for most families. The patients' relatives volunteer to look after them and prepare home-cooked meals. The meals in hospitals are served three times a day, but in most cases the food is low in calories and tasteless.

Dominance Patterns: According to the Constitution of Ukraine, men and women have equal rights. Women constitute about 75% of all the workers in the health system (e.g., hospital attendants, paramedics, nurses, doctors).

Eye-Contact Practices: Direct eye contact is acceptable.

Touch Practices: Ukrainians have no religious or sexual restrictions relating to touch during medical examinations. Shaking hands is common when men greet each other.

Perceptions of Time: In general, punctuality depends on where people live and their social status. In urban areas, people try to be on time, whereas in rural areas the notion of time is often quite flexible.

Pain Reactions: People accept analgesics and usually try to relieve their pain. Narcotic analgesics for patients with cancer are paid for by the state fund.

U

Birth Rites: The infant mortality rate is 10 deaths per 1,000 live births, and the fertility rate is 1.7 children born per woman. Many families hope that the first-born child will be a boy and the second child will be a girl. In maternity hospitals, doctors and midwives assist women during childbirth, and it is not common for fathers to be present. Mothers and infants are usually placed in different wards. Recently, many maternity hospitals are offering rooming-in post-delivery, where the mother and newborn can stay together. During pregnancy and while breastfeeding, most mothers do not drink alcohol, smoke, or eat chocolate or citrus fruit. They avoid taking medications unless they are absolutely necessary. Life expectancy is 65 for men, 76 for women.

Death Rites: The dominant religion in Ukraine is Christianity, and people accept the inevitability of death. If a person dies in a hospital, an autopsy is usually performed to identify the cause. If a person dies at home, family members are usually present. The hospice system is in the very beginning of its development. Death is followed by funerals with a priest, relatives, and neighbors. Ukraine has not yet legalized the sale of cadavers' organs.

Food Practices and Intolerances: The main meals are breakfast (until 9:00 AM), lunch (from 1:00 to 2:00 PM), and dinner (after 7:00 PM). Lunch usually consists of a first course (borscht, or soup), a second course (meat with potatoes) with a salad (of cabbage, tomatoes, or cucumbers), and a third course of tea or coffee and dessert. Traditionally, people eat a lot of bread, potatoes, and dairy products. Borscht with dumplings, *varenyky* (pirogy) with cottage cheese, and pork lard are all national Ukrainian dishes. Of the meat products, Ukrainians seem to prefer pork. Apples are the preferred fruit. Sugar is made from sugar beets that are grown in large quantities. Of the alcoholic drinks, *horilka* (40% vodka) is the most popular.

Infant-Feeding Practices: Approximately 20% of mothers breastfeed during the first year. Most women begin bottle-feeding after several weeks or months of breastfeeding.

Child-Rearing Practices: Children are reared by their families and in school. From early childhood, children are taught to be disciplined and obedient. From 1 to 6 years, children attend kindergarten, where they are cared for by teachers (from 8:00 or 9:00 AM to 5:00 or 6:00 PM). They are given food four times a day and have a nap after lunch. Teachers read books, tell fairytales, organize games, and take children for outdoor walks. The number of kindergartens has drastically decreased because of the economic crisis.

National Childhood Immunizations: BCG at birth and at 7 and 14 years; DTwP at 3, 4, 5, and 18 months; OPV at 5 and 18 months and at 3, 6, and 14 years; measles at 1 and 6 years; DT at 6 years; MMR at 6 years; Td at 14 and 18 years; HepB at 1 day and at 1 and 6 months; IPV at 3 and 4 months; mumps at 15 years (young men); rubella at 15 years (girls only); and TT at 60 years. The percent of the target population vaccinated, by antigen, is: BCG and HepB3 (98%); DTP1 (96%); and DTP3, MCV, and Polio3 (99%).

Other Characteristics: The pollution in industrial regions is 6.5 times higher than it is in the United States and 3.2 times higher than it is in other European countries. It is estimated that the polluted environment causes 21% of all diseases in Ukraine, and another 13% are directly attributed to polluted drinking water.

BIBLIOGRAPHY

Central Intelligence Agency: *2006: The world factbook, Ukraine*. Retrieved September 21, 2006, from https://www.cia.gov/cia/publications/factbook/print/up.html.

Ponomarenko VM, ed: Health protection in Ukraine: the problems and perspectives, Ternopil, *"Ukrmedknyha,"* 1999.

Ukrainian Institute for Social Research: The socio-economic outcomes of HIV/AIDS epidemy in Ukraine: new prognoses. The British Council; DFID,— 2003, Kyiv.

UNAIDS: 2006 Ukraine: Retrieved September 21, 2006, from http://www.unaids.org/en/Regions_Countries/Countries/ukraine.asp.

Voronenko YV, Moskalenko VF, eds: Social medicine and management of health protection, Ternopil, *"Ukrmedknyha,"* 2000.

World Health Organization: 2006: Immunization, vaccines and biologicals. Retrieved September 21, 2006, from http://www.who.int/immunization_monitoring/en/globalsummary/countryprofileresult.cfm?C='ukr'.

http://www.britannica.com/Ukraine, 2005 (retrieved February 18, 2006).

◆ UNITED ARAB EMIRATES

MAP PAGE (802)

Abdulbari A. Bener

Location: Situated on the eastern side of the Arabian Peninsula, the country is primarily desert and rich in oil. Its boundaries are the Persian Gulf to the north, Gulf of Oman to the northeast, Oman to the east, Saudi Arabia to south and west, and a short frontier with Qatar to the northwest. In 1968, Britain announced that they intended to leave the Gulf in 1971, which led to the independence of Bahrain and Qatar and the formation of a new federation—the United Arab Emirates (UAE)—in 1971. The UAE is a federation of the seven emirates of Ajman, Abu Dhabi, Dubai, Fujairah, Ras Al-Khaimah, Sharjah, and Umm Al Quwain. The total area is 83,600 km^2 (32,269 square miles). The emirate of Abu Dhabi comprises 85% of the total area, and the smallest emirate, Ajman, measures only 259 km^2 (100 square miles). The UAE has undergone rapid economic development since the discovery of oil and has become a center for commercial and financial activities in the region, especially Dubai Emirate. The population is 2.6 million; the capital is Abu Dhabi. The gross domestic product (GDP) per capita is $43,400. Literacy rates are 76% for men, 82% for women.

Major Languages	Ethnic Groups	Major Religions
Arabic (official)	Emirati 19%	Islam 55%
Farsi (Persian)	Other Arab and Iranian 23%	Christianity 35%
English	South Asian 43%	Hinduism 10%
Hindi	Westerners and East	
Urdu	Asians 7%	
	Other 8%	

The UAE's vast economic development attracts thousands of expatriate workers each year. The population grew from 200,000 in the 1960s to 4.7 million in 2005; 65% are non-nationals. Compared with other societies that have experienced rapid transformations because of oil wealth, the desert, oases, wadis, mountains, and sea all provide opportunities for city dwellers to physically recapture the old way of life and reestablish contact with members of their family or tribe. The landscape is very dry, with little vegetation or animal life.

Health Care Beliefs: The government is committed to the World Declaration on Health and the constitution of the World Health Organization (WHO). They stipulate that health is a basic human right and an ultimate objective for social and economic development, and that all countries shall be committed to reform their health systems in a suitable manner and take collective action against dangers to the health and well-being of the world community. The community is multicultural and multiethnic and has many different health beliefs. Individuals of higher status who can afford health care are more aware of health promotion and prevention programs, whereas by necessity, the poor are more crisis oriented. The UAE has a ministerial Preventive Medicine Department at the Ministry of Health that is responsible for prevention programs such as vaccinations and public health education (e.g., antismoking and anticancer campaigns). The ministry also runs school health programs and conducts surveys on various diseases, such as diabetes mellitus and asthma. Early screening programs for children and adults, promotion of occupational health and safety, and promotion of healthy lifestyles are gaining ground. Efforts should concentrate on health education for reducing mortality and morbidity of communicable and noncommunicable diseases. Early detection and efficient management of diseases should also be stressed.

Predominant Sick-Care Practices: Biomedical. Economic development has been accompanied by improvement in the health infrastructure and services. The Primary Health Care Clinics (PHC) is a package of comprehensive care offered to individuals, UAE citizens, expatriate workers, families, and the community. The Ministry of Health has made great efforts to develop the services of PHC to make them more equitable and accessible to all residents. The number of centers increased from 45 clinics in 1977 to 106 health centers by the end of 2002. Health status and socioeconomic conditions of the population have markedly improved. Prosperity and modernization in recent years has made many urban individuals more sensitive toward pain and disease. Their reactions to minor illnesses of loved ones, relatives, or members of their own tribe tend to be exaggerated and more expressive. Gravely morbid or terminal illnesses are fought relentlessly, and occasionally extraordinary measures are taken to prolong life merely to satisfy family or tribal members. The steady decline in childhood diseases is a positive indicator of the effectiveness of prevention and control strategies.

Ethnic-/Race-Specific or Endemic Diseases: Endemic diseases include hepatitis A and B, α- and β-thalassemia, cystic echinococcosis, and malaria (endemic or imported from Oman). People are at risk for brucellosis, Crimean Congo fever, and viral hemorrhagic fever. The incidence of cardiovascular disease is increasing fairly rapidly; in addition to accidents and cancer, cardiovascular disease is one of the major causes of death. Other noncommunicable diseases such as diabetes mellitus and congenital abnormalities have recently emerged as major causes of mortality. A major decrease in rates of all infectious diseases in all age groups has evolved, especially among children, but noncommunicable diseases have become the leading causes of morbidity and mortality. Overall, the proportional mortality rates of the top five causes of death in 2002 give a clear indication of trends: cardiovascular (29%), motor-vehicle crashes and injuries (13%), cancer (8%), congenital anomalies (6%), and respiratory diseases (4%). Signs, symptoms, and ill-defined conditions constitute a proportion (11%), as do unknown causes (10%). The WHO has no reports on the prevalence of human immunodeficiency virus (HIV) and acquired immunodeficiency syndrome (AIDS); however, the Joint United Nations Programme on HIV/AIDS (UNAIDS) reports an estimate of 0.2%. There is a comprehensive national plan that has screened three million people over the last 6 years. To reduce the spread of the disease, expatriates who are tested and found to be infected are deported to their home countries.

Health-Team Relationships: Public hospitals have facilities for handling medical emergencies and accidents as well as programs to handle disasters resulting in numerous casualties. Health services are available throughout the country, although standards vary. In large hospitals, the number of medical staff members seems adequate, but they have proportionally fewer health professionals than in Western countries. The inequitable geographic distribution of health care resources has long been recognized as a problem, despite immense progress. Health care personnel, like many other professionals, tend to move to cities and large towns in numbers that exceed their need. Those who specialize in medicine, nursing, or one of many other health care professions have to be located in places with larger populations to ensure they have an adequate patient base. Nurses have recently begun migrating to Western countries because they offer better conditions overall.

Families' Role in Hospital Care: Family members or close friends stay with hospitalized patients and expect to participate in care or take on a vigilant, supervisory role.

U

Dominance Patterns: For all practical purposes, the role of men is frequently that of decision maker for all members of the family. The male head of the family is its provider, spokesman, and representative, although the women are often the primary decision makers. The man who heads the household upholds the Islamic norms of conduct for the outside world and embodies the social standing of the family within the community. If he is a true local, his children will never be considered anything less than full members of the local tribal society, even if their mother is foreign. The social standing of an individual man—and consequently of his entire family—depends first and foremost on the purity of his tribal Arab lineage. This does not mean, however, that a man of pure tribal stock is invariably in a higher position than a wealthy man of uncertain tribal background. Social standing based on a man's wealth is determined by the level at which he can expect to arrange marriages for the members of his family. A woman has no position in the world outside the home, whereas her position within the family circle is a confined environment to develop her abilities. Neither man nor woman has an identity other than in the context of the family to which they belong. In the Arab world, men marry their paternal uncle's daughter (i.e., cousin) so often that another name for a wife is "my uncle's daughter," even when couples are not related. A cross-sectional population study showed that the frequency of consanguineous marriages in Al-Ain City, Abu Dhabi Emirate, and Dubai Emirate is very high and has increased (about 51%). Consanguinity is more common among women with educated husbands (with secondary or university educations) than among women with less educated husbands. Mothers, even educated ones, tend to stay at home, raise the children, and conform to the traditional role of women in an Islamic society. Regardless, changes have taken place in the last decade, and more and more women are developing careers. With better education, it is expected that cultural habits such as consanguineous marriages will decrease. Arranged marriages are common, and there are few opportunities for members of the opposite sex to meet and socialize. When a husband and wife divorce or the husband dies, the sons are expected to support their mother by providing a house and money if necessary or to take her into their own homes.

Eye-Contact Practices: About 15% of adult women cover their faces with a veil. Most women do not cover their eyes; therefore, direct eye contact is possible during conversations, although it must stay within the boundaries of modesty.

Touch Practices: Touch during professional examinations of patients has no gender restrictions. In general, however, female patients prefer female doctors, and male patients often feel more comfortable with male doctors.

Perceptions of Time: People are fairly relaxed about punctuality.

Pain Reactions: Religious and socioeconomic issues and cultural background seem to have an important influence on how people react to pain. Individuals of *pathan* background (i.e., mountain people) seem to be more tolerant of pain than are individuals in other communities. It has been observed that some Arabs tend to be more expressive than others, as if they have a genetically determined pain threshold.

Birth Rites: The high quality and accessibility of health services are reflected by sharp decreases in infant mortality: from 15 to 8 deaths per 1,000 live births. The fertility rate is 2.88 children born per woman. Birth is a celebrated occasion, and Muslim parents usually read verses of the holy Koran to their infants. Immediate bathing after birth is discouraged if the infant is covered with vernix caseosa and is delayed for 12 to 24 hours. Life expectancy has reached 73 for men, 78 for women.

Death Rites: Muslims who have a strong belief in Islamic teaching tend to be less emotionally expressive when in despair. They also consider death as not only the ultimate fate of each and every soul but also as an absolute surrender to Allah's will. Death is a test of the strength of their faith, so they should try to bear its pain with strength. Muslim doctors may recommend transfusions to save lives, and organ donations are permitted. Autopsies are uncommon because the deceased person must be buried intact; cremations are not permitted. For Muslim burials, the body is wrapped in special pieces of cloth and buried without a coffin in the ground immediately after death.

Food Practices and Intolerances: Pork, carrion, and blood are forbidden. The cuisine consists of *falafel* (balls of chickpea paste that are deep-fried and served in flat bread), *fuul* (fava beans, garlic, and honey paste), *hummus* (chickpeas with garlic and lemon), and *shawarma* (chicken or lamb served in flat bread). Food tends to be spicy. Alcohol is sold only in restaurants and bars of three-star hotels. Ramadan fasting is practiced by all except children or those who are sick.

Infant-Feeding Practices: The importance of colostrum is well known, and breastfeeding within 30 minutes after delivery is highly encouraged. A recent prospective cohort study of 221 infants described factors affecting initiation, patterns, and supplemental feeding in the UAE. None of the mothers opted not to breastfeed, but only 4% exclusively breastfed during the first month (although 51% initiated breastfeeding on the first day of life). Factors associated with delaying initiation of breastfeeding after the first day of life included low birth weight, complicated delivery, ignorance about the advantages of colostrum, and young maternal age. Non-milk supplements included water, tea, juice, and *yansun* and *babunj* (local herbal drinks).

Child-Rearing Practices: Child rearing is no longer as strict as it was. Although the UAE is a patriarchal society, boys and girls seem to do what they like, although the attitudes and gestures of girls are more closely observed by other members of the family. Both parents seem to share responsibility for disciplining their children, but the father has the upper hand.

National Childhood Immunizations: BCG at birth; DTwP at 18 months; DTwPHibHep at 2, 4, and 6 months; DT at 6 years; Hib at 18 months; OPV at 2, 4, 6, and 18 months and at 6 years; measles at 9 months; MMR at 15 months and 6 years; Td 15 years; and rubella at 12 years (girls). The percent of the target population vaccinated, by antigen, is: BCG (98%); DTP1 (96%); HepB3 (92%); and DTP3, Hib3, MCV, and Polio3 (94%).

Other Characteristics: The Ministry of Public Health has made a great effort to develop the services of primary health care to make them more equitable and accessible to all residents in the country. Strengthening public health is one of the WHO's regional office's priorities, and the UAE in collaboration with countries in the region is aiming to achieve this.

BIBLIOGRAPHY

Al-Mazroui MJ, Oyejide CO, Bener A, Cheema MY: Breastfeeding and supplemental feeding for neonates in Al-Ain, the United Arab Emirates, *J Trop Pediatr.* 43:304–306, 1997.

Bener A, Abdulrazzaq YM, Al-Gazali LI, Micallef R, Al-Khayat AI, Gaber T: Consanguinity and associated socio-demographic factors in the United Arab Emirates, *Hum Heredity.* 46:256–264, 1996.

Bener A, Crundall D: Road traffic accidents in the United Arab Emirates compared to Western Countries, *Adv Transport Stud.* 6:5–12, 2005.

Bener A, Denic S, Al-Mazrouei M: Consanguinity and family history of cancer in children with leukemia and lymhomas, *Cancer.* 92:1–6, 2001.

Central Intelligence Agency: 2006: *The world factbook, United Arab Emirates.* Retrieved September 21, 2006, from https://www.cia.gov/cia/publications/factbook/print/ec.html.

Sabri S, Bener A, Eapen V, Abu zaeid MSO, Al-mazrouei AM, Singh J: [Socio-economic status lifestyle habits and the risk of hypertension in a developing country.] *Eastern Mediterranean Health J. (WHO Bull)* 10:610–619, 2004.

UNAIDS: 2006 United Arab Emirates. Retrieved September 21, 2006, from http://www.unaids.org/en/Regions_Countries/Countries/united_arab_emirates.asp.

World Health Organization: 2006: Immunization, vaccines and biologicals. Retrieved September 21, 2006, from http://www.who.int/immunization_monitoring/en/globalsummary/countryprofileresult.cfm?C='are'.

World Health Organization: 2005: WHO vaccine-preventable diseases: monitoring system, Geneva. Retrieved December 30, 2005, from http://www.who.int/vaccines/.

◆ UNITED KINGDOM (UNITED KINGDOM OF GREAT BRITAIN AND NORTHERN IRELAND)

MAP PAGE (798)

Angela Ellis

Location: The United Kingdom, which comprises England, Scotland, Wales, and Northern Ireland, is an island nation off the coast of France in the northern Atlantic Ocean. The total area is 244,820 km² (94,525 square miles). The population is 60.6 million. The capital, London, has about eight million people. Thanks to the moderating effects of the Gulf

Stream, the United Kingdom enjoys a temperate climate despite its northern latitude. The gross domestic product (GDP) per capita is $30,300. About 17% live below the poverty line.

Major Languages	Ethnic Groups	Major Religions
English	English 81%	Church of England
Welsh	Scottish 10%	Church of Wales
Scottish Gaelic	Irish, Welsh, Ulster 6%	Church of Scotland
	West Indian, Indian,	Church of Ireland
	Pakistani, Other 3%	Roman Catholic,
		Presbyterian,
		Methodist
		Muslim, Sikh,
		Hindu, Jewish

Although Welsh and Scottish Gaelic are also officially recognized by the government, all adult Welsh or Scottish Gaelic speakers also know English. Some recent immigrants, many of whom come from former colonies of the United Kingdom, have yet to learn English. Literacy rates are 99% for both men and women.

Health Care Beliefs: Modern; increasingly active role in health prevention. In general, Britons understand the need for prevention of disease through healthy living, but many fail to act on that knowledge. The temptations of smoking, drinking, unhealthy eating, and physical inactivity can overwhelm people's will to maintain healthy lifestyles. Although Britons are coming to consider mental illness as less shameful, a certain stigma is still attached to diseases such as depression and schizophrenia.

Predominant Sick-Care Practices: Biomedical and complementary. Most consult doctors when they are ill or injured. The National Health Service (NHS) provides medical care for all residents, but concerns about the quality and availability of treatment remain a major topic of debate in British politics. The last few decades have witnessed a growing interest in alternative forms of health care. Popular choices include massage, aromatherapy, acupuncture, and herbal remedies. Perhaps a better term for this kind of treatment is complementary medicine because although Britons have become more willing to consider new techniques, most also continue to rely simultaneously on more orthodox treatment options.

Ethnic-/Race-Specific or Endemic Diseases: The leading killer of Britons is cardiovascular disease. In 2003, more than one third of British deaths resulted from diseases of the heart and circulatory system. Moreover, Scotland has one of the highest heart-disease levels in the world. Experts often attribute this dubious distinction to widespread smoking, poor eating habits, and a sedentary yet stressful lifestyle among the Scots. Furthermore, poor treatment by the National Health Service and long waits for its services aggravate the problem for all populations. Tooth decay plagues the British, especially in the poorer north. Fluoridation of drinking water has yet to become standard, and only 10% of Britons benefit from this method of strengthening teeth. Arguments that fluoride causes health problems such as Alzheimer's disease, Down syndrome, and cancer still carry weight among many Britons. Ethnic minorities, usually defined by the British Department of Health as coming from the Black Caribbean, Pakistan, Bangladesh, India, China, and Ireland, face health problems specifically related to their minority status. Cardiovascular disease, diabetes, and obesity all affect members of immigrant groups at higher rates. Poverty is probably mostly to blame for ill health among ethnic minorities, but racism and lack of education about health also play a part. For example, on average, members of ethnic minority groups such as Bangladeshi men smoke cigarettes more, which clearly is associated with the high rates of heart disease in this group. In addition, South Asian men develop oral cancer at a higher rate because of the cultural tradition of chewing tobacco and betel leaves. On a more positive note, other than the Irish, British ethnic minorities drink less alcohol than the average Briton. The Joint United Nations Programme on HIV/AIDS (UNAIDS) reports the prevalence rate for human immunodeficiency virus (HIV) in adults (aged 15 to 49 years) to be 0.2%, with 68,000 people living with HIV, including 21,000 women. Deaths from acquired immunodeficiency syndrome (AIDS) are fewer than 1,000. The percentage of infections through heterosexual sex has increased, but it is probable that in some of those cases infection occurred abroad. The percentage of infections from intravenous drug use and homosexual sex has decreased.

Health-Team Relationships: As part of an attempt to modernize the perennially overburdened NHS, the United Kingdom's Department of Health has implemented new programs to break down traditional barriers between doctors, nurses, and other health care providers. For instance, to ameliorate the chronic shortage of doctors in the NHS system, nurses and pharmacists already have, or soon will receive, broader prescription powers. Specially trained nurse and pharmacist supplementary prescribers can order drugs to treat minor injuries and ailments such as cuts, ear and bladder infections, and acne; medications that promote healthier living, such as vitamins for pregnant women; and (once a doctor has provided the initial diagnosis), drugs that provide palliative care for chronic illnesses such as asthma and diabetes. In turn, nurses hope to shift some of their more routine responsibilities to health care assistants. Unfortunately, nurses, in addition to doctors, remain in short supply, partly because they receive low pay and insufficient recognition considering the highly trained, professional nature of their work. Furthermore, doctors often criticize changes that would allow other health care professionals to take on responsibilities formerly reserved for doctors.

Families' Role in Hospital Care: Britons tend to consider health care as a service best provided by professionals. Families generally offer emotional support to hospitalized relatives but do not provide actual physical care. For example, despite widespread concern about the quality of hospital food, most patients in British hospitals still expect to eat food provided by the hospital rather than meals brought in by family members.

Dominance Patterns: Most Britons would agree that equality between men and women is desirable, but reality fails to achieve the ideal. Moreover, socioeconomic class distinctions are more fixed than they are in the United States. Nonetheless, younger generations are becoming less deferential toward their supposed social superiors, as the growing disinterest in and resentment of the royal family demonstrates.

Eye-Contact Practices: People do not avoid direct eye contact because of status or gender. Looking directly at a speaker indicates that the listener is paying attention, and not doing so suggests inattention.

Touch Practices: The British prefer to maintain an area of personal space. They also tend to reserve deliberate physical touching, other than shaking hands, for those they know well. British culture allows women and men and women and women to touch each other more freely than men and men. Younger generations are also more open to expressing physical affection. Most Britons allow health care providers to touch them as needed for diagnosis and treatment.

Perceptions of Time: The British place a high value on punctuality. Generally, they strive to arrive at appointments on time and expect others to do the same.

Pain Reactions: The British tend to expect stoic toleration of physical and emotional pain. Outward displays of discomfort make others uncomfortable.

Birth Rites: The United Kingdom has the highest teen pregnancy rate in Western Europe. The vast majority of British mothers deliver their children in hospitals under the care of doctors. During the last few years, some have expressed concern that 25% of British infants are delivered via cesarean section. Numerous critics of the practice have suggested that perhaps British mothers have become "too posh to push," meaning that they prefer the convenience of a scheduled cesarean to the pain and unpredictability of natural delivery. At the same time, the country has experienced an increasing demand for midwives, so at least some pregnant women are hoping for less routine medical intervention in their deliveries. Unfortunately, this increasing demand comes at a time when the number of midwives working for the NHS is falling dramatically, which has required more than one maternity unit to close temporarily. In 2004, the NHS employed just fewer than 28,000 midwives, whereas in 1994 there were more than 35,000. The Royal College of Midwives claims that the country needs to recruit another 10,000 midwives to guarantee adequate care. On the whole, British parents wish for healthy infants regardless of sex, and most have their wish granted because the United Kingdom's infant mortality rate of 5 per 1,000 has decreased to an all-time low. The fertility rate is 1.66 children born per woman, and life expectancy is 76 for men, 81 for women.

U

Death Rites: About three fourths of Britons now choose cremation over burial, partly because it is less expensive. No widespread opposition to organ donation and autopsy exists. Still, not enough organs are donated to meet the needs of those who need them. Many British doctors argue for a system of presumed consent, which means people who do not want to donate their organs must deliberately opt out. Today, potential donors must register as such with the NHS and carry donor cards that identify them as willing donors. Even then, family members can block harvest after the potential donor's death.

Food Practices and Intolerances: The British enjoy the questionable privilege of being able to eat too much food with too many calories and too much fat, and obesity rates have tripled over the last 2 decades. In 2003, 23% of adult Britons were obese. At the same time, during the last 3 decades, Britons have cut their consumption of red meat and solid fats and increased their intake of poultry, fruits, and vegetables. Concern over developing Creutzfeldt-Jakob disease from eating tainted beef is partly, but not entirely, responsible for the decrease in beef consumption. Not surprisingly, those of higher educational and socioeconomic levels often eat more balanced diets than their less educated and poorer compatriots. Overall, Britons enjoy fried foods, such as the famous meal of fish and chips and lesser known favorites such as deep-fried Mars candy bars. Typically, if they are right-handed, they put a knife in the right hand and the fork in the left and use both simultaneously when eating.

Infant-Feeding Practices: A slight but growing majority of mothers try breastfeeding their infants at least once. According to the most recently available statistics, only 64% of mothers in England and Wales nursed their infants in 1990, but the percentage climbed to 68% in 1995 and to 71% in 2000. Scotland had a similar increase, from 50% to 55% to 63%, and Northern Ireland's rate increased from 36% to 45% to 54%. Overall, older and better educated women from higher social classes are more inclined to breastfeed.

Child-Rearing Practices: British child-rearing practices are becoming more permissive. Nevertheless, British law still permits parents to strike or "smack" their children as "reasonable chastisement." A 2004 amendment, however, forbids parents to create any cuts, bruises, or even reddening of the skin through corporal punishment; violators face up to 5 years in prison. Teachers may not smack pupils under any circumstances. Still, the idea of a total ban on physical punishment of children by parents remains widely unpopular. Most children sleep in their own beds from birth, and even infants often sleep in a different room than their parents. Ideally, at least among Britons who can afford it, children do not share bedrooms, especially beds, with siblings of the opposite sex.

Naional Childhood Immunizations: Dtap/IPV/Hib and MenC at 2, 3, and 4 months; MMR at 13 months; dTaP/IPV or DtaP/IPV and MMR between 3 years, 4 months and 5 years; and Td/IPB between 13 and 18 years. The percent of the target population vaccinated, by antigen, is: DTP1 (90%); Hib3 and Polio3 (91%); and MCV (81%). Childhood immunizations are not mandatory. A growing number of parents have expressed concern about the combined vaccination for measles, mumps, and rubella and the possibility that it may cause autism and bowel disease. Because of these fears, by 2003, the immunization rate for these diseases had fallen, and outbreaks of measles, mumps, and rubella continue to occur.

U

BIBLIOGRAPHY

BBC News: news.bbc.co.uk (retrieved March 20, 2006).
British Heart Foundation Statistics: www.heartstats.org (retrieved March 20, 2006).
Central Intelligence Agency: 2006: *The world factbook, United Kingdom.* Retrieved September 21, 2006, from https://www.cia.gov/cia/publications/factbook/print/uk.html.
Department of Health: www.doh.gov.uk (retrieved March 20, 2006).
Guardian Unlimited: www.guardian.co.uk (retrieved March 20, 2006).
National Statistics: www.statistics.gov.uk (retrieved March 20, 2006).
Royal College of Midwives: www.rcm.co.uk (retrieved March 20, 2006).
Royal College of Nursing: www.rcn.co.uk (retrieved March 20, 2006).
Royal College of Physicians: www.rcplondon.co.uk (retrieved March 20, 2006).
UNAIDS: 2006: United Kingdom. Retrieved September 21, 2006, from http://www.unaids.org/en/Regions_Countries/Countries/united_kingdom.asp.
World Health Organization: 2006: Immunization, vaccines and biologicals. Retrieved September 21, 2006, from http://www.who.int/immunization_monitoring/en/globalsummary/countryprofileresult.cfm?C='gbr'.

◆ URUGUAY (ORIENTAL REPUBLIC OF)

MAP PAGE (797)

Hamlet Suarez and Ximena Carrera Garese

Location: Uruguay is situated in the Southern Cone of South America. It borders Brazil on the northeast, Argentina on the west and south, the River Plate to the south, and the Atlantic Ocean to the east. Its total area is 176,215 km^2 (68,019 square miles). The population is 3.4 million; 92% in urban areas. Montevideo, the capital city, has 2.9 million people. The gross domestic product (GDP) per capita is $9,600, and 22% live below the poverty line.

Major Languages	Ethnic Groups	Major Religions
Spanish	White 88%	Catholic 66%
	Mestizo 8%	Protestant 2%
	Black 4%	Jewish 1%
		Unaffiliated, Other 31%

English, French, Italian, and Portuguese are taught in public secondary schools. Literacy rates are 98% for both men and women. Uruguay is a cosmopolitan society with successive European migration, primarily from Spain and Italy but also from England, Eastern Europe, and Germany.

U

Health Care Beliefs: Western; limited herbal therapy; active role. Most people go to a doctor or a hospital when they are ill. The use of alternative medicine such as homeopathy and herbs is only marginal. Some groups promote the use of herbs for digestive or kidney function problems, and herbs are commonly used as therapies for obesity and asthma. Uruguay was created by European immigration and has no indigenous population, which explains the absence of witch doctors. The beliefs that relate health problems and their solutions to religious phenomena, which are more common in rural populations in Latin America, are not significant, although some semi-religious practices used in Brazilian culture are found on the Uruguay-Brazil border. Uruguay has many major initiatives for health promotion: *Promocion para la Salud de la Edad Adulta* ("Promotion of Health for Adults"), the Vascular Disease Prevention Program, the Hidatidosis Prevention Program, the Breast Cancer Prevention Program, the Mental Illness Prevention Program, *Programa Materno-Infantil* (the "Mother-Infant Program," which includes the Pregnancy and Lactation Program), Health Care for Children and the Newborn, the HIV Prevention Program, and the *Comision Honoraria de Lucha Contra el Cancer* (the "Honorary Commission for Policy Against Cancer"). All these programs focus on various approaches to disease prevention, such as diet, exercise, and general lifestyle measures. In March 2006, by presidential decree, smoking was forbidden in public places—the first step of its kind taken in Latin America.

Predominant Sick-Care Practices: Biomedical. Middle and upper-class Uruguayans have private insurance, the most extensive health service in the country. Those in the lower classes are assisted by the public health system, which maintains a hospital network in the main cities and inland. Uruguay also has a form of extended health insurance coverage and the Fondo Nacional de Recursos, a national program for high-technology medicine, such as heart surgery and organ transplantation, that provides these procedures for the entire population as needed. Uruguayans are at significant risk for developing cancer, especially lung and colon cancers; smoking and diet are contributing factors.

Ethnic-/Race-Specific or Endemic Diseases: Hidatidosis is the most characteristic endemic disease in the rural population. The disease is found in sheep and is transmitted to humans through contact with dogs, which are fed raw animal organs on farms. Fortunately, the country's hidatidosis program was responsible for achieving a significant decrease in the annual number of cases in the last decade. Influenza is an endemic problem in winter, but the country has a free vaccination program for older adults. Dengue, malaria, and cholera have not colonized the country. Vaccination against hepatitis A and B is encouraged by the Public Health Ministry and is compulsory for high-risk populations such as health care professionals and workers. The major health problems in the population, in decreasing order of importance, are vascular disease (34%), cancer (23%), accidents (4%), infectious diseases (2%), and diabetes (2%). The Joint United Nations Programme on HIV/AIDS (UNAIDS) reports the prevalence rate for HIV in adults (aged 15 to 49 years) to be 0.5%, with 9,600 people living with human immunodeficiency virus (HIV), including 5,300 women. Deaths from acquired immunodeficiency syndrome (AIDS) are fewer than 500. About 19% of pregnant women are receiving treatment to reduce mother-to-child transmission. The most prevalent modes of transmission are sexual (71%), blood (25%), and perinatal (4%).

Health-Team Relationships: Doctors have good working relationships with nurses but have always had the dominant position. Doctors are well respected and have high standards. Ethical issues are addressed by a committee from the Association of Doctors *(Sindicato Medico de Uruguay)*. The professional role of the nurse has expanded in the last 20 years, and nurses complete 5 years of coursework at the University of the Republic School of Nursing. Plans for a doctoral nursing program were implemented 2 years ago.

Families' Role in Hospital Care: Families actively participate in the care of hospitalized relatives and usually stay with them throughout the day and night to assist as needed. The practice of a family taking food to a hospitalized relative is more common in public hospitals. The poorest individuals are cared for by public hospitals; they have no costs other than the cost of transportation for family members traveling from other parts of the country. Doctors tend to be protective of their patients. In cases of devastating illnesses such as cancer, doctors consult with families about prognosis and tend to avoid giving patients bad news so that they can remain hopeful.

Dominance Patterns: Although Uruguay has a Latin culture, male dominance is not very strong. Because most women work, decision making about finances and other issues involves both men and women. Women actively participate in political activities, and Uruguay has a legislative commission that is currently considering the rights of female workers. Women continue to receive less pay than men for the same job.

Eye-Contact Practices: Direct eye contact is acceptable in social and medical environments.

Touch Practices: Because Uruguay has a Latin society, touch is an important way to express acceptance and friendship. A handshake during a formal greeting or kissing on the cheek when greeting families and friends is the norm.

Perceptions of Time: Punctuality is not a characteristic of Uruguayans, and arriving late to social events is common. For example, even weddings are expected to start at least 45 minutes later than their scheduled time. Time is more of an issue in the workplace, and people tend to be punctual for business appointments. Uruguayans focus heavily on past traditions.

Pain Reactions: Pain is expressed freely and usually elicits feelings of empathy and concern. In lower socioeconomic groups, controlling expressions of pain is valued for men. In general, men and women are very verbal about pain. Love and support from family and friends are highly valued in painful situations.

Birth Rites: The health care system is heavily involved in pregnancy and childbirth. Uruguayans are equally happy when sons and daughters are born. The fertility rate is 1.89 children born per woman. The infant mortality rate is 12 deaths per 1,000 live births. Life expectancy is high for the region: 73 for men, 80 for women.

Death Rites: The family relationship is strong, and family members support each other when a loved one dies. Funerals are not particularly formal occasions, and people do not wear special clothes when attending. Women rarely wear black mourning clothes; this is common only among older women who emigrated from Spain or Italy. The funeral is carried out immediately after death, generally at funeral parlors, and lasts 18 to 24 hours. Family and friends express sympathy by sending flowers. Organ donations are encouraged.

Food Practices and Intolerances: Meat has a significant role in the diet, although during the last 30 years, the consumption of vegetables and fruits has increased. The most typical food is *parrillada* ("barbecue"), which is roasted beef or lamb with sausages and offal (animal organs such as kidneys and certain glands) that are cooked on red-hot coals. The typical hot beverage is *mate,* an herbal infusion imported from Brazil and Paraguay that contains xanthine and is similar to tea and coffee. Uruguayans drink mate from a dry, empty pumpkin. Herbs and occasionally sugar are added through a hole in the top of the pumpkin. Hot water is added, and the individual drinks from a special silver tube called a *bombilla* ("small pump").

Infant-Feeding Practices: Breastfeeding is usual during the first 6 months of life, and many women continue for an additional 4 months. After 6 months, foods are introduced gradually. The first food is usually mashed fruit, followed by mashed vegetables and then ground beef and chicken. Most mothers work outside the home and continue to receive their salaries from the government during a 3-month leave after the birth. After 3 months, they must return to work on a part-time basis, and after 6 months they must return to full-time work. This arrangement was designed to encourage breastfeeding in the first 6 months of life as recommended. Working mothers generally put their children in nurseries while they work or leave them with family members, often grandparents. Mothers with better-paying positions may hire sitters to stay in their homes.

Child-Rearing Practices: The society is quite permissive with children. Public education is secular, free, and compulsory at the primary and secondary levels. Children usually live with their parents for financial reasons until they marry or have a family of their own. They become independent considerably later than do children in North America and Europe.

National Childhood Immunizations: BCG at birth; DT at 2, 4, 6, and 12 months (special groups); DTwP at 5 years; DTwPHibHep at 2, 4, 6, and 12 months; HepA first contact + 6 months (at-risk groups); HepB 12 years, +1, +6 months; Hib at 2, 4, 6, and 12 months (immunocompromised); influenza at 6 to 23 months; IPV at 2, 4, 6, and 12 months (immunocompromised); MMR at 12 months and 5 years; OPV at 2, 4, 6, and 12 months; Td at 12 years (every 10 years); and varicella at 12 months. The percent of the target population vaccinated, by antigen, is: BCG and DTP1 (98%); DTP3, MCV, and Polio3 (95%); and HepB3 and Hib3 (94%).

BIBLIOGRAPHY

Asociación Panamericana de Infectología (SLIPE): *Manual de Vacunas*, 2005, SLIPE. Montevideo, Uruguay.

Central Intelligence Agency: 2006: The World Factbook, Uruguay. Retrieved September 21, 2006 from https://www.cia.gov/cia/publications/factbook/print/uy.html.

Instituto Nacional de Estadistica (INE): http://www.ine.gub.uy (retrieved March 10, 2006).

Miglionico A: *Analysis and tendencies of health in Uruguay.* Montevideo, 1999, Department of Statistics, Ministry of Public Health.

Ministry of Public Health, General Office of Health: *The health system in Uruguay, tendency and perspectives.* 1999. FIS, DELPHI Report.

Ministerio de Salud Publica: http://www.msp.gub.uy (retrieved March 10, 2006).

UNAIDS: 2006 Uruguay. Retrieved September 21, 2006, from http://www.unaids.org/en/Regions_Countries/Countries/uruguay.asp.

World Health Organization: 2006: Immunization, vaccines and biologicals. Retrieved September 21, 2006, from http://www.who.int/immunization_monitoring/en/globalsummary/countryprofileresult.cfm?C='ury.

◆ UZBEKISTAN (REPUBLIC OF)

MAP PAGE (799)

Lori Rosenstein and Nodira Ochilova

Location: Formerly a part of the Soviet Union, Uzbekistan is located in central Asia between the Amu Darya and Syr Darya Rivers, Aral Sea, and the Tien Shan Mountains. It is bordered by Kazakhstan to the north and northwest, Kyrgyzstan and Tajikistan to the east and southeast, and Turkmenistan to the southwest. It includes the Karakalpakstan Autonomous Republic. The most southern tip of Uzbekistan borders Afghanistan. The total area is 447,400 km^2 (172,741 square miles). The capital is Tashkent. Two thirds is desert or semi-desert. The population is 27.3 million. Literacy rates are 100% for men and 99% for women. The gross domestic product (GDP) per capita is $1,800, and about 28% live below the poverty line.

Major Languages	Ethnic Groups	Major Religions
Uzbek	Uzbek 80%	Sunni Muslim 88%
Russian	Russian 6%	Eastern Orthodox 9%
Tajik	Tajik 5%	Other 3%
Other	Kazak 3%	
	Karakalpak, Tatar,	
	Korean, Other 6%	

U

Health Care Beliefs: Traditional; acute sick care. Common colds, including sore throats and stomachaches, are generally believed to be caused by chilled drinks, ice cream, and cold drafts (including those from fans and air conditioners). It is rare to see people chill water; most beverages are served at room temperature. During the hot summer, many people do not roll down windows while using public transportation because they fear becoming ill. A cure for a cold and fever is considered to be a hot bowl of oily soup, and food is also used to cure stomach flu. Abrasions, cuts, and scrapes are often treated with vodka, which is used as an antiseptic. People who have a chest cold and cough may receive a vodka rub on the chest. Newborn infants wear a bracelet with a black and white eye-shaped bead, which is worn to protect the child from the "evil eye" (others who can harm people merely by looking at them). A girl who becomes a "woman" before marriage (i.e., has premarital sex) may have difficulty being "married off" by her father, a terrible situation for a woman. Young girls and women are discouraged from sitting on cement steps or curbs without a handkerchief or piece of paper because it is believed doing so can make her infertile. Therefore, strongly held attitudes toward hygiene and the causes of illness are, not infrequently, based on inaccurate information. For example, many families use only cold water and no soap to clean dirty dishes because they do not want to heat the water, and dish and laundry soap are expensive and strong. Some complain they can taste dish soap on clean dishes. In addition, after eliminating, people wash their hands with water but do not always use soap. These hygiene practices increase the risk of infection with bacteria and parasites.

Predominant Sick-Care Practices: Biomedical; magical-religious. The health care system provides "first-aid" hospitals in every region. Some health care is provided free, which is indicated on documents signed by patients; however, the government allows the patient to receive free medical treatment for only up to 5 days. The remaining expenses are paid by the patient. Occasionally, a hospital stay is very expensive. Hospitals tend to have Western medical equipment, but some hospitals and clinics are very unsanitary. It is not uncommon to see cockroaches crawling on the floors and walls. Medications are widely available in the pharmacies and at the local markets, and people can buy what they need without a prescription, even drugs that are strong and have serious side effects. Western health professionals working in Uzbekistan have found potent antibiotics that require prescriptions in the United States and most European countries being sold at pharmacies. Because of pervasive economic corruption, if a patient needs any type of surgery, he or she will have to bribe the doctors (in U.S. dollars) to get the surgery they need.

Ethnic-/Race-Specific or Endemic Diseases: Endemic diseases include leishmaniasis, hepatitis B and E, echinococcosis, and goiter. The Uzbek people are at risk for poliomyelitis, malaria, tuberculosis, and childhood anemia. The country had an epidemic of diphtheria from 1993

U

to 1996. According to the Muslim religion, alcohol cannot be consumed; however, alcoholism is a significant health problem because heavy alcohol consumption permeates Uzbek society. Many men also smoke cigarettes and chew tobacco. The diet consists of high amounts of starch, meat, fat, salt, and cottonseed oil. According to the Joint United Nations Programme on HIV/AIDS (UNAIDS), the estimated prevalence rate for HIV in adults (aged 15 to 49 years) is 0.2%, with 31,000 people living with human immunodeficiency virus (HIV), including 4,100 women. Deaths from acquired immunodeficiency syndrome (AIDS) number fewer than 500. The dominant mode of transmission is injecting drug use (59%), followed by heterosexual contact (11%) and sex between men (less than 1%). Most citizens refuse to believe that AIDS exists in Uzbekistan, although AIDS education is becoming more prevalent. For example, a television commercial about AIDS shows prostitutes approaching cars and getting in them. Homosexuality is considered taboo, and the slang term "blue" is often used to refer to homosexuals. Those who even believe that homosexuality exists are often negative and sometimes hostile about the topic, and most people discuss it only in private. When people speak about homosexual relationships, they are referring primarily to gay men.

Health-Team Relationships: Doctors are highly respected, although their salaries are very low. Only doctors diagnose and inform patients about their illnesses. Nurses assist the doctors with treating patients by speaking with families, giving information about health issues, and occasionally providing food for patients.

Families' Role in Hospital Care: Families are responsible for preparing food for their hospitalized relatives. If a child needs surgery, the mother is allowed to stay overnight.

Dominance Patterns: The head of the family and the central decision maker in most Uzbek families is the father or patriarch. In more traditional social situations, men and women sit and eat in separate rooms. When women cannot get pregnant, the assumption is always that she has the fertility problem. It is rare for a doctor to suggest that a man may have fertility issues. Infertility has serious cultural consequences: women are shunned by in-laws and overall by society. Because girls and women are expected to be virgins when they marry, after the first night as a married couple, most traditional families display the bed sheets to demonstrate that the woman's hymen has been broken. If there is no blood, the assumption is that the woman was not a virgin.

Eye Contact and Touch Practices: It is acceptable to make direct eye contact with everyone. In some very traditional areas, however, women are not permitted to make eye contact with men or shake their hands. When younger men or women greet an older woman, they place their right hand on their heart, and the older woman pats them on the back. If a younger woman greets an older man, she may shake his hand if he offers his. If he does not, she shows respect by placing her right hand on her heart. Women greet each other by kissing two or three times on alternating cheeks.

Perceptions of Time: People often plan for the future, especially for the future of their children. In fact, they spend their lives preparing for their children's future. People are on time for doctor's appointments. There are no such things as transportation (i.e., bus or taxi) schedules. It is not uncommon for drivers to stop at friends' or families' houses, en route, for a meal and tea. Therefore, one can never say with certainty the exact time they can be expected.

Pain Reactions: It is acceptable for women to express pain, as it is for men with severe injuries. People believe that men are strong, so it is relatively uncommon for a man to openly express his pain. Many women have abortions without anesthesia, and it is excruciatingly painful; not surprisingly, women are known to scream out loud. Abortion is used primarily as birth control and is not considered an ethical issue.

Birth Rites: The fertility rate is three children born per woman. Most women give birth in a hospital, but some very religious families prefer to give birth at home. The delivery practices are similar to Western ways, and if a woman is in intense pain, she can request pain medication. It was once customary for women to give birth without family members present, but their presence has become more acceptable. The mother stays in the hospital for at least 3 days after birth but may stay 5 days if the delivery was abnormally difficult. Uzbek people circumcise boys at 5 years of age. Some traditional families arrange marriages within the family; for example, it is not uncommon for first cousins to marry. Recently, doctors have been educating families about the potential dangers of close familial marriages. Children born with severe abnormalities may die; in rare cases, they are killed. Women may have at least five abortions in their lifetimes. One 55-year-old woman known by the author has had 12 abortions. Until 5 years ago, abortions were performed without anesthetics, but this is changing. The infant mortality rate is high at 70 deaths per 1,000 live births. Life expectancy is 61 years for men, 68 for women.

Death Rites: To prepare a body for burial, family members wash and dress the body in new clothes. Only family members are allowed to see the body before the burial, and it is against customary laws to place anything inside the coffin. After 1 full day, a procession goes to the burial site; only men carry the coffin. Women and children are not permitted to be in the procession or at the burial site. The length of mourning depends on the age of the deceased. If the person was young, the family mourns and does not work for 40 days. If the relative was older, the family mourns for 1 year. People gather at the house of the deceased to pay their respects. They greet the mourning relatives, who stay outside the house crying and wailing, openly and loudly. Women dress in white and cover their heads with a white scarf. People who come to pay their respects enter the house, sit down, eat the national dish (osh), and reminisce about the deceased. Men and women sit in separate rooms or areas.

U

Food Practices and Intolerances: Most people eat three meals a day. Breakfast consists mostly of nuts, fruit, bread, jam, rice pudding, or sweet cheese. Dinner is the largest meal of the day. The national dish, *osh*, consists of rice, meat, fat, and carrots cooked in heavy cottonseed oil. The flat, round bread that is served is considered very holy, and breaking the bread into pieces indicates that a meal has begun. Pieces of bread are passed around to each person. If a guest is at the table, most of the bread is placed in front of the person as a sign of respect. It is unacceptable for the bread to be upside down or for a bottom part of the bread to be showing—this is considered very rude and an insult to the family and Allah.

Infant-Feeding Practices: Breastfeeding is common. Women know that it is healthier to feed an infant with the mother's breast milk than with formula, and it is cheaper as well. It is not uncommon for women to breastfeed until the child is 4 years old.

Child-Rearing Practices: Boys are coddled and given a lot of freedom, and if the youngest child is a boy, he is given the most physical affection from the mother. Young girls often do not get physical affection from their parents. In Western cultures, parents are encouraged, at a particular development stage, not to pick up or coddle infants every time they cry, so that they will not suffer from separation anxiety. In Uzbek culture, one can observe women picking up or holding infants almost all the time.

National Childhood Immunizations: BCG at birth and at 7 and 14 years; DT at 2, 3, and 16 months (in case of contraindication with DTP); DTwP at 2, 3, 4, and 16 months; OPV at birth and at 2, 3, 4, and 16 months and at 7 years; measles at 12 months and 6 years; mumps at 16 months; Td at 7, 16, 26, and 46 years; and MMR at 12 months and at 6 years (part of country). The percent of the target population vaccinated, by antigen, is: BCG, Polio3, DTP1, DTP3, and HepB3 (99%); and MCV (98%).

BIBLIOGRAPHY

Beutels P, Musabaev EI, VanDamme P, and Yasin T: The disease burden of hepatitis B in Uzbekistan, *J Infect.* 40(3):234, 2000.

Carr JK, Nadai Y, Eyzaguirre L, Saad MD, Khakimov MM, and Yakubov SK: Outbreak of a West African recombinant of HIV-1 in Tashkent, Uzbekistan, *J Acquir Immune Defic Syndr.* 39(5):570–575, 2005.

Central Intelligence Agency: 2006: *The world factbook, Uzbekistan.* Retrieved September 21, 2006, from https://www.cia.gov/cia/publications/factbook/print/uz.html.

Niyazmatov BI, Shefer A, Grabowski M, and Vitek CR: Diphtheria epidemic in the Republic of Uzbekistan, 1993–1996, *J Infect Dis.* 181(suppl 1):S104–S109, 2000.

UNAIDS: 2006 Uzbekistan. Retrieved September 21, 2006, from http://www.unaids.org/en/Regions_Countries/Countries/uzbekistan.asp.

World Health Organization: 2006: Immunization, vaccines and biologicals. Retrieved September 21, 2006, from http://www.who.int/immunization_monitoring/en/globalsummary/countryprofileresult.cfm?C='uzb'.

◆ VENEZUELA (BOLIVARIAN REPUBLIC OF)

MAP PAGE (797)

Marino J. González

V

Location: Venezuela is located on the southern Caribbean coast of South America, north of Brazil and east of Colombia. The climate is tropical but is influenced by changes in altitude from the coastline, to the plains and high plateaus, and to the Andes Mountains. The capital is Caracas. The total area is 912,050 km^2 (352,144 square miles), with only 5% devoted to agriculture. The Orinoco River (2150 km) divides the country into the more densely inhabited north and the mostly uninhabited rain forests and savannas to the south that extend into the Amazon Basin north of Brazil. The population is estimated at 25.7 million, and 88% live in urban areas. The gross domestic product (GDP) per capita is $6,100, and about 47% live below the poverty line. Literacy rates are 94% for men, 93% for women.

Major Languages	Ethnic Groups	Major Religions
Spanish	Mestizo 67%	Roman Catholic 96%
Indigenous	White 21%	Protestant 2%
	Black 10%	Other, none 2%
	Amerindian 2%	

Various indigenous languages are spoken in the remote interior. Venezuela has African, Amerindian, Arab, and European (primarily Spanish, Portuguese, and Italian) influences. Venezuela has three distinct classes (rich, middle class, and poor). According to recent estimates, the distribution of classes was 2% wealthy, 31% middle class, and 67% poor.

Health Care Beliefs: Western and traditional; active and passive roles. The health services provided by the Ministry of Health and Social Development (MSDS) place more emphasis on primary and secondary health care, whereas the social security system, which also attends non-secured citizens, covers more specialized treatments, such as renal dialysis, transplantation, and antiretroviral drugs, among others. Health agents and public health monitors provide some community interventions. The number of private health care providers is growing, and providing service to most of the middle class. A large majority of Venezuelans (including Amerindians) believe in Western, or science-based, medicine. Alternative medicine is, for the most part, practiced by witches *(brujos)*. In addition to prayers, chants, and ceremonies, witches use herbs to cure their clients. Amulets and religious articles are used as protection against bad luck or bad influences from other people. Belief in astrology is widespread among all social classes.

Predominant Sick-Care Practices: Biomedical and magical-religious. The Venezuelan health system can be divided according to its two major sources of financing and methods of delivery: public and private. The public system is financed through fiscal revenues and payroll taxes, and the private system is primarily financed through community and personal insurance plans. The public sector comprises national hospitals, social security institutions, and decentralized services (hospital and outpatient care services) at the state level. The major public institution is the Ministerio de Salud (Ministry of Health) of Venezuela (MSDS), which accounts for about 63% of total public health expenditures. The prevalence rate for human immunodeficiency virus (HIV)/acquired immunodeficiency syndrome (AIDS) was last reported as 0.7% in 1999, but country-specific models are not available. The Joint United Nations Programme on HIV/AIDS (UNAIDS) and the Pan American Health Organization (PAHO) provide limited data on HIV; it is estimated that 110,000 adults and children are living with HIV/AIDS, including 32,000 women.

Health-Team Relationships: The term *doctor* is used indiscriminately as an expression of respect and affection. Nurses are addressed by the title *enfermera* or their first name. *Brujos* and *comadronas* are male or female healers who often serve rural populations and sections of suburban populations.

Families' Role in Hospital Care: The family is responsible for direct care, and family members may bring food or take turns staying with the patient 24 hours a day. It is common for the family to take part in decisions about procedures such as surgery and referrals.

Dominance Patterns: The extended family can include godparents (*compadres*), who are occasionally chosen according to their social status in the community and as a form of recognition. Godparents are expected to help provide medical care for their godchildren if needed, although it is common for godparents and godchildren never to see each other after the baptism. The tradition of asking for the parents' blessing for marriage is less prominent in the younger generation but remains popular in some parts of Venezuela. When more than one last name is used, the mother's name follows the father's. Having the same last name gives families a sense of belonging.

Eye-Contact Practices: Direct eye contact is common between sexes and social classes.

Touch Practices: Use of the body and touch during social contacts is the "tropical" way of relating. Two women greet each other by kissing on one cheek, as do men and women and men and men. The *abrazo* ("embrace") is a common greeting among males. Handshaking occurs primarily with foreigners and on formal occasions. Touching while talking is common.

Perceptions of Time: Venezuelans are casual about punctuality and live in the present. The future is a very ambiguous and heterogeneous concept, and definitions of *early* and *late* are flexible. Arriving late can be a sign of a higher social standing. Immediate rewards for activity are preferred to delayed gratification.

Pain Reactions: Pain is expressed vocally through moans and groans, although men tend to be stoic. It is much more common for women to express emotional problems by referring to a physical entity such as headaches.

V

Birth Rites: Fathers are not usually present during labor and delivery, although the presence of a family member is common. Childbirth is often by cesarean section. Girls may have their ears pierced soon after birth, frequently while they are still in the hospital. A rest period of 45 days after birth is typical, and fathers usually take several days off from work. Working parents continue to collect their salaries, and working mothers usually have flexible hours, including time off to breastfeed. The extended family may assume the role of primary caregiver when parents return to work. Tubal ligations after women have had two children (one boy and one girl) are common among those in the middle and upper class. This procedure is more difficult to obtain for those in the lower class. The fertility rate is 2.23 children born per woman, and the infant mortality rate is 21.54 deaths per 1,000 live births. Life expectancy is 71 for men, 78 for women.

Death Rites: The poor often carry their dead to a cemetery in a cardboard casket. In small towns, the funeral may involve the entire community, and many people join the procession. Small businesses may be closed and activities suspended as a sign of sympathy and respect. Children often lead the procession by carrying a crown or a cross of natural flowers. Male relatives are the pallbearers and are followed by close relatives and friends. Family and friends pray. Middle- and upper-class individuals are buried in wooden caskets. Family graves, in which several people may be buried, are becoming less common. Cremation is slowly becoming more popular but is not widely practiced. During a funeral service, the body is surrounded by flowers, and only the head shows; burial is usually the day after death. In the middle and upper classes, the procession is done in cars. Cremation is becoming available in larger cities.

Food Practices and Intolerances: *Arepas* ("cornbread"), or bread with eggs, meat, cheese, and black beans are common for breakfast, although cereals and fruit are becoming popular. The main meal at noon consists of rice, black beans, mashed bananas, pasta, and meat or fish. The consumption of vegetables and salads is increasing. The trend in middle-class families in which mothers and fathers work is to eat the noon meal at a self-service restaurant or in a luncheonette, although going back home is a popular choice because of the 2-hour lunch break allowed by most employers. Away from home, *arepa, empanada* ("cornbread sandwich"), or a sandwich is common. Supper is a light meal (of soup or leftovers from lunch) and is eaten in the evening, although it is not uncommon to eat a two- or three-course dinner.

Infant-Feeding Practices: Breastfeeding is generally short term, and the attitude of the father can be the most significant factor in its duration. A filling formula made of a thickening agent (e.g., flour of manioc, corn, or rice) and water is often used, especially by poor families, to fill the stomach of a hungry infant or toddler. Slight obesity in infants or children is considered a sign of health.

Child-Rearing Practices: Children are treated affectionately. Warm embraces by all family members are common. Grandmothers and friends play an active role in caregiving, especially in families in which the mother works outside the home. Middle- and upper-class children are enrolled in private or parochial schools. Lower-class students receive a public school education. Young children are enrolled in a *crèche* (day care) or kindergarten. Children in the lower socioeconomic class often work instead of going to school. Homeless children are a concern in large cities.

National Childhood Immunizations: BCG at birth; DTwP at 18 months; DTwPHibHep at 2, 4, and 6 months; OPV at birth, 2, 4, and 6 months; HepB at birth and at 1 and 6 months; MMR at 1 year; TT/Td CBAW first contact, +2 months, +1, +2, and +3 years; and YFV at 6 months. The percent of the target population vaccinated, by antigen is: BCG (95%); DTP1 (98%); OPV (83%); DTP3 and HepB3 (88%); Hib3 (87%); MCV (76%); Polio3 (81%); TT2plus (87%); and YFV (94%).

BIBLIOGRAPHY

Central Intelligence Agency: *2006: The world factbook, Venezuela.* Retrieved September 21, 2006 from https://www.cia.gov/cia/publications/factbook/print/ve.html.

González R, Marino J: *Gasto del componente de salud del Ministerio de Salud y Desarrollo Social,* Caracas, 2004, Universidad Simón Bolívar, Unidad de Políticas Públicas (mimeo).

González R, Marino J: *Reformas del sistema de salud en Venezuela 1987–1999: Balance perspectivas.* Santiago de Chile, 2001, CEPAL. Serie Financiamiento del desarrollo. No. 111.

Riutort M: *El costo de erradicar la pobreza.* In UCAB-Asociación Civil para la Promoción de Estudios Sociales, Vol 1. Caracas, 2001, UCAB-ACPES, pp. 15–26.

Instituto Nacional de Estadística: Retrieved February 5, 2006, from http://www.ine.gov.ve.

Pan American Health Organization: OPS. Retrieved February 5, 2006, from http://www.paho.org/.

UNAIDS: *2004 Report on the global AIDS epidemic.* Geneva, 2004, UNAIDS.

World Health Organization: 2006: Immunization, Vaccines and Biologicals. Retrieved September 21, 2006 from http://www.who.int/immunization_monitoring/en/globalsummary/countryprofileresult.cfm?C='ven'.

◆ VIETNAM (SOCIALIST REPUBLIC OF)

MAP PAGE (805)

Lien Quach, Hoa L. Nguyen, and Huong T.N. Nguyen

Location: Vietnam is located on the Indochina peninsula in South East Asia overlooking the Tonkin Gulf in the north and South China Sea in the south. The total area is 330,000 km^2 (127,243 square miles). Vietnam borders China to the north and Laos and Cambodia to the west. Most of the country is mountains and plateaus with the marshy Mekong River delta in the south. The population is 84.4 million: the capital is Hanoi. Most people are concentrated along the coast and delta river ways. The gross domestic product (GDP) per capita is $2,800, with 20% below the poverty line. Literacy rates are 94% for men, 87% for women.

Dominant Languages	Ethnic Groups	Dominant Religions
Vietnamese (official)	Vietnamese 87%	Buddhist 60%
French	Chinese 3%	Confucianism 13%
Chinese	Other 10%	Taoist 12%
English		Catholic 3%
Khmer		Other 12%

The Kinh ethnic group accounts for five of every six people. The rest include Chinese and other minorities such as the Muong, Thai, Meo, Khmer, Man, and Cham. Most Vietnamese practice some form of Buddhism; however, there are also Christian, Cao Dai, Hoa Hao, and other local religious sects.

Health Care Beliefs: Vietnamese from different regions of the country have different beliefs about illness. Some popular beliefs include that illness is a curse or punishment from the gods, or an imbalanced *yin-yang* ("principle of two mutually interdependent and constantly interacting polar energies that sustain all living organisms") or blocked *chi* ("the circulating life energy thought to be inherent in all things"). Herbs are considered important for staying healthy, and herbal treatment may result in undesirable interactions with Western medications. Stigma against mental illness is highly prevalent, and emotional disturbances may warrant health-seeking efforts only when they manifest somatically.

Predominant Sick-Care Practices: Magical-religious, Eastern medicine and biomedical. Self-medication and the use of many drugs simultaneously are customary. Usually, Western methods are used for acute diseases. For chronic and lifelong diseases, people often prefer Eastern medicine because they believe it is safe and has no side effects. Most Eastern medicine is thought as "cool," whereas most Western medicine is considered "hot." Water is a "cold" substance, so it may be restricted when a person is sick (they cannot drink it or wash themselves in it). Folk remedies include acupuncture, massage, herbal remedies, and dermabrasive practices such as cupping, pinching, rubbing, and burning. Coin rubbing and cupping are used to draw illness out of the body. In rubbing, a heated coin or one smeared with oil is vigorously rubbed over the body, producing red welts. Cupping *(moxibustion)* is the process of placing heated cups on the body to suck out "bad winds" or unhealthy air currents. The resulting red marks are thought to be evidence of the illnesses being brought to the surface of the body. The Vietnamese believe that the marks will develop only in people who are ill. It is important to take medicine that can restore the yin-yang and hot-cold balances. More than half of Vietnamese seek health care in the private sector, for either Western or Eastern remedies. There is no consistent pattern to suggest that wealth is associated with the use of the private sector. Medication costs account for a substantial percentage of household expenditures.

Ethnic-/Race-Specific or Endemic Diseases: The leading causes of morbidity are pneumonia, acute bronchial conditions, diarrhea and gastroenteritis, transportation accidents, primary hypertension, influenza, and pulmonary tuberculosis (TB). Malaria is prominent, and there is high risk of TB. In 2004, there were 82,944 pulmonary TB cases. Women are at higher risk than men and are less likely to be diagnosed. The current cure rate is 90%. The human immunodeficiency virus (HIV)/acquired immunodeficiency syndrome (AIDS) epidemic is concentrated among high-risk groups, with a national adult prevalence of around 0.4%. According to sentinel surveillance in 2003, prevalence was 32% for injecting drug users, 7% for female sex workers, 2% for sexually transmitted disease (STD) patients, 0.34% for pregnant women, and 4% for TB patients. The Ministry of Health projected that by 2005, HIV infections would reach between 198,000 and 256,000. It was estimated that 52,000 to 66,000 would develop AIDS, and 47,000 to 60,000 would die as result. Up to December 2004, there were 90,360 cases of HIV in all provinces, 14,428 cases of AIDS, and 8,398 deaths. About 96% of those living with HIV/AIDS are aged 15 to 49. Antiretroviral therapy was introduced recently, but about 1,000 people received antiretroviral treatment in 2004—of 22,000 who needed it.

Health-Team Relationships: Health care providers are expected to be altruistic when they are practicing medicine: working with their hearts with little concern for money. Young or recently qualified doctors may be considered incompetent and are often asked about the year they completed their training. Older health professionals with 20 years' experience are considered authority figures and experts. Patients are told little about their conditions, medications, or diagnostic procedures, so patients often do not understand their medical treatment. Educating patients and families is not a role nurses play. Sparing a person's feelings is more important than telling the truth, so "yes" may actually mean "no." In traditional families, the oldest male makes the important health care decisions.

Families' Role in Hospital Care: When a family member is sick, the immediate family is responsible for seeking traditional treatment first, including coining, cupping, pinching, steaming, acupuncture, or herbs. If the person needs to be treated in a hospital, the family then provides company and support to their loved one. They reside at the bedside and sleep in the patient's bed or on thin straw mats. It is expected that food, assistance with hygiene, and personal comfort will be provided 24 hours a day by family members or someone hired by the family.

Dominance Patterns: Vietnamese families consist of extended networks of three or four generations living together, especially in rural areas. Nuclear families make up 71% of all households. Although men are typically the head of the household, the economic and emotional power that women provide is an important dynamic. Women frequently influence family decisions regarding health care, child education, and other domestic issues. Decision-making is influenced by astrological beliefs and the lunar calendar. Children are expected to care for their aging parents until they die. To convey respect for others, it is customary to stand when speaking; and it is considered disrespectful to point a finger at another person.

Eye-Contact Practices: In urban settings, direct eye contact is accepted, but in rural settings looking directly at another while talking is considered disrespectful. In traditional settings, women are often afraid of direct eye contact, particularly with men, as it may be interpreted as passion and should not be displayed in public. Blinking means that a message has been received.

Touch Practices: A person's head is considered the center of the soul and is not touched by others, except by older adults who may touch the heads of young children. Touching persons of the same sex is acceptable, and touching between women can be very affectionate. It is unacceptable for a man to touch a woman he does not know. The female breast is accepted dispassionately as an infant's food source; however, the lower torso is extremely private. The area between the waist and knees is kept covered, even in private. Handshaking has gained wide acceptance with men. A man does not extend his hand to a woman or superior. Sisters and brothers do not touch or kiss each other.

Perceptions of Time: Time is thought to move in a recurring circle rather than in a linear direction; important events are scheduled according to the lunar cycle. Cycles of development, and magic numbers, are commonly held beliefs about luck and misfortune. For example, it is thought that 49 and 53 are deadly years for men, and those ages should be avoided by women when marrying. Many people believe in reincarnation.

Pain Reactions: Stoic reactions are the norm, and pain may be severe before a person requests relief. People may remain quiet or even smile when in pain. Pain is considered an emotional problem which people do not want to talk about with their physicians; they prefer to show they are strong and enduring. This characteristic may create barriers to diagnosis and treatment.

Birth Rites: The fertility rate is two children born per woman, and the infant mortality rate is 25 deaths per 1,000 live births. The timing of a child's birth is often calculated because it is believed to affect the baby's destiny. Some pregnant women avoid weddings and funerals and abstain from sexual intercourse because they believe they could harm themselves or the infant. The squatting position is preferred for delivery. The presence of a close female relative may be desired. Regardless of the temperature of the room or the outdoors, women in labor drink only warm or hot water and keep themselves warm by wearing socks and using blankets. Men, unmarried women, young girls, and husbands are usually not present during birth. In rural areas, delivery at home with a midwife is preferred. At birth, the child is considered 1 year old. After delivery, women following traditional Chinese practices do not bathe or wash their hair in order to keep their yin-yang balanced. Some women believe they should not shower or be exposed to cold wind during the first month. They are often urged to eat a lot of food to breastfeed. Some do not leave the house for a month, whereas others (in rural areas) begin working immediately after delivery. Circumcision is generally not done. Newborns are not given compliments (i.e., are not called beautiful, healthy, or smart) for fear that they will be captured by evil spirits. Out-of-wedlock pregnancy is considered shameful and is usually hidden from the family. In fact, the mother might secretly abort the fetus using Chinese herbs or conventional methods. Life expectancy is 68 for men, 74 for women.

Death Rites: Dying people are helped to recall their past good deeds so that they will be in the proper mental state for their next life. Cremation is new and is practiced only in urban areas. Death at home is preferred. After death in some regions, a coin, jewels (in a wealthier family), or rice (in a poorer family) is put into the mouth. The family believes these items may help the soul during its encounters with gods and devils and might help the deceased to be reincarnated into a rich person in the next life. During the first night, monks or psychic masters are invited to the house to perform rituals, believed to help the deceased leave mortal life. The coffin is brought back to the deceased person's hometown so that he or she can be buried next to the family. Open expressions of grief include crying, moaning, and even self-beating. Following the funeral, an altar is set up for the dead in the house, where the family will worship at the first week, the 49th day, and the 100th day. After a few years, the family may remove the coffin, wash the bones, and put them in a small ceramic box. Then they either bury them again or cremate them and send them to a pagoda. Only after this ceremony can the ceremonies be considered complete. Usually worship of the deceased continues for many years.

Food Practices and Intolerances: Vietnamese prefer chopsticks. The diet consists primarily of rice and also meat, seafood, fruit, and vegetables. Meals are eaten together, with all the foods in the center of the table, and everyone shares. Lactose intolerance is not unusual. Vietnam has a higher prevalence of childhood malnutrition than other countries with similar levels of human development, even though poverty has been reduced. The prevalence of underweight, stunting, and wasting was 27%, 31%, and 8%, respectively, for children under 5 years of age in 2004. Overweight and obesity have increased, with the estimated prevalence of overweight (including obesity) as 10% to 20%. Children between ages 6 and 11 and adults aged 40 to 50 seem to be at the highest risk, particularly in cities.

Infant-Feeding Practices: Breastfeeding is encouraged for infants and children younger than 2 years. About 82% breastfeed up to age 1 year; only 28% breastfeed exclusively for 3 months. Introduction of complementary food is very early because mothers believe that breast milk alone is not enough for strong growth. Most families wean their infants during the third month with rice porridge sweetened with sugar, condensed milk, or rice porridge with fish sauce and a small portion of meat. After that, solid foods such as rice powder with a modest amount of meat or eggs are introduced.

Child-Rearing Practices: Parents are relaxed about and enjoy the development of young children. The extended family is often involved; grandparents play an important role because they are considered experienced and wise. In many families, especially in rural areas, young children never go to childcare centers; instead, they stay with grandparents when parents go to work. When grandparents are not available, the oldest child, regardless of gender, is often responsible for the care of younger siblings. If the parents are either dead, too old, or too ill to care for the children, extended family or older children will take up the responsibility. In Vietnamese culture, children are expected to obey and comply with the family's expectations rather than to make independent decisions. At age 6, a child starts school, and parents now place great emphasis on the child's good performance at school.

National Childhood Immunizations: BCG at birth and 1 month; DTP at 2, 3, and 4 months; OPV at 2, 3, and 4 months; HepB at birth and at 2 and 4 months; measles at 9 to 11 months. The percent of the target population vaccinated, by antigen, is: BCG, DTP3, MCV (95%); OPV (96%); DTP1, HepB, Polio3 (94%); measles (97%); and pregnant women vaccinated by TT2 (92%).

Other Characteristics: Putting feet on the furniture, photographing three people in a group, and voicing dissent are often considered offensive. It is considered better to be silent than to disagree. Names are listed in order by family name, middle name, and given name, so the family is the primary source of a person's identity. Women retain their own names after marriage. Age, associated with wisdom and experience, is valued and respected. Education is considered more important than wealth by most. Vietnamese are polite and guarded. The signal commonly used around the world to beckon someone, that is, moving the index finger with the palm of the hand up, is offensive, because it is the motion used to call a dog.

BIBLIOGRAPHY

Central Intelligence Agency: *2006: The world factbook, Vietnam*. Retrieved September 21, 2006, from https://www.cia.gov/cia/publications/factbook/print/vm.html.

Nguyen TH, Nguyen TL, Trinh QH: HIV/AIDS epidemics in Vietnam: evolution and responses, *AIDS Education & Prevention.* 16(3 suppl A):137–154, 2004.

Thang NM, Popkin BM: Patterns of food consumption in Vietnam: effects on socio-economic groups during an era of economic growth, *Eur J Clin Nutr.* 58(1): 145–153, 2004.

Thang NM, Popkin B: Child malnutrition in Vietnam and its transition in an era of economic growth, *J Hum Nutr Dietetics.* 16(4):233–244, 2003.

UNAIDS: Retrieved March 9, 2006, from http://www.unaids.org/en/Regions_Countries/Countries/viet_nam.asp.

UNDP: Retrieved February 15, 2006, from http://www.undp.org.vn/undp/docs/2004/briefing04/briefing04.pdf.

World Health Organization: Retrieved March 9, 2006, from http://www.wpro.who.int/NR/rdonlyres/57C15C23-A8BE-4EA0-BC27-3226A64F9128/0/vtn.pdf.

World Health Organization: 2006: Immunization, vaccines and biologicals. Retrieved September 21, 2006, from http://www.who.int/immunization_monitoring/en/globalsummary/countryprofileresult.cfm?C='vnm'.

◆ YEMEN (REPUBLIC OF)

MAP PAGE (802)

Yahia Ahmed Raja'a

Location: The Republic of Yemen is located in the southern part of the Arabian Peninsula. The capital is Sana'a. It is bordered by Yahia Ahmed Raja'a Saudi Arabia to the north, the Arabian Sea to the south, the Red Sea to the west, and Oman to the east. Yemen has a total area of about 550,000 km^2 (212,355 square miles), and the population is 21.4 million, with 46% aged between 0 and 14 years. The mountainous areas run parallel to the Red Sea and the Gulf of Aden. The coastal area extends along a strip approximately 2,000 km long. The plateau area runs parallel to and lies to the east and north of the mountainous highlands. Yemen also has a desert area (Al-Ruba Al-Khali, or "the empty quarter") and 112 islands. The gross domestic product (GDP) per capita is $900, with 45% below the poverty line. Yemen is one of the poorest countries in the Arab world.

Major Languages	Ethnic Groups	Major Religions
Arabic	Arab 95%	Sunni and Shia Muslim 98%
	East Indian,	Other (Jewish, Christian,
	African 5%	Hindu) 2%

A minority of the population speaks the Mahri language, a Himyarite descendent language that was predominant more than 2,000 years ago. Literacy rates are 71% for men, 30% for women.

Health Care Beliefs: Both modern and traditional; acute sick care. The vast majority seek modern medical care, especially for physical illnesses. Some people use herbs exclusively, whereas others combine herbs with modern medicine. It is not uncommon for people to have strong traditional beliefs about disease causation and treatment while simultaneously embracing modern medicine if they are not cured. Preventive care is valued, but financial constraints dictate that more crisis-oriented care is sought only after a person is extremely ill.

Predominant Sick-Care Practices: Indigenous; magical-religious; and biomedical if available. *Markh* (neck, back, and abdomen massage) is used for headaches and backaches and to encourage pregnancy. Highly experienced persons (mostly women) practice *markh* combined with *essab* to treat infants with persistent diarrhea and vomiting. *Essab* is the practice of binding a child's abdomen with a piece of cloth to open blocked bowels. *Mysam,* placing a very hot metallic rod on a part of the body, is used to treat a wide range of conditions, such as epilepsy, jaundice, or fear. The type of condition determines where the rod is placed. *Hijamah* is sucking out blood (using a vacuumed animal horn or tin can) from puncture points in the back or joints and is usually done to promote health in older adults and to treat general fatigue. Many people attend holy Koran treatment sessions in the rapidly increasing numbers of treatment centers. These centers are used mainly to treat *muss,* a condition caused by a satanic soul's possession of the body. This soul orders people to commit sins and inhibits them from doing good deeds and achieving their ambitions; it also impairs many bodily functions. Another widely spread belief is that *fag'ah* (fear) affects many psychosomatic functions. For example, it can hemolyze blood and lead to jaundice. Mild *fag'ah* is managed by unexpected contact with a small piece of a hot coal, such as that on a lit cigarette, or with very cold water. It is thought that severe *fag'ah* must be treated with iron supplements (either in pharmaceutical preparations or home-extracted iron water).

Ethnic-/Race-Specific or Endemic Diseases: Diarrheal diseases, acute respiratory tract infections, and undernutrition in children younger than 5 are the most common health problems. Drug resistant *Falciparum* malaria, schistosomiasis (intestinal and urinary), and helminthiasis (especially the soil-transmitted form) are all highly endemic. The Joint United Nations Programme on HIV/AIDS (UNAIDS) reports the estimated prevalence rate for human immunodeficiency virus (HIV) in adults (aged 15 to 49 years) to be less than 0.2%. According to UNAIDS, there is no reliable surveillance information, although the limited information available indicates a steadily growing epidemic since 1990, when the first case of acquired immunodeficiency syndrome (AIDS) was reported. The major mode of transmission appears to be heterosexual; however, homosexuality is considered rare, socially rejected, and punished by law, so transmission between men who have sex with men may be particularly underreported.

Health-Team Relationships: The doctor is usually the health team leader. Nurses, pharmacists, and laboratory technicians are subordinate to doctors, although the whole team is respected. Pharmacists are more likely to be considered businessmen rather than health professionals.

Families' Role in Hospital Care: A family member is expected to stay with and help care for hospitalized relatives. The family usually purchases drugs, brings food, assists with personal hygiene, and calls the medical staff when necessary.

Dominance Patterns: Males are dominant. Extended families are prevalent primarily in the rural areas, where 75% of the population resides. About 60% of women are full-time housewives, but a considerable number, primarily in rural areas (24%), are actively engaged in cultivation and raising animal herds in addition to their household activities. Many women marry young, at about 16. At the dinner table, the best foods are kept for the men.

Eye-Contact Practices: Direct eye contact is customary with everyone, including parents and authority figures. The given name is generally used during discussions. During professional meetings, the term *brother* precedes the first name.

Touch Practices: Physical touching is acceptable, but only between members of the same sex.

Perceptions of Time: Punctuality is not a very important value, and being 15 minutes late to a rendezvous is not even mentioned. People are generally present oriented, but the future is also of considerable concern.

Pain Reactions: People react to pain expressively, and complaining to friends is encouraged. Illnesses, such as psychiatric disorders, that involve cultural stigmas are mentioned only to close friends.

Birth Rites: A common saying is that "Two wedding ceremonies are easier than one birth." If the delivery occurs at home, which is common (84%), more than half involve the assistance of the mother or a relative; or, if these individuals are absent, a trained birth attendant steps in. Only 22% of women have trained medical assistants during childbirth. The infant mortality rate is high at 60 deaths per 1,000 live births. Births to mothers younger than 20 years of age and first births are more likely to include help from health professionals. Medically assisted deliveries are more common among women living in urban areas, coastal regions, or plateau regions. When a newborn is a boy, three shrills are heard by the people waiting outside the delivery room. If only one shrill is heard, the newborn is a girl. A new razor blade is used to cut the umbilical cord in two thirds of the home deliveries. One quarter use clean scissors, and only 5% use sterile medical instruments. The most common dressing used on the cord stump is a thread. Cauterization of the stump is involved in 15% of births, application of kohl in 8%, use of hot oil in 5%, and use of cotton or sterile dressings in 4%; 6% have no treatment. Mothers are expected to be still for several hours after delivery, and water and spicy foods are not allowed; only hot drinks are consumed. An entire hen is cooked for the new mother daily for 40 days, and friends and relatives visit her during this period. On day 40, a celebration is held, and the mother can resume sexual relations. Male children are usually circumcised on the seventh day after birth by the barber, who usually performs the operation at home. The occasion is celebrated by slaughtering one or two sheep, and neighbors and relatives are either invited for lunch or given the meat. About 19% of girls were previously circumcised, but this practice is decreasing. The median age of female circumcision is 8 days, and it is performed by birth attendants 68% of the time, grandmothers 19% of the time, and barbers and others 5% of the time. Razor blades are used for 75% of the procedures. The fertility rate is 6.58 children born per woman. Life expectancy is 60 for men, 64 for women.

Death Rites: Yemenis believe in an afterlife. Close relatives are called to spend the last hours with a dying person, and the head of the dying person is directed toward Mecca. The dead body is washed and perfumed, wrapped in one continuous piece of hand-sewn white cloth, and buried in the ground without a coffin. The period between death and burial is only a few hours. Autopsies are uncommon, but organ donations are allowed, provided they are done for free. Mourning lasts from 3 to 10 days. The wife of a deceased husband dresses in black clothes and does not leave the husband's home for 4 months and 10 days. After this mourning period, she is free to marry again.

Food Practices and Intolerances: Yemenis commonly say that "All foods call bread Sir." Bread is available at every meal. Various other grains, oils, ghee, butter, other dairy products, and eggs are also consumed. Fish or the meat of hens, sheep, or cows is usually eaten once or twice per week. Foods are usually cooked fresh daily and served very hot with many spices; three meals per day is the norm. The family eats from the same dishes using the fingers of the right hand. Spoons are used when eating rice dishes. Drinking tea at breakfast and dinner is common. Animals are slaughtered according to Islamic requirements; wine, blood, pork, donkeys, mules, canines, and birds with claws are forbidden.

Infant-Feeding Practices: Most Yemeni mothers breastfeed their children for long periods. Giving colostrum to a newborn is common, and about half of all infants begin breastfeeding within 1 hour of birth.

Child-Rearing Practices: Attitudes towards child rearing are exemplified by the saying "If your son becomes older, treat him as a brother." Children younger than 5 years usually sleep with their parents, and older boys and girls sleep in separate rooms. Both parents (primarily the mother) participate in child rearing and discipline. During adolescence the mother predominantly takes care of the daughters and the father takes care of the sons.

National Childhood Immunizations: BCG at birth; DTwP at 6, 10, and 14 weeks; DTwPHibHep at 6, 10, and 14 weeks; OPV at birth and 6, 10, and 14 weeks; measles at 9 and 18 months; vitamin A at 9 and 18 months; TT at first contact, +1 month, +6 months, +1 year, +1 year. The percent of the target population vaccinated, by antigen, is: BCG (66%); DTP1 (99%); DTP3 and HepB3 (86%); Hib3 (57%); MCV (76%); and Polio3 (87%).

Other Characteristics: Seven percent of currently married women are involved in polygamous marriages. Most men chew the soft leaves of the khat plant *(Katha edulis)*, which is a stimulant. Khat is chewed and stored in the left side of the mouth under the cheek for approximately 3 hours per session. Friends usually attend khat-chewing sessions, and most of the houses in Yemen are prepared to receive the chewers. Khat sessions are held during every social event, at the end of the week, and occasionally daily. The practice of khat chewing is associated with many health problems: hypertension, duodenal ulcers, hemorrhoids, and mental disorders.

BIBLIOGRAPHY

Al-Hadrani AM: Khat induced hemorrhoidal diseases in Yemen, *Saudi Med J.* 21:475, 2000.

Central Intelligence Agency 2006: The world factbook, Yemen. Retrieved September 21, 2006, from https://www.cia.gov/cia/publications/factbook/print/ym.html.

Raja'a YA et al: *A decade study on birth outcomes in Al-Thawra hospital, Sana'a—Yemen,* The second Yemeni-Italian Medical Conference, Al-Mukalla, Yemen, 2001.

Raja'a YA et al: Khat chewing is a risk factor of duodenal ulcer, *Saudi Med. J* 21:887, 2000.

UNAIDS: 2006 Yemen. Retrieved September 21, 2006, from http://www.unaids.org/en/Regions_Countries/Countries/yemen.asp.

World Health Organization: 2006: Immunization, vaccines and biologicals. Retrieved September 21, 2006, from http://www.who.int/immunization_monitoring/en/globalsummary/countryprofileresult.cfm?C='yem'.

✦ ZAMBIA (REPUBLIC OF)

MAP PAGE (801)

Charles Michelo

Location: Zambia shares borders with Tanzania to the northeast, Malawi and Mozambique to the east; Botswana, Zimbabwe, and Namibia to the south; Angola to the west; and Democratic Republic of Congo to the north. Zambia's total area is 752,614 km^2 (290,583 square miles); the capital is Lusaka. It lies on the Central African high plateau with an average altitude of 1,200 m above sea level. The Rift Valley formations in the eastern and southern parts of the country have produced escarpment systems and valley troughs. Zambia has a subtropical climatic setting that comprises semiarid and tropical conditions as well as a mixture of the two. There are three distinct seasons: the warm rainy (November-April), the cool dry (May-July), and the hot dry (August-October). The major rivers are the Zambezi, Kafue, Luangwa, Kabompo, Luapula, and Chambeshi. Zambia's population has grown rapidly, to more than 12 million, with 51% aged 0 to 16 years. The gross domestic product (GDP) per capita is $900, with 86% living below the poverty line.

Major Languages	Ethnic Groups	Major Religions
English (official)	Bantu 98%	Christian 50%-75%
Local dialects:	Other (Europeans) 2%	Islam, Hindu 24%-49%
Bemba,		Indigenous beliefs 1%
Tonga, Lozi,		
Kaonde, Lunda,		
Luvale, and Nyanja		

Zambia has at least 72 tribes and 20 distinct languages, of which Bemba, Tonga, Lozi, Kaonde, Lunda, Luvale, and Nyanja are the major ones. However, no strong ethnic feelings exist, as indicated by intertribal marriages and other associations. English is the official language, but most Zambians speak more than one local language. Literacy rates are 87% for men, 75% for women.

Health Care Beliefs: Indigenous and modern; active and passive roles. Information on health issues, national campaigns, and promotions have helped most people understand the causes of various diseases, largely the result of improved literacy. As a result, national campaigns against cholera and poliomyelitis as well as vitamin A supplementation programs and general immunizations have been well received. Although people previously believed that poisoning or witchcraft was responsible for human immunodeficiency virus (HIV)/acquired immunodeficiency syndrome (AIDS), this belief has changed, and even traditional herbalists who once claimed they could treat HIV now refer clients to conventional medical facilities. Certain psychiatric conditions continue to be associated with spirits (e.g., *mashawe*), and people resort to their ancestral spirits for help with a cure.

Predominant Sick-Care Practices: Traditional; religious; biomedical. A comprehensive network of health institutions, hospitals, clinics, and health posts is widely used; however, a parallel traditional health care service also exists. Zambia has thousands of traditional healers of different levels who use various practices and provide care to about 40% of the population. For chronic diseases such as HIV, people invariably consult traditional healers when they lose hope in conventional medicine. They may simultaneously consult and receive treatment from traditional healers and conventional medical doctors. Traditional healers have generally responded positively to education about cross-infections among their patients by modifying some of their practices; for example, they ask each patient to bring a new razor blade for any skin-piercing procedures. The country has also trained traditional birth attendants, who provide care where health centers are not accessible, a particular problem in rural areas. Zambia has three main tertiary level referral hospitals: Ndola, Kitwe and a university teaching hospital in Lusaka; but the provincial hospitals also serve as referral facilities. Secondary level care is provided in district hospitals, whereas rural health centers and urban clinics serve as primary care points. Church-run hospitals and health centers also provide primary as well as secondary level care and are often the sole provider of health care services in their localities. These facilities are complemented by a wide range of privately owned surgery centers, clinics, and a growing number of private hospitals. All blood products used in these institutions are screened for HIV and syphilis, as well as hepatitis B. Spiritual healing is also increasingly becoming a major option of health care, particularly among the charismatic and Pentecostal churches.

Ethnic-/Race-Specific or Endemic Diseases: Malaria, acute respiratory infections, diarrheal diseases, anemia, malnutrition, hypertension, HIV and tuberculosis are major health problems. In addition, worm infestation, sporadic outbreaks of cholera (especially during the rainy season), sickle cell disease, and tetanus still burden the health care system. Traditional healers are thought to be very effective in treating epileptic seizures and mental illnesses, some sexually transmitted illnesses, and infertility. They attempt to treat opportunistic infections in those with HIV/AIDS. Most people use home remedies based on information passed from generation to generation or obtained from neighbors. Some home remedies are effective and have been trusted for years. Zambia is one of the sub-Saharan countries most affected by HIV. The country has established antenatal care (ANC)-based surveillance and population-based surveys measuring infection and risk. The Joint United Nations Programme on HIV/AIDS (UNAIDS) reports the prevalence rate of HIV in adults (aged 15 to 49 years) as 17%, with 1.1 million people living with HIV, including 570,000 women and 130,000 children aged 0 to 14 years. About 98,000 deaths are attributed to AIDS. There are 710,000 children aged 0 to 17 who are orphans due to parental AIDS. Urban rates are currently 25% of the population, and rural areas are 12%. There has been a marked decline in HIV among educated young people (aged 15 to 24). Widespread denial continues to exist within families.

Health-Team Relationships: Doctors with various specialties are available in hospitals, although there is a critical shortage of doctors and nurses. Clinics and rural health centers are run primarily by clinical officers and nurses. Patients prefer to be cared for by doctors but are willing to accept treatment by clinical officers and nurses on duty. The doctor-patient ratio is estimated to be 1:11,000, and the nurse-patient ratio is 1:1,571. All health care workers are poorly remunerated and are forced to seek greener pastures elsewhere—hence the provider-patient ratios remain poor and worsen over time.

Families' Role in Hospital Care: The critical shortage of nursing staff makes care from family members essential. Families perform nursing tasks, purchase all needed medicines, provide personal patient hygiene, and counsel patients. Family members also supplement meals by bringing in food supplies. Home-based care has become a prominent aspect of care for AIDS patients. To supplement this role, the Roman Catholic Church has introduced the concept of hospices. Terminal care is provided within local areas, so family ties may be maintained when care at home becomes too difficult.

Dominance Patterns: Zambia is a male-dominated country, although demands for gender equality are growing. The responsibilities of caring for those who are ill, orphans, and other vulnerable people fall on the shoulders of women. Clan patterns vary from matrilineal to patrilineal systems. However, almost all tribes still practice the system of paying *lobola* (a bride price) by the groom as an official marriage rite. This takes various forms, such as money, livestock, clothing, or tools.

Eye-Contact Practices: It is generally accepted that lowering the eyes is a sign of respect to older adults, and when young people do the opposite, it is condemned by society. Eye contact among young peers is deemed to be correct behavior and is often a useful tool when communicating a message of affection to a member of the opposite sex.

Touch Practices: Physical touching in public between members of the opposite sex is unacceptable; however, physical touching among friends of the same sex is acceptable and has no sexual connotations. Physical touching by children is not an issue. Most greet others with a handshake. A handshake is also used as a symbol of reconciliation when there has been a quarrel, dispute, or disagreement.

Perceptions of Time: Punctuality is not important, and this is taking an economic toll. Even at important gatherings, the norm is for people to arrive late. Past traditions and ceremonies are freely practiced and celebrated with no time in mind. Tribe-specific ceremonies are becoming more important in the culture and have restored pride in tribal heritage and customs.

Pain Reactions: Pain and grief are openly expressed, and the community is supportive of those in pain or those who are grieving. Like most

Bantu cultures, men are not expected to show pain and grief in public. Similarly, women in labor are expected to endure the pain as a sign of growing up.

Birth Rites: In urban areas, it is estimated that more than 90% of women use antenatal services. Most births occur in clinics. Mothers are referred to the hospital only if there is a bad obstetric history or an impending complication requiring closer supervision. Some clinics in high-density residential areas are specifically designated as maternity clinics and are run by qualified midwives. In rural areas, geographic and financial access to antenatal services is a challenge because doctors and midwives prefer not to serve there. To solve this problem, Zambia has trained traditional birth attendants to serve primarily in these rural areas, although experienced women also assist in deliveries. When the delivery is conducted by such people, their names may be given to the baby as recognition of their role. In some rural areas where traditions are still held in high esteem, herbs are used to bathe the infant or are tied around the infant's neck or arm for protection against evil. The umbilical cord has tremendous significance because the infant is considered strong and mature after the umbilical stub withers and drops off, and most tribes do not name an infant until this happens. Cutting the cord in a traditional way may cause infection; neonatal tetanus is still a major problem. The infant mortality rate was 89 deaths per 1,000 in 2005. The fertility rate is six children born per woman. Life expectancy decreased from 54 years in the mid-1980s to 37 years in 1998 at the peak of HIV epidemic, but it is estimated to be about 40 years for both men and women at present.

Death Rites: Death is not readily accepted, so people usually blame others for the event. The HIV epidemic has made death an everyday occurrence. This fact, combined with the harsh economy, has forced people to shorten the mourning period. When a person dies, relatives, friends, and neighbors assemble at the funeral house until after the burial to give both physical and emotional support to the family. In some tribes like the Tongas in the south, this is also a time to eat meat because livestock is killed only for such events, especially if the deceased was an adult man. At the end of the mourning period, property is disbursed as inheritance, and a child is selected to be named after the deceased to ensure that his spirit lives on in the family. If he was married and his wife or wives are still alive, a nephew is selected to inherit as well.

Food Practices and Intolerances: *Nshima,* a thick cornmeal preparation, is a staple food for most Zambians; however, cassava and sorghum are used in some parts of the country. These dishes are eaten with a relish of some form and meat, vegetables, or fish. Most people use their hands to eat.

Infant-Feeding Practices: Working mothers are given a statutory 3 months of paid maternity leave. Health care instruction encourages breastfeeding for at least 6 months. Most working mothers use breast and bottle-feeding. Weight gain, immunizations, and general development are closely monitored by a countrywide comprehensive "younger-than-5 clinic" initiative.

Child-Rearing Practices: Working mothers employ maids to supervise their infants while they work. Fortunately, numerous centers have been established to train these maids. It is not uncommon for young women, often relatives who have dropped out of school, to be called on to help with an infant's care. Children mix freely and play with other children in nearby neighborhoods. Generally, children are loved and protected by everyone in the neighborhood.

National Childhood Immunizations: BCG at birth or first contact; DTPHibHep at 6, 10, and 14 weeks; DTwPHib at 6, 10, and 14 weeks; measles at 9 months; OPV at birth and 6, 10, and 14 weeks; vitamin A at 6 + 6 months; TT at first contact, +1, +6 months, and +1, +1 year. The percent of the target population vaccinated, by antigen, is: BCG, and DTP1 (94%); DTP3, HepB3, Hib3, and Polio3 (80%); and MCV (84%). In some areas of the country, sporadic outbreaks of measles have occurred in older children, and so some local health posts give a measles booster at 15 months.

BIBLIOGRAPHY

Central Intelligence Agency: *2006: The world factbook, Zambia.* Retrieved September 21, 2006, from https://www.cia.gov/cia/publications/factbook/print/za.html.

Central Statistical Office (CSO): Zambia: *Zambia demographic and Health Survey 2001–2002.* CSO (Zambia). CBoH (Zambia), and ORC Macro, Lusaka, and Maryland, 2003.

Dzekedzeke K, Fylkesnes K: Reducing uncertainties in global HIV estimates-the case of Zambia, *BMC Public Health.* 6(1):83, 2006.

Hjortsberg C, Mwikisa C: Cost of access to health services in Zambia, *Health Policy and Planning.* 17(1):71, 2002.

Kwalombota M: The effect of pregnancy in HIV-infected women, *AIDS-Care.* 14(3):431, 2002.

Michelo C, Sandøy IF, Fylkesnes K: Marked HIV prevalence declines in higher educated young people: evidence from population-based surveys (1995–2003) in Zambia, *AIDS.* 20:1031–1038, 2006.

Ministry of Health: Zambia and World Health Organization: National 10-year human resources plan for public health in WHO country cooperation strategy, Zambia 2002–2005. Retrieved August 26, 2006, from http://www.who.int/countryfocus/cooperation_strategy/countries/ccs_zmb_final_en.pdf.

Sandøy IF, Kvåle G, Michelo C, Fylkesnes K: Antenatal clinic-based HIV prevalence in Zambia—declining trends but sharp local contrasts in young women, *Trop Med Int Health.* 11(6):917–928, 2006.

UNAIDS: 2006: Zambia. Retrieved September 21, 2006, from http://www.unaids.org/en/Regions_Countries/Countries/zambia.asp.

Yokona J: Non-communicable disease in sub-Saharan Africa, *Lancet.* 351(9249):74, 2001.

Wikipedia: Retrieved August 25, 2006, from http://en.wikipedia.org/wiki/Demographics_of_Zambia.

World Health Organization: 2006: Immunization, vaccines and biologicals. Retrieved September 21, 2006, from http://www.who.int/immunization_monitoring/en/globalsummary/countryprofileresult.cfm?C='zmb'.

◆ ZIMBABWE (REPUBLIC OF)

MAP PAGE (801)

Thubelihle Mathole

Location: The Republic of Zimbabwe is a landlocked country located in south central Africa. The total area is more than 390,000 km² (156,000 square miles) of grassland and high plateau. The capital is Harare. It borders Zambia to the northwest, Botswana to the southwest, South Africa to the south, and Mozambique to the east and northwest. Zimbabwe enjoys a temperate climate with hot, rainy summers and warm, dry winters. It has a population of 12.2 million, 65% of whom live in rural areas; 41% of the population is aged 0 to 14 years. The gross domestic product (GDP) per capita is $2,300, with 80% living below the poverty line. Literacy rates are 94% for men, 87% for women.

Major Languages	Ethnic Groups	Major Religions
Shona (major)	Shona 71%	Christianity 61%
English (official)	Ndebele 16%	Traditional/indigenous
Si'Ndebele	Mixed race ("colored"),	beliefs 32%
	Asians 1%	Muslims 2%
	White less than 1%	Nonreligious 5.0%
	Other indigenous	
	Africans 11%	

Health Care Beliefs: Indigenous; acute sick care; active or passive role. In indigenous care, illness or other misfortunes are considered the result of the breakdown of social relations, and care includes biomedical, social, psychological, and spiritual aspects. Diseases (*zvirwere* in Shona, or *izifo* in Si'Ndebele) are believed to be transmitted by *mamhepo*, air that is in a state of imbalance. Illness is explained by two types of bad air. First, diseases that cause minor problems, such as coughing or headaches, are believed to originate from bad air in the physical environment, and such diseases are considered normal. An example is *nhova*, which is a sunken fontanel in infants. Although actually caused by dehydration, it is treated in traditional communities with *muti* ("African medicine"). The second type of bad air is considered unnatural because grave health problems result. These diseases are considered to be caused by evil—because God, in His infinite goodness, would not allow such ills to hurt humanity. It is believed that those who are immoral or unhygienic—physically, spiritually, or socially—have lost the mediation with God provided by ancestors' spirits. Therefore, they are more susceptible to bad airs and their consequences, such as sexually transmitted diseases (e.g., *runyoka*, or hepatitis B). Most believe that the cause of mental illness is supernatural, whether it is possession by a spirit or the result of witchcraft and spells. Good spirits are known as *vadzimu*, or family spirits, and are considered friendly. Evil spirits can be angry spirits, or *ngozi*, or may manifest as *mashara*, which are alien spirits. Mental illness engenders shame, so the help of a *nganga* ("traditional healer"), is usually sought. Nganga are believed to have the ability to identify the person responsible or to exorcise the alien spirit.

Predominant Sick-Care Practices: Traditional, magical-religious, biomedical. Since 1980, the government has undertaken an almost complete restructuring of the health sector, providing free care to all and building hundreds of hospitals and clinics in both urban and rural settings. Access to modern facilities increased from 14% before 1980 to 87% a decade later. Although general health status was improved, use of available resources has been less than ideal because most seek help from traditional healers first. People who live in urban areas tend to use Western services for their initial attempts at resolving illness given that traditional healers are situated primarily in rural settings. Healers may be sought by city dwellers only when Western treatments have failed or when an affliction is thought to have a supernatural cause. Traditional medicine continues to be used even when biomedical care is readily available because it is more familiar and culturally acceptable. Women combine biomedical and traditional care during pregnancy. They use clinics for the assurance that the pregnancy is progressing well and also consult persons with supposed supernatural powers.

Ethnic-/Race-Specific or Endemic Diseases: Government spending has decreased from $35 per capita in the 1980s to $11 in 2000, mostly because of the burden of human immunodeficiency virus (HIV)/acquired immunodeficiency syndrome (AIDS). Communicable diseases such as schistosomiasis and intestinal parasites affect both adults and children. Significant problems among adults include tuberculosis (often in combination with HIV), chloroquine-resistant malaria (in rural areas), and cholera (although fairly well controlled). HIV has devastated the health of Zimbabweans, impacting the economic, social, and cultural landscape of the country. It is estimated that 1.8 million people, including 900,000 women, are living with HIV; the estimated prevalence rate in adults (aged 15 to 49 years) is 25%. Most of those infected are the most economically productive of the country's citizens, reducing overall life expectancy by 26 years. About 1.1 million have died since 1995, about 56,000 children aged 0 to 15 years are living with HIV/AIDS, and almost one million children are orphans as the result of parental AIDS. The number of people who go for voluntary counseling and testing is low but improving. The number of sick clients or those with sick partners who visited testing centers also has increased, partly attributed to awareness of the need for previously unavailable antiretroviral drugs. About 171,000 people need antiretrovirals, but only 42,000 are currently receiving them because of the lack of drugs.

Health-Team Relationships: In Shona culture, the medical doctor is thought to be the only one with the authority and knowledge to treat illness. This tends to negate the talents of nurses and trained community health care workers, who outnumber doctors and provide the bulk of general care. It also affects the efficiency of the referral system because patients sometimes bypass local clinics and go directly to referral centers, resulting in congestion, frustration among health care providers, and poor-quality care. Nurses are usually the first point of contact, and the roles they play vary according to location and the number of doctors available. Community health workers (trained lay individuals) form an important part of the network in rural areas. Budget cuts for the health sector have resulted in shortages of drugs; high hospital fees; and the rapid exodus of doctors, nurses, and other health professionals. In 2002, about 2,297 of qualified staff (77 doctors and 1,920 nurses) left the country. The remaining medical staff in government institutions was 742 instead of the required 1,200 and 713 nurses instead of the required 1,200. Most hospitals demand cash payment up front, and so the poor have little access to care other than traditional medicine.

Families' Role in Hospital Care: When a family member is ill, it is usual for extended family to travel from distant cities and rural areas to provide help. Those who are able donate funds to defray the costs of the hospital stay. Often, large numbers of family members, old and young, keep watch at the bedside for hours. Relatives often bring herbal treatments, secretly given with food. Integration of traditional medicine into formal health services remains a challenge. Relatives may request a patient's discharge to enable them to use traditional care at home. The role of families has expanded as essential drugs, intravenous solutions, and latex gloves have been scarce. Many families are told to purchase saline drips and prescriptions from an outside source or to bring in all the patients' meals because food and other resources are no longer provided. The government is encouraging home-based care for terminally ill patients such as those with AIDS. The lack of resources results in such patients being discharged early to be taken care of by relatives and neighbors.

Dominance Patterns: Traditional society is primarily patriarchal. If a woman bears only female children and her husband is very traditional, he may take a second wife to produce a son to continue the family name. Women are expected to marry and produce many children, all of whom belong to the husband and his family. Children take the father's surname and his *mutupo* (or "totem," the sacred family animal) and remain with the husband's family should the marriage fail. The man and his family are expected to pay *roora* or *lobola* (a "bride price") in the form of cattle, money, or furniture to the prospective bride's family. Today the bride price has become more symbolic than binding. During times of illness, women are expected to care for the sick at home and in the hospital. Men provide support but seldom take an active a role. The situation has worsened during the HIV era. Women take care of their husbands and relatives when they are ill, but they may be left alone when they have the disease.

Eye-Contact Practices: Children avoid eye contact with authority figures. Children who look into the eyes of a parent directly, particularly when being chastised, are considered defiant and disrespectful: they are expected to look down. Eye contact is avoided between inferiors and superiors (employer and maids or gardeners, students and teachers). Western medical practitioners may misinterpret this lack of eye contact as disinterest, when in actuality the patient is trying to be respectful.

Touch Practices: Maintaining personal space is not a concern because Zimbabweans grow up in an extended family constantly surrounded by other people. Touching among relatives is acceptable, but not by non-relatives. Although women are free to hug one another in greeting, as are men, it is inappropriate for men and women to hug in public. Some exceptions exist, such as when a mother welcomes her son or husband home after a long absence. The usual mode of greeting between men and women and members of the same gender is a handshake.

Perceptions of Time: Zimbabwe has adopted punctuality, especially in business situations; however, a popular saying, "There is no rush in Africa," highlights the underlying nonchalance about timeliness. People are expected to be late for engagements, which may affect business interactions and deadlines for payment. A friend would be reluctant to offend another friend by reminding them about an outstanding debt.

Pain Reactions: Men are expected to bear pain in silence with minimal expression, whereas women may react more openly. During childbirth, it is considered natural to express feelings verbally, but women are taught that pain leads to joy, so it behooves them to endure it. After a death, especially that of a child or close family member, societal rules are relaxed somewhat, and men may express their emotional pain more openly, if only for a short time.

Birth Rites: The fertility rate is three children born per woman. Childless women are often treated as social outcasts because a popular belief is that infertility is caused by witchcraft. The help of a nganga may be sought, for the social stigma can be overwhelming. Husbands are allowed to divorce an infertile woman or take a second wife. Social wealth is measured in large part by a family's number of offspring. Prenatal care is provided by nurses to those who have access to medical facilities. Traditional midwives (trained or untrained) are used in underserved areas where women give birth at home. It is believed that a difficult labor is an indication of previous adultery; so the woman must confess her indiscretions to ease the passage of the infant. Out of respect for the woman's privacy, it is rare for a husband to be present. The umbilical cord is buried in the ground ceremoniously. The infant is considered vulnerable to evil and natural illnesses, so protection is provided with medications and by observing taboos. An amulet may be tied around the infant's waist or wrist with a piece of string to ward off evil spirits. A first bath may be given in an herbal concoction with protective powers obtained from a nganga. Infants are kept away from strangers the first few weeks to protect them from infections and to shield them from those who might have bad thoughts about them or the family. The infant mortality rate is very high at 69 deaths per 1,000 live births. The primary causes of death in children younger than 5 years include respiratory tract infections, malnutrition, diarrhea, and especially, HIV. Life expectancy is 40 for men, 38 for women.

Death Rites: Death is due to one of five causes: natural causes such as illness, supernatural causes such as *ngozi* ("angry spirits"), violence or accidents, behavioral indiscretions, and the ill will of other people. The women, wearing wraps around their waists and head scarves, sit on the floor in a central room of the home, wailing and singing, taking turns preparing food in the kitchen, and comforting one other. The men sit on chairs in the same room or another, speaking among themselves. This ritual can go on for several days, and few people get any sleep. Men are usually buried at their rural homes, whereas women are buried at their husband's home. Children, who belong to the father, are buried at his home. The ceremony at the graveside is conducted by a priest for Christian families, and others follow traditional rituals. The worldly possessions of the deceased are distributed to the extended family, so that each will receive at least one item as a remembrance. Autopsies and organ donations are considered acceptable but unusual. Cremation is infrequent.

Food Practices and Intolerances: At funerals and weddings, relatives and friends usually contribute in cash or kind. Many people in urban areas grow their own vegetables, and subsistence farming is the norm in rural areas. A staple of the traditional diet is *sadza*, a thick paste made from maize meal cooked with water and eaten with the hands. When maize meal is scarce, bulrush millet, finger millet *(rapoko)*, or sorghum are alternatives. Sadza may be consumed with fermented milk but is usually eaten with meat and leafy green vegetables such as covo, pumpkin leaves, mbowa, or derere-munda. A meal is not considered complete without meat, especially beef or chicken. In rural areas, families raise goats for food for celebrations, and dried beans and bambara nuts are popular. Various types of fruit are wild and grown domestically: guavas, mangoes, pawpaw, mazhanje, and baobab. Lactose intolerance is widespread, especially among children, although it is not often recognized.

Infant-Feeding Practices: Most women breastfeed for 18 to 20 months, either because they appreciate the value of breast milk or because formula is too expensive or unavailable. The first supplemental food at about 3 months is cornmeal porridge given in a cup with a spoon or on the mother's fingertips. Peanut butter *(dovi)*, sugar, margarine, or oil may be added to improve palatability and nutritional value. Adult foods are introduced by 4 to 9 months of age, although breastfeeding may continue. Some believe that traditional drinks such as *mahewu* are good for children because they increase the amount of blood, whereas foods such as groundnuts, boiled maize, and meat are believed to be difficult to digest and able to cause diarrhea. Weaning begins by giving the child sweet or adult foods or by putting bitter substances such as hot pepper on the nipples. It is believed that breast milk becomes poisonous once a woman becomes pregnant again. If the child consumes the milk of a pregnant woman, an emetic is provided by a traditional healer to cleanse the infant's gut.

Child-Rearing Practices: Child rearing is the responsibility of the entire community, particularly in rural areas, where most people reside. Discipline is meted out by adults who witness mischievous behavior, and parents are informed. Important traditions are taught early, such as respect for older adults, the importance of showing deference for those in authority, and how to act when people visit. The men and women in the community are models of conduct, and corporal punishment is considered essential and necessary. The disciplinarian is usually the father, but another male relative takes on the role when the father is absent. Since 1980, girls and boys have reaped the benefits of expanded opportunities for education: considered essential for all children regardless of gender.

National Childhood Immunizations: BCG at birth; DT at 5 years; DTwP at 3, 4, 5 and 18 months; HepB at 3, 4 and 5 months; measles at 9 months; OPV at 3, 4, 5, and 18 months and 5 years; TT at first contact, +6 months, +1, +1, +5 years; vitamin A at 6, 12, 18, 24, 30, and 36 months. The percent of the target population vaccinated, by antigen, is: BCG (98%); DTP1 (95%); DTP3 and Polio3 (90%); and MCV (85%).

Z

BIBLIOGRAPHY

Central Intelligence Agency: 2006: The world factbook, Zimbabwe. Retrieved September 21, 2006, from https://www.cia.gov/cia/publications/factbook/print/zi.html.

Chinowaita M: Doctors, nurses in mass exodus, *The Daily News*, 20-11-2002. Harare, Zimbabwe, 2002.

Government of Zimbabwe: *The 2002 National Census: national census report.* Harare, 2002, Central Statistical Office.

The Herald: 30 July 2006, Zimbabwe, Some hospitals ignore government directives: patients turned away for lack of cash up-front. Harare, 2006, Zimbabwe.

Mathole T, Lindmark G, Ahlberg BM: Competing knowledge claims in the provision of antenatal care: a qualitative study of traditional birth attendants in rural Zimbabwe, *Health Care for Women Int.* 26:937–956, 2005.

UNAIDS: 2006 Zimbabwe: Retrieved September 21, 2006, from http://www.unaids.org/en/Regions_Countries/Countries/zimbabwe.asp.

UNAIDS: Evidence for HIV decline in Zimbabwe: a comprehensive review of the epidemiological data. Retrieved July 28, 2006, from http://data.unaids.org/publications/irc-pub06/zimbabwe-epi-reportnovos-en.pdf.

World Health Organization (2001): WHO welcomes OAU declaration on traditional medicine (WHO/AFRO Press Release). Retrieved on April 3, 2003, from http://www.afro.who.int/press/2001/pr20010820.html.

World Health Organization: 2006: Immunization, vaccines and biologicals. Retrieved September 21, 2006, from http://www.who.int/immunization_monitoring/en/globalsummary/countryprofileresult.cfm?C='zwe'.

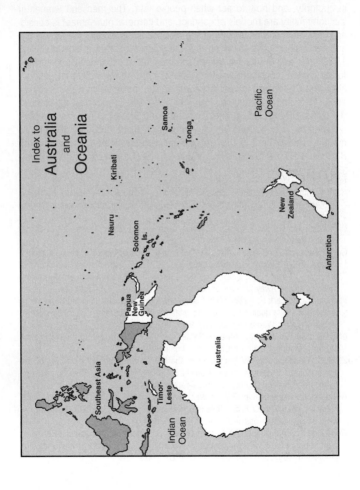

Index to
Australia
and
Oceania

Pacific
Ocean

Samoa

Tonga

Kiribati

New
Zealand

Nauru

Antarctica

Solomon
Is.

Papua
New
Guinea

Australia

Southeast Asia

Timor-
Leste

Indian
Ocean

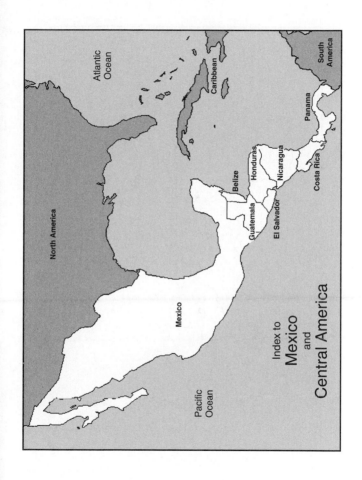

Index to Mexico and Central America

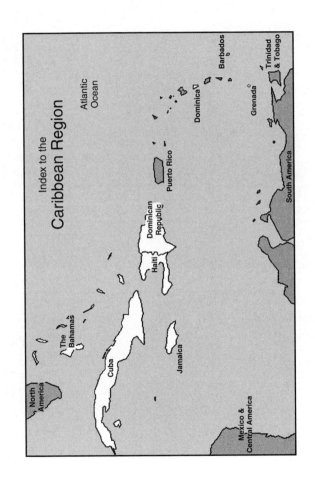

Index to the
Caribbean Region

Atlantic
Ocean

Barbados

Trinidad
& Tobago

Dominica

Grenada

Puerto Rico

Dominican
Republic

Haiti

South America

The
Bahamas

Cuba

Jamaica

North
America

Mexico &
Central America

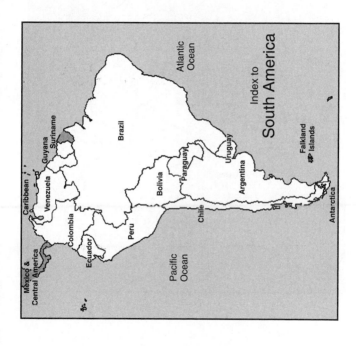

Index to
South America

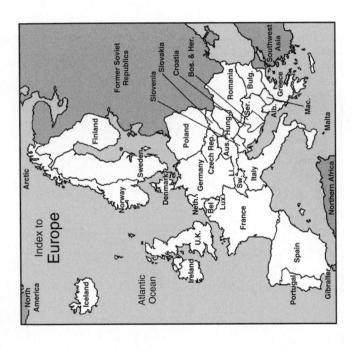

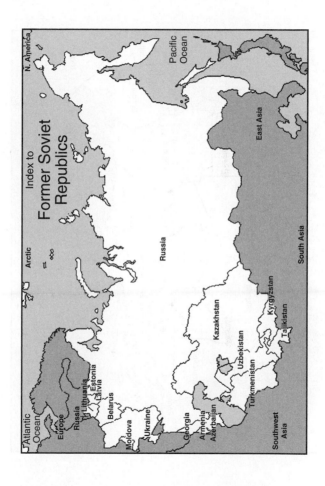

Index to
Former Soviet
Republics

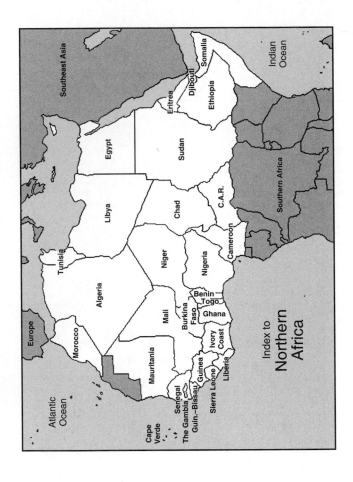

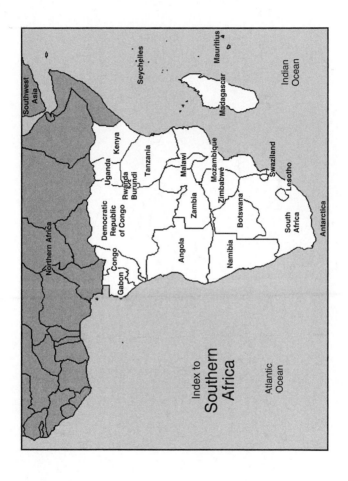

Index to
Southern
Africa

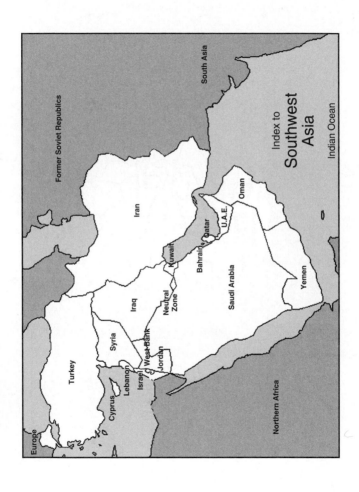

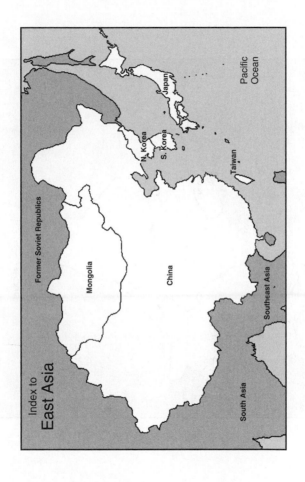

Index to East Asia

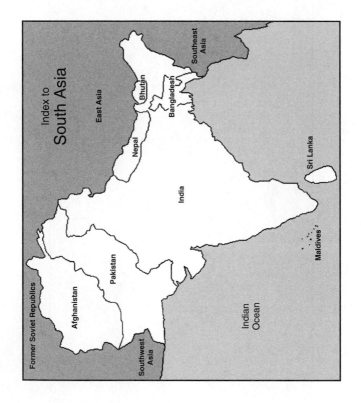

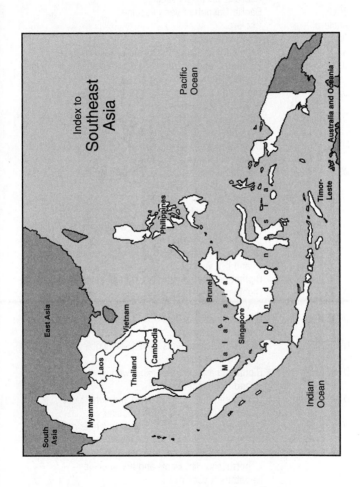

Index to Southeast Asia

aP	Acellular pertussis vaccine
BCG	Bacille Calmette-Guérin vaccine
Cholera	Cholera
Dip	Diphtheria vaccine
DT	Tetanus and diphtheria toxoid children's dose
DTaP	Diphtheria and tetanus toxoid with acellular pertussis vaccine
DTaPHep	Diphtheria and tetanus toxoid with acellular pertussis and HepB vaccine
DTaPHepIPV	Diphtheria and tetanus toxoid with acellular pertussis, HepB, and IPV vaccine
DTaPHib	Diphtheria and tetanus toxoid with acellular pertussis and Hib vaccine
DTaPHibHep	Diphtheria and tetanus toxoid with acellular pertussis, Hib and HepB vaccine
DTaPHibHepIPV	Hexavalent diphtheria, tetanus toxoid with acellular pertussis, Hib, hepatitis B and IPV vaccine
DTaPHibIPV	Diphtheria and tetanus toxoid with acellular pertussis, Hib and IPV vaccine
DTaPIPV	Diphtheria and tetanus toxoid with acellular pertussis and IPV vaccine
DTIP	Diphtheria and tetanus toxoid vaccine and IPV vaccine
DTwP	Diphtheria and tetanus toxoid with whole cell pertussis vaccine
DTwPHep	Diphtheria and tetanus toxoid with whole cell pertussis and HepB vaccine
DTwPHiB	Diphtheria and tetanus toxoid with whole cell pertussis and Hib vaccine
DTwPIPV	Diphtheria and tetanus toxoid with whole cell pertussis and IPV vaccine
DTwPHibHep	Diphtheria and tetanus toxoid with whole cell pertussis, Hib and HepB vaccine
DTwPHibIPV	Diphtheria and tetanus toxoid with whole cell pertussis, Hib and IPV vaccine
DTwPHibHepIPV	Hexavalent diphtheria, tetanus toxoid with whole cell pertussis, Hib, HepB and IPV vaccine
HepA	Hepatitus A vaccine
HepB	Hepatitis B vaccine
HepBIG	Hepatitis B immune globulin
HIB (Hib)	Haemophilus influenzae type b vaccine
HPV	Human papillomavirus vaccine
IPV	Inactivated polio vaccine

JapEnc	Japanese encephalitis
MCV	Meningococcal conjugate vaccine
Measles	Measles vaccine
MenAC	Meningococcal AC
MenACWY	Meningococcal ACWY
MenC_conj	Meningococcal C conjugate vaccine
MM	Measles and mumps vaccine
MR	Measles and rubella vaccine
MMR	Measles, mumps and rubella vaccine
Mumps	Mumps vaccine
Neisvac-C	Meningococcal Group C, tetanus toxoid conjugate
OPV	Oral polio vaccine
Penta	Combined diphtheria-tetanus-acellular pertussis (DTPa), Hepatitis B, and inactivated poliovirus vaccine
Pneumo_conj	Pneumococcal conjugate vaccine
Pneumo_ps	Pneumococcal polysaccharide vaccine
Pig-Bel	Fatal enteritis necroticans vaccine
PNC	Pneumococcal polysaccharide conjugate
Rabies	Rabies vaccine
Rotavirus	Rotavirus vaccine
Rubella	Rubella vaccine
TBC	Anti-tubercular vaccine
TBE	Tick borne encephalitis
Td	Tetanus and diphtheria toxoid for older children/adults
TT	Tetanus toxoid
TT/Td	Tetanus toxoid/Tetanus and diphtheria toxoid for older Children/adults
Typhoid	Typhoid fever vaccine
TyphoidHepA	Typhoid fever and Hepatitis A vaccine
Varicella	Chickenpox vaccine
VitA	Vitamin A supplementation
YF	Yellow fever vaccine